Rob & Smith's

Operative
Cardiac Surgery

SIXTH EDITION

Rob & Smith's Operative Surgery

Other volumes available in the series

Operative Surgery of the Colon, Rectum and Anus 6th Edition

P. Ronan O'Connell, Robert D. Madoff, Michael Solomon

Operative Thoracic Surgery 6th Edition

Larry R. Kaiser, Glyn Jamieson, Sarah K. Thompson

Operative Oral and Maxillofacial Surgery 3rd Edition

John D. Langdon, Mohan F. Patel, Robert Ord, Peter A. Brennan

Operative Pediatric Surgery 7th Edition

Lewis Spitz and Arnold G. Coran

ART EDITOR

Gillian Lee FMAA, HonFIMI, AMI, RMIP
Gillian Lee Illustrations, 15 Litle Plucketts Way, Buckhurst Hill, Essex, UK

Contributing medical artists

Kelly Cassidy BA(Hons), MMAA
28 Belton Hill, Fullwood, Preston,
Lancashire PR2 3SU

Emily Evans BSc (Hons), PGCE, MMAA
21A Stanley Road, London E4 7DB

Debbie Maizels BSc(Jt Hons), BA(Hons), CBiol, MRSB, MMAA
Tregerry Cottage, Treneglos, Launceston,
Cornwall PL15 8UF

Amanda Williams BA(Hons), FMAA
86 Hadley Road, Barnet
Hertfordshire EN5 5QR

Philip Wilson FMAA
Tregerry Cottage, Treneglos, Launceston,
Cornwall PL15 8UF

Thanks and acknowledgement is also given to Beth Croce for use of her drawings in Chapter 7: Expanded use of arterial conduits.

Rob & Smith's
Operative
Cardiac Surgery

SIXTH EDITION

Edited by

Thomas L. Spray, MD
Chief, Division of Cardiothoracic Surgery
Mortimer J. Buckley Jr MD Endowed Chair in Cardiothoracic Surgery
The Children's Hospital of Philadelphia
Professor of Surgery
Perelman School of Medicine, University of Pennsylvania
The Children's Hospital of Philadelphia
Division of Cardiothoracic Surgery
Philadelphia, PA

Michael A. Acker, MD
Chief, Division of Cardiovascular Surgery
Director, Penn Medicine Heart and Vascular Center
Julian Johnson Professor of Surgery
Perelman School of Medicine, University of Pennsylvania
Hospital of the University of Pennsylvania
Philadelphia, PA

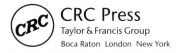

CRC Press
Taylor & Francis Group
Boca Raton London New York

CRC Press is an imprint of the
Taylor & Francis Group, an **informa** business

CRC Press
Taylor & Francis Group
6000 Broken Sound Parkway NW, Suite 300
Boca Raton, FL 33487-2742

© 2019 by Taylor & Francis Group, LLC
CRC Press is an imprint of Taylor & Francis Group, an Informa business

No claim to original U.S. Government works

Printed and bound in India by Replika Press Pvt. Ltd.

Typeset by Evolution Design & Digital Ltd (Kent)

Printed on acid-free paper

International Standard Book Number-13: 978-1-4441-3758-3 (Pack: Hardback and ebook)

Library of Congress Cataloging-in-Publication Data

Names: Spray, Thomas L., editor. | Acker, Michael A. (Michael Andrew), editor.
Title: Operative cardiac surgery / edited by Thomas L. Spray, Michael A. Acker.
Description: Sixth edition. | Boca Raton : CRC Press, 2018. | Includes bibliographical references and index.
Identifiers: LCCN 2018032584| ISBN 9781444137583 (hardback : alk. paper) | ISBN 9781351175975 (ebook).
Subjects: | MESH: Cardiac Surgical Procedures--methods | Heart Diseases—surgery.
Classification: LCC RD598 | NLM WG 169 | DDC 617.4/12--dc23
LC record available at https://lccn.loc.gov/2018032584

Visit the Taylor & Francis Web site at
http://www.taylorandfrancis.com

and the CRC Press Web site at
http://www.crcpress.com

Contents

SECTION IV   SURGERY FOR HEART FAILURE

SECTION V   THORACIC AORTIC DISEASE

SECTION VI   SURGERY FOR CARDIAC RHYTHM DISORDERS AND TUMORS

SECTION VII   SURGERY FOR CONGENITAL HEART DISEASE

Contributors

David H. Adams, MD
Professor and Chairman
Department of Cardiothoracic Surgery
The Mount Sinai Medical Center
New York, New York, USA

Gabriel S. Aldea, MD, FACS, FACC
William K. Edmark Professor
Chief, Adult Cardiac Surgery
Co-Director, Regional Heart Center
University of Washington Medical Center
Seattle, Washington, USA

Zohair Y. Al Halees, MD, FACC, FRCSC, FACS
Senior Consultant Cardiac Surgeon
Heart Center
Advisor to the CEO
King Faisal Specialist Hospital & Research Center
Riyadh, Saudi Arabia

Nelson Alphonso, MD, FRACS
Director of Cardiac Surgery
Queensland Paediatric Cardiac Service
Lady Cilento Children's Hospital
Brisbane, Australia

Robert H. Anderson, BSC, MD, FRCPATH
Visiting Professor
Institute of Genetic Medicine
Newcastle University
Newcastle, UK

George J. Arnaoutakis, MD
Assistant Professor of Surgery
Division of Thoracic and Cardiovascular Surgery
University of Florida
Gainesville, Florida, USA

Marvin D. Atkins, MD
Methodist DeBakey Cardiovascular Surgery Associates
Houston Methodist Hospital
Houston, Texas, USA

Pavan Atluri, MD
Associate Professor of Surgery
Director, Cardiac Transplantation and Mechanical Circulatory Assist
Program;
Director, Minimally Invasive and Robotic Cardiac Surgery Program
Division of Cardiovascular Surgery
Department of Surgery
University of Pennsylvania
Philadelphia, Pennsylvania, USA

Erle H. Austin III, MD
Professor and Vice-Chairman
Department of Cardiovascular and Thoracic Surgery
University of Louisville;
Former Chief, Cardiovascular Surgery
Norton Children's Hospital
Louisville, Kentucky, USA

Emile Bacha, MD
Professor and Chief
Cardiac, Thoracic and Vascular Surgery
Columbia University Medical Center
NewYork-Presbyterian Hospital
New York, New York, USA

Carl Lewis Backer, MD
Division Head, Cardiovascular-Thoracic Surgery
Ann & Robert H. Lurie Children's Hospital of Chicago;
A.C. Buehler Professor of Surgery
Department of Surgery, Feinberg School of Medicine
Northwestern University
Chicago, Illinois, USA

David J. Barron, MD FRCP FRCS(CT)
Consultant Cardiac Surgeon
Birmingham Children's Hospital
Birmingham, UK

Joseph E. Bavaria, MD
Past-President (2016–17)
Society of Thoracic Surgeons (STS)
Brooke Roberts-William M. Measey Professor of Surgery
Vice-Chief, Division of Cardiovascular Surgery
Surgical Director, Heart and Vascular Center
Director, Thoracic Aortic Surgery Program
University of Pennsylvania
Philadelphia, Pennsylvania, USA

Christian A. Bermudez, MD
Director of Thoracic Transplantation
Surgical Director, Lung Transplantation and ECMO
Associate Professor of Surgery
Division of Cardiovascular Surgery
University of Pennsylvania Health System
Philadelphia, Pennsylvania, USA

Pierre-Luc Bernier, MD, CM, MPH, FRCSC
Cardiac Surgeon
The Montreal Children's Hospital & The Royal Victoria Hospital
McGill University Health Centre;
Assistant Professor of Surgery
McGill University
Montreal, Canada

David P. Bichell, MD
Chief
Pediatric Cardiac Surgery
Vanderbilt University Medical Center
Monroe Carrel Jr Children's Hospital
Nashville, Tennessee, USA

Steven F. Bolling, MD
Professor of Cardiac Surgery
Department of Cardiac Surgery
The University of Michigan Hospitals
Ann Arbor, Michigan, USA

Johannes Bonatti, MD, FETCS
Chief
Heart and Vascular Institute
Cleveland Clinic Abu Dhabi
Abu Dhabi, UAE

Michael A. Borger, MD, PhD
Chief Physician
Helios Heart Center
Leipzig, Germany

Edward L. Bove, MD
Professor of Surgery
Department of Cardiac Surgery
University of Michigan School of Medicine
Ann Arbor, Michigan, USA

Jack H. Boyd, MD
Clinical Assistant Professor
Department of Cardiothoracic Surgery
Stanford University School of Medicine
Stanford, California, USA

Alexander A. Brescia, MD
Fellow in Cardiac Surgery
Department of Cardiac Surgery
University of Michigan Medicine
Ann Arbor, Michigan, USA

Julie Brothers, MD
Assistant Professor of Pediatrics
Perelman School of Medicine at University of Pennsylvania;
Attending Cardiologist
Department of Pediatrics
The Children's Hospital of Philadelphia
Philadelphia, Pennsylvania, USA

Chase R. Brown, MD
Cardiothoracic Surgery Resident
Division of Cardiovascular Surgery
Hospital of the University of Pennsylvania
Philadelphia, Pennsylvania, USA

Brian F. Buxton, MB MS, FRCS, FACS, FRACS, AM
Professor of Cardiac Surgery
University of Melbourne
Melbourne, Australia;
Epworth Research Institute
Richmond, Australia

Duke E. Cameron, MD
Co-director of Thoracic Aortic Surgery Center
 and Co-director Adult Congenital Surgery Heart Program
Division of Cardiac Surgery
Massachusetts General Hospital
Boston, Massachusetts, USA

Edward Cantu, MD, MSCE
Assistant Professor of Surgery
Associate Director of Lung Transplantation
Director of Lung Transplant Research
Director of Ex Vivo Perfusion
Department of Surgery
Division of Cardiovascular Surgery
Hospital of the University of Pennsylvania
Philadelphia, Pennsylvania, USA

Javier G. Castillo, MD
Assistant Professor of Cardiovascular Surgery
Director, Hispanic Heart Center;
Executive Director, Mitral Foundation
Department of Cardiothoracic Surgery
The Mount Sinai Medical Center
New York, New York, USA

Paul Chai, MD
Associate Professor of Surgery
Division of Cardiac, Thoracic and Vascular Surgery
Columbia University Medical Center
New York-Presbyterian Hospital
New York, New York, USA

Edward P. Chen, MD
Professor of Surgery
Division of Cardiothoracic Surgery
Emory University Hospital
Atlanta, Georgia, USA

W. Randolph Chitwood Jr, MD
Emeritus Professor of Cardiothoracic Surgery
Emeritus Director of East Carolina Heart institute
Department of Cardiovascular Sciences
East Carolina Heart Institute at East Carolina University
Greenville, North Carolina, USA

Gordon A. Cohen, MD, PhD, MBA
Professor and Chief
Pediatric Cardiothoracic Surgery
Benoff Children's Hospital
University of California San Francisco
San Francisco, California, USA

James L. Cox, MD
Surgical Director, Center for Heart Rhythm Disorders
Bluhm Cardiovascular Institute
Professor of Surgery
Feinberg School of Medicine
Northwestern University
Chicago, Illinois, USA

Jose P. da Silva, MD
Visiting Professor of Cardiothoracic Surgery
Surgical Director
Center for Valve Therapy
Children's Hospital of Pittsburgh
Pittsburgh, Pennsylvania, USA

William M. DeCampli, MD, PhD
Chief, Pediatric Cardiovascular Surgery
Arnold Palmer Hospital for Children;
Professor of Surgery
University of Central Florida College of Medicine
Orlando, Florida, USA;
Managing Director, Data Center
Congenital Heart Surgeons Society
The Hospital for Sick Children
Toronto, Ontario, CA

Joseph J DeRose Jr, MD
Chief, Division of Cardiothoracic Surgery
Professor, Cardiothoracic Surgery
Albert Einstein College of Medicine
Montefiore-Einstein Medical Center
Broynx, New York, USA

Nimesh D. Desai, MD PhD
Associate Professor of Surgery
Division of Cardiovascular Surgery
University of Pennsylvania
Philadelphia, Pennsylvania, USA

Nhue L. Do, MD
Assistant Professor of Surgery
Johns Hopkins University School of Medicine
Johns Hopkins Hospital
Baltimore, Maryland, USA

Daniel-Sebastian Dohle, MD
Aortic Surgery Fellow
Division of Cardiovascular Surgery
University of Pennsylvania
Philadelphia, Pennsylvania, USA;
Head of Aortic Arch Surgery
Department of Cardiothoracic and Vascular Surgery
Johannes-Gutenberg University
Mainz, Germany

Aaron Eckhauser, MD
Associate Professor of Surgery
Pediatric Cardiothoracic Surgery
University of Utah
Primary Children's Hospital
Salt Lake City, Utah, USA

Martin J. Elliott, MD, FRCS
Professor of Cardiothoracic Surgery at University College London;
Emeritus Professor of Physic at Gresham College, London;
Consultant Cardiothoracic Surgeon
The Cardiac Unit
The Great Ormond Street Hospital for Children NHS FT
London, UK

Jared W. Feinman, MD
Assistant Professor
Department of Anesthesiology and Critical Care
Perelman School of Medicine
University of Pennsylvania
Philadelphia, Pennsylvania, USA

Andrew C. Fiore, MD
Professor
Division of Cardiovascular Surgery
St Louis University School of Medicine
St Louis, Missouri, USA

Charles D. Fraser Jr, MD, FACS
Professor of Surgery and Pediatrics
University of Texas, Dell Medical School;
Director, Texas Center for Pediatric and Congenital Heart Disease
Dell Children's Medical Center
Austin, Texas, USA

Stephanie Fuller, MD, MS
Thomas L. Spray Endowed Chair in Congenital Cardiothoracic
Surgery
Associate Professor of Surgery
Perelman School of Medicine
University of Pennsylvania
Division of Cardiothoracic Surgery
The Children's Hospital of Philadelphia
Philadelphia, Pennsylvania, USA

Shinichi Fukuhara, MD
Thoracic and Cardiac Surgeon
University of Michigan Cardiovascular Center
Ann Arbor, Michigan, USA

Sean D. Galvin, MB ChB, FCSANZ, FRACS
Adjunct Professor
Cardiothoracic Surgeon
Department of Cardiothoracic Surgery
Wellington Regional Hospital
Wellington, New Zealand

J. William Gaynor, MD
Professor of Surgery
Perelman School of Medicine at University of Pennsylvania;
Department of Cardiothoracic Surgery
The Children's Hospital of Philadelphia
Philadelphia, Pennsylvania, USA

Thomas G. Gleason, MD
Ronald V. Pellegrini Professor and Chief
Division of Cardiac Surgery
Department of Cardiothoracic Surgery
University of Pittsburgh School of Medicine
Pittsburgh, Pennsylvania, USA

László Göbölös, MD, FESC
Associate Staff Physician
Heart and Vascular Institute
Cleveland Clinic Abu Dhabi
Abu Dhabi, UAE

Michael Grushko, MD
Director, Clinical Cardiac Electrophyisology
Jacobi and North Central Bronx Hospitals
Montefiore Einstein Heart Center;
Assistant Professor of Medicine
Albert Einstein College of Medicine
Bronx, New York, USA

T. Sloane Guy, MD
Chief, Division of Cardiovascular Surgery
Chief, Robotic Surgery
Temple University School of Medicine
Philadelphia, Pennsylvania, USA

Ismail El-Hamamsy, MD PhD
Associate Professor
Division of Cardiac Surgery
Montreal Heart Institute
Université de Montréal
Montreal, Quebec, Canada

G. Chad Hughes, MD
Director, Duke Center for Aortic Disease
Surgical Director, Duke Center for Structural Heart Disease
Associate Professor
Division of Thoracic and Cardiovascular Surgery
Duke University Medical Center
Durham, North Carolina, USA

Frank L. Hanley, MD
Professor of Cardiothoracic Surgery
Stanford University School of Medicine;
Executive Director
Betty Irene Moore Children's Heart Center
Lucille Packard Children's Hospital
Stanford, California, USA

W. Clark Hargrove III, MD
Clinical Professor of Surgery
Division of Cardiovascular Surgery
Penn Presbyterian Medical Center
University of Pennsylvania
Philadelphia, Pennsylvania, USA

Philip A.R. Hayward, BM(Oxon), MRCP, FRCS, FRACS
Associate Professor of Cardiac Surgery
University of Melbourne
Melbourne, Australia;
Department of Cardiac Surgery
Austin Hospital
Heidelberg, Australia

Charles B. Huddleston, MD
Thoracic and Cardiac Surgeon
Department of Surgery
St Louis University School of Medicine
St Louis, Missouri, USA

Valluvan Jeevanandam, MD
Professor of Surgery
Section of Cardiac and Thoracic Surgery
Department of Surgery
University of Chicago
Chicago, Illinois, USA

Tara Karamlou, MD, MSc
Division of Pediatric Cardiac Surgery and the Heart Vascular Institute
Cleveland Clinic
Cleveland, Ohio, USA

Tom R. Karl, MD, MS, FRACS
Professor of Surgery
Johns Hopkins All Children's Hospital
St Petersburg, Florida, USA

Arman Kilic, MD
Assistant Professor of Cardiothoracic Surgery
University of Pittsburgh Medical Center
Philadelphia, Pennsylvania, USA

Elgin Kocyildirim, MD
Assistant Professor
University of Pittsburgh
Department of Cardiothoracic Surgery
McGowan Institute of Regenerative Medicine
Pittsburgh, Pennsylvania, USA

Irving L. Kron, MD
Senior Associate Vice President for Health Affairs
Interim Dean
University of Arizona School of Medicine
Pheonix, Arizona, USA

Andrew Krumerman, MD
Associate Professor
Department of Medicine (Cardiology)
Albert Einstein College of Medicine
New York, New York, USA

Murray H. Kwon, MD, MBA
Associate Clinical Professor
Division of Cardiothoracic Surgery
Department of Surgery
David Geffen School of Medicine at UCLA
Los Angeles, California, USA

Francois Lacour-Gayet, MD
Professor of Surgery
Royal Hospital National Heart Center
Muscat, Sultanate of Oman

Maxime Laflamme, MD, MSc, FRCSC
Surgeon
Heart and Lung Institute
Quebec, Canada

Yves Lecompte, MD
Honorary Consultant Surgeon
Department of Pediatric Cardiac Surgery
APHP Sick Children Hospital
Paris, France

Timothy Lee, MD
Surgeon
Department of General Surgery
University of California - San Francisco
San Francisco, California, USA

Patrick M. McCarthy, MD
Chief, Division of Cardiac Surgery
Director, Bluhm Cardiovascular Institute
Department of Cardiac Surgery
Bluhm Cardiovascular Institute
Northwestern Memorial Hospital;
Heller-Sacks Professor of Surgery
Feinberg School of Medicine
Northwestern University
Chicago, Illinois, USA

Edwin C. McGee Jr, MD, FACS
Professor of Surgery
Executive Medical Director, Solid Organ Transplant Programs
Surgical Director, Heart Transplantation and LVAD Program
Department of Thoracic and Cardiovascular Surgery
Loyola University Medical Center
Chicago, Illinois, USA

Kaushik Mandal, MD
Cardiac Surgeon
Division of Cardiac Surgery
Johns Hopkins University School of Medicine
Baltimore, Maryland, USA

Peter B. Manning, MD
Pediatric Cardiothoracic Surgeon
Section of Pediatric Cardiothoracic Surgery
St Louis Children's Hospital
Professor of Surgery
Washington University School of Medicine
St Louis, Missouri, USA

Christopher E. Mascio, MD
Alice Langdon Warner Endowed Chair
Pediatric Cardiothoracic Surgery
Children's Hospital of Philadelphia;
Associate Professor of Clinical Surgery
Perelman School of Medicine, University of Pennsylvania
Philadelphia, Pennsylvania, USA

Bonnie L. Milas, MD
Professor of Clinical Anesthesiology and Critical Care
Department of Anesthesiology and Critical Care
Perelman School of Medicine
University of Pennsylvania
Philadelphia, Pennsylvania, USA

David Luís Simón Morales, MD
Professor of Surgery and Pediatrics
Clark-Helmsworth Chair of Pediatric Cardiothoracic Surgery
Director of Congenital Heart Surgery
The Heart Institute
Cincinnati Children's Hospital Medical Center
The University of Cincinnati College of Medicine
Cincinnati, Ohio, USA

Victor O. Morell, MD
Co-Director
University of Pittsburgh Medical Center Heart and Lung Institute;
Vice Chair and Director of Cardiovascular Services
Department of Cardiothoracic Surgery;
Chief, Pediatric Cardiothoracic Surgery
Children's Hospital of Pittsburgh
Pittsburgh, Pennsylvania, USA

Michael O. Murphy, MA, MD, MRCP, FRCS
Cardiothoracic Registrar
Guy's & St Thomas' Hospital
London, UK

Takeyoshi Ota, MD, PhD
Assistant Professor of Surgery
Co-Director, Center for Aortic Disease
Section of Cardiac and Thoracic Surgery
Department of Surgery
The University of Chicago Medical Center
Chicago, Illinois, USA

Massimo A. Padalino, MD, PhD
Staff Pediatric Cardiac Surgeon
Pediatric and Congenital Cardiac Surgery Unit
Department of Cardiac Thoracic Vascular Sciences and Public Health
University of Padua
Padua, Italy

Albert J. Pedroza, MD
Cardiothoracic Surgery Resident
Department of Cardiothoracic Surgery
Stanford University School of Medicine
Stanford, California, USA

Louis P. Perrault, MD, Ph.D, FRCSC, FACS, FECS
Head
Department of Surgery
Montreal Heart Institute;
Professor of Surgery and Pharmacology
Université de Montréal
Montreal, Quebec, Canada

Ryan Plichta, MD
Assistant Professor
Division of Cardiothoracic Surgery
Duke University Medical Center
Durham, North Carolina, USA

Alberto Pochettino, MD
Professor of Surgery
Division of Cardiovascular Surgery
Mayo Clinic
Rochester, Minnesota, USA

Jeffrey Poynter, MD
Cardiothoracic Surgery Fellow
Division of Cardiovascular Surgery
University of Pennsylvania Health System
Philadelphia, Pennsylvania, USA

John D. Puskas, MD, MSc, FACS, FACC
Professor, Icahn School of Medicine at Mount Sinai;
Chairman, Department of Cardiovascular Surgery
Mount Sinai Saint Luke's
Mount Sinai Beth Israel and Mount Sinai West System;
Director, Surgical Coronary Resvascularizarion
Mount Sinai Heath System
New York, New York, USA

James A. Quintessenza, MD
Professor of Surgery
Cincinnati's Children's Hospital Medical Center
University of Cincinnati;
Kentucky Children's Hospital
University of Kentucky
Kentucky, USA

Olivier Raisky, MD, PhD
Professor of Cardiac Surgery
University Paris Descartes
Sorbonne Paris Cité;
Consultant Surgeon
Department of Pediatric Cardiac Surgery
APHP Sick Children Hospital
Paris, France

V. Mohan Reddy, MD
Professor of Surgery
UCSF School of Medicine;
Chief
Division of Pediatric Cardiothoracic Surgery
University of California, San Francisco
Benioff Children's Hospital
San Francisco, California, USA

J. Mark Redmond, MD, FRCSI
Consultant Pediatric Cardiac Surgeon
Our Lady's Childrens' Hospital Crumlin
Dublin, Ireland

Jennifer C. Romano, MD, MS
Associate Professor
Pediatric Cardiac Surgery
Department of Cardiac Surgery
University of Michigan School of Medicine
Ann Arbor, Michigan, USA

Matthew A. Romano, MD
Assistant Professor of Cardiac Surgery
Department of Cardiac Surgery
The University of Michigan Hospitals
Ann Arbor, Michigan, USA

Joshua M. Rosenblum, MD, PhD
Resident
Division of Cardiothoracic Surgery
Emory University Hospital
Atlanta, Georgia, USA

Nishant Saran, MBBS
Fellow
Department of Cardiovascular Surgery
Mayo Clinic
Rochester, Minnesota, USA

Joseph S. Savino, MD
Professor
Department of Anesthesiology and Critical Care
Perelman School of Medicine
University of Pennsylvania
Philadelphia, Pennsylvania, USA

Erin M. Schumer, MD, MPH
Trainee Cardiothoracic Surgeon
Department of Cardiothoracic Surgery
University of Louisville
Louisville, Kentucky, USA

Mahesh S. Sharma, MD
Assistant Professor of Surgery
Department of Cardiothoracic Surgery
Pediatric Cardiothoracic Surgeon
Children's Hospital of Pittsburgh
Pittsburgh, Pennsylvania, USA

Richard J. Shemin, MD
Robert and Kelley Day Professor
UCLA David Geffen School of Medicine;
Chief, Division of Cardiac Surgery
Vice Chairman, Department of Surgery
Co-Director of Cardiovascular Center
Ronald Reagan UCLA Medical Center
Los Angeles, California, USA

Irving Shen, MD
John C. Hursh Chair
Pediatric Cardiac Surgery
Doernbecher Children's Hospital
Portland, Oregon, USA

Mark S. Slaughter, MD
Professor and Chair
Department of Cardiovascular and Thoracic Surgery
University of Louisville;
Editor-in-Chief
ASAIO Journal
Louisville, Kentucky, USA

Nicholas G. Smedira, MD
Heart and Vascular Institute
Department of Thoracic and Cardiovascular Surgery
Cleveland Clinic
Cleveland, Ohio, USA

Diane E. Spicer, BS, PA(ASCP)
University of Florida
Department of Pediatric Cardiology
Congenital Heart Center
Gainesville, Florida, USA

Thomas L. Spray, MD
Chief, Division of Cardiothoracic Surgery
Mortimer J. Buckley Jr MD Endowed Chair in Cardiothoracic Surgery
The Children's Hospital of Philadelphia;
Professor of Surgery
Perelman School of Medicine
University of Pennsylvania;
The Children's Hospital of Philadelphia
Division of Cardiothoracic Surgery,
Philadelphia, Pennsylvania, USA

Robert J. Steffen, MD
Heart and Vascular Institute
Department of Thoracic and Cardiovascular Surgery
Cleveland Clinic
Cleveland, Ohio, USA

Giovanni Stellin, MD, PhD
Professor of Cardiac Surgery
Chief of Pediatric and Congenital Cardiac Surgery
Department of Cardiac Thoracic Vascular Sciences and Public Health
University of Padua
Padua, Italy

Elizabeth H. Stephens, MD, PhD
Cardiothoracic Surgeon
Lurie Children's Hospital
Northwestern University
Chicago, Illinois, USA

Ibrahim Sultan, MD
Assistant Professor of Cardiothoracic Surgery
Division of Cardiac Surgery
Department of Cardiothoracic Surgery
University of Pittsburgh
Pittsburgh, Pennsylvania, USA

Wilson Y. Szeto, MD
Professor of Surgery
University of Pennsylvania School of Medicine;
Vice Chief of Clinical Operations and Quality
Division of Cardiovascular Surgery;
Chief, Cardiovascular Surgery at Penn Presbyterian Medical Center;
Surgical Director, Transcatheter Cardio-Aortic Therapies
Philadelphia, Pennsylvania, USA

Christo I. Tchervenkov, MD, FRCSC
Division Head
Division of Pediatric Cardiovascular Surgery;
Department of Surgery
The Montreal Children's Hospital of the McGill University Health
Center
Montreal, Canada

Gianluca Torregrossa, MD
Associate Director of Robotic Heart Surgery
Department of Cardiac Surgery
Mount Sinai Saint Luke
Mount Sinai Health System
New York, New York, USA

Victor T. Tsang, MD, FRCS
Professor of Cardiac Surgery UCL
Great Ormond Street Hospital
St Bartholomew's Hospital
London, UK

Ross M. Ungerleider, MD, MBA
Medical Director, Heart Center;
Chief, Pediatric Cardiac Surgery
Driscoll Children's Hospital
Corpus Christi, Texas, USA

Prashanth Vallabhajosyula, MD, MS
Associate Professor of Surgery
Division of Cardiovascular Surgery
Hospital of the University of Pennsylvania
University of Pennsylvania
Philadelphia, Pennsylvania, USA

Edward D. Verrier, MD
Professor of Surgery
Department of Surgery
University of Washington
Seattle, Washington, USA

Vladimiro L. Vida, MD, PhD
Associate Professor of Cardiac Surgery
Pediatric and Congenital Cardiac Surgery Unit
Department of Cardiac Thoracic Vascular Sciences and Public Health
University of Padua
Padua, Italy

Pascal R. Vouhé, MD, PhD
Professor of Cardiac Surgery
University Paris Descartes
Sorbonne Paris Cité;
Head Surgeon
Department of Pediatric Cardiac Surgery
APHP Sick Children Hospital
Paris, France

Luca A. Vricella, MD, FACS
Professor of Surgery and Pediatrics
Director, Pediatric Cardiac Surgery and Heart Transplantation
Johns Hopkins University
Baltimore, Maryland, USA

Cynthia E. Wagner, MD
Resident Physician
Cardiothoracic Surgery Residency Program
University of Virginia
Charlottesville, Virginia, USA

Sarah T. Ward, MD
Fellow in Cardiac Surgery
Department of Cardiac Surgery
The University of Michigan Hospitals
Ann Arbor, Michigan, USA

Richard D. Weisel, MD, FRCSC
Professor of Cardiac Surgery
University of Toronto;
Senior Scientist
Toronto General Research Institute;
Surgeon
Division of Cardiovascular Surgery
Toronto General Hospital
Toronto, Canada

Matthew L. Williams, MD
Assistant Professor of Surgery
Perelman School of Medicine
University of Pennsylvania
Philadelphia, Pennsylvania, USA

Terrence M. Yau, MD, CM, MSc, FRCSC
Angelo and Lorenza DeGasperis Chair in Cardiovascular
Surgery Research;
Director of Research
Division of Cardiovascular Surgery
University Health Network;
Professor of Surgery
University of Toronto
Toronto, Canada

Farhan Zafar, MD
Assistant Professor
Pediatric Cardiothoracic Surgery
Cincinnati Children's Hospital Medical Center
University of Cincinnati College of Medicine
Cincinnati, Ohio, USA

Prologue

The Rob & Smith's Operative Surgery series established a legacy of texts focusing on the critical element of all surgical fields — the operative procedure itself. Specialization and even sub-specialization of surgery practice has led to growing number of editions in the Operative Surgery series, resulting in a broad dissemination of texts from experienced surgeon-leaders sharing their surgical skills by demonstrating how they perform the subject operation. This central goal continues to be the focus of Operative Surgery texts: thoroughly described and carefully illustrated major surgical procedures.

Even in the current multi-media environment with access to videos of surgical procedures, the unique value of these Operative Surgery texts persist. Individual chapters on all major operations performed in the particular specialty area provide the reader with exposure to leading surgeons' full clinical and technical skills and experience. This expert commentary combined with precise and detailed illustrations maintain the special relevance of Operative Surgery texts.

This 6th Edition of Operative Cardiac Surgery, being published only 14 years after the previous edition, reflects the continued swift refinement and evolution of adult and congenital heart surgery. Progress, improvement and the development of new procedures in cardiac surgery are marked by single decades. The rapid progress that challenges cardiac surgeons to learn, enhance and refine their surgical skills has been incorporated in this 6th Edition.

While the role of the surgeon encompasses the full span of the encounter with the patient, including diagnostic, peri- and post-operative management, the singular essential role he or she plays is in the performance of the operation. How to carry out the operation safely and effectively is the essential element of the surgeon's responsibility. This new Operative Cardiac Surgery textbook is an invaluable volume by expert surgeons for the benefit of other surgeons. It is intended for surgeons who aspire to the best surgical outcomes for their patients, based on the most current and successful surgical techniques. Congratulations to the Editors, Michael Acker and Thomas Spray, for this updated 6th Edition. The many contributors deserve special acknowledgement and thanks for their efforts and expertise. The entire cardiac surgery community, and our patients, are the beneficiaries of this outstanding text.

Timothy J. Gardner

Preface

It has been 14 years since the publication of the 5th Edition of *Operative Cardiac Surgery* by Gardner and Spray. The 5th Edition contained 60 separate chapters dealing with the full spectrum of adult and pediatric cardiac surgery techniques and procedures that encompassed the specialty in the early 2000s. In order to encompass the entire range of adult and pediatric cardiac surgery today, the 6th Edition contains 68 chapters reflecting the progress of cardiac surgery in multiple areas over the past 14 years.

The section on surgery for ischemic heart disease now includes a new chapter on robotic total endoscopic coronary artery grafting (TECAB). The section on valvular heart disease has been expanded to include new chapters on TAVR, valve sparing aortic root replacement and tricuspid valve surgery. The section on heart failure has been expanded to include a new chapter on temporary mechanical assistance, including ECMO for the treatment of cardiogenic shock, and surgery for hypertrophic cardiomyopathy. We have also decided to include a chapter on lung transplantation since lung transplantation is done largely by cardiothoracic surgeons today. The section on thoracic aortic disease has been expanded to include new chapters on thoracic endovascular aortic repair (TEVAR), hybrid aortic arch repair, as well as including a discussion on Type B aortic dissections. Finally, the section on cardiac rhythm disorders now includes a separate chapter on the Maze procedure for the treatment of atrial fibrillation. In addition to these many new chapters, all our chapters have been largely rewritten with new illustrations and by a new set of authors who are currently experts in the field.

In the section on congenital heart disease, the previous chapters from the 5th Edition have remained and new chapters have been added on aortic pulmonary window; cardiac transplantation for congenital heart disease; lung and heart/lung transplantation for congenital heart disease; ventricular assist devices for congenital heart disease; congenital mitral valve repair and aortic valve repair.

The new edition continues to distinguish itself in its outstanding illustrations that accompany every chapter with detailed descriptions of the operative procedures. This addition continues the tradition of utilizing brilliant art work and illustrations that clearly reflect the anatomic and technical features of each operative procedure.

Dr. Spray and I are honored to have had the opportunity to edit the 6th Edition with such a renowned and respected group of authors. We thank all our editors and contributors to this work knowing that it has been a long time in coming. I specifically want to thank Miranda Bromage for her superb leadership in shepherding this large project to the finish line.

Thomas L Spray, MD
Michael Acker, MD

Perioperative management

Echocardiography for cardiac surgery

JARED W. FEINMAN, BONNIE L. MILAS, AND JOSEPH S. SAVINO

HISTORY

The ability to perform real-time cardiovascular imaging in the operating room using transesophageal echocardiography (TEE) has been the most important diagnostic advancement in cardiac surgery over the past 30 years. TEE was developed in the mid 1970s but did not enter widespread use until the early 1980s when flexible TEE probes with manipulatable tips became available. The early probes were only capable of imaging along a single plane (monoplane), which somewhat limited their utility. The technology behind ultrasound image acquisition has moved forward rapidly, however, to the point that modern TEE probes can image along a 180 degree axis, display multiple imaging planes simultaneously (x plane imaging) and acquire large pyramids of data that allow real-time, three-dimensional (3D) rendering of cardiac structures. As intraoperative TEE use has become commonplace, there has been a joint effort by the American Society of Echocardiography (ASE) and the Society of Cardiovascular Anesthesiologists (SCA) to standardize the perioperative TEE examination through the issuance of joint guideline statements as well as the establishment of a board certification process administered by the non-profit National Board of Echocardiography. The first set of guidelines on performing a comprehensive TEE exam was issued in 1999, and consisted of 20 standard echocardiographic views. This was expanded to 28 two-dimensional (2D) views and a focused 3D exam in the most recent 2013 update. Current recommendations state that an intraoperative TEE should be performed (barring a contraindication) in all patients undergoing open heart, thoracic aorta, or catheter-based cardiac surgery, in most patients having coronary artery bypass grafting (CABG), and in any patients having non-cardiac surgery with known or suspected cardiac pathology that may impact outcomes.

PRINCIPLES AND JUSTIFICATION

A few general principles regarding image generation, interpretation of data, and limitations of the ultrasound system are useful in understanding TEE in the operating room. In basic terms, the ultrasound transducer uses piezoelectric crystals to convert electrical energy into high-frequency acoustic energy (ultrasound waves) and vice versa. The ultrasound waves that are emitted from the transducer travel through tissue planes where they can be absorbed (converted into heat), refracted (if crossing between objects with different propagation speeds), or reflected (if adjacent media have different acoustic impedances) back towards the probe where they are converted by the ultrasound system into an image. Since reflection occurs best at a 90-degree angle, 2D imaging will be most effective when the ultrasound beam is orthogonal to the tissue being imaged. Also, any material that causes a lot of reflection (e.g. prosthetic valves and calcium deposits) will not allow the ultrasound beam to pass beyond it, impairing the ability to image more distant structures. The data being reflected back to the ultrasound probe can be expressed in two different imaging formats. The most common is 2D B-mode imaging, where a line of echo data is moved back and forth in an arc through a section of tissue and displayed so that a continuous 2D image is generated. Alternatively, in M-mode imaging a single scan line is displayed over time, which allows for a very high frame rate and accuracy of linear measurements. Modern, full matrix array transducers have about 3000 independent piezoelectric elements that can be fired in a phased manner to generate a radially propagating scan line. The scan line can be steered in three planes to generate a true 3D volume of data, which can either be displayed in real time or stitched together with adjected volumes using ECG-gating to produce an even larger volume of 3D data.

Doppler ultrasound can be used to assess the velocity of blood flow or tissue movement within the heart and vascular structures. Since this form of imaging relies on the Doppler shift equation:

$$\text{Doppler shift} = \frac{(2 \times \text{velocity of object} \times \text{incident frequency} \times \text{cosine } \theta)}{\text{Propagation speed of ultrasound}}$$

a calculated velocity will be most accurate when the ultrasound beam is perfectly aligned with the blood flow being assessed (cosine 0° = 1), and should only be used if θ is <20 degrees. This stands in contrast to the aforementioned 2D imaging, which will achieve the best resolution when the structure being imaged is orthogonal to the ultrasound beam. Doppler imaging is used in three common modes: pulsed-wave Doppler, continuous-wave Doppler, and color-flow Doppler. Pulsed-wave and continuous-wave Doppler imaging both assess the velocity of the object being imaged over time, but differ in that the former is limited in the maximum velocity that can be assessed (Nyquist limit) but has range specificity, while the latter is not limited by a maximum velocity but has range ambiguity. Thus, pulsed-wave Doppler is used to assess low-velocity flow in a specific location (e.g. pulmonary vein flow, transmitral inflow in a non-stenotic valve) while continuous-wave Doppler is useful in assessing high-velocity flow through a stenotic or regurgitant valve. Color-flow Doppler imaging overlays pulsed-wave Doppler data on a standard 2D image to generate a color map that provides information on the direction of blood flow as well as semi-quantitative information on the mean velocities of flow. Traditionally, blue denotes movement away from the ultrasound probe and red movement towards the probe.

The TEE probe itself is essentially a modified gastroscope with a matrix array of piezoelectric crystals at the tip in place of a camera. Probe insertion and manipulation may lead to significant injury, and precautions are necessary to minimize the risk. Most perioperative TEEs are performed in anesthetized and intubated patients who cannot respond to pain or discomfort caused by excessive probe impingement of soft tissue. Before insertion, the TEE probe is inspected for damage or any break in the encasement. Then the probe is lubricated, inserted into the mouth, and passed posteriorly into the esophagus, and most imaging occurs at the level of the midesophagus, upper esophagus, or stomach. Manufacturers' recommendations for probe cleaning and maintenance should be followed with a systematic approach to instrument processing. Complications from probe insertion are uncommon (0.2% in one case series of 7200 patients reported by Kallmeyer et al.), and range from minor trauma to the teeth or pharynx to esophageal perforation, which carries with it a high risk of mortality.

Contraindications to TEE are disorders of the mouth, esophagus, or stomach that could preclude safe passage of the probe. These include esophageal strictures, diverticula, or webs, cancerous masses, or an active esophageal perforation or bleed. Abnormal displacement of the esophagus, such as may occur with a large aortic aneurysm, is not a contraindication, but is associated with increased risk. In patients where there is a question of esophageal disease, the risks and benefits of TEE for that specific procedure must be weighed. If TEE is to be performed, it may be prudent to first have an esophagogastroduodenoscopy (EGD) done in the operating room to make sure that placement is safe, and/or to use a pediatric TEE probe, which is much smaller in diameter than a standard adult probe but comes with significant imaging limitations.

COMPREHENSIVE TEE EXAMINATION

The current ASE/SCA guideline statement on performing a comprehensive TEE examination lists 28 standard views with additional 2D and 3D imaging performed as needed (see **Figure 1.1**). The TEE probe is initially inserted to a depth of approximately 30 cm and the entirety of the examination is performed by adjusting the rotation of the beam within the probe (omniplane angle), rotating the probe itself to the left or right, or moving the probe farther into or out of the esophagus/stomach. The views and the corresponding approximate omniplane angle (between 0° and 180°) for each view are illustrated in the figure. The order in which a TEE exam is conducted varies between individual providers. While there is no "ideal" order of imaging, it is important for an echocardiographer to choose a protocol and follow it in every case, as this will prevent any unanticipated findings from being missed. When discussing standard TEE views, the nomenclature is such that each view is named for the location of the probe in space (e.g. upper esophageal (UE), midesophageal (ME), or transgastric (TG)) followed by what is being imaged (four-chamber, two-chamber, etc.). Figure 1.1 has been reproduced with permission from Hahn RT, Abraham T, Adams MS, et al. Guidelines for performing a comprehensive transesophageal echocardiographic examination: recommendations from the American Society of Echocardiography and the Society of Cardiovascular Anesthesiologists. *J Am Soc Echocardiogr.* 2013; 26: 921–64.

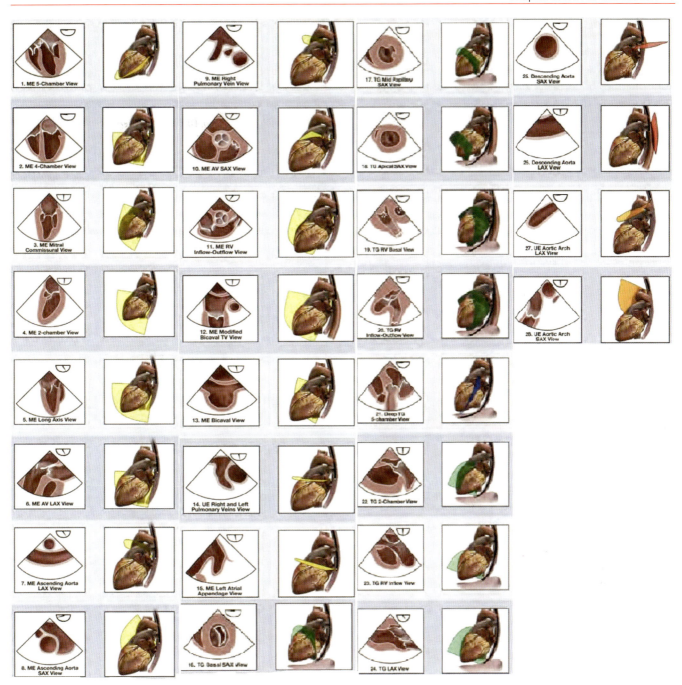

1.1 TEE examination standard views.

Left ventricle

The left ventricle (LV) can be divided into a series of segments that allows correlation of regional wall motion with abnormalities in coronary blood flow. There are currently two commonly used models of left ventricular anatomy: the 16-segment model and the 17-segment model. The only difference between the two is that the former divides the apex of the heart into anterior, lateral, inferior, and septal regions, while the latter adds a fifth segment, the apical cap, made up of the myocardium beyond the end of the LV cavity.

The longitudinal axis of the LV is described as basal, mid, or apical. The midesophageal four-chamber view shows the three inferoseptal and three anterolateral segments (**Figure 1.2a**). Midesophageal two-chamber views show the three anterior and three inferior segments (**Figure 1.2b**) and midesophageal long-axis (LAX) views show the two anteroseptal and two inferolateral segments (**Figure 1.2c**). TG short-axis (SAX) views show all six segments at the mid (**Figure 1.2d**) and basal (**Figure 1.2e**) levels, and all four segments at the apical level. These figures have been reproduced with permission from Shanewise JS, Cheung AT, Aronson S, et al. ASE/SCA guidelines for performing a comprehensive intraoperative multiplane transesophageal echocardiography examination: recommendations of the American Society of Echocardiography Council for Intraoperative Echocardiography and the Society of Cardiovascular Anesthesiologists Task Force for Certification in Perioperative Transesophageal Echocardiography. *Anesth Analg.* 1999; 89: 870–84, and *J Am Soc Echocardiogr.* 1999; 12: 884–900.

See also **Figures 1.3–1.7**.

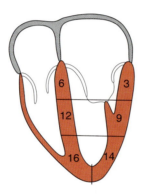

a. ME four-chamber view

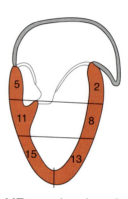

b. ME two-chamber view

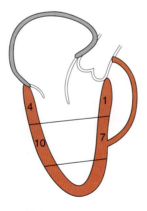

c. ME long-axis view

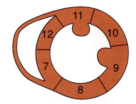

d. TG mid-short-axis view

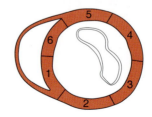

e. TG basal short-axis view

Key

Basal segments	Mid segments	Apical segments
1 = Basal anteroseptal	7 = Mid anteroseptal	13 = Apical anterior
2 = Basal anterior	8 = Mid anterior	14 = Apical lateral
3 = Basal anterolateral	9 = Mid anterolateral	15 = Apical inferior
4 = Basal inferolateral	10 = Mid inferolateral	16 = Apical septal
5 = Basal inferior	11 = Mid inferior	
6 = Basal inferoseptal	12 = Mid inferoseptal	

1.2a–e

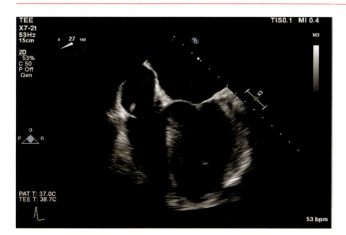

1.3 LV midesophageal four-chamber view.

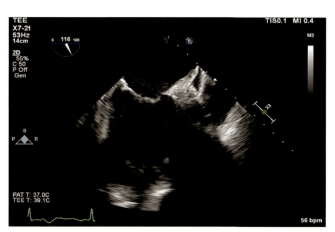

1.4 LV midesophageal two-chamber view.

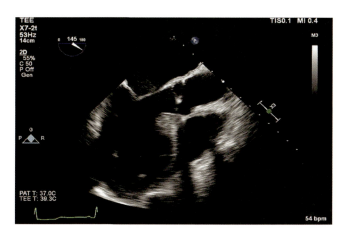

1.5 LV midesophageal long-axis view.

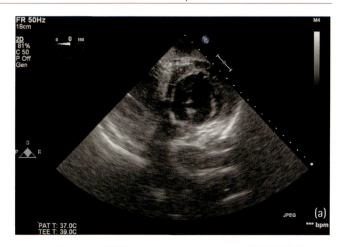

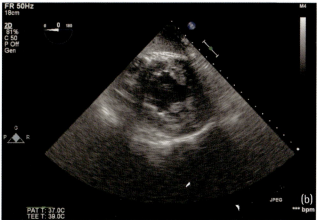

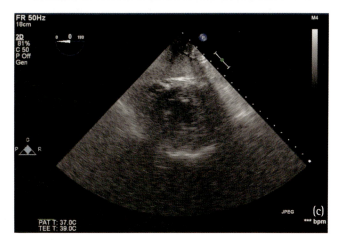

1.6a–c LV transgastric short-axis views: (a) basal, (b) mid papillary, and (c) apical.

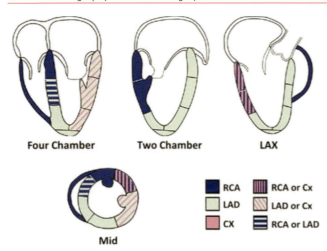

Four Chamber   **Two Chamber**   **LAX**

Mid

■ RCA	▦ RCA or Cx
☐ LAD	▨ LAD or Cx
▦ CX	▤ RCA or LAD

1.7 Coronary perfusion pattern of the LV. This figure has been reproduced with permission from Lang RM, Badano LP, Mor-Avi V, et al. Recommendations for cardiac chamber quantification in adults: an update from the ASE and EACVI. *J Am Soc Echocardiogr.* 2015; 28: 1–39.

Left ventricular wall motion is scored based on wall thickening and the degree of endocardial excursion using the following scale: normal (wall thickening greater than 30%), mild hypokinesis (10–30%), severe hypokinesis (<10%), akinesis (no thickening), and dyskinesis (paradoxical motion). Wall motion can be abnormal globally (as in dilated cardiomyopathy) or regionally. The latter is usually related to myocardial ischemia or infarction, but may accompany less common diagnoses such as sarcoidosis, myocarditis, and takotsubo cardiomyopathy. Over time, ischemic segments

may become thinned and echogenic due to fibrosis and scarring and can even progress to aneurysm formation. In addition to regional function, the global function of the LV is assessed, most commonly by ejection fraction (EF), which is equivalent to:

(LV end-diastolic volme – LV end-systolic volume) / (LV end-diastolic volume) × 100%

An EF of <50% is considered abnormal, although a normal EF does not exclude reduced cardiac function in the setting of significant mitral regurgitation (MR) or isolated regional wall motion abnormalities. LV global function is frequently assessed qualitatively via "eye-balling" an EF, but quantitative measurements of LV function are possible. These include simple 2D measurements such as fractional area change (FAC) (end diastolic area - end systolic area / end diastolic area) or more complex volumetric assessments like the Simpson's method of disks, in which the endocardial border of the LV is traced in systole and diastole and the volume of blood in the LV and EF are calculated automatically by dividing the LV into a bullet-shaped stack of disks whose volumes are summed.

Three-dimensional echocardiography (3D TEE) (**Figure 1.8**) has allowed for increasingly accurate calculations of LV volumes and EF compared with 2D TEE, as well as made detecting regional wall motion abnormalities more quantitative. The use of global longitudinal strain also shows promise as a quantitative measure of LV function and may even have a role in unmasking problems with LV function before there is a decrement in EF. However, more studies are still necessary to understand when strain measurement is most useful, especially in TEE as opposed to transthoracic echocardiography (TTE).

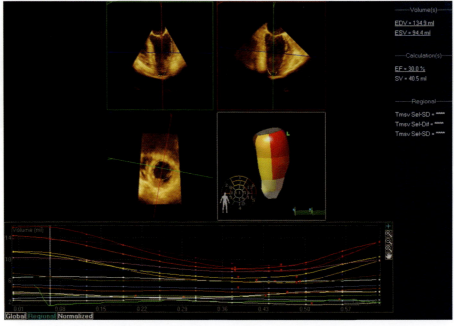

1.8 3D LV analysis using the QLab software from Philips, Inc.

Right ventricle

The right ventricle (RV) has a crescentic shape and is located anteriorly (farther from the imaging probe in TEE), which makes both qualitative and quantitative assessments of its function difficult. Standard TEE views for interrogating the RV include the midesophageal four-chamber view (see **Figure 1.3**), the midesophageal RV inflow–outflow view (**Figure 1.9**), the transgastric RV basal view, and the transgastric RV inflow view. RV function is commonly assessed qualitatively as normal or mildly, moderately, or severely hypokinetic based on looking at the motion of the RV free wall, the RV outflow tract, the RV septal wall, and the movement of the tricuspid annulus during the cardiac cycle. There are a few quantitative measurements that can be made to assess RV contractility, including RV FAC and the tricuspid annular plane systolic excursion (TAPSE), but these have not been well studied in TEE. 3D echocardiographic assessment of the RV is possible using offline software that allows recreation of the crescentic shape of the RV and semi-automates calculation of RV EF, which has been shown in a few studies to correlate well with cardiac MRI imaging, but this software is not yet widely available in the operating room. In a similar way to the LV, RV strain has been looked at in some TTE studies and demonstrated good reproducibility and predictive ability, but much more work remains to be done before this methodology is widely adopted.

Aortic valve, aortic root, and left ventricular outflow tract

The aortic valve (AV) is examined in long-axis (**Figure 1.10**) and short-axis (**Figure 1.11**) views with and without color Doppler in all patients. This allows the echocardiographer to visualize all three cusps and determine if any aortic regurgitation (AR) or aortic stenosis (AS) is present. While most AVs are trileaflet, bicuspid valves are present in about 2% of the population, and unicuspid and quadricuspid valves are possible. From the long-axis view, the diameter of the AV annulus, the sinuses of Valsalva, the sinotubular junction (STJ), and the left ventricular outflow tract (LVOT) are measured. These are helpful for surgical planning and sizing of the AV prosthesis during aortic valve replacement (AVR). The deep TG view permits the echocardiographer to align the ultrasound Doppler beam with the flow of blood through the AV and LVOT so that velocities, and thus peak and mean gradients, can be calculated to grade the severity of AS.

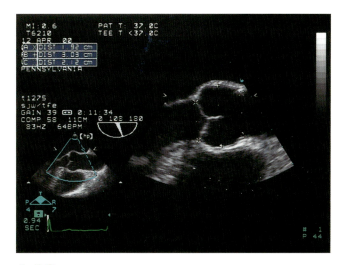

1.10 Long-axis view of the aortic valve.

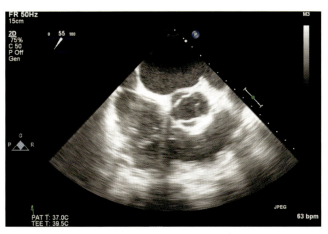

1.9 Midesophageal RV inflow–outflow view.

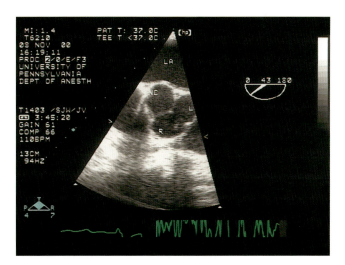

1.11 Short-axis view of the aortic valve.

AORTIC STENOSIS

Echocardiographic imaging in AS typically reveals areas of increased echogenicity representing leaflet calcification, immobile leaflets, and a small systolic orifice. Congenitally bicuspid valves develop stenosis at a higher rate and earlier in life than trileaflet valves, so are frequently seen in the OR (**Figure 1.12**). These valves have an elliptical, "fish-mouth" pattern appearance during systole in short axis. Patients may also have an "acquired" bicuspid valve, where one of the commissures has become calcified and fused, appearing similar to a raphae. Senile calcific AS and rheumatic AS appear similarly on TEE, and cannot be differentiated easily based on imaging alone. A close examination must also be made of the LVOT to rule out subaortic stenosis from a subvalvular membrane, systolic anterior motion (SAM) of the mitral valve, other congenital anomaly.

The severity of valvular stenosis (**Figure 1.13**) is determined by measurement of the transvalvular gradient and calculation of an aortic valve area. The maximum transaortic pressure gradient is calculated from the modified Bernoulli equation:

$$\text{Maximum gradient} = 4v^2$$

where v is the maximum velocity through the valve. This formula assumes that there is no flow acceleration in the LVOT from obstruction, SAM, or other etiology. If this is not the case, then the maximum velocity through the LVOT, obtained via pulsed-wave Doppler in the LVOT, must be factored into the equation. The presence of LVOT obstruction will also change the waveform of the continuous-wave velocity curve through the valve, giving it a dagger shape. The mean gradient is calculated by tracing the spectral envelope of the velocity curve and averaging the instantaneous gradients over the whole systolic ejection period. Pressure gradients are flow-dependent, and will be elevated when stroke volume is increased (e.g. pregnancy, exercise, AR) and reduced when stroke volume is decreased (e.g. hypovolemia, LV dysfunction, under general anesthesia).

The AV area (AVA) can also be calculated from Doppler measurements using the continuity equation:

$$\text{AVA} = (\text{Area}_{\text{LVOT}} \times \text{VTI}_{\text{LVOT}}) / (\text{VTI}_{\text{AV}})$$

Error can easily be introduced into this calculation by misalignment of the Doppler flow with blood flow across the AV or LVOT, as well as in measurement of the LVOT diameter, where small errors will become large errors once squared to obtain the LVOT cross-sectional area. To overcome this, the LVOT area can be measured directly using 3D TEE. The AVA can also be directly measured using planimetry of the valve orifice in the midesophageal AV short-axis view, but this is not a very accurate measurement due to the elliptical nature of the AV. 3D planimetry of the AV orifice has been shown to be more accurate and reproducible than 2D planimetry (**Figure 1.14**).

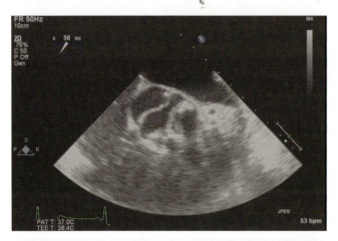

1.12 Midesophageal AV short-axis view of a stenotic bicuspid valve.

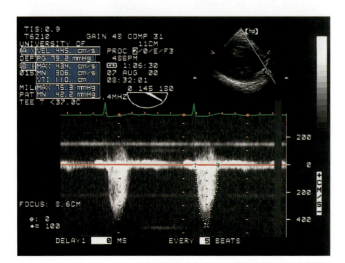

1.13 Continuous-wave Doppler through a stenotic AV.

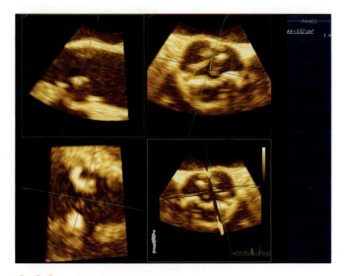

1.14 3D planimetry of a stenotic aortic valve area.

Traditionally, AS has been treated surgically by open AVR. This is rapidly changing, however, as more and more patients are treated endovascularly using transcatheter aortic valve replacement (TAVR). A wire is placed across the AV (**Figure 1.15a**), most commonly retrograde via the femoral artery (although transapical, transaxillary, and transaortic approaches are also used), and a valve is moved into position within the native, stenotic AV along this wire and finally deployed (**Figure 1.15b**), crushing the native leaflets between the new valve and the aortic wall. Paravalvular leaks are relatively common following TAVR, and must be assessed echocardiographically in the operating room via TTE or TEE.

Preoperative annular sizing is also essential in TAVR, as direct valve sizing during the procedure is impossible. This is often done using either 3D echocardiography or contrast-enhanced CT (**Figure 1.16**).

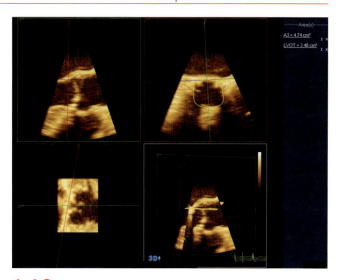

1.16 3D sizing of the aortic annulus.

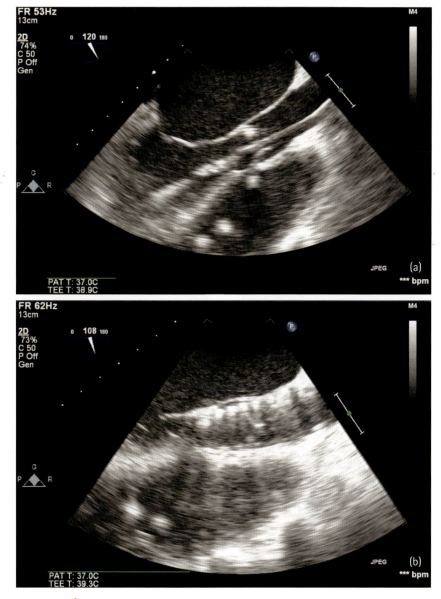

1.15a, b Transcatheter aortic valve replacement (TAVR).

AORTIC REGURGITATION

The echocardiographic assessment of aortic regurgitation (AR) includes determination of the severity and etiology of the regurgitation, the effect of the regurgitant lesion on ventricular size and function, and the presence of associated findings. AR may be due to abnormalities of the aortic root, ascending aorta, or the valve cusps. AR is often seen in the setting of AS, as calcified, restricted leaflets have difficulty coapting during diastole.

Myxomatous AV disease produces redundant, often prolapsing, cusps (**Figure 1.17**). Endocarditis produces AR through cusp or annular destruction and may be accompanied by vegetations and/or root abscesses (**Figure 1.18**).

Dilation of the aortic root and/or ascending aorta with normal cusp morphology can lead to AR owing to a lack of normal supporting structures (**Figure 1.19**). Causes of aortic root dilation include hypertension, collagen vascular disorders (e.g. Marfan syndrome, Ehlers–Danlos syndrome, Loeys–Dietz syndrome), rheumatoid arthritis, syphilitic aortitis, and poststenotic dilation associated with AS.

Aortic dissection produces an intimal flap in the lumen of the aorta and may produce AR by dilation of the aortic root, interruption of normal coaptation of the cusps by the intimal flap, or separation of one or more cusps from the aortic wall if the valve is involved in the dissection (**Figure 1.20**). In chronic AR, the LV responds to the volume load by slow, progressive dilation that eventually leads to a decrement in LV function. In acute AR (aortic dissection or AV endocarditis) the LV size may be normal but LV end-diastolic pressure may be elevated.

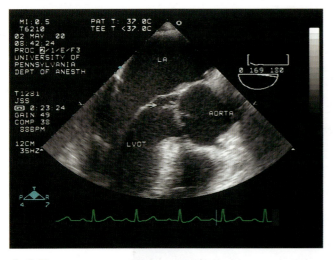

1.17 Midesophageal AV long-axis view demonstrating a prolapsing AV with vegetation (arrow).

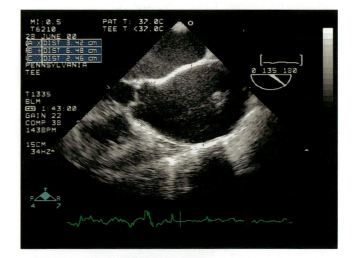

1.19 Midesophageal AV long-axis view demonstrating AR owing to aortic dilation.

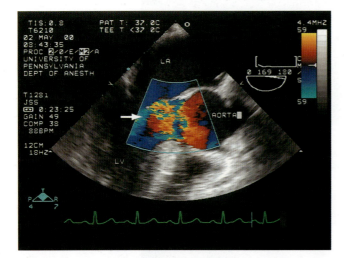

1.18 Midesophageal AV long-axis view demonstrating severe AR (arrow).

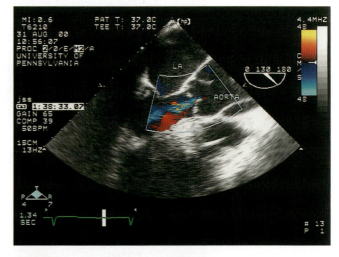

1.20 Midesophageal AV long-axis view of AR in the setting of a Type A aortic dissection.

AR severity is assessed in several ways, the simplest being the use of color Doppler across the LVOT and AV (**Figure 1.21**). The width of the AR jet can be compared to the width of the LVOT. If the jet is <25% of the LVOT width, then the AR is mild, 25–65% is moderate, and >65% of the LVOT width is severe AR. Additionally, the vena contracta, or smallest width of the AR jet at the level of the valve leaflets, can be measured, with a value of >0.6 cm corresponding to severe AR.

The continuous-wave Doppler spectral recording of AR typically reveals an increased velocity flow of 3–5 m/s (**Figure 1.22**). The rate of deceleration of the regurgitant jet corresponds to severity of AR, with aortic diastolic pressure decreasing more rapidly as AR worsens. Thus, the Doppler tracing can be used to calculate a pressure half-time (PHT) in milliseconds, with mild AR having a value of >500 ms and severe <200 ms. These measurements, however, can be affected by LV compliance and aortic pressure. Finally, pulsed-wave Doppler can be used in the proximal descending thoracic aorta (DTA) to look at blood flow during diastole. If there is holodiastolic reversal of flow in the DTA, this is pathognomonic for severe AR.

Mitral valve and left atrium

The move towards mitral valve (MV) repair in the majority of patients with degenerative MV disease was made possible, in part, by the widespread use of intraoperative TEE. TEE often provides a better view of the MV and left atrium (LA) than TTE due to the proximity of both structures to the esophagus. TEE allows for the rapid identification of annular calcification, prolapsing or restricted scallops, annular dilation, and the integrity of the subvalvular apparatus with high precision, which allows for better surgical planning before the initiation of cardiopulmonary bypass.

MITRAL REGURGITATION

The most common etiologies of mitral regurgitation (MR) are myxomatous (degenerative) MV disease, ischemic heart disease, rheumatic heart disease, and endocarditis. Surgical correction of MR is guided primarily by the severity of the regurgitation, the etiology of the MR, and the anatomy of the leaflets and annulus. Severity of MR is assessed through several methods, most of which attempt to find an easily measurable surrogate for the effective regurgitant orifice area (EROA) of the valve. These include the vena contracta width and proximal isovelocity surface area (PISA) of the regurgitant jet, the ratio of jet area to LA area, and the presence or absence of systolic reversal of the pulmonary venous inflow. Determining the etiology of MR consists largely of looking for prolapsing or tethered (restricted) leaflets, as well as assessing for annular and LV dilation or the presence of perforations or clefts in the MV leaflets (**Figure 1.23**). Etiology has a big impact on the repairability of the valve. An isolated P2 prolapse can be repaired in nearly all cases, while a complex lesion with prolapse of multiple scallops on both leaflets and a cleft should only be repaired by a surgeon with sufficient experience in complex MV repairs; otherwise, valve replacement should probably be pursued.

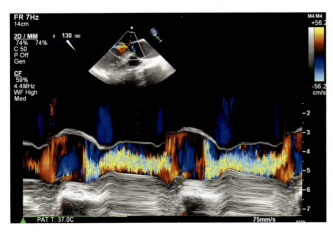

1.21 M-mode of the AR jet in the LVOT.

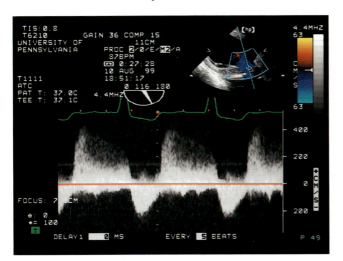

1.22 Transgastric long-axis view with continuous-wave Doppler producing high-velocity diastolic flow signal.

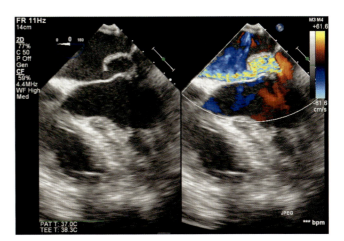

1.23 Midesophageal four-chamber view showing posterior (P2) leaflet flail and severe MR.

2D TEE assessment of the MV consists of four midesophageal views (shown in **Figure 1.24**) which cut the MV in such a way that, between these views, the six anterior (A1-3) and posterior (P1-3) scallops can be seen. The TG basal short-axis view (**Figure 1.25**) and TG two-chamber view are also useful in assessing MV pathology and examining the subvalvular apparatus.

3D TEE has been a major advance in the evaluation of MV disease. Using 3D echo, the entirety of the MV as well as the subvalvular apparatus can be visualized in real time from any angle. This allows for more rapid and accurate identification of prolapsing segments with less interobserver variability than 2D TEE. This is especially true for more complex valvular lesions. Color Doppler can also be added to 3D echo of the MV to help better identify the etiology of MR and more accurately grade the severity of MR using methods like vena contracta area and 3D PISA. Finally, there

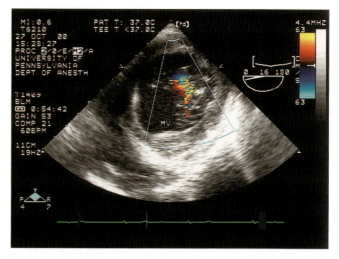

1.25 Transgastric basal short-axis view.

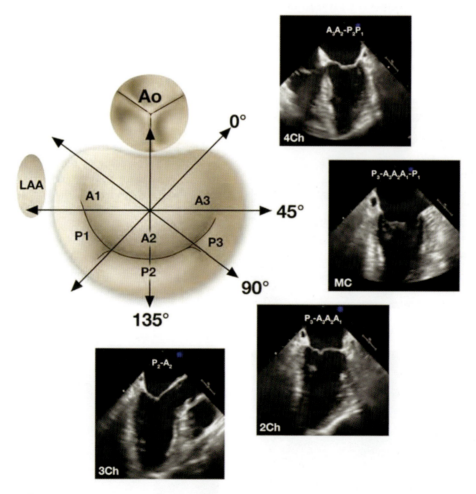

1.24 2D TEE midesophageal views of the mitral valve.

is software available from several manufacturers that allows for 3D quantitative assessment of the MV structure, which has helped elucidate many more details about MV function in both degenerative and especially ischemic MR. Examples are shown in **Figure 1.26**.

Residual MR after mitral repair is not uncommon. Mild to moderate MR detected under the influence of general anesthetics might revert to severe MR and symptomatic pulmonary edema in the exercising patient. The mechanisms of failed repair include persistent excessive leaflet motion, prolapse, perforation, and a spectrum of disorders producing malcoaptation of the anterior and posterior leaflets.

SAM of the MV tends to occur in patients with an excessively long (i.e. edge-to-annulus) posterior leaflet. SAM produces MR and obstruction of the LVOT (**Figure 1.27**). Hypovolemia and vasodilatation exacerbate SAM. Treatment includes volume administration as well as medications to increase afterload and decrease heart rate (i.e. phenylephrine). If persistent, reinitiation of cardiopulmonary bypass and a sliding posterior valvuloplasty or MV replacement may be necessary. The maximum allowable MR after repair is controversial. Many clinicians will accept 1+ MR, especially

if reinitiation of cardiopulmonary bypass and recrossclamping poses a significantly increased risk (e.g. elderly, concomitant ischemic disease, decreased EF).

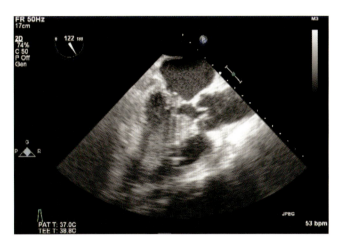

1.27   Systolic anterior motion (SAM) of the mitral valve can produce MR.

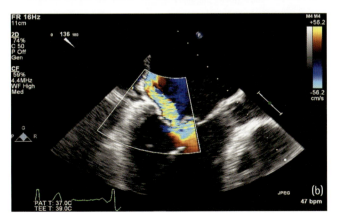

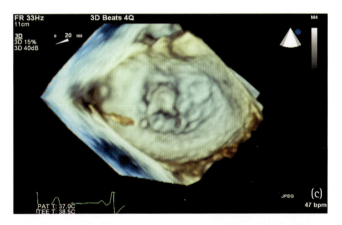

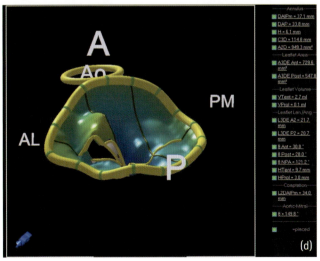

1.26a–d   Anterior leaflet (A1) flail in (a) 2D and (b) with color Doppler. (c) 3D TEE of the same lesion and (d) a quantitative map of the MV.

MITRAL STENOSIS

The most common etiologies of mitral stenosis (MS) are rheumatic heart disease and senile calcific disease. As the MV leaflets become increasingly thickened and calcified, their free movement in both diastole and systole becomes limited, resulting in stenosis and often accompanying regurgitation. The decision of when to operate on a patient with MS is determined by the severity of the MS and accompanying symptoms (i.e. LA dilation, arrhythmias, shortness of breath). The severity of MS can be assessed in several ways. The first is by assessment of transvalvular gradients. The obstructed filling of the LV results in an elevated transmitral flow velocity and elevated peak and mean gradients. Mean gradient is used for the grading of MS severity with values of 5–10 mmHg for moderate MS and >10 mmHg for severe MS. PHT can also be used to assess MS severity, with a value of >220 ms corresponding to severe MS and an MV area of <1.0 cm^2.

3D TEE can also be beneficial when assessing MS. Aside from being able to better see the movement of the leaflets from both the LA and the LV, MVA can be measured from a 3D data set of a stenotic valve using planimetry with greater accuracy and reproducibility than from 2D echo alone. The reason for this is that the likelihood of a 2D live, TG short-axis view of the MV being perfectly in plane with the minimum valve area is remote while, with 3D TEE, the image can be post-processed so that an en face view of the smallest valve area is easily obtained and measured (**Figure 1.28**).

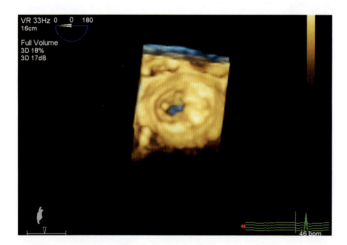

1.28 3D TEE of a stenotic mitral valve.

Tricuspid valve, right atrium, interatrial septum, and pulmonary artery

TEE of the right atrium and tricuspid valve is a reliable method of detecting atrial septal defects, sinus venosus defects, anomalous insertion of pulmonary veins, dilated coronary sinus (i.e. persistent left-sided vena cava), and abnormalities of the tricuspid valve (**Figures 1.29 and 1.30**). Insertion of a coronary sinus cardioplegia cannula can also be facilitated by direct imaging. Patent foramen ovale are common and diagnosis is established using 2D color Doppler and/or contrast echocardiography.

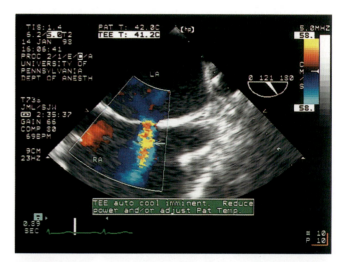

1.29 Midesophageal bicaval view with blood flow through a patent foramen ovale (arrow).

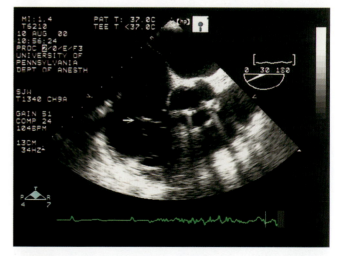

1.30 Midesophageal AV short-axis view. Dilated right atrium with flail portion of tricuspid valve (arrow).

Tricuspid regurgitation (TR) is becoming a more widely recognized problem in cardiac surgery patients (**Figure 1.31**), and severe TR has been shown in some studies to be an independent predictor of mortality. The decision of whether to repair a tricuspid valve during concomitant cardiac surgery is often made in the operating room based upon TEE findings. The severity of TR is based on the size of the regurgitant jet in the right atrium, the vena contracta width of the TR, and the presence or absence of systolic flow reversal in the hepatic veins. Tricuspid valve replacement is much less common than repair and is most frequently due to endocarditis, although damage to the valve from carcinoid heart disease or iatrogenic injury from EP or other procedures is also seen.

TEE views of the main pulmonary artery (PA) include the midesophageal RV inflow–outflow view, the midesophageal ascending aorta SAX view (**Figure 1.32**), and the UE aortic arch SAX view. These allow for the assessment of pulmonary arterial dilation as well as the presence of any large thrombi that may necessitate embolectomy or AngioVac procedure.

The presence of a large PE is often accompanied by acute RV dilation and failure, and RV free wall akinesis with apical sparing may be seen (McConnell's sign). The pulmonic valve is not always seen clearly with TEE due to its anterior position in the chest, but a basic interrogation for regurgitation and/or stenosis with color Doppler is usually possible. In those patients with pulmonic valve disease, a TTE may provide more information for diagnosis and surgical planning.

Thoracic aorta

AORTIC ANEURYSM

Patients presenting with an aortic aneurysm for elective repair have generally had their diagnosis confirmed by a variety of imaging modalities, including TTE, CT, MRI, and/or angiography before arriving in the operating room. Patients may, however, present for emergent surgery in the setting of rupture or dissection of a known aneurysm. The decision of when to operate on a dilated thoracic aorta depends largely on the diameter of the aneurysm and the rate of expansion, and varies between normal patients and those with a family history of thoracic aortic disease, bicuspid AV, or known collagen vascular disease. The pre-procedure TEE in aortic aneurysm repair should focus on measurement of the aneurysm itself as well as the adjacent normal aortic tissue for graft sizing, interrogation of the AV to determine whether concomitant AVR is necessary, and evaluation of ventricular function (**Figure 1.33**). The post-procedure TEE is aimed at assessing the repair and detecting infrequent complications, like malperfusion, dissection, residual intracavitary air or debris, and worsened AR. New regional wall motion abnormalities may suggest ischemia from air emboli or a technical issue with the anastomosis of the coronary ostia onto the graft if the aortic root was replaced.

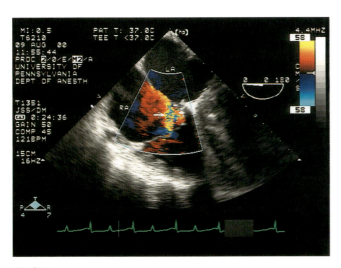

1.31 Midesophageal four-chamber view demonstrating moderate tricuspid regurgitation (arrow).

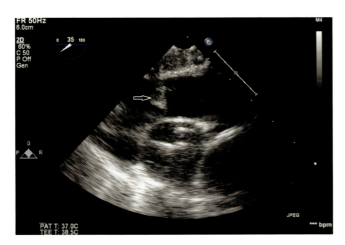

1.32 Mobile thrombus seen in the right main pulmonary artery in the midesophageal ascending aorta short-axis view.

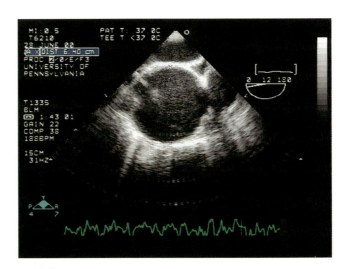

1.33 Midesophageal ascending aorta short-axis view demonstrating an aneurysm.

AORTIC DISSECTION

TEE offers several distinct advantages in the diagnosis of an acute aortic dissection. These include a high sensitivity and specificity (98% and 95% respectively according to a meta-analysis by Shiga et al.), expediency, and the ability to simultaneously assess LV function and look for AR or a pericardial effusion. The major disadvantage of TEE when compared to CT or MRI is the inability to image the distal portion of the ascending aorta and proximal arch due to the location of the air-filled trachea, so a dissection isolated to this location may be missed if TEE is the sole imaging modality. Given TEE's utility in aortic dissection, it is common to have patients admitted straight to an operating room from the emergency department or an outside hospital if a dissection is suspected based on history, physical exam, or imaging. Once in the operating room, general anesthesia is carefully induced and a TEE probe is placed, where the diagnosis of aortic dissection can be confirmed and a decision can be made about whether to proceed emergently with surgery or if the patient should be sent to the ICU for medical management and possible eventual open (TAAA repair) or endovascular (TEVAR) repair. The major deciding factor between emergent surgery or the ICU is whether the dissection involves the ascending aorta (Type A) or is isolated to the DTA (Type B). The former is a surgical emergency, while the latter may be managed medically unless there are signs of malperfusion, rupture, or hemodynamic instability. Bypassing the delay and risk associated with obtaining CT or MRI scans, often in isolated, poorly monitored locations, can be life-saving. See **Figures 1.34** and **1.35**.

Color-flow Doppler may detect blood flow within a true (endothelial/atherosclerotic lined) and/or false lumen. An entry site (fenestration) between the true and false lumen is often identified. The absence of a discrete flap does not exclude the diagnosis of dissection. Intramural hematoma is never a normal finding and implies significant injury to the integrity of the aortic wall (e.g. dissection, transection, or disruption). Hematoma may appear as an echogenic mass within the media or adjacent to the aorta, contained by echogenic adventitia. Caution should be used to avoid misinterpretation due to ultrasound artifacts such as reverberation artifact and beam-width artifact in oblique image planes. Transthoracic imaging of the suprasternal notch may reveal a limited dissection in the portion of the aortic arch that is not readily accessible by TEE. Ultrasound examination of the carotid arteries may also be useful to detect extension of the dissection into the carotid arteries, as well as confirm bilateral flow post-repair.

Extension of the dissection flap into the aortic root can result in a flail aortic cusp and severe AR or can propagate down one or both coronary ostia, producing severe ventricular dysfunction. Aortic rupture into the pericardium or pleural space is often fatal. However, if the rupture is contained by adjacent structures, a pericardial effusion/tamponade or pleural effusion can be detected and tolerated by the patient until emergency surgery corrects the defect.

Initial echocardiographic assessment should focus on a detailed examination of all parts of the thoracic aorta with and without color Doppler to detect an intimal flap and confirm the diagnosis of aortic dissection. A transgastric short-axis view of the LV determines whether the pericardium contains blood and permits assessment of regional and global ventricular function. The midesophageal AV short-axis and long-axis views provide images of AV integrity and allow the detection of AR as well as measurement of the aortic annulus and root to guide valve repair or replacement if necessary. Color-flow Doppler imaging can be used to verify flow within the proximal right and left coronary arteries. On initiation of cardiopulmonary bypass, the adequacy of arterial inflow into the true lumen should be confirmed, and flow in the carotid arteries can be assessed using a handheld transducer.

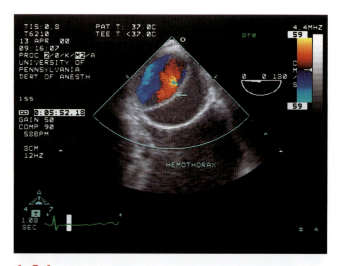

1.34 Descending aorta short-axis view. Aortic dissection with pleural effusion, probably hemothorax. The hallmark of aortic dissection is a linear, mobile echogenic density (i.e. intimal flap [arrow]) within the lumen of the aorta. Undulating motion of the flap can be associated with systole.

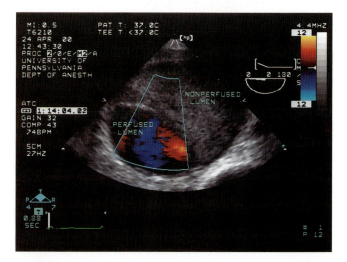

1.35 Descending aorta short-axis view. Aortic dissection with thrombosed false lumen.

Prosthetic valves

The interrogation of a prosthetic valve, either in the setting of a fresh valve replacement or redo surgery, presents a unique set of challenges to the echocardiographer. There are two main types of prosthetic valves, each with their own unique imaging characteristics. Bioprosthetic valves consist of animal-derived leaflet tissue (often bovine or porcine) with a metallic and fabric stent structure and sewing ring (although stentless valves also exist). Mechanical valves are most often bileaflet in construction, but other designs may be seen, especially in older patients. Both valves produce a number of imaging artifacts due to their structure, including shadowing, mirroring, side-lobe artifacts, and others, which can make accurate assessment of function difficult. Mechanical valves also have physiologic washing jets (the number and characteristics of which vary by valve) which can make the detection of paravalvular leaks difficult.

Generally, paravalvular leaks typically produce high-velocity, high-variance jets external to the sewing ring that extend farther into the adjacent cardiac chamber than a typical washing jet. In **Figure 1.36**, a deep transgastric long-axis view demonstrates a paravalvular leak from a prosthetic valve in the aortic position.

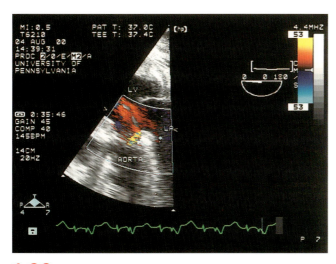

1.36 Deep transgastric long-axis view showing a paravalvular leak from a prosthetic valve in the aortic position.

Intravalvular leaks may also be seen in prosthetic valves, and are due to leaflet dysfunction or destruction or impingement of leaflet movement by valve malposition, pannus formation, or some other structure. Prosthetic valve stenosis may be detected via Doppler measurements of transvalvular peak and mean gradients. 3D TEE may be especially useful when assessing for paravalvular leak, as it allows visualization of the entire valve and sewing ring in one image, facilitating rapid localization of the leak and guidance of surgical or transcatheter closure.

FURTHER READING

Andrawes M, Feinman J. 3-dimensional echocardiography and its role in preoperative mitral valve evaluation. *Cardiol Clin.* 2013; 31: 271–85.

Baumgartner H, Hung J, Bermejo J, et al. Echocardiographic assessment of valve stenosis: EAE/ASE recommendations for clinical practice. *J Am Soc Echocardiogr.* 2009; 22: 1–23.

Hahn, RT, Abraham T, Adams MS, et al. Guidelines for performing a comprehensive transesophageal echocardiographic examination: recommendations from the American Society of Echocardiography and the Society of Cardiovascular Anesthesiologists. *J Am Soc Echocardiogr.* 2013; 26: 921–64.

Kallmeyer IJ, Collard CD, Fox JA, et al. The safety of intraoperative transesophageal echocardiography. *Anesth Analg.* 2001; 92: 1126–30.

Lang RM, Badano LP, Mor-Avi V, et al. Recommendations for cardiac chamber quantification in adults: an update from the ASE and EACVI. *J Am Soc Echocardiogr.* 2015; 28: 1–39.

Mathew JP, Swaminathan M, Ayoub CM. *Clinical manual and review of transesophageal echocardiography.* 2nd edn. New York: The McGraw-Hill Companies; 2010.

Shiga T, Wajima Z, Apfel CC, et al. Diagnostic accuracy of transesophageal echocardiography, helical computed tomography, and magnetic resonance imaging for suspected thoracic aortic dissection. *Arch Int Med.* 2006; 166: 1350–6.

Zoghbi WA, Enriquez-Sarano M, Foster E, et al. Recommendations for evaluation of the severity of native valvular regurgitation with two-dimensional Doppler echocardiography. *J Am Soc Echocardiogr.* 2003; 16: 777–802.

2

Cardiopulmonary bypass: access, technical options, and pathophysiology

JACK H. BOYD AND ALBERT J. PEDROZA

HISTORY

The development of cardiopulmonary bypass (CPB) can be largely attributed to the pioneering work of John Gibbon, who demonstrated its first successful use in animals in the 1930s and performed the first successful human open heart operation in 1953, when he repaired an atrial septal defect using CPB. This initial success was unfortunately followed by several deaths, and he became discouraged by the results and postponed its subsequent human use. At around the same time, C. Walton Lillehei began using controlled cross-circulation from parent to child to allow intracardiac repairs. In 1965, John Kirklin used a modified Gibbon heart–lung machine for intracardiac repair in a series of patients, heralding the era of CPB. Since this early work, progressive developments have occurred in materials used and in surgical techniques to improve the safety, reliability, and efficacy of CPB.

PRINCIPLES AND JUSTIFICATION

CPB is utilized when an empty heart is required for intracardiac repair, when cardiac mechanical arrest is needed, when cardiac manipulation requires circulatory support, and when deep hypothermia is needed to allow for a period of systemic and/or cerebral circulatory arrest. During CPB, systemic deoxygenated venous blood drains into the extracorporeal circuit and passes via a venous reservoir to a pump, which propels blood through a membrane oxygenator for gas exchange before return to the systemic arterial circulation (**Figure 2.1**). This circuit diverts blood flow from the patient's cardiopulmonary circulation while maintaining blood oxygenation and organ perfusion. The circuit also includes a heat exchanger for body temperature manipulation and access ports for the administration of perfusate and drugs and for acquisition of intraoperative blood samples. Additional components of the bypass circuit enable the administration of cardioplegia solution, venting of cardiac chambers, and blood salvage from the surgical field.

Systemic anticoagulation is required during CPB to prevent blood clotting within the circuit. A systemic bolus of 300 units/kg of unfractionated heparin is administered prior to cannulation to maintain an activated clotting time (ACT) of greater than 400 seconds during bypass. The ACT is routinely monitored in 20–30-minute intervals throughout the bypass run, and heparin is readministered to maintain adequate anticoagulation. A fraction of patients exhibits heparin resistance, defined by failure to achieve the ACT goal despite escalated heparin dosing. This process is mediated at least in part by deficiency of antithrombin III and is rectified by administration of either fresh frozen plasma or antithrombin concentrate, which is more expensive but curbs transfusion risks. Patients who are unable to receive heparin (e.g. patients with heparin-induced thrombocytopenia) can safely be anticoagulated with a direct thrombin inhibitor such as bivalirudin or by utilizing a protocol with intravenous epoprostenol in addition to heparin.

Adequate pump flow rates on CPB depend on the temperature and body surface area of the patient. At physiologic temperatures, a minimum of $2.2 \, \text{L/m}^2$ should be maintained. The use of therapeutic hypothermia can reduce flow requirements. As a general principle, systemic oxygen consumption decreases about 10–12% for every 2 °C reduction in body temperature. In practice, this concept allows for up to 20–40 minutes of safe circulatory arrest with selective cerebral perfusion and systemic cooling to 24 °C. There is considerable variability in the practice of surgeons regarding optimal temperature management during CPB. Multiple clinical trials have demonstrated that routine cardiac operations can be safely performed under only mild hypothermia without active cooling through the bypass circuit. Rewarming should be timed to allow for normothermia at the end of the bypass run to minimize time on pump.

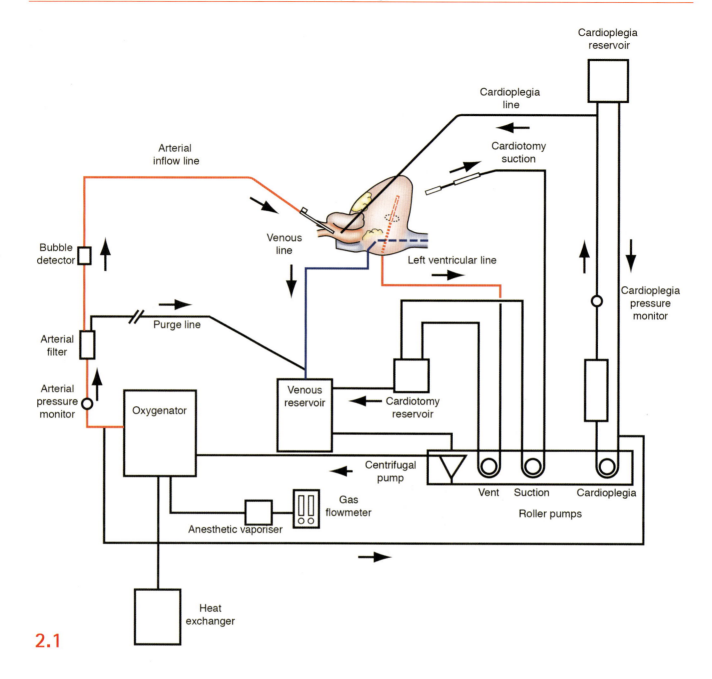

2.1

While limited data exist on optimal systemic perfusion pressures on bypass, experimental models suggest maintenance of a mean arterial pressure no less than 40 mmHg is sufficient. In practice, maintaining a more physiologic mean pressure of 60 mmHg is a safe approach, and relatively higher pressures should be targeted in the setting of known atherosclerotic cerebrovascular disease. Systemic blood pressure is highly dynamic in the cardiac operating room due to fluid shifts, variable pump flow rates, and the vasodilatory properties of anesthetics. Accordingly, constant communication between the surgeon, anesthesiologist, and perfusionist is necessary to maintain adequate perfusion, minimize blood loss from the extracorporeal circuit, and optimize working operative conditions.

PREOPERATIVE ASSESSMENT AND PREPARATION

In the modern era of cardiac surgery, an expanding array of available cannulation and perfusion strategies enables the surgeon to optimize the operative field for the planned operation. The surgeon must develop a preferred plan as well as contingencies for both suspected and unforeseen complicating factors. The preoperative assessment for any cardiac case should include consideration of venous and arterial cannulation strategies, the need for venting cannulae, and myocardial protection. The selection of an appropriate arterial cannula is made based on the body surface area of the patient and vascular anatomy. A 20-French aortic cannula is generally sufficient for most adult cardiac operations.

Preoperative history and physical exam should identify history or stigmata of cerebrovascular disease, ventricular dysfunction, renal disease, and peripheral vascular disease. All preoperative imaging should be reviewed, including assessment for calcification of the aorta to ensure safe central cannulation and for atherosclerotic disease that may complicate peripheral cannulation or placement of an intra-aortic balloon pump.

ANESTHESIA

General anesthesia with neuromuscular blockade and endotracheal intubation is required for cardiac surgical cases. If operative strategy dictates thoracotomy with single-lung ventilation, either a dual-lumen tube or bronchial blocker is used for bronchial isolation. Multimodal invasive and external monitoring devices should be routinely employed to guide intraoperative decision-making (**Table 2.1**). At a minimum, surface ECG, pulse oximetry, radial and/or femoral arterial catheters, and a Foley catheter should be in place prior to commencing a cardiac operation. Transesophageal echocardiography is routinely employed. Cerebral near-infrared spectroscopy (NIRS), traditionally used in aortic procedures, should be considered for all cases. A pulmonary artery catheter provides real-time monitoring of hemodynamic parameters but is not necessarily required in all cases.

In particularly high-risk cases with elevated concern for cardiovascular collapse during induction of anesthesia (e.g. severe aortic stenosis, critical coronary lesions, severely reduced ejection fraction) the surgeon should consider pre-induction placement of an intra-aortic balloon pump or femoral arterial and venous access to enable rapid cannulation for bypass. Appropriate access for the administration of vasoactive drugs and volume resuscitation generally necessitates large-diameter central venous catheter placement.

OPERATION

Access for central cannulation

Although employment of minimally invasive operations is constantly increasing, most cardiac operations are still performed via median sternotomy (**Figure 2.2a**). Adequate access is feasible through a skin incision starting 3 cm below the sternal notch and ending above the inferior tip of the xiphoid process. For a standard sternotomy, the sternum is completely divided in the midline with a reciprocating sternal saw.

Table 2.1 Multimodal monitoring

Monitoring modality	Parameters
Surface ECG	Heart rhythm, ischemia
Arterial catheter	Blood pressure, arterial blood gas
Pulmonary artery (Swan–Ganz) catheter	CVP, PA pressure, cardiac output
Transesophageal echocardiology (TEE) probe	Ventricular function, valvular disease, cannula/wire placement
Foley catheter	Core temperature, urine output
Cerebral near-infrared spectroscopy (NIRS)	Cerebral oximetry (oxygenation)

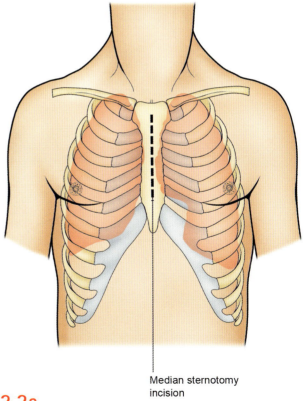

Median sternotomy incision

2.2a

Mini-sternotomy permits limited access to the superior pericardium. The length of the skin incision can be limited to 6–8 cm. The manubrium and sternum are divided inferiorly to the 3rd or 4th intercostal space and horizontally in a J or T shape, enabling partial sternal division and mediastinal access (**Figure 2.2b**).

Following sternal division, a retractor is placed with the ratchet directed superiorly (**Figure 2.2c**). The thymic tissue is mobilized by separating its lobes. After identification of the crossing left innominate vein, the pericardium is entered in the midline. Absence or hypoplasia of the left innominate vein raises suspicion for a persistent left superior vena cava (SVC). The pericardiotomy is extended inferiorly to the diaphragm and laterally in either direction to develop an inverted-T incision, taking care not to enter into the pleural spaces. Pericardial stay sutures are placed bilaterally along the length of the divided pericardium to aid exposure. Heparin is given in anticipation of cannulation.

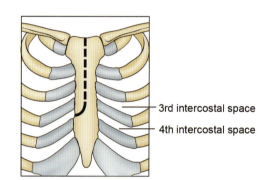

AORTIC CANNULATION PURSESTRINGS

Following sternotomy, the aortopulmonary window is minimally developed via lateral retraction of the aorta and division of the intervening connective tissue to permit placement of an aortic cross-clamp (**Figure 2.3**). The ascending

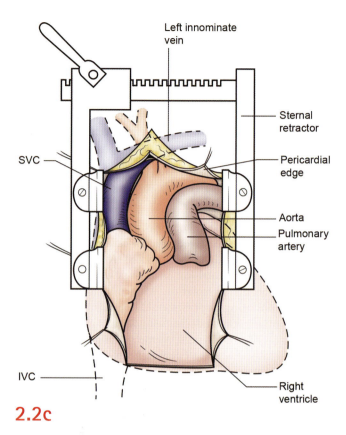

2.2c

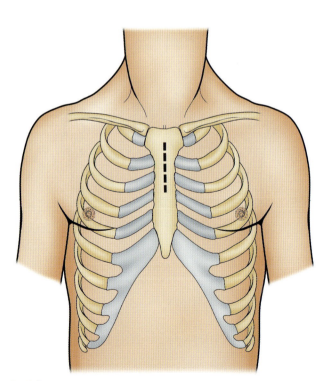

2.2b

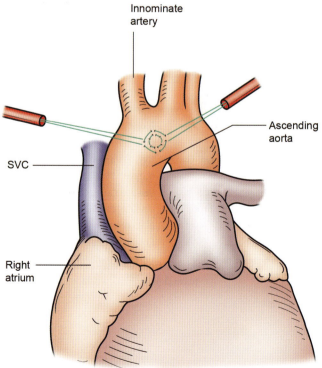

2.3

aorta is inspected and palpated. If there is concern for atheroma or calcification, epiaortic ultrasound should be used to identify a safe cannulation site. The cannulation site is prepared at the level of the aortic pericardial reflections below the innominate artery. Two concentric, diamond-shaped pursestring sutures are placed via partial-thickness (into the tunica media but not through the intimal layer) bites of 3-0 non-absorbable braided suture. The pursestrings should be made sufficiently large to accommodate the aortic cannula. The sutures are secured with tourniquets.

VENOUS CANNULATION PURSESTRING

Venous cannulation strategies are selected to suit operative indications. For many cardiac operations, a single, dual-stage venous cannula placed via the right atrial appendage will provide adequate drainage (**Figure 2.4a**). A single, 3-0 pursestring suture is placed encircling the tip of the right atrial appendage and secured with a tourniquet.

Bicaval venous cannulation is typically preferred for right-sided intracardiac cases and may be desirable for access to the interatrial groove for left atriotomy. An oval pursestring suture (greater height than width) is placed in the SVC above the cavoatrial junction with 3-0 non-absorbable braided suture and secured with a tourniquet. Similarly, a pursestring suture is placed at the base of the right atrium approximately 2 cm above the junction of the inferior vena cava (IVC) (**Figure 2.4b**).

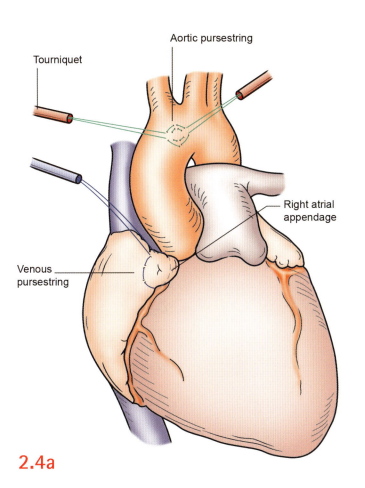

Tourniquet

Aortic pursestring

Right atrial appendage

Venous pursestring

2.4a

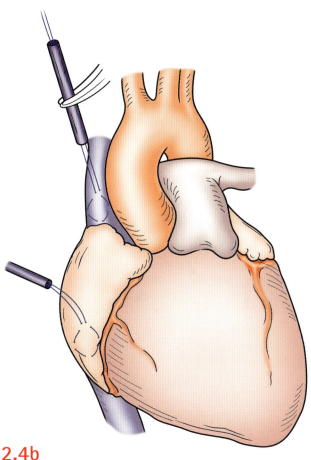

2.4b

ARTERIAL CANNULATION

Once an adequate ACT is reached, the ascending aorta is cannulated for bypass. The surgeon should ensure that the systolic blood pressure is below 100 mmHg prior to proceeding. A number 11 blade is used to create a transverse aortotomy of adequate size to accommodate the cannula at the center of the pursestring sutures (**Figure 2.5a**). The incised adventitia is held over the aortotomy with forceps to prevent excess blood loss while the surgeon inserts the aortic cannula, directed initially perpendicular to the aorta and then towards the descending thoracic aorta. The pursestrings are tightened and secured to the cannula, which should be anchored to the surgical field with a stay suture. TEE evaluation confirms the intraluminal position of the cannula. The aortic cannula is carefully de-aired and connected to the bypass circuit on the field. After connection, the arterial pressure and pulse in the circuit are checked by the perfusionist. Poor pulse amplitude or high pressure in the arterial cannula raises suspicion for malposition of the aortic cannula including placement against the aortic wall, into an arch vessel, or iatrogenic aortic dissection.

Alternatively, the aorta can be accessed with a large bore needle followed by a flexible J-tipped wire advanced into the descending thoracic aorta (**Figure 2.5b**). After TEE visualization of the wire in the descending aorta, the needle is removed and serial dilators are advanced over the wire into the aorta via Seldinger technique, followed by the aortic cannula. This technique may be used in the setting of Stanford type A aortic dissection to allow central access with reliable cannulation of the true lumen, as verified by TEE visualization of the wire within the true lumen of the descending thoracic aorta (**Figure 2.5c**).

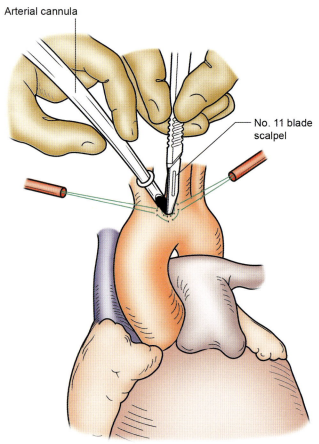

2.5a

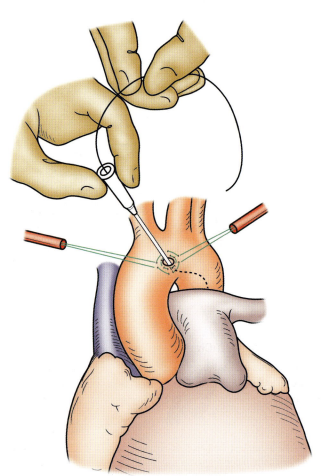

2.5b

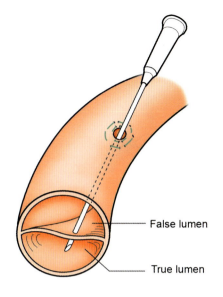

False lumen

True lumen

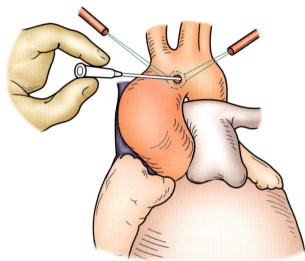

2.5c

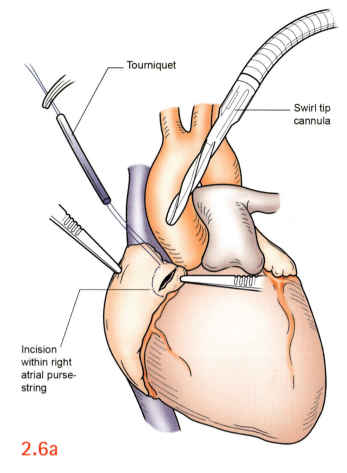

Tourniquet

Swirl tip cannula

Incision within right atrial purse-string

2.6a

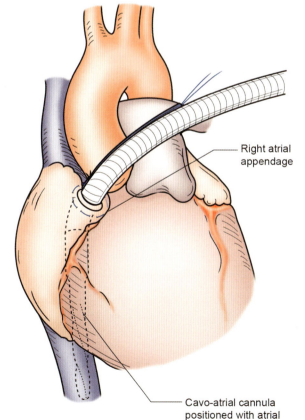

Right atrial appendage

Cavo-atrial cannula positioned with atrial portion in right atrium and caval position (tip) in IVC

2.6b

VENOUS CANNULATION

Dual-stage cannulation of the right atrium is performed via amputation of the tip of the appendage and division of atrial trabeculations with scissors. The cannula is placed into the atrium, directed inferiorly and posteriorly towards the IVC, and secured (**Figure 2.6a and b**). TEE visualization ensures that the cannula has not advanced into the hepatic veins, which will hinder venous drainage. The venous cannula is de-aired and connected to the bypass circuit.

Right-angled or straight cannulae are placed separately in the SVC and IVC positions (**Figure 2.7a**) and connected via a Y-connector to the venous line. Right-sided operations are aided by the placement of caval snares to minimize blood return into the operative field and air entrainment into the bypass circuit (**Figure 2.7b**). The SVC is circumferentially mobilized by dividing the pericardial reflection superiorly and laterally. The medial aspect is mobilized, taking care to avoid damage to the underlying right pulmonary artery. The IVC is easily mobilized by dividing the thin pericardial reflection between the right inferior pulmonary vein and the IVC.

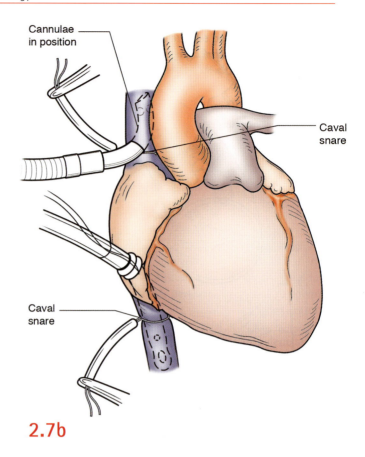

2.7b

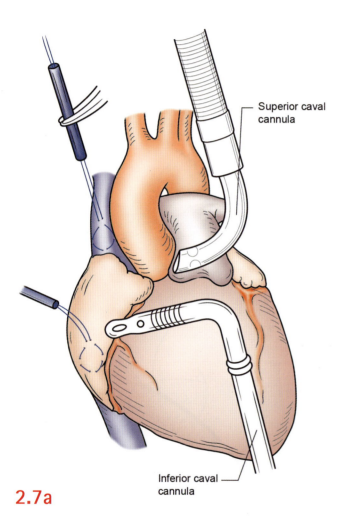

2.7a

Peripheral cannulation

AXILLARY ARTERY CHIMNEY GRAFT

Systemic perfusion via the right axillary artery may be desirable for certain operations (e.g. aortic dissection or aortic arch replacement, porcelain aortas, some minimally invasive operations). A 4 cm incision is made parallel to and just below the lateral one-third of the right clavicle, and the pectoralis major fibers and clavipectoral fascia are divided longitudinally (**Figure 2.8a**). The axillary vein is encountered first, and may be retracted medially to expose the underlying artery. Proximal and distal vessel control is secured with vessel loops. A side-biting clamp or two straight clamps can alternatively be used to minimize this dissection. A bolus of 5000 units of heparin is administered prior to arteriotomy.

Once proximal and distal control is obtained, a longitudinal arteriotomy is prepared for end-to-side anastomosis of an 8 mm Dacron graft with running 5-0 polypropylene suture (**Figure 2.8b**). This "chimney-graft" method is preferred to direct axillary cannulation due to the risk of vascular injury and/or malperfusion to the distal upper extremity with direct cannulation. The perfusion graft can then be de-aired and connected to the bypass pump by inserting an aortic cannula into the graft or attaching standard tubing connectors to the graft.

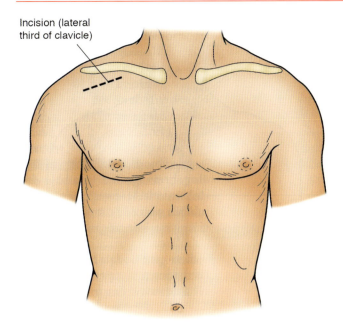

Incision (lateral third of clavicle)

FEMORAL VESSEL ACCESS

Peripheral cannulation may be preferred to enable minimally invasive operations via right or left anterolateral thoracotomy, thoracoscopic, or robotic approaches. Extrathoracic placement of arterial and venous lines maximizes operative exposure while maintaining a small incision. The femoral vessels are accessed via a 2 cm oblique incision midway between the inguinal ligament and inguinal crease to ensure exposure of the common femoral artery proximal to its bifurcation (**Figure 2.9a**). After oblique division of the subcutaneous tissues, the femoral sheath is identified and opened longitudinally, exposing the femoral vessels.

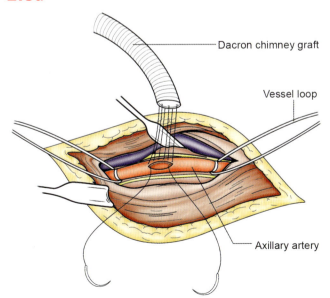

Clavicular fibres of pectoralis major

Axillary vein retracted

Brachial plexus

Clavipectoral fascia

Sternal fibres of pectoralis major

Axillary artery

2.8a

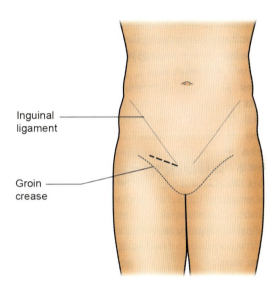

Inguinal ligament

Groin crease

Dacron chimney graft

Vessel loop

Axillary artery

2.8b

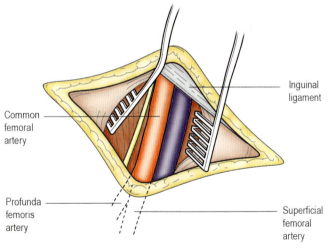

Common femoral artery

Profunda femoris artery

Inguinal ligament

Superficial femoral artery

2.9a

The artery is circumferentially dissected and a single, 4-0 polypropylene pursestring suture is placed midway between the umbilical ligament and the takeoff of the superficial femoral artery (SFA) (**Figure 2.9b**) and secured with a tourniquet. The anterior aspect of the femoral vein can also be easily exposed for cannulation with this dissection. The femoral artery is cannulated peripherally via needle arteriotomy. A wire is advanced into the descending thoracic aorta in retrograde fashion and visualized with TEE. Serial dilation with Seldinger technique is performed and the tapered arterial cannula is advanced into the abdominal aorta.

Alternatively, percutaneous arterial puncture and serial dilation may be used in conjunction with a variety of percutaneous closure devices to cannulate the femoral artery without surgical cutdown. When possible, arterial puncture should be performed under ultrasound guidance to avoid SFA cannulation.

Peripheral venous cannulation via open exposure or percutaneous access is performed with Seldinger technique and TEE verification of cannula placement (**Figure 2.9c**). The femoral cannula is advanced into the right atrium enabling adequate drainage for CPB. Bicaval cannulation can be performed with extrathoracic cannulae for minimally invasive operations. The addition of a second cannula placed percutaneously in the right internal jugular vein produces excellent venous drainage. Venous suction may be used to obviate the need for caval snares.

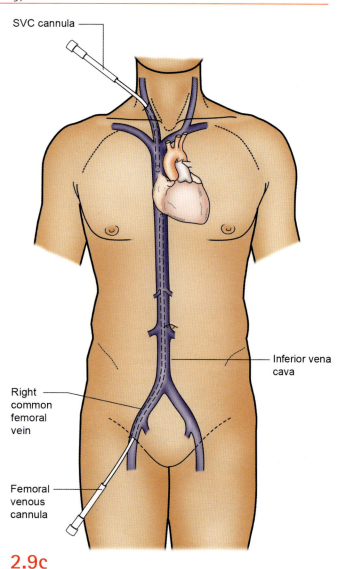

2.9c

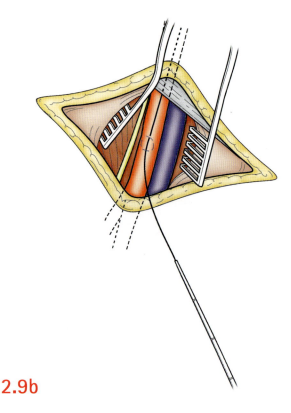

2.9b

Cardioplegia line cannulation

ANTEGRADE CARDIOPLEGIA

An antegrade cardioplegia cannulation site is selected proximal enough to the aortic cannula to allow for placement of an aortic cross-clamp placement. A pledgeted 4-0 polypropylene horizontal mattress suture is placed allowing for puncture with the cardioplegia needle-catheter (**Figure 2.10a**). The inner needle is withdrawn, allowing blood to flush and de-air the cannula, and the catheter is secured with a tourniquet. The aortic root catheter, which also serves as an aortic root vent for de-airing purposes, is then connected to the bypass circuit with a Y-connector to enable connection to both suction and cardioplegia lines from the pump. Delivery of antegrade cardioplegia allows for rapid induction of cardiac arrest and ensures perfusion of cardioplegia solution into both the right and left circulation. The surgeon must be aware of flow-limiting coronary stenoses, which may limit

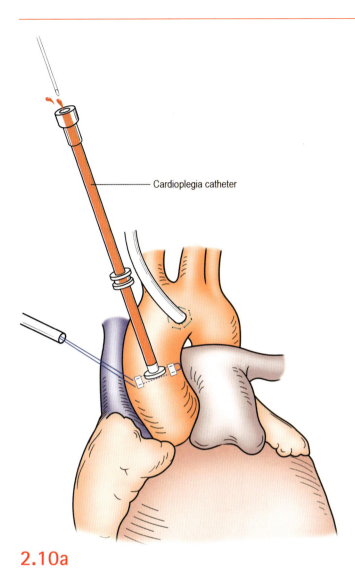

Cardioplegia catheter

2.10a

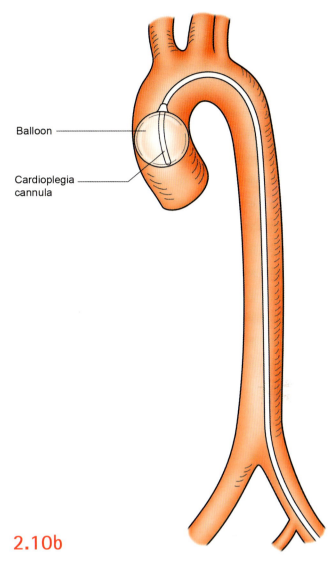

Balloon

Cardioplegia cannula

2.10b

distal circulation of cardioplegia. The presence of aortic valve insufficiency raises the risk of left ventricular distention with antegrade cardioplegia administration. Additionally, procedures requiring aortotomy (aortic valve, aortic aneurysm repair) or significant cardiac retraction which may distort aortic root geometry (e.g. mitral valve) will require an alternative cardioplegia strategy for re-dosing, and either retrograde cardioplegia or direct ostial perfusion with handheld catheters should be considered to supplement myocardial protection.

The use of an endoaortic occlusion balloon catheter obviates the need for transthoracic aortic cross-clamp (Chitwood clamp) placement during minimally invasive operations. The balloon catheter is advanced peripherally over a wire from the femoral arterial catheter side port access into the ascending aorta (**Figure 2.10b**). Inflation of the balloon distal to the sinotubular junction and proximal to the innominate artery

enables occlusion of flow, permitting delivery of antegrade cardioplegia via the tip of the catheter proximal to the balloon. The catheter tip can also be used as a root vent when not administering cardioplegia. Proper positioning and appropriate inflation of the balloon are crucial. Positioning can be directed by TEE and/or fluoroscopy. Maintaining proper position throughout the procedure is aided by the use of bilateral radial arterial lines. If the left arterial line dampens or decreases compared to the right, the balloon is likely obstructing the origin of the innominate artery, potentially causing cerebral hypoperfusion. Ensuring there is no slack or redundancy in the length of the catheter after positioning will prevent the balloon from migrating too proximally during the case. A bolus of adenosine at the initiation of cardioplegia and the resultant asystole allows the cardioplegia to be instilled with limited cardiac output, stabilizing the balloon and ensuring adequate myocardial protection.

RETROGRADE CARDIOPLEGIA

Placement of a coronary sinus cannula enables administration of retrograde cardioplegia through the venous circulation (**Figure 2.11**). A non-pledgeted mattress stitch is placed in the anterior and inferior aspect of the right atrium, which is incised with a number 11 blade. The balloon-tipped cannula is conformed to a slight bend by its inner stylet and guided through the atriotomy into the coronary sinus by directing the tip posteriorly and slightly medial to the IVC–RA junction. TEE visualization, direct palpation of the balloon within the coronary sinus, and the return of dark, highly deoxygenated blood verify proper cannula placement. The catheter can then be secured with a tourniquet, de-aired, and connected to the cardioplegia line and pressure-monitoring lines. A right ventricle tracing on the pressure monitoring line further confirms proper placement. While retrograde cardioplegia administration allows for intermittent delivery without disrupting operative workflow, the surgeon must remain cognizant that right ventricle myocardial protection is relatively reduced with retrograde delivery.

Left ventricle vent

Intraoperative venting of the left ventricle (LV) is utilized to facilitate surgical exposure, prevent LV distention, and reduce myocardial rewarming. Contributors of LV filling on bypass include venous return from the bronchial circulation, cardiac Thebesian veins, and blood not suctioned by venous cannulae and circulated through the lungs. Most commonly, a pursestring suture is placed in the right superior pulmonary vein, which is incised for placement of a semi-flexible cannula (**Figure 2.12**). The cannula is advanced across the mitral valve into the LV and secured with a tourniquet. Placement of a pulmonary artery vent reduces circulation from the right heart, but does not address additional sources of LV filling. The use of ventricular apical vents has been largely abandoned due to the risk of myocardial injury or hemorrhage, but they can be used to emergently empty a distended ventricle.

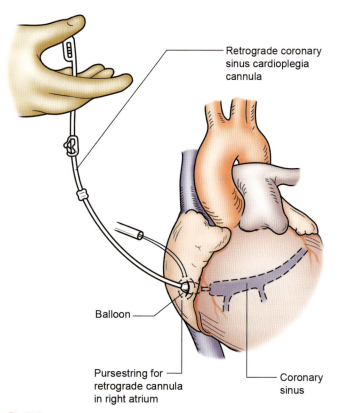

Retrograde coronary sinus cardioplegia cannula

Balloon

Pursestring for retrograde cannula in right atrium

Coronary sinus

2.11

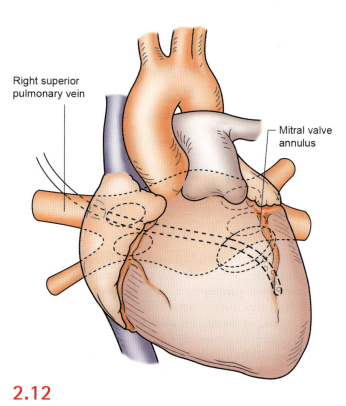

Right superior pulmonary vein

Mitral valve annulus

2.12

INITIATION OF BYPASS

CPB is commenced at the discretion of the surgeon. Prior to initiation, the circuit should be primed with both retrograde and antegrade autologous blood via the bypass cannulae to minimize hemodilution with crystalloid solution priming. Autologous blood may also be sequestered from the circuit for subsequent autotransfusion of blood with limited exposure to the coagulopathic effects of the circuit surface.

CPB is initiated with gradually increasing antegrade flow. The pressure gradient across the arterial cannula is assessed. An unexpectedly high gradient (classically greater than 100 mmHg, though this is highly variable depending on cannula size and placement strategies) raises suspicion for malpositioning or obstruction of the cannula outflow. As the flow rate is gradually increased, right ventricular emptying can be assessed visually in the field. Loss of pulsatility with the cardiac cycle on the arterial line tracing also verifies an empty LV, though this may be obscured by aortic valve insufficiency or significant bronchial return to the LV. This transition period is commonly associated with transient hypotension that may require vasopressor support. Once satisfactory flows are achieved and cardiac decompression is ensured the surgeon can proceed with placement of an aortic cross-clamp and cardioplegia administration, if indicated.

SEPARATION FROM BYPASS

At the completion of the planned surgical intervention, separation from bypass requires physiologic optimization. Prior to weaning, the patient must achieve normothermia, a stable, perfusable rhythm, complete de-airing, removal of extra cannulae, and adequate hemostasis of surgical suture lines and cannula sites. Timed, active warming during the final portions of the operation minimizes extraneous bypass time for rewarming. Atrial and/or ventricular pacing wires may be placed at the surgeon's discretion for rhythm management purposes. The heart and aortic root should be actively de-aired via the aortic root vent. Ventilation is resumed at this stage, and Valsalva maneuvers to recruit the lung parenchyma aid de-airing of the pulmonary veins. Venting and cardioplegia cannulae are removed and their placement sutures tied down and oversewn. Once these requirements are met, cardiac contractility is optimized with administration of inotropic agents and calcium prior to separation from bypass.

Weaning from bypass commences with partial occlusion of the venous cannula, allowing the right heart to fill. Careful attention must be paid to avoid ventricular distention during this time. The preload conditions should be continuously assessed and volume administered from the pump reservoir via the arterial cannula as needed to optimize mechanics. Once adequate hemodynamic status is assured, the venous line is clamped and bypass is ceased. The venous cannula is then removed, and the pursestring suture is resecured but not tied down in case bypass needs to be recommenced. Additional pump reservoir volume can be incrementally administered via the arterial cannula based on ongoing assessment of preload via CVP, pulmonary artery diastolic pressure, and TEE visualization. Once hemodynamic stability is confirmed, a test dose of protamine is administered. Vasopressor administration is frequently needed to treat transient hypotension with protamine administration. The arterial cannula is then removed and the remainder of the protamine dose administered. Additional residual volume in the pump may be hemoconcentrated and salvaged for subsequent transfusion.

POSTOPERATIVE CARE

Initial postoperative care commences upon transfer of the patient from the operating room to the intensive care unit (ICU). Basic laboratory studies (blood count, general chemistry panel, coagulation studies), an arterial blood gas, and a chest radiograph are obtained. Multimodal monitoring is resumed via surface ECG, arterial pressure line, and frequently a pulmonary artery catheter with continuous cardiac output monitoring. Urine output and chest tube drainage are closely monitored, and adjunct laboratory assays (lactic acid, central venous oxygen saturation) may assist in the continuous evaluation of the patient's physiologic status in the ICU.

Exposure to the bypass circuit simultaneously activates several modes of systemic inflammation and induces common clinical manifestations observed in the postoperative patient – coagulopathy, vasodilation, interstitial edema, and end-organ injury. Management following on-pump cardiac surgery is directed towards minimizing the physiologic sequelae of these processes and myocardial insult following arrest and reperfusion.

Coagulopathy

Postoperative bleeding is an independent risk factor for morbidity and mortality following cardiac surgery. Both the intrinsic and extrinsic coagulation cascades are activated by exposure to the foreign surface of the pump and the inherent tissue damage of surgery, resulting in the generation of thrombin and underscoring the necessity of systemic heparinization on bypass (**Figure 2.13**). While heparin inhibits thrombus formation through antithrombin activation, the upstream coagulation cascades remain constitutively activated throughout the bypass run with concomitant fibrinolysis driven by thrombin and inflammatory mediators, resulting in consumption of coagulation proteins that contributes to postoperative coagulopathy. Furthermore, platelet destruction and activation by exposure to the circuit tubing leads to a 30–50% reduction in platelet counts and dysfunction of the remaining platelet pool. Hypothermia further contributes to bleeding in the ICU. Clinical trials

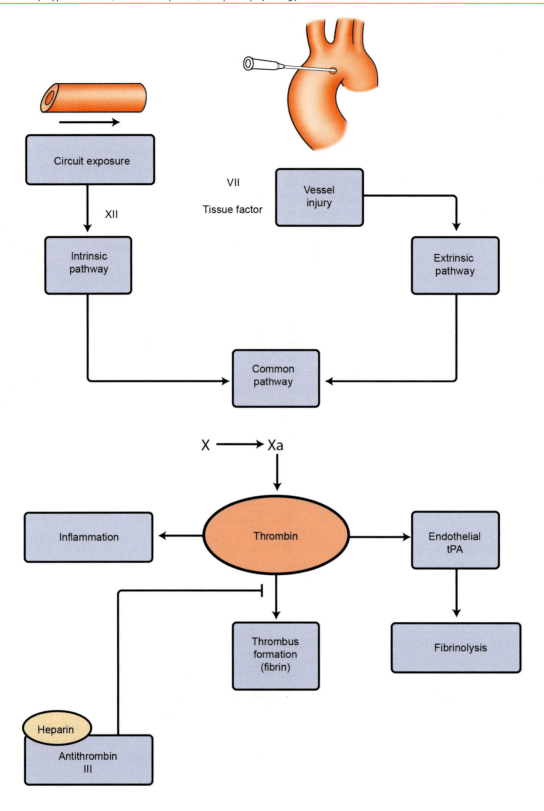

2.13

utilizing minimized extracorporeal circuit surface area and circuit coating with biocompatible materials have demonstrated reductions in inflammatory changes following bypass and modest improvements in neurologic and respiratory complications but have largely failed to produce clinically relevant differences in outcomes. The synthetic lysine analogue antifibrinolytics ε-aminocaproic acid (amicar) and tranexamic acid (TXA) have been studied in postoperative cardiac surgery patients with reduction in postoperative blood loss. Desmopression, a synthetic vasopressin analogue, has also demonstrated some efficacy in reducing bleeding after CPB via stimulation of endothelial factor VIII and von Willebrand factor.

Bleeding must be closely monitored following cardiac surgery. Following most routine operations, less than 100 mL of blood loss per hour is expected immediately after surgery, with steady decline with time. Chest tube drainage in excess of 100 mL per hour prompts assessment of blood counts and coagulation studies to guide the administration of blood products. Elevated PTT may indicate residual heparin effect and prompt additional protamine, while elevated INR may be reversed with fresh frozen plasma. Cryoprecipitate should be considered in the setting of reduced fibrinogen levels. Thromboelastography (TEG) is a clinical assay that assesses both coagulation and thrombolysis and may further guide therapy. In patients with refractory bleeding in excess of 200 mL per hour, empiric treatment of coagulopathy and anemia can be instituted prior to the return of laboratory valuations. The administration of recombinant factor VII or factor VIII inhibitor bypass activity (FEIBA) can be considered. These products rapidly and effectively reduce coagulopathies but significantly increase the likelihood of subsequent venous and even arterial thrombotic complications. Persistent or excessive bleeding after correction of coagulopathy mandates return to the operating room for exploration.

Inflammatory response

The profound systemic inflammatory response to CPB results from activation of both cell-mediated and humoral pathways and manifests in a biphasic fashion. This response is observed clinically as vasodilation, interstitial edema, and end-organ injury. In the early phase, five interrelated plasma protein systems (contact, complement, intrinsic and extrinsic coagulation, and fibrinolytic) are systemically activated in concert with leukocytes upon exposure to the foreign surface of the CPB circuit. The late phase results from reperfusion injury following heart and lung ischemia during aortic cross-clamp time and potentially by endotoxin translocation in the gut. The clinical manifestations of these inflammatory changes range from subclinical biochemical changes to overt organ failure, and vary among patients based on preoperative characteristics, the length of the bypass run, and the use of circulatory arrest.

Factor XII (Hageman factor), a critical activator of the contact pathway, is activated by the presence of the non-endothelial surface of the circuit and autocleaved into its active form, XIIa. Factor XIIa subsequently activates the intrinsic coagulation cascade and drives the conversion of high-molecular-weight kinogen (HK) to bradykinin and its subsequent prostacyclin-mediated vasodilatory response. Factor XIIa also activates kallikrein, leading to activation of neutrophils, fibrinolysis, and positive feedback upregulation of factor XII activation. The process is represented in **Figure 2.14**.

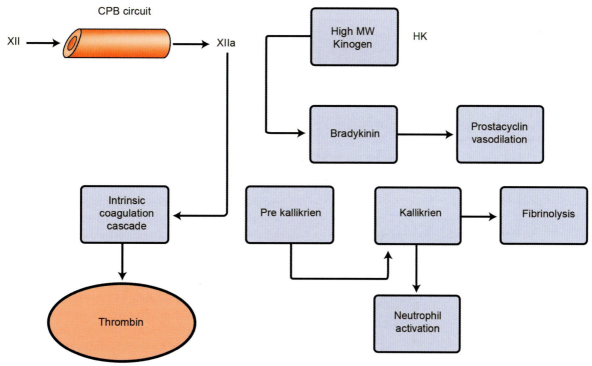

2.14

The complement system, illustrated in **Figure 2.15**, serves as a biologic adjuvant to antibody-mediated response to pathogens via inflammatory amplification and assembly of the cytotoxic membrane attack complex (MAC). Complement may be activated via antibody-dependent (classic) and independent pathways (alternative), ultimately resulting in activation of the C3 protease via cleavage into C3a and C3b components. Activation of the alternative pathway during CPB results from exposure to the foreign surface of the circuit, leading to C3 cleavage, plasma protein factor B activation and cleavage of C5 to C5a and C5b. These components drive the physiologic responses of the complement pathway: direct neutrophil activation by C5a and formation of the MAC, a cytotoxic transmembrane channel composed of C5b and C6, C7, C8, and C9 polymers. Clinically, these processes contribute to direct end-organ injury via MAC-mediated cell lysis as well as vasodilation and tissue edema mediated by activated complement proteins.

Complex interactions between the vascular endothelium and white blood cells govern many of the clinical sequelae following CPB (**Figure 2.16**). Neutrophil activation by contact and complement systems results in both cell-mediated tissue injury and the release of toxic granules containing reactive oxygen species (ROS), proteases, and arachidonic acid metabolites. Monocyte activation following bypass results in excretion of pro- and anti-inflammatory cytokines including TNF-α. In response to activated plasma inflammatory pathways and cytokines, endothelial cells upregulate expression of selectins and integrins to promote neutrophil adhesion. Recruited neutrophils aggregate within microvasculature leading to occlusion and microischemic changes. Aggregation of activated platelets in complexes with fibrin and/or leukocytes creates intravascular microemboli that further contribute to end-organ damage. Neutrophils also facilitate late-phase tissue damage via transmigration across the endothelial layer into the interstitial space and release of toxic granules.

END-ORGAN MANIFESTATIONS OF SYSTEMIC INFLAMMATORY RESPONSE

Generalized tissue edema represents one of the most immediate indicators of the post-CPB inflammatory syndrome, reflecting microvascular permeability and fluid loss into the interstitial space reflecting on a large scale. In the immediate postoperative setting, fluid administration is frequently required to combat this third-space fluid loss. Nearly all patients will require subsequent diuresis in the subacute recovery period to mobilize this peripheral fluid.

Edema affects every organ system, but it is most prominently apparent in the acute lung injury frequently observed in the ICU. Increased alveolar–arterial oxygen gradient, decreased lung compliance, pulmonary shunting, and pulmonary edema may be encountered, posing threats to successful extubation. Renal injury is also common and is an independent risk factor for poor surgical outcomes. The etiology for renal insults in cardiac surgery is multifactorial, resulting from relative hypotension and non-pulsatile perfusion on pump as well as inflammatory injury. Up to 20% of patients will manifest acute kidney injury (AKI), defined as an increase in serum creatinine greater than 50% above baseline, and roughly 1–2% will require renal replacement therapy at least temporarily.

Neurologic injury, which probably occurs on at least a subclinical basis in every patient who undergoes cardiac surgery, is similarly affected by inflammatory changes resulting in tissue edema as well as hemodynamic insults on CPB. Overt neurologic sequelae, ranging from temporary neurocognitive deficits and delirium (25–50% of patients) to the entire spectrum of cerebrovascular events (1–3% of patients) are unfortunately common following cardiac surgery. While strokes after cardiac surgery can be attributed to mechanical causes, intracerebral swelling is likely to contribute to other common neurologic insults postoperatively. Cardiac injury resulting from ischemia, reperfusion injury, and inflammation manifests with tissue edema, myocardial cellular injury and apoptosis. Clinically, these insults are observed in the form of reduced cardiac contractility frequently requiring inotropic support, susceptibility to arrhythmia, and conduction system abnormalities.

2.15

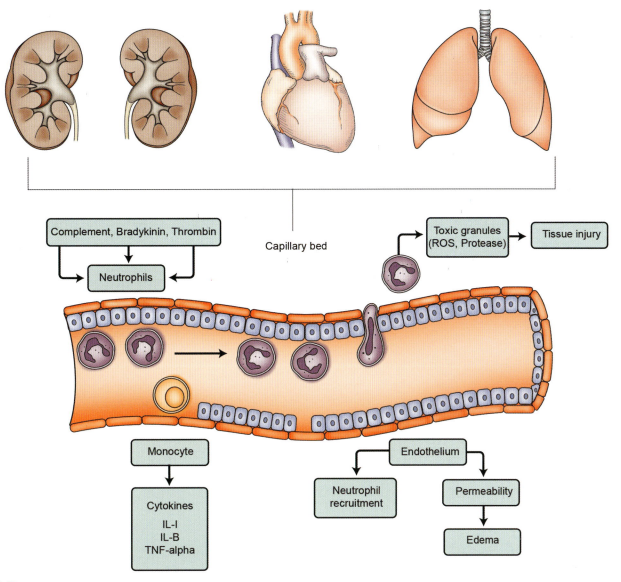

2.16

Postoperative care related to the systemic inflammatory syndrome following CPB is largely supportive. Systemically reduced vascular tone resulting from circulating cytokines is combatted with titration of vasopressors and inotropes to simultaneously support afterload and cardiac performance. Efforts to curb CPB-related insults after cardiac surgery have targeted multiple drivers of inflammation without great clinical success. Trials of systemic corticosteroid therapy reliably reduced inflammatory markers but collectively failed to demonstrate a significant clinical benefit. The use of leukocyte-depleting filters in the bypass circuit effectively reduced leukocyte counts but resulted in enhanced inflammatory markers and minimal clinical benefit. Complement inhibitors were studied in a large, multicenter trial (PRIMO CABG trial) but yielded significant improvement in 30-day mortality for only the highest risk group of patients. Trials of ultrafiltration to remove plasma inflammatory mediators were largely ineffective and yielded no significant benefit.

There is limited evidence for the preoperative use of high-dose statins as a modifier of inflammation, with a suggestion of reduced serum cytokines. Trials of neutrophil elastase inhibitors have yielded some benefit in respiratory endpoints, attributed to reduction of neutrophil-mediated lung injury. Interestingly, trials comparing off-pump coronary surgery to on-pump have not consistently demonstrated improvement in inflammation or clinical measures.

Collectively, the lack of significant clinical improvement with these single interventions speaks to the complexity of physiologic insults following CPB and cardiac surgery in general. Nevertheless, the countless advances in surgical technique, perfusion strategies, anesthesia, and postoperative care in the brief six decades since the introduction of CPB have led to reduction of mortality rates of just 1–3% for routine operations despite the tremendous physiologic insults required to arrest and intervene upon the diseased heart. Ongoing advances in endovascular and hybrid procedures promise to further minimize the collateral damage inflicted en route to durable surgical repair.

FURTHER READING

Chitwood WR (ed.). *Atlas of robotic cardiac surgery.* London: Springer-Verlag; 2014.

Ghosh S, Falter F, Perrino AC (eds). *Cardiopulmonary bypass.* Cambridge: Cambridge University Press; 2015.

Landis RC, Brown JR, Fitzgerald D, et al. Attenuating the systemic inflammatory response to adult cardiopulmonary bypass: a critical review of the evidence base. *J Extra Corpor Technol.* 2014; 46: 197–211.

Mora CT (ed.). *Cardiopulmonary bypass: principles and techniques of extracorporeal circulation.* New York: Springer-Verlag; 1995.

Warren OJ, Smith AJ, Alexiou C, et al. The inflammatory response to cardiopulmonary bypass. Part 1: mechanisms of pathogenesis. *J Cardiothorac Vasc Anesth.* 2009; 23: 223–31.

3

Circulatory arrest: retrograde vs antegrade cerebral protection

JOSHUA M. ROSENBLUM AND EDWARD P. CHEN

HISTORY

Management of the whole body's metabolic demands during cardiac surgery has been a process in evolution since the initial work by Bigelow in 1950 demonstrating the feasibility of hypothermia as a strategy for end-organ protection. In 1975, Griepp and colleagues reported the first successful use of hypothermic circulatory arrest (HCA) for aortic arch reconstruction. In the ensuing decades, clinical work has focused on techniques to improve neurologic protection during the period of cerebral ischemia. Despite advances in surgical technique for arch reconstruction, the ability to overcome the metabolic demands of the brain and the edema associated with ischemia-reperfusion injury has been challenging. Most centers now employ some method of cerebral protective adjunct at the time of HCA by maintaining perfusion to the brain via retrograde cerebral perfusion (RCP) or selective antegrade cerebral perfusion (SACP), either unilateral (uSACP) or bilateral (bSACP). Currently, data conflict over the ideal method for cerebral protection during circulatory arrest and the optimum temperature for hypothermia, but randomized trials are in progress.

PRINCIPLES AND JUSTIFICATION

Although "clamp and sew" techniques for aortic reconstruction may be feasible for distal segments, the unique anatomy of the aortic arch and direct perfusion of the brain from the great vessels, with its poor tolerance to ischemia, makes operations involving arch reconstruction nearly impossible without circulatory arrest. The vascular pathologies that result in a need for proximal aorta replacement also affect the great vessels; in the setting of acute dissection or aneurysmal disease, fragile innominate and carotid arteries are at risk of further irreparable damage with extensive manipulation and clamping, so HCA allows for meticulous reconstruction of the aortic arch in a blood-free operative field. As a protective adjunct to cerebral ischemia, hypothermia is a relatively intuitive concept as decreased temperature results in reduction of metabolic demand. The brain is highly metabolically active and sensitive to ischemic insult, so hypothermia effectively reduces this metabolic need, attenuates the ischemia-reperfusion injury, and helps to limit cerebral edema. More recently, increased use of SACP has further refined the protective strategies for brain protection by initiating circulatory arrest at more moderate levels of hypothermia and avoiding deep hypothermia. Due to the fact that end-organ systems outside the brain can tolerate ischemia at warmer temperatures, moderate hypothermia has been shown to be safe and effective when utilized in conjunction with SACP.

Despite significant improvement in perioperative care and surgical techniques, serious complications during aortic arch surgery are substantially more prevalent than in cases that do not require circulatory arrest. Neurologic injury in the form of permanent stroke, temporary neurologic dysfunction, or spinal cord injury is perhaps the most feared complication of circulatory arrest. In some series, although still relatively rare, permanent stroke is 2–2.5 times higher in cases requiring circulatory arrest compared to standard cardiopulmonary bypass. Furthermore, sensitive measures of neurocognitive function after arch surgery often demonstrate subtle deficits that can last for months despite normal imaging. These findings highlight the importance of adequate cerebral protection and optimal temperature management during arch surgery with either RCP or SACP.

Finally, the well-studied coagulopathy common with cardiopulmonary bypass operations is magnified by the hypothermia utilized during circulatory arrest for aortic arch operations. Although modest improvements in surgical technique have helped to combat bleeding, aortic operations requiring circulatory arrest carry non-trivial rates of significant postoperative chest tube drainage and need for reintervention for bleeding. Hypothermic coagulopathy can be seen at temperatures as warm as 35 °C but significantly worsens with progressive hypothermia. This profound medical coagulopathy often cannot be reversed with pro-tamine administration alone and requires transfusion of cryoprecipitate and thawed plasma to replete coagulation cascade factors. Ongoing studies to examine the neurological effects of warmer circulatory arrest temperatures using SACP or RCP will additionally help to ameliorate associated hypothermia-induced coagulopathy. Despite these known increased risks for major morbidity and mortality, many cases requiring HCA are often emergent and/or life-saving, thus elective use must carefully acknowledge this risk/benefit ratio.

PREOPERATIVE ASSESSMENT AND PREPARATION

Preoperative assessment and workup for cases requiring circulatory arrest are similar to any other major cardiac surgery operation. By nature of the disease processes bringing these patients to thoracic aorta and arch surgery, cross-sectional imaging of the chest and great vessels with either contrast-enhanced CT or MRI has generally been completed. Careful attention to patency of the carotids, jugulars, and right axillary artery must be paid, and one must take note of significant atherosclerotic burden as this may limit bypass circuit flow to the brain and body during critical portions of the case. Carotid duplex ultrasonography is routinely employed in the preoperative workup to identify any significant flow-limiting stenosis; however, unless pre-existing symptoms or events suggest a discontinuous Circle of Willis, we no longer perform transcranial Doppler studies routinely. Finally, it should be obvious that specific arch anatomy and known great vessel anomalies must be identified in the preoperative period to allow for efficient operative conduct.

ANESTHESIA

Conduct of anesthesia delivery during cases requiring circulatory arrest is not markedly different than other major cardiac surgery cases, using a combination of opiate-, propofol-, and volatile anesthetic-based sedation after induction. Anesthetic doses are halved during the period of HCA. Levels of sedation to maintain brain electrical silence are critical to ensure reduced cerebral metabolism. All patients receive high-dose corticosteroids, which are re-dosed every 6–8 hours. Mannitol is given in the prime for the cardiopulmonary bypass circuit as well as when rewarming is initiated.

Monitoring

Standard arterial, central venous, and pulmonary artery catheter access and monitoring are required for circulatory arrest operations regardless of the technique of cerebral protection employed (**Figure 3.1**). For all cases, both elective and emergent, a left radial arterial line should be placed and femoral arterial monitoring lines should be placed in cases of dissection to alert to the possibility of distal malperfusion as a result of false lumen perfusion. In addition, pre-bypass femoral arterial pressure lines are routinely placed in older patients or those with depressed cardiac function to allow for easy access and placement of intra-aortic balloon pump support on separation from CPB. Additionally, pressure monitoring in the inflow circuit at the right axillary artery cannulation site should be used in order to monitor cerebral perfusion pressure at the time of SACP.

Several methods of cerebral monitoring have been used throughout the last few decades. Neuronal electrical activity can be measured by electroencephalographic (EEG) monitors or somatosensory evoked potentials (SSEPs) as well as motor evoked potentials (MEPs). Modern bispectral index (BIS) monitors are single-channel EEG processors which give an easy-to-interpret and reliable measure of cerebral activity, while MEPs and SSEPs are more challenging and time-consuming when utilized on a routine basis. Cerebral perfusion can be measured directly with a jugular bulb venous saturation catheter; however, more centers, including our own, are moving towards bilateral transcranial non-invasive cerebral oximetry monitoring. Although there was initial concern over the reliability of these monitors, interventions based on saturation trends from baseline throughout the case can be valuable to maintenance of adequate cerebral perfusion and oxygenation.

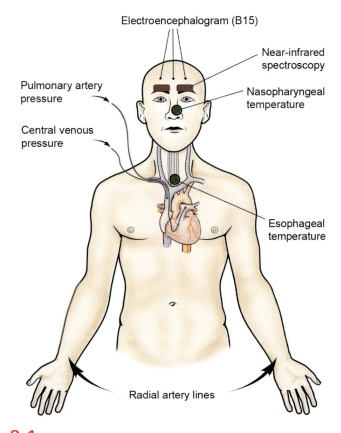

3.1

pH management

The solubility of CO_2 increases with cooling, thereby reducing the partial pressure of CO_2 with concomitant alkalinization of blood and an increase in the hemoglobin affinity for oxygen. Two main strategies can be employed to manage patients during this time: either add CO_2 to the system to maintain a pH of 7.4 and $PaCO_2$ of 40 mmHg (pH-stat), or allow the $PaCO_2$ to remain low thus keeping the temperature-corrected pH unchanged (alpha-stat). Well-designed studies comparing these methods are sparse, although both are employed in modern practice with some evidence for pH-stat superiority in pediatric populations. In our institution, alpha-stat management is preferred as it best complements the brain's autoregulatory mechanisms and helps to prevent overcirculation. Vasoconstriction and subsequent reduction in cerebral blood flow is the natural response to hypothermia-induced decrease in PCO_2. By keeping this mechanism intact, we believe that the alpha-stat method helps to prevent cerebral edema and loss of autoregulation of cerebral blood flow.

OPERATION

Operative details are described in other chapters, but certain points should be addressed.

- In acute type A dissection, femoral arterial cannulation is generally reserved for patients in extremis upon induction of anesthesia. Given the relative ease of axillary artery exposure and cannulation, and the vast improvement in outcomes with SACP during circulatory arrest in non-randomized consecutive series, we prefer this technique even in emergent type A dissection cases.
- In degenerative aneurysms and in cases where the integrity of the axillary and femoral arteries is in question, direct cannulation of the arch under TEE guidance can be used for cooling with post-DHCA perfusion being resumed via a graft side arm.
- Given the questionable benefit of RCP for providing nutritive blood flow, particularly during extended periods of circulatory arrest, we reserve this technique for young patients who require expected short circulatory arrest times.
- Sites for venous drainage are at the surgeon's discretion but, when RCP is planned, bicaval cannulation with snaring of the superior vena cava (SVC) is required.

Cooling

Once arterial and venous cannulation is achieved based on the planned strategy for cerebral protection (DHCA ± RCP or SACP), cardiopulmonary bypass is initiated with flow rates of ~2–2.5 L/min/m² (**Figure 3.2**). Perfusion pressure of 65 mmHg is generally targeted, but is kept higher if concerns for renal or cerebral perfusion predominate, with liberal use of alpha-agonists as needed. Minimal dissection and manipulation of the aortic tissue is performed prior to initiation of CPB. Cooling using the integrated heat exchanger is commenced immediately, with a maximum 10 °C gradient between blood inflow and water bath temperature. Target temperature is determined based on nasopharyngeal temperature, as this is the closest measure of true cerebral temperature. Bladder temperature is another useful measure of core temperature, but this is reliant on adequate urine production and does not correlate well with cerebral temperature. Goal cooling for DHCA is <18 °C with or without RCP which often requires 45 minutes of cooling, and for cases using SACP we generally cool to nasopharyngeal temperature of 26 °C. Complete EEG silence should be achieved prior to initiation of circulatory arrest, particularly if using DHCA alone or in combination with RCP.

Arrest period

Once target temperature is reached, corporeal inflow from the bypass circuit is stopped, the aortic cross-clamp (if present) is removed, and the distal ascending aorta is transected, thus marking the beginning of the arrest period. At this point, RCP or SACP if being used, as discussed below, is begun to maintain cerebral protection. All diseased aortic tissue is resected, and the distal aortic anastomosis is completed. It is our practice to use felt only for acute dissection

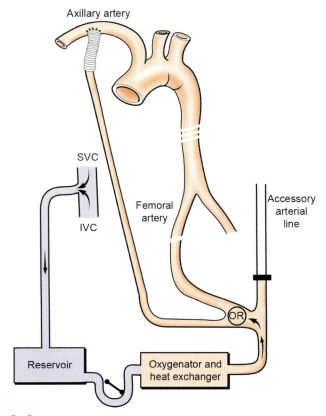

3.2

cases wherein a strip of felt is sandwiched between the adventitia and intima to create a neomedia layer.

For total arch reconstruction, a multi-branched graft should be used to reconstruct the arch vessels, with the left subclavian reconstruction being done during the arrest period and left carotid and innominate reconstruction being done during rewarming (**Figure 3.3**). Access to suture lines can be challenging once the anastomosis is complete, so we generally reinforce both anterior and posterior running portions with interrupted sutures as well. Upon completion of the distal anastomoses, air and debris are evacuated under pressure from the bypass circuit either via a graft sidearm or through the axillary cannulation site. Once satisfactory de-airing is complete, a cross-clamp is placed on the proximal graft and full cardiopulmonary bypass flow is resumed.

Retrograde cerebral perfusion

In retrograde cerebral perfusion (RCP), flow in the SVC is reversed to provide cerebral protection utilizing a bridge between the arterial and venous circuits in the bypass setup.

RCP can be set up with bicaval venous cannulation and essentially any arterial cannulation site (femoral, axillary, or ascending aortic) (**Figure 3.4a**). The arterial circuit is Y-branched to allow for eventual side-arm cannulation and

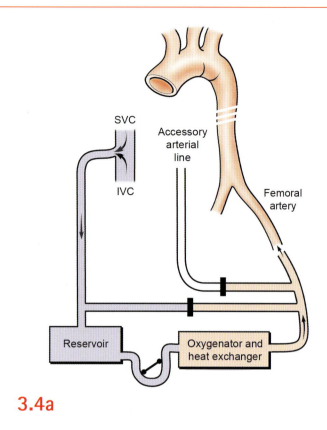

3.4a

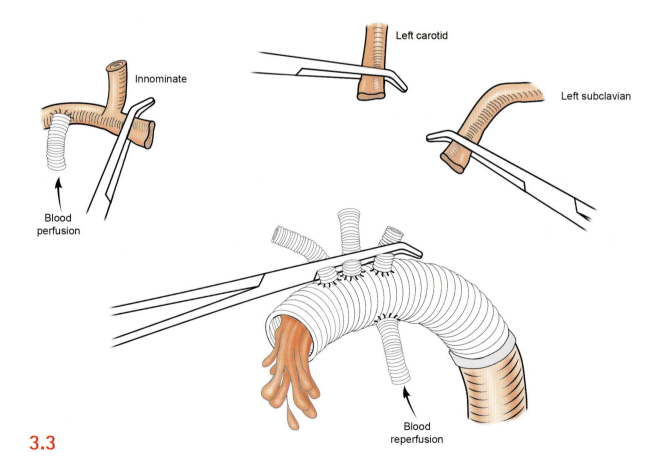

3.3

one branch of the "Y" is connected to the SVC cannula. A 3/8-inch bridge is placed connecting the arterial and venous lines of the SVC cannula and is occluded during the cooling and warming periods.

Upon initiation of circulatory arrest once the temperature nadir is reached, pump outflow lines are clamped, and the clamp on the arteriovenous bridge is removed (**Figure 3.4b**). Venous drainage from the SVC is stopped, and the inferior vena cava (IVC) line is clamped after partially exsanguinating the patient into the pump reservoir. Pump outflow, now retrograde through the venous line into

the SVC, is initiated at a slow rate and gradually increased to 500 mL/min at a maximum pressure of 25–30 mmHg. Pump suction lines are used to scavenge blood emanating from the head vessels during this period.

If necessary during circulatory arrest, RCP flow can be interrupted to aid in visualization for construction of the distal aortic anastomosis. Once complete, normal venous drainage is resumed, arterial inflow through a side arm of the aortic graft is commenced, and the arteriovenous bridge is clamped (**Figure 3.4c**). Standard cardiopulmonary bypass is thus resumed, and rewarming begins.

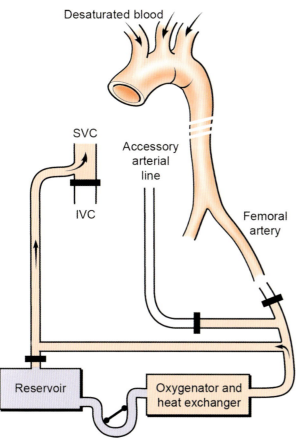

3.4b

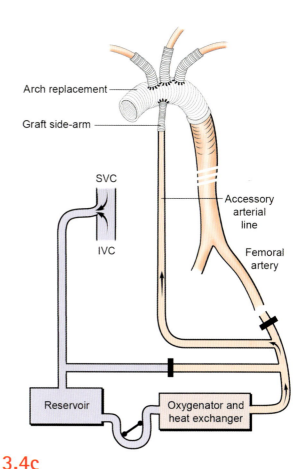

3.4c

Selective arterial cerebral perfusion

Selective arterial cerebral perfusion (SACP) is a technique to perfuse the brain with antegrade blood flow during lower body circulatory arrest, allowing for longer periods of safe arrest at warmer corporeal temperatures.

Some groups cannulate the innominate artery after sternal entry. We find that using the axillary artery provides the added benefit of keeping the arterial cannula out of the operative field. The axillary artery is approached through a separate incision in the right deltopectoral groove. An 8 mm gortex graft is sewn to the axillary artery and a perfusion cannula is inserted (**Figure 3.5a**). Venous drainage is achieved with a two-stage right atrial cannula, and cooling is initiated upon institution of CPB. During cooling, the innominate and left carotid artery origins must be isolated and prepared for

clamping. The innominate vein can be transected for better visualization, but this is rarely necessary.

Once target temperature is reached, arterial inflow is lowered to 10 mL/kg/min. The aorta is transected, and the innominate artery is clamped (**Figure 3.5b**). We routinely also clamp the left carotid artery to improve cerebral perfusion pressure through extracranial collaterals; alternatively, the left carotid can be left open while monitoring the cerebral oximeter and then clamped if the left-sided cerebral oximetry saturations diminish. Upon completion of arch reconstruction, the innominate clamp is removed as the CPB flow is slowly increased to full flow. Once de-airing is complete, the proximal graft is clamped and the distal suture line is checked for hemostasis after pressurization. Rewarming is then commenced.

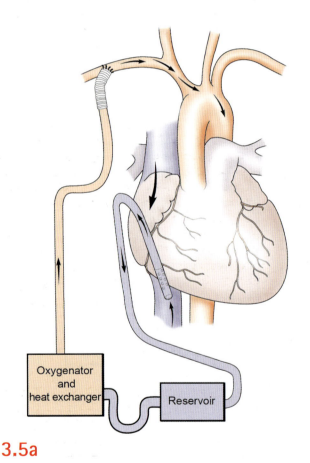

3.5a

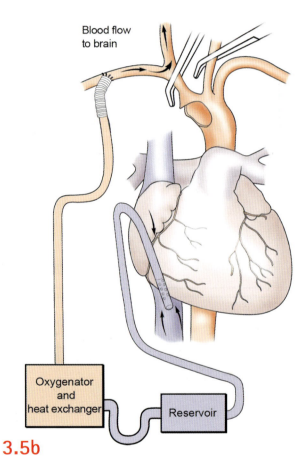

3.5b

Rewarming

Rewarming to near-normothermia is as critical a step as cooling and circulatory arrest. Careful attention to all parameters of mean arterial pressure, pH, glycemia, hematocrit, and cerebral oximetry is necessary to avoid further cerebral ischemia-reperfusion injury. In the case of RCP or DHCA, antegrade perfusion is recommenced through a cannula in a side arm of the distal aortic graft used for arch reconstruction (**Figure 3.6**) and, in cases using SACP, perfusion is resumed at full flow through the axillary artery cannulation site once the innominate artery clamp is removed. Larger patients or those with small arch vessels may require an additional cannula placed in an aortic graft side arm to provide adequate bypass circuit flows for optimum cardiac output.

At this point, the distal aortic suture line is inspected for hemostasis. For total arch reconstruction (as opposed to hemi-arch replacement), we tend to favor utilization of a multi-branched aortic graft and leave the left carotid artery and innominate artery reconstruction until after rewarming has occurred, thus necessitating the additional arterial perfusion cannula in a graft side arm. During this rewarming period, any additional proximal aortic procedures (valve replacement, root reconstruction, etc.) are completed. Since avoidance of cerebral hyperthermia is important, the arterial

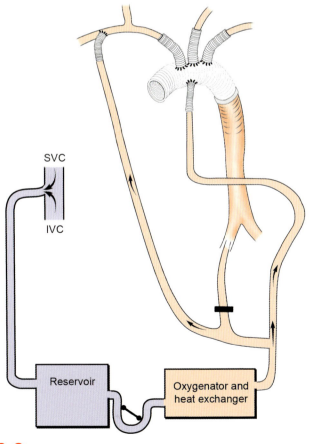

3.6

SVC

IVC

Reservoir

Oxygenator and heat exchanger

inflow temperature from the bypass circuit does not exceed 37°C. As a result, it is generally not possible to reach whole-body normothermia, so bypass is discontinued at a core temperature of 35–36°C.

Hemostasis

As mentioned above, hemostasis can be challenging after completion of bypass during aortic operations requiring hypothermia. Clearly, meticulous surgical technique and attention to detail is needed throughout all phases of these operations. This premise starts with skin incision and sternal entry, which should remain as bloodless as possible, especially in the case of reoperative surgery. Each anastomosis must be checked after completion with flow from the pump or pressurized cardioplegia. We avoid topical hemostatic agents when possible as some of these have been known to cause suture-line pseudoaneurysms and can make any reoperation more challenging. All patients in our institution receive thromboxane A2 infusion at the completion of cardiopulmonary bypass, and we utilize aggressive blood product resuscitation strategies. Data from trauma registries and massive transfusion protocols clearly show a benefit to balanced transfusion with equal utilization of platelet apheresis units, thawed cryoprecipitate, and thawed plasma. Aortic surgery, especially those cases requiring circulatory arrest, is akin to trauma management, thus nearly all patients receive equal parts of these blood products in addition to protamine to achieve adequate hemostasis prior to chest closure. Finally, as many of these patients do not have violation of either pleural space, the risk for tamponade is considerable, so we place several large-bore silastic drainage tubes around all anastomoses and in the posterior pericardium.

POSTOPERATIVE CARE

There are no significant differences in postoperative care for patients after aortic surgery with circulatory arrest as compared to other open cardiac operations, with a few caveats. Standard cardiac output, filling pressures, and arterial pressures are monitored frequently, and methods to maintain normothermia, including fluid warmers and forced air heating blankets, should be employed. Hypoxemia, hypotension, and hypoperfusion should be avoided at all costs as these can contribute to and exacerbate cerebral ischemia-reperfusion injury. Liberal use of vasopressors and inotropes as well as colloid resuscitation to maintain supraphysiologic mean arterial pressure and cardiac output in the first 12–24 hours postoperatively is critical to promote cerebral perfusion. Although several randomized trials have proven the safety of conservative blood transfusion strategies in cardiac surgery, there are no randomized trials for aortic surgery with circulatory arrest.

Thus, we encourage red blood cell transfusion to maintain a serum hemoglobin around 9–10 g/dL. Once normothermia is reached, sedation is lightened to perform a full neurological exam, and when cardiorespiratory parameters are improved, stable, and acceptable, patients are weaned from ventilator support.

OUTCOMES

Profound (<14 °C) and deep hypothermia (14–20 °C) made aortic arch reconstruction safe while providing a means of cerebral protection during circulatory arrest. Although profound hypothermia has essentially been abandoned due to its modest benefit over DHCA with substantially increased risk profiles, DHCA is used routinely and has been proven safe, especially when the circulatory arrest time is expected to be shorter than 30–40 minutes. Large series of arch reconstruction using DHCA alone have shown excellent outcomes, with mortality and permanent stroke rates less than 5% and 10-year survival of up to 70%, but some have shown that rates of subtle temporary neurological dysfunction are as high as 30%, even when circulatory arrest times are shorter than 30 minutes. For this reason, we reserve this technique for special circumstances when adjunct measures are not available as a result of anatomic issues with difficult vascular access prior to circulatory arrest and those with tenuous anatomy, such as a contained rupture or pseudoaneurysm formation.

RCP was the first adjunct to HCA proposed to improve cerebral protection during the arrest phase. Even with long arrest times (60 minutes), RCP was shown in large initial series to reduce both stroke and mortality over HCA alone. Mounting clinical and experimental evidence, however, suggests equivocal benefits and even potential harm of RCP. Animal models demonstrate that the SVC and cerebral circulation has numerous venovenous collaterals, which result in blood being shunted away from the brain during RCP, thus impairing cerebral cooling. Furthermore, recent clinical studies found that, while RCP utilization may improve mortality and stroke risk, it does not appear to reduce the rate of temporary neurological dysfunction. Thus, in our institution, RCP is used sparingly, specifically for those young patients who need hemi-arch reconstruction with presumed short circulatory arrest times.

SACP, whether unilateral or bilateral, has provided a substantial improvement in cerebral protection during circulatory arrest over DHCA or RCP alone, particularly with prolonged periods of circulatory arrest for complex arch reconstruction. Initial descriptions of the technique used individual catheters for perfusion directly into the ostia of the head vessels, but most institutions now cannulate the axillary or innominate artery for arterial return. Many clinical series have shown excellent results with SACP, with rates of mortality, stroke, and temporary neurological dysfunction as low as 5%. While we use uSACP in over 90% of aortic arch cases, bSACP predominates in Europe. Clinical data conflict over whether bSACP is superior to uSACP, but some studies suggest a benefit, especially with prolonged HCA times. Perhaps most importantly, SACP has allowed for utilization of warmer ischemic temperatures at the time of HCA, and reliable, safe results have been reported with SACP and moderate (20–28 °C) hypothermia. In our center, we routinely use SACP at 26 °C for hemi-arch and total arch reconstruction and reserve deep hypothermia for more complex cases. Randomized trials aimed at demonstrating the efficacy and safety of moderate hypothermia with SACP as compared to DHCA with RCP or SACP are currently underway.

FURTHER READING

Bonser RS, Wong CH, Harrington D, et al. Failure of retrograde cerebral perfusion to attenuate metabolic changes associated with hypothermic circulatory arrest. *J Thorac Cardiovasc Surg.* 2002; 123: 943–50.

Ergin MA, Uysal S, Reich DL, et al. Temporary neurological dysfunction after deep hypothermic circulatory arrest: a clinical marker of long-term functional deficit. *Ann Thorac Surg.* 1999; 67: 1887–90.

Gega A, Rizzo JA, Johnson MH, et al. Straight deep hypothermic arrest: experience in 394 patients supports its effectiveness as a sole means of brain preservation. *Ann Thorac Surg.* 2007; 84: 759–66.

Kayatta MO, Chen EP. Optimal temperature management in aortic arch operations. *Gen Thorac Cardiovasc Surg.* 2016; 64: 639–50.

Leshnower BG, Myung RJ, Kilgo PD, et al. Moderate hypothermia and unilateral selective antegrade cerebral perfusion: a contemporary cerebral protection strategy for aortic arch surgery. *Ann Thorac Surg.* 2010; 90: 547–54.

Sundt TM 3rd, Orszulak TA, Cook DJ, Schaff HV. Improving results of open arch replacement. *Ann Thorac Surg.* 2008; 86: 787–96.

4

Intraoperative myocardial protection

RICHARD D. WEISEL AND TERRENCE M. YAU

HISTORY

Bigelow in Toronto introduced hypothermia to protect the heart for cardiac surgery in the 1950s. Deep hypothermia and circulatory arrest facilitated the repair of complex congenital cardiac defects. The initial attempt at induced cardiac arrest to facilitate intracardiac procedures was performed by Melrose in 1955. Unfortunately, the high potassium concentrations produced myocardial necrosis, which resulted in the early abandonment of induced cardioplegic arrest. Direct coronary perfusion and induced ventricular fibrillation were employed to protect the heart, but poor visualization and reports of myocardial injury encouraged cardiac surgeons to discover alternate approaches. For coronary surgery, sequential aortic cross-clamping was employed for the construction of distal coronary anastomoses, but the need for the intra-aortic balloon pump or fatal subendocardial necrosis were concerning.

In the 1970s, crystalloid cardioplegia was introduced to cool and protect the heart during intracardiac repair and a variety of formulations were supported by Tyers, Roe, Gay, and Bretschneider. In the 1980s, Follette and Buckberg suggested that blood provided the best vehicle for potassium cardioplegia based on animal studies. Blood cardioplegia delivered nutrients and oxygen to the ischemic myocardium with better osmotic, buffering, and antioxidant capability than crystalloid cardioplegia. In Toronto, Fremes and colleagues demonstrated better clinical outcomes with blood compared with crystalloid cardioplegia. In the 1990s, warm blood cardioplegia was introduced in Toronto and evaluated worldwide. In addition, antegrade, retrograde, and combined techniques of blood cardioplegia were evaluated in a variety of clinical trials. This experience provided cardiac surgeons with a variety of techniques to individualize myocardial protection to the needs of patients with different challenges.

This chapter reviews current concepts of myocardial protection and the metabolic and physiological rationale behind them. The advantages and disadvantages of differing delivery methods are discussed and the relative merits of various cardioplegic additives are reviewed. The cardiac surgeon has a unique opportunity not only to prevent damage during cardiac arrest but also to resuscitate the ischemic myocardium and restore myocardial metabolism and ventricular function to normal following the cardiac surgical procedure.

CARDIOPLEGIA

Evolution of potassium cardioplegia

Potassium cardioplegia was introduced by Melrose and colleagues in 1955 and their formulation contained nearly 240 mEq/L of potassium. In 1957, Donald Effler was one of the first surgeons to use potassium citrate to induce cardioplegic arrest in patients. Unfortunately, the technique was soon abandoned when pathological evidence of severe myocardial injury was demonstrated. In 1973, Gay and Ebert reintroduced hyperkalemic cardioplegic arrest using concentrations of potassium which were one-tenth of those used by Melrose and Effler. Not surprisingly, the focal myocardial inflammatory lesions noted with earlier cases were eliminated. Thereafter, low-dose potassium cardioplegia administered in a crystalloid solution became the most commonly used clinical method of achieving mechanical arrest during cardiac surgical procedures.

Blood and crystalloid cardioplegia

Initial approaches to optimize crystalloid cardioplegia included oxygenation of the crystalloid solution. This approach was soon followed by the introduction of blood as the primary cardioplegic vehicle. In addition to functioning as a more efficient oxygen carrier, whole blood offered the added benefits of a more efficient buffering capacity, a reduction in myocardial edema (due to increased oncoticity) and less hemodilution. Furthermore, whole blood contained a number of endogenous free-radical scavengers which may aid in the attenuation of ischemia-reperfusion injury.

These properties led many surgeons to adopt blood-based cardioplegia in the early 1980s. One of the first supportive studies was a randomized clinical trial of blood vs crystalloid cardioplegia performed by Fremes and colleagues in

Toronto. In patients undergoing elective coronary artery bypass graft (CABG) surgery, blood cardioplegia was associated with the maintenance of aerobic myocardial metabolism during the cross-clamp period and a decrease in lactate production during reperfusion. Although the improved metabolic activity did not translate into significantly improved clinical outcomes in low-risk patients, higher-risk patients with unstable angina who received blood cardioplegia demonstrated a decreased incidence of perioperative myocardial infarction, low output syndrome, and death compared to those who received crystalloid cardioplegia.

Conversely, some surgeons have reported good outcomes with the use of single-dose crystalloid cardioplegic formulations including del Nido cardioplegia (an extracellular solution) and Custodial (an intracellular solution). These solutions have been used primarily in pediatric surgery or for valvular surgery in adults, but there is as yet little data on their safety and efficacy in patients with coronary artery disease, where suboptimal protection or delivery may have greater consequences.

Dilution of blood cardioplegia

Using separate rolling pumps and heat exchangers, the original blood cardioplegic techniques combined cold oxygenated blood from the bypass circuit with a crystalloid solution at a 2:1, 4:1, or 8:1 ratio. Since the early 1990s, blood cardioplegic solutions with even higher concentrations of blood have been used as the level of hypothermia decreased. Indeed, some surgeons currently use a blood-only cardioplegic solution supplemented with essential electrolytes, including potassium and magnesium. Menasche demonstrated that this technique of undiluted blood cardioplegia effectively reduced the volume of crystalloid administration from 750 mL to less than 100 mL. Moreover, the intrinsic buffering capacity of blood-only cardioplegia precluded the need for additional buffering agents. Since Menasche reported his results, the crystalloid component of cardioplegia has been simplified, now consisting of only potassium, magnesium, and dextrose.

Yau in Toronto compared the results with 8:1 blood cardioplegia with microplegia (66:1) during isolated CABG. A propensity matching of 1980 patients in each group revealed a significant reduction in the amount of crystalloid delivered (437 ± 88 mL in the 8:1 group and 45 ± 32 mL in the microplegia group). Reducing the crystalloid load may have reduced the amount of cardiac edema because the microplegia group had a significant independent reduction in the need for high-dose inotropes or intra-aortic balloon pumps (low cardiac output syndrome) following CABG surgery.

Metabolic substrate-enhanced cardioplegia

Preclinical investigations found that prolonged ischemic arrest resulted in depletion in Krebs-cycle intermediates (including **glutamate and aspartate**). This metabolic depletion may contribute to the delayed recovery of postoperative myocardial metabolism and function seen with cold blood cardioplegia. In a trial by Rosenkranz and colleagues, hearts arrested with glutamate- and aspartate-supplemented cardioplegia achieved earlier metabolic recovery. However, other reports found that glutamate and aspartate supplementation was not associated with improved recovery of myocardial metabolism or ventricular function in patients undergoing CABG.

The addition of **lactate** to blood cardioplegia is another metabolic intervention which has been studied in clinical trials. During cardioplegic arrest, myocardial oxidation of fatty acids and glucose (the predominant substrates for aerobic metabolism) is impaired, and lactate, which is readily metabolized to pyruvate, is the preferred substrate for aerobic metabolism during reperfusion. In a randomized clinical trial, the infusion of Ringer's lactate prior to and during cardioplegic arrest was associated with improved cardiac metabolic and functional recovery and a reduction in perioperative ischemic injury compared to controls. Although many metabolic additives have been investigated over the years with varying results, metabolic additives in general have not been widely adopted due to a lack of unequivocal clinical benefit.

CARDIOPLEGIC TEMPERATURE

Normothermic cardioplegia

Traditional cardioplegic methods employed intermittent infusions of hypothermic (less than 10 °C) blood or crystalloid cardioplegic solutions during aortic cross-clamping. Cold cardioplegia, in addition to minimizing myocardial metabolic requirements, enabled an immediate assessment of cardioplegic delivery based on the degree of regional cooling. Some surgeons preferred to augment myocardial cooling with the direct application of topical saline slush or with a cooling jacket apparatus. However, the benefits of additional topical cooling have been difficult to demonstrate and were occasionally associated with postoperative phrenic nerve palsy or an increased incidence of respiratory compromise.

Although hypothermia provides excellent protection to the arrested heart, functional recovery with reperfusion is often delayed, presumably due to the hypothermic inhibition of myocardial enzymes that may remain inactive for hours following cardioplegic arrest. In 1982, Rosenkranz demonstrated that an initial warm induction of cardioplegic arrest prior to administration of hypothermic cardioplegia improved myocardial metabolic and functional recovery. Similarly, Teoh demonstrated that a terminal infusion of warm blood cardioplegia just prior to cross-clamp removal (the cardioplegic "hot shot") facilitated early myocardial metabolic recovery while maintaining electromechanical arrest. Presumably, normothermic reperfusion enables an early resumption of temperature-dependent mitochondrial enzymatic function and a quick return to aerobic metabolism with a resultant increase in adenosine triphosphate (ATP) generation.

Moreover, the persistent non-contractile state of the heart enables the use of available ATP for the repair of cellular injury and the repletion of energy stores rather than the maintenance of unnecessary contractile activity. By the late 1980s, the standard technique of myocardial protection in Toronto consisted of intermittent cold blood cardioplegia with a terminal hot shot. In cases of severe preoperative ischemia, warm induction with a substrate-enhanced cardioplegic solution was used.

Development of warm heart surgery

As early as 1978, Behrendt demonstrated that the basic cardioprotective effects of cardioplegia were independent of hypothermia. Lowering the heart temperature did not reduce myocardial oxygen requirements much beyond that observed with hyperkalemic arrest alone. In 1991, Lichtenstein and colleagues in Toronto extrapolated the benefits of initial and terminal warm cardioplegia to introduce the concept of warm heart surgery. Citing the well-documented deleterious effects of hypothermic cardioplegia (including impairment of mitochondrial energy generation, poor substrate utilization and membrane injury), Lichtenstein suggested that the heart could be maintained at a temperature of 37 °C throughout the cross-clamp period to facilitate the recovery of myocardial metabolism and function following cross-clamp removal. In turn, the metabolic needs of the heart would be met by near-continuous infusions of blood cardioplegia. Buckberg and colleagues demonstrated the feasibility and potential efficacy of this approach in a canine heart model. Myocardial oxygen consumption was reduced from 5.6 mL/min/100 g to 1.1 mL/min/100 g when the heart was arrested at 37 °C. Lowering the heart temperature to 18 °C provided little additional benefit, with a reduction in myocardial oxygen consumption from 1.1 mL/min/100 g to 0.31 mL/min/100 g.

In 1991, Lichtenstein and colleagues presented the results of surgery in 121 consecutive patients receiving normothermic antegrade blood cardioplegia during CABG. In comparison to a historical cohort of 133 patients receiving hypothermic antegrade blood cardioplegia, warm heart patients had a lower incidence of perioperative myocardial infarction and fewer patients required the intra-aortic balloon pump after surgery. Although mortality was also lower in the normothermic group (0.9% versus 2.2% in the hypothermic group), this difference did not reach statistical significance. In 1994, Naylor in Toronto reported the results of a prospective clinical trial involving nearly 2000 CABG patients randomized to receive either normothermic or hypothermic cardioplegia. Although no difference in mortality or myocardial infarction was found between groups, patients in the normothermic group had a significantly lower incidence of postoperative low cardiac output syndrome. Similarly, Yau and colleagues in Toronto demonstrated improved early postoperative myocardial end-systolic elastance, preload recruitable stroke work, and postoperative early diastolic relaxation in patients receiving normothermic compared to hypothermic cardioplegia.

Optimal cardioplegic temperature

Normothermic cardioplegia offered the promise of resuscitating the ischemic heart while facilitating early postoperative recovery of myocardial metabolism and function. Unfortunately, inadequate distribution of cardioplegia and the necessity to interrupt the cardioplegic infusion during distal anastomoses resulted in substantial anaerobic metabolic activity and warm ischemic injury. To avoid these detrimental effects, Yau and colleagues compared the results of tepid (29 °C) blood cardioplegia to those of warm (37 °C) and cold (4 °C) blood cardioplegia (producing myocardial temperatures of 37 °C or 18 °C, respectively) in 72 patients undergoing isolated CABG. Myocardial oxygen consumption and anaerobic lactate release were greatest during warm, intermediate during tepid, and least during cold cardioplegic arrest. They also found that warm retrograde and tepid retrograde techniques resulted in greater lactic acid washout during reperfusion. Left ventricular stroke work indices were best after warm antegrade and tepid antegrade in comparison to cold antegrade cardioplegia. Thus, both warm and tepid techniques were beneficial. However, unlike warm cardioplegia, tepid antegrade cardioplegia offered additional protection during cardioplegic interruptions. Moreover, by preventing cold-related injury, myocardial functional recovery with tepid infusions was more rapid than with cold cardioplegia. Based on these studies, most surgeons have not attempted to cool the heart as much during cold blood cardioplegic arrest. Instead, warmer heart temperatures have been tolerated. Those surgeons who prefer warmer blood cardioplegia currently allow the heart temperatures to drift. These compromises may simultaneously optimize both cerebral and myocardial protection.

CARDIOPLEGIC DELIVERY

Antegrade cardioplegic delivery

Standard cardioplegic delivery involves the administration of antegrade infusions into the aortic root at perfusion pressures of 70–100 mmHg. Delivery is accomplished through a 12-gauge cardioplegia cannula positioned in the mid ascending aorta. The same cannula can be used for aortic venting between cardioplegic infusions. To achieve electromechanical arrest, initial doses of 500–1000 mL are usually required (more if left ventricular hypertrophy is present). Thereafter, arrest is maintained by intermittent antegrade infusions into the aortic root as well as through each completed vein graft at the completion of each distal and/or proximal anastomosis. During valvular surgery, maintenance doses are generally administered every 15–20 minutes.

The concern with antegrade cardioplegia, however, is the possibility of hypoperfusion of distal vascular beds due to severe proximal obstructions of the coronary arteries (when vein grafts have yet to be completed or when internal mammary arterial grafts are anastomosed to the left anterior descending artery last). Moreover, antegrade cardioplegia may be detrimental in reoperative coronary bypass surgery because of the risk of saphenous vein graft embolization when cardioplegia is delivered via the aortic root. Additional limitations may exist during valvular operations. In patients with significant aortic regurgitation, antegrade cardioplegic delivery via the aortic root may be ineffective, leading to ventricular distention. In these patients, the aorta must be opened soon after cross-clamp application to enable direct cardioplegic administration via the coronary ostia. Subsequent ostial infusions, however, may obscure the operative field and be cumbersome during valve implantation.

Retrograde coronary sinus cardioplegia

Retrograde cardioplegic delivery via the coronary sinus was first introduced in the early 1980s. Experimental studies demonstrated the feasibility of this approach, which has since been widely adopted, especially for patients undergoing valve replacement or reoperative CABG surgery. In aortic valve surgery, retrograde cardioplegia may obviate the need for antegrade cardioplegic delivery via the coronary ostia. In mitral valve surgery, retrograde cardioplegia is not impeded by mitral retraction, as is often the case with antegrade cardioplegic delivery. For reoperative CABG surgery, retrograde cardioplegia is believed to be beneficial because embolization from old vein grafts may be prevented.

For effective retrograde coronary sinus cardioplegia, a catheter is introduced through a right atrial pursestring and directed into the coronary sinus. Catheter position is confirmed by palpation and by direct measurement of coronary sinus pressures. Maintenance of acceptable perfusion pressures (40 mmHg or less) is achieved with a soft self-inflating occlusive balloon designed to maintain adequate myocardial perfusion while preventing perivascular hemorrhage, edema or coronary sinus rupture. If the right atrium is opened and the coronary sinus directly cannulated, placement of a pursestring suture at the base of the coronary sinus prevents catheter dislodgement and minimizes reflux into the right atrium.

Combined antegrade and retrograde cardioplegia

Although delivery of antegrade cardioplegia may be limited by native coronary stenoses, distribution of retrograde cardioplegia may be unreliable to the right ventricle and inhomogeneous to the left ventricle. To overcome such inherent limitations, a combined antegrade and retrograde approach has been demonstrated to be effective in a number of randomized clinical trials. Another approach is to combine antegrade and retrograde cardioplegic delivery. Retrograde cardioplegia can be administered continuously throughout the cross-clamp period or stopped when necessary to facilitate visualization. At the completion of each

proximal anastomosis, antegrade cardioplegia can be given into the native coronary circulation as well as all completed vein grafts. The disadvantage of this approach is the need to de-air the aortic root before each antegrade bolus, an added step that can be time-consuming and potentially hazardous if air is incompletely removed from the aorta.

Another technique is to combine continuous retrograde cardioplegia with infusions down each completed vein graft. Determination of the adequacy of cardioplegic delivery can be accomplished with contrast transesophageal echocardiography. Real-time assessment and quantification of myocardial perfusion permits the surgeon to modify the technique to ensure homogeneous cardioplegic distribution. In one study with this imaging technique, antegrade cardioplegic delivery provided more homogeneous perfusion compared to retrograde delivery at similar flow rates. Right ventricular perfusion was poor regardless of the direction of cardioplegic administration. In this study, simultaneous delivery provided the most consistent results and offered the best perfusion of the anterior left ventricle and right ventricle in comparison to antegrade or retrograde routes alone.

Technical aspects of cardioplegia administration

Following aortic and venous cannulation, a simple 4-0 polypropylene pursestring suture is placed either at the midlevel of the right atrium (2–3 cm lateral to the atrioventricular groove) or at the base of the right atrial appendage to anchor the retrograde cardioplegia cannula. Another 4-0 polypropylene mattress or figure-eight suture is placed on the anterior aspect of the mid ascending aorta to secure the antegrade cardioplegia cannula. The typical antegrade cannula is a 12-gauge device with a two-limbed connector enabling both cardioplegic delivery and aortic root venting. The aortic root vent provides for effective decompression of the left heart during CABG procedures with either antegrade or retrograde infusions. During valve procedures, either the LA or the LV is usually vented directly.

After insertion of the antegrade cannula and preferably prior to initiation of cardiopulmonary bypass, the retrograde cardioplegia cannula can be inserted through the atrial pursestring. The catheter is advanced carefully into the coronary sinus orifice with the position of the cannula tip verified by digital palpation behind the heart. Elevating the heart slightly anteriorly (with the inferior vena cava fixed in place by the previously positioned venous cannula) can facilitate this catheter-positioning maneuver. Once the catheter is positioned appropriately, irrigation of the pressure lumen expands the self-inflating balloon near the tip of the catheter. The central catheter lumen is then aspirated, flushed through a tubing extension which is connected to a pressure transducer, and zeroed in preparation for subsequent use. If the cannula is placed too deeply into the coronary sinus, the balloon may occlude the orifice of the posterior interventricular vein and lead to poor regional perfusion. When the catheter is properly deployed, coronary sinus pressures typically range between 25 cm and 35 cm H$_2$O. Care must be taken when displacing the heart, particularly when accessing the lateral LV for grafting, not to dislodge the coronary sinus cannula. Continuous monitoring of coronary sinus pressures and attention from the perfusionist are required to ensure reliable retrograde cardioplegic delivery.

When the aorta is opened for aortic valve or root procedures, cardioplegia may be delivered via flexible cannulae, ranging in size from 4 Fr to 7 Fr, directly into the coronary ostia. Frequently this is given intermittently, which requires attention from the surgeon but which avoids prolonged cannulation of the coronaries. Prolonged cannulation has been associated with a very low incidence of coronary injury, usually presenting several months later with a new proximal coronary artery stenosis just at or beyond where the tip of the cannula would have been. Nonetheless, for complex and lengthy operations, and particularly aortic root operations where coronary buttons are excised and mobilized, cannulae can be placed into the coronary ostia, snared or tied in with a 5-0 polypropylene suture, and left in place to facilitate continuous low-flow-rate antegrade cardioplegia. This permits excellent myocardial protection, requires no further attention from the surgeon, and keeps cardioplegic effluent out of the operative field.

Alternatively, many surgeons prefer to use retrograde cardioplegia for aortic valve or root operations, as it obviates the need for direct coronary cannulation and keeps the surgical field free of additional cannulae, with the only caveat being that of the effluent from the coronary arteries into the operative field.

During CABG, particularly in patients with ongoing ischemia, vein grafts may be connected to a cardioplegic perfusion system after completion of the distal anastomoses, facilitating rapid antegrade reperfusion. While the optimal cardioplegic flow rate to reperfuse an acute infarction is not known, low pressures and flow rates may limit the no-reflow phenomenon.

ADJUNCTIVE STRATEGIES FOR MYOCARDIAL PROTECTION

Early methods aimed at minimizing the risks associated with coronary bypass surgery primarily involved the manipulation of the conditions of ischemia and reperfusion. Parameters such as cardioplegic composition, temperature, flow direction, and flow rate have been extensively evaluated resulting in near-optimal conditions for current myocardial protection. Not surprisingly, healthy patients presenting for elective coronary bypass surgery face a very low risk of perioperative cardiac morbidity and mortality. Despite such advances, however, conventional cardioplegic techniques may be insufficient in high-risk patients undergoing cardiac surgery. Improvements in the management of such patients may require pharmacologic manipulation as well as the application of cardioplegic additives to further improve cardiac protection.

Myocardial preconditioning

Ischemic preconditioning describes the phenomenon whereby brief episodes of myocardial ischemia afford protection against the adverse effects of a subsequent, more prolonged episode of ischemia. Ischemic preconditioning is the most powerful endogenously mediated form of myocardial protection. Preconditioning can be induced prior to coronary bypass surgery by intermittently cross-clamping the aorta. However, this approach has not been shown to be beneficial and may be dangerous.

Remote ischemic conditioning (RIC) has been demonstrated to induce the cardioprotective effects of preconditioning by producing brief periods of ischemia of the arm or leg before cardiac surgery. The discovery that the RIC stimulus could be induced non-invasively with a standard blood pressure cuff placed on the upper arm or leg has permitted the clinical application of this approach. Importantly, the timing of the RIC stimulus can accommodate most clinical settings of acute ischemia and reperfusion injury, as it has been reported to protect the heart whether applied prior to (termed remote ischemic preconditioning), after the onset of ischemia (termed remote ischemic perconditioning), or even at the time of reperfusion (termed remote ischemic postconditioning). Commercial devices are now available to produce RIC automatically before cardiac surgery. The mechanisms responsible for the benefits of RIC have not been identified. A blood-borne factor conveying the cardioprotective signal from the site of the RIC to the organ protected has been supported by two observations: (1) coronary effluent from the ischemic conditioned heart or blood from a conditioned animal was shown to protect a native recipient heart from ischemic and reperfusion injury, suggesting the transfer of protective humoral factors; and (2) a period of reperfusion of the remote conditioned organ was required for protection suggesting that protective stimulus required the washout of protective blood-borne humoral factors generated in the conditioned site and transported through the circulation to the organ protected. Studies have also demonstrated that RIC was able to recruit endogenous endothelial progenitor cells as well as mesenchymal and hematopoietic stem cells to the infarcted myocardium resulting in a reduction in infarct size, increased angiogenesis and improved cardiac function in animal models. Future studies will be required to identify the mechanisms responsible for the beneficial effects of RIC in humans.

An early clinical trial demonstrated that RIC (three 5 min inflations and deflations of a cuff placed on the upper arm to 200 mmHg) administered prior to cardiac surgery reduced perioperative myocardial injury (43% less troponin T release) in adults undergoing elective CABG surgery. Subsequent studies reported mixed results and large-scale randomized trials will be required to establish the benefits of RIC.

Several **pharmacological agents** have been shown to

mimic the beneficial effects of preconditioning without the need for an ischemic stimulus. Such agents include adenosine, adrenergic agonists, bradykinin, amiloride, and opioids. Unfortunately, many of these agents are either toxic or produce unwanted side effects.

Adenosine, believed to be an intermediary in the ischemic preconditioning phenomenon, may afford significant myocardial protection during ischemia and reperfusion by multiple mechanisms. Adenosine reduces experimental myocardial infarct size by activating cardiac myocyte A1 and A3 receptors, improving postischemic myocardial energetics and reducing platelet and neutrophil adherence to the coronary endothelium. In clinical studies, adenosine added to blood cardioplegia during CABG in a dose which did not lower vascular resistance increased postoperative cardiac ATP concentrations, improved cardiac function and reduced creatine kinase MB isoenzyme release in comparison to randomized controls. A large multi-institutional randomized, double-blinded, placebo-controlled trial reported that adenosine cardioplegia reduced the incidence of perioperative myocardial infarction and the requirement for intra-aortic balloon pump assistance. However, adenosine cardioplegia did not reduce the need for inotropic agents, the prespecified primary endpoint for the trial. Adenosine cardioplegia may improve the recovery from cardiac ischemia, but the appropriate dose and delivery circumstances have not been determined.

Adenosine-lidocaine and **adenosine-procaine** cardioplegia have been suggested to improve myocardial protection in small single-center clinical trials. Polarized arrest has been proposed to reduce Na^+ and Ca^{2+} loading, vasoconstriction, endothelial dysfunction, reperfusion arrhythmias and contractile stunning. However, large controlled trials will be required to determine the benefit of these approaches.

Acadesine is an adenosine-regulating agent which protects the heart by increasing adenosine concentrations only in ischemic tissues. The RED-CABG trial was a multinational, randomized, double-blind, placebo-controlled investigation in 3080 high-risk CABG patients which evaluated the cardioprotective effect of acadesine. This agent did not reduce mortality, non-fatal stroke or severe left ventricular dysfunction.

Preventing calcium overload may reduce ischemic and reperfusion injury. A purinergic (P2) receptor antagonist was evaluated in the MEND-CABG II trial, which did not reduce mortality or non-fatal MI (a creatine kinase MB isoenzyme fraction of at least 100 ng/mL or new Q waves) in 3023 high-risk patients undergoing CABG. Although this approach to prevent calcium accumulation during reperfusion showed great promise in preclinical studies, the appropriate dose and delivery of the agent to protect the heart during cardiac surgery has not been established.

Insulin cardioplegia

Aortic cross-clamping induces anaerobic metabolism, and persistent lactate release during reperfusion indicates a delay in the recovery of aerobic metabolism which is predictive of postoperative ventricular dysfunction. By stimulating the rate-limiting enzyme pyruvate dehydrogenase, **insulin** has been demonstrated in experimental studies to facilitate the conversion from anaerobic to aerobic metabolism early during reperfusion enabling rapid recovery of myocardial ATP synthesis. A placebo-controlled randomized trial of insulin (10 IU/L) cardioplegia in 56 elective CABG patients demonstrated rapid conversion to aerobic cardiac lactate extraction in the insulin group compared to persistent lactate release in the placebo group. Two hours postoperatively, left ventricular stroke work indices were higher in the insulin cardioplegia patients at similar filling pressures. In a placebo-controlled randomized trial in 1126 patients undergoing urgent CABG for unstable angina, the primary composite outcome of low output syndrome and/or enzymatic myocardial infarction was not different between groups (insulin 30%, placebo 26%, $p = 0.2$). Although insulin to control glucose levels has become routine, the appropriate dose and method of delivery to protect the heart has not been established.

Cariporide

Cariporide inhibits the sodium–hydrogen exchanger (NHE-1 isoform) which limits intracellular Na accumulation, prevents calcium overload following ischemic injury, reduces infarct size and accelerates the recovery of ventricular function. The Expedition trial was a multinational, double-blind, placebo-controlled randomized investigation of cariporide during CABG in 5761 high-risk patients. The study was terminated early by the Data and Safety Monitoring Board because of a marked reduction in the incidence of MI. At 5 days, the incidence of MI declined from 19% in the placebo group to 14% in the treatment group ($p = 0.000005$). However, more focal persistent cerebrovascular events were observed with cariporide (4.5%) than with placebo (2.5%, $p = 0.02$) and were associated with an increase in mortality. Cariporide reduced ischemic injury but increased the risk of stroke. The reasons were not determined and sodium–hydrogen exchange inhibitors are unlikely to be employed clinically for myocardial protection.

Reducing Inflammation

Complement activation during cardiac surgery (via complement components C3 and C5) contributes to perioperative inflammation, vasoconstriction, vascular leakage, leukocyte activation, and cardiac injury. The inhibition of complement activation can modulate inflammation and the resultant tissue damage. **Pexelizumab** is an anti-C5 antibody fragment that effectively blocks C5, thus blocking the formation of C5a and C5b-9 (membrane attack complex). The PRIMO-CABG I trial demonstrated that the use of pexelizumab yielded an 18% risk reduction in death or myocardial infarction ($p = 0.07$) compared with placebo in patients undergoing CABG surgery. Subgroup analysis showed that patients with two or more risk factors derived the greatest benefit. The PRIMO-CABG II trial randomized 4254 patients with two or more risk factors undergoing CABG with or without valve replacement. The investigators found no significant difference between the groups for the incidence of the combined endpoint of death and MI (15% vs 16%, respectively; $p = 0.2$) or for any of the individual endpoints.

ALTERNATIVE METHODS OF MYOCARDIAL PROTECTION

The evolution of myocardial protection over the past three decades has focused primarily on the optimization of cardioplegia-induced electromechanical arrest. Despite remarkable advances, however, alternative, more traditional techniques are still used by some surgeons and have merit under circumstances where cardioplegic arrest may not be feasible.

Intermittent ischemic arrest

Cardiac surgery can be accomplished with intermittent cross-clamping of the aorta for short periods without the use of cardioplegia. Although a relatively dry operative field may result, complete mechanical arrest is seldom achieved. During coronary bypass surgery, the cross-clamp is applied for construction of distal anastomoses. Then the cross-clamp is removed and reperfusion is undertaken for a period equal to that of the cross-clamp time. This practice facilitates repayment of the oxygen debt. Systemic hypothermia may be employed as an adjunctive measure to further reduce myocardial oxygen demands during the periods of ischemia. Proximal anastomoses are usually constructed during periods of reperfusion with the help of a partial occluding clamp applied to the anterior ascending aorta.

Although this technique may also afford ischemic precon-ditioning by virtue of the multiple brief ischemic episodes, the technique has some disadvantages. Despite the use of systemic hypothermia, ventricular fibrillation usually ensues during cross-clamping, resulting in increased myocardial oxygen demands and exacerbation of ischemia in regions distal to severe coronary obstructions. Moreover, exposure of the heart to repeated episodes of ischemia-reperfusion injury may be increase ischemic injury. The requirement for repeated aortic cross-clamping may also be hazardous in patients with diffuse atherosclerotic disease of the aorta, due to the risk of cerebral atheroemboli. Nonetheless, despite such potential drawbacks, some surgeons report excel-lent results even in high-risk patients comparable to those observed with cardioplegic arrest.

Hypothermic fibrillatory arrest

Experimental evidence suggests that subendocardial ischemia can be minimized if the hypothermic, vented, spontaneously fibrillating heart is perfused at pressures of 80–100 mmHg. In these circumstances, coronary bypass surgery can be per-formed with local vessel control thus avoiding the potential complications of cardiac arrest. A study by Akins and col-leagues reported the results of hypothermic fibrillatory arrest in 3085 patients who underwent cardiac operations between 1980 and 1993. The overall mortality in this series was 1.6%, with a 2.5% incidence of perioperative myocardial infarction, and a requirement for intra-aortic balloon pump support of 2.5%. Of note, this series also included 371 patients (12%) who underwent emergent surgery for complications of cardiac catheterization. Hypothermic fibrillatory arrest provides a viable option for patients at high risk of aortic cross-clamping due to severe atherosclerotic disease. Distal anastomoses can be performed during fibrillatory arrest, whereas proximal anastomoses can be constructed to pedi-cled mammary arterial grafts, the innominate artery, the aortic arch, or the subclavian artery.

CONCLUSIONS

Current techniques of intraoperative myocardial protection are constantly evolving. To date, changes in cardioplegic composition, temperature and delivery have been success-ful in optimizing intraoperative myocardial protection, such that stable patients presenting for elective cardiac surgery face a remarkably low risk of perioperative morbid-ity or mortality. Although such patients likely have little to gain from additional intraoperative protective measures, future improvements may be crucial in reducing the mor-bidity and mortality in high-risk patients presenting with poor ventricular function and/or persistent preoperative ischemia. A variety of cardioplegic additives have been tested in large number of patients undergoing cardiac sur-gery. Unfortunately, the ideal approach to resuscitate the ischemic heart and restore myocardial metabolism and ventricular function has not yet been determined. However, investigations continue with the hope that soon the heart can be returned to normal during cardioplegic arrest.

FURTHER READING

Development of cardioplegia

Cohen G, Borger MA, Weisel RD, Rao V. Intraoperative myocardial protection: current trends and future perspectives. *Ann Thorac Surg.* 1999; 68: 1995–2001.

Fremes SE, Christakis GT, Weisel RD, et al. A clinical trial of blood and crystalloid cardioplegia. *J Thorac Cardiovasc Surg.* 1984; 88: 726–41.

Guru V, Omura J, Alghamdi AA, et al. Is blood superior to crystalloid cardioplegia? A meta-analysis of randomized clinical trials. *Circulation.* 2006; 114(Suppl I): 331–8.

Lichtenstein SV, Abel JG, Slutsky AS and the Warm Heart Investigators. Randomised trial of normothermic versus hypothermic coronary bypass surgery. *Lancet.* 1992; 339(8804): 1305.

Yau TM, Ikonomidis JS, Weisel RD, et al. Ventricular function after normothermic versus hypothermic cardioplegia. *J Thorac Cardiovasc Surg.* 1993; 105: 833–44.

Refinements of cardioplegic techniques

Algarni KD, Weisel RD, Caldarone CA, et al. Microplegia during CABG was associated with less low cardiac output syndrome: a propensity matched comparison. *Ann Thorac Surg.* 2013; 95: 1532.

Menasche P, Subayi J, Piwnica A. Retrograde coronary sinus cardioplegia for aortic valve operations: a clinical report on 500 patients. *Ann Thorac Surg.* 1990; 49: 556–64.

Yau TM, Ikonomidis JS, Weisel RD, et al. Which techniques of cardioplegia prevent ischemia? *Ann Thorac Surg.* 1993; 56: 1020–8.

Preconditioning

Hausenloy DJ, Mwamure PK, Venugopal V, et al. Effect of remote ischaemic preconditioning on myocardial injury in patients undergoing coronary artery bypass graft surgery: a randomised controlled trial. *Lancet.* 2007; 370(9587): 575–9.

Ramzy D, Rao V, Weisel RD. Clinical applicability of preconditioning and postconditioning: the cardiothoracic surgeon's view. *Cardiovasc Res.* 2006; 70: 174–80.

Cardioplegic enhancements

Adenosine cardioplegia trial: Mentzer RM Jr, Birjiniuk V, Khuri S, et al. Adenosine myocardial protection: preliminary results of a phase II clinical trial. *Ann Surg.* 1999; 229: 643–9.

Insulin cardioplegia trial: Rao V, Christakis GT, Weisel RD, et al. The insulin cardioplegia trial: myocardial protection for urgent coronary artery bypass grafting. *J Thorac Cardiovasc Surg.* 2002; 123: 928–35.

Preventing calcium overload – MEND-CABG trial: MEND-CABG II Investigators, et al. Efficacy and safety of pyridoxal 5′-phosphate (MC-1) in high-risk patients undergoing coronary artery bypass graft surgery: the MEND-CABG II randomized clinical trial. *JAMA.* 2008; 299: 1777–87.

Cariporide – the Expedition trial: Mentzer RM Jr, Bartels C, Bolli R, et al. Sodium-hydrogen exchange inhibition by cariporide to reduce the risk of ischemic cardiac events in patients undergoing coronary artery bypass grafting: results of the EXPEDITION study. *Ann Thorac Surg.* 2008; 85: 1261–70.

Terminal complement blockade – Primo CABG I: Verrier ED, Shernan SK, Taylor KM, et al. Terminal complement blockade with pexelizumab during coronary artery bypass graft surgery requiring cardiopulmonary bypass: a randomized trial. *JAMA.* 2004; 291: 2319–27.

Terminal complement blockade – Primo CABG II: Smith PK, Shernan SK, Chen JC, et al. Effects of C5 complement inhibitor pexelizumab on outcome in high-risk coronary artery bypass grafting: combined results from the PRIMO-CABG I and II trials. *J Thorac Cardiovasc Surg.* 2011; 142: 89–98.

Acadesine – RED-CABG trial: Newman MF, Ferguson TB, White JA, et al. Effect of adenosine-regulating agent acadesine on morbidity and mortality associated with coronary artery bypass grafting: the RED-CABG randomized controlled trial. *JAMA.* 2012; 308: 157–64.

Surgery for ischemic heart disease

5

On-pump coronary artery bypass grafting

MARVIN D. ATKINS AND MATTHEW L. WILLIAMS

Ischemic heart disease remains the leading cause of death throughout the developed world. The incidence of death from cardiovascular disease, however, continues to decline due to improved preventative strategies and better medical therapies. The development of coronary artery bypass grafting (CABG) surgery remains one of the greatest surgical achievements in medicine. Since the last edition of this book, CABG has seen a significant change in utilization in the United States. A review of the National Inpatient Sample reveals that the number of CABG procedures in the US decreased from 337 400 in 2003 to 202 900 in 2012, a 40% decrease. The rate of interventional therapy for coronary disease (percutaneous transluminal coronary angioplasty; PTCA) also has been decreasing since 2004, with an annual rate of decline of 2.5%. Explanations for the decrease in CABG and PTCA utilization include more aggressive risk factor reduction including decreasing rates of smoking and increased statin and antiplatelet usage. Although performed less frequently, and in higher risk patients than decades past, CABG will continue to be a routine part of the practice of cardiothoracic surgery. The surgical outcomes with coronary artery bypass (CAB) are carefully watched by patients, national and state regulators, insurance providers, and hospital administrators. National standards leave little room for error in the performance of CABG. Many states report individual surgeon risk-adjusted outcomes, and risk aversion may be an unintended consequence of well-intentioned transparency.

HISTORY

A variety of surgical procedures have been developed over the last 70 years to treat the symptoms of obstructive coronary artery disease (CAD).[1] Myocardial revascularization began in the early 1900s with extracardiac operations, such as sympathetic denervation and thyroid ablation. Initial attempts by Beck and others abraded the exposed pericardial surface to induce inflammatory adhesions and neovascularization between the epicardium and the parietal pericardium. More than 60 years ago, an operation was developed by Vineberg in which the transected internal mammary artery (IMA) was implanted in the myocardium. In the late 1950s and early 1960s, a few attempts at direct coronary endarterectomy were made. The question of who performed the first CAB is a subject of great debate, with claims of the first such operations reported decades later. Goetz performed the first well-documented CAB operation utilizing the right IMA and the right coronary artery employing a metal tube to connect the two in 1960. CABG began in earnest, however, in the late 1960s along two parallel paths that included bypassing coronary artery obstructions using either the IMA as the bypass conduit or reversed saphenous vein grafts from the leg. Each approach had early proponents, but the use of saphenous vein grafts became the dominant approach by the majority of cardiac surgeons in the 1970s. This preference was based on the perceived ease of use with the larger and technically less demanding saphenous vein graft. Saphenous veins could be used to graft any coronary artery site, including arteries on the lateral and inferior wall of the heart. The IMA graft, however, especially the pedicled graft, was limited to anterior and proximal coronary artery sites.

Although many of the earliest CABG procedures were limited to one or two distal coronary artery targets, multiartery grafting was performed increasingly frequently as the procedure grew in popularity and effectiveness. By the late 1970s, just 10 years after the initiation of direct CABG, most patients were receiving multiple bypass grafts with anastomoses to the distal right and circumflex systems in addition to the left anterior descending and proximal right coronary arteries. Some early proponents of the IMA graft persisted in the use of this conduit as a pedicled graft to the left anterior descending coronary artery (LAD).

By the mid 1980s, with CABG being carried out increasingly often throughout the world and with 10- to 15-year follow-up experience available from the early group of bypass recipients, two extremely important observations were made. Many of the earliest patients to receive bypass grafts were returning 5–10 years after their operation, with recurrent angina and symptoms similar or even worse than the original complaints that had led to their initial bypass operation. On repeat catheterizations, many were found to have marked progression of atherosclerosis in their native coronary arteries and, even more alarming, severe obstructive atherosclerosis in the vein grafts that were used in the original procedure. A second unexpected observation was that, in patients who had IMA bypass grafts performed previously, graft atherosclerosis and premature graft occlusion were rarely encountered. This observation was even true in patients whose accompanying saphenous vein grafts were severely diseased and/or obstructed.

These findings led to changes in the approach that was taken to CABG in the mid to late 1980s, which have resulted in the current standard approach to CAB surgery. The majority of patients who undergo CABG surgery today receive a pedicled left IMA (LIMA) graft to the LAD. Other required bypasses are constructed using reversed saphenous vein grafts, with proximal aortic anastomoses. This combination of LIMA plus two or more saphenous vein grafts can be described as the traditional, and most common, configuration for patients who have multiple coronary bypass grafting still today. That paradigm, however, is slowly changing based upon favorable data with the use of total arterial revascularization. The use of bilateral internal mammary grafts, skeletonized mammary arteries, radial artery grafts, as well as the techniques of sequential anastomoses allows for complete arterial revascularization. The use of bilateral mammary grafts, however, does increase the risk of sternal wound infection, especially in diabetic patients. This subject is discussed further in Chapter 7, "Expanded use of arterial conduits."

The technique of hybrid coronary revascularization involves the use of minimally invasive techniques for the LIMA graft to the LAD and then the use of angioplasty/stenting to lesions in the right and circumflex artery distributions. This can be done at the time of CABG in a hybrid suite or in a staged fashion. The role of hybrid revascularization remains to be defined. Recent data from the Cardiothoracic Surgical Trials Network revealed no major adverse clinical event differences between multivessel percutaneous coronary intervention (PCI) and hybrid coronary revascularization at 12 months. Long-term follow-up of this study and others is needed as the patency benefits of a LIMA-to-LAD graft occur beyond a year. This topic is discussed further in Chapter 10, "Robotic total endoscopic coronary artery bypass grafting."

A key feature in the current therapeutic approach to patients who undergo coronary bypass is the initiation of specific medications postoperatively to reduce progression of native artery and especially vein graft atherosclerosis. This secondary preventive approach includes the use of aspirin and other antiplatelet agents, lipid-lowering medications, and a variety of other drugs that affect baseline coronary artery tone and degree of vasodilation, heart rate, blood pressure, and even endothelial inflammatory susceptibility. Other important components of secondary prevention for patients who have a coronary bypass grafting procedure are weight loss and stress reduction, dietary compliance, exercise programs, and smoking cessation, whenever applicable.

PRINCIPLES AND JUSTIFICATION

The guidelines for surgical revascularization established by the American Heart Association, American College of Cardiology, American Association for Thoracic Surgery, Society of Thoracic Surgeons and others were last updated in 2014.[2] The most common indications for CABG in symptomatic patients include:

- left main stenosis >50%
- stenosis >70% in three major coronary arteries (especially in patients with diabetes) or two-vessel CAD with involvement of the proximal LAD
- stenosis >70% in two major coronary arteries with extensive myocardial ischemia based upon stress testing
- significant (>70%) multivessel disease and mild to moderate LV systolic dysfunction
- significant (>70%) proximal LAD stenosis and extensive ischemia
- survivors of sudden cardiac death with presumed ischemia mediated ventricular arrhythmia caused by >70% in a major coronary artery
- patients with severe angina refractory to medical therapy and one or more severe (>70%) coronary artery stenoses
- failed PCI or anatomy not amenable to PCI
- mechanical complications of myocardial infarction such as ventricular septal defect (VSD), papillary muscle rupture, or myocardial rupture.

A surgical consultation for CAD involves an in-depth discussion with the patient and their family members about the indications, risks, and typical outcomes associated with the operation. In order to provide informed consent for the surgical procedure, we use a preprinted, standardized consent form to ensure coverage of the typical risks. We routinely calculate an individual morbidity and mortality risk for each patient using the online STS risk calculator (http://riskcalc.sts.org).[3]

Contraindications to coronary bypass surgery include any coexisting conditions that significantly limit life expectancy such as malignancy, severe chronic obstructive pulmonary disease (COPD), or severe decompensated liver disease. Advanced age, frailty, morbid obesity, end-stage renal disease, and cerebrovascular disease increase the risk with surgery but are not in and of themselves absolute contraindications. Depending upon such comorbid conditions, some patients may be better treated with high-risk PCI.

Overall, the average risk of 30-day perioperative death is low at approximately 2%. This mortality risk is <1% for elective patients who are <65 years of age with normal LV function. Although mortality is low, associated non-fatal complications are significant. The most common postoperative complications include perioperative MI, early graft thrombosis from technical issues (5–10%), low cardiac output syndrome, atrial fibrillation (15–40%), stroke (1.5%), cognitive dysfunction, bleeding (2–5% requiring reoperation), deep sternal wound infection (1%), acute kidney injury

(3–5%), aortic dissection (<0.05%), pneumonia, prolonged mechanical ventilation, and gastrointestinal complications (bleeding, ileus).

PREOPERATIVE ASSESSMENT AND PREPARATION

All patients who are referred to a surgeon for consideration of CABG will have had a coronary angiogram performed. Often, however, the patient who is referred for CABG will require one or more additional studies. Assessment of global left ventricular function with calculation of the ejection fraction as well as assessment of regional ventricular function, using a perfusion study or 2D echocardiogram, may be helpful. Regional wall motion assessment may be especially important in situations in which coronary arterial branches are completely occluded and not visualized on coronary angiography. The presence of retained regional contractile function, as well as other signs of viability, should prompt an attempt at coronary artery identification and grafting in these areas. The surgeon should assess these studies and discuss his or her plans for bypass grafting with the patient before the procedure. Requests by cardiologists for consideration of bypass grafting should be seen as actual consultations for assessment of suitability for surgery, not prescriptions to perform specific operations according to the judgments made exclusively by the cardiologists or other physicians.

Another important component of preoperative assessment that requires the input of the surgeon is the availability of suitable conduits. Few CABG candidates have such severe peripheral vascular disease that the IMA is not suitable for use as a bypass conduit. A complete occlusion of the proximal left subclavian artery, however, such that a subclavian "steal" might occur, can be determined by the absence or marked reduction of blood pressure in the left arm. The diagnostic cardiologist should be expected to visualize the LIMA during coronary artery studies in patients with severe brachiocephalic arterial obstructive disease. A more common problem that causes unsuitability of the LIMA for grafting is seen in patients who have had prior anterior thoracic irradiation, especially those who have been radiated for mediastinal lymphoma. In some instances, the LIMA is encased in dense fibrous scarring from post-irradiation inflammation. This situation may also occur in some female patients after mastectomy with post-resection chest wall irradiation. A frequent problem that is overlooked when referring patients for multivessel coronary artery grafting, however, is the absence of saphenous veins in those who have had saphenous vein stripping because of severe varicosities. In addition, varicosed saphenous veins may pose problems. In either situation, physical examination and ultrasound venous mapping should be undertaken preoperatively. The expanded use of arterial conduits make this less of a problem today than in years past.

The presence of significant peripheral vascular disease can alter the approach to lower-extremity vein harvesting. Leg testing with calculation of arterial brachial indices is indicated. Evaluation for concomitant carotid artery disease by ultrasound is indicated in those with physical exam findings of a carotid bruit or a history of transient ischemic attack (TIA) or stroke. Significant COPD should be evaluated with preoperative pulmonary function tests and an attempt at smoking cessation and medical optimization is paramount. An Allen's test and/or ultrasound of the radial artery in the non-dominant arm can be performed.

ANESTHESIA

The standard for on-pump CAB has been general endotracheal anesthesia. Large-bore intravenous access, typically with a central line, is routine. Our practice has been to place a Swan–Ganz catheter for postoperative management, although many institutions will forgo this in the setting of a normal preoperative ejection fraction and normal postop echo. In 2010, the American Society of Anesthesiologists and the Society for Cardiac Anesthesia Task Force on Transesophageal Echocardiography (TEE) updated the practice guidelines for the use of TEE. These guidelines recommend the routine use of TEE in adult patients undergoing cardiac or thoracic aortic procedures. A complete TEE examination should be performed with the following intent:

1. to confirm and refine the preoperative diagnosis
2. to detect new or unsuspected pathologic conditions
3. to adjust the anesthetic and surgical plan accordingly
4. to assess the results of the surgical intervention.

We have found the routine use of TEE to be essential in the performance of CABG. Following induction and prior to scrubbing in for the procedure, the attending surgeon goes over the TEE with the anesthesiologist, noting the preoperative cardiac function of the RV and LV, evidence of aortic insufficiency, atheroma in the ascending aorta, and any other unexpected valvular findings. Evidence of aortic insufficiency mandates placement of a left ventricular vent and a retrograde cardioplegia catheter. Following successful CABG, a postoperative TEE exam confirms the ventricular function. Any evidence of worsening ventricular function mandates continued reperfusion on pump and consideration of a technical error in the bypass grafts. Air embolism typically occurs down the right-sided grafts and is treated with increased perfusion pressure and reperfusion to push the air through the coronary circulation. RV dysfunction will typically improve by echo and plans for discontinuation of bypass can begin. Evidence of LV dysfunction, especially in the setting of preoperative dysfunction, can signal difficulty weaning from bypass. In such patients, a femoral arterial line is placed prior to incision for possible use of an intra-aortic balloon pump to separate from cardiopulmonary bypass.

OPERATION

Incision

The incision is made from the midpoint of the sternal notch and sternal angle down to the tip of the xyphoid (**Figure 5.1**). Retraction in the sternal notch allows careful division of the clavicular–clavicular ligament. Careful attention is paid to the position of the innominate artery, which is typically superior and deep to this. Dissection is stopped when a finger carefully goes under the table of the sternum. The sternal saw should be inserted from the top, with the saw guard facing the patient's neck and the saw blade on the caudal side. After division and retraction of the sternum, it is occasionally necessary to extend the incision cephalad to avoid undue tension on the midline skin and subcutaneous tissue when the sternum is fully retracted. The edges of the sternum are carefully cauterized for hemostasis. A minimal amount of bone wax is used to stop bleeding in the marrow. The thymic tissues, subcutaneous tissue, and any muscle is divided up to the inferior edge of the brachiocephalic vein.

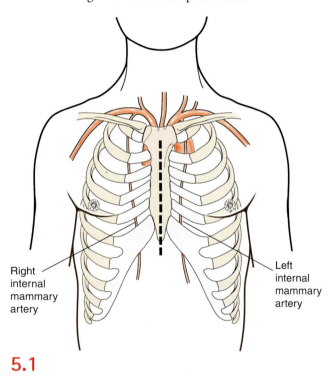

Right internal mammary artery

Left internal mammary artery

5.1

Isolation of the internal mammary artery

The mammary artery arises from the left subclavian artery close to the thyrocervical trunk and under the sternal end of the clavicle (**Figure 5.2**). It extends on the inside of the anterior chest wall just lateral to the sternum and costosternal cartilages from the clavicle down to the costochondral junction. The IMA branches form the intercostal arteries and, at the fifth or sixth interspace, the mammary artery divides into the musculophrenic and superior epigastric branches. The IMA is accompanied by two veins with tributaries from

the intercostal vascular pedicle and adjacent chest wall. These veins enter the left subclavian vein just below the origin of the mammary artery from the subclavian artery. The phrenic nerve enters the thorax close to the origin of the IMA and traverses behind the subclavian vein. This nerve can be injured by electrocautery near the origin of the IMA.

Prior to heparinization, a mammary retractor is placed to lift the left hemisternum. The proximal blade is placed under the manubrium and the distal blade is placed just above the xyphoid (**Figure 5.3**). The hemisternum is slowly

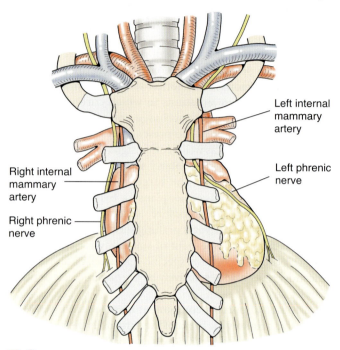

Right internal mammary artery

Right phrenic nerve

Left internal mammary artery

Left phrenic nerve

5.2

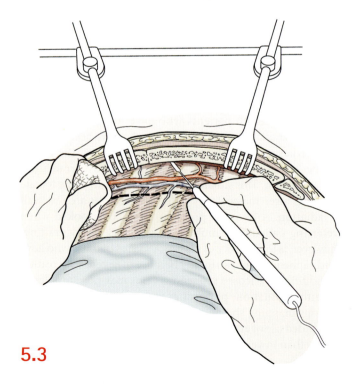

5.3

elevated and the table is rotated to the left for improved visualization. We like to open the left pleural space wide at this time. This allows for the pedicled IMA graft to fall away from the midline. A 1 cm wide pedicle that includes the IMA and accompanying veins is isolated using cautery and metal clips. With the left chest wall elevated, parallel cuts are made in the endothoracic fascia medial and lateral to the visualized or palpated mammary artery. We begin the dissection plane proximally, at the level of the third rib.

Once the first portion of the pedicle, including the artery and vein, is gently separated from the chest wall, traction placed on the pedicle allows visualization of the venous and arterial side branches (**Figure 5.4**). Care is taken not to grasp the mammary artery. Downward retraction with closed forceps is useful. Side branches on the arterial side are clipped with small hemaclips and the chest wall side is carefully cauterized on low power. The pedicle is mobilized proximally to the level of the subclavian vein and distally past the IMA bifurcation for sufficient length. We carefully check the chest wall and bed of the IMA pedicle for hemostasis. The patient is heparinized at this point and the distal pedicle is divided after placing large clips across the IMA bifurcation. The flow in the IMA is assessed at this point. A soft-jaw bulldog retractor is placed on the distal end of the IMA pedicle and papaverine is injected on the pedicle. The pedicle is carefully placed in the left chest cavity, avoiding twisting. Some surgeons occlude the pedicled graft at its cut end with a hemaclip, allowing for flow throughout the length of the mammary artery to avoid distal artery vasospasm and, hopefully, to dilate the artery.

Saphenous vein harvest

Both lower extremities are circumferentially prepped and draped into the field for harvesting of the saphenous vein. Many find it useful to use ultrasound preoperatively to evaluate the size of the saphenous vein and mark its location. The legs are placed in a frog-leg position to expose the vein. An assistant is typically harvesting the saphenous vein at the same time as mobilization of the IMA pedicle. It is important to convey to the assistant the anticipated number of venous bypasses to be used. A good rule of thumb is that a sufficient length of vein extends from the tip of the thumb to the tip of the little finger with the fingers extended. The greater saphenous vein courses along the medial thigh and leg in a sufficiently constant pattern that, once the vein is identified either distally or proximally, skip incisions can be made to avoid a long and deforming scar down the entire length of the lower extremity (**Figure 5.5**). If multiple incisions and tunneling are used, it is important to avoid traction injury to the vein. A vessel loop placed around the vein can be used for careful traction. The vein should be irrigated and flushed so that it does not dry out and injure the endothelium.

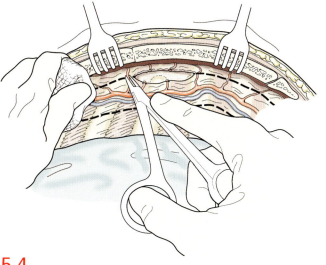

5.4

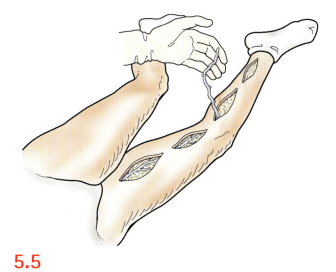

5.5

Endoscopic vein harvest

Endoscopic saphenous vein harvesting (**Figure 5.6a–c**) has supplanted open vein harvesting in most practices. A variety of devices, retractors, and maneuvers has been described and used clinically. In many patients, it is possible to make two small incisions, one in the medial thigh just above the knee and the other in the infrainguinal upper thigh area, to harvest a long segment of saphenous vein. A long tubular scope is placed in the lower incision and CO_2 insufflation is used for visualization. Through the use of a combination of blunt dissection and gentle traction, the venous side branches can be divided as far away from the saphenous as allowed. The scope can be reversed and dissection continued down the lower leg if necessary. Once adequate vein is mobilized, the vein is divided proximally and distally. A vein cannula is placed in the proximal portion and secured to orient the flow in the vein (**Figure 5.6b and c**).

The vein is prepared by double-clipping the side branches directly against the saphenous vein wall. Any leaking spots are repaired with 6-0 Prolene at this time. The vein harvest site is irrigated and hemostasis achieved. A drain is typically left in the tract and the leg wrapped in an elastic bandage. When performed successfully, endoscopic vein harvest results in a marked reduction in wound morbidity and discomfort for the patient. Some data do suggest, however, that endoscopic vein harvest is associated with worse vein graft patency, MI, repeat revascularization, and even death. A large VA-sponsored multi-institutional randomized controlled trial (REGROUP) is currently underway and hopes to answer this question in the future.

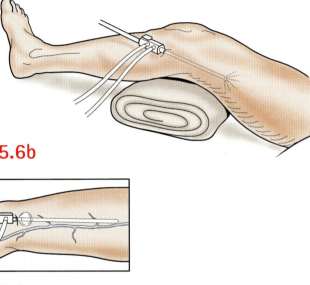

5.6b

5.6c

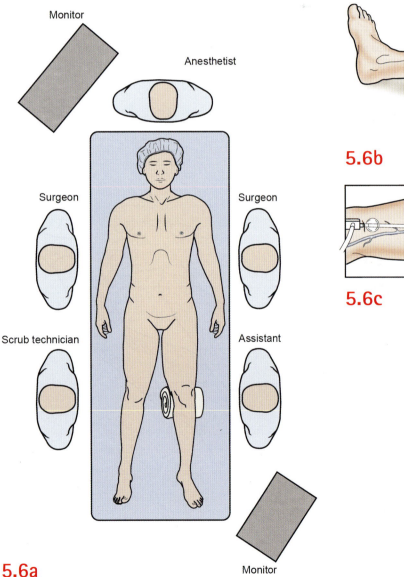

5.6a

Cardiopulmonary bypass

In preparation for cardiopulmonary bypass (CPB) (**Figure 5.7**), pericardial traction sutures are placed bilaterally to elevate and expose the heart. The phrenic nerve is visualized on the outer surface of the pericardium and a T-shaped incision or window is made to allow the IMA pedicle to come through under no tension. The ascending aorta is carefully palpated for calcium, plaque, or wall thickening. Two pursestring sutures are placed in the proximal aortic arch at the level of the innominate artery. If there is concern for plaque in the ascending aorta via TEE or manual palpation, epiaortic ultrasound can be used to find an acceptable spot for cannulation. Rarely, the innominate artery or axillary artery must be used for arterial cannulation in this setting. Single venous cannulation is performed through the right atrial appendage with a dual-stage cannula, the tip of which is placed in the inferior vena cava. It is important at this point to think about the placement of the cross-clamp and leaving enough room for the cardioplegia cannula and proximal graft sites. A combined antegrade cardioplegia/root vent cannula is placed in the mid ascending aorta. A retrograde coronary sinus catheter is not routinely placed in patients with well-compensated left ventricular function and no evidence of aortic insufficiency but can be easily added. A temperature monitoring probe can be inserted into the septum, to the right of the LAD.

Assessment of targets

It is easier to evaluate bypass targets prior to cardioplegic arrest. A careful review of the coronary angiogram immediately before the start of the case is standard. Visual inspection and palpation of possible distal targets for calcium can help one determine a safe area for bypass. Intramyocardial targets can be difficult to find. These are suspected when the angiogram reveals a very straight segment of artery. Typically, intramyocardial targets are free of atherosclerosis. In rare instances a small probe can be advanced via the very distal LAD retrograde from the apex to define the intramyocardial LAD portion. Once a distal target site is identified, we will typically score the epicardial surface with a sharp knife and expose the superficial surface of the vessel without entering it. Once all distal targets have been marked and cannulation has been completed, cardioplegic arrest is begun.

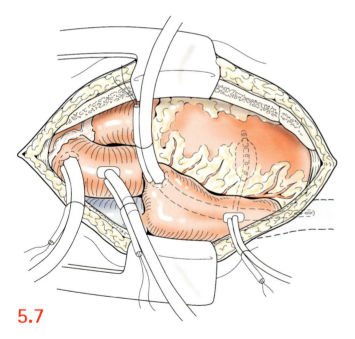

5.7

Distal anastomoses

VEIN GRAFT ANASTOMOSES

In conventional CABG, construction of the venous bypass is performed first so that undue tension is not placed on the LIMA to LAD anastomosis. In addition, placing the distal vein grafts sequentially allows for direct cardioplegia administration into areas of obstructed arterial flow. For visualization of the distal right coronary artery, right posterior descending artery or distal right posterolateral branches, the patient can be placed in a slight Trendelenburg position with traction applied to the acute margin of the heart. Options for improved exposure include the use of silastic tapes placed under the artery, use of the HeartNet, or use of an assistant for retraction (**Figure 5.8a**). Once the anastomotic area is stabilized, the epicardium overlying the artery is incised and the artery entered (**Figure 5.8b**). We use CO_2 insufflation to help distend the artery and help visualize entry into the vessel. The arteriotomy is extended for a distance of 6–8 mm. The vein graft is beveled approximately 30 degrees. The arteriotomy should match the beveled conduit diameter and be at least 1.5 times the diameter of the distal coronary artery. The anastomosis is completed with a single 7-0 Prolene suture (**Figure 5.8c**).

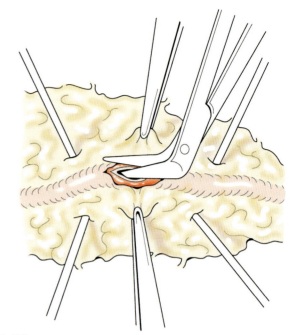

5.8b

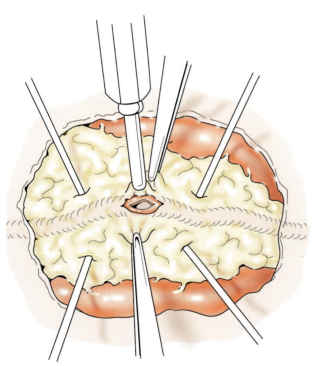

5.8a

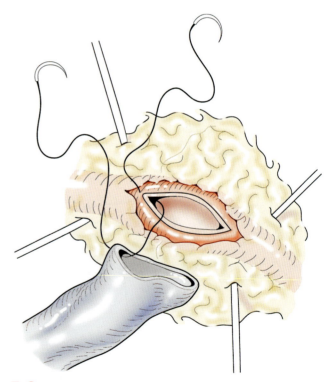

5.8c

With the distal end of the vein held open by the assistant with two fine forceps, a continuous anastomosis is constructed beginning either at the toe or the heel. Four or five suture throws are placed through the vein and the coronary artery, after which the vein is lowered into place and the anastomosis completed (**Figure 5.8d and e**). A fine nerve hook can be used to snug up the continuous suture to avoid leaking. A small probe (1.5 mm) can be placed prior to completion of the suture line to evaluate the toe of the anastomosis. The vein graft is filled with 50 mL cold blood cardioplegia to evaluate for anastomotic leakage as well as for myocardial protection. The vein graft can then be occluded distally with a soft-jaw bulldog clamp, filled with heparinized saline, and sized appropriately for a tension-free graft. We typically fill the heart by partial occlusion of the venous return line when sizing the vein graft. The proximal vein graft anastomosis can be completed at this point or saved for the end. Additional antegrade or retrograde cardioplegia can be given while the heart is repositioned for additional inferior wall or lateral wall targets.

For lateral wall grafts, a cold lap pad is placed behind the heart to retract the apex of the left ventricle gently to the right, exposing the vessels of the lateral wall. Exact positioning is dependent on the sites that are chosen for distal anastomoses and, using either gentle manual traction or

silastic tapes, the portion of the obtuse marginal or other lateral arterial branches are stabilized and incised. The anastomoses are completed in a similar heel-to-toe fashion as described above.

INTERNAL MAMMARY ANASTOMOSIS TO THE LAD CORONARY ARTERY

Following completion of all the distal vein graft anastomoses, the pedicled IMA is retrieved from the lateral pericardial space or left pleural cavity. Care is taken to ensure no twisting of the mammary pedicle. The distal clip or proximal clamp is removed and flow is assessed. The soft clamp is then replaced to the very proximal IMA and the arterial graft is brought through the pericardial window or T incision into the surgical field. An appropriate graft site is chosen on the LAD and stabilized with silastic tapes or a spring retractor (**Figure 5.9a**). The IMA pedicled graft is brought down to the proposed graft site to ensure a tension-free anastomosis. If there is any concern for stretch, the fascia and muscle of the pedicle can be incised in several spots, gaining an additional 5–10 mm of length for each fascial incision (**Figure 5.9b**).

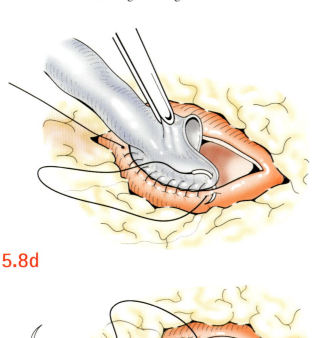

5.8d

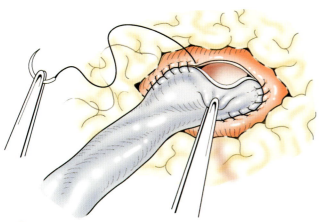

5.8e

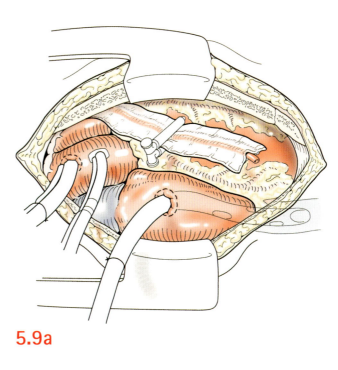

5.9a

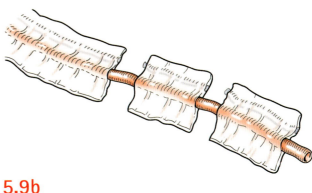

5.9b

Once an adequate pedicle length is determined, the LAD is incised and the mammary artery incised on an angle at an appropriate distal site (**Figure 5.10a**). Every attempt should be made to transect the mammary artery as proximal as possible where the caliber is largest. We tend to leave a small segment of distal mammary artery attached to use as a handle to grasp the artery. This small segment is transected when completing the toe of the anastomosis (**Figure 5.10b and c**).

Avoiding any direct contact with the endothelial surface of the mammary artery or the LAD, the assistant retracts the pedicle and the small handle of the mammary to allow exposure for the operative surgeon. A 7-0 Prolene suture is used to construct a parachuted anastomosis of 4–5 mm in length (**Figure 5.11a**). After between three and five suture throws, the heel of the anastomosis is brought down onto the surface of the heart, the suture line is gently snugged up, and the remainder completed (**Figure 5.11b**). The suture line is tied and the proximal clamp removed to evaluate for hemostasis. Our practice is to secure both sides of the mammary pedicle to the epicardial surface with a 6-0 suture to prevent movement and take tension off the suture line.

5.10a

5.10b

5.10c

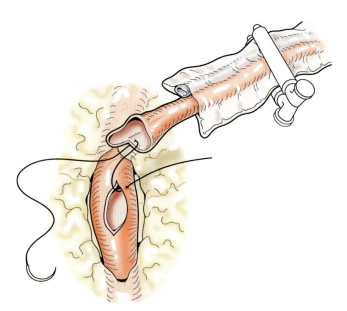

5.11a

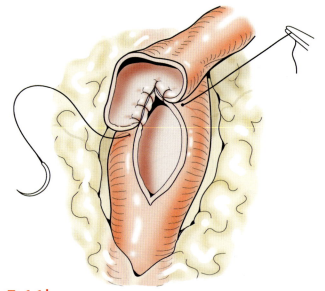

5.11b

Proximal vein graft anastomoses

Systemic cooling is reversed during construction of the IMA to LAD anastomosis. The proximal vein graft anastomoses are constructed at this point if not already done (**Figure 5.12a–c**). This can be done with the cross-clamp still in place or with a side-biting aortic clamp. We prefer to perform the proximals with the original cross-clamp in place to avoid aortic manipulation and risk stroke. This also allows for reperfusion of the entire heart at the same time once the cross-clamp and IMA clamp are removed. The aortotomy is made with a 3.5 mm or 4 mm aortic punch. If the aortic wall appears excessively thick, another site is chosen and the aortotomy closed with a 4-0 Prolene suture. The proximal anastomoses are completed with a 5-0 Prolene suture starting at the outside three o'clock position of the vein graft (if looking at the end down the vein graft opening) and then a back-handed suture at the three o'clock position on the aorta. This is parachuted counterclockwise and brought down once the nine o'clock position is reached. The suture at the nine o'clock position is then brought around and tied to the three o'clock suture.

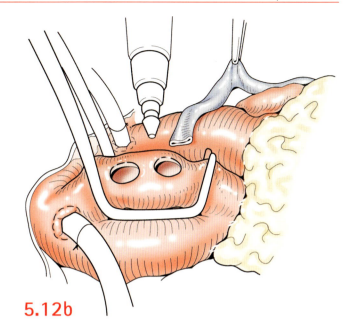

5.12b

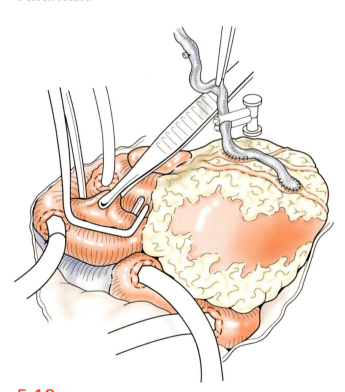

5.12a

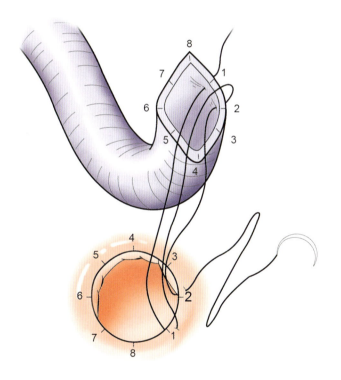

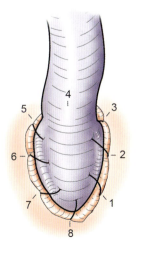

5.12c

Sequential distal vein graft anastomoses

In instances where vein graft length is limited or when there is concern for multiple anastomoses on the ascending aorta, one can construct two or more distal touchdown sites with a single vein graft (**Figure 5.13a–e**). The optimal spatial relationships of vein graft to artery may be difficult to assess in the decompressed arrested heart. One should avoid tension or excessive length between the end vein segment to the distal coronary artery anastomosis site and the side-to-side vein graft coronary artery anastomotic site that creates the second or third touchdown point for a single vein graft. The distal end-to-side anastomosis is typically created first. The easiest orientation for the more proximal side-to-side anastomosis is with the vein parallel to the artery. The anastomosis is begun at the heel and the far wall is completed open. It is then parachuted down and the front wall is completed. Others prefer a technique of perpendicular sequential side-to-side anastomosis. Care must be taken not to make the arteriotomy or vein graftotomy too long or a gull-wing deformity can occur.

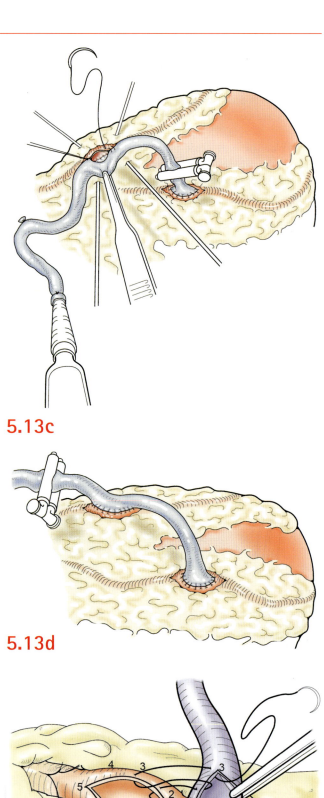

5.13c

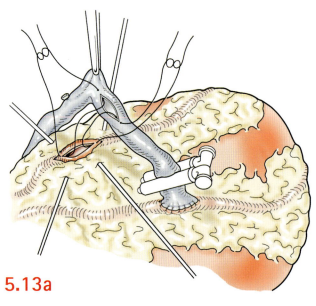

5.13a

5.13d

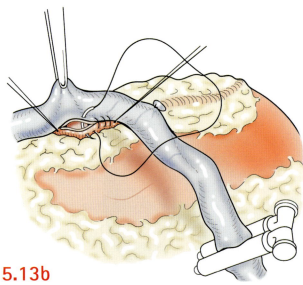

5.13b

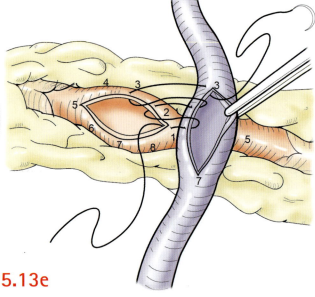

5.13e

In the somewhat uncommon situation in which it is necessary to construct more than one distal touchdown site with the pedicled IMA, the order of grafting is reversed and the side-to-side anastomosis is completed first, so that the mammary artery pedicle that remains attached to its origin can be freely manipulated (**Figure 5.14a and b**). Again the artery is carefully measured, the overlying fascia on the pedicle is freed up and a 3–4 mm longitudinal side-to-side anastomosis is completed. The major concern with this technique is that, if not measured correctly, the distal end to side IMA to LAD anastomosis can be under tension. Given the importance of this anastomosis, we only use this technique under extenuating circumstances.

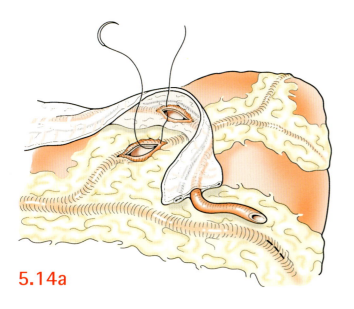

5.14a

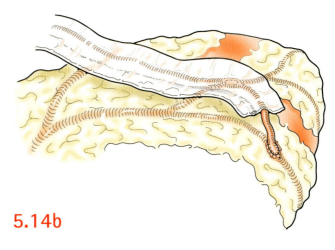

5.14b

Coronary endarterectomy

Occasionally, one encounters such a diffusely diseased coronary artery that coronary endarterectomy appears to be the only option for a satisfactory distal anastomosis. In general, coronary endarterectomy should be reserved for those rare situations in which an adequate touchdown site for the distal anastomosis cannot be identified. Achieving a good distal endpoint with the endarterectomy can be difficult and therefore this technique is associated with increased graft failure. Endarterectomy of the right coronary artery is more commonly performed than the LAD or lateral wall vessels.

The endarterectomy technique (**Figure 5.15a–e**) is begun by establishing a dissection plane between the hard luminal

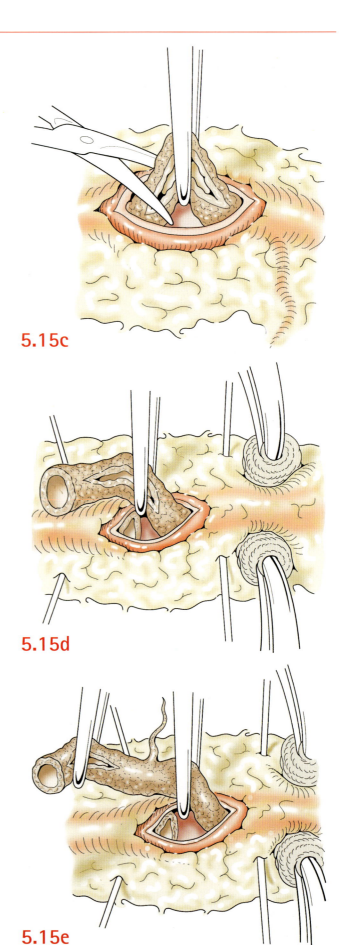

5.15c

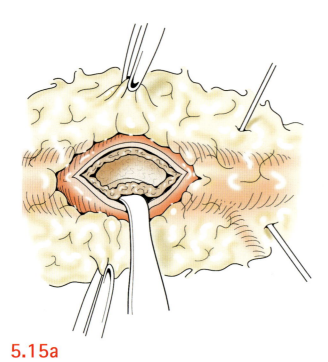

5.15a

5.15d

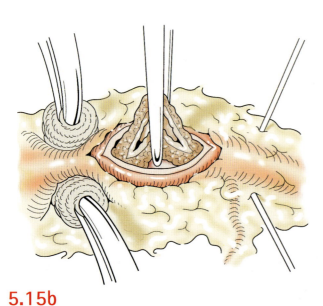

5.15b

5.15e

plaque and the outer media of the arterial wall. A fine tissue elevator can be used to initiate the plaque dissection, with care being taken to avoid disrupting the outer arterial wall. Once the atheromatous luminal plaque is encircled bluntly, the core is grasped firmly and peanut dissectors can be used laterally to provide countertraction as the plaque is being gently retracted. On the proximal end, once a reasonable portion of core plaque is retracted or resistance met, the core should be transected and the proximal plaque allowed to retract up into the artery. Distally the same process is performed, with the hope of removing a tapered distal cast of the artery. After the endarterectomy core is removed, the arterial wall is carefully inspected for injury or residual plaque. At this point an anastomosis can be constructed to a relatively disease-free artery.

Following completion of all vein graft anastomoses, the pump flow is decreased and the aortic cross-clamp or side-biting aortic clamp is removed. Next, the vein graft, which should be occluded distally, is de-aired by fine-needle puncture to avoid entrapped air. Blood flow is then established into the distal coronary arteries. The aortic root vent is started for de-airing. We typically place both arterial and venous wires for pacing at this point. After appropriate reperfusion and return of a normal, stable cardiac rhythm, CPB is discontinued. The venous cannula is removed and snared down in case of the need to go back on bypass. The root vent and retrograde cardioplegia or LV vent are removed and the sites oversewn. Right-angle 32 Fr chest tubes are placed posterior to the heart and in the left pleural space overlying the diaphragm. The angled tube posterior to the heart is angled out of the way of any inferior graft sites. The aortic cannula is then removed and the site oversewn. A 28 Fr straight chest tube is placed in the left pleural apex and one in the anterior mediastinum prior to closure.

POSTOPERATIVE CARE

Separation from CPB, reversal of heparinization, wound closure, and general physiologic management should be expeditiously and simply managed. In some situations, the patient's hemodynamic stability is sluggish, especially if the ischemic period was protracted because of the construction of multiple grafts. Low-dose inotropic stimulation may be helpful, but excessive inotropic administration may inappropriately increase the energy demands on the post-ischemic heart and may contribute to a low cardiac output state several hours after surgery. In patients with extensive and diffuse CAD, especially older patients, maintenance of an adequate perfusion pressure may also be an important component of early postoperative management, particularly because vasodilatation may develop from hemodilution, rewarming, or other post-cardiotomy changes. Such pathological vasodilatation may be easily reversed with low-dose alpha-adrenergic stimulation.

Complete systemic rewarming should be achieved to avoid hypothermia-induced myocardial depression or excessive vasoconstriction. After systemic cooling during CPB, the patient's extremities may remain cold. Despite attaining a normal core body temperature near the end of the CPB run, the patient may quickly become hypothermic in the immediate post-bypass period. In this case, topical rewarming should be carried out once the patient is in the ICU.

OUTCOME

From the mid 1980s until recently, patients who underwent CABG were warned by their physicians and surgeons that late failure of vein grafts should be expected. Various estimates of the scope of graft failure have been that 50% or more of grafts would occlude between 5 and 10 years after surgery. On the other hand, most estimates of late functioning of the LIMA graft to the LAD were for a 90% or greater probability.

The LIMA graft is now being constructed to the LAD in the great majority of patients who have a CABG procedure. The use of this graft approaches 100% in patients younger than 65–70 years old who undergo CABG and have disease present in the LAD system. As a result of this shift to continue mammary artery grafting over the last 10–15 years, and in recognition of the fact that this particular graft configuration remains functional for many years in more than 90% of patients and conveys clear survival benefit for most patients because of sustained patency and flow to the LAD system, the number of patients who present for reoperation and repeat CABG has declined in the last few years. When a patient has had the traditional operation and is referred for repeat CABG today, frequently the LIMA-to-LAD graft is found to be functioning, whereas one or more of the vein grafts have occluded.

Even this finding, however, is occurring less frequently because intensive secondary preventive measures have been applied to patients who present with severe CAD that requires bypass grafting. Strong evidence that antiplatelet agents such as aspirin and lipid-lowering medications enhance the resistance of native arteries and bypass conduits to progressive atherosclerosis has fostered the long-term pharmacological treatment of post-CABG patients.

To what extent the expanded use of arterial conduits in younger patients who require bypass grafting enhances the durability of the coronary bypass procedure remains to be established. For the majority of patients who present in need of bypass grafting, especially those in the older age range, and particularly those who can be expected to follow secondary preventive protocols carefully, this traditional procedure of a LIMA graft to LAD and saphenous vein grafts to the remaining obstructed coronary arteries is quite reliable. This improvement in durability of benefit from the traditional CABG procedure should be conveyed to the prospective patient, who may have been subjected to faulty information about excessively frequent coronary artery bypass graft failures based on outdated follow-up information.

REFERENCES

1. Mueller RL, Rosengart TK, Isom OW. The history of surgery for ischemic heart disease. *Ann Thorac Surg.* 1997; 63(3): 869–78.
2. Fihn SD, Blankenship JC, Alexander KP, et al. 2014 ACC/AHA/AATS/PCNA/SCAI/STS focused update of the guideline for the diagnosis and management of patients with stable ischemic heart disease: a report of the American College of Cardiology/American Heart Association Task Force on Practice Guidelines, and the American Association for Thoracic Surgery, Preventive Cardiovascular Nurses Association, Society for Cardiovascular Angiography and Interventions, and Society of Thoracic Surgeons. *J Am Coll Cardiol.* 2014; 64(18): 1929–49.
3. Online STS Adult Cardiac Surgery Risk Calculator: http://riskcalc.sts.org.

6

Off-pump coronary revascularization

GIANLUCA TORREGROSSA, TIMOTHY LEE, AND JOHN D. PUSKAS

HISTORY

Coronary artery bypass grafting (CABG) represents the gold standard treatment for complex coronary artery disease. The efficacy of this procedure for survival, symptom improvement, and quality of life has been well documented.

While outcomes with conventional bypass grafting using cardioplegic arrest continue to improve over time across the Society of Thoracic Surgeons (STS) National Cardiac Database, CABG is still associated with complications that may negate an otherwise successful coronary revascularization, in particular periprocedural stroke, which in all randomized trials of CABG vs PCI has been more frequent after CABG than after PCI.

Renewed interest in off-pump bypass grafting (OPCAB) and refinement of surgical techniques for multi-vessel OPCAB in the mid 1990s presented surgeons with the option of revascularization without the potential complications of extracorporeal support, in particular avoiding or minimizing the manipulation on the ascending aorta and decreasing the incidence of stroke. Although many centers have adopted this technique, in North America OPCAB procedures peaked at 25% in 2004 and have declined since then. For most surgeons, the lack of a mortality benefit for OPCAB over conventional on-pump coronary artery bypass (ONCAB) in randomized trials has diminished enthusiasm for implementing this strategy in routine practice. Furthermore, many surgeons consider an off-pump approach a more technically demanding procedure which may result in less complete revascularization. There is growing concern that OPCAB, especially in the hands of inexperienced operators, may be associated with reduced long-term graft patency and increased need for repeat revascularization procedures, which may potentially result in inferior long-term survival compared with traditional on-pump CABG surgery. Nonetheless, numerous retrospective comparisons of risk-adjusted outcomes between OPCAB and ONCAB within large institutional or national databases have consistently supported the belief that OPCAB is associated with reduced morbidity and mortality, especially in higher-risk patients.

Despite the hundreds of studies investigating off-pump surgery, many of the results reported in the literature have been inconclusive or contradictory as to the overall benefit of the technique. Most studies have suffered from the fact that they have been retrospective reviews with perceived patient selection bias, despite many times including sophisticated statistical risk adjustment. And while newer prospective studies continue to be published, questions regarding the ultimate benefit of this technique remain unanswered in the minds of many surgeons.

PRINCIPLES AND JUSTIFICATION

The challenge of off-pump CABG is to construct a coronary anastomosis on a 1.25–2.5 mm internal diameter moving vessel. The accuracy of off-pump CABG is based on 3D stabilization of the target site segment without affecting the myocardial function. The motion of the target is complex and consists of slow and fast components, the latter particularly in the end-diastolic filling phase of the heart. This motion makes accurate microvascular suturing without mechanical stabilization impossible. Therefore, proper local cardiac wall stabilization to minimize myocardial movement and to optimize presentation of the target coronary artery is the cornerstone of beating-heart surgery.

Currently, three methods of tissue stabilization exist:

- suction fixation
- pressure fixation
- vessel loop-plate fixation.

The stabilizer may be retractor-based or operation table rail-based.

The suction-based 'Octopus' (**Figure 6.1a**) was developed at Utrecht University Medical Center. Suction fixation allows tissue stabilization and presentation in a neutral plane so as not to compress the myocardium. The Octopus I two-pod stabilizer (Medtronic, Minneapolis, MN) is mounted on the operation table rail and has the advantage of being able to be used in all access routes including port access. The Octopus I also enables unlimited spreading of the epicardial fatty tissue and therefore further immobilization in the z-direction, as most coronaries are embedded in a discrete groove in the fatty tissue. The Octopus II one-arm stabilizer (Medtronic, Minneapolis, MN) is (sternal) retractor-based, like most current stabilizers today, and is easier to use. Spreading of the tip of the pods is still possible. Suction fixation requires additional measures such as management of tubing and suction, separate for left and right in the Octopus I and combined in the Octopus II.

Tissue stabilization by pressure is easier to apply but exerts more pressure on the heart. However, compared to suction fixation, the technique has less grip on the heart, and slipping may occur (**Figure 6.1b**).

Vessel loop-plate fixation uses a combination of simultaneous foot plate stabilization and a vessel loop under the target vessel for stabilization, leading to segmental occlusion simultaneously (**Figure 6.1c**). The foot plate, however, is more difficult to use in sequential grafting because of its size.

The adoption of OPCAB into clinical practice requires a commitment to learning a unique skill set that has been associated with improved outcomes in certain patient subgroups. We consider that this is best achieved by routine adoption of OPCAB techniques such that the surgeon can employ this approach in patients likely to derive the most benefit. OPCAB surgery poses unique challenges to a surgeon who is accustomed to operating in a motionless and bloodless field. Furthermore, OPCAB requires adept first and second assistants to provide exposure on a beating heart as well as excellent anesthesia management to maintain hemodynamics and alert the surgical team of potential hemodynamic problems. Thus, the commitment to OPCAB is usually tied to a belief that the technical challenges inherent in the procedure are worth overcoming so that the patient may benefit from the avoidance of cardiopulmonary bypass. The inexperienced OPCAB surgeon embarking on the learning curve is best advised to choose his or her initial patients carefully and pay close attention to coronary anatomy as well as other important patient variables.

The surgeon must come to the operating room with an operative plan that is flexible enough to change as operative findings mandate. Unlike ONCAB, in which graft sequence and hemodynamic management are relatively straightforward, OPCAB requires careful consideration of coronary anatomy, confounding patient variables, and attention to hemodynamic fluctuations. Early in a surgeon's experience, it is probably prudent to exclude patients with difficult lateral wall targets, especially multiple lateral wall targets, severe left ventricular dysfunction, left main disease, or other complex cases. Ideal early candidates for OPCAB include those undergoing elective primary coronary revascularization with

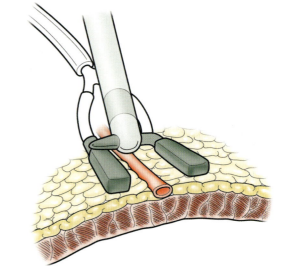

6.1a

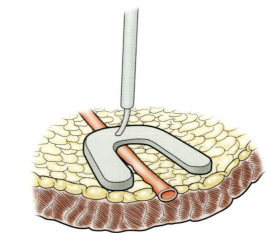

6.1b

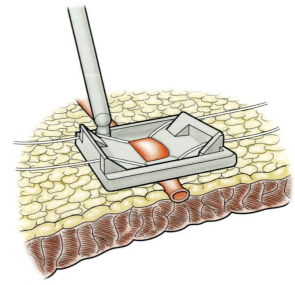

6.1c

good target anatomy, preserved ventricular function, and one to three grafts with easily accessible or no lateral wall targets. When teaching OPCAB to residents, the left anterior descending coronary anastomosis is usually the easiest, given its anterior location. This is usually followed by easily accessible diagonal branches, then inferior wall vessels, and, finally, lateral wall targets, which are the most difficult to expose and perform off-pump.

As experience is gained in OPCAB, higher-risk and technically more challenging procedures can be undertaken. These include procedures on patients with marginal hemodynamics but who are otherwise stable, those requiring multiple grafts to the posterior and lateral walls or the atrioventricular groove, and those with enlarged right or left ventricles. Difficult patients most likely to benefit from off-pump surgery include those with severe left ventricular dysfunction, renal insufficiency, atherosclerotic disease of the ascending aorta, or severe chronic obstructive pulmonary disease, and those grafted emergently after an acute myocardial infarction. Patients presenting the most significant technical challenge for OPCAB include those requiring reoperations, those with small and diffusely diseased vessels, and those with cardiomegaly, ischemic arrhythmias, ischemic mitral regurgitation, and pectus excavatum.

PREOPERATIVE ASSESSMENT AND PREPARATION

The preoperative evaluation of patients for OPCAB demands careful planning and consideration for certain risk factors. We routinely perform screening carotid duplex ultrasonography on all patients over the age of 65, smokers, those with a carotid bruit, history of transient ischemic attack or stroke, left main coronary disease, peripheral vascular disease, or history of prior carotid intervention. The remainder of the preoperative evaluation is similar to ONCAB. In patients with a murmur, dyspnea, aortic or mitral regurgitation, or ventricular dysfunction on cardiac catheterization, preoperative echocardiography is also warranted. It is important to be aware of right ventricular dysfunction, valvular regurgitation, or pulmonary hypertension because positioning during OPCAB can result in dramatic changes in these parameters. Computed tomography (CT) scan of the chest without contrast is particularly helpful in the preoperative assessment to magnify any aortic calcification that can mandate an anaortic clampless OPCAB strategy. Overall, the clinical condition of the patient, the urgency of the operation, and ventricular function need to be carefully assessed to determine whether an off-pump approach will be practical.

Although patients operated on more acutely may benefit from an off-pump approach, it is important to have a backup plan explicitly prepared should an OPCAB approach be poorly tolerated. Patients with left ventricular dysfunction from a recent infarct pose a more difficult challenge than those with chronic ventricular dysfunction, with the former being much more sensitive to cardiac manipulation and displacement and more likely to develop intraoperative arrhythmias.

OPERATIVE PLANNING

General principles

At the time of surgery, as in other cardiac operations, all patients require invasive monitoring with an arterial line, Foley catheter, and central venous line. We use comprehensive transesophageal echocardiography to provide valuable information about valvular regurgitation, regional myocardial function, and pulmonary hypertension; pulmonary artery catheters are placed selectively.

In our experience, a well-experienced anesthesia team is essential for maintaining stable hemodynamics and ensuring a smooth and uneventful operation. Unlike ONCAB, which requires active coordination among surgeon, anesthesiologist, and perfusionist, the anesthesiologist and surgeon must work especially closely to maintain hemodynamic stability during OPCAB. Instead of relying on cardiopulmonary bypass to ensure adequate perfusion, other maneuvers are required to avoid dramatic fluctuations in hemodynamic status that can have detrimental consequences. Subtle changes in hemodynamic status, gradual elevation in pulmonary artery pressures, frequent boluses or increased requirement of inotropes and vasopressors to maintain hemodynamic stability, and rhythm changes can herald cardiovascular collapse. Such an event can reliably be avoided if these changes are verbalized and discussed between anesthesiologist and surgeon pre-emptively. When manipulating the heart, it is important for the surgeon to communicate these abrupt maneuvers to the anesthesia team so that appropriate action can be taken proactively and inappropriate reactions (bolusing vasopressors) avoided. Changes in table position (e.g. Trendelenburg position) can provide dramatic volume changes that affect cardiac output and blood pressure. Indeed, autotransfusion of intravascular volume from the lower extremities by Trendelenburg positioning should be the first maneuver to maintain hemodynamic stability. Placing the patient in steep Trendelenburg can provide a rapid increase in preload and subsequent cardiac output and blood pressure, whereas reverse Trendelenburg can be helpful in lowering blood pressure if partial aortic clamping is required for proximal anastomoses.

We prefer to avoid giving massive volumes of intravenous fluids which requires later postoperative diuresis. Instead, aggressive use of Trendelenburg positioning and judicious use of alpha-adrenergic agents provides stable hemodynamics in the large majority of patients undergoing OPCAB. This includes patients with pulmonary hypertension, mild or moderate ischemic mitral regurgitation, or left ventricular dysfunction in which cardiac manipulation and displacement as well as regional myocardial ischemia may be poorly tolerated without inotropic support. If preload conditions have been optimized, then vasopressor agents such as norepinephrine may be used to assist with maintaining adequate blood pressure during distal anastomoses.

Maintaining normothermia is critically important and requires more effort during OPCAB procedures, because the luxury of the cardiopulmonary bypass circuit for rewarming does not exist. This usually can be accomplished by infusing intravenous fluids through warmers, warming inhalational anesthetic agents, maintaining warm room temperatures before and during the procedure, and using convective forced-air warming systems. These can be placed around the patient before draping the patient to maintain normothermia, but sterile systems can also be placed on the lower body and extremities after graft harvesting.

Anticoagulation

At our institution, anticoagulation regimens vary according to surgeon preference. For surgeons in their early experience, a full "pump" dose of heparin is reasonable in the event that conversion to cardiopulmonary bypass becomes necessary. Some of our surgeons continue to implement a full dose with 400 IU/kg to maintain an activated clotting time (ACT) of greater than 400 seconds; others use a half dose or 180 IU/kg, whereas others start with 10 000 IU and administer additional doses (3000 IU every half hour) to maintain an ACT of 275–350 seconds. Reversal of anticoagulation with varying doses of protamine is usually administered to facilitate hemostasis.

OPERATION

Access

The most commonly used access (**Figure 6.2**) is currently the sternotomy (A) because it offers wide access to all major coronary artery segments. In addition, better understanding of the pump function of the displaced heart and particularly the advent of new "tricks" to subluxate the beating heart without compromising the pump function favor this approach. Currently, the anterior thoracostomy (B), the subxiphoid laparotomy (median) (C), and the posterior thoracotomy (E) are used for subsets of patients with limited one-vessel disease. In favorable topography, the anterior thoracostomy (B), the distal sternotomy (D), the transverse curved laparotomy (F), and the left posterior thoracotomy allow multiple grafting, provided that the vessels are nearby and, in the case of the anterior thoracotomy, no wide-angled diagonal–left anterior descending (LAD) fork is present.

A second, major advantage of the sternotomy is that the internal mammary arteries (IMAs) can be harvested in the usual familiar way using a table-based retractor (Rultract, Cleveland, OH) (**Figure 6.3a–c**). Our preference is to skeletonize the internal thoracic arteries (ITAs) in order to maximize the length, favor Y- and T-anastomosis, and preserve the vein drainage of the thoracic wall minimizing the risk of wound infection.

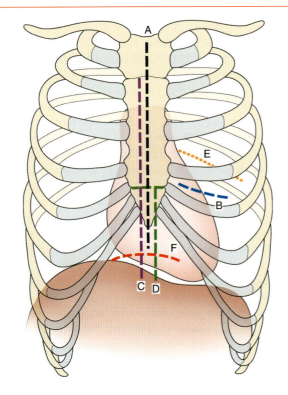

6.2

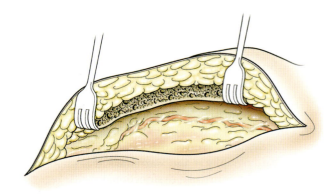

6.3a

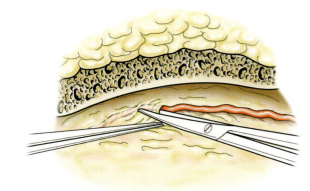

6.3b

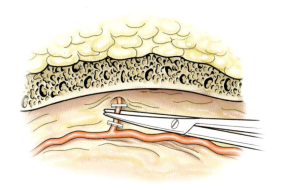

6.3c

Preferentially, grafts are used as an *in situ* graft. T- and Y-anastomoses are constructed with free IMA and radial artery or 5–10 cm saphenous vein on a stable pulmonary artery (folded towel or suction stabilizer on the common pulmonary artery can serve as a stable platform) (**Figure 6.4a**). The T- or Y-anastomosis may be constructed at first or as a final anastomosis. It is constructed preferably using a two-needle technique, the back suture first (**Figure 6.4b**). This technique enables economic use of graft material (skeletonization favors jump grafting) and reduces or may avoid touching the ascending aorta. In practice, complete arterial revascularization in OPCABG can be achieved in almost all patients, using up to five-vessel arterial revascularization with intense use of both IMAs.

In the sternotomy approach the procedure should always start with a deep pericardial stitch 3 cm laterally from the confluence of the two pulmonary veins, using a braided-two stitch. With this stitch, a long sling is lowered with a snugger so that a tripod retractor is created to improve stability of displacement (**Figure 6.5a and b**).

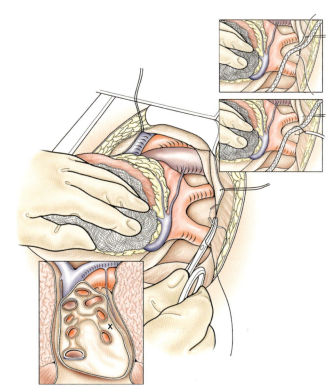

6.5a

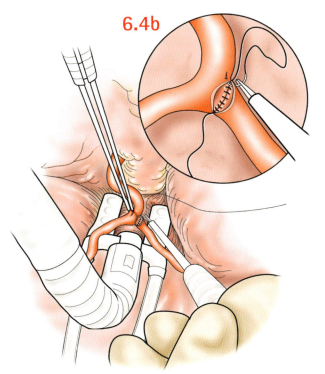

6.4b

6.4a

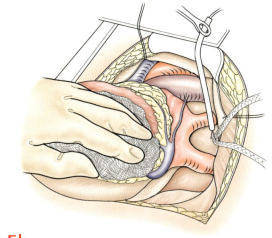

6.5b

The stabilizer is mounted on the sternotomy-retractor. The heart is displaced, and the stabilizer is positioned to the target and fixed. Suction-fixation takes ±15 seconds before it is effective. The three parts of the tripod are then fixed to the towel dressing. Finally, the target exposure can be adjusted to expose the three major territories: the anterior wall (**Figure 6.6a**), the inferior wall (**Figure 6.6b**), and the posterior wall (**Figure 6.6c**). The distal right coronary artery (RCA) itself can be exposed, leaving the heart in its cradle. An additional suction device on the apex can support the positioning of the heart for lateral and inferior wall exposure. It stabilizes the upright position of the heart and helps to maintain the geometry of the beating heart. This is an important tool to support hemodynamics in off-pump revascularization in the impaired and dilated ventricle (**Figure 6.6d**).

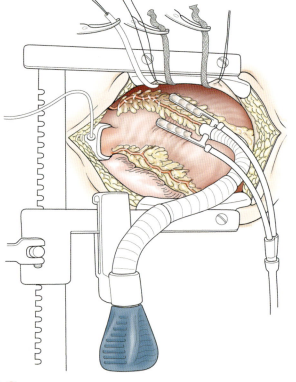

6.6a

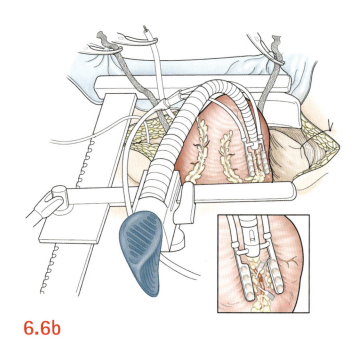

6.6b

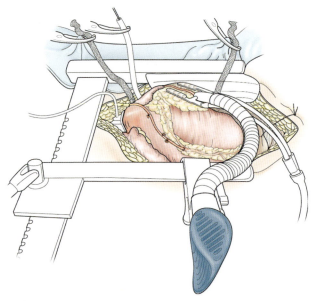

6.6c

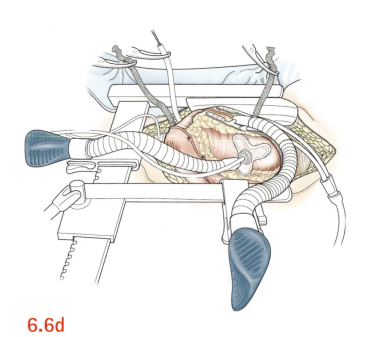

6.6d

Displacement should always be preceded by intravenous volume supplementation to achieve a right atrial pressure in the range of 8–10 cm H_2O and to increase the preload by head-down and right lateral tilt of the operating table (Trendelenburg maneuver) to avoid inflow obstruction (**Figure 6.7**). The thin-walled right atrium and ventricle may "kink" or "get compressed" easily. Transesophageal echocardiography is an ideal monitor of this inflow obstruction. If compression of the heart is the main problem, the right pericardium can be incised towards the inferior caval vein and the pleura opened to allow the heart to drop in the right pleural cavity. However, slackening of the right pericardial stay suture can be tried at first. Unless the ventricle is impaired, hemodynamic stabilization can usually be obtained within 1–2 minutes without any inotropes. A mean arterial blood pressure of 60–80 mmHg is recommended. If necessary, inotropic support of first choice is phenylephrine as a bolus dose, because it is non-chronotropic. When continuous support is anticipated, dopamine in low dosage, i.e. 2–4 µg/kg per minute, is started before displacement. This stage of the procedure requires close cooperation between surgeon and anesthetist. If the circulation does not improve promptly, the heart must be repositioned. Too much inotropic drug support should also be avoided because the stabilizer will lose its grip on the "hard" myocardium. Volume load of 1000–1500 mL causes approximately the same "water damage" as on-pump surgery.

Management of anastomosis site

After the conduits are routed intrapericardially, their length to the target site is measured. In the case of free grafts, proximal anastomosis on the ascending aorta is usually done last. The question arises: which vessel first? The LAD is best done first if the RCA is not totally occluded. The LAD requires only moderate displacement, which is well tolerated. This advantage is especially true when the anastomosis site is distal to a big diagonal branch, thus keeping more myocardium perfused.

If the RCA is dominant and totally occluded while the LAD has a moderate stenosis, preference is to graft the RCA first, completing the bypass with both distal and proximal site in order to supply the heart with blood while occluding the LAD for the distal anastomosis.

Marginal targets are generally left until last due to the manipulation of the heart required to expose them.

We found that in almost all vessels the "clamp and sew" technique is warranted. If hemodynamic instability occurs, a prompt use of shunt with releasing of the proximal snare is the best next step to adopt (**Figure 6.8a**). Routine use of the shunt is not our standard because this increases the surgical complexity and compromises the quality of the distal target.

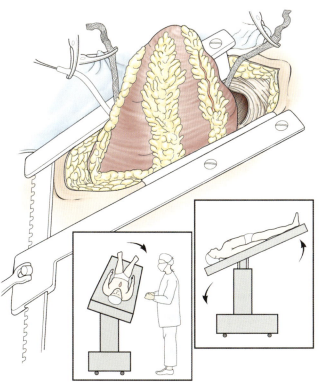

6.7

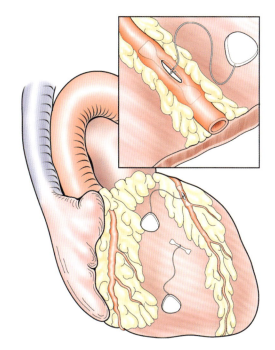

6.8a

Temporary occlusion can be performed in several ways: an atraumatic microvascular clamp (Acland [Landmark Surgical Instrumentation and Equipment, Merseyside, UK]; **Figure 6.8b**), Silastic snare (**Figure 6.8c**), buttressed suture (**Figure 6.8d**), or disposable clip (**Figure 6.8e**). Occluding the vessel also distally using atraumatic microvascular clamps (Acland) produces a dry anastomosis site and imitates clean

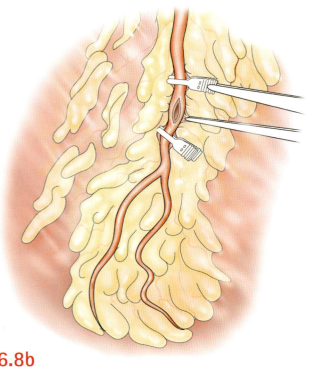

6.8b

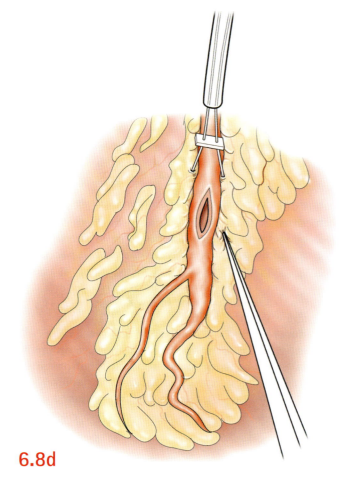

6.8d

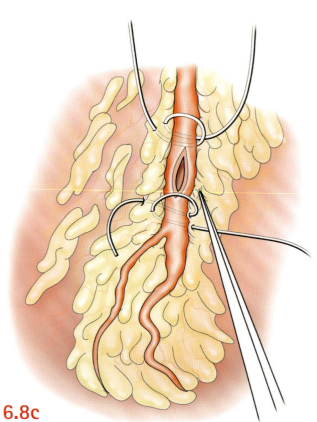

6.8c

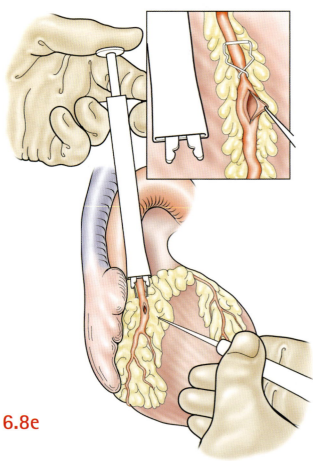

6.8e

globally arrested heart surgery. Preferably, the clamps should be positioned from aside in order not to compromise the suture-loop handling. This has an additional advantage of preserving the collateral flow to the distal myocardium. Alternatively, a blower/mister should be used to maintain a clear view (**Figure 6.8f**).

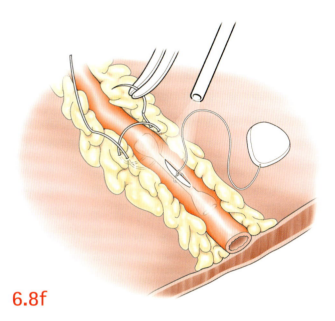

6.8f

Anastomosis

A single, running 8-0 or 7-0 suture is used, usually with a one-needle technique. In grafting of the diagonal sequential to the LAD, the side anastomosis is performed using a two-needle technique, starting with the back wall first, suturing the coronary artery from outside to inside (**Figure 6.8g**). This method is used because of the orientation of the vessel to the surgeon. In the distal RCA anastomosis, the toe is most distal and therefore is done first, using the two-needle technique.

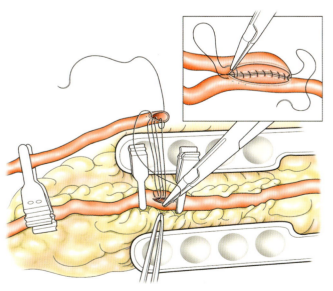

6.8g

Quality assessment

Intraoperative quality assessment can be performed by angiography or, more practically, transit-time ultrasound graft flow measurement. In combination with simultaneous assessment of additional parameters, such as the qualitative flow pattern, the ratio flow–mean arterial blood pressure, and – before tying the knot – assessment of free graft flow, native coronary flow, and distal stump pressure, transit-time ultrasound graft flow measurement has additional value.

Alternative access routes

LEFT ANTERIOR THORACOTOMY

Isolated revascularization of the most important coronary artery, the LAD, is most suitable via a small left anterior thoracotomy in the fourth or fifth intercostal space. The patient is intubated using a double-lumen tube. Through this incision the left IMA can be harvested either directly or video-assisted (**Figure 6.9a**).

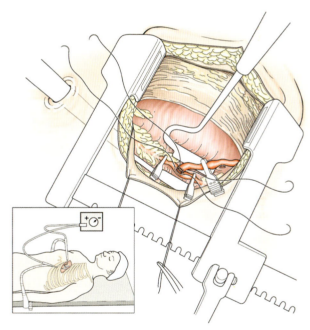

6.9a

Usually, the pleura is opened, and the left lung is deflated. In the incision the left IMA is identified carefully. The left accompanying vein is clipped and cut. More length is gained caudally and craniad by meticulous dissection while the wound is gradually opened with a small retractor (**Figure 6.9b**). Harvesting in the skeletonized way using fine DeBakey forceps and the cautery spatula is preferred. The endothoracic fascia is gradually opened, and small strands are cauterized using low-energy coagulation ("coagulation/fulgurate"). All branches are clipped and cut in between to avoid thermal damage. By hoisting the craniad ribs by a retractor attached to the table rail or by a thoracic wall tilting device which in turn is attached to the wound retractor, dissection can be completed up to the level of the first intercostal space. High dissection is particularly necessary in planned jump grafts to the diagonal branch and LAD. If additional length is necessary distally, the cartilage of the caudal rib is cut with a knife from the inside to enable easy healing and to avoid damaging the IMA. The cartilage is sutured at closure. The least invasive technique is the Cohn "H-graft" preparation. In this technique a graft is used as an interposition graft without dissection of the IMA (**Figure 6.9c**). Resection of cartilage may be necessary in this H-graft. Careful wound closure is important to prevent lung herniation.

After heparinization, the IMA is distally cut between clips. The pericardium is opened longitudinally, and the lateral rim is suspended, after which two-lung ventilation can usually be resumed. The LAD is identified. A peanut swab may help to identify its position by assessing the right ventricle transition to the more solid septum from right to left. Then a retractor or table rail-based stabilizer is positioned. When the Octopus I suction paddles are used, the paddle to the left side of the LAD (straight right paddle) is positioned through a separate stab wound, and the paddle to the right side of the LAD (left preformed paddle) is positioned aside in the wound. Suction (-400 mmHg) is activated, and dissection is started, followed by spreading of the pods. Microvascular clamps are used for local segmental occlusion. The already prepared IMA is then grafted to the LAD. Before and after tying, quality assessment is performed.

In sequential grafting, which is only feasible in a narrow-angled diagonal–LAD fork, the diagonal side-to-side anastomosis is always performed first. Exposure is feasible with suction fixation by median displacement of the anterolateral myocardium. In this anastomosis, a two-needle technique is performed, whereas in end-to-side anastomosis, the parachute down the heel technique is preferred (see "Anastomosis", above).

The Cohn graft may be particularly suitable to perform a salvage revascularization of the LAD in a poor-risk patient. This graft is a short interposition between the IMA and the LAD with radial artery or saphenous vein graft (Cohn H-graft; see **Figure 6.9c**). Therefore, cartilage is resected to expose only a short segment of the LAD. The anastomosis is usually performed first on the LAD and then to the IMA. Competition or steal phenomenon seems not to be an issue, as little diastolic flow augmentation may relieve angina (**Figure 6.9c**).

Alternatively, for off-pump single LAD grafting in redo cases or in the absence of an IMA, the subclavian artery or preferably the proximal axillary artery can be used as the inflow conduit, utilizing a saphenous vein graft or radial artery (**Figure 6.9d**). The artery is exposed via an infraclavicular incision, retracting the pectoralis major muscle and pectoralis minor muscle, median to the deltoid muscle. The artery is identified above the vein, encircled, and segmentally

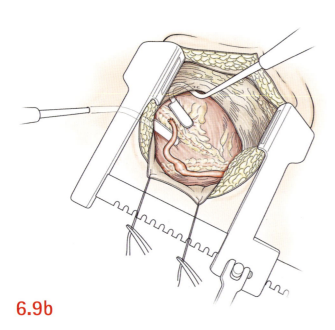

6.9b

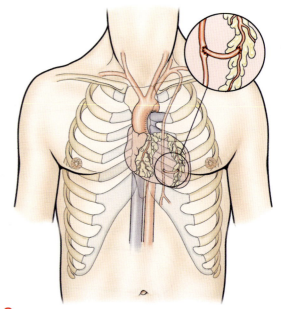

6.9c

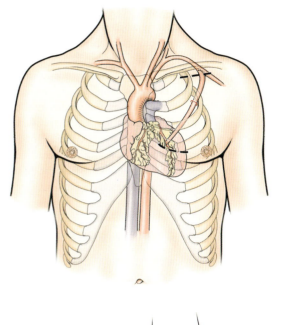

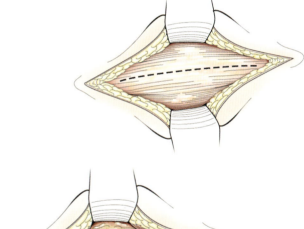

clamped. After the proximal anastomosis at the caudal–dorsal aspect (to prevent kinking) has been completed, the left lung is deflated. The adjacent intercostal space is opened with a curved forceps for 2–3 cm (in case of a narrow space through the bed of the locally resected second or third rib). Using a long-grasping forceps, the surgeon passes the graft to the small left anterior thoracotomy. A light cable may help with this, and also to check for hemostasis of the intercostal space. The LAD anastomosis is then performed as described (see **Figure 6.9a**).

Graft flow is measured, preferably with the stabilizer removed, as this may affect distal myocardial tissue perfusion. Protamine is given, starting with 25 mg. The pericardium is closed, leaving 4 cm IMA intrapericardially to facilitate redo surgery. The thoracotomy wound is closed, leaving a pleuradrain via the stab wound.

LEFT POSTERIOR THORACOTOMY

Left posterior thoracotomy is useful for redo surgery. The patient is in the right lateral position. Double-lumen intubation is recommended. A 15 cm posterior thoracotomy in the fifth or sixth intercostal space exposes the circumflex artery branches well (**Figure 6.10**). The pericardium is opened posterior to the phrenic nerve. For the diagonal branch and the LAD grafting, the thoracotomy incision should be extended anteriorly and the pericardium also opened ventrally to the phrenic nerve. The quality of the descending aorta as the inflow conduit is sometimes disappointing. Alternative inflow conduits have been discussed previously. The radial artery and saphenous vein can be used. Tissue stabilization can be retractor-based (thoracotomy retractor) or table rail-based.

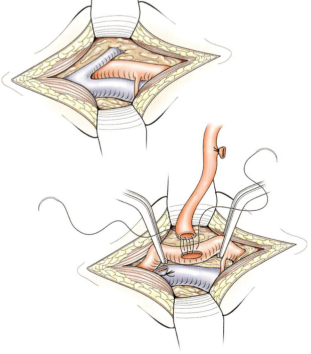

6.9d

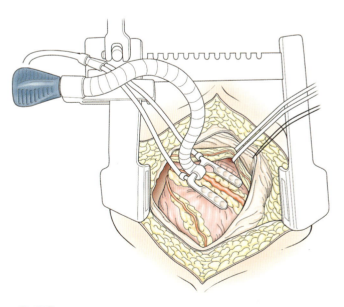

6.10

OTHER NON–STERNOTOMY OPCABG APPROACHES

The competitive status of percutaneous transluminal coronary angioplasty and stenting has stimulated an interest in minimally invasive direct CABG. This is allowed by absence of cardiopulmonary bypass, permitting surgeons to pursue a less invasive approach that spares the sternum, expedites the postoperative course, and decreases the length of stay. A left thoracotomy was adopted in the 1990s as an alternative route to offer OPCAB LITA-to-LAD grafting. Initially, specialized retractors and instruments simplified the LITA harvesting and allowed surgery through a minimally invasive direct thoracotomy (MIDCAB). Internal thoracic artery harvesting was further improved by the creation of the da Vinci® surgical system (Intuitive Surgical, Inc.), which facilitates harvesting of single or double ITAs, and also allows completion of anastomosis to the anterior and lateral wall of the heart. We note that the left thoracotomy approach is also used in patients undergoing a reoperation CABG as an alternate route of access to the lateral wall, thereby avoiding a repeat sternotomy and a potential injury to patent grafts.

POSTOPERATIVE CARE

The postoperative care of patients undergoing OPCAB is similar to that of ONCABG patients. It is important in OPCAB patients to maintain an appropriate temperature soon after surgery. Aspirin (162 mg postoperatively, then 81 mg/day) and clopidogrel (150 mg postoperatively, then 75 mg/day) are routinely administered early in the postoperative period after mediastinal drainage decreases below 100 mL/h for 4 hours. This has not been associated with an increased risk of mediastinal re-exploration. Because of the absence of cardiopulmonary bypass-related coagulopathy, patients may have a relative hypercoagulable perioperative state, which theoretically may jeopardize early graft patency. Bednar and colleagues demonstrated a significantly higher expression of P-selectin, a marker of platelet activity, in the OPCAB patients compared with ONCAB patients, suggesting a procoagulant state. For this reason, we administer aspirin and clopidogrel early postoperatively, and then continue dual antiplatelet therapy in the postoperative period for at least 6 months. Aspirin is continued for life, unless contraindicated.

OUTCOME

Clinical outcomes after OPCAB and ONCAB have been compared for more than a decade, with enrollment across many centers and including hundreds of thousands of patients. Despite the abundance of literature, there is still no consensus regarding the optimal bypass strategy, especially in low-risk patients. In higher-risk patients, it appears in recent studies that OPCAB may reduce both morbidity and mortality.

Studies may be divided into prospective randomized trials and observational retrospective analyses. Prospective trials provide the most accurate comparison between groups and avoid the selection bias and confounding inherent to retrospective and observational analyses. However, due to resource constraints, these studies are smaller and thus statistically underpowered to detect incremental differences in morbidity or mortality rates following CABG. This remains true despite the recent completion and publication of three large, multicentered randomized trials – ROOBY, GOPCAB, and CORONARY – as the patient sample sizes required to demonstrate a significant difference in mortality would be more than 50 000 patients, and similar sample sizes would be required to detect differences in stroke and myocardial infarction. Retrospective and observational analyses provide the necessarily large cohort size and long duration of follow-up to power these studies sufficiently to detect small but important differences in outcomes. However, retrospective studies are inherently limited by biases, the most important of which is selection bias, which persists despite the use of propensity matching and other advanced statistical methodologies designed to control for confounding. Taken together, both types of studies can provide valuable information to guide clinical practice.

CONCLUSIONS

OPCABG avoids the morbidity and mortality associated with cardiopulmonary bypass, but it is more technically demanding. In the hands of experienced surgeons and teams early clinical outcomes are equivalent to OPCABG for most patients and superior for high-risk patients. Indeed, the relative benefit of OPCAB is greatest for those patients who are at greatest risk of adverse events caused by conventional CABG on CPB. It is important to emphasize that OPCAB enables anaortic techniques and minimally invasive approaches that reduce perioperative morbidity, and it may be combined with multiple arterial or all-arterial grafting to optimize long-term outcomes. The authors believe that the current state-of-the-art surgical coronary revascularization for most patients is anaortic OPCAB with multiple or all-arterial grafts. However, the benefits of OPCAB require that completeness of revascularization and precision of anastomoses are not compromised; this is achievable in most patients by scrupulous attention to detail and experienced application of the technical principles discussed here.

FURTHER READING

Calafiore AM, Di Giammarco G, Teodori G, et al. Left anterior descending coronary artery grafting via left anterior small thoracotomy without cardiopulmonary bypass. *Ann Thorac Surg.* 1996; 61: 1658–65.

Dewey TM, Mack MJ. Myocardial revascularization without cardiopulmonary bypass. In: Cohn LH (ed.). *Cardiac surgery in the adult.* 3rd edn. New York, NY: McGraw-Hill; 2008: pp. 633–54.

Diegeler A, Borgermann J, Kappert U, et al., for GOPCABE Study Group. Off-pump versus on-pump coronary artery bypass grafting in elderly patients. *N Engl J Med.* 2013; 368: 1189–98.

Halkos ME, Puskas JD, Yanagawa B. Myocardial revascularization without cardiopulmonary bypass. In: Cohn LH (ed.). *Cardiac surgery in the adult.* 5th edn. New York, NY: McGraw-Hill; 2011: pp. 519–38.

Head SJ, Davierwala PM, Serruys PW, et al. Coronary artery bypass grafting vs. percutaneous coronary intervention for patients with three-vessel disease: final five-year follow-up of the SYNTAX trial. *Eur Heart J.* 2014; 35: 2821–30.

Keeling WB, Williams ML, Slaughter MS, et al. Off-pump and on-pump coronary revascularization in patients with low ejection fraction: a report from The Society of Thoracic Surgeons National Database. *Ann Thorac Surg.* 2013; 96: 83–9.

Lamy A, Devereaux PJ, Prabhakaran D, et al., for the CORONARY Investigators. Off-pump or on-pump coronary artery bypass grafting at 30 days. *N Engl J Med.* 2012; 366: 1489–97.

Lamy A, Devereau PJ, Prabhakaran D, et al., for the CORONARY Investigators. Five-year outcomes after off-pump or on-pump coronary-artery bypass grafting. *N Engl J Med.* 2016; 375: 2359–68.

Lytle BW, Sabik JF. On-pump and off-pump bypass surgery: tools for revascularization. *Circulation* 2004; 109: 810.

Ricci M, Karamanoukian HL, Abraham R, et al. Stroke in octogenarians undergoing coronary artery surgery with and without cardiopulmonary bypass. *Ann Thorac Surg.* 2000; 69: 1471.

Shroyer AL, Grover FL, Hallter B, et al., for the Veterans Affairs Randomized On/Off Bypasss (ROOBY) Study Group. On-pump versus off-pump coronary-artery bypass surgery. *N Engl J Med.* 2009; 361: 1827–37.

Stevens LM, Noiseux N, Avezum A, et al., on behalf of the CORONARY Investigators. Conversion after off-pump coronary artery bypass grafting: the CORONARY trial experience. *Eur J Cardiothorac Surg.* 2017; 51: 539–46.

Van Dijk D, Spoor M, Hijman R, et al., for the Octopus Study Group. Cognitive and cardiac outcomes 5 years after off-pump vs. on-pump coronary artery bypass graft surgery. *JAMA.* 2007; 297: 701–8.

Yanagawa B, Nedadur R, Puskas JD. The future of off-pump coronary artery bypass grafting: a North American perspective. *J Thorac Dis.* 2016; 8: S10.

7

Expanded use of arterial conduits

PHILIP A.R. HAYWARD, SEAN D. GALVIN, AND BRIAN F. BUXTON

HISTORY

Evolution in techniques for the correction of coronary artery disease coupled with an improved understanding of basic pathophysiologic mechanisms (in grafts and in native coronary arteries) have led to an improvement in the quality of life and survival for patients undergoing surgical revascularization. The internal thoracic artery (ITA) was used clinically by Vineberg as early as 1946 when he implanted it into an intramyocardial tunnel in the left ventricle. Green and colleagues reported the early experience with direct anastomosis of the ITA in 1966 but it took 30 years until Loop showed superior outcomes with ITA use. Subsequent reports by Lytle confirmed that bilateral ITA grafting is associated with survival benefit of 10% at 10 years.

Carpentier used the radial artery (RA) initially with poor results; however, in 1992 his colleague Acar reintroduced it with the understanding that atraumatic handling and pharmacological dilatation of the RA could lead to excellent patency. Other arterial conduits have been used but none of these has had wide acceptance. Today, extended (two or more arterial grafts) and total arterial grafting are possible in the majority of patients using a variety of conduits and facilitated by sequential, T- or Y- and extension grafting techniques.

PRINCIPLES AND JUSTIFICATION

The fundamental principle behind using arterial grafts is to provide durable conduits deployed with low morbidity and mortality. Current evidence suggests that arterial conduits have an equivalent or improved long-term patency and offer reduced long-term cardiovascular morbidity compared to saphenous vein (SV) grafts. Survival analysis of bilateral compared to single ITA grafting in non-randomised studies suggests that two ITA grafts are superior to one and are associated with a decreased risk of death, reoperation and angioplasty. Similarly, addition of the RA as a second or third arterial graft also appears to improve outcomes, with a number additional benefits compared to the SV. Characteristics of the RA that make it suitable for use as a bypass conduit and preferable to SV graft as the second or third conduit of choice are:

- ability to reach all coronary territories
- size match with the coronary arteries
- uniform caliber along length of graft
- ease of harvest
- low rate of wound complication including infections
- earlier patient ambulation
- improved patient satisfaction.

A potential complication of arterial graft harvesting is tissue ischemia. There are a number of relative contraindications to bilateral internal thoracic artery (BITA) harvesting which may increase a patient's risk of sternal ischemia and wound complications:

- obesity (BMI > 35)
- severe airways disease
- poorly controlled diabetes
- chest wall radiotherapy.

While skeletonization of the ITA can reduce this risk, some of these patients may only safely receive a single ITA supplemented with one or both RAs. Hand ischemia following RA harvest is rare with adequate preoperative assessment. In a study of 2417 patients who underwent RA removal, fingertip ischemia developed in only two individuals, one of whom suffered from scleroderma, a probable contraindication.

Despite the perceived increase in surgical complexity with extended and total arterial grafting techniques, early morbidity and mortality are low and there are increasing data that maximal arterial grafting improves long-term survival and reduces long-term cardiovascular morbidity.

PREOPERATIVE ASSESSMENT AND PREPARATION

General

Patients who present for coronary artery bypass surgery may have extensive medical comorbidity. Preoperative assessment should include special attention paid to the presence of peripheral vascular disease, which may predict calcification and atheroma in extrathoracic arterial conduits. A chest radiograph may identify chronic airways disease or other pulmonary pathology. Pulmonary function tests should be performed if there is a history of respiratory disease and bilateral ITA use is contemplated. Computed tomography (CT) scanning of the chest is helpful if aortic calcification is suspected and, if combined with CT coronary angiography in cases of reoperative surgery, can assess the relationship of major cardiac structures to the sternum and the location of previous bypass grafts.

Assessment of conduits

INTERNAL THORACIC ARTERY

The ITA is rarely affected by atherosclerosis, although mild intimal hyperplasia is common. The ITA is rarely discarded and in our experience can be used in 99% of patients. A major contraindication to the use of an *in situ* ITA is the presence of an aortic arch or subclavian artery atheroma. Patients who present for reoperation usually have their ITAs studied by CT angiography to exclude the possibility of injury from previous surgery.

RADIAL ARTERY

The RA has a relatively high prevalence of intimal disease compared with the ITA. Intimal atherosclerotic calcification may be seen in older patients, diabetics, and those with peripheral vascular disease. A modified Allen's test is used for screening all patients who are undergoing RA harvesting. When abnormal (>10 s) or borderline (5–9 s), Doppler ultrasound assessment of hand collateral circulation can be performed. Radial access coronary angiography (RA-CA) is becoming more common and may cause structural and functional damage to the RA. Whether it can be used as a bypass conduit after several months' delay is currently unknown. If its use is mandated due to a deficit of conduit, then ultrasound examination of the artery preoperatively may exclude stenosis or sites of occlusion and recannalization but does not exclude wall fibrosis and scarring.

SAPHENOUS VEIN

Although arterial grafting is preferred, all patients should have at least one leg prepared for SV harvesting in case suitable arterial grafts are not available.

Grafting strategy

Extended or total arterial grafting requires accurate preoperative planning. Compared with SV, there is a more limited supply of conduit and a greater degree of morbidity or potential risk attributable to conduit harvesting. Careful preoperative review of the angiogram is mandatory, for identification of targets, assessment of lesion severity to ensure that any composite Y or sequential grafts are bypassing balanced stenoses, and to estimate approximate distances between aorta and probable anastomotic sites (gauged by left ventriculography or echocardiographic measurements of heart size). Lesions in the left with more than 70% and right coronary systems more than 90% stenosis are suitable for arterial grafting.

Aortic calcification is also noted to predict whether it is appropriate to place proximals to the aorta, and any abnormality may be confirmed by intraoperative epiaortic scanning. In patients who have a severely diseased or calcified aorta, off-pump coronary bypass surgery using one or both *in situ* ITA grafts and an RA graft minimizes the risk of cerebral atheroembolism (**Figure 7.1**). The grafting strategy will depend upon all of these assessments, although the preoperative plan formulated is subject to change on examination of the epicardial vessels and the conduits which have been prepared.

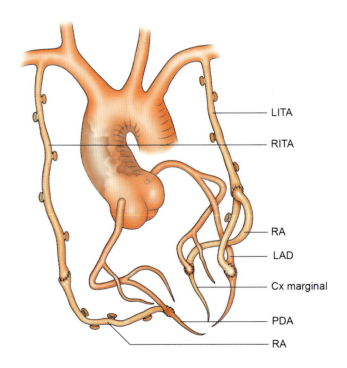

7.1

ANESTHESIA

A number of different anesthetic techniques can be used in patients who are being treated for coronary artery disease. The basic principles are to provide a narcotic-based relaxant anesthesia, with an inhalation agent supplemented as required. Heart rate control is particularly important, as intraoperative tachycardia is associated with myocardial ischemia. Cardiac output monitoring and transesophageal echocardiography inform the surgeon and anesthesia team to optimize managements, but these are not specific to arterial grafting techniques, except when use of a postoperative vasodilator (such as a phosphodiesterase inhibitor) is employed to prevent graft spasm.

OPERATION

Techniques for harvesting arteries

INTERNAL THORACIC ARTERY

Anatomy

The ITA arises from the first part of the subclavian artery in the root of the neck just above and behind the sternal end of the clavicle and descends anteromedially behind the internal thoracic, jugular and brachiocephalic veins. The phrenic nerve crosses the ITA obliquely from its medial to its lateral side, the nerve usually passing in front of the artery. The artery descends vertically 1 cm lateral to the sternal border, behind the first six costal cartilages, between the anterior intercostal membranes and internal intercostal muscles (**Figure 7.2a**). Down to the level of the second or third costal cartilage, the ITA is separated from the pleura by a strong layer of endothoracic fascia and inferiorly by the transversus thoracis muscle (**Figure 7.2b**). The ITA is accompanied by venae comitantes, which join to form a single vein at the level of the third costal cartilage; the internal thoracic vein ascends medial to the artery and terminates in the brachiocephalic vein; note that the right internal thoracic vein terminates at a lower level than the left internal thoracic vein. At the level of the sixth intercostal space, the ITA divides into terminal branches: the musculophrenic artery and the superior epigastric artery.

The pericardiacophrenic artery is the first branch of the ITA and usually divides near the upper limit of the mobilization of the ITA. This branch lies immediately behind the lateral or inferior border of the subclavian vein, where it accompanies and supplies the phrenic nerve. Several other branches arise from the upper ITA to supply the manubrium, the sternothyroid muscle, and the mediastinum.

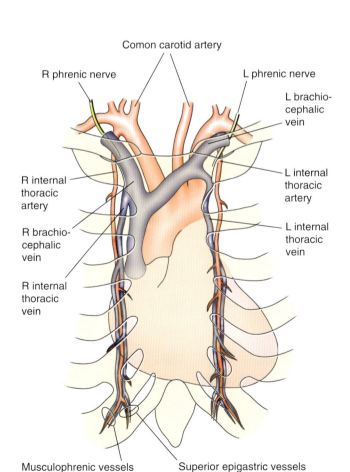

7.2a

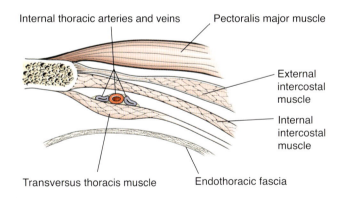

7.2b

In the anterior intercostal spaces, the perforating, sternal, and intercostal branches of the ITA form a rich anastomosis that supplies the sternum (**Figure 7.3**, modified from de Jesus RA, Acland RD. Anatomic study of the collateral blood supply of the sternum. *Ann Thorac Surg.* 1996; 59(1): 163–8). The ITA branches are connected with the posterior intercostal arteries and terminal branches of the superior, epigastric, and musculophrenic arteries. Branches should be divided near the ITA to preserve the collateral supply of the sternum and minimize the risk of sternal ischemia.

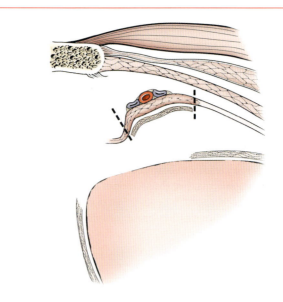

7.4a

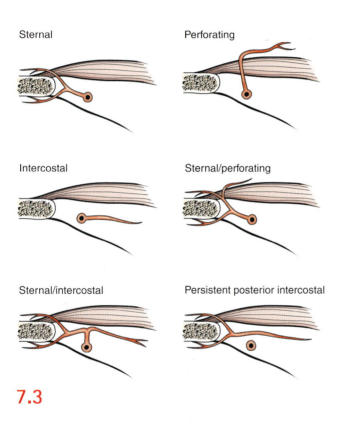

Sternal

Perforating

Intercostal

Sternal/perforating

Sternal/intercostal

Persistent posterior intercostal

7.3

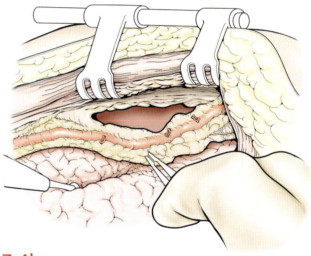

7.4b

Surgical technique

The ITA can be harvested using a pedicled, semiskeletonized or skeletonized technique. The hemisternum is elevated and the pleura separated from the chest wall to a point lateral to the ITA (**Figure 7.4a and b**). Skeletonization or semiskeletonization provides additional length compared to the pedicled method, with the added advantage of preserving the collateral blood supply of the chest wall (**Figure 7.5**). Our preference is skeletonization, which is particularly important in elderly and diabetic patients, in whom sternal ischemia is more likely to cause infection.

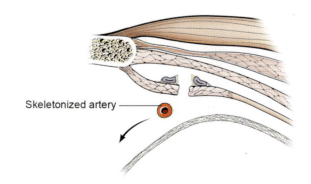

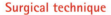
Skeletonized artery

7.5

Using low-power cautery, the fascia between the medial internal thoracic vein and the ITA is scored along its length and the ITA is exposed. The vein is pushed upwards to allow the development of a plane between it and the ITA (**Figure 7.6**). Grasping the lateral edge of the divided endothoracic allows for atraumatic retraction of the ITA while cautery is used to free its fibrous attachments and branches are divided with fine scissors between proximally and distally placed hemoclips.

The proximal extent of dissection is the upper border of the subclavian vein, at least above the branch to the first intercostal space (**Figure 7.7**). In the upper two intercostal spaces the ITA is separated from the pleura only by endothoracic fascia and, if the ITA is harvested carefully, the technique can be performed entirely extrapleurally. The dissection is extended distal to the level of the bifurcation into the musculophrenic or superior epigastric artery, and the latter ideally may be left intact if length is adequate.

The right ITA (RITA) is normally mobilized after the left side has been completed (**Figure 7.8a and b**). Because of the asymmetry of the heart, achieving the maximum length of the RITA is desirable so that left-sided coronary arteries or distal right coronary artery (RCA) branches can be anastomosed directly. The technique proceeds in a similar fashion to that of the left; however, at the proximal end, additional dissection is required to obtain maximal length. After the second and first perforating branches are divided, the ITA dissection is continued proximally until it disappears beneath the inferior border of the right brachiocephalic vein. Division of the right internal thoracic vein may be necessary for improved exposure of the proximal RITA. Division of the pericardiacophrenic, manubrial, sternothyroid, and mediastinal branches in the triangle formed by the ITA and internal thoracic vein and the phrenic nerve is important. Division of these branches and mobilization of the ITA above and behind the lower border of the brachiocephalic vein provides an additional 1 cm in length.

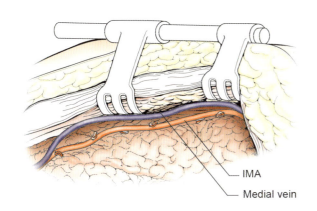

7.6

IMA
Medial vein

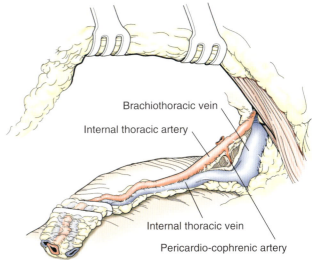

7.8a

Brachiothoracic vein
Internal thoracic artery
Internal thoracic vein
Pericardio-cophrenic artery

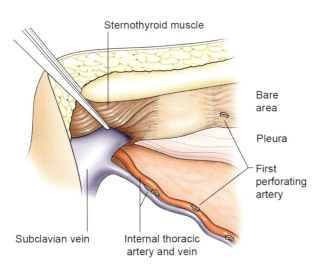

7.7

Sternothyroid muscle
Bare area
Pleura
First perforating artery
Subclavian vein
Internal thoracic artery and vein

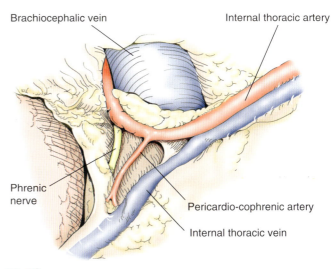

7.8b

Brachiocephalic vein
Internal thoracic artery
Phrenic nerve
Pericardio-cophrenic artery
Internal thoracic vein

Following harvest of the left ITA (LITA) and/or RITA and after systemic heparinization, the ITA may be divided distally. The distal end is clipped to allow the artery to distend under systemic arterial pressure, a vasodilating solution is applied and we store the ITA in a warm blood-based solution in a syringe or soaked swab until required. A vasodilator solution is used topically and for storage of arterial grafts and can be mixed 50/50 with heparinized blood or Ringer's lactate solution if required:

- Ringer's lactate 150 mL
- heparin 5000 IU
- papaverine 120 mg (1 mM).

RADIAL ARTERY

Anatomy

The RA arises from the bifurcation of the brachial artery in the cubital fossa and terminates by forming the deep palmar arch in the hand. It lies immediately beneath the deep fascia, surrounded by collateral veins. The brachioradialis muscle and the lateral cutaneous nerve of the forearm cover its proximal portion. The terminal sensory branch of the radial nerve lies immediately lateral to the proximal third of the RA (**Figure 7.9**).

The RA has a number of anatomical variations. The most common and important variation is the high origin of the RA, which occurs in 14% of upper limbs. In these patients, the RA is found to originate from the proximal half of the brachial artery in 11%, with 2% arising from the axillary artery and 1% from the distal brachial artery above the cubital fossa. In the forearm, the position of the artery is usually constant.

Anastomoses at the wrist and hand vary. In a previous anatomical study, the superficial palmar arch of the ulnar artery was found to provide the blood supply to all fingers in 67% of hands. The "classic" type of superficial palmar arch, in which the superficial branch of the RA joins the superficial palmar arch of the ulnar artery, was found to be relatively uncommon (12.5%). The complete deep palmar arch, in which continuity exists between the deep palmar branches of the radial and ulnar arteries, was found in 87.5% of hands. However, every hand had at least one major branch connecting the radial and the ulnar arteries.

Three structures may be damaged during harvesting: the lateral cutaneous nerves of the forearm, the superficial branch of the radial nerve, and the deep branch of the radial nerve. Damage to this latter structure, although rare, can cause serious complications, as it provides the motor supply to the extensor muscles of the forearm. Care should be taken when dissecting the proximal part of the RA to avoid deep retraction proximally toward the brachial artery.

Surgical technique

The artery is exposed through an incision overlying and slightly medial to the RA (**Figure 7.10a**). After the deep fascia is divided, the RA can be seen with its paired venae comitantes. To mobilize the RA, the deep fascia should be divided just lateral to the tendon of the flexor carpi radialis muscle (**Figure 7.10b**). A few small branches pass vertically

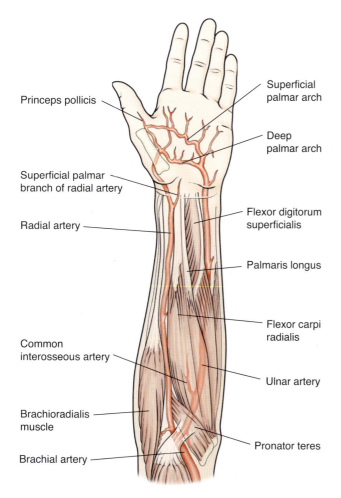

Princeps pollicis

Superficial palmar arch

Deep palmar arch

Superficial palmar branch of radial artery

Radial artery

Flexor digitorum superficialis

Palmaris longus

Common interosseous artery

Flexor carpi radialis

Ulnar artery

Brachioradialis muscle

Pronator teres

Brachial artery

7.9

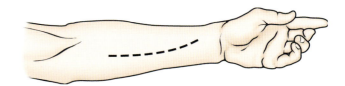

7.10a

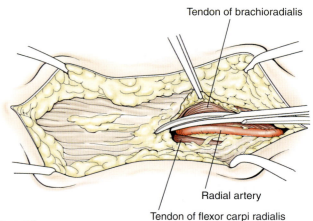

Tendon of brachioradialis

Radial artery

Tendon of flexor carpi radialis

7.10b

and supply the brachioradialis muscle. These branches may cause a hematoma if damaged. The RA is semiskeletonized and is mobilized with its venae comitantes. Side branches are divided between metal clips and clipped close to the artery, whereas smaller branches can be cauterized. Experience with ultrasonic shears (Harmonic Focus®; Ethicon Endo-Surgery Inc., Cincinnati, OH) to harvest the RA has been encouraging, being both expeditious and atraumatic. The use of endoscopic RA harvesting is also becoming more common and, while we have limited experience with this technique, non-randomized observational reports have suggested that this is a safe alternative to open harvest.

The distal end of the RA is divided approximately 2 cm above the wrist, after the distal end of the wound is elevated. The proximal end of the RA can be followed to the bifurcation of the brachial artery (**Figure 7.11**). The bifurcation is heralded by the presence of the radial recurrent artery and a complex of large veins. Once the distal end has been divided, a solution of papaverine mixed with an equal amount of blood or Ringer's lactate may be injected into the distal end of the artery. The distal end is then clipped and allowed to dilate under arterial pressure while the upper end of the dissection is completed. The RA is usually divided approximately 1 cm distal to the bifurcation of the brachial artery; if extra length is required, the recurrent branch can be divided. The RA is then flushed with and subsequently stored in the papaverine solution until required.

ULNAR ARTERY

Occasionally, when we have had no other choice, we have used the ulnar artery as a bypass conduit. The ulnar artery has been found to be a satisfactory alternative in a few patients. The major concern with removing the ulnar artery is its proximity to the ulnar nerve, which supplies the intrinsic muscles of the hand. Direct trauma or ischemia may cause an ulnar nerve palsy. For this reason, use of the ulnar artery has been discontinued.

GASTROEPIPLOIC ARTERY

The gastroepiploic artery is sometimes used as a third *in situ* arterial graft when the ITA cannot reach the posterior surface artery of the heart or when other conduits are not available.

Anatomy

The right gastroepiploic artery (RGEA) is the largest terminal branch of the gastroduodenal artery. The RGEA lies between the posterior surface of the duodenum and the anterior surface of the pancreas and travels along the greater curvature of the stomach between the two layers of the greater omentum, along with the gastroepiploic veins. The RGEA terminates by anastomosing with the left gastroepiploic artery, which arises from the splenic artery near the hilum of the spleen (**Figure 7.12**).

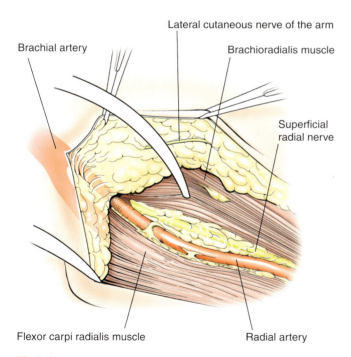

Brachial artery
Lateral cutaneous nerve of the arm
Brachioradialis muscle
Superficial radial nerve
Flexor carpi radialis muscle
Radial artery

7.11

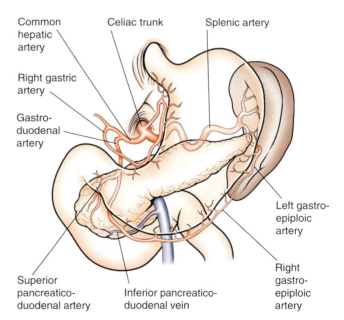

Common hepatic artery
Celiac trunk
Splenic artery
Right gastric artery
Gastro-duodenal artery
Left gastro-epiploic artery
Superior pancreatico-duodenal artery
Inferior pancreatico-duodenal vein
Right gastro-epiploic artery

7.12

Surgical technique

The median sternotomy incision is extended inferiorly for a further 5 cm. Following ITA harvesting, the peritoneum is opened to expose the stomach. The RGEA is seen along the greater curvature of the stomach. A nasogastric tube is used to empty the stomach. The gastroepiploic artery is palpated so that its size can be evaluated. The RGEA and pedicle, including the veins, are detached from the omentum, and the branches are ligated with silk, a metal clip or with the use of an ultrasonic scalpel. Usually, the RGEA is removed from the lower two-thirds of the greater curvature of the stomach, extending distally but not beyond the pylorus. Further dissection may cause injury to the superior pancreaticoduodenal artery. The RGEA pedicle can be introduced into the pericardial cavity anteriorly or by a posterior route through a 2–3 cm hole in the diaphragm. The posterior or retrogastric approach has been advocated to reduce the risk of graft injury at reoperation for a cardiac or abdominal procedure. The RGEA artery is usually grafted to an artery on the inferior wall of the heart.

INFERIOR EPIGASTRIC ARTERY

The size and length of the inferior epigastric artery (IEA) vary and, in many patients, when it is used alone, the length is not sufficient for an independent graft. The IEA is probably best used as a composite graft with the LITA, either as a Y- or extension graft. This is a very rarely used conduit.

Grafting procedure

The final plan of how best to deploy the arterial grafts is made after harvesting, following assessment of the epicardial targets. **Figure 7.13a–e** summarizes the principle grafting configurations. Assuming triple-vessel disease, the configuration depends upon the selection of the best conduit for the LAD. Traditionally, the LITA has been regarded as the gold-standard graft for the left anterior descending (LAD). The LITA may also form the basis for a sequential or Y-graft to a diagonal branch if the latter is separately diseased, or in order to backfill the mid LAD where tandem LAD lesions

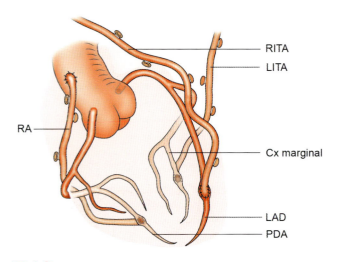

7.13a

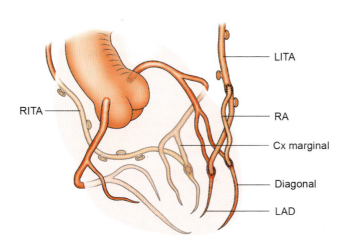

7.13b

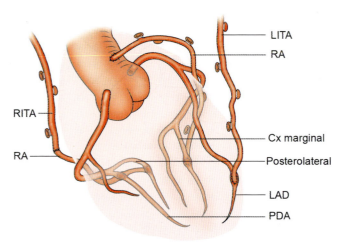

7.13c

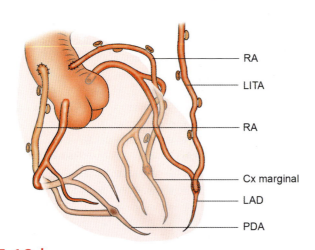

7.13d

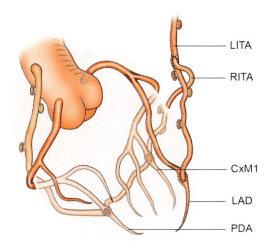

LITA

RITA

CxM1

LAD

PDA

7.13e

exist. Under this standard configuration, a mid or distal circumflex (Cx) marginal branch may be grafted with an *in situ* RITA passed posteriorly through the transverse sinus, a relatively complex maneuver. Alternatively, it may be passed across the midline deep to the thymic fat, lying on the innominate vein, to reach the left side where it then runs into the pericardium adjacent to the LITA to run to a proximal marginal branch lying close to the left atrial appendage. Any second obtuse marginal branch may be grafted with an aortocoronary RA graft, or as a Y-graft off the RITA using an RA fragment. Finally, the posterior descending or posterolateral branch of the RCA may be grafted with an aortocoronary RA graft, or with an *in situ* gastroepiploic artery in centers with expertise in this.

Our preference is to utilize a simpler configuration, grafting the LAD with the *in situ* RITA (**Figure 7.13a**). The RITA has the same patency as the LITA in our and others' published experience when grafted to the LAD, is histologically identical, and is commonly larger in caliber and flow. It may be passed across the midline deep to the thymic fat, as described above. From here it may graft to the mid LAD singly, or a Y-graft may be run from it to a diagonal branch. Using this configuration, the *in situ* LITA may now be used to graft one or more marginal branches of the Cx singly, sequentially, or using a Y-graft of RA off it to the second target. The revascularization is completed with an aortocoronary RA graft to the terminal branch of the RCA or, more rarely, an *in situ* gastroepiploic artery may serve this role.

A third configuration is to graft the LAD with the *in situ* LITA in a standard manner and use the *in situ* RITA to graft the RCA. However, use of this conduit *in situ* to the main RCA has been associated with disappointing patency of around 60% in our experience, likely due to competitive flow in the large-bore native RCA. An alternative is to use a fragment of RA anastomosed end to end to the RITA to extend the *in situ* conduit, in order to reach the posterior descending artery, where there is less risk of competitive flow. However, we believe that the reported prognostic advantage afforded by use of bilateral *in situ* internal thoracic arteries arises when used to graft the left coronary circulation, so the RITA may not be used to its best effect in this configuration.

When use of bilateral internal thoracic arteries is contraindicated, total arterial revascularization may still be achieved by use of LITA and bilateral radial arteries. Using this complement, the LAD will be grafted with the *in situ* LITA and aortocoronary radial arteries may be run to the obtuse marginal branch or branches of the Cx and the terminal branch of the RCA. If additional arterial conduit is required to provide an extra Y limb to a supplementary target, a short segment of distal RITA may be removed proximal to the bifurcation into musculophrenic arteries and superior epigastric arteries and, provided its length is limited to 2–3 cm, this should not significantly affect perfusion of the right hemisternum from the proximal subtotal RITA.

Fourth-order targets include diagonal branches, or individually diseased obtuse marginal branches of the Cx, or terminal branches of the RCA, all of which may require supplementary grafting. This can sometimes be easiest achieved with a separate aortocoronary graft using a fourth arterial conduit where both ITAs and radial arteries are available. However, when only three conduits are available, supplementary grafts may be performed via sequential or composite grafting techniques. The advantages of the sequential method include conduit preservation and the requirement for fewer anastomoses and possibly therefore shorter operative time or cross-clamp time. This may be offset by the relative technical difficulty of the side-to-side anastomosis, with the potential to compromise two targets if a technical error is made. Importantly, sequential grafts, with fixed locations mid graft rather than just at the proximal and distal ends, are less able to find their own lie within the chest and may be liable to kinking at the side-to-side anastomosis unless the length and orientation of the graft segments on the beating, closed-chest heart are near perfect, which can be difficult to gauge on an arrested elevated heart. Proponents of Y-grafting techniques argue that the proximal anastomosis can be performed prepump, and therefore the number of anastomoses under cross-clamp is not increased, and there are the advantages of being able to check satisfactory flow in both limbs thereafter prior to commencement of the revascularization procedure. Furthermore, the Y-graft has greater capacity to find its own optimal lie within the chest, and kinking is less likely unless lengths and lie are significantly distorted. Finally, all distal anastomoses can be performed as a standard end-to-side in-line manner, which is less liable to technical error.

In the Y-graft the fragment of conduit is implanted in line with the main trunk, while in the T-graft implantation is perpendicular to it. Each has its proponents, but it is important that the length of the segment being implanted into the main trunk is measured so that it is appropriate to the angle of the anastomosis. In general, a Y configuration will employ a more proximal Y anastomosis and a longer limb, which takes a lazy lie. A T-graft usually has a shorter limb emerging more distally on the common stem opposite its target, running perpendicular to the main trunk and coursing directly to its distal anastomosis. The lengths and lie must be adjusted accordingly.

Irrespective of whether the procedure is performed on or off pump, it may be possible and advantageous to construct composite grafts prior to commencement of the revascularization stage. However, such preparatory construction of composite grafts requires some familiarity with the optimum lie of grafts and some experience to judge the distances, so that Y limbs are not too short (placing anastomoses or the common trunk under tension) nor too long (encouraging kinking). For off-pump surgery it may be desirable to construct any proximal anastomoses on the aorta via a partial occlusive clamp or occlusive device such as the Heartstring (Maquet Getting Group, Germany) prior to the

revascularization, in order to gain immediate reperfusion following completion of each distal anastomosis, but again this requires some familiarity to judge lengths appropriately, particularly when composite or sequential grafts are employed.

Anastomosis techniques

DISTAL ANASTOMOSIS (END-TO-SIDE TECHNIQUE)

A 4–5 mm coronary arteriotomy (two or three times the diameter of the native coronary artery) is placed at the point that is free from disease. The end of the arterial graft is fashioned so that the circumference of the graft just exceeds that of the native coronary artery (**Figure 7.14a–c**).

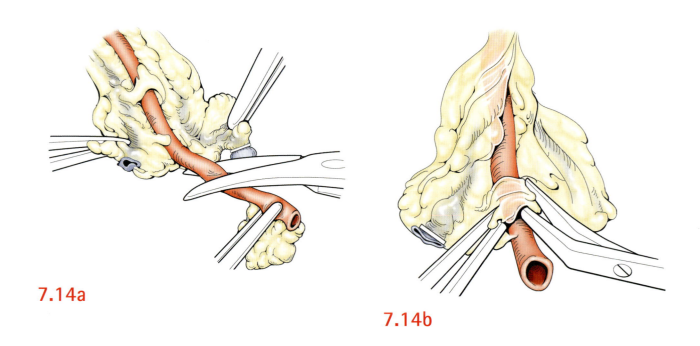

7.14a

7.14b

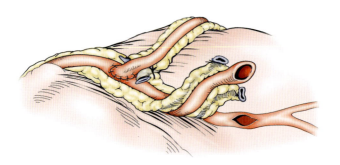

7.14c

The native coronary artery is orientated away from the surgeon. Through the use of a two-arm suture the anastomosis is commenced at the proximal end of the coronary arteriotomy at the point furthest from the surgeon (**Figure 7.15a**). One suture is passed from the lumen to the exterior of the coronary artery and clipped (**Figure 7.15b**); the other arm is placed through the heel of the arterial graft (**Figure 7.15c**). After two or three sutures have been inserted, the graft is then approximated to the native vessel. Suturing, using a forehand technique, is then continued from outside to inside the lumen of the coronary artery until the distal end

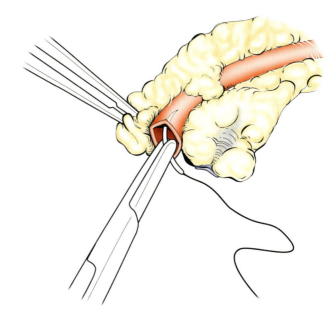

7.15b

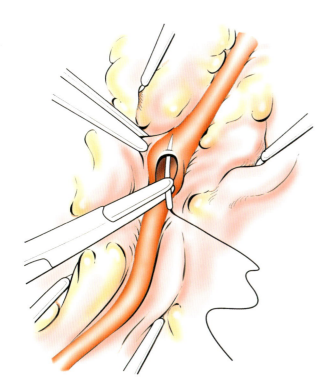

7.15a

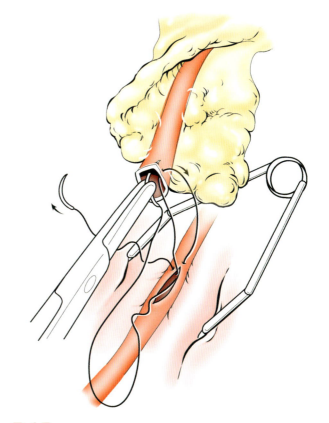

7.15c

of the arteriotomy is reached (**Figure 7.15d**). The apex of the graft is rotated to expose the distal end of the arteriotomy. Commencing proximally, the surgeon sews the second suture from outside the graft through the anastomosis to the outside of the coronary artery. This suture is continued to the distal end of the anastomosis (**Figure 7.15e**). Placement of the apical sutures at the distal end is facilitated by traction on the last loop of the first suture.

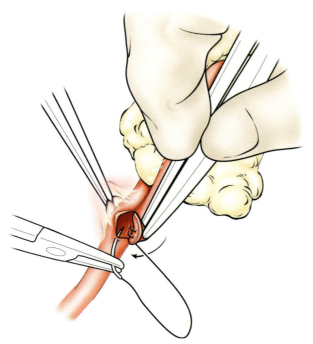

7.15d

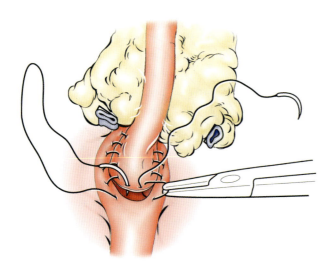

7.15e

SEQUENTIAL ANASTOMOSIS (SIDE-TO-SIDE TECHNIQUES)

Sequential anastomoses conserve the length of arterial conduits by increasing the number of distal anastomoses. This may be performed in line (parallel) for a diagonal target or at 30, 60, or 90 degrees off the axis of the coronary target (diamond anastomosis) for sequential grafts to the Cx or right coronary branches.

Parallel technique

The technique of a parallel anastomosis is almost identical to the standard technique used for an end-to-side anastomosis. This technique is suited to anastomosing the LAD with its diagonal branch, when the latter is closely aligned to the LAD. A parallel anastomosis may require an additional length of conduit to avoid tension between the anastomotic points, and to allow the conduit to take a lazy S lie. This technique is not suitable for proximal or laterally placed diagonal branches where angulation may occur at the site of the side-to-side anastomosis. In these cases Y-grafting is preferable.

The site for anastomosis of the LITA with the diagonal branch is chosen with the heart distended and lying in its normal position. Sufficient length of ITA proximal to the side-to-side anastomosis should be left so that the heart can be elevated without putting tension on the graft. The first sutures are placed from within the native vessel and graft and are continued using a forehand technique down the left side of the anastomosis to the heel (**Figure 7.16**). The distal (free) end of the ITA graft is elevated to facilitate placement of the

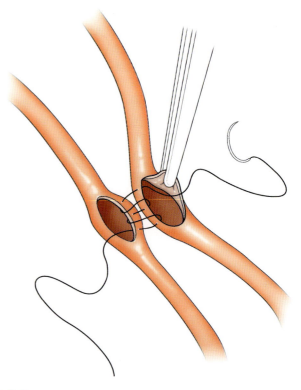

7.16

heel sutures. The second suture is then continued down the medial side of the anastomosis to the heel, where the two ends are tied. A stay suture is placed distal to the side-to-side anastomosis to maintain the alignment of the LITA graft. The end-to-side anastomosis between the distal LITA and the LAD completes the sequential graft.

Diamond technique

The diamond technique is useful for grafting the Cx marginal coronary artery branches, which lie parallel and are close to one another, and also for grafting the posterolateral and posterior descending branches of the RCA. Diamond-shaped anastomoses are necessary when graft length is insufficient to create the loops that are required for the parallel technique. The distance between the end-to-side and end-to-end anastomoses is judged by either distending the heart or grasping the pericardium with forceps and stretching it to its natural limit. A few extra millimeters of length in the graft allow space for inspecting the end-to-end and the end-to-side anastomoses and provide additional length if the left ventricle becomes overdistended.

The arteriotomies should be small to avoid distortion of the native artery or the graft at the site of the anastomosis. In general, the length of the arteriotomies should be similar to or only marginally greater than the diameter of the native coronary artery or conduit. The side-to-side anastomosis can be performed before or after the end-to-side technique.

Our preference when grafting the marginal branches is to perform the distal anastomosis first and then to allow the graft to rotate away from the surgeon to expose the site for the side-to-side anastomosis (**Figure 7.17**). The proximal anastomosis is performed last. Suturing is commenced at a point farthest from the surgeon, at the apex of the native coronary artery. Three or four sutures are placed before the graft and native vessels are approximated. The lateral side of the anastomosis is sutured to the distal end of the native arteriotomy. Elevation of the graft as the suture is continued around the right-hand side of the anastomosis, finishing at the point nearest the surgeon, facilitates this maneuver. The other suture is used to complete the anastomosis. The suture is tied after the graft is distended with blood to minimize the risk of stricture or narrowing of the anastomosis. Occluding the vessel beyond the anastomosis checks hemostasis. Additional tacking sutures are not usually required with a diamond technique.

PROXIMAL ANASTOMOSIS

Aortic anastomosis

The anastomosis is commenced on the aorta at a point furthest from the surgeon, using a monofilament suture and a forehand technique. The heel sutures are placed through the aorta and the graft. The right side of the anastomosis is completed using a forehand technique. The left side is then completed and the anastomosis tied at its apex.

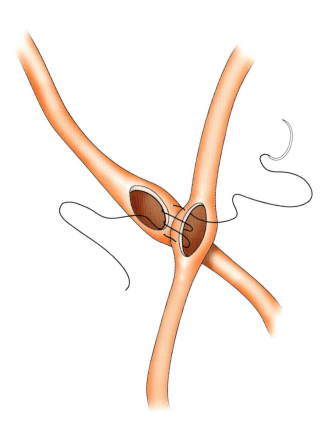

7.17

Left internal thoracic artery: Y-graft

The anastomosis is performed on the chest wall side of the LITA, at a point just distal to its entry into the pericardial cavity. With experience it is possible to construct such composite grafts prior to establishment of cardiopulmonary bypass (CPB). The LITA is placed on the left side of the skin incision. A 4–5 mm incision is made in the ITA and the arterial free graft (AFG; e.g. RA or a segment of distal ITA) is then cut obliquely and the arteriotomy matched to that of the ITA. Suturing is usually commenced at the distal end of the ITA and the free graft (the heel of the anastomosis) and continued proximally using a forehand technique (**Figure 7.18**). The proximal sutures are placed more accurately if the free graft is elevated to expose the toe. The suture line is completed using a forehand technique down the opposite side of the anastomosis to the toe, where the sutures are tied.

Graft extension

If the length of the RITA is insufficient to reach the terminal branches of the RCA, a segment of AFG can be used to extend the RITA graft to the distal target artery. The technique of extension grafting often only requires a short length of an AFG to reach either the posterior descending or posterolateral branch of the RCA without tension.

The distal end of the RITA and proximal end of the AFG are transected at an approximate 45-degree angle after having been dilated previously with the papaverine solution. Suturing is usually commenced at the apex of the AFG, which is joined to the heel of the *in situ* ITA graft (**Figure 7.19**). Sutures continue around the left side of the anastomosis to the apex. Rotating the anastomosis through 180 degrees exposes the sutures in the heel of the free graft. The second suture is placed along the opposite side of the anastomosis, and the sutures are tied after release of the clamp to distend the pedicle. Additional stay sutures are placed on either side of the anastomosis to prevent rotation at the anastomotic site. Distal flow is checked before the terminal end-to-side anastomosis is commenced.

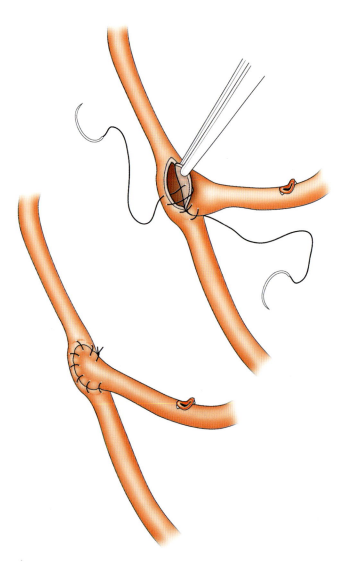

7.18

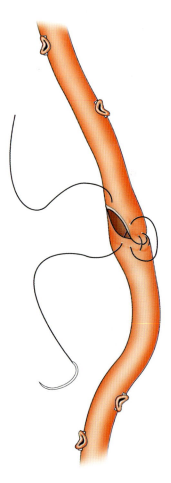

7.19

POSTOPERATIVE CARE

In patients who have arterial grafts, it is important to maintain a mean systemic blood pressure of greater than 70 mmHg with a cardiac index in excess of 2.5 L/m^2. In those patients in whom the cardiac index is low (less than 2.5 L/m^2), our preference, after satisfactory volume loading, is to use a low-dose inodilator such as milrinone (phosphodiesterase III inhibitor), which enhances myocardial contractility and arterial dilatation. Alternatively, nitroglycerin, which also relaxes vascular muscle, can be used. We have not observed any graft spasm in patients who have been given topical as well as systemic vasodilators. In patients who are excessively vasodilated and have a high cardiac index, or cannot increase their cardiac output sufficiently to compensate, noradrenaline (norepinephrine) may be required to achieve a mean arterial pressure of 70–80 mmHg and a normal systemic vascular resistance.

OUTCOME

The *in situ* left or right ITA, when grafted to the LAD or Cx marginal, has reported patency of 90–95% at 10 years. When grafted to the distal main RCA or posterior descending branch, patency of the *in situ* RITA is reduced (80% and 89% at 10 years respectively). Studies comparing the RITA with the RA as a second arterial conduit have yielded conflicting results, reflecting the difficulty in controlling for all variables and bias. The Arterial Revascularization Trial (ART), a multicenter international randomized controlled trial, is in progress and, once completed, will provide the definitive comparison of long-term outcomes of single vs bilateral ITA grafting. Patency of AFGs including the RA has been reported to be 92.5% at both 5 and 7 years. Several randomized trials comparing combinations of RA, free RITA, and SV have shown encouraging early results but, until the 10-year results of the Radial Artery Patency and Clinical Outcomes (RAPCO) randomized trial become available, no direct comparisons of the late patency of AFG and SV grafts exist. Recent metanalysis however does suggest the superior medium term patency and clinical outcomes in favour of RA over SVG. Importantly, follow-up angiography in our unit and elsewhere suggests that the use of arterial conduits may be associated with reduced native vessel disease progression when compared to the use of vein grafts, which may be the primary benefit in terms of improved long-term survival.

Arterial grafting techniques have been in use in our unit for over 20 years. We have performed coronary artery bypass grafting using one or more arterial grafts in 11 700 patients with excellent results. Three-vessel disease was present in 6059 patients. Among 11 700 patients, 3167 received a RITA graft and over 10 300 received one or more RA grafts. Just 23 ulnar arteries were employed. Mortality overall has been 1.6%, perioperative myocardial infarction 0.8%, sternal infection 1.1% and harvest site complication 0.9%, confirming that a strategy of complex arterial grafting need not increase perioperative risk. In our experience extended or total arterial grafting techniques have resulted in superior graft patency, fewer harvest site complications and, most importantly, superior event-free survival.

Extended and total arterial grafting using one or both ITAs supplemented with RAs is achievable in most patients. It requires careful preoperative planning, meticulous harvesting and anastomotic techniques, and some skill and experience in judging optimum length, lie, and orientation of conduits, particularly when combined together. Once mastered, these techniques will lead to improved long-term survival and cardiovascular outcomes.

ACKNOWLEDGEMENTS

The authors wish to acknowledge the help of Dr William Shi and Beth Croce in preparing this chapter.

FURTHER READING

Athanasiou T, Saso S, Rao C, et al. Radial artery versus saphenous vein conduits for coronary artery bypass surgery: forty years of competition – which conduit offers better patency? A systematic review and meta-analysis. *Eur J Cardiothorac Surg.* 2011; 40: 208–20.

Buxton BF, Galvin SD. The history of arterial revascularization: from Kolesov to Tector and beyond. *Ann Cardiothorac Surg.* 2013; 2(4): 419–26.

Hayward PA, Buxton BF. Mid-term results of the Radial Artery Patency and Clinical Outcomes randomized trial. *Ann Cardiothorac Surg.* 2013; 2(4): 458–66.

Lytle BW. Bilateral internal thoracic artery grafting. *Ann Cardiothorac Surg.* 2013; 2(4): 485–92.

Taggart DP, Altman DG, Gray AM, et al. Randomized trial to compare bilateral vs. single internal mammary coronary artery bypass grafting: 1-year results of the Arterial Revascularisation Trial (ART). *Eur Heart J.* 2010; 31(20): 2470–81.

Tatoulis J, Buxton BF, Fuller JA. The right internal thoracic artery: forgotten conduit, 5,766 patients and 991 angiograms. *Ann Thorac Surg.* 2011; 92: 9–17.

8

Reoperative coronary artery bypass grafting

MURRAY H. KWON AND RICHARD J. SHEMIN

HISTORY

Since its inception during the late 1950s, coronary artery bypass grafting (CABG) has become commonplace. Given the vast number of these procedures performed over the last half century and the known limitations of vein graft patency, it is surprising to find that reoperative CABG has declined in the modern era to as low as 2.2% of all CABGs performed.[1] There are multiple reasons for this including the increased use of arterial grafts, the effectiveness of percutaneous coronary intervention (PCI), and the availability of newer and better antilipid and antiplatelet drug options. An important factor driving the growth of PCI is that the risks of reoperative CABG remain high. Operative mortality, myocardial infarction, and prolonged ventilation occur at significantly higher rates in this group. The risks of injury to the heart as well as patent bypass grafts are always a concern and the presence of scar tissue as well as the progression of native coronary artery disease (CAD) can make the technical feasibility of reoperative CABG challenging.

PRINCIPLES AND JUSTIFICATION

Given the above, there are distinct considerations that must be made when evaluating a candidate for reoperative CABG that are not present when considering first-time operations. This chapter will highlight key points in patient evaluation, selection, operative technique, and postoperative management to maximize chances for a favorable risk–benefit ratio in this challenging group.

PREOPERATIVE ASSESSMENT AND PREPARATION

Every operation must be approached with the following strategic objectives in mind:

1. What are the prospects that successful revascularization will alleviate the chief complaint?

2. What precautions need to be taken to ensure safe sternal re-entry?
3. What is the quality of target vessels for bypass?
4. What is the adequacy of conduits, i.e. internal mammary artery (IMA) if it was not previously utilized as well as remaining vein and arterial vessels?
5. What is the plan for old saphenous vein grafts (SVGs) with varying levels of patency?

It is helpful to know the indications for which revascularization is being considered. Most patients will present for surgical evaluation following coronary angiogram. This study may have been obtained following non-invasive studies for patient complaints of recurrent angina. It may also have been performed emergently in a patient suffering acute coronary syndrome. Or it may be the final workup in a patient presenting with worsening ischemic cardiomyopathy and heart failure symptoms. This latter group is particularly high risk.

Thus, while the coronary angiogram is of critical importance to all CABG cases, certain patients may require further workup to ascertain myocardial viability. Institutional and surgeon preferences will dictate whether positron emission tomography (PET), cardiac magnetic resonance imaging (CMR), and/or dobutamine stress echo are utilized. It is important to become familiar and adept with reading the study of choice as there are few situations as futile as bypassing non-viable myocardium.

One must assess from the angiogram any potential clues as to why a graft may now be occluded. If the patient has exceedingly poor targets with minimal run-off, there is little to indicate that reattempting bypass will be successful. Alternatively, the appearance of a stricture at the anastomotic site, with an otherwise patent target vessel, is a reassuring finding. Know the options for conduits. Was a left internal mammary graft already utilized? If so, and it is now occluded, or exhibiting the so-called "string sign," would a right IMA be available and considered for usage on the left anterior descending (LAD)?

One may find that certain parts of the heart are exceedingly difficult to access due to adhesions. Having knowledge with regards to which vessels are collateralizing and which are collateralized may be helpful when the prospects of full revascularization become less likely due to intraoperative difficulties with scar tissue. Bypassing the former may be a judicious compromise in these circumstances.

One must know whether there are suitable remaining vein and arterial conduits that can be utilized. Vein and radial arterial ultrasound to assess vessel caliber and quality in addition to flow in the palmar arch (Allen's test) in the latter are helpful in delineating the conduit options.

An echocardiogram will be critical towards establishing myocardial function and the presence of concomitant valvular pathology. We routinely obtain non-contrast CT scans of the chest to ascertain anatomy and highlight any specific concerns that may be present on re-entry, such as proximity of the aorta or other cardiac structures. When the angiogram does not give sufficient clarity with respect to the trajectory of the LIMA graft, a CT scan is often helpful as, even in a non-contrast enhanced image, it is possible to follow the surgical clips present on the vessel to make sure they are remote from the midline. In summary, when evaluating a patient for reoperative CABG, it is critical to note the patient's condition, myocardial viability, targets, conduits, and anatomy.

OPERATION

Redo sternotomy

Safe sternal re-entry is critical to success and every measure must be employed to avoid beginning a complex procedure with a divergent path to address injury associated with the redo sternotomy. The preoperative imaging will have documented important details such as the proximity of the ascending aorta, innominate vein, right ventricle, and/or pedicled mammary artery in addition to detailing any calcifications which might render aortic manipulation or cross-clamping perilous.

It is the authors' strong belief that plans for alternate cannulation need to be formulated *a priori* to avoid catastrophe associated with either bleeding or intractable arrhythmias that are best managed with expeditious institution of cardiopulmonary bypass (CPB).

Draping of the patient must be wide and extensive to fully reflect this philosophy. Both the common femoral and axillary arteries provide excellent alternatives and the selection of which to use must be made according to the patient's anatomy. The benefit of groin cannulation (**Figure 8.1**) is relative expediency as the vessel merely needs to be exposed. Severe peripheral vascular disease, or the presence of bulky mural thrombus in the descending thoracic aorta which might embolize into the cerebrovascular tree with retrograde flow from below, might prompt one to consider an axillary

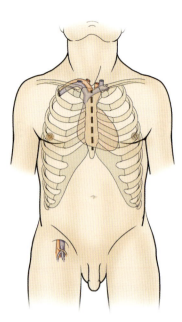

8.1

approach. The disadvantages of an axillary cannula are that many feel most comfortable with the placement of a Dacron graft versus direct cannulation of the vessel itself. This takes additional time and does require the initiation of some level of anticoagulation up front to prevent graft thrombosis possibly leading to increased bleeding. Preferential flow to the ipsilateral upper extremity is also something to be aware of when considering this approach.

In rare cases, such as adherence of an aorta to the posterior table of the sternum, it may be necessary to heparinize the patient and initiate CPB as well as cooling to prepare for hypothermic circulatory arrest prior to sternal opening. As this greatly extends the CPB time as well as bleeding risk associated with earlier systemic heparinization, the decision to employ this strategy must be made carefully, especially if there is any degree of aortic insufficiency.

If an axillary arterial cannulation approach is selected, an incision is made one finger breadth below the clavicle extending approximately 7 cm medial to the deltopectoral groove. The pectoralis major muscle fibers are divided and the pectoralis minor is partially divided. Care must be taken to avoid injury to the brachial plexus, which must be handled gently. In obese patients, a deep self-retaining retractor and a hand-held Doppler can be useful in locating the vessel. Once it is dissected free and encircled, 5000 units of intravenous heparin are administered and, after 3 minutes, a C-clamp is placed. The vessel is opened longitudinally and an 8 mm Dacron graft is sewn end to side, which will later accommodate the arterial cannula of choice. After decannulation, the graft can be clamped and oversewn, thus patching the axillary artery.

Once cannulation preparations have been made, the old scar is incised (**Figure 8.2**). Clipped wires are left in place to provide tactile feedback when the oscillating saw breaches the posterior table of the sternum. Another approach is to divide up to the posterior table and then utilize heavy scissors to gently divide this final layer under direct vision. It is very important in this approach that the scissor tips are not directed down into the myocardium to avoid injury.

Upon successful sternal division, the process of dissection of the mediastinal contents off the posterior table can begin (**Figure 8.3a and b**). Either electrocautery or sharp dissection can be utilized. We perform electrocautery to have a dry surgical field and reduce postoperative bleeding.

Blunt dissection has absolutely no role in cardiac surgery at any time. The assistant must be careful not to inadvertently tear the underlying structures with overexuberant anterior retraction. Success begets success and one will find as the dissection proceeds laterally that the heart and other structures will fall away out of the immediate area of risk. Knowledge of where the IMA lies is critical to avoid injury. While many feel only a few centimeters are needed to place a retractor, it is our belief that further mobilization, when safe, is advantageous as it reduces the risk of tearing upon opening a retractor and often makes subsequent exposure of the remote lateral wall easier. At other times, however, the extent of adhesions makes early CPB followed by dissection the safer and more expeditious choice.

Should one encounter myocardial bleeding it is imperative to avoid the temptation to open the retractor further as this will only exacerbate the injury. In fact, one of the first maneuvers should be to counterintuitively close the retractor a few turns as this will allow for less traction on the tear. Success of repair is then contingent upon mobilizing adhesions adjacent to the injury which will allow for a tension-free suture. The use of Hegar dilators is often helpful to tamponade bleeding and allow time for accurate and effectual suture placement. It is very important, however, to know when repair attempts are futile and when one must quickly establish CPB to enable safe repair and resumption of the original intended operation.

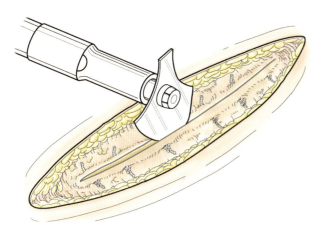
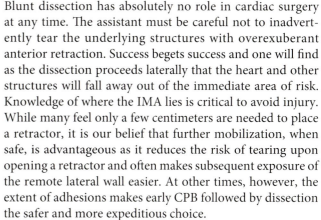

8.2

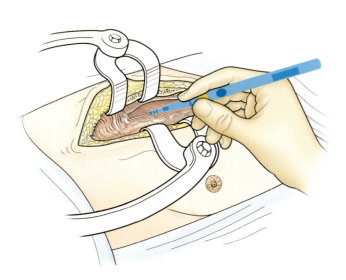

8.3a

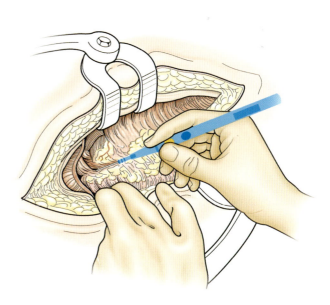

8.3b

A cautionary word when dissecting free the ascending aorta is warranted (**Figure 8.4**). Beware the overly "clean" dissection plane as this often connotes an exarterectomization of the vessel. This leaves behind an exceedingly fragile partial medial and intimal layer that can rupture either at that time or with subsequent minimal manipulation. A true plane is usually identified by its rather tenacious nature. One should know which of the vein grafts originating off the aorta are patent to avoid their injury or the risk of distal embolization of thrombotic material. In certain cases, when atheromatous vein graft disease is known to exist, transecting them early to avoid potential distal embolization of debris with their manipulation should be considered. Enough aorta needs to be dissected to allow ample room for safe cannulation, aortic root vent/cardioplegia needle placement, and cross-clamping.

the left internal mammary artery (LIMA) has been utilized and is patent, one must be able to isolate and clamp it to prevent washout of cardioplegia and early myocardial recovery in between arresting doses (**Figure 8.5**). In those rare situations where the patent LIMA is inaccessible, deep hypothermia along with systemic hyperkalemia and intermittent retrograde cardioplegia administration may be employed.[3] It has been documented that, when the risk of graft injury precludes the safe mobilization and clamping of the LIMA, alternative strategies such as these have met with equal outcomes.[4] A useful technique to control flow in the IMA is to encircle the vessel with an elastic vessel loop with a blunt needle. Tightening the double loop will control flow through the vessel without the need to dissect it completely free circumferentially.

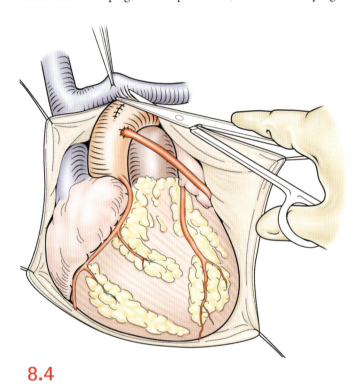

8.4

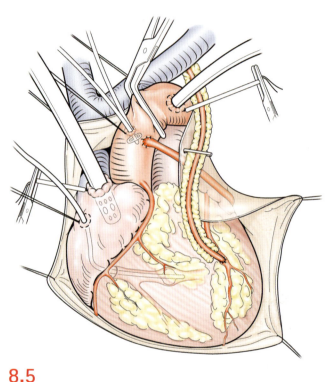

8.5

Cannulation and myocardial protection

Upon completion of dissection, one can usually cannulate above the original operation cannulation site, taking into account any areas of calcification or existing vein grafts. For myocardial protection, both antegrade and retrograde cardioplegia cannulae are placed in the ascending aorta and coronary sinus, respectively. Because of the variability in perfusion afforded from antegrade delivery alone, not to mention the risks of embolization of atheroma, the utility of effective retrograde cardioplegia is widely accepted as a crucial adjunct. Proximally dividing very diseased patent vein grafts prior to retrograde cardioplegia can prevent atheroembolization.[2] It is very important to have enough of the aorta dissected free posteriorly to allow full cross-clamping as anything less will assure the inability to achieve and maintain cardiac arrest. If

Revascularization

With the heart in full diastolic arrest, one can now commence revascularization. The atretic remnants of occluded grafts are a helpful roadmap to the target vessels which are often obscured by scar tissue. One area of emerging consensus is what to do with a patent vein graft at the time of reoperative CABG. The surgical dogma has been to mandate replacement of a vein graft older than 5 years. However, lack of supporting evidence in addition to the known risks of such a strategy have caused this approach to fall out of favor. For most, recognition that certain vein grafts are "privileged" has led many to select judiciously which grafts to replace and which to leave alone.[5]

Distal anastomoses

There are many options for distal anastomoses. If the hood of the previous saphenous bypass graft is open, one can sew to the original hood (**Figure 8.6a**) or a remnant of the vein graft left behind after it is transected (**Figure 8.6b**). If disease involves the previous anastomosis, then a site distally is selected and bypassed using conventional techniques. In the setting of a patent but diseased vein conduit, ligation of the old graft should be considered to prevent potential atheromatous embolization (**Figure 8.6c**).

A dilemma exists, however, when a LIMA was not used during the original operation and is now being utilized to replace a diseased vein graft (**Figure 8.7**). The same survival advantage seen in first-time CABGs of the LIMA to LAD has been documented in the reoperative cohort as well.[6] The compelling data behind IMA usage even extend to recycling a LIMA conduit that may have developed disease at the distal anastomosis but is otherwise patent. Its successful usage, however relies on a tension-free anastomosis to a target vessel with adequate run-off.

One important consideration is that flow down an immature IMA conduit may be insufficient in the immediate peri- and postoperative periods. It is therefore recommended that an existing vein graft is not ligated in these situations. If the previous venous conduit must be ligated, a new vein graft may be placed proximally or on a diagonal branch to bridge a patient until such time when the new IMA can provide adequate blood flow. It is unknown, however, what deleterious effect on IMA patency may be seen with competitive flow with this strategy.

Proximal anastomoses

The proximal orifices of vein grafts are rarely occluded. Therefore the hood of previous vein grafts is often a convenient area to situate the proximal anastomoses to the new vein conduits. When there is insufficient conduit, a concession is often made by performing the proximal anastomosis to the midbody of an existing SVG in an end-to-side fashion (**Figure 8.8**). Sequential grafting also provides an option to deal with inadequate conduit and to reduce the number of proximal anastomoses.

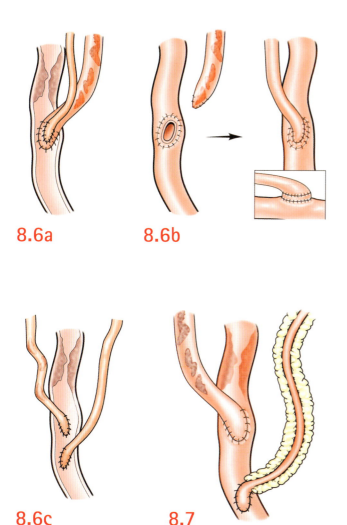

8.6a   **8.6b**

8.6c   **8.7**

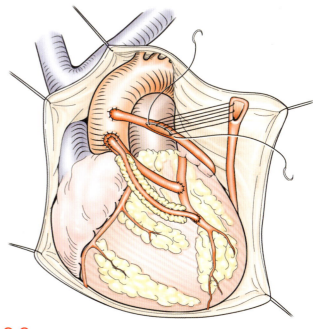

8.8

POSTOPERATIVE CARE

The postoperative management of patients undergoing reoperative CABG is in many ways not unlike that of first-time surgical patients. Still, standards of care must reflect that these patients are at higher risk for death, respiratory failure, renal failure, stroke, reoperation for bleeding, and deep sternal wound infections. Appropriate vigilance and scrutiny of these patients is therefore critical.

OUTCOME

A recent review of the Society of Thoracic Surgeons Adult Cardiac Surgery Database shows that, as a percentage of overall CABGs, reoperative surgery is declining, from 6.0% in 2000 to 3.4% in 2009. Despite the fact that patients undergoing reoperative surgery are sicker with more left main disease, history of myocardial infarction, and heart failure, mortality has also declined during this same period.[7] These improvements are attributed to better pre-, intra-, and postoperative management. That being said, reoperative CABG still represents a mortality risk 3.5 times that seen in first-time CABG patients. Thus, while employing the various strategies detailed in this chapter are helpful, perhaps the most critical variable remains careful patient selection. Taking the time to fully ascertain the potential benefit to derive from a known risky procedure will be very important in ensuring that the positive trends in reoperative CABG outcomes continue.

REFERENCES

1. Spiliotopoulos K, Maganti M, Brister S, Rao V. Changing pattern of reoperative coronary artery bypass grafting: a 20-year study. *Ann Thorac Surg.* 2011; 92(1): 40–7.
2. Fazel S, Borger MA, Weisel RD, et al. Myocardial protection in reoperative coronary artery bypass grafting. *J Card Surg.* 2004; 19(4): 291–5.
3. Kaneko T, Nauta F, Borstlap W, et al. The "no-dissection" technique is safe for reoperative aortic valve replacement with a patent left internal thoracic artery graft. *J Thorac Cardiovasc Surg.* 2012; 144(5): 1036–41.
4. Smith RL, Ellman PI, Thompson PW, et al. Do you need to clamp a patent left internal thoracic artery–left anterior descending graft in reoperative cardiac surgery? *Ann Thorac Surg.* 2009; 87(3): 742–7.
5. Mehta ID, Weinberg J, Jones MF, et al. Should angiographically disease-free saphenous vein grafts be replaced at the time of redo coronary artery bypass grafting? *Ann Thorac Surg.* 1998; 65(1): 17–22.
6. Sabik JF, Raza S, Blackstone EH, et al. Value of internal thoracic artery grafting to the left anterior descending coronary artery at coronary reoperation. *J Am Coll Cardiol.* 2013; 61(3): 302–10.
7. Ghanta RK, Kaneko T, Gammie JS, et al. Evolving trends of reoperative coronary artery bypass grafting: an analysis of the Society of Thoracic Surgeons Adult Cardiac Surgery Database. *J Thorac Cardiovasc Surg.* 2013; 145(2): 364–72.

Repair of postinfarction ventricular septal defect

CYNTHIA E. WAGNER AND IRVING L. KRON

HISTORY

With the universal implementation of early reperfusion therapies after myocardial infarction (MI), postinfarction ventricular septal defect (VSD) has become an uncommon complication after transmural MI. The first successful surgical repair was reported by Cooley and colleagues in 1956.[1] Early approaches emphasized delayed repair, based on the tenet that necrotic tissue would organize over time, allowing sutures to be more securely placed around a fibrous margin. However, it is now recognized that potential surgical candidates are at risk of rapid clinical deterioration from the effects of multi-organ failure, and early repair prior to the onset or worsening of cardiogenic shock is now the recommended practice. In recent years, the majority of patients are initially managed with intra-aortic balloon pumps (IABP). There will be an increasing role for percutaneous VSD closure devices, either as a definitive treatment or as a stabilizing measure, in select patients based on anatomic considerations and hemodynamic stability at the time of presentation.

PRINCIPLES AND JUSTIFICATION

Perfusion of the anterior two-thirds of the interventricular septum is supplied by the left anterior descending artery (LAD), while blood supply to the posterior third of the septum is from the posterior descending artery, arising from the right coronary artery (RCA) in 80% of the population. Postinfarction VSDs are therefore classified as anterior or posterior following occlusion of these respective coronary arteries. Postinfarction VSDs are also classified as simple or complex, with simple VSDs consisting of a single site of rupture across the interventricular septum and complex VSDs consisting of multiple serpiginous tracts across the septum. Depending on the size and location of the infarction, which dictates flow across the shunt and ventricular function, clinical symptoms range from a benign murmur to cardiogenic shock, defined as failure to maintain systolic blood pressure above 80 mmHg or cardiac index above 1.8 L/min/m^2 despite optimal support with intravenous inotropes or an IABP.

Posterior VSDs are often complex and can be associated with a ruptured posteromedial papillary muscle and mitral regurgitation, as the posteromedial papillary muscle has a single source of blood supply (RCA or circumflex artery). Posterior VSDs are associated with increased mortality. In a prospective study corroborating this observation, preoperative predictors of poor prognosis were independent of infarct or shunt size, left ventricular function, or extent of coronary disease, and instead were based on cardiogenic shock and right ventricular dysfunction (as measured by free wall motion index, end-diastolic pressure, and right atrial pressure). In this study, mortality among patients with posterior VSDs was directly related to size of right ventricular infarction.[2] The likely explanation for this finding is that occlusion of the RCA compromises perfusion to a volume-overloaded right ventricle, resulting in decreased right ventricular function and therefore decreased left ventricular preload, decreased cardiac output, multi-organ failure, and death.

The GUSTO-I trial (Global Utilization of Streptokinase and TPA for Occluded Coronary Arteries), a prospective randomized multicenter trial, was the first study to analyze postinfarction VSD after early reperfusion. Of 41 021 patients enrolled in the study, 84 patients were diagnosed with postinfarction VSD, resulting in a lower incidence of 0.2% than previously reported. Prior to early reperfusion, postinfarction VSDs developed 4–6 days after transmural MI in 2% of this patient population. The majority of patients in the GUSTO-I trial were diagnosed by echocardiography alone at a median time of 1 day after symptom onset, considerably earlier than prior to early reperfusion. Alternative diagnostic modalities included left heart catheterization (left-to-right shunt by ventriculography) or right heart catheterization (step-up in oxygen saturation from the right atrium to the pulmonary artery). Of those patients who underwent cardiac catheterization, 50% had single-vessel disease and the majority had total occlusion of the infarct artery, found to be the LAD in nearly two-thirds of patients. As such, anterior infarction, as well as advanced age and female gender, were associated with postinfarction VSD. Patients without a history of angina or prior MI were also more likely to develop postinfarction VSD, likely as a result of total occlusion in a single-vessel disease system without extensive collaterals. Importantly, the GUSTO-I trial reported lower 30-day mortality rates (47% vs 94%) and lower 1-year mortality rates (53% vs 97%) for those patients with postinfarction VSD who underwent operative repair vs medical management, a significant finding that influences practice today.[3]

PREOPERATIVE ASSESSMENT AND PREPARATION

Physical examination findings of a new holosystolic murmur and signs of new-onset heart failure in a patient with a history of a recent MI should prompt emergent bedside transthoracic echocardiography. Patients diagnosed with postinfarction VSDs are initially managed with inotropic support and IABP counterpulsation in efforts aimed at afterload reduction, increased systemic perfusion, and decreased flow across the shunt.

Most patients will have undergone cardiac catheterization at the time of presentation, facilitating the planning of concomitant coronary artery bypass grafting (CABG) at the time of postinfarction VSD repair. However, while some studies have shown improved early and late survival after concomitant CABG, other studies have failed to show this survival benefit. Complete revascularization, which improves collateral blood flow, has also been associated with decreased mortality as compared to revascularization of the culprit artery alone. Therefore, the potential benefit of concomitant CABG and the risk of longer cardiopulmonary bypass time must be considered for each individual patient based on the extent of coronary artery disease and hemodynamic stability at the time of repair. Cardiac catheterization should not delay early operative intervention. Similarly, while some patients may have mitral regurgitation from a ruptured papillary muscle or tethered cord, the decision to perform concomitant mitral valve repair should be made on an individual basis. In those patients with significant ventricular impairment (decreased left ventricular ejection fraction or right ventricular dysfunction), the possibility of requiring a ventricular assist device in the immediate postoperative period is real and should be considered prior to postinfarction VSD repair. In a subset of these patients in cardiogenic shock and multi-organ failure, percutaneous VSD closure devices may represent a bridge to surgical repair. Unfortunately, our experience with this modality has been poor.

ANESTHESIA

Standard monitoring includes surface electrocardiography, pulse oximetry, capnography, and placement of nasal and bladder temperature probes. An arterial line to monitor continuous blood pressure and frequent arterial blood gas analysis is most commonly placed in the left radial artery, though site of placement will depend on cannulation strategy and plans for concomitant CABG. A central line with a pulmonary artery catheter is essential to monitor cardiac output, pulmonary artery pressure, central venous pressure, and oxygen saturation step-up from the right atrium to the pulmonary artery. Also essential in the repair of postinfarction VSD is transesophageal echocardiography with color flow Doppler, which allows quantitation of shunt size (Qp/Qs) as well as precise identification of shunt location, potential valvular involvement (mitral regurgitation from a ruptured papillary muscle or a tethered leaflet), and preoperative ventricular function, which will guide operative decisions.

OPERATION

High-flow cardiopulmonary bypass is established under mild systemic hypothermia. Constant attention to myocardial protection is critical. Venous cannulation strategy is dependent on the location of the VSD, the extent of free wall infarction, and the planned surgical approach. Postinfarction VSDs are exposed by a left ventriculotomy through an area of necrosis along the anterior or posterior free wall, with the transinfarct incision made parallel to the interventricular septum and the corresponding adjacent LAD or posterior descending artery. Alternatively, small VSDs may be approached through a right atriotomy. Methods of VSD closure include patch repair or infarct exclusion.

Anterior VSDs

Anterior VSDs are approached through a left ventriculotomy parallel to the LAD. We favor patch repair for anterior VSDs (**Figure 9.1a**). Thorough debridement of necrotic tissue along the free wall and septum is completed until viable myocardium is visualized. An oversized pericardial or synthetic patch is positioned along the left ventricular side of the septal defect and secured in place with felt-reinforced 2-0 polypropylene mattress sutures placed several centimeters away from the defect. Avoiding tension, the patch is trimmed anteriorly and anchored to the left and right ventricular free wall using felt-reinforced mattress sutures.

If extensive infarctectomy of the anterior left ventricular free wall is required, a separate patch to restore normal ventricular geometry is secured in place along the free wall and anchored to the septal patch.

Alternatively, postinfarction VSD closure with multiple patches has been reported, as well as the use of various sealants in an effort to decrease residual shunting or VSD recurrence.

When technically possible, the free wall infarct may be excluded with a 2-0 polypropylene pursestring suture placed around the endocardial base of the infarcted myocardium, similar to a Dor procedure for left ventricular aneurysmectomy (**Figure 9.1b**). Viable myocardium is reapproximated with felt-reinforced mattress sutures. Large defects are covered with a pericardial or synthetic patch. The septal defect is closed separately.

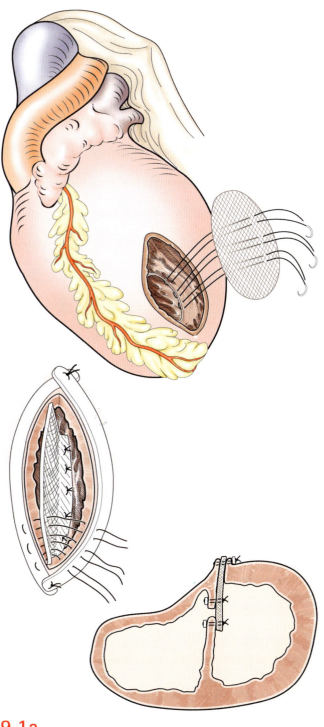

9.1a

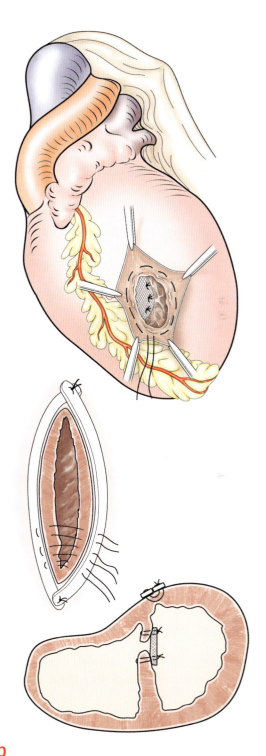

9.1b

Posterior VSDs

Posterior VSDs are approached through a left ventriculotomy parallel to the posterior descending artery near the base of the heart (**Figure 9.2**). These repairs are more complex, due to the challenging nature of the exposure and the close proximity of the mitral valve annulus, subvalvular apparatus, and posteromedial papillary muscle. We favor infarct exclusion as the method of repair for posterior VSDs. Initially reported by David et al., this method of repair consists of limited debridement and placement of an entirely intracardiac pericardial or synthetic patch circumferentially along the left ventricular endocardium, thus excluding the septal defect from the reconstructed left ventricular cavity.[4] Meticulous care is taken to maintain normal ventricular dimensions and to prevent distortion of adjacent structures. This technique offers the potential advantage of decreased manipulation of the right ventricle and often friable septum.

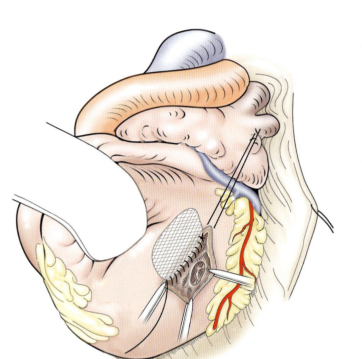

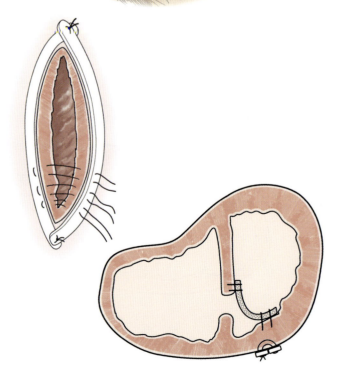

9.2

POSTOPERATIVE CARE

Some patients will have residual shunting across the VSD, which may be monitored with serial echocardiography or pulmonary artery catheter measurements. Patients should also be monitored for VSD recurrence in the immediate postoperative period. Depending on symptom severity and ventricular function, open or percutaneous reintervention may be required. Some patients will require dialysis postoperatively, and intravascular volume status may be adjusted to allow ventricular recovery. Inotropic support and IABP counterpulsation may be weaned as guided by measurements of cardiac output and systemic perfusion as well as by ventricular function on serial echocardiography. Due to the presence of multiple vascular access sites and potential for sepsis, patients should be frequently assessed for signs of infection and started on broad-spectrum antibiotics as clinically indicated.

OUTCOME

Despite advances in perioperative management and intraoperative technique, mortality after repair of postinfarction VSD remains the highest among all cardiac surgeries performed today. A retrospective review of the Society of Thoracic Surgeons National Database was recently completed in the largest study to date examining outcomes after surgical repair. Among 2876 patients who underwent repair between 1999 and 2010 at 666 centers across North America, overall operative mortality was 43%, with major morbidity or death occurring in 77% of patients within 30 days of surgery. Postoperative dialysis was the most common complication, required in 12% of patients.

In this study, 65% of patients were supported preoperatively with an IABP and more than 50% of patients were in cardiogenic shock at the time of repair. Surgical status was classified as emergent in 50% and urgent in 35% of patients. As expected, mortality increased with surgical acuity and was greater than 50% following emergent operations. Interestingly, mortality was found to vary inversely with the time interval between MI and surgical repair, with mortality approaching 70% if repair was within 6 hours of the MI, 60% if within 24 hours, greater than 50% if within 7 days, and less than 20% if operative intervention occurred more than 7 days after the MI. This finding may reflect a relationship between infarct size (and ventricular function) and time to VSD development, or more likely be explained by earlier repair being offered to unstable patients in cardiogenic shock with increased mortality.

Preoperative use of beta blockers and lipid-lowering agents was associated with decreased mortality. Of the patients in this study, 33% had undergone prior percutaneous coronary intervention and less than 10% had undergone prior CABG, which resulted in a survival advantage among this small group of patients. On cardiac catheterization, 33% were found to have triple-vessel coronary artery disease, and concomitant CABG was performed in 64%, which was not associated with increased operative mortality but did not confer a protective effect.

In this study, the average age of patients undergoing postinfarction VSD repair was 68 years, and there was a slight male predominance. Risk factors associated with increased mortality included advanced age, female gender, cardiogenic shock, elevated creatinine (with preoperative dialysis showing the largest effect on multivariate analysis), emergency status, longer cardiopulmonary bypass times and aortic cross-clamp times, as well as posterior location of the VSD.[5]

In an initial study examining long-term outcomes after postinfarction VSD repair in the elderly, the majority of hospital survivors were in New York Heart Association functional class I or II at follow-up, with no difference observed between patients younger than age 70 and patients age 70 or older (83% vs 92%). There was also no difference in long-term survival between these two groups. The majority of late deaths in both groups were attributed to cardiac causes, including recurrent MI or heart failure.[6]

In a recent study examining early and late morbidity and mortality after postinfarction VSD repair, in-hospital deaths occurred at a median time of 3.5 days postoperatively (range 0–27 days). Over 50% of the subset of patients requiring dialysis postoperatively died within 30 days. Five percent of patients had permanent neurologic deficits and 5% had transient neurologic deficits. Actuarial survival and freedom from major adverse cardiac events among 30-day survivors was 95% and 91% at 1 year, 88% and 61% at 5 years, 73% and 40% at 10 years, and 51% and 19% at 15 years. Risk factors for the development of ventricular tachyarrhythmia, which occurred in 27% of patients at a median time of 5.9 years postoperatively, included occlusion of the LAD and concomitant left ventricular aneurysmectomy. The majority of these patients underwent placement of an automatic implantable cardiac defibrillator. Risk factors for the development of heart failure, which occurred in 46% of patients at a median time of 3.9 years postoperatively, included hypertension, preoperative left ventricular ejection fraction less than 40%, posterior location of the VSD, and residual interventricular

communication after repair. A residual or recurrent shunt was detected in 35% of patients, and half of these patients underwent reintervention at a time interval ranging from the immediate postoperative period up to 10 years after the original repair, depending on symptom severity and ventricular function. In all patients who presented for reintervention, the shunt was found to be the result of dehiscence between the patch and infarcted septum.[7]

Throughout the past decade, the number of postinfarction VSD repairs has remained constant at 0.1% of total cardiac surgeries performed annually, yet operative mortality has not decreased in a linear trend over this period. The average number of repairs performed annually at any individual institution has ranged from 0.09 to 3.7 during this time (among participating centers in the Society of Thoracic Surgeons National Database). Our field will continue to be challenged to make the further refinements in perioperative care and surgical technique necessary to improve outcomes after repair of this high-risk yet infrequent complication of ischemic heart disease.

REFERENCES

1. Cooley DA, Belmonte BA, Zeis LB, et al. Surgical repair of ruptured interventricular septum following acute myocardial infarction. *Surgery* 1957; 41: 930–7.
2. Moore CA, Nygaard TW, Kaiser DL, et al. Postinfarction ventricular septal rupture: the importance of location of infarction and right ventricular function in determining survival. *Circulation* 1986; 74: 45–55.
3. Crenshaw BS, Granger CB, Birnbaum Y, et al. Risk factors, angiographic patterns, and outcomes in patients with ventricular septal defect complicating acute myocardial infarction. GUSTO-I (Global Utilization of Streptokinase and TPA for Occluded Coronary Arteries) Trial Investigators. *Circulation* 2000; 101: 27–32.
4. David TE, Dale L, Sun Z. Postinfarction ventricular septal rupture: repair by endocardial patch with infarct exclusion. *J Thorac Cardiovasc Surg* 1995; 110: 1315–22.
5. Arnaoutakis GJ, Zhao Y, George TJ, et al. Surgical repair of ventricular septal defect after myocardial infarction: outcomes from The Society of Thoracic Surgeons National Database. *Ann Thorac Surg.* 2012; 94: 436–44.
6. Muehrcke DD, Blank S, Daggett WM. Survival after repair of postinfarction ventricular septal defects in patients over the age of 70. *J Card Surg.* 1992; 7: 290–300.
7. Fukushima S, Tesar PJ, Jalali H, et al. Determinants of in-hospital and long-term surgical outcomes after repair of postinfarction ventricular septal rupture. *J Thorac Cardiovasc Surg.* 2010; 140: 59–65.

10

Robotic total endoscopic coronary artery bypass grafting

LÁSZLÓ GÖBÖLÖS AND JOHANNES BONATTI

HISTORY

The common aim of any minimally invasive surgical procedure is to result in the smallest trauma possible and to perform an intervention by a port-only approach rather than large exposing incisions. Following numerous unsuccessful attempts to undertake endoscopic coronary bypass surgery utilizing long-shafted thoracoscopic instrumentation, the first total endoscopic coronary artery bypass grafting (TECAB) was carried out in 1998 with the aid of a surgical robot. Since then the technique has gradually progressed from a single-vessel to a multi-vessel surgical approach and is performed both on the beating heart and in cardioplegic conditions. TECAB can also be combined with percutaneous coronary intervention (PCI) techniques in what are commonly called integrated or hybrid procedures. Further updated surgical robot generations are available on the medical market and procedure-specific robotic adapters (perhaps better termed "end effectors") have significantly improved vision, ease of exposure of target vessels, and overall ergonomic features of the operation.

PRINCIPLES AND JUSTIFICATION

According to our current opinion any patient with clear indication for coronary bypass surgery can be considered for TECAB. However, it is crucial to keep the major contraindications in mind, as listed in **Table 10.1**. Hence TECAB is rather an elective form of surgery, not well suited to redo procedures that would expose the surgeon to a technical challenge resulting in a long and tedious operation with extensive time demand on taking down adhesions in the endoscopic setting. Any factor that causes reduction or distortion of the pleural space (i.e. chest wall deformities, bovine heart or reduced lung volume) has to be respected. Thorough preoperative analysis of pros and cons has to be undertaken, whether to expose the patient to a potentially longer cardiopulmonary bypass (CPB) time, myocardial ischemia, and overall procedural duration in contrast to the benefits of the minimally invasive approach. This dilemma is especially valid for patients who have additional comorbidities. Respecting the listed contraindications, 25–30% of current CABG patients in our center can be approached in

Table 10.1 TECAB contraindications

Absolute contraindications	Relative contraindications
Cardiogenic shock	Unstable patient on IABP
Hemodynamic instability	Severe left venticular function (EF < 30%)
Severe lung function impairment (FEV1 < 70%, VC < 2.5 L)	Bovine heart (<25 mm between LV and chest wall)
Pulmonary hypertension	Previous heart surgery
Chest deformities (e.g. pectus excavatum)	Previous severe chest trauma
Multimorbid patient	Previous chest irradiation
Significant generalized vasculopathy	
Diffusely diseased or small coronaries	
Intramyocardial coronaries for beating heart–TECAB	
Ascending aortic diameter > 3.8 cm and severe aortoiliac calcification for arrested heart–TECAB	

robotic endoscopic fashion. As TECAB necessarily involves a significant surgical learning curve, we strongly recommend starting with simple operative procedures, strictly in low-risk patients. Simulator models and wet-lab sessions are also key elements of shortening the learning curve.

PREOPERATIVE ASSESSMENT AND PREPARATION

All patients should undergo the same preoperative workup process as for conventional coronary artery bypass grafting (CABG). The usual preoperative assessment consists of past medical and current clinical history, physical examination, standard blood tests (complete blood count, kidney and liver function tests, clotting profile, blood group analysis and cross-match procedure), carotid Doppler study, ankle-brachial-index (ABI), pulmonary function test, and echocardiography. In order to evaluate TECAB suitability, computed tomographic (CT) angiography of the chest, abdomen, and pelvis are carried out. All necessary CT parameters to be assessed by the surgeon, the surgical team, and the radiologist are listed in **Table 10.2**.

ANESTHESIA

Standard cardiac anesthesia principles are also valid for TECAB cases, although an experienced anesthesiologist with special interest in minimally invasive procedures should supervise the operation. Specific anesthetic aspects to consider include:

- double lumen intubation or bronchial blocker
- percutaneous defibrillator pads
- constant transesophageal echocardiography (TEE) follow-up during procedure
- near-infrared spectroscopy (NIRS) monitoring for both cerebral and lower extremity.

Transesophageal echocardiography (TEE) is an essential tool for monitoring overall cardiac function and regional wall motion, and also for checking the position of the endoballoon throughout the cardioplegic TECAB. Maintaining good bilateral communication with the anesthetic team during the procedure is vital:

- to determine when to initiate single-lung ventilation
- for setting the level of CO_2 inflation pressure
- for monitoring leg ischemia, if femoral arterial CPB is applied
- for detecting incidental migration of the endoballoon during cardioplegic TECAB
- for providing sufficient heart rate control, assessment for eventual regional wall motion abnormalities at beating heart TECAB, and respiratory management after a longer CPB run utilizing single-lung ventilation.

OPERATION

Hardware requirements and procedural versions

There is currently only one surgical robot available on the market which provides sufficient performance to undertake TECAB (please see www.intuitivesurgical.com). Surgeons performing TECAB mainly use the third-generation da Vinci® surgical system (Si version). **Figure 10.1** shows the surgeon's position behind the robotic console. Using so-called "masters," the surgical manual maneuvers are translated into intrathoracic robotic instrument movements and robotic 3D camera positions. Foot pedals allow switching between camera and instrument control as well as for electrocautery. Surgical vision is provided by a 3D binocular system. Not all TECAB instruments are yet available for the fourth-generation system (Xi version).

As discussed above, TECAB can be performed with or without the aid of CPB and on the non-beating or beating

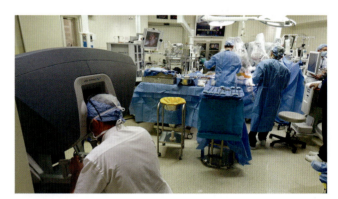

10.1

Table 10.2 CT angiography chest/abdomen/pelvis parameter assessment prior to TECAB

Heart	Lungs	Vascular
Heart dimensions (cardiothoracic ratio, LV distance to chest wall)	Lung size (intrathoracic workspace)	Ascending aortic diameter at right pulmonary artery crossing
LIMA and target vessel distance	Lung pathology	Atherosclerotic significance at all aortic levels
Target vessel course (epimyocardial vs intramyocardial)	Pleural pathology (e.g. adhesions, plaques)	Iliofemoral anatomy and pathologic changes
Pericardial fat pad size		Other vascular pathologies (e.g. aneurysm, dissection, etc.)

heart. The first procedure is commonly described as AH (arrested heart)-TECAB, the latter is also known as BH (beating heart)-TECAB. We strongly recommend developing skills for both methods as they add an optimal level of flexibility for the robotic surgical team and enable the tailoring of the operative efficacy to the patient's requirements.

BH-TECAB has the benefit of avoiding the side effects of CPB, although target vessel exposure and anastomotic suturing are technically more demanding in BH-TECAB than in AH-TECAB. Surgeons should initially master anastomotic techniques on the arrested heart before moving to the beating-heart procedure. We also recommend stand-by cannulation for CPB even in BH-TECAB, which might be a life-saving measure if there is limited intrathoracic space and the patient develops sudden myocardial ischemia, hemodynamic instability, or severe ventricular arrhythmia, for example. Establishing perfusion in these acute life-threatening situations is extremely challenging with a robot docked to the patient. It also may require extra time, if there is significant hemodynamic compromise, and might result in additional, otherwise avoidable vascular complications. Having instant peripheral CPB access available has proven to be a very valuable add-on in our experience.

In cardioplegic TECAB the anastomotic suturing is easier, although AH-TECAB requires specific skill sets in remote-access perfusion and the application of an endoballoon or transthoracic cross-clamping. All these skills should be developed initially in procedures other than TECAB (e.g. mini thoracotomy ASD II repair or mitral valve repair) before employing them in total endoscopic CABG. Our experience is that grafting the right or distal circumflex coronary artery territory is reliable only on arrested heart as the target is completely flaccid and can be adequately rotated and positioned.

Operative steps

1. PATIENT POSITIONING, OPERATIVE LAY–UP

The patient is placed on the operating table in the standard supine position. The arms are positioned beside the trunk and the left side of the chest is slightly elevated with the aid of an antidecubitus jelly roll. Conversion to an open procedure always has to be an available option, therefore the patient is prepared and draped as for conventional coronary bypass surgery and the equipment for open CABG should always be also on site.

2. PORT INSERTION AND ROBOT DOCKING

The ports are inserted into the patient's left chest and ideally should be placed by the most experienced team member as the correct port access is essential for the operation. Port access requires complete left lung deflation to avoid organ injury and must be confirmed by the anesthetic team before placement attempt. The camera port is situated in the fifth intercostal space at the anterior axillary line and CO_2 is insufflated at a pressure of 8 mmHg. In case

of hemodynamic compromise (e.g. sudden hypotension) during this phase, the CO_2 pressure should be adequately adjusted to avoid further disturbance in the venous return. The thoracic cavity is then inspected, and under scope vision the right and left instrument ports are placed cranially and caudally four fingerbreadths away from the camera port, midway between the anterior axillary line and the midclavicular line. Next the surgical robot is docked to the patient and a robotic cautery spatula is inserted by the right manipulator arm and DeBakey forceps via left arm. **Figure 10.2** indicates the port arrangement and correct placement of the instruments in the chest, and in the photograph in **Figure 10.3** the robotic arms can be seen docked to the patient.

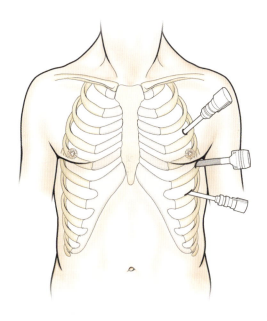

10.2

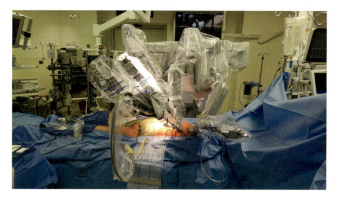

10.3

3. HARVESTING THE INTERNAL MAMMARY ARTERY

In the "camera up" position of the 30-degree angled robotic camera, the internal mammary artery (IMA) can be identified by the visible pulsations in the usual vessel run-off. The electrocautery is set to 15–20 watts, and the endothoracic fascia and muscle layer over the IMA are removed. The superficially freed IMA is harvested with the skeletonizing technique, applying mild mechanical traction and concomitant cauterization of side branches on the adjacent chest wall (**Figure 10.4**). Liga-clipping is seldom necessary to close up large branches, although sometimes it is required to settle side-branch bleeding. If both IMAs have to be harvested, the right pleura can be accessed for opening following generous robotic endoscopic retrosternal dissection. The easier approach in double IMA harvesting settings is for the right IMA to be taken down prior to the left; in a reverse sequence the left artery could compromise vision and access. Following heparin administration the IMA distal end can be clipped, then divided by robotic Potts scissors, and dropped into the left thoracic cavity, allowing autodilation.

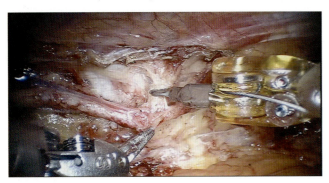

10.4a

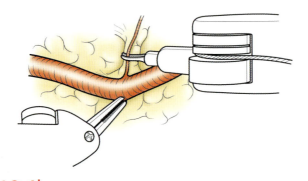

10.4b

4. UTILITY PORT PLACEMENT

The next step after IMA harvesting is to insert a 5 mm utility port under scope control in the left parasternal region, just opposite the camera port. Since introduction of this step significant operative time reductions were noted in the literature. This port allows the supply and removal of materials required during the operative procedure (e.g. suture material, bulldogs, suction tubing, silastic tapes).

5. ACCESS THROUGH THE MEDIASTINAL FAT AND PERICARDIUM

In "camera down" mode the pericardial fat pad and the pericardium itself can be sufficiently visualized. With the aid of an electrocautery spatula on the right and long-tip forceps on the left, the fat pad is removed in a craniocaudal direction. If the pericardial fat pad is grossly enlarged, initiating CPB can facilitate the resection process, providing more intrathoracic space by decompressing the heart. Following fat pad removal the pericardium is opened just above the right ventricular outflow tract, further incised heading towards the substernal part of the pericardial reflection, and then conducted laterally. In the cranial direction the aperture moves towards the phrenic nerve, which must be positively identified beyond doubt. Care must be taken to avoid both the nerve and the left atrial appendage due to their vicinity.

6. PERIPHERAL ACCESS CARDIOPULMONARY BYPASS AND APPLICATION OF THE ENDOCLAMP (BALLOON OCCLUSION)

A preoperative CT angiogram is essential to determine the eventual atherosclerotic changes of the aorta and iliofemoral system. In case of non-existent or mild grades of aortoiliac atherosclerosis, the femorofemoral cannulation for CPB can be commenced at low risk. The standard vascular exposure target is the left groin. Dissection of the femoral vessels should be limited as much as possible in order to prevent lymphatic leaks. To avoid malperfusion of the distal limb, an additional perfusion line is inserted in every case and the peripheral blood supply is monitored by near-infrared spectroscopy (NIRS) throughout the whole procedure. The venous drainage is provided by a 25 Fr cannula forwarded to the superior vena cava under TEE guidance. A 21 Fr or 23 Fr arterial perfusion cannula equipped with a side arm is placed into the femoral artery and the CPB circuit is closed.

Safe application of the ascending aortic endoballoon for cardioplegic procedures requires lack of ascending, arch, and descending thoracic aortic atherosclerosis; the maximal acceptable ascending aortic diameter is 38 mm. The aortic valve should be functionally competent and also structurally intact. The completely deflated endoballoon is progressed via the side arm of the arterial perfusion cannula with the aid of a guide wire. The guide wire is advanced into the aortic root under constant TEE follow-up, then the endoballoon is positioned just right above the aortic valve. The cardioplegia line is connected to the heart–lung machine tubing; pressure monitoring of the aortic root and endoballoon commences via corresponding manometers. It is vital to avoid accidental injection of air through the plegia catheter into the aortic root.

The heart–lung machine has to be initiated gradually for TECAB and the descending thoracic aorta should be visualized during initiation of CPB so as to detect any signs of retrograde aortic dissection at the earliest opportunity. When sufficient venous drainage is achieved, at low blood pressure and lack of ventricular ejections, the endoballoon is inflated and the correct position in the aortic root is echocardiographically confirmed. Following endoballoon inflation the cardioplegic solution is administered. Rapid cardioplegic induction can be established by the administration of adenosine (6 mg/20 mL of normal saline). If a stable balloon position is confirmed, the cooling can be initiated, and cardioplegia has to be repeated every 20 minutes. A percutaneous retrograde cardioplegic cannula can also be placed as necessary; in this case both ante- and retrograde cardioplegia can be commenced according to customized protocols.

If moderate to severe aortoiliac atherosclerosis is present, we strongly advise abandoning the femoral approach. Instead, the left subclavian artery is targeted as the arterial perfusion site in the infraclavicular region and an 8 mm prosthetic "chimney anastomosis" is created to connect the arterial line without compromise of the peripheral limb perfusion. Axillary cannulation ensures antegrade perfusion from the descending thoracic aortic level downstream and may also reduce the risk of retrograde aortoiliac dissection. The endoballoon catheter can still be inserted in most cases via a separate 19 Fr cannula placed into the common femoral artery.

If severe aortoiliac calcification is present or a descending or arch protruding/mobile aortic atheroma is detected on TEE, the endoballoon application is contraindicated. In these cases we choose a BH-TECAB procedure. As mentioned earlier, BH-TECAB patients should all be cannulated for safety reasons and the cannulae are placed at an activated clotting time (ACT) level of 300 s and are flushed with heparin saline solution. Should CPB become necessary, the ACT is raised to 480 s. CPB backup is extremely helpful in beating-heart multivessel TECAB when, for example, ischemia occurs during target vessel occlusion, if intrathoracic space is limited, or if bleeding occurs. During supportive pump runs significant diffuse bleeding might be encountered through portholes, the IMA bed, and other structures, which may require intermittent transthoracic suction to evacuate the pool of blood in the left pleural space.

7. IDENTIFICATION AND EXPOSURE OF THE TARGET VESSELS

To expose different structures on the heart surface, the robotic endostabilizer provides an effective support in both BH-TECAB and AH-TECAB. This device is fed through a 12 mm port situated on the left subcostal space two finger-breadths lateral to the xiphoid angle. The insertion process is guided by the robotic camera in "up facing" view. The subcostal port is connected to the fourth arm of the da Vinci® system.

To gain an optimal view and optimal access to the targeted coronary arteries the camera is set "face down". With the aid of the subcostal endostabilizer device the left anterior descending (LAD) and circumflex (Cx) coronary artery branches can be reached sufficiently. The endostabilizer is activated by a dedicated foot pedal and the suction pods are lined up alongside the target area; local immobilization is achieved in this fashion in beating heart-TECAB and the target vessel is moved into a comfortable work position in both BH-TECAB and AH-TECAB.

The right coronary artery system can be accessed by inserting the endostabilizer through the 12 mm left-sided instrument port. With this port arrangement the subcostal port can be used as the left robotic instrument arm. The acute margin of the right ventricle is lifted up using the endostabilizer and excellent access to the posterior descending artery or posterolateral artery can be gained. To this point, we have applied this method only in arrested heart-TECAB. In the beating heart setting the endostabilizer has to be applied carefully on the right ventricular surface as accidental perforation poses a potential challenge.

As appropriate exposure of the target vessel is achieved, the epicardium is opened with robotic Potts scissors.

8. ROBOT–FACILITATED ENDOSCOPIC CORONARY ANASTOMOSIS

Prior to commencing on the coronary anastomotic process, final fashioning is undertaken on the bypass graft material. The bulldog occluded graft facet is shaped in an oblique manner and further opened to a total length of 4 mm to create a "cobra head" type anastomotic profile. Simultaneously the free flow of the vessel has to be ensured.

In a similar way to conventional bypass grafting, DeBakey forceps and a robotic lancet beaver knife open the target area of the vessel. The incision is then enlarged to approximately 4 mm in length by robotic Potts scissors to match the previously fashioned graft. A 7 cm long double-armed polypropylene suture is supplied via the parasternal utility port. A pair of robotic black diamond micro forceps facilitate the coronary artery suture process.

The initial stitch is placed back-hand on the toe of the coronary artery in an inside-out fashion. The needle is parked safely away in the epicardium. The suture line is continued with the contralateral needle, but now from the toe of the graft inside-out and the coronary artery site will follow as outside-in. After the first three throws the graft is parachuted down to the coronary level and the stitching procedure becomes easier. It is essential to apply adequate suture line tension in order to avoid leaks on the back wall, which are more challenging to correct than on the facing front side. **Figure 10.5** shows the back-wall suturing process.

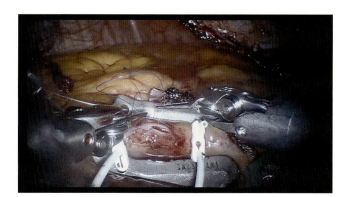

10.5a

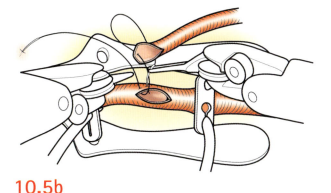

10.5b

Figures 10.6 and 10.7 show the suturing sequence and its completion.

After going around the heel, the needle is parked away and the first needle is taken to carry on from the toe of the anastomosis again to complete the suture line. Lumen patency can be checked gently with the tips of micro forceps. The completed suture line has to be meticulously inspected for slings. Slings can be corrected with the aid of suture needles. A useful video demonstration of the robotic coronary anastomotic technique is available at http://www.youtube.com/watch?v=l6DiBz2JUnY.

It has recently become possible for all coronary territories to be robotically revascularized without any compromise. The most common TECAB procedures are left internal mammary to the left anterior descending artery (LIMA to LAD), right internal mammary artery (RIMA) to LAD combined with LIMA to the diagonal, Cx territory bypasses, and LIMA to LAD combined with RIMA to the RCA territory. The last procedure requires a Y-graft construct.

Some specific issues have to be borne in mind when completing anastomoses on an arrested or a beating heart. In AH-TECAB the target vessel can already be opened at the end stage of cardioplegic solution administration to reduce the risk of coronary back-wall injury. Back bleeding from the target vessel might occur as a result of either inadequate venous drainage or retrograde aortic root flow as a consequence of low endoaortic balloon pressure. Repositioning of the venous cannula improves the overall drainage; additional controlled inflation of the endoballoon or silastic tape application around the target vessel will provide instant improvement of the operative field flooding. Safe suturing should only be carried on if a clear operative view is obtained.

To achieve a bloodless operative field in BH-TECAB, silastic tapes are placed proximal and distal to the graft landing zone, despite the fact that in most instances only the proximal one is going to be occluded. Following this, the target vessel is opened and an appropriately sized intraluminal shunt is forwarded initially into the distal segment of the aperture. The contralateral shunt side is then guided through the proximal vessel and the silastic tape is loosened. In BH-TECAB, the stitching maneuvers must be very gentle and well controlled in order to avoid accidental laceration of the coronary wall. Reducing the heart rate to facilitate the anastomotic process can be obtained by temporary administration of esmolol. It is a surgical challenge to manage the procedure on magnified bouncing operative field, therefore intense simulation training in dry- and wet-lab settings is strongly recommended prior to moving into the clinical setting.

9. FINAL TASKS

Bypass graft transit time ultrasound flow is measured in all cases by a specifically designed endoscopic flow probe to warrant standard operative outcome. This specific probe is delivered through the subcostal port.

Blood retention in the left pleural space is evacuated by a flexible suction tube via the utility port.

On completion of the surgical procedure the patient is

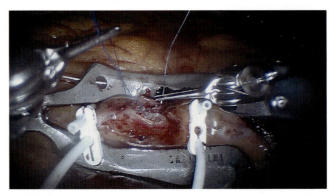

10.6a

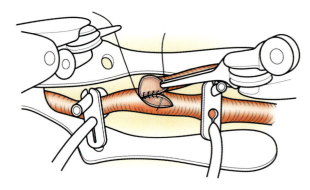

10.6b

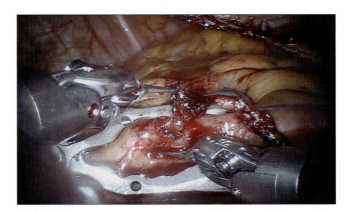

10.7a

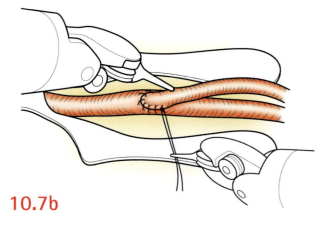

10.7b

weaned off CPB, leaving the robot docked and the instruments parked in the IMA bed. This step is necessary as the heart is filled after decannulation and the eventual reinsertion of instruments might be challenging, if required.

As a result of the combination of single-lung ventilation and application of CPB, a significant transient respiratory compromise might occur as a temporary phenomenon.

Once the patient's oxygenation is stabilized and the pump function is adequate, protamine is administered. At this stage the last robotic inspection of the thoracic cavity commences, where close attention of both the console surgeon and the tableside team is required. Once sufficient hemostasis is achieved, the robotic system is undocked. The ports are still left in position as it is important to avoid CO_2 loss for the last manual inspections with the robotic camera. The ports are then removed in a stepwise fashion under scope supervision, and the portholes are cauterized and packed with surgical hemostat (e.g. Fibrillar™, Surgicel™). A chest drain is inserted via the camera porthole. This procedure should be undertaken with left lung inflation in order to avoid graft injuries at the last phase of the operation. Infiltration of the portholes with local anesthetics supports postoperative pain control.

POSTOPERATIVE CARE

TECAB postoperative care basically follows the principles of standard post-sternotomy bypass surgery. As a result of single-lung ventilation, atelectasis might develop, which usually resolves with respiratory therapy. Special attention should be paid to regular peripheral arterial and venous circulation assessment during the postoperative course following remote access cannulation. Postoperative pain might be quite intense, especially alongside the camera port area, but it generally diminishes within the early postoperative days. Sternal precautions do not have to be considered after minimally invasive procedures.

OUTCOME

Minimally invasive TECAB is feasible utilizing robotic technology. In the early development of the technique,

TECAB was restricted to single bypass grafts to the LAD only. As most patients require multiple CABG, further development of complex robotic procedures were initiated. Successful innovative multi-vessel TECAB procedures in the early 21st century have enabled us to convert the experiences to a clinical reality. Further emerging technological progress in the robotic technology has led to feasibility of multi-vessel bypass grafting in both arrested- and beating-heart settings. The ultimate leap in the procedure to enable multi-vessel TECAB for beating-heart surgery is the availability of the robotic endostabilizer, albeit this device also expands surgical performance in cardioplegic robotic settings. The spectrum of multi-vessel endoscopic surgical revascularization can also be extended by PCIs in advanced hybrid coronary procedures. We have to bear in mind that multi-vessel TECAB requires significantly higher time investment than single-vessel procedures and conversion rates are also higher due to the technical complexity. However, clinical short- and long-term outcomes match the standards of traditional open CABG via a sternotomic approach. The main advantages of multi-vessel TECAB include a completely preserved sternum, utilization of double IMA even in high-risk groups, and a remarkably short recovery time.

FURTHER READING

Bonatti J, Lee JD, Bonaros N, et al. Robotic totally endoscopic multivessel coronary artery bypass grafting: procedure development, challenges, results. *Innovations* 2012; 7: 3–8.

Bonatti J, Lehr E, Vesely M, et al. Hybrid coronary revascularization: which patients? When? How? *Curr Opin Cardiol.* 2010; 25: 568–74.

Bonatti J, Schachner T, Bonaros N, et al. Robotic assisted endoscopic coronary bypass surgery. *Circulation* 2011; 124: 236–44.

Bonatti J, Wehman B, De Biasi AR, et al. Totally endoscopic quadruple coronary artery bypass grafting is feasible using robotic technology. *Ann Thorac Surg.* 2012; 5: 111–12.

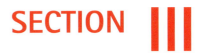

Surgery for valvular heart disease

11

Aortic valve replacement

ISMAIL EL-HAMAMSY, MAXIME LAFLAMME, AND LOUIS P. PERRAULT

SURGICAL ANATOMY

The aortic valve (AV) sits at the outlet of the left ventricle. The normal AV is a trileaflet structure, with three semilunar cusps. The AV cannot be described as an independent entity since it is a part of the functional aortic root (AR). The AR has four main structural components: the aortic annulus, the aortic cusps, the sinuses of Valsalva, and the sinotubular junction (STJ). The right and left coronary ostia arise from the right and left sinuses, while the sinus without coronary orifice is called the non-coronary sinus. The aortic annulus (AA) is the anchoring point of the AV leaflets. It is a crown-shaped structure. The plane connecting the three tips, also known as commissures, represents the STJ.

Subcommissural triangles are important contributors to optimal aortic root dynamics. They are also important anatomical landmarks within the aortic root. The triangle between the non-coronary and the right coronary sinuses is in direct continuity with the membranous part of the ventricular septum. The bundle of His is normally located at the junction between the membranous and ventricular septa. The membranous septum is crossed by the hinge of the tricuspid valve, dividing it into an atrioventricular and an interventricular component. It is also in direct contact with the right fibrous trigone. Extending from the right to the left fibrous trigone, the AV is contiguous to the anterior leaflet of the mitral valve. Separating these two structures is the aortic–mitral curtain, a fibrous structure which can measure 5–10 mm in height. The fibrous trigones act as a hinge mechanism during the cardiac cycle, allowing both valves to share the same orifice, while expanding in systole (aortic valve) and diastole (mitral valve). Finally, the basal ring is a virtual plane which lies approximately 1–2 mm below the nadir of each cusp and is relevant in valve-conserving operations.

AORTIC VALVE PATHOLOGY

Aortic stenosis

Aortic stenosis (AS) is most often observed in elderly patients due to degenerative calcific changes of AV cusps.

Atherosclerosis-related risk factors are commonly found in patients with degenerative AS. Nearly 2–7% of the population over 65 years will develop varying degrees of AS. The second most frequent etiology, mostly in younger patients, is congenital bicuspid AVs, present in 1–2% of the population. Rheumatic disease has been largely eradicated in the western world, but it remains a common cause of AV disease in developing countries.

In AS there is obstruction to blood flow across the AV during systole. The left ventricle (LV) initially compensates through concentric hypertrophy secondary to systolic pressure overload. The classic symptoms of AS are angina, syncope, and dyspnea, and they may appear after many asymptomatic years of slowly progressing AV stenosis. Once these symptoms develop, they result in a significantly decreased survival if no surgical correction is performed. Severe AS is defined by a mean aortic gradient greater than 40 mmHg, a jet velocity greater than 4.0 m/s and an aortic valvular area (AVA) of less than 1.0 cm^2 or 0.6 cm^2/m^2 when indexed to BSA.

Aortic insufficiency

Aortic insufficiency (AI) results from primary diseases of AV cusps (e.g. congenital AV malformations, endocarditis, rheumatic disease, autoimmune diseases) or secondary to dilatation of the aortic root at the level of the STJ or the basal ring (e.g. aortic aneurysms, aortic dissections, aortitis, connective tissue disorders). Acute AI results from aortic dissection, endocarditis or trauma. In AI, there is abnormal regurgitation of blood from the aorta into the LV during diastole. In acute AI, the LV is of normal size and relatively non-compliant. The volume overload causes LV end-diastolic pressure to rise substantially and is transmitted to the left atrium and pulmonary circulation, resulting in acute pulmonary edema and congestive heart failure. In chronic AI, the LV undergoes adaptation in response to the long-standing regurgitation. The LV reacts to volume overload through compensatory dilatation (eccentric hypertrophy), and to a lesser degree with concentric hypertrophy. Progressive LV dilatation limits the increase in diastolic pressure transmitted to the left atrium and pulmonary vasculature. However, dilatation leads to LV interstitial fibrosis, which may result in irreversible changes in structure and function.

INDICATIONS FOR SURGERY

Aortic stenosis

Classical ACC/AHA Class I indications for aortic valve replacement (AVR) in AS are:

- severe symptomatic AS
- severe (asymptomatic) AS in patients undergoing cardiac surgery for other indications (CABG, other valve, ascending aorta)
- severe (asymptomatic) AS with LV systolic dysfunction.

ACC/AHA Class IIa indications for AVR include:

- asymptomatic severe AS with a positive exercise test
- moderate AS in patients undergoing cardiac surgery for other indications (CABG, other valve, ascending aorta).

Aortic insufficiency

Acute AI is a surgical emergency and requires immediate AVR or repair.

In chronic AI, ACC/AHA Class I indications for AVR or repair are:

- symptomatic severe AI
- asymptomatic severe AI with LV systolic dysfunction (<50%)
- severe AI while undergoing cardiac surgery for another reason (CABG, other valve, ascending aorta).

ACC/AHA Class IIa indications for AVR or repair include asymptomatic patients with normal LV function but with severe LV dilatation (end-systolic diameter greater than 50 mm or indexed end-systolic diameter greater than 25 mm/ m^2).

VALVE SUBSTITUTES

In AI, AV repair should always be considered if feasible to preserve the native valve and avoid prosthetic replacement. Multiple AV repair techniques exist and are beyond the scope of this chapter. Prosthetic AVR exposes the patient to several potential morbidities: structural valve deterioration (SVD), non-structural dysfunction (pannus formation, paravalvular leak and patient–prosthesis mismatch (PPM)), valve thrombosis, thromboembolism, bleeding, and prosthetic endocarditis.

Available options for AVR fall into two categories: mechanical valves and biological valves. Biological valve options can be subdivided into stented prostheses (either porcine or bovine), stentless prostheses, homografts, and pulmonary autografts (Ross procedure). Stentless bioprostheses are especially useful in patients requiring aortic root replacement with a biological valve or in patients with small aortic annuli, in order to avoid PPM. These valves are not widely used because implantation is more complex than stented AVR. The main indication for aortic homograft use is extensive aortic valve endocarditis with involvement of the aortic–mitral continuity. In these instances, the mitral flange on the aortic homograft can be used for anterior mitral leaflet reconstruction. Though the risk of recurrent endocarditis was thought to be lower with homografts than prosthetic valves, several series have failed to demonstrate any differences between different surgical options. The Ross procedure (pulmonary autograft in the aortic position) is a surgical option for AVR. It offers excellent long-term survival, low rates of valve-related complications, and good hemodynamics, and does not necessitate anticoagulation. However, because of its technical complexity and the risk of late reintervention, its use is limited to high-volume centers of expertise.

When selecting between mechanical and biological valves, the surgeon must discuss with the patient the risks and benefits of each option. Biological valves are more likely to undergo SVD and reoperation than mechanical valves. In contrast, mechanical valves are more thrombogenic than bioprosthetic valves and necessitate lifelong warfarin anticoagulation. Although some newer valve models now require lower international normalized ratio (INR) targets (1.5–2.0) and home INR monitoring kits are more widely available, the linearized risk of bleeding remains higher than in patients on no anticoagulants. In addition to considerations of valve durability and bleeding risk, patient age should be foremost in the choice of prosthesis. In younger patients, the Ross procedure should be considered in selected patients as it has been shown to translate into significant improvements in long-term outcomes. In addition, the availability and expanding field of valve-in-valve technology using transcatheter aortic valve implantation (TAVI) should be weighed into the decision-making algorithm.

OPERATIVE TECHNIQUE

Surgical approach

Aortic valve replacement can be performed through a median sternotomy with standard or limited skin incision, through an upper midline sternotomy extending to the right third or fourth intercostal space, or through an anterior right thoracotomy in the second or third intercostal space. Although less invasive incisions are being increasingly applied, median sternotomy remains the surgical approach of choice for AVR.

Cardiopulmonary bypass and myocardial protection

Except for the Ross procedure, where the right side cavity is opened for harvesting the pulmonary autograft, AVR is performed with a single two-stage venous cannula in the right atrium for venous return. The distal ascending aorta is cannulated for systemic perfusion. A cannula for antegrade cardioplegia is inserted in the aortic root and a preshaped catheter is inserted in the coronary sinus through the right atrium for retrograde cardioplegia in selected cases. Left ventricular venting is performed through the right superior pulmonary vein.

Once all cannulae are in place, an activated clotting time (ACT) of >480 seconds is necessary before cardiopulmonary bypass (CPB) is initiated. Attention should be given at this time to proper venous drainage and absence of LV distension. The plane between the aorta and the pulmonary artery is divided for secure and proper positioning of the aortic cross-clamp.

We use mild systemic hypothermia (34 °C). Cold blood cardioplegia (4 °C) is used with antegrade induction followed by intermittent retrograde perfusion, in selected cases. When the procedure is prolonged and the aortic root open, additional protection can be obtained with intermittent antegrade direct cardioplegia administration into the coronary ostia with a soft, undersized cannula to avoid microtrauma and subsequent iatrogenic stenosis.

Exposure of the aortic valve

For stentless AVR or the Ross procedure, complete transection of the aorta above the sinotubular junction (STJ) offers ideal aortic root exposure. For stented AVR, transverse or oblique (hockey-stick) aortotomy is preferred (**Figure 11.1**). In both techniques, the incision is started anteriorly 1 cm above the STJ. In cases where the STJ is narrow, extending the incision obliquely into the non-coronary sinus allows easier passage of a large valve prosthesis. This incision can be extended into the aortic annulus or further into the anterior mitral leaflet in cases requiring aortic root enlargement. Commissural sutures are pulled outward to improve valve and root exposure.

Valve excision, debridement, and sizing

Valve leaflets excision is started at the commissures. Using scissors, the aortic valve leaflets are resected en bloc at their hinge point (**Figure 11.2**). Further debridement is carefully performed using a rongeur. The aim is to remove all calcium at the level of the annulus in order to suture the prosthesis into pliable tissues, which reduces the risk of paravalvular leaks. Care should be taken to avoid disruption of the annulus in cases of generous debridement, as well as preventing calcium fragments from falling into the left ventricle, as these may embolize systemically or into the coronary ostia.

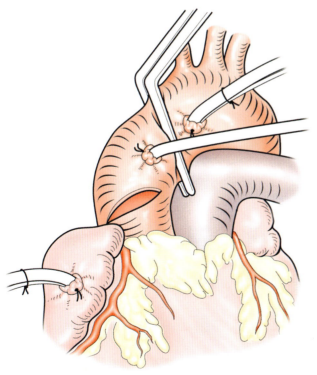

11.1

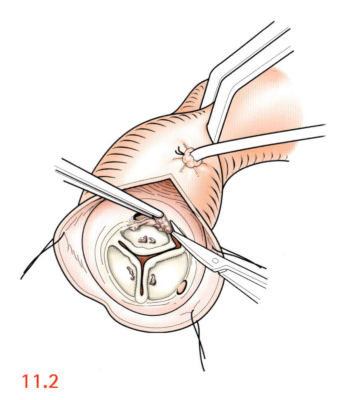

11.2

The annulus is then sized (**Figure 11.3**) and an appropriate prosthesis chosen. Patient body surface area (BSA) and valve effective orifice area (EOA) characteristics should be considered to avoid PPM. If PPM is anticipated, a root enlargement procedure should be performed to fit a larger prosthesis. An alternative to root enlargement procedures is full root replacement using a stentless bioprosthetic root, which eliminates the risk of PPM. In addition, the importance of implanting a large stented bioprosthesis at first operation is increasingly important should a valve-in-valve procedure be considered.

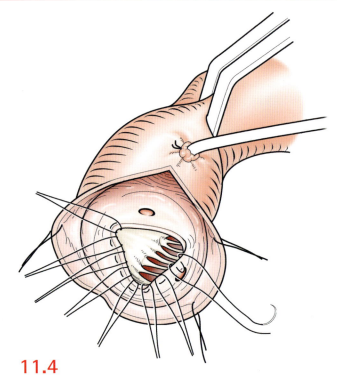

11.4

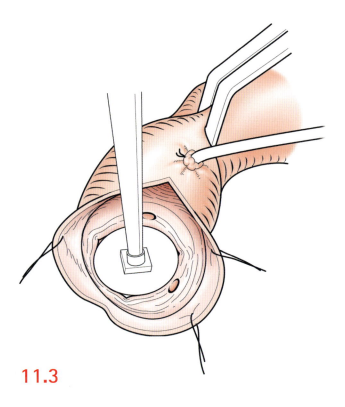

11.3

Valve implantation

STENTED PROSTHESIS

Pledgeted Ticron 2-0 U-stitches are used to secure the prosthesis to the annulus (**Figure 11.4**). Typically, four or five pledgeted sutures are needed per sinus. The sutures should be strong enough but not include too much annular tissue to avoid crowding the space beneath the prosthesis, which may cause turbulence and favor pannus formation. Attention should be given when placing the sutures at the level of the right and non-coronary cusp commissure to avoid injury to the conduction tissue. These sutures should follow the crown shape of the annulus instead of a straight line in the subcommissural triangle. Pledgets can be placed on the aortic side or ventricular side. We prefer placing them on the ventricular side because it allows a larger prosthetic valve in a supra-aortic position. However, when implanting mechanical prostheses, pledgets are placed on the aortic side to ensure proper placement of the prosthesis and avoid losing any pledgets in the ventricular cavity.

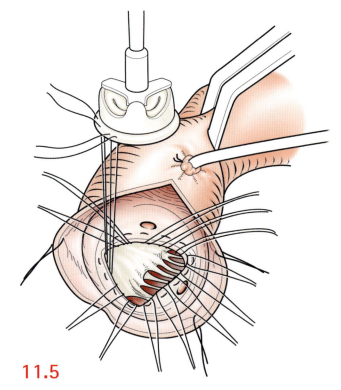

11.5

Once all sutures are placed in the sewing ring, the prosthesis is lowered onto the annulus (**Figure 11.5**). Care should be taken not to force the prosthesis to avoid aortic tearing or prosthesis deformation. Sutures are tied at the nadir of each sinus first to ensure proper placement of the prosthesis and avoid obstruction of the coronary ostia.

After the prosthesis is tied in place, the coronary ostia should be visible (**Figure 11.6**). In case of doubt about potential paravalvular leaks, a small right-angle clamp is used to probe the spaces between the sutures.

In patients with a small aortic annulus, annular enlargement should be considered. To do this, the aortotomy is extended toward the nadir of the non-coronary sinus. Depending on the targeted degree of annular enlargement, the incision can be continued into the aortic annulus, or further into the anterior leaflet of the mitral valve (**Figure 11.7**).

Once the incision has been prolonged, the space is filled with a diamond-shaped patch of Dacron or bovine pericardium, sutured first to the anterior leaflet of the mitral valve (**Figure 11.8**). When both limbs of the suture have passed beyond the native aortic annulus, the prosthesis is sutured into place as previously described. The non-coronary sinus is then sutured to the interposition graft (**Figure 11.9**), before the aortotomy is fully closed. Extending the incision into the anterior leaflet of the mitral valve allows the placing of a prosthesis one or two sizes larger than the original measurement.

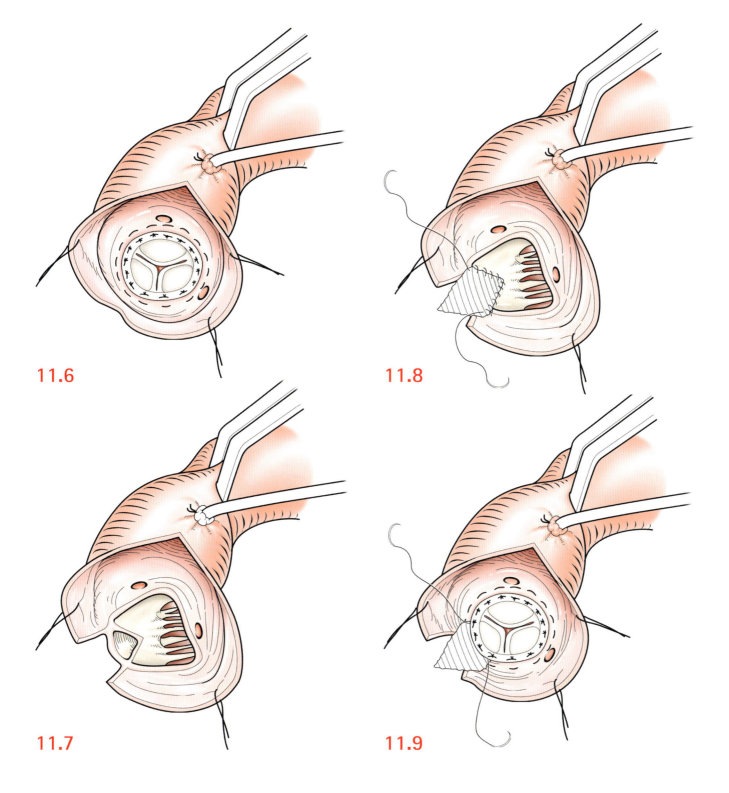

11.6

11.8

11.7

11.9

STENTLESS PROSTHESIS

Stentless AVR can be performed using the total root or the subcoronary techniques. We prefer using total root replacement to minimize leaflet distortion and ensure an even distribution of stresses on the leaflets. A continuous running suture or interrupted single 4-0 polypropylene sutures are used to suture the prosthesis to the aortic annulus. Suturing is started at the commissure between the right and left coronary sinuses. The prosthesis is placed in its anatomical position. However, because the angle between the pig coronary ostia is significantly narrower than in humans, the xenograft buttons should be ligated and the patient coronaries alternately positioned within the sinus wall. Alternatively, the stentless root can be placed in a subcoronary position.

First, the sinuses of Valsalva from the xenograft root are resected, leaving 2–3 mm of sinus wall at the attachment of the leaflets (**Figure 11.10**). Three 4-0 polypropylene sutures are then placed at each commissure, and through the stentless root (**Figure 11.11**). The stentless root is lowered and the proximal suture line is performed at the level of the aortic annulus (**Figure 11.12**). The second suture line is then performed following the crown shape of the xenograft onto the native sinus wall (**Figure 11.13**), ensuring coronary ostial permeability (**Figure 11.14**).

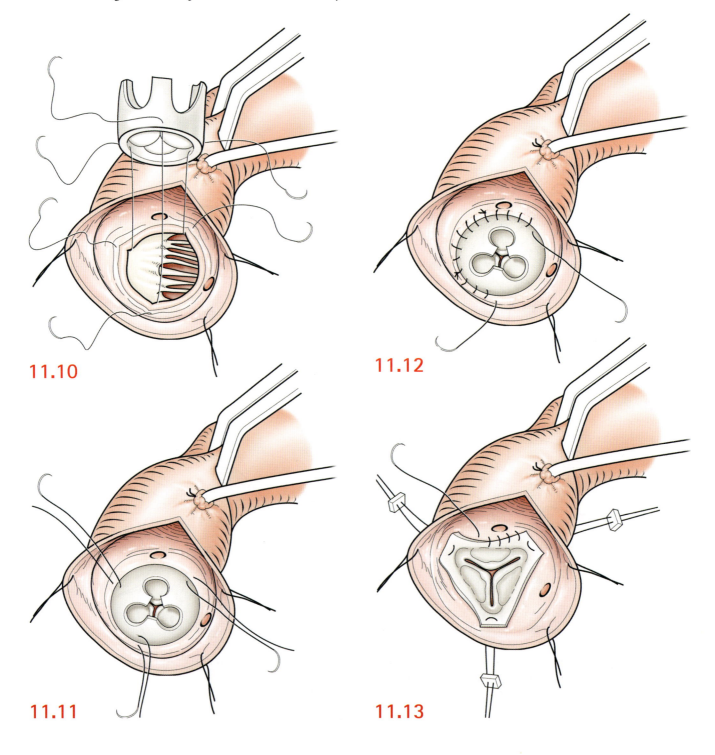

11.10

11.12

11.11

11.13

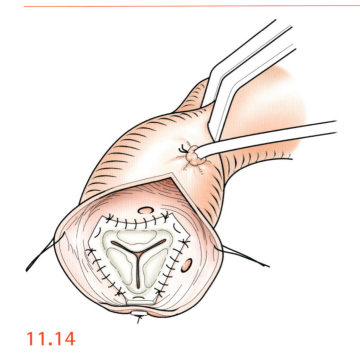

11.14

ROSS PROCEDURE

Pulmonary autograft harvesting

Once the decision to replace the aortic valve has been confirmed, a transverse incision is made on the main pulmonary artery (PA) 5 mm proximal to the origin of the right PA. The pulmonary valve is inspected and will be used only if it has a normal-appearing trileaflet configuration with no major fenestrations. The PA is transected and freed from the aortic root down to the right ventricular muscle. Using a right-angle clamp through the pulmonary valve, the right ventricle is poked approximately 5 mm below the nadir of the non-facing cusp. The pulmonary root is then carefully harvested, leaving no more than 5 mm of infundibular muscle under the insertion line of the leaflets. By staying close to the leaflets, injury to the first septal artery is greatly minimized. After harvesting the pulmonary autograft, the infundibular muscle is trimmed leaving 2 mm below the insertion of the cusps and cut 2–3 mm above the level of the STJ to avoid exposing the PA to systemic pressures.

Pulmonary autograft implantation

As with stentless roots, both total root replacement and subcoronary implantation techniques can be used. We favor the total root technique. The autograft is implanted in a subannular position using single interrupted 4-0 polypropylene sutures, while ensuring symmetrical spatial distribution of the commissures. Distal autograft anastomosis to native aorta or Dacron graft is performed using 5-0 polypropylene sutures. The coronary buttons are reimplanted in their corresponding sinuses using 6-0 polypropylene sutures. If the aortic annulus is more than 2 mm larger than the pulmonary annulus, an extra-aortic ring annuloplasty is performed to reduce the size of the native aortic annulus. The coronary ostia are anastomosed to their respective sinuses. Following surgery, strict blood pressure control is immediately instituted and maintained for the first 6–12 months to allow adaptive remodeling of the autograft. Maximum target systolic blood pressure should be 100–110 mmHg.

Pulmonary homograft implantation

The largest pulmonary homograft available is always used to replace the pulmonary root (28–30 mm), irrespective of the original pulmonary annulus diameter. Proximal and distal implantation is made with a standard running suture. Care is taken to avoid purse-stringing the distal suture line between the pulmonary homograft and the main PA.

Aortotomy closure and de-airing

The aorta is closed using a running 4-0 polypropylene suture. Before unclamping the aorta, de-airing maneuvers are performed. The venous cannula is partially clamped to allow blood to fill the heart, the left ventricular vent is stopped, Valsalva maneuvers are initiated, and root suction is started while manually shaking the heart to dislodge air bubbles from the left-sided chambers. If a retrograde cardioplegia cannula is in place, it is used to de-air the coronary arteries. The cross-clamp is then removed. If residual air is observed on transesophageal echocardiography, suction on the aortic root is continued until it can no longer be observed.

FURTHER READING

Anderson RH. Clinical anatomy of the aortic root. *Heart.* 2000; 84(6): 670–3.

Ashikhmina EA, Schaff HV, Dearani JA, et al. Aortic valve replacement in the elderly: determinants of late outcome. *Circulation.* 2011; 124(9):1070–8.

Brennan JM, Edwards FH, Zhao Y, et al. Long-term safety and effectiveness of mechanical versus biologic aortic valve prostheses in older patients: results from the Society of Thoracic Surgeons Adult Cardiac Surgery National Database. *Circulation.* 2013; 127(16):1647–55.

Carrier M, Pellerin M, Perrault LP, et al. Aortic valve replacement with mechanical and biologic prosthesis in middle-aged patients. *Ann Thorac Surg.* 2001; 71(5 Suppl): S253–6.

Chiang YP, Chikwe J, Moskowitz AJ, et al. Survival and long-term outcomes following bioprosthetic vs mechanical aortic valve replacement in patients aged 50 to 69 years. *JAMA.* 2014; 312(13):1323–9.

Coutinho GF, Correia PM, Paupério G, et al. Aortic root enlargement does not increase the surgical risk and short-term patient outcome? *Eur J Cardiothorac Surg.* 2011; 40(2): 441–7.

Egbe AC, Pislaru SV, Pellikka PA, et al. Bioprosthetic Valve Thrombosis Versus Structural Failure: Clinical and Echocardiographic Predictors. *J Am Coll Cardiol.* 2015; 66(21): 2285–94.

El-Hamamsy I, Eryigit Z, Stevens LM, et al. Long-term outcomes after autograft versus homograft aortic root replacement in adults with aortic valve disease: a randomised controlled trial. *Lancet.* 2010; 376(9740): 524–31.

El-Hamamsy I, Clark L, Stevens LM, et al. Late outcomes following freestyle versus homograft aortic root replacement: results from a prospective randomized trial. *J Am Coll Cardiol.* 2010; 55(4): 368–76.

Ganapathi AM, Englum BR, Keenan JE, et al. Long-Term Survival after Bovine Pericardial Versus Porcine Stented Bioprosthetic Aortic Valve Replacement: Does Valve Choice Matter? *Ann Thorac Surg.* 2015; 100(2): 550–9.

Glaser N, Jackson V, Holzmann MJ, et al. Aortic valve replacement with mechanical vs. biological prostheses in patients aged 50–69 years. *Eur Heart J.* 2016; 37(34): 2658–67.

Head SJ, Çelik M, Kappetein AP. Mechanical versus bioprosthetic aortic valve replacement. *Eur Heart J.* 2017; 38(28): 2183–91.

Korteland NM, Etnel JRG, Arabkhani B, et al. Mechanical aortic valve replacement in non-elderly adults: meta-analysis and microsimulation. *Eur Heart J.* 2017; 38(45): 3370–77.

McClure RS, McGurk S, Cevasco M, et al. Late outcomes comparison of nonelderly patients with stented bioprosthetic and mechanical valves in the aortic position: a propensity-matched analysis. *J Thorac Cardiovasc Surg.* 2014;148(5): 1931–9.

Mazine A, Ghoneim A, El-Hamamsy I. The Ross Procedure: How I Teach It. *Ann Thorac Surg.* 2018; 105(5): 1294–1298.

Nguyen DT, Delahaye F, Obadia et al. Aortic valve replacement for active infective endocarditis: 5-year survival comparison of bioprostheses, homografts and mechanical prostheses. *Eur J Cardiothorac Surg.* 2010; 37(5): 1025–32.

Puskas J, Gerdisch M, Nichols D, Quinn R, et al.Reduced anticoagulation after mechanical aortic valve replacement: interim results from the prospective randomized on-X valve anticoagulation clinical trial randomized Food and Drug Administration investigational device exemption trial. *J Thorac Cardiovasc Surg.* 2014; 147(4):1202–1210; discussion 1210–1.

Stassano P, Di Tommaso L, Monaco M, Iorio F, Pepino P, Spampinato N, Vosa C. Aortic valve replacement: a prospective randomized evaluation of mechanical versus biological valves in patients ages 55 to 70 years. *J Am Coll Cardiol.* 2009; 54(20): 1862–8.

12

Minimal access aortic valve surgery

ELIZABETH H. STEPHENS AND MICHAEL A. BORGER

HISTORY

Aortic valve replacement (AVR) is the second most common cardiac surgery procedure currently performed in developed countries. Although AVR has been performed for more than 50 years, the first description of a minimally invasive surgery (MIS) approach was not published until 1996 by Cosgrove and Sabik[1] and this method is currently employed in only 10% of isolated AVR patients. The slow development and acceptance of MIS AVR surgery is difficult to explain, given the relatively small and focused surgical field required for aortic valve procedures. One reason for its slow adoption is that MIS AVR is more technically challenging than conventional AVR, which is reflected by the increased myocardial ischemic and cardiopulmonary bypass (CPB) times associated with these procedures. However, numerous studies have shown that MIS AVR can be performed with equal safety and efficacy compared to conventional surgery. In addition, several clinical benefits have been demonstrated, including shorter ventilation times, shorter intensive care unit stays, decreased blood loss and transfusions, faster patient recovery, and improved cosmesis. Although MIS AVR is performed by the minority of cardiac surgeons, interest seems to be increasing within the cardiac surgery community. Increasing patient demand and the rapid proliferation of transcutaneous aortic valve procedures are two factors that may be factors driving this trend.

The term minimal(ly) invasive surgery is not consistently defined within the literature, but a key element is that the AVR procedure is performed without the use of a full sternotomy. Various approaches have been described including upper hemisternotomy, right lateral mini-thoracotomy, parasternal, and transverse sternotomy. The first approach is used by the majority of surgeons performing MIS AVR, although the right lateral mini-thoracotomy approach is slowly gaining in popularity. A MIS approach can also be used for aortic valve repair, aortic root replacement, replacement of the ascending aorta, and proximal aortic arch replacement, but these topics will not be discussed in this chapter.

Several recent technological developments have been made with the goal of increasing the proportion of patients undergoing MIS AVR surgery. Specialized equipment including retractors, cannulae for CPB, surgical instruments, and novel suturing techniques may improve the feasibility of these procedures. One of the most interesting advancements has been the development of sutureless or rapid deployment valves. Several studies have demonstrated that these novel bioprostheses are associated with a marked reduction in myocardial ischemic times, evidence that they facilitate the performance of MIS AVR.[2]

PRINCIPLES AND JUSTIFICATION

The main principle of MIS AVR surgery is to perform a safe and effective aortic valve procedure, without an increase in complication rates. The key to this goal is a well-planned approach that will lead to good exposure of the aortic valve. Speed of the procedure should not be the primary concern of the surgeon, particularly early in his/her experience. The increased operative times associated with MIS are not clinically relevant in the majority of patients requiring isolated AVR surgery. Although a definite learning curve exists for MIS AVR surgery, it is less than for many other cardiac operations (e.g. MIS mitral valve surgery, complex aortic procedures, high-risk reoperative surgery). In addition, improvements in low- and high-fidelity surgical models, increased surgical mentoring, and establishment of peer-to-peer MIS learning centers should help mitigate the learning curve effect for future cardiac surgeons.

Several lines of evidence justify the performance of MIS AVR surgery. As stated above, several studies have demonstrated clinical benefits associated with this operation. A meta-analysis of 4667 patients demonstrated a statistically significant reduction in ventilation time, blood loss, ICU stay, supraventricular arrhythmia rate, hospital stay, and early mortality rate in patients undergoing MIS AVR procedures.[3] However, myocardial ischemic and CPB times were longer in the MIS group, with an average of 9 and 11 minutes, respectively. A large retrospective study from Leipzig also suggested improved long-term survival in propensity-matched MIS AVR patients, although the mechanism behind this observation is unclear.[4]

Several other reasons may justify the performance of MIS AVR surgery.

- Some studies have demonstrated additional clinical benefits other than those listed above, including decreased transfusion rates, decreased pain, decreased sternal infection rate, better quality of life, and shortened return to work times.
- The history of cardiovascular interventional medicine demonstrates that patients prefer less invasive procedures. Increased acceptance by patients and their family members may result in better psychological preparation for their cardiac operation, as well as increased motivation for a faster postoperative recovery.
- The decreased surgical exposure (particularly of the right atrium and ventricle) leads to decreased postoperative adhesions and easier re-entry in the case of future reoperation.
- The additional technical skills that surgeons acquire during MIS AVR surgery are similar to those required for many other types of less invasive cardiovascular interventions, which are likely to increase in number in the future.
- Establishment of a successful MIS program may result in increased patient referrals and increased recognition from referring cardiologists and surgical peers.

PREOPERATIVE ASSESSMENT AND PREPARATION

Preoperative assessment for patients undergoing an upper hemisternotomy MIS procedure is similar to that for all patients undergoing AVR surgery including transthoracic echocardiography (TTE), chest X-ray (CXR), routine blood work, pulmonary function tests in symptomatic patients, and cardiac catheterization for patients over 40 years of age or those with risk factors for coronary artery disease. The CXR should be examined closely in order to examine the relation of the calcified aortic valve to sternal landmarks. If the surgeon suspects an elongated ascending aorta or a "horizontal heart," then a computed tomography (CT) scan should be performed. Inferior displacement of the aortic valve may result in suboptimal surgical exposure, which must be avoided in order to ensure a safe operation.

Preoperative pulmonary function tests should be performed in all patients undergoing a right anterolateral mini-thoracotomy MIS approach. In addition, a preoperative CT exam should be performed in order to rule out a leftward shift of the ascending aorta for such procedures. At least part of the ascending aorta should lie right of the sternal border at the level of the pulmonary bifurcation (**Figure 12.1**). In addition, the distance from the right second intercostal space to the aortic valve should be 10 cm or less at the level of the pulmonary bifurcation in the sagittal view.

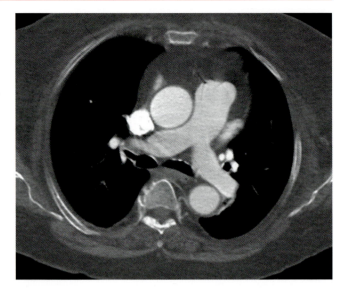

12.1 Preoperative computed tomography examination confirming that the ascending aorta lies at least partially to the right of the sternum at the level of the pulmonary bifurcation.

An MIS approach can be applied in virtually any patient requiring isolated AVR, once the surgeon has sufficient experience with the procedure. MIS AVR should probably be avoided in the early part of the surgeon's experience in patients with marked obesity or an inferiorly displaced aortic valve. The MIS approach can also be used for reoperative surgery, aortic root replacement, and replacement of the ascending aorta with or without the proximal arch once the surgeon has sufficiently mastered the technique.

ANESTHESIA

Anesthetic considerations for MIS AVR surgery are no different than for conventional full sternotomy procedures. A single lumen endotracheal tube is sufficient for both of the most common MIS AVR approaches (i.e. upper hemisternotomy and right anterior mini-thoracotomy). If the lung interferes with exposure during the mini-thoracotomy approach, then a moist sponge placed in the right pleura will suffice. Some surgeons request that the anesthesiologist insert a percutaneous retrograde cardioplegia catheter in the coronary sinus prior to starting the procedure, but we find this to be unnecessary and cumbersome. We prefer antegrade cardioplegia via the aortic root or coronary ostia (see step 3 below).

Patients can be extubated according to institutional protocol. Although extubation in the operating room is possible, we prefer fast-track management of all isolated AVR patients with short-acting anesthetic agents and extubation in the recovery room or shortly after arrival in the intensive care unit.

OPERATION

1. A skin incision 6–8 cm in length is made starting 1–2 cm above the sternal manubrium junction and extending 5–7 cm toward the xiphoid (**Figure 12.2**). The incision is continued from the skin down to the sternum with electrocautery. An oscillating sternal saw is used to divide the sternum midline from the sternal notch to the level of the fourth intercostal space. Division of the sternum is then either continued as a "J" or "T" to the fourth intercostal space.

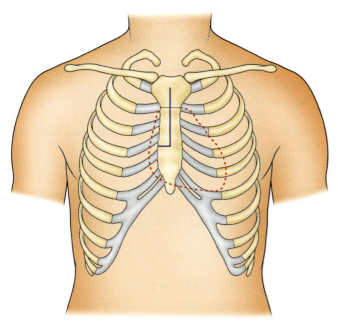

12.2

Four pericardial stay sutures are placed at the four "corners" of the incision, then pulled up with force in order to bring the mediastinal structures closer to the skin. The position of the right atrial appendage (RAA) relative to the exposed operative field is then carefully examined, in order to decide on the optimal venous cannulation technique (**Figure 12.3**).

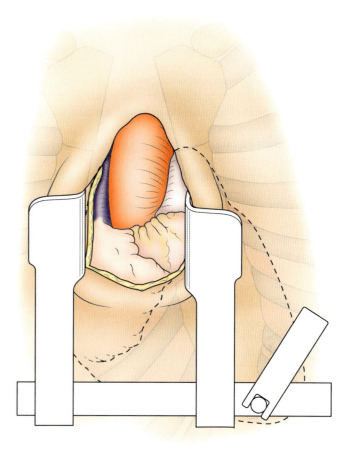

12.3

The venous cannula can be carefully tunneled between the pericardium and posterior sternum, prior to insertion in the RAA (**Figure 12.4**). Other options include direct cannulation of the atrial appendage through the incision, or percutaneous cannulation of the femoral vein under echocardiographic guidance.

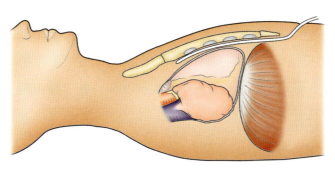

12.4

2. A Finochietto retractor is inserted, pericardial stay sutures are placed, and the exposure of the RAA is assessed. If the RAA is adequately exposed, it can be directly cannulated via the incision. If this option is chosen, then a low-profile, oval-shaped, wire-reinforced cannula should be used in order to minimize obstruction of the surgical field. If the RAA cannot be completely visualized (because of inferior displacement of the heart or mistaken division of the sternum at the third intercostal space), the venous cannula can be tunneled between the sternum and pericardium (subxiphoid) and inserted into the right atrium. Care must be taken to ensure that the tunnel remains above the pericardium with this technique, in order to avoid injuring the right ventricle. Once the cannula has been successfully tunneled, the proximal end must be clamped with a heavy tubing clamp in order to avoid its slippage into the subcutaneous tissue, and to avoid blood loss during RAA cannulation. The tunneling technique has the advantage of the cannula being removed from the surgical field, but it is more technically challenging than direct cannulation via the incision. Alternatively, the femoral vein can be used for venous cannulation. Percutaneous femoral venous cannulation has the advantage of completely eliminating the cannula from the surgical field, but risks the complications of peripheral cannulation (i.e. injury to the deep venous structures or local groin complications). We prefer a 32/40 French Medtronic two-stage venous cannula with wire reinforcement (Medtronic, Minneapolis, MN) when cannulating the RAA. Once CPB has been initiated, venous drainage is assisted with vacuum pressure (-30 to -50 mmHg).

3. Two pursestring sutures are placed on the distal ascending aorta or aortic arch, while the assistant gently retracts the aorta inferiorly using a curved Adson retractor (**Figure 12.5**). Aortic cannulation is performed in the standard manner thereafter, while the assistant continues to apply gentle downward traction. We prefer an 18 Fr or 20 Fr FemFlex cannula (Edwards Lifesciences, Irvine, CA), although caution must be employed in order to avoid damaging the posterior aortic wall with the tip of the obturator. A needle vent (DLP 14 g Aortic Root Cannula, Medtronic, Minneapolis, MN) is used for administering antegrade cardioplegia, as well as to assist in de-airing the heart at the conclusion of the case. In patients with more than mild aortic regurgitation, we prefer to fibrillate the heart with a fibrillator, followed by transverse aortotomy and direct cardioplegia delivery via the coronary ostia. Direct antegrade cardioplegia can be administered via indwelling Polystan catheters (Vitalcor,

Medical Technology in Motion, Westmont, IL) or temporary placement of "hockey sticks" (Sorin, Mirandola, Italy). We do not use retrograde cardioplegia because of difficulties in positioning the catheter via the MIS approach, as well as obscuring of the operative field from blood that runs out of the coronary ostia.

We prefer to administer one dose of antegrade cold crystalloid cardioplegia (Custodiol, Essential Pharmaceuticals, Ewing, NJ) or Del Nido cold blood cardioplegia, both of which can safely provide myocardial protection for up to 90 minutes of ischemia. The initial dose consists of 1.5 L of Custodiol or 1.0 L of Del Nido cardioplegia, whereby larger doses may be considered for patients with extreme left ventricular hypertrophy. A second dose (500 mL) may be given after 60–90 minutes if the surgeon expects a prolonged cross-clamp time. Alternatively, standard blood antegrade cardioplegia can be administered via the coronary ostia every 20 minutes.

Placement of the left ventricular vent via the right superior pulmonary vein can be challenging using the MIS approach. We prefer to insert the vent immediately following cross-clamping of the ascending aorta, in order to prevent entrapment of air into the left atrium. If difficulty is encountered with the right superior pulmonary vein approach, three other options can be considered:

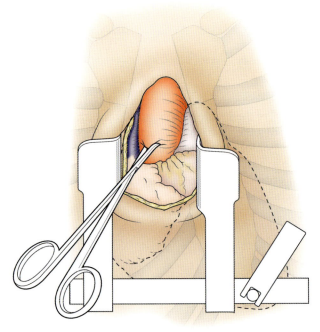

12.5

- across the aortic valve (although cannula in the operative field throughout the case)
- via the main pulmonary artery (although not as effective in venting the left ventricle)
- through the dome of the left atrium (approached between the aorta and right atrium) (**Figure 12.6**).

4. Once the patient is on CPB, the distal ascending aorta is clamped using a standard aortic cross-clamp, although a low-profile, flexible clamp (Cygnet, Vitalitec, Plymouth, MA) may result in less obstruction of the surgical field. An aortotomy is performed according to the surgeon's preference. We prefer a transverse aortotomy 1 cm superior to the ostium of the right coronary artery. Cardioplegia is given down the ostia using mushroom-tip or hockey-stick catheters in patients with aortic insufficiency (**Figure 12.7**). Once the aorta is opened, the surgical field is continuously flooded with carbon dioxide in order to lower the risk of subsequent air embolization.

5. Standard resection of the aortic valve cusps is performed using valve scissors (**Figure 12.8**). The aortic annulus is thoroughly debrided of calcium using a rongeur. At this point, we prefer to flush the left ventricle of any debris

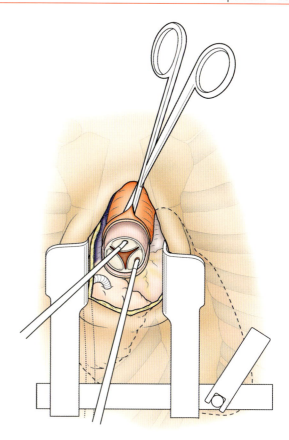

12.7

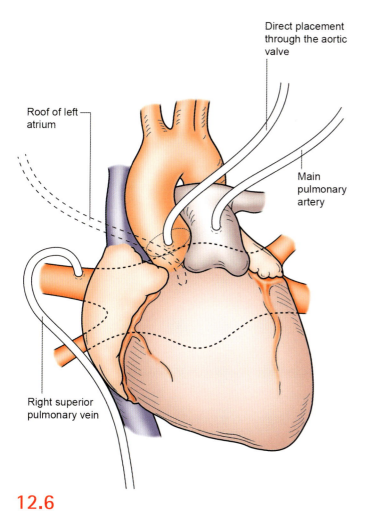

Direct placement through the aortic valve

Roof of left atrium

Main pulmonary artery

Right superior pulmonary vein

12.6

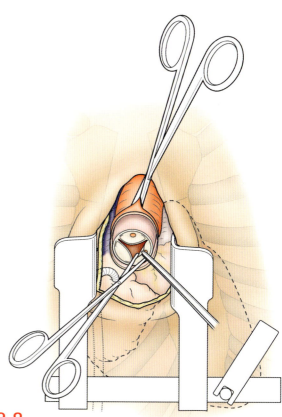

12.8

using a bulb syringe. The left ventricular vent should be stopped and a wall sucker positioned in front of the left main ostium during flushing of the ventricle. Three stay sutures may be placed at the top of each commissure in order to improve valve exposure, but we do not find this necessary. Annular non-everting pledgeted mattress sutures are placed in a standard fashion, with the pledgets on the ventricular side of the annulus (**Figures 12.9 and 12.10**). The valve prosthesis is lowered into place using a "shoehorn" technique, then force is applied with the

fingertip to the sewing ring between each strut, while maintaining upward tension on the annular sutures. Once the valve sutures have been tied, the coronary ostia are gently probed with a medium right-angle clamp to ensure patency (**Figure 12.11**). The space between the annulus and the sewing ring is also probed circumferentially, in order to assess for a possible paravalvular leak. The use of sutureless aortic valves and automatic knotting devices may simplify these stages of the procedure.

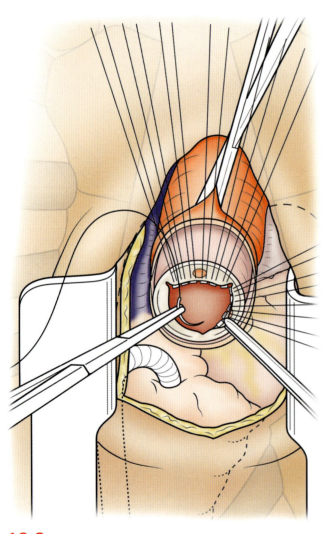

12.9

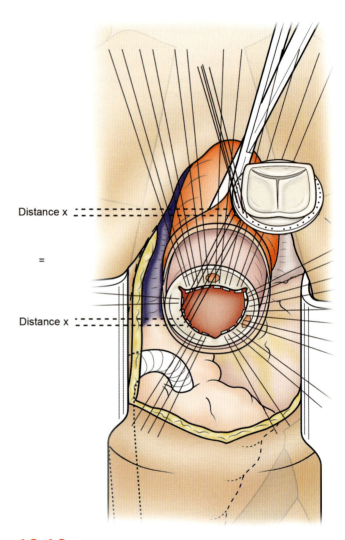

Distance x

=

Distance x

12.10

6. The aortotomy is closed with a double layer in order to ensure hemostasis. We prefer a 4-0 polypropylene suture with a horizontal mattress technique for the first layer, followed by an over-and-over running baseball stitch (**Figure 12.12**).

Prior to removal of the aortic cross-clamp, de-airing techniques are performed. The heart is filled with venous blood, the left ventricle is compressed with a sponge stick, and the lungs are inflated with sustained positive pressure. In addition, manual compression over the left ventricular apex may be applied externally. The left ventricular vent is stopped prior to these maneuvers, and the needle vent is applied to high suction immediately prior to opening of the cross-clamp. The left ventricular vent is applied to gentle suction following cross-clamp removal (**Figure 12.13**). Once the aortic cross clamp is removed, intracavitary air is assessed by transesophageal echocardiography (TEE). Pacing wires should be placed on the

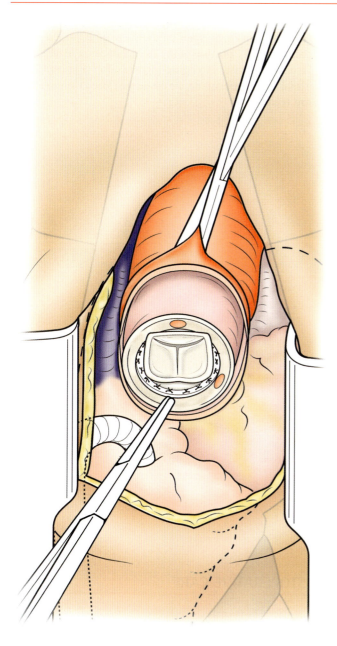

12.11

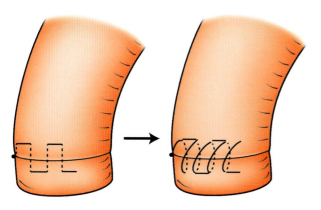

12.12

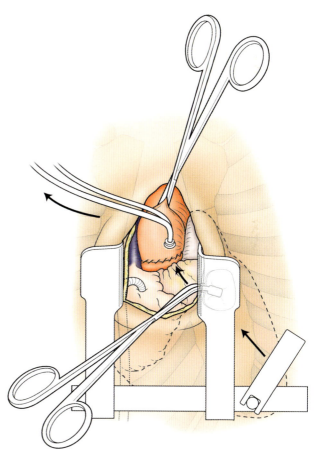

12.13

right ventricle while it is completely decompressed, prior to coming off CPB. Care must be taken in avoiding the mammary vessels when passing the pacing wires through the parasternal space and skin (**Figure 12.14**). When TEE confirms adequate de-airing of the left ventricle, the patient is weaned from CPB in a standard fashion.

8. The sternum is closed using six sternal wires: one pair at the manubrium, one pair below the manubrium, and one pair at the "T" portion of the sternal incision. Each pair is fastened together in a figure-eight fashion (**Figure 12.16**). The skin and subcutaneous tissue are closed using a standard technique.

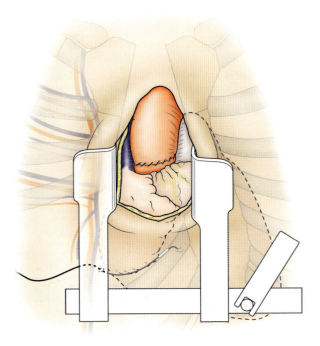

12.14

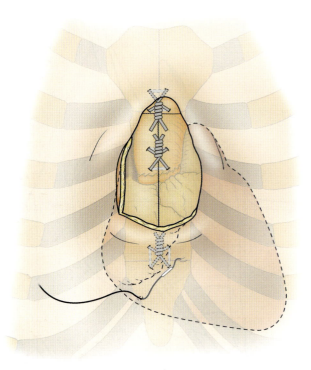

12.16

7. Once surgical hemostasis has been confirmed, protamine is administered. In those patients in whom the venous cannula was tunneled through the subxiphoid space, the chest tube is sutured to the end of the venous cannula with a heavy stitch. The chest tube is then exteriorized by pulling on the subxiphoid portion of the venous cannula (**Figure 12.15**). Pacing wires can also be tunneled in the same fashion.

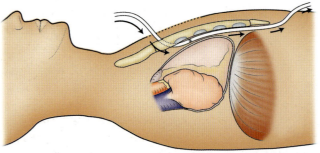

12.15

POSTOPERATIVE CARE

The patient is transferred to the cardiothoracic intensive care unit, although a cardiac recovery room can be used when available. Patients are fast-tracked and weaned to extubation 2–6 hours after leaving the operating room, although intraoperative extubation can be performed in select cases. Patients are typically transferred to the cardiothoracic step-down unit the following morning. Aggressive chest physical therapy, frequent use of incentive spirometry, and early mobilization are encouraged. We prefer to remove mediastinal chest tubes within 24 hours if output is less then 250 mL/12 hour or consistently <20 mL/hour and serosanguinous. The patient remains on telemetry until discharge, and pacer wires are removed prior to discharge echocardiography (in order to rule out resultant pericardial effusion). We do not routinely anticoagulate patients who receive bioprosthetic valves.

OUTCOME

The evidence to date shows that MIS AVR can be performed safely and effectively and is associated with several clinical advantages. Potential drawbacks of MIS AVR, however, include increased operative, bypass, and cross-clamp times, particularly during the early portion of the surgeon's experience.

Multiple studies have compared outcomes of conventional versus MIS AVR in a prospective and retrospective fashion. Doll et al.[5] retrospectively compared 175 patients who underwent MIS AVR to 258 patients who underwent conventional AVR via full sternotomy. Patients who underwent MIS AVR had decreased morbidity and mortality, lower incidence of respiratory failure, shorter ICU and hospital length of stay, and less transfusion requirements at the expense of slightly longer cross-clamp time (5 minutes) and operating room time (14 minutes), but no significant difference in CPB time. Patient selection bias limits the interpretation of such retrospective studies, but subsequent small, randomized controlled trials have largely confirmed their results.

A large, single-center study by Tabata et al.[6] involving 1005 patients showed excellent short-term and long-term outcomes for MIS AVR out to 11 years postoperatively. Of note, this study also included 130 patients (13%) who underwent reoperative AVR and 62 patients (6%) who had concomitant ascending aortic surgery, highlighting the potential for this technique in more complex procedures. The authors achieved excellent results with a median length of stay of 6 days, operative mortality rate of 1.9%, and reoperation for bleeding rate of 2.4%. In addition, pneumonia was observed in only 1.3% of patients and deep sternal wound infection in 0.5%. Also notable was a significant decrease in CPB time, incidence of bleeding, and operative mortality over time, confirming the presence of a learning curve associated with this approach.

Bakir et al.[7] also reviewed their results of 506 patients who underwent MIS AVR compared to conventional AVR and found that the MIS patients had shorter cross-clamp and CPB times, less blood loss, and shorter hospital stay. Similarly, Glauber et al.[8] used propensity matching to compare their results of 192 MIS AVR patients (using a right anterior minithoracotomy approach) to patients undergoing conventional AVR. The MIS patients had a lower incidence of atrial fibrillation and blood transfusions, shorter ventilation duration, shorter length of stay, and no difference in mortality. A recent large propensity-matched study by Merk et al.[4] compared 479 MIS AVR patients to matched controls. MIS patients had better medium-term survival compared to matched conventional AVR patients (5-year survival 89.3 ± 2.4% vs 77.7 ± 4.7%) with a hazards ratio of 0.47 on Cox-regression analysis. The study also demonstrated less bleeding in MIS patients while cross-clamp times were slightly longer (3 minutes), similar to the results of previous studies.

Few randomized controlled trials examining MIS AVR compared to conventional approach exist to date. However, Bonacchi et al.[9] randomized a total of 80 patients to the two techniques and demonstrated no significant differences in CPB or cross-clamp times between groups but longer total operating time in the MIS patients. MIS patients also had fewer transfusions, shorter ventilation times, decreased pain at 1 hour and 12 hours postoperatively, and better lung function 5 days postoperatively. Machler et al.[10] randomized 120 patients to MIS or conventional AVR and showed no difference in cross-clamp, CPB, or operating times. However, MIS AVR patients had shorter ventilation times, less blood loss, and less analgesic use. A smaller randomized control study of 40 patients by Aris et al.[11] comparing MIS and conventional AVR results found MIS patients had longer cross-clamp times but no difference in transfusion requirements, pain, forced expiratory pressure, or CPB time.

A meta-analysis by Murtuza et al. from 2008[3] showed marginal benefits in perioperative mortality (odds ratio, OR, 0.72 [range: 0.51–1.0], $p = 0.05$), but statistically significant shorter ICU and lengths of hospital stay, decreased ventilation duration, and decreased transfusion requirements, at the potential expense of longer cross-clamp, CPB, and total operating times in MIS AVR patients.

In conclusion, MIS AVR surgery is associated with an improved cosmetic result and decreased bleeding, pain, and ICU/hospital length of stay, but it is associated with longer cross-clamp and CPB times. Although MIS AVR can be performed safely, a learning curve exists and surgeons should be aware of potential pitfalls in both patient selection and operative techniques.

REFERENCES

1. Cosgrove DM 3rd, Sabik JF. Minimally invasive approach for aortic valve operations. *Ann Thorac Surg*. 1996; 62: 596–7.
2. Borger MA, Moustafine V, Conradi L, et al. A randomized multi-center trial of minimally invasive rapid deployment versus conventional full sternotomy aortic valve replacement. *Ann Thorac Surg*. 2015; 99(1): 17–25.
3. Murtuza B, Pepper JR, Stanbridge RD, et al. Minimal access aortic valve replacement: is it worth it? *Ann Thorac Surg*. 2008; 85: 1121–31.
4. Merk DR, Lehmann S, Holzhey DM, et al. Minimal invasive aortic valve replacement surgery is associated with improved survival: a propensity-matched comparison. *Eur J Cardiothorac Surg*. 2015; 47(1): 11–17.
5. Doll N, Borger MA, Hain J, et al. Minimal access aortic valve replacement: effects on morbidity and resource utilization. *Ann Thorac Surg*. 2002; 74(4): S1318–22.
6. Tabata M, Umakanthan R, Cohn LH, et al. Early and late outcomes of 1000 minimally invasive aortic valve operations. *Eur J Cardiothorac Surg*. 2008; 33: 537–41.
7. Bakir I, Casselman FP, Wellens F, et al. Minimally invasive versus standard approach aortic valve replacement: a study in 506 patients. *Ann Thorac Surg*. 2006; 81: 1599–604.
8. Glauber M, Miceli A, Gilmanov D, et al. Right anterior minithoracotomy versus conventional aortic valve replacement: a propensity score matched study. *J Thorac Cardiovasc Surg*. 2013; 145: 1222–6.

9. Bonacchi M, Prifti E, Giunti G, et al. Does ministernotomy improve postoperative outcome in aortic valve operation? A prospective randomized study. *Ann Thorac Surg.* 2002; 73: 460–5.

10. Machler HE, Bergmann P, Anelli-Monti M, et al. Minimally invasive versus conventional aortic valve operations: a prospective study in 120 patients. *Ann Thorac Surg.* 1999; 67: 1001–5.

11. Aris A, Camara ML, Montiel J, et al. Ministernotomy versus median sternotomy for aortic valve replacement: a prospective, randomized study. *Ann Thorac Surg.* 1999; 67: 1583–7.

13

TAVR: transfemoral and alternative approaches

CHASE R. BROWN AND WILSON Y. SZETO

HISTORY

In 1960, the first aortic valve replacement was performed on cardiopulmonary bypass with a mechanical prosthesis. Five years later, the first tissue aortic valve made of porcine pericardium was successfully implanted. During the following 40 years, valve design was slow and iterative and the aortic valve procedure remained hostage to cardiopulmonary bypass. However, in 2002, the field was disruptively transformed when Cribier performed the first transcatheter aortic valve replacement (TAVR) in a patient who was inoperable for surgical aortic valve replacement (SAVR). This demonstration illustrated that acutely sick, high-risk patients with severe aortic valve stenosis could benefit from a minimally invasive catheter-based approach without cardiopulmonary bypass support. Since then, multiple randomized controlled trials have revealed the safety and efficacy of TAVR in high- and intermediate-risk patients. As patient populations around the world continue to age, TAVR will continue to be refined and increasingly used to treat aortic valve pathologies. Consequently, mastery of this procedure is paramount for all cardiothoracic surgery trainees and is a technique that should be embraced for appropriately selected patient populations.

PRINCIPLES AND JUSTIFICATION

All patients considered for TAVR should have severe symptomatic aortic stenosis (AS) or Stage D aortic valve disease. The 2014 American Heart Association/American College of Cardiology (AHA/ACC) Guideline for the management of patients with valvular heart disease defines severe AS based on valve hemodynamics, valve anatomy, and patient symptoms. There are three types of Stage D disease and a unifying characteristic is that all patients have symptomatic disease with reduced leaflet motion due to calcific or rheumatological valve changes. Most commonly, symptoms include chest pain, syncope, exertional dyspnea, and decreased exercise tolerance. Stage D1 is in symptomatic patients with an aortic valve area $\leq 1.0\,cm^2$ (index area of $\leq 0.6\,cm^2/m^2$), aortic velocity $\geq 4.0\,m/s$, and a mean transaortic gradient $\geq 40\,mmHg$.

Stage D2 is found in symptomatic patients with an aortic valve area $\leq 1.0\,cm^2$ but with low-flow low-gradient AS due to a depressed ejection fraction <50%. In Stage D2 disease, while aortic valve velocity is <4.0 m/s at rest, it increases to $\geq 4.0\,m/s$ with a low-dose dobutamine stress echocardiography. Lastly, Stage D3 is a challenging diagnosis and found in symptomatic patients with an aortic valve area $\leq 1.0\,cm^2$ and a normal ejection fraction (>50%) but with a low aortic valve velocity (<4.0 m/s). Additional criteria to confirm the diagnosis are an index valve area $\leq 0.6\,cm^2/m^2$ and a stroke volume index $<35\,mL/m^2$ when the patient is normotensive and no other causes explains symptoms.

First approved in 2011, TAVR indications have been rapidly evolving as trials for the balloon-expandable (Edwards Sapien, Edwards Lifesciences, Irvine, CA) and self-expanding valves (CoreValve, Medtronic, Minneapolis, MN) have demonstrated safety and efficacy in patients in lower-risk patient populations. Currently in the United States, TAVR is commercially approved for the Edwards Sapien 3 and the Medtronic Evolut PRO for patients considered intermediate risk, high risk, and extremely high risk for SAVR with a life expectancy greater than 1 year after the procedure. While these valves comprise the majority of implantations worldwide, there are several other commercially available TAVR devices internationally. As these other devices remain in clinical trials in the United States, they will not be discussed here.

Once a patient is diagnosed with severe AS (Stage D), the first step is risk stratification to determine if the patient is an optimal candidate for either SAVR or TAVR. Risk assessment and evaluation should be completed by the structural heat team, comprising cardiac surgeons, cardiologists, structural interventional cardiologists, imaging specialists, and cardiac anesthesiologists. Risk stratification is based on a validated algorithm to predict 30-day mortality after SAVR known as the Society of Thoracic Surgeons risk score (STS score). In addition, the frailty index, patient comorbidities, and procedure-related complications are evaluated. Intermediate-risk patients have an STS score of 4–8%, with mild frailty or one major organ system dysfunction, and minimal procedure-specific impediments. High-risk cohorts are those patients with an STS score >7%, moderate to severe frailty, dysfunction of two or more major organ systems, and a possible procedure-specific impediment. Prohibitive risk/ inoperable is classified as >50% mortality at 1 year or three or more major organ system dysfunctions, or severe frailty, or severe procedure-related impediments. Frailty index is determined by a patient's cognitive function, activities of daily living, physical fitness, and nutritional status. The discussion with the patient to pursue SAVR vs TAVR also involves patient preference, ≤60–65 years old and would benefit from a mechanical valve, and need for concurrent cardiac procedures such as coronary artery bypass graft (CABG) or additional valve intervention. The main contraindication for TAVR is a life expectancy of less than 1 year despite a successful procedure and less than 25% survival over 2 years. In general, it is reasonable for younger patients less than 80 years old who are low to intermediate risk without multiple comorbidities and have never had cardiac surgery to undergo SAVR. Older patients (greater than 80 years old) who are intermediate or high risk with multiple comorbidities and have had a previous sternotomy are probably better candidates for TAVR. However, long-term follow-up data and valve durability for more than 10 years with TAVR remains unknown.

PREOPERATIVE ASSESSMENT AND PREPARATION

Every TAVR evaluation begins with a transthoracic echocardiogram (TTE). Based on this test, aortic valve morphology (tricuspid vs bicuspid), valve function, aortic sinus/root anatomy and size can be determined. It is not absolutely necessary to obtain a transesophageal echocardiogram (TEE) unless the TTE is inadequate due to body habitus or valve calcification. While the TTE can provide some details in determining aortic annular size, the standard of care is to use a gated cardiac computed tomography angiogram (CTA) for annular sizing. The area, circumference/perimeter, and the major and minor axes of the annulus are calculated. Sapien valves are determined based on the annular area whereas Evolut R valves are based on annular perimeter measurements (**Figure 13.1**). In addition to the annular dimensions, the sinus of Valsalva, sinotubular junction, and coronary ostia heights above the annulus should be measured. For access planning, a CTA of the chest, abdomen, and pelvis is also indicated to evaluate the entire aorta and aortobifemoral anatomy for tortuosity and should be completed at the same time as the gated cardiac CTA. The iliofemoral vessels should be assessed for the location and morphology of calcification, degree of vessel tortuosity, and minimum diameters. Patients must also undergo coronary angiography to determine the presence of coronary artery disease. Flow-limiting stenosis in one or more coronary arteries should be discussed with the heart

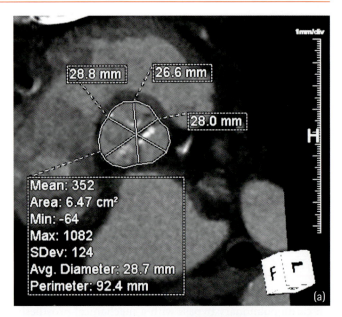

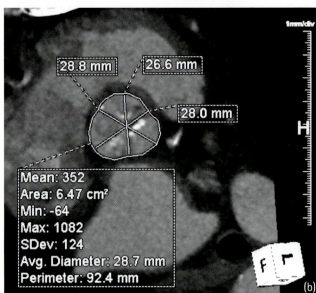

13.1a,b Standard of care is to use a gated cardiac computed tomography angiogram (CTA) for annular measurements to determine correct valve size. (a) Device size is determined from annular area for Edwards Sapien valves and from annular circumference for CoreValve devices. (b) Coronal view to measure the aortic annulus, sinotubular junction, and ascending aortic diameters.

team to determine treatment options, including percutaneous coronary intervention pre/post TAVR, CABG, and SAVR, or hybrid options. Currently, there is a lack of evidence to direct decision-making in regards to revascularization approach and TAVR.

DETERMINING ACCESS AND APPROACH

Multiple studies have demonstrated that transfemoral TAVR has the best outcomes and least complications when iliofemoral anatomy is suitable. As delivery devices have decreased in size, approximately 75–85% of patients undergoing TAVR evaluation have suitable anatomy for a transfemoral approach via percutaneous or direct femoral cutdown. In the transfemoral approach, mild to moderate (non-circumferential) calcifications of the iliofemoral arteries are acceptable and diameters must be at least 5.5–6.0 mm, depending on device. Moderate to severe tortuosity of the iliac arteries with significant calcification is prohibitive to sheath advancement due to risk of arterial rupture, and alternative access sites are indicated. However, severely tortuous iliac arteries without calcifications can usually be straightened with a stiff guidewire (**Figure 13.2**).

If the iliofemoral arteries are severely calcified, tortuous, and too small for safe access, patients should be evaluated for alternative access. At our institution, we prefer the left or right transaxillary approach with a direct cutdown. If the axillary arteries are severely calcified with small diameters (<6 mm) as seen on the CTA, then a transapical or transaortic approach is our third preferred option. In patients with a porcelain aorta, severe ascending tortuosity, or history of prior sternotomy, a transapical approach may be a more appropriate option. The transapical route is not ideal in patients with chronic obstructive pulmonary disease (COPD) or low ejection fractions. Lastly, transcarotid and transcaval approaches have been described and used when other access is contraindicated. However, these alternative access routes account for less than 2% of all TAVR cases, and they will not be discussed here.

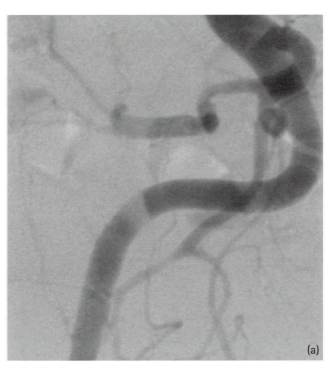

(a)

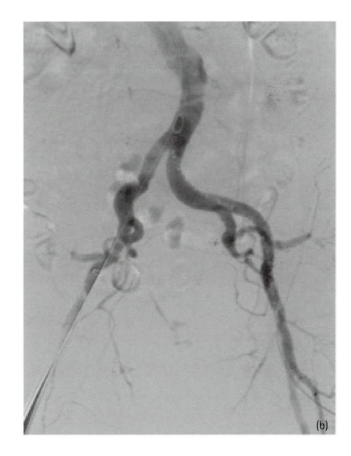

(b)

13.2a,b Transfemoral access. (a) Significant right iliac tortuosity (without calcifications) is not a contraindication to transfemoral access. (b) After advancing a stiff guidewire, the right iliac artery is straightened and allows for device placement.

Valve device choice

There are several considerations for valve choice. In the United States, there are two TAVR valves commercially available: the balloon-expandable Sapien family (S3) (Edwards Lifesciences, Irvine, CA) made of bovine pericardium mounted in a cylindrical, short cobalt chromium stent (**Figure 13.3**), and the self-expanding CoreValve Evolut PRO (Medtronic, Minneapolis, MN) made from porcine pericardium and mounted in a tall nitinol stent (**Figure 13.4**). There are few absolute reasons for device preference and decision-making should be based on valve characteristics in reference to various anatomical considerations and user experience. The balloon-expandable Sapien S3 valve is generally preferable in patients with a severely angulated ascending aorta (>70 degrees) or a dilated ascending aorta (>43 mm). Additionally, the Sapien valve is the only commercially available valve approved in the United States for the transapical approach. The self-expanding CoreValve Evolut PRO is preferred in a heavily calcified aortic annulus due to theoretical risk of rupture with a balloon-expandable valve, the ability to recapture the valve prior to final deployment, and its smaller 14 Fr access sheath, which accommodates femoral arteries ≥5.5 mm (as compared to the 16 Fr sheath used for the Sapien valve that mandates vessels ≥6.0 mm).

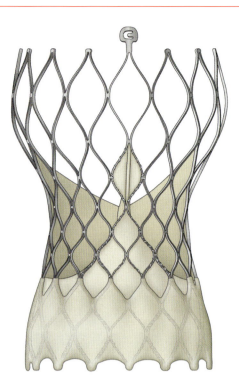

13.4 Self-expanding CoreValve Evolut PRO valve.

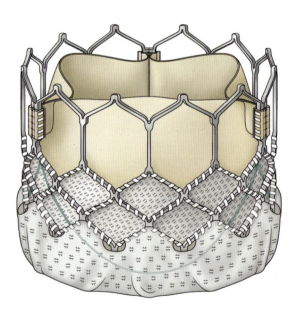

13.3 Balloon-expandable Edwards Sapien 3 valve.

ANESTHESIA

Anesthesia for TAVR procedures has evolved. In the early experience, TAVR was performed in patients under general anesthesia with pulmonary artery (PA) catheters and intraoperative TEE; the modern procedure is now safely performed in a "fast-track and minimalistic" approach with monitored anesthesia care (MAC) and conscious sedation without a PA catheter or TEE. In our center, even in high- and prohibitive-risk patients, all transfemoral TAVR patients, with a rare exception, undergo MAC with conscious sedation. Intraoperative TEE has been replaced with a TTE performed after valve deployment to evaluate position and function. These patients are transported directly to a step-down unit within 6–12 hours if hemodynamically stable and no evidence of post-procedure cardiac conduction abnormalities. In the transaxillary, transaortic, and transapical approaches, general anesthesia is used with a single lumen endotracheal tube. PA catheters are generally reserved for patients with poor left ventricular (LV) function or severe pulmonary hypertension. In the transapical approach, TEE is used to assist with identification of LV apex, valve placement, and cardiac function at case completion. Nonetheless, when general anesthesia is used during TAVR, every attempt is made to extubate in the operating room or within the first 6 hours postoperatively.

One of the main complications of TAVR intraoperatively is hemodynamic collapse or prolonged hypotension once the valve is positioned across the aortic annulus or after rapid ventricular pacing. When the device is inserted across the aortic annulus, this can induce worsening stenosis with aortic insufficiency resulting in significant hemodynamic collapse that may need to be treated with inotropes, pressors, and rarely with emergent cardiopulmonary bypass. Additionally, it is imperative that all patients have defibrillation pads as, occasionally, wire manipulation in the left ventricle or rapid ventricular pacing can induce ventricular fibrillation that requires electrocardioversion. At our institution, due to these potential intraoperative catastrophes, we remain committed to performing these procedures in the hybrid operating room with the heart team approach intact.

OPERATION

Transfemoral approach

Transfemoral access is the least invasive and should be the preferred approach with suitable anatomy. Based upon the CTA or aortobifemoral angiogram, the femoral artery with less calcification and tortuosity should be used for the device and the contralateral femoral artery for diagnostic catheters. After the patient is prepped and draped, the fluoroscopic C-arm should be positioned over the patient. The first step is to obtain femoral arterial access with a 6 Fr sheath and femoral venous access and 7 Fr sheath on the non-device side. A temporary pacing wire is advanced through the femoral vein to the apex of the right ventricle, and pacing thresholds and capture should be verified. Next, with fluoroscopic guidance, a 6 Fr pigtail catheter is advanced through the femoral arterial sheath into the right coronary cusp for balloon expandable valves or the non-coronary cusp for self-expanding valves. Aortography is then performed to determine the optimal fluoroscopic working angle for device deployment (**Figure 13.5**). It is critical to obtain a coplanar

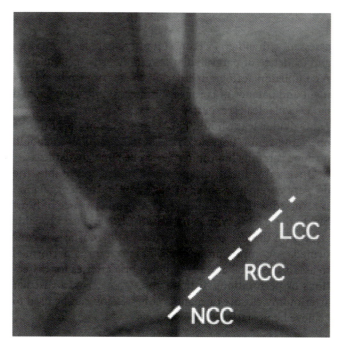

13.5 An aortogram is performed to determine the optimal viewing angle. It is critical to obtain a coplanar view with the inferior aspect of all three coronary cusps on the same plane. (LCC, left coronary cusp; RCC, right coronary cusp; NCC, non-coronary cusp.)

view where the inferior aspects of all three coronary cusps are on the same plane. Femoral access on the device side is then obtained with a 6 Fr sheath. An ultrasound can be used to locate the common femoral artery, ensuring the artery is entered above the profunda and areas of calcification are avoided. Single arterial puncture in the common femoral artery on the device side cannot be overemphasized and is the most important step to minimize arterial complications and the need for surgical cutdown. Percutaneous access approaches are always favored at our institution unless there is significant atherosclerotic disease and calcification. If percutaneously accessed, two Perclose ProGlide (Abbot Vascular, Santa Clara, CA) devices are used to pre-close the puncture site. Alternatively, a surgical cutdown to obtain femoral arterial access can be performed. A 160 cm 0.35-inch J wire is inserted into the femoral artery and serial dilators are used to accommodate a 16 Fr sheath for the Sapien S3 and a 14 Fr sheath for the CoreValve Evolut R valve. Heparin is then administered to achieve an activated clotting time (ACT) of 250–300 seconds.

Attention is then focused on crossing the aortic valve. An Amplatz Left-1 (AL1) catheter is inserted over the wire to the ascending aorta. The wire is then exchanged for a 160 cm 0.35-inch straight-tipped guidewire and used to cross the valve. The AL1 catheter is advanced into the left ventricle and the wire is exchanged for a 260 cm 0.35-inch diameter Amplatz Extra Stiff J guidewire with broad pigtail coil at the proximal end. Sometimes it is necessary to use a pigtail catheter to seat the pigtail coil properly in the LV. At this point, a balloon aortic valvuloplasty (BAV) can be performed under rapid pacing, but this can generally be avoided as it may induce severe aortic regurgitation and increase the risk for embolization. BAV is most useful when the aortic valve is heavily calcified or when undecided between two valve sizes. Contrast seen leaking around the balloon into the LV during inflation indicates that the larger-sized valve should be implanted.

Next, the valve-delivery system is inserted over the wire and advanced to the aortic annulus using smooth, short movements. It is important to watch the valve under fluoroscopy while it navigates areas of tortuosity and angulation in the iliac arteries, aorta, and aortic arch. While one operator is advancing the device over the wire, another should be carefully observing the wire position in the LV so it does not advance and cause a perforation. Additionally, gentle backpressure should be applied on the wire when crossing the aortic annulus as this helps to center the device within the commissures.

The optimal landing zone is dependent on the type of valve being used and it is important to follow each manufacturer's instructions for use. Positioning is done using fluoroscopic guidance and TEE if available. The CoreValve Evolut PRO should be positioned 3–5 mm below the annulus (**Figure 13.6**), while the Sapien S3 valve is positioned so that 20% of the valve is below the annulus in the LV and 80% of the valve is on the aortic side after deployment (**Figure 13.7**). An aortogram is generally performed to verify correct placement before deployment is started.

Once the valve is correctly positioned, one operator should be holding on to the device to make microadjustments while another begins to deploy the device. It is a good habit to use valve calcification on fluoroscopy as a reference point while the valve is being deployed to keep the position stable. For balloon-expandable valves, rapid ventricular pacing should be initiated to a rate of 180–220 beats/minute so that the systolic blood pressure drops to less than 70 mmHg and pulse pressure to less than 20 mmHg. A slow, controlled inflation helps to stabilize the valve and prevent large movements. The balloon is held inflated for 4 seconds then quickly deflated. With self-expanding valves, rapid pacing is less important but can be initiated at a ventricular rate of 100–120 beats/min. The CoreValve Evolut PRO is deployed slowly, allowing for additional aortograms if necessary. Once the valve is two-thirds deployed, it is functional but it can still be recaptured and its position adjusted.

Immediately following device deployment, the delivery device is retreated through the deployed valve but coiled wire is kept in the LV. The valve position and function should be

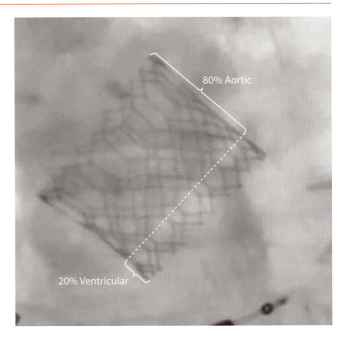

13.7 Proper positioning of the Sapien S3 valve after deployment. The dashed line represents the aortic annulus.

assessed with either TTE or TEE to evaluate leaflet motion and evidence of paravalvular leak and aortic insufficiency. A completion aortogram is performed to confirm the placement and patency of coronary arteries. While trace or mild paravalvular leak is expected after TAVR, moderate to severe paravalvular leak should be addressed before leaving the operating room. Post-deployment balloon dilation should be done carefully but can resolve some paravalvular leaks.

Once valve function and position are acceptable, the delivery system is removed over the wire and anticoagulation is reversed with protamine. If there is no evidence of heart block, the pacing wire is removed. The Perclose ProGlide strings on the device side are tied and hemostasis is confirmed. A completion bifemoral aortogram is performed to assess the distal aorta and iliofemoral arteries for dissections or perforations. If there are no concerns, a vascular arteriotomy closure or manual compression can be used to achieve hemostasis.

Transaxillary approach

The transaxillary approach is the second preferred option as it is the least invasive of the alternative routes and is ideal in frail patients with prior sternotomy, a porcelain aorta, and low ejection fractions when femoral access is contraindicated.

First, a femoral artery is accessed and a pigtail catheter is placed for an aortogram catheter, and a transvenous pacing wire is placed through the femoral vein into the apex of the right ventricle. The left or right axillary artery can be used but the left provides more stability for the delivery system with less concern for carotid occlusion with the

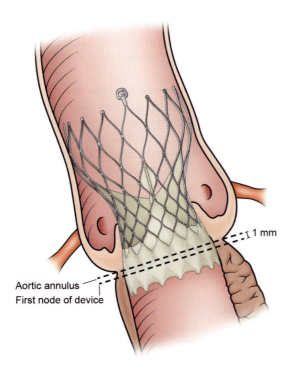

13.6 Proper positioning at final deployment of the CoreValve Evolut PRO valve.

delivery sheath. The incision should be approximately one fingerbreadth below the clavicle in the midclavicular line. Surgical cutdown is performed by separating the pectoralis major muscle fibers longitudinally and then retracting the pectoralis minor laterally or dividing it for optimal exposure. It is critical to avoid injury to the medial and lateral cords of the brachial plexus, which usually are superior to the artery. There are perforating pectoral nerves from the brachial plexus that can be excised with minimal morbidity if necessary. Vessel loops are placed proximally and distally around the axillary artery and a pursestring suture without felt pledgets is placed around the expected arteriotomy site. Heparin is given for an ACT greater than 250 seconds. Using the Seldinger technique, the axillary artery is accessed and a 7 Fr sheath inserted. As aforementioned, the aortic valve is crossed with a 6 Fr AL1 catheter and then a 0.35-inch diameter Amplatz Extra Stiff J guidewire with a broad pigtail coil is placed within the LV. The 7 Fr sheath is then removed and exchanged for the valve manufacturer's device sheath, which is 14 Fr for the CoreValve system or 16 Fr for the

Edwards Sapien device. The valve is then advanced over the stiff wire under fluoroscopic guidance (**Figure 13.8**). When the left axillary artery is used, the most proximal end of the sheath should be positioned in the aorta at the origin of the innominate artery. When the right axillary artery is used, it is possible to occlude the right carotid with the delivery sheath and the sheath should only be advanced to the ostium of the right subclavian artery. Once the valve is positioned across the annulus, deployment is similar as described previously. **Figure 13.9** illustrates device deployment for the Edwards Sapien valve.

When the valve function and position are acceptable based on echocardiography and aortography, the delivery system can be removed and the axillary arteriotomy closed by tying the pursestring. It is important to perform a completion angiogram to verify no dissection or stenosis of the axillary artery.

13.8 Fluoroscopy of the left transaxillary approach. The CoreValve Evolut PRO is advanced over a stiff guidewire across the aortic annulus to be deployed.

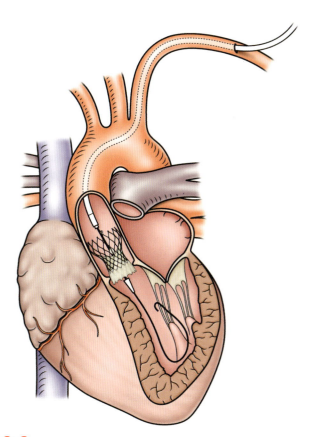

13.9 Left transaxillary device deployment with a CoreValve Evolut PRO.

Transaortic approach

A transaortic approach is a good option when the femoral and axillary arteries are unsuitable. It should be avoided in patients with a hostile mediastinum, bypass grafts overlying the aorta, or a severely calcified ascending aorta. While it leads to a more difficult dissection, a previous sternotomy is not an absolute contraindication.

The patient is positioned supine with a shoulder roll to provide neck extension. As previously described, the femoral artery and vein are accessed for an aortogram and right ventricular pacing wire, respectively. A 5 cm skin incision (3 cm above the sternomanubrial junction to 2 cm below) is made and a mini-sternotomy is performed as a "J" into the right second intercostal space (**Figure 13.10**). A child's chest retractor is inserted, the aorta is exposed and the pericardium is sutured to the skin for optimal exposure. The innominate vein is identified and mobilized to expose the distal ascending aorta. Heparin is administered to achieve an ACT above 250 seconds. After digital palpation of the aorta to avoid areas of calcification, two aortic pursestrings are placed near the base of the innominate artery. An 18-gauge needle is used to enter the aorta within the center of the pursestring, and a 7 Fr sheath is inserted over a short 0.35-inch J wire. A soft-tipped straight 0.35-inch wire and 6 Fr AL1 catheter are used to cross the aortic valve. The wire is then exchanged for a 0.35-inch Amplatz Extra Stiff J guidewire with a broad pigtail coil. The valve manufacturer's specific transaortic sheath should be inserted 2 cm into the aorta and the valve should be slowly advanced to cross the aortic annulus and deployed (**Figure 13.11**).

Figure 13.12 shows the Edwards Sapien 3 valve being deployed under fluoroscopy. It is important to verify that the balloon is completely outside the sheath before inflation. For this reason, when using a balloon-expandable valve, it is important to have at least 6 cm from the aortic annulus to the access site on the ascending aorta. Valve positioning, deployment, and post-deployment evaluation are then completed as described previously in the transfemoral approach. Anticoagulation is reversed, and the wires and sheath are removed. The pursestring sutures are then tied and a chest tube is inserted through the right third intercostal space and placed anterior to the aorta. Two or three sternal wires are placed in the sternum and the chest and skin are closed.

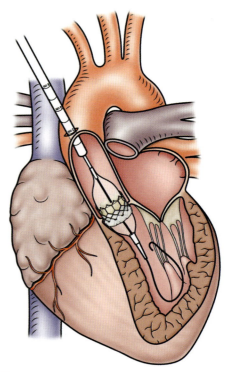

13.11 Deployed Edwards Sapien 3 valve.

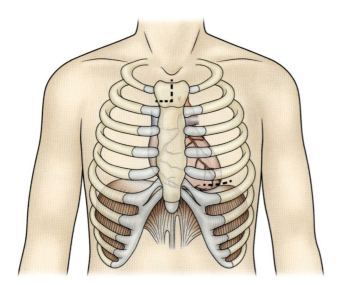

13.10 Incision locations and access to transaortic and transapical approaches. A "J" mini-sternotomy is made for the transaortic approach and a 5 cm left thoracotomy is made in the fifth intercostal space.

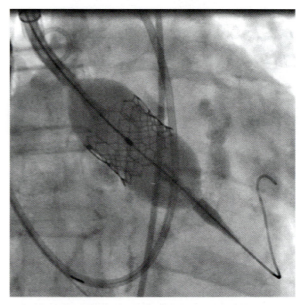

13.12 Transaortic deployment of a balloon–expandable Edwards Sapien 3 valve under fluoroscopy. Note that the balloon must be outside the delivery sheath before deployment.

Transapical approach

The transapical approach is the fourth access route and recent meta-analyses have revealed worse outcomes compared to the others. In frail, elderly patients the myocardium can disrupt after a TA approach and LV bleeding is a major complication. However, due to its antegrade deployment technique, it has the lowest risk for stroke and least amount of paravalvular leak. Main contraindications to this approach are severe COPD and a low ejection fraction. At this time, only the Edwards Sapien 3 valve is approved for the transapical approach in the United States.

As mentioned above, aortogram is completed from the femoral artery and a transvenous pacer is passed and secured in the RV apex from the femoral vein. A 5 cm left thoracotomy is made in the fifth intercostal space to expose the LV apex (as seen in **Figure 13.10**). The exact location of LV apex access is critical to the success of this technique and fluoroscopic guidance and TEE are very useful. Two 3-0 Prolene perpendicular large pledgeted mattress sutures are placed deep within the myocardium but not full-thickness, making sure to avoid the left anterior descending artery (**Figure 13.13**).

A new FDA-approved device called Permaseal (Micro Interventional Devices, Newtown, PA) simplifies transapical closure. After obtaining ventricular access, this device is placed over a wire and instantaneously delivers eight anchored 2-0 braided polyester sutures with pre-tied knots into the myocardium (**Figure 13.14**). To obtain access, an 18-gauge needle is inserted into the apex, centered within

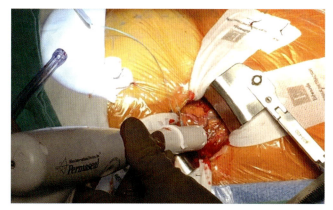

13.14 Permaseal device to simplify transapical access. This device delivers eight 2-0 braided polyester sutures with pre-tied knots.

the pursestrings, and a 0.35-inch soft J wire is used to cross the aortic valve under fluoroscopy. Heparin is administered to achieve an ACT of greater than 250 seconds. A 7 Fr right Judkins catheter is used to direct the wire into the descending aorta, and the wire is advanced to the abdominal aorta. The wire is exchanged for a 260 cm 0.35-inch Extra Stiff Amplatz wire with a soft J tip. The Judkins catheter is exchanged for the Edwards transapical sheath and is inserted into the left ventricular cavity approximately 4 cm. The valve should be inspected under fluoroscopy before insertion to check that it has been placed on the delivery device for antegrade deployment, as this valve orientation is different from the other approaches. **Figure 13.15** shows the device sheath through

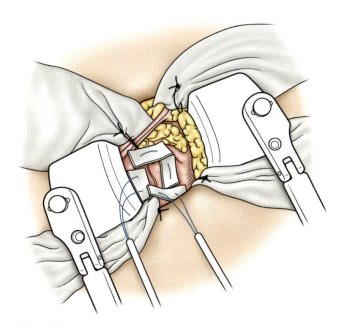

13.13 Left thoracotomy through the fifth intercostal space with rib retractors. Two large pledgeted mattress sutures are placed through the LV apex.

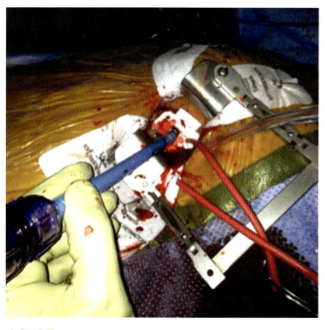

13.15 The valve is inserted through the LV apex into the LV and through the aortic annulus.

the center of the pledgeted sutures on the LV apex. The valve is then inserted antegrade across the annulus (**Figure 13.16**).

Valve positioning, deployment, and post-deployment evaluation are completed as described previously for the transfemoral approach (**Figure 13.17**). Anticoagulation is reversed, and the wires and sheath are removed. Rapid-rate ventricular pacing is initiated to a rate of 120–160 beats/minute to decompress the LV while tying the mattress sutures on the apex. A chest tube is placed in the left pleural space through a separate stab incision and, if possible, the pericardium is closed over the LV. The ribs are reapproximated with a 2-0 pericostal suture and thoracotomy incision closed in the normal fashion.

POSTOPERATIVE CARE

Early identification of cardiac conduction defects is critical and occurs in approximately 10–20% of patients. Patients who present with heart block in the operating room or in recovery should have a temporary pacemaker placed via the right internal jugular vein, and, if arrhythmias are persistent, will need a permanent pacemaker before discharge. As the transfemoral approach is the most common access route, groin hematomas are the main complications, and ultrasound should be used when there is concern for a pseudoaneruysm. If a pseudoaneruysm is present and greater than 1 cm, thrombin injection can be completed with excellent results. Only rarely does a pseudoaneruysm require surgical repair.

Due to the ongoing concern for leaflet thrombus formation, patients should be started on antithrombotic therapy. The current standard after TAVR is 75 mg clopidogrel daily for 3–6 months with lifelong 81 mg aspirin daily. Patients with Afib can be resumed on Coumadin and aspirin without clopidogrel. All patients should undergo a TTE before discharge and a repeat echocardiogram at 1 month and again annually. Even high-risk patients with multiple comorbidities can be discharged within 3–5 days postoperatively.

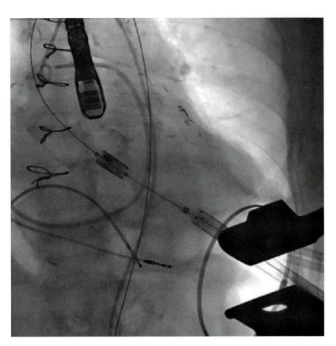

13.16 Fluoroscopy of the Edwards Sapien 3 valve in the aortic annuls through a transapical approach.

OUTCOME

Transfemoral TAVR is the safest access route, and this cannot be overemphasized. In a recent meta-analysis of approximately 17 000 patients undergoing TAVR, patients with transfemoral access had a 30-day and 1-year mortality of 4.7% and 16.4% compared to 8.1% and 24.8% in those with alternative access routes. Within this study, transapical access had the worst 30-day and 1-year outcomes when compared directly to transfemoral and transaxillary approaches. This has been confirmed in multiple studies. It is therefore important to consider every TAVR patient first for transfemoral access.

FURTHER READING

Chandrasekhar J, Hibbert B, Ruel M, et al. Transfemoral vs non-transfemoral access for transcatheter aortic valve implantation: a systematic review and meta-analysis. *Can J Cardiol.* 2015; 31: 1427–38.

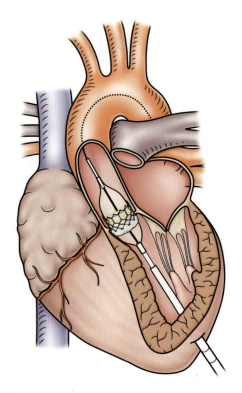

13.17 Edwards Sapien 3 valve through a transapical approach.

Holmes DR Jr, Mack MJ, Kaul S, et al. 2012 ACCF/AATS/SCAI/ STS expert consensus document on transcatheter aortic valve replacement. *J Am Coll Cardiol.* 2012; 59: 1200–54.

Leon MB, Smith CR, Mack MJ, et al. Transcatheter or surgical aortic-valve replacement in intermediate-risk patients. *N Engl J Med.* 2016; 374: 1609–20.

Mack MJ, Leon MB, Smith CR, et al. 5-year outcomes of transcatheter aortic valve replacement or surgical aortic valve replacement for high surgical risk patients with aortic stenosis (PARTNER 1): a randomized controlled trial. *Lancet.* 2015; 385: 2477–84.

Nishimura RA, Otto CM, Bonow RO, et al. 2014 AHA/ACC Guideline for the management of patients with valvular heart disease: executive summary. *Circulation.* 2014; 10: 2438–88.

Otto CM, Kumbhani DJ, Alexander KP, et al. 2017 ACC expert consensus decision pathway for transcatheter aortic valve replacement in the management of adults with aortic stenosis. *J Am Coll Cardiol.* 2017; 69(10): 1313–46.

14

Aortic valve repair

GEORGE J. ARNAOUTAKIS AND JOSEPH E. BAVARIA

HISTORY

Theodore Tuffier is recognized to have performed the first aortic valve repair in a patient with aortic stenosis in 1913. The operation involved digital invagination of the anterior ascending aorta wall and "tearing" of the stenotic valve. Prior to the popularization of Gibbon's and Lillehei's methods for extracorporeal circulation in the mid 1950s, efforts to correct aortic regurgitation surgically were limited to closed correction. As aortic regurgitation was not very amenable to these approaches, refinements in cardiopulmonary bypass (CPB) and myocardial protection enabled the development of open valvular procedures. Since then, a variety of reports have been published on repair of aortic insufficiency (AI) by suturing two adjacent cusps together to correct prolapse or by excising the non-coronary cusp and its aortic sinus and narrowing the aortic root and proximal ascending aorta, thereby converting the aortic valve into a bicuspid valve.

However, until recently, aortic valve repair has not been widely embraced. This is largely due to excellent published outcomes with aortic valve replacement coupled with technical complexity of valve repair and concerns over repair durability. The development of aortic valve-sparing root replacement operations in the 1990s and refined knowledge of the functional anatomy of the aortic valve and aortic root complex have renewed interest in aortic valve repair. To standardize valve repair approaches, a functional classification scheme for aortic regurgitation, akin to the Carpentier classification for mitral valve regurgitation, was developed. Aortic valve repair avoids endocarditis risk and the bleeding and thromboembolic complications associated with mechanical prostheses. Thus, repair represents an attractive alternative to aortic valve replacement, especially in younger patients.

PRINCIPLES AND JUSTIFICATION

Surgical anatomy

The aortic root complex operates as a unit, and understanding the surgical anatomy and intricate geometric relationships is necessary for successful aortic valve repair and aortic root reconstruction. The aortic root consists of four distinct anatomic components: the aortic annulus (AA), the aortic leaflet cusps, the aortic sinuses of Valsalva, and the sinotubular junction (STJ). The entire circumference of the ventriculoaortic junction (VAJ) is defined by a band of connective tissue, which is referred to as the *aortic annulus*. The AA joins the aortic root to the left ventricle (LV) outflow tract. The annulus is attached to interventricular muscle for approximately 45% of the circumference and to fibrous structures for 55%. Histology demonstrates that the aortic root has a fibrous continuity with the anterior leaflet of the mitral valve and membranous septum, whereas it is attached to the muscular interventricular septum by fibrous strands. The anatomic AA does not remain in the same horizontal plane, but rather has a scalloped shape. The recently defined concept of "functional aortic annulus" has been considered to include the STJ, the VAJ, and the anatomic crown-shaped annulus demarcated by the insertion point of each of the aortic valve leaflets (**Figure 14.1**).

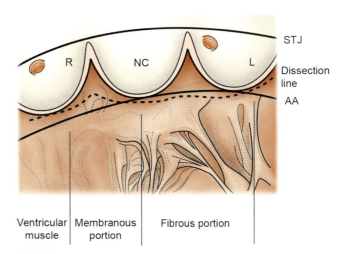

14.1 Proper aortic valve function relies on important anatomic relationships between the valve annulus and leaflets. For purposes of aortic valve repair strategies, the aortic annulus (AA) is considered as a unit, the "functional aortic annulus," and consists of the ventriculoaortic junction, the anatomic crown-shaped annulus where each leaflet inserts on the aortic wall, and the sinotubular junction (STJ). R, right; L, left, NC, non-coronary.

The *aortic leaflets, or cusps*, possess a semilunar shape, with the base of each leaflet attached to the AA in a scalloped fashion. The center of each leaflet inserts on the AA at the lowest point of the scallop, or nadir. Following the scalloped shape, the leaflet insertion point becomes higher in each direction away from the nadir and toward the neighboring leaflet. The location where two leaflets come in contact is the highest point of the scallop and is referred to as the commissure. This anatomical configuration delineates three distinct triangles below the annulus and between neighboring leaflets. These triangles are part of the LV. The triangle beneath the right and left cusps is composed of interventricular myocardium, while the other two are composed of fibrous tissue. The plane connecting the superior edge of each commissure defines the STJ. The STJ demarcates the border where the aortic root ends and the ascending aorta begins. The segments of arterial wall that are delineated by the AA proximally and by the STJ distally are called the *sinuses of Valsalva*.

The geometric relationships and function of the various components of the aortic root are intimately connected. Aortic leaflet area principally determines the size of the aortic root. The length of the base of an aortic leaflet is approximately 1.5 times longer than the length of its free margin. The free margin of an aortic leaflet extends from one commissure to the other. Thus, the free margin lengths of the aortic leaflets are determined both by the diameters of the AA and the STJ.

The ratio of the transverse diameter of the AA at the level of each nadir to the diameter of the STJ is approximately 1.2 in children and young adults. These diameters tend to equalize in older patients, approaching a ratio of 1. The lengths of the free margins of the aortic leaflet must exceed the diameter of the aortic orifice because, when the aortic valve is closed, each leaflet extends from one commissure to the center of the aortic root and to the other commissure.

The aortic sinuses are important to maintain coronary artery blood flow throughout the cardiac cycle as well as to create eddies to close the aortic cusps during diastole. The aortic root is very elastic in young patients, expanding considerably during systole and contracting during diastole. However, the amount of elasticity declines with age, and the aortic root becomes less compliant in older patients.

Pathophysiology

Efforts at aortic valve repair have been hampered by the lack of a standardized approach to classify mechanisms of AI. Analogous to the Carpentier classification for mitral valve disease, El Khoury devised a classification system to categorize the etiology of aortic insufficiency (**Figure 14.2**). This classification scheme offers a mechanistic understanding for all causes of AI while also establishing a common nomenclature. Furthermore, the classification provides a systematic approach to guide repair techniques.

Type I AI occurs in the presence of normal leaflet structure and mobility, and it is attributable to dilation of one or more components of the functional aortic annulus or cusp perforation, as seen with endocarditis or trauma. In type Ia insufficiency, aneurysms of the ascending aorta cause

AI class	Type 1 Normal cusp motion with FAA dilation or cusp perforation				Type II Cusp prolapse	Type III Cusp restriction
	Ia	Ib	Ic	Id		
Mechanism						
Repair techniques (primary)	STJ remodeling *Ascending aortic graft*	Aortic valve sparing: *Reimplantation or remodelling with SCA*	Annuloplasty	Patch repair *Autologus or bovine pericardum*	Prolapse repair *Plication Triangular resection Free margin Resuspension Patch*	Leaflet repair *Shaving Delcalcificato Patch*
(Secondary)	SCA		STJ Annuloplasty	Annuloplasty	Annuloplasty	SCA

14.2   The El Khoury classification system categorizes the etiology of aortic insufficiency and systematically guides repair strategies. AI in the setting of normal leaflet motion is labeled as type I; further categorization into subtypes is predicated on specific pathologic conditions. Type II AI is attributed to excessive cusp motion, and type III AI is a result of restrictive cusp motion. Reprinted from Boodhwani M, de Kerchove L, Glineur, et al. Repair-oriented classificiation of aortic insufficriency: impact on surgical techniques and clinical outcomes. *J Thorac Cardiovasc Surg.* 2009; 137: 286–94 with permission from Elsevier.

outward displacement of the commissural posts at the level of the STJ, which impairs central coaptation of valve leaflets. This is the mechanism of AI in patients with ascending aortic aneurysm, mega-aorta syndrome, and long-standing hypertension causing a dilated and elongated ascending aorta. Type Ib insufficiency involves dilation of the sinuses of Valsalva and the STJ. Type Ic arises from dilation of the VAJ. In types Ia–c without concomitant type II or type III insufficiency, the jet of AI will be directed centrally. In types Id, II, or III, the AI jet will have an eccentric direction. It is important to bear in mind that multiple simultaneous pathogenic mechanisms may occur in a given patient, leading to a component of both central and eccentric regurgitation.

MARFAN SYNDROME

Dilation of the sinus of Valsalva segments does not cause AI if there is no dilation at the VAJ or STJ. In patients with Marfan syndrome who experience more advanced degenerative disease of the media, the AA at the level of the VAJ will often dilate, creating so-called annuloaortic ectasia. In this condition, the fibrous components of the LV outflow tract become enlarged. Thus, the normal relationship between muscular (45% of the circumference) and fibrous (55% of the circumference) components is altered in favor of the fibrous component.

BICUSPID AORTIC VALVE SYNDROME

Patients with bicuspid aortic valve (BAV) syndrome have multiple possible etiologic factors for AI, based on one of three BAV phenotypes: ascending aorta aneurysm and mild root dilation (type Ia AI); isolated ascending aorta aneurysm (type Ia AI); and isolated root aneurysm with normal ascending diameter (type Ib AI).

Patients with BAV may also have isolated dilation of the VAJ without ascending aorta or sinus of Valsalva aneurysm, thereby causing type Ic insufficiency. Finally, there may be leaflet prolapse or type II insufficiency. The free margin of the larger of the two cusps, usually the one that contains a raphe, becomes elongated and develops leaflet prolapse.

TYPE A AORTIC DISSECTION

In type A aortic dissection, AI is often a result of detachment of one or multiple commissures, most commonly the commissures relating to the non-coronary cusp. This detachment leads to leaflet prolapse or type II insufficiency. Many patients with acute type A aortic dissection have pre-existing aortic root or ascending aorta dilatation, which contributes in the form of type I AI.

OTHER CONDITIONS

Ankylosing spondylitis, Reiter's syndrome, osteogenesis imperfecta, rheumatoid arthritis, systemic lupus erythematosus, and idiopathic giant cell aortitis are connective-tissue disorders that can be associated with AI, usually because of scarring of the aortic cusps and subsequent restriction. These often result in type III insufficiency. Subaortic membranous ventricular septal defect causes aortic insufficiency because of

down-and-outward displacement of the AA along the right cusp, which may become elongated and cause leaflet prolapse.

Indications and patient selection

Except in rare circumstances, aortic valve repair operations should be undertaken in accordance with current guidelines for aortic valve surgery. Current recommendations include symptomatic patients with severe aortic regurgitation or asymptomatic patients with severe AI and left ventricular dysfunction (ejection fraction less than 50%) or progressive left ventricular dilation. Earlier operation may be justifiable in patients with severe AI if the aortic valve is reparable. Aortic valve repair can be satisfactorily performed only in a small proportion of patients with aortic valve disease. Aortic valve repair is a valuable operative procedure for patients with AI due to prolapse of an aortic cusp or due to dilation of the aortic root with normal aortic cusps.

Repair is seldom indicated in patients with aortic stenosis. Mechanical debridement of mildly calcified tricuspid aortic valves is sometimes performed in elderly patients in whom the primary indication for cardiac surgery is coronary artery disease. The calcific deposits should be confined to the AA and leaflet base and should be removed manually. If calcium extends on to leaflet body or free margin, the aortic valve should be replaced.

Transesophageal echocardiography (TEE) remains the best diagnostic modality to study the aortic root and mechanism of AI. While the performance of TEE is the purview of cardiologists and cardiac anesthesiologists, to successfully perform aortic valve repair it is imperative for the cardiac surgeon to be proficient in independent image interpretation. Each component of the aortic root must be carefully investigated to assess the cause of aortic valve dysfunction. The number of leaflets, leaflet thickness, free margin appearance, and leaflet excursion during the cardiac cycle represent the most important information to determine reparability of the aortic valve. Information regarding the morphology of the aortic sinuses, STJ, and ascending aorta is also important. Diameters of the VAJ, sinus of Valsalva segments, STJ, and leaflet heights should be measured. The lengths of the free margins of the cusps should be estimated if possible. Dilation of the STJ is easily diagnosed by echocardiography. If the aortic sinuses, leaflets, and annulus appear normal, and the AI is central, reduction of the STJ diameter will restore valve competence. This situation is frequently the case in patients with ascending aortic aneurysm and mega-aorta syndrome.

Individuals with dilated STJ and aortic sinuses but with normal aortic cusps by echocardiography may also be candidates for aortic valve repair, although a more complex reconstruction of the aortic root is needed. This scenario occurs in patients with Marfan syndrome. The probability of repairing the aortic valve successfully decreases as the diameter of the STJ increases because, when this junction exceeds 50 mm, the aortic cusps become attenuated, overstretched, and develop stress fenestrations in the commissural areas.

While debated, the presence of multiple large fenestrations along each commissural area may be cause to abandon efforts at aortic valve repair and proceed to replacement.

Patients with aortic insufficiency due to prolapse of a BAV are also candidates for aortic valve repair, providing that echocardiography demonstrates pliable, thin, and mobile cusps without calcification. Children with subaortic ventricular septal defect and AI are also candidates for aortic valve repair. Rheumatic valvulitis and other non-rheumatic inflammatory diseases of the aortic valve are less suitable for valve repair. Finally, patients with significantly depressed ventricular function or multiple medical comorbidities are not optimal candidates for repair. If the repair is unsatisfactory upon release of the aortic cross-clamp, such patients without physiologic reserve to withstand additional myocardial ischemia are not ideal candidates to perform aortic valve repair.

PREOPERATIVE ASSESSMENT AND PREPARATION

Patients younger than 40 years of age and without coronary artery risk factors do not routinely require coronary angiography before surgery, but it should be performed in older patients. It is important that patients undergoing attempted aortic valve repair understand in advance of surgery that repair may not be feasible. Ultimately, the determination of reparability occurs in the operating room after valve inspection. For this reason, the possibility of valve replacement, including prosthesis options, must be discussed with the patient before surgery. As with all valve operations, poor dental hygiene and other potential sources of postoperative bacteremia must be addressed prior to elective operations.

ANESTHESIA

Anesthetic agents and techniques are the same as for any cardiac surgical operation requiring CPB. Intraoperative TEE should be used to confirm the diagnosis, and also to evaluate the valve for reparability. TEE is indispensable to assess for a satisfactory repair.

OPERATION

There are several overarching technical objectives to achieve a durable aortic valve repair:

- annular stabilization (and reduction when necessary)
- correction of leaflet abnormalities
- optimization of effective leaflet height and coaptation zones. Effective leaflet height is defined as the highest point of coaptation and the annular plane in long axis on TEE. The coaptation zone is the length of aortic leaflets that are touching during the midpoint of diastole (**Figure 14.3**).

Aortic valve repair is performed via median sternotomy. While less invasive approaches such as upper partial

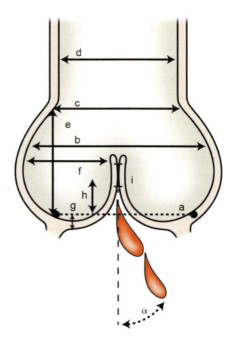

14.3 Important echocardiographic measurements to guide repair strategies. a, Aortic annulus; b, sinuses of Valsalva; c, sinotubular junction; d, ascending aorta; e, height of the sinus of Valsalva; f, distance from coaptation tips to aortic wall; g, leaflet billowing defined as distance from the aortic annulus to the belly of the lowest cusp; h, distance from the tip of the leaflet coaptation to the aortic annulus (effective height); i, coaptation zone. This figure was published in JACC: Cardiovascular Imaging, Vol 2, , Jean-Benoît le Polain de Waroux, MD, et al., Mechanisms of recurrent aortic regurgitation after aortic valve repair, pp. 931–939, Copyright Elsevier, 2009.

sternotomy have been described for aortic valve and aortic root operations, adequate visualization is critical to successful repair. CPB is established by cannulating the distal ascending aorta or transverse aortic arch, venous cannulation, retrograde cardioplegia cannulation, and LV vent placement. Multiple approaches are described for adequate LV venting but we prefer a catheter via the right superior pulmonary vein. Regardless of the aortic valve or aortic root pathology, the optimal approach to expose the aortic valve for repair is through a generous transverse aortotomy at least 1 cm above the commissures. Even in the absence of aortic aneurysm, we prefer to transect the aorta completely to facilitate aortic root mobilization. The selection of cardioplegia solution is generally institution-specific. In the setting of severe insufficiency, we achieve electromechanical arrest by providing an initial dose of retrograde cardioplegia, topical hypothermia, and then ostial antegrade coronary perfusion after opening the aorta. Myocardial protection during the period of myocardial ischemia is accomplished using a combination of retrograde cardioplegia and intermittent doses of cold blood cardioplegia delivered directly into the coronary artery orifices. We prefer handheld ostial cardioplegia catheters, but soft, self-inflating balloon cannulae can be used by securing them to the adjacent aortic wall.

Valve analysis

The components of the aortic root are carefully assessed. The key determinant of aortic valve repair is the quality of the aortic leaflets. The number of leaflets, their tissue quality, thickness and pliability, and the presence of fenestrations are observed. Leaflet mobility is best determined by suspending each commissure to a normal position. To accomplish this, individual pledgeted 4-0 polypropylene horizontal mattress sutures are placed at the top of each commissure, and retracted using clamps (**Figure 14.4**). This permits application of gentle traction as well as a dynamic evaluation of valve anatomy. If leaflet prolapse exists, this can be corrected by one of the methods described below. The lengths of the free margins of the cusps are measured (**Figure 14.5**). Free margin

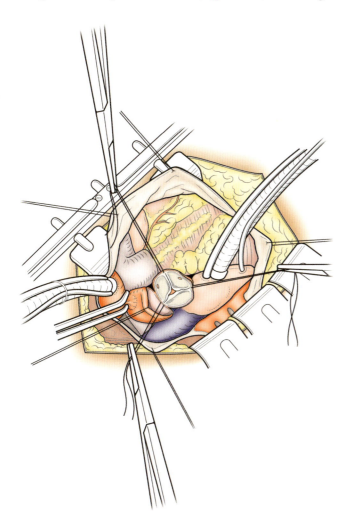

14.4 After establishing cardiopulmonary bypass and myocardial arrest, a generous transverse aortotomy is performed 1 cm above the sinotubular junction. The posterior 2–3 cm of aortic wall may be left intact, or the aorta can be completely transected for additional exposure. Separate commissural traction sutures are placed at the top of each commissural post using 4-0 polypropylene. Gentle traction is applied, thus allowing an assessment of valve anatomy. The valve leaflets should be examined for geometry, coaptation, fenestrations, mobility, and calcification.

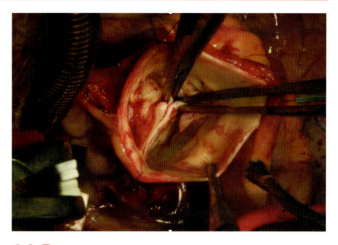

14.5 Non-prolapsing leaflets are identified as reference leaflets. Traction is exerted on leaflets in both directions to identify free margin lengths and a leaflet with excessive free margin length compared to a reference leaflet requires plication to increase the effective height.

equalization is conceptually critical in order to address leaflet prolapse. The diameters of the VAJ and STJ should be smaller than the average length of the free margins of the aortic cusps. If not, surgical reduction should be part of the valve repair.

Type Ia lesions arise in the setting of supracoronary ascending aortic aneurysm and are treated using ascending aorta replacement. To size the ascending prosthetic graft properly, the normal physiologic closed position of the valve should be reproduced by applying traction to each of the commissural stay sutures. Any valve-sizing system will suffice, with our preference being the Freestyle porcine root sizer system. Care must be taken when sizing the prosthesis. An oversized prosthesis can lead to residual aortic insufficiency, whereas an undersized prosthesis may cause supravalvular stenosis or induce leaflet prolapse. It is also important to maintain proper spacing of the suture line when completing this anastomosis because uneven spacing between commissures may also lead to leaflet prolapse.

Repair of leaflet prolapse

Prolapse of an aortic leaflet is corrected by shortening the free margin. This maneuver involves plicating the central portion of the cusp with full-thickness fine polypropylene (Prolene) or Gore-Tex sutures. To delineate the amount of prolapsed leaflet requiring plication, a 7-0 polypropylene suture is placed in the middle of the reference cusps which are not prolapsed. Light axial traction is applied, and the prolapsed leaflet is stretched gently in the parallel direction to the reference cusp. A 5-0 polypropylene suture is placed from the aortic to the ventricular side of the prolapsed leaflet, at the site where it meets the center of the reference leaflet. The angle of traction is then reversed and the same suture is placed from the ventricular to the aortic side of the leaflet where it is aligned with the center of the reference leaflet. The leaflet distance spanning the two ends of this 5-0 suture represents the amount of excess free margin. This excess leaflet is plicated upon tying this suture (**Figure 14.6**). Additional plication sutures are placed as needed until the leaflet free margin lengths have equalized.

If the leaflet is very thin, horizontal mattress sutures with a fine strip of pericardial pledget on each side can be used. The degree of free margin shortening depends on the lengths of the free margins of the other cusps. Minor prolapse of a thinned-out cusp or of a cusp with a fenestration along its commissural attachment can be corrected by weaving

a double layer of a 6-0 expanded polytetrafluoroethylene (PTFE) suture along the free margin from commissure to commissure (**Figure 14.7**).

In BAV disease, the anterior leaflet is usually the one that prolapses. That leaflet often contains a raphe, which should be released. If there is insufficient leaflet tissue at the site of a cleft, patch augmentation of the leaflet has been described, although concerns remain about the durability of this approach. After the length of the free margin of the prolapsing leaflet is corrected, the subcommissural triangles

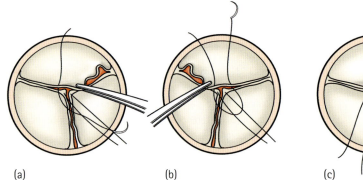
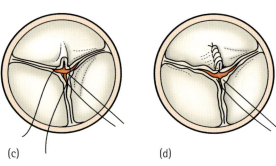

(a)   (b)   (c)   (d)

14.6a–d   (a) A fine 7-0 polypropylene suture is placed in the center of two reference leaflets for alignment. A prolapsed leaflet is gently pulled parallel to the reference leaflet and a 5-0 polypropylene suture is passed through the prolapsed leaflet at the site where it lines up with the center of the reference leaflet. (b) Traction is then applied in the opposite direction, and the same 5-0 suture is placed through the edge of the prolapsed leaflet at the location where it is aligned with the middle of the reference leaflet. (c, d) This 5-0 suture is tied with excess tissue on the aortic side, thus plicating the excess leaflet tissue. The plication can be extended as needed.

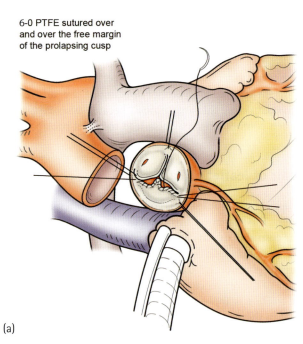
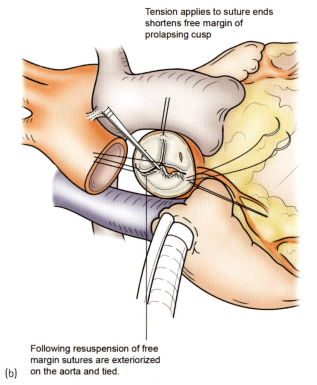

6-0 PTFE sutured over and over the free margin of the prolapsing cusp

Tension applies to suture ends shortens free margin of prolapsing cusp

Following resuspension of free margin sutures are exteriorized on the aorta and tied.

(a)   (b)

14.7   (a) Minor prolapse of an attenuated leaflet or a leaflet with fenestration along its commissural attachment can be repaired by placing a double layer of a 6-0 PTFE suture along the free margin from commissure to commissure. (b) The free margin length is shortened by applying gentle traction on each branch of the PTFE suture while simultaneously applying opposite resistance using a forceps positioned in the center of the free margin. After achieving the desired length of free margin shortening, the two suture ends at each commissure are tied. PTFE, polytetrafluoroethylene.

can be plicated to increase the coaptation area of the cusps. This plication is accomplished by passing a horizontal mattress suture from the outside of the aortic root to the inside, including the AA immediately beneath the commissural areas. There are emerging mid- and long-term repair durability data that subcommissural annuloplasty is inferior to external or internal ring annuloplasty. Thus, the indications for subcommissural annuloplasty are limited to patients with isolated leaflet prolapse and a small VAJ diameter.

Aortic valve annuloplasty

Early reports on aortic valve repair suggested that patients with subcommissural annuloplasty had less favorable results compared with patients who underwent circumferential annular stabilization. There is still a limited role for subcommissural annuloplasty in patients with mildly dilated aortic annulus measuring less than 27 mm. In patients with root aneurysm, we perform valve sparing root replacement using the reimplantation technique described by Tirone David (see **Chapter 22**). Details of that procedure are discussed elsewhere in this text, but the proximal suture line serves to accomplish circumferential external annular reduction and stabilization. Some surgeons prefer the remodeling technique described by Yacoub, with the premise that this root reconstruction yields a more compliant aortic root with long-term left ventricular benefits. However, this approach does not accomplish a sufficient annular reduction and stabilization, and thus many surgeons combine the remodeling technique with a circumferential external annuloplasty ring.

In patients with non-aneurysmal ascending aorta or sinus of Valsalva segment but dilated VAJ annuloplasty alone should achieve the desired annular reduction and stabilization. There are various options for annuloplasty including both internal and external approaches. The HAART 300 aortic annuloplasty device (BioStable Science & Engineering, Austin, TX) is a commercially available internal annuloplasty device designed to restore root geometry and provide annular stabilization. In Europe, a commercially manufactured external annuloplasty ring is available (Extra-Aortic™, CORONEO Inc., Montreal, Canada). However, we prefer to perform external annuloplasty by determining the desired size annuloplasty ring and selecting a woven straight Dacron graft in that size. Four or five rings of the graft are cut and serve as the ring. A deep root dissection is performed using electrocautery, with particular emphasis to dissect down along the interventricular muscle region, taking care not to enter the right ventricular chamber. It is important to carry dissection down low to the level of the VAJ so that adequate annular stabilization is accomplished with placement of the external ring. A deep subcoronary dissection is also performed and vessel loops are placed around each coronary artery. Several 2-0 Tycron horizontal mattress sutures are then placed in subannular fashion from inside to outside the LV outflow tract, approximately 2 mm below the VAJ. We avoid placing sutures immediately below both coronary arteries. Care should also be taken in the region

of the membranous system to avoid the conduction system. The cut ends of the selected Dacron graft are then tunneled underneath each coronary artery, and the integrity of the ring re-established using a 5-0 polypropylene suture to join the cut ends. Both ends of each subannular suture are then sequentially placed through the Dacron ring and tied down (**Figure 14.8a–d**). The ring can be tied down over a Hegar

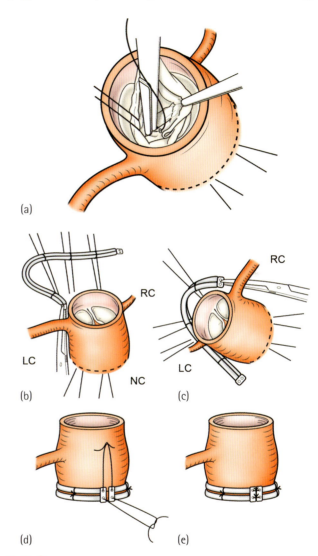

14.8a–e (a, b) Between five and nine horizontal mattress sutures placed in a subannular location serve to anchor the external ring annuloplasty. Deep aortic root mobilization is necessary for proper placement of the subannular sutures. Five or six sutures are usually placed in bicuspid valve pathology, with seven to nine in tricuspid aortic valves. The sutures are placed approximately 2–3 mm below the leaflet insertion point, with caution to avoid the conduction system in proximity to the membranous septum. (c) The ring is cut to enable passage beneath each coronary artery, and (d) circumferential integrity is then re-established with 5-0 polypropylene sutures. (e) The subannular stitches are then placed through the ring and tied down. If there is concern for over-narrowing of the annulus, the sutures can be tied down over a Hegar dilator. LC, left coronary; NC, non-coronary; RC, right coronary.

dilator (Jarit Instruments, Hawthorne, NY) positioned in the LV outflow tract in order to prevent a narrowed VAJ. Once this has been completed, the valve leaflets are reassessed to ensure that the annuloplasty has not induced prolapse.

Selection of the appropriate graft size is important to achieve effective annular reduction without overly narrowing the LV outflow tract or inducing leaflet prolapse. A general rule is that the internal aortic diameter will be approximately 5–7 mm smaller than the selected size of Dacron graft. The targeted final AA diameter should consider the patient's body surface area. Prior to restoring aortic continuity with a continuous suture line, valve competence is again assessed. Static saline testing is used by irrigating the aortic root and increasing LV vent flow to very high. A competent valve will be evident by a static column of saline.

Another strategy for annular reduction and stabilization is a suture annuloplasty. This technique also requires extensive root mobilization, with dissection carried down to the nadir of the non-coronary sinus. A PTFE suture is placed in the septal myocardium external to the commissure between the right and left leaflets. This suture is placed at the level of the basal plane. The needle is tunneled underneath the left coronary artery and the other end of the suture is placed through the right ventricular myocardium underneath the right coronary artery. Both ends of the suture are fixed in the aortic adventitia at the nadir of the non-coronary sinus. This suture is tied down over a Hegar dilator to avoid an overly constrictive annuloplasty.

An additional technique for external annular stabilization in the setting of root aneurysm is the Florida sleeve procedure. An extensive root mobilization is performed; however, the aortic sinus segments and coronary buttons are left intact to the level of the STJ. Any concomitant leaflet pathology is addressed. Six subannular sutures are placed 2 mm below the level of the leaflet insertion points from the ventricle side to the aorta, and then passed through the woven Dacron graft. These are tied with a presized dilator across the annulus to prevent excessive narrowing of the annulus. Openings in the graft to accommodate the coronary arteries are created with slits below them to create "keyholes" (**Figure 14.9**). These slits are then repaired by simple sutures below the coronary arteries. At the distal part of the sleeve graft at the level of the STJ a horizontal mattress suture secures the aorta to the graft, again taking care to recreate proper commissural alignment. The appeal of this procedure is a simplified technique without the need for coronary reimplantation, although long-term data are not yet available.

Assessment

Aortic valve repair must be performed with intraoperative TEE. At the completion of the procedure, trace aortic insufficiency is acceptable. In addition, the morphology of the repaired valve is very important. Persistent prolapse of one cusp may progress with time and cause recurrent aortic insufficiency. It is better to correct the prolapse with a second

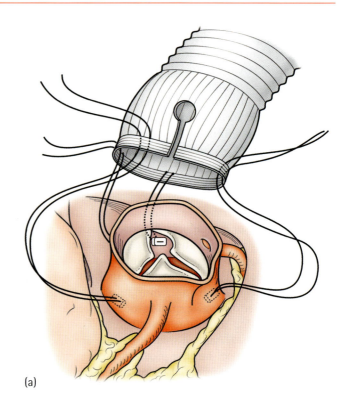

(a)

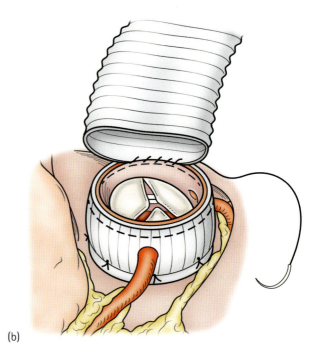

(b)

14.9a–b (a) Subannular anchoring sutures are placed in a similar fashion to the external ring annuloplasty. A left coronary artery keyhole is fashioned after the graft sleeve is temporarily seated. The vertical slits in the graft below each coronary keyhole are repaired after the sleeve is seated with 5-0 polypropylene suture. (b) A running horizontal mattress suture resuspends the aorta and aligns the posts of the commissures. A running suture line is used to complete the distal anastomosis with either native aorta or a straight Dacron graft if ascending or hemi-arch replacement has been performed, thus recreating the sinotubular junction.

pump run and further shortening of the free margin of the cusp. Central aortic insufficiency without prolapse is usually due to inadequate coaptation of the cusps. This situation can be corrected by further reduction of the diameter of the STJ without placing the patient back on CPB and with echocardiographic guidance. A temporary plication of the graft at the level of the STJ is done and the valve function assessed by Doppler echocardiography.

In addition, there are several TEE-based measurements that are known to be predictive of long-term durability. A post-repair annulus measurement at the level of the VAJ greater than 28 mm is independently associated with worse long-term durability. In addition, an effective height less than 9 mm has been independently shown to predict repair failure. Systematic use of dedicated leaflet calipers (Fehling Instruments, Karlstein, Germany) to measure effective leaflet height during repair is extremely important to ensure a durable repair.

POSTOPERATIVE CARE

Patients who undergo aortic valve repair receive the same care as any patient who undergoes cardiac surgery using CPB. Patients are aggressively weaned from the ventilator. Most patients are cared for in an intensive care setting during the first day. They are then discharged to a cardiac surgical ward. They receive analgesic and cardiac medications as needed. We do not routinely anticoagulate these patients beyond use of aspirin. Most patients are discharged from the hospital within 5–7 days.

OUTCOME

Early outcomes of aortic valve repair operations in experienced centers have been excellent. Several published series have documented that these operations can be performed safely with relatively low hospital mortality (1%) and morbidity. There are fewer published reports on long-term durability. The multicentre international AVIATOR registry (AorticValve repair InternATiOnal Registry) analyzed 232 consecutive patients operated on with a standardized approach to aortic valve repair. Subvalvular external aortic annuloplasty was systematically used for annulus reduction and stabilization. Leaflet repair was performed in 75.4% (175) of patients. The 30-day operative mortality rate was 1.4% and actuarial survival at 7 years was 90%. Freedom from reoperation was 90.5% for root aneurysms, 100% for tubular aortic aneurysms, and 97.5% for isolated AI. There were no outcomes differences with respect to valve morphology. The use of systematic effective height assessment improved freedom from reoperation from 86% to 99%. Ongoing surveillance is necessary to accumulate additional long-term data. Follow-up studies have identified predictors for a durable repair such as establishing an effective leaflet height of greater than 9 mm. Use of prosthetic material for patch leaflet repair, annular measurement above 28 mm, and commissural orientation have all been shown to negatively affect durability of repair. Long-term data will further delineate modes of failure, thus paving the way for further refinement in surgical technique.

REFERENCES

Boodhwani M, de Kerchove L, Glineur D, et al. Repair-oriented classification of aortic insufficiency: impact on surgical techniques and clinical outcomes. *J Thorac Cardiovasc Surg.* 2009; 137(2): 286–94.

Boodhwani M, El Khoury G. Aortic valve repair: indications and outcomes. *Curr Cardiol Rep.* 2014; 16(6): 490.

David TE, Coselli JS, Khoury GE, et al. Aortic valve repair. *Semin Thorac Cardiovasc Surg.* 2015; 27(3): 271–87.

Lansac E, Di Centa I, Sleilaty G, et al. Long-term results of external aortic ring annuloplasty for aortic valve repair. *Eur J Cardiothorac Surg.* 2016; 50(2): 350–60.

Le Polain de Waroux JB, Pouleur AC, Robert A, et al. Mechanisms of recurrent aortic regurgitation after aortic valve repair: predictive value of intraoperative transesophageal echocardiography. *JACC Cardiovasc Imaging.* 2009; 2(8): 931–9.

Schneider U, Feldner SK, Hofmann C, et al. Two decades of experience with root remodeling and valve repair for bicuspid aortic valves. *J Thorac Cardiovasc Surg.* 2017; 153(4): S65–S71.

Vallabhajosyula P, Szeto WY, Habertheuer A, et al. Bicuspid aortic insufficiency with aortic root aneurysm: root reimplantation versus Bentall root replacement. *Ann Thorac Surg.* 2016; 102(4): 1221–8.

15

Mitral valve replacement

T. SLOANE GUY

HISTORY

The early history of surgery for mitral valve disease began with closed commissurotomy without heart bypass, first performed successfully by Elliot Cutler of Boston in 1923 and Souttar of England in 1925. The procedure was largely abandoned due to high mortality rates although subsequent development of the operation by Dwight Harken of Boston and Charles Bailey of Philadelphia resulted in limited success in the 1940s and 1950s.

Replacement of the mitral valve began with the use of the heart–lung machine and the Starr–Edwards ball and cage valve, first implanted in 1960. This valve is still in use today in some countries, but it has largely been abandoned for low-profile tilting-disk valves due to their lower incidence of thromboembolism and reduced noise.

Bioprosthetic valves were developed in the 1970s to allow patients to avoid the use of warfarin. The first such available valve was the Hancock valve followed by the Carpentier–Edwards valve.

PRINCIPLES AND JUSTIFICATION

Valve repair has been clearly shown to be superior to replacement in most circumstances, when it is possible. However, there remain many patients for whom replacement is superior, such as those with severely damaged and calcified leaflets due to rheumatic disease. Another subset of patients that may be considered for replacement include those with functional Carpentier Type I or Type IIIB disease with a dilated ventricle in whom repair has a significant rate of recurrence. Complex mitral disease challenging to repair but that is repairable (such as bileaflet prolapse) should probably be treated in high-volume centers by surgeons with experience and success in treating such valves.

Mitral stenosis

Intervention on the mitral valve for stenosis is general indicated when the valve area is less than $1.5 \, \text{cm}^3$, the mean gradient is >10 mmHg, and the patient has elevated filling pressures (pulmonary artery and wedge pressures) and/or symptoms. If the valve morphology is amenable to percutaneous balloon valvuloplasty, this is the preferred option. However, many patients do not have appropriate morphology due to leaflet calcification or left atrial appendage clot and are therefore better surgical candidates. Open mitral commissurotomy is an option, especially in young patients, however the durability is highly dependent on the morphology of the valve and replacement is often a superior option, especially if a mechanical valve can be used.

Mitral regurgitation

Most patients undergoing surgery for mitral regurgitation today can and should have a valve repair rather than replacement, especially for myxomatous disease which should have a >95% repair rate in expert hands. Surgery of the mitral valve in patients with symptoms, an enlarged heart, elevated pulmonary artery pressures, or new onset of atrial fibrillation is clearly indicated. Patients without these characteristics should only undergo surgery when the predicted rate of repair is high and surgery performed at a high-volume center.

Mitral valve endocarditis with regurgitation, heart failure, large vegetation, failure of medical management, or annular abscess often requires replacement.

Indications for bioprosthetic valves

Bioprosthetic valves are indicated for patients over age 65 or in those for whom anticoagulation is contraindicated. Bioprosthetic valves degenerate more quickly in younger patients, who often have the strongest desire to avoid warfarin. Women who desire children should receive a bioprosthetic valve, as should non-compliant patients. Endocarditic valves can be replaced with either bioprosthetic or mechanical valves although patients with a recent history of i.v. drug abuse often are deemed unable to manage warfarin due to non-compliance and receive a tissue valve. There is no difference in recurrence rates for endocarditis based on type of valve implanted.

Indications for mechanical valves

Mechanical mitral valve replacement is indicated for patients requiring replacement (rather than repair) who are younger than age 65, have no contraindications to anticoagulation (such as non-compliance), are willing to have a mechanical valve placed, already have a mechanical valve in the aortic position, and do not require Coumadin for other reasons such as atrial fibrillation. Patients who are on Coumadin for other reasons but have a significant chance of bleeding can still be considered for a tissue valve. Patients with left ventricular outflow tract obstruction due to hypertrophic obstructive cardiomyopathy (HOCM) are also candidates for a mechanical valve and this virtually eliminates the obstruction in most cases.

PREOPERATIVE ASSESSMENT AND PREPARATION

Cardiac catheterization is indicated for most patients over age 40 or with a strong family history of coronary disease or other major risk factors. In addition to identifying coronary disease, other important findings would include severe mitral annular calcification (MAC) and a left-dominant coronary system. MAC can dramatically increase the complexity of what is an otherwise simple operation. A left-dominant coronary system may put the patient at increased risk of a large myocardial infarction with injury to the circumflex with too deeply placed sutures in the annulus. Anticipating these challenges prior to the entry into the operating room is critical to managing them appropriately. Severe MAC can usually be seen easily on the cardiac catheterization films.

Preoperative echocardiography is indicated in all patients. A transesophageal echocardiogram (TEE) with or without 3D reconstruction might be considered in complex valve pathologies to estimate the chance of repair versus replacement. Non-contrast CT scan of the chest should be considered in patients who have evidence of aortic calcification on chest X-ray or catheterization.

ANESTHESIA

Patients undergo mitral valve replacement under general anesthesia using standard inhalational techniques. Patients should have an arterial line placed, a Foley bladder catheter with temperature probe inserted, and usually a pulmonary artery catheter inserted as well. An intraoperative TEE probe is placed to confirm the pathology prior to incision and to assess the valve function postoperatively including looking for perivalvular leaks. The TEE is also helpful for assessing the presence of air prior to separation from bypass and evaluating cardiac function after coming off bypass. In addition, the TEE can detect acute postoperative wall motion abnormalities that are suggestive of a circumflex coronary artery injury.

OPERATIVE PROCEDURE

Incisions

COMPLETE MEDIAN STERNOTOMY

There are several different incisions that can be used to replace the mitral valve. The standard incision is complete median sternotomy. Many surgeons use this routinely. In our practice, its use is limited to those with a contraindication to minimally invasive approaches (very low ejection fraction, dense right chest adhesions, severe MAC, concomitant CAD requiring bypass, ascending aorta >40 mm). **Figure 15.1a** demonstrates the incision and **Figure 15.1b** the associated

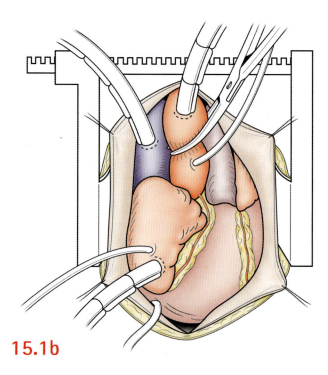

15.1a

15.1b

exposure. Also demonstrated is standard bicaval cannulation along with antegrade and retrograde cardioplegia.

UPPER MINI-STERNOTOMY

An upper mini-sternotomy incision, as illustrated in **Figure 15.2**, can also be used to approach the mitral valve. Access to the valve must be obtained via the left atrial dome as will be detailed later in this chapter. Cannulation can be performed either directly through the incision or peripherally. Bicaval cannulation is unnecessary with this approach given that the right atrium is not entered and the superior vena cava is not occluded by retraction.

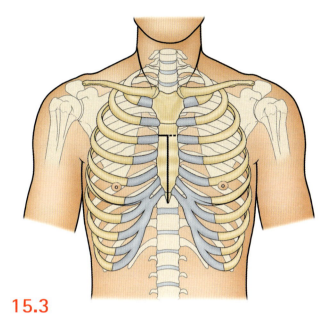

15.3

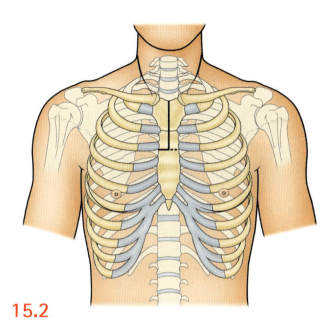

15.2

INTERSPACE THORACOTOMY

Mitral valve surgery was performed in the 1960s through a standard generous right anterior–lateral fourth or fifth interspace thoracotomy (**Figure 15.4**) as this approach afforded the easiest access to the mitral valve based on the angle of the valve. Although largely abandoned in favor of median sternotomy, it still has a valuable role for patients with prior surgery, particularly with patent bypass grafts, at centers without experience in advanced minimally invasive right chest approaches to the valve. A Waterston's groove approach is used and cold fibrillatory arrest may be employed with this technique in redo patients (26 °C). Cannulation can be peripheral or central.

LOWER MINI-STERNOTOMY

A lower mini-sternotomy incision (**Figure 15.3**) may be used to perform a minimally invasive mitral valve replacement. A 6–8 cm skin incision is employed over the lower sternum. The lower mini-sternotomy is executed by cutting the sternum from the xiphoid up to the second intercostal space combined with a "T" or upside-down "L", leaving the manubrium intact. Access to the left atrium is gained via Waterston's groove or transseptally and is aided by use of a "McCarthy" mini-sternotomy mitral retractor (Kapp Surgical Instruments, Cleveland, OH). Cannulation can be peripheral or central.

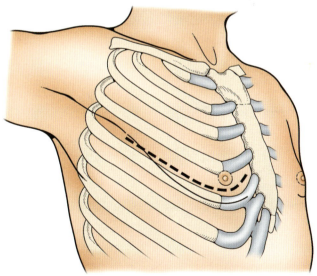

15.4

MINI-THORACOTOMY

Alternatively, a "mini"-thoracotomy (**Figure 15.5a**) into the right anterior–lateral chest may be employed (fourth or fifth interspace). These incisions are typically 5–10 cm in size although frequently a much larger rib interspace incision is employed to allow for greater rib spreading, improving exposure. Soft-tissue retractors such as the Alexis retractor (Applied Medical, Rancho Santa Margarita, CA) or the CardioVations soft-tissue retractor (Edwards Lifesciences, Irvine, CA) are usually employed. Adjunctive techniques to assist with these smaller incisions are numerous. Long endoscopic instruments are usually used. An endoscopic camera is often employed to improve valve visualization. Peripheral cannulation (femoral artery and vein) is fairly standard in this approach although some centers still employ central cannulation with this technique. Cardiac arrest may be obtained with either a transthoracic aortic clamp or use of the CardioVations Intraclude catheter (Edwards Lifesciences) along with percutaneous coronary sinus retrograde cardioplegia. In addition,

many surgeons employ robotic assistance in combination with these "mini"-thoracotomies in order to make the valve portion of the procedure easier, given the increased range of motion of the robotic instruments over standard straight-shafted endoscopic instruments. **Figure 15.5b** demonstrates the positions of incisions.

"TOTALLY ENDOSCOPIC ROBOTIC" APPROACH

Select centers such as ours routinely employ a "totally endoscopic robotic" approach to isolated mitral valve replacement (**Figure 15.6a and b**) in which an extremely small working

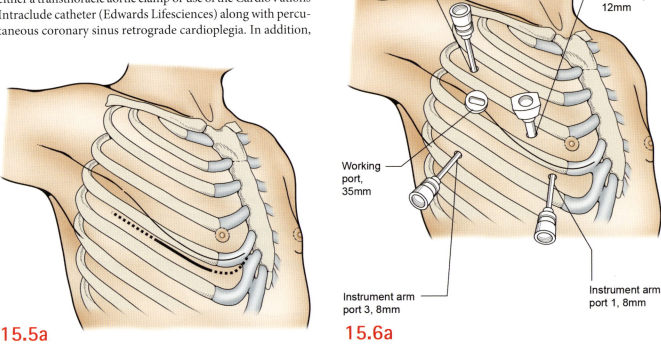

Instrument arm port 2, 8mm

Camera port, 12mm

Working port, 35mm

Instrument arm port 3, 8mm

Instrument arm port 1, 8mm

15.6a

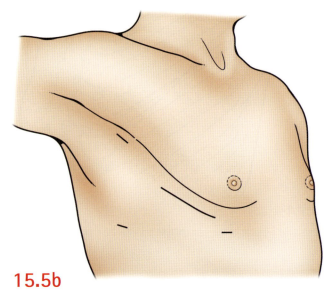

15.5a

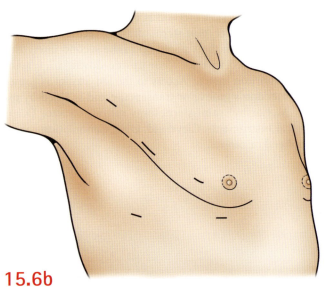

15.5b

15.6b

port (35 mm in length) is used in conjunction with the robot, peripheral cannulation, and the endoclamp and percutaneous retrograde system. The port size is larger than that used for repair (15 mm) in order to fit the prosthetic valve into the chest. This procedure requires extensive training and team preparation.

Sutures are placed in the annulus and exteriorized in a linear fashion at the bottom of the wound in strict order and placed in two linear suture guides. They are then placed through the valve, which is then lowered into the view of the camera where the console surgeon lowers it into place while the bedside assistant tightens up the sutures. Sutures may then be secured using either endoscopic knot-tying or the Cor-Knot device (LSI Solutions, Rochester, NY), which is much faster. Direct knot-tying by the console surgeon is generally too slow compared to these techniques.

Approaches to the mitral valve

The classic intracardiac exposure (**Figure 15.7**) of the mitral valve is performed through the intra-atrial groove. Either limited dissection with lateral entry into the left atrium may be performed or the groove can be more extensively dissected medially, which may improve exposure and reduce the risk of pulmonary vein narrowing.

Although not commonly employed in most centers, a simple way to expose the mitral valve is via the left atrial dome (**Figure 15.8**) between the superior vena cava and the aorta, approximately 1 cm away from the base of the aorta. The aorta is completely encircled and retracted leftward by silastic tubing and by rotation of the aortic cross-clamp leftward. The dome incision is started in the middle then carried toward the superior vena cava then lateral (away from the ventricle) to the left atrial appendage. Stay sutures are placed and handheld "spoon" or "nerve root" retractors are used to expose the valve. This approach does not require bicaval cannulation. It can be used through an upper mini-sternotomy.

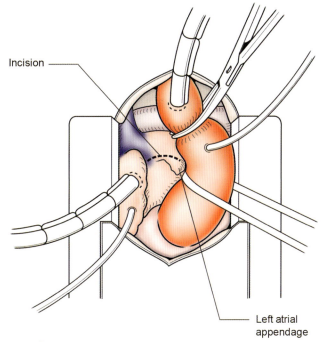

Incision

Left atrial appendage

15.8

The mitral valve can easily be exposed via an incision into the atrial septum after making a right atriotomy (transeptal incision, **Figure 15.9**). Bicaval cannulation is performed in combination with caval tapes. The right atrial incision is a standard one starting near the right atrial appendage then carried down to the inferior vena cava (IVC) lateral to the cannula. An incision is then made in the fossa ovalis (never medial to it) and extended superiorly and inferiorly, making sure not to approach the tricuspid valve or coronary sinus/triangle of Koch. Stay sutures are used in four quandrants on both the right atriotomy and the septotomy with hand-held "spoon" retractors as an adjunct.

In cases where exposure is anticipated to be difficult, there is no open technique with better exposure to the

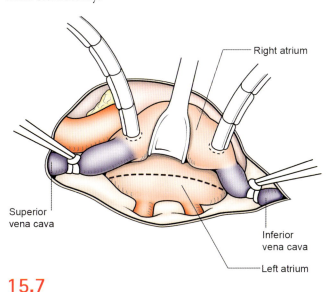

Right atrium

Superior vena cava

Inferior vena cava

Left atrium

15.7

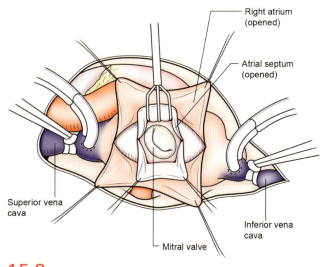

Right atrium (opened)

Atrial septum (opened)

Superior vena cava

Inferior vena cava

Mitral valve

15.9

mitral valve than the extended superior transeptal approach (**Figure 15.10**). It is essentially a combination of the transeptal approach (see **Figure 15.9**) and the dome approach (see **Figure 15.8**). A right atrial incision is made extending from lateral to the IVC cannula inferiorly up into the right atrial appendage. Stay sutures are placed. A transeptal incision is made into the fossa ovalis of the septum then carried superiorly up and through the middle of the right atrial appendage onto the dome of the left atrium 1 cm lateral to the aorta and then just lateral to the left atrial appendage. Additional stay sutures are then placed into the left atrial/septal incision. Limited manual traction with "spoon" retractors is applied by the assistant.

We employ this approach in cases where exposure is anticipated to be difficult and the mitral replacement may be more challenging, such as with severe MAC or in redo cases with a patent internal mammary artery (IM) graft where the heart cannot "flop" over to the left as easily. Some concern has been raised over a slightly increased risk of heart block with extended superior trans-septal approaches given interruption of the artery to the sinoatrial (SA) node. There are groups who use this approach routinely for mitral valve surgery given its excellent exposure of the mitral valve.

Valve implant techniques

The surgeon must be aware of the important structures surrounding the mitral valve (**Figure 15.11**), particularly when placing sutures in those areas. The challenge is that one cannot see the structures directly but must "know" where they are generally located and avoid them. A common complication is injury or kinking of the circumflex coronary artery (particularly dangerous in right-dominant coronary circulation. This can be caused by the valve sutures as well as the sutures used to close the left atrial appendage. Also seen is massive aortic insufficiency after removal of the aortic cross-clamp caused by catching the non-coronary or left coronary leaflet of the aortic valve. Placing suture bites to high above the anterior leaflet and aortomitral continuity is the usual cause. Less common complications include sewing-in a retrograde coronary sinus cardioplegia cannula or injuring the conducting system.

When feasible, mitral valve replacement should be performed using "chordal sparing" techniques (**Figure 15.12a–c**). The advantage of this is that it preserves the mechanical scaffolding of the left ventricle, which has been shown to reduce long-term dilatation of the ventricle as well as improve

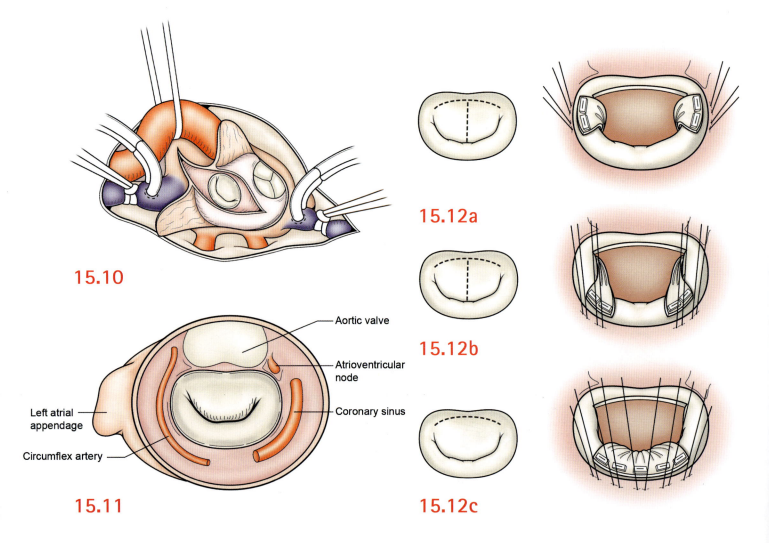

15.10

15.11

Aortic valve

Atrioventricular node

Coronary sinus

Left atrial appendage

Circumflex artery

15.12a

15.12b

15.12c

short- and long-term survival. Additionally, incorporating anterior and posterior leaflet tissue into the annular suture line of a replacement likely helps to prevent perivalvular leaks and atrioventricular disruption. There are a variety of ways to accomplish this, as detailed in the figure. Our preferred approach is simply to detach the anterior leaflet off the annulus, drop it on top of the posterior leaflet (where it belongs and end-systole), and incorporate anterior and posterior leaflet tissue into the posterior valve sutures (non-everting, pledgets on ventricular side). The anterior leaflet tissue is trimmed if necessary.

Mitral valve replacement may be performed with either everting (intra-annular, with pledgets on the atrial side, **Figure 15.13**) or non-everting (supra-annular, with pledgets on the ventricular side, **Figure 15.14**). Each has advantages and disadvantages. Advantages of the everting technique include a decreased chance of residual valve tissue interfering with mechanical valve function. Different types of mechanical valves may be more or less prone to this problem. The everting technique may be more protective of a perivalvular leak, although this is highly debatable. The everting technique does put much more stress on the atrioventricular groove and may have the disadvantage of being more likely to be associated with atrioventricular disruption, although this is unproven. Also, a smaller valve may be required with an intra-annular technique. On the other hand, the non-everting technique is simple, reduces stress on the atrioventricular groove, and is applicable to either bioprosthetic or mechanical valves.

POSTOPERATIVE CARE

The postoperative care of patients is essentially the same as for other cardiac surgical procedures. Immediate postoperative issues include observing for bleeding, maintenance of adequate filling pressures and cardiac output, use of inotropes when needed (especially in patients with severe mitral regurgitation and decreased ejection fraction preoperatively), and observation of neurological status.

Postoperative atrial fibrillation is common. The incidence is reduced through the use of perioperative beta blockers and some centers use prophylactic amiodarone as well. Maintenance of a normal potassium level is very important. Cardioversion may be performed when appropriate.

All patients receive Coumadin anticoagulation postoperatively no matter what type of valve is implanted, with a goal international normalized ratio (INR) of 2.5–3.5. We usually start Coumadin on postoperative day 1 or 2 and, if this is not therapeutic by day 3 or 4, unfractionated heparin is instituted. Patients with mechanical mitral valves will require Coumadin for life. Patients with bioprosthetic valves not in atrial fibrillation may have the Coumadin stopped at 3 months after the sewing ring is well endothelialized.

OUTCOME

Early mortality for mitral valve replacement in the absence of coronary disease remains less than 5%. Hospital mortality

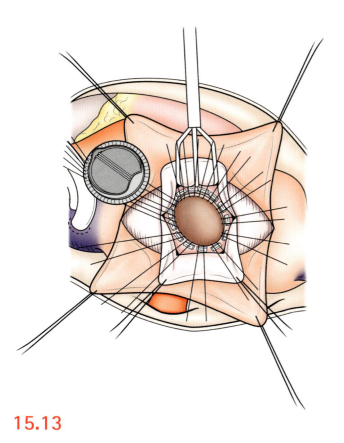

15.13

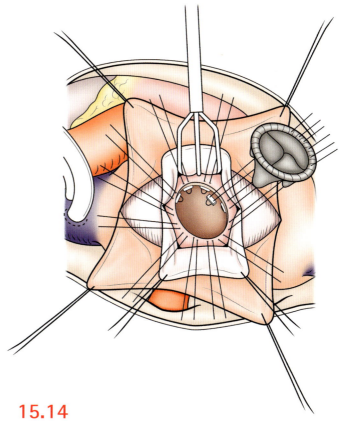

15.14

for patients undergoing combined mitral valve replacement and coronary bypass is in the region of 9% in most studies. Operative mortality is mostly secondary to comorbidities rather than technical failures. Mortality rates have fallen in recent years likely due to better myocardial protection, improved postoperative care, and the use of chordal sparing techniques, which have clearly been shown to reduce even short-term mortality. Patients requiring urgent surgery (torn chordae with florid pulmonary edema, acute infarction with papillary muscle rupture) have a much higher risk of death or complications. Long-term (10-year) survival after mitral valve replacement ranges from 50% to 75%. Freedom from reoperation at 15 years ranges from 30% to 80% and likely depends on the age of patients in a given study in addition to the prosthetic valve used.

The incidence of thromboembolism and stroke with mechanical valves reported is highly variable but is around 2% for each per year. These rates are much lower for tissue valves but both can still occur. Endocarditis occurs in less than 1% of patients.

Mitral valve replacement remains an important tool in the treatment of mitral valve disease. Although repair is possible in most patients, there remains a subset that should undergo replacement. Surgical priorities should always be kept in mind:

1. avoid a mortality
2. fix the patient's problem effectively
3. minimize complications.

Under this algorithm, mitral replacement remains the best option for many patients.

FURTHER READING

Bonow RO, Carabello BA, Chatterjee K, et al. Focused update incorporated into the ACC/AHA 2006 guidelines for the management of patients with valvular heart disease: a report of the American College of Cardiology/American Heart Association Task Force on Practice Guidelines (Writing Committee to Revise the 1998 Guidelines for the Management of Patients With Valvular Heart Disease): endorsed by the Society of Cardiovascular Anesthesiologists, Society for Cardiovascular Angiography and Interventions, and Society of Thoracic Surgeons. *Circulation.* 2008; 118(15): e523–661.

Enriquez-Sarano M, Sundt TM 3rd. Early surgery is recommended for mitral regurgitation. *Circulation.* 2010; 121(6): 804–11; discussion 812.

Fedak PW, McCarthy PM, Bonow RO. Evolving concepts and technologies in mitral valve repair. *Circulation.* 2008; 117(7): 963–74.

Gudbjartsson T, Absi T, Aranki, S. Mitral valve replacement. In: Cohn L (ed.). *Cardiac surgery in the adult.* 4th edn. New York: McGraw-Hill Medical; 2011: pp. 1031–68.

Maltais S, Schaff HV, Daly RC, et al. Mitral regurgitation surgery in patients with ischemic cardiomyopathy and ischemic mitral regurgitation: factors that influence survival. *J Thorac Cardiovasc Surg.* 2011; 142(5): 995–1001.

Murphy DA, Miller JS, Langford DA, et al. Endoscopic robotic mitral valve surgery. *J Thorac Cardiovasc Surg.* 2006; 132(4): 776–81.

16

Mitral valve repair

JAVIER G. CASTILLO AND DAVID H. ADAMS

HISTORY

The first documented mitral valve operation was performed by Elliot Cutler at the Peter Bent Brigham Hospital (Boston) in 1923. Cutler used a tenotomy knife to access the left ventricle and partially incised both mitral leaflets on a patient with rheumatic disease and consequent severe mitral stenosis (MS). Two years later, in 1925, Henry Souttar performed the first digital dilation of the mitral valve on a patient with a similar clinical profile at the London Hospital. Unfortunately, although successful, the procedure was not well received by the medical community due to its significant perioperative complications and the skepticism around this surgery did not trigger further referrals. In 1948, after multiple failed attempts, Charles Bailey introduced the modern era of mitral commissurotomy at the Episcopal Hospital in Philadelphia. Soon after, other surgeons including Charles Dubost in Paris and Dwight Harken in Boston perfected the technique and launched mitral valve repair as a therapeutic alternative for mitral valve disease. In 1957, Walton Lillehei performed the first open mitral annuloplasty under extracorporeal circulation.

At that time, although mitral valve repair had an exponentially increasing acceptance among cardiovascular specialists, the advent of prosthetic valves in the early 1960s led most to consider valve replacement as the primary therapy for mitral valve disease. However, early publications reported mortality rates as high as 30% as well as numerous perioperative complications. Pioneering surgical leaders including Dwight McGoon, Robert Frater, and Alain Carpentier continued to research and work on the development of mitral valve repair. Carpentier, considered by most to be the "father of mitral reconstructive surgery," described the principles of mitral valve repair, combining leaflet resection, ring annuloplasty, and chordal techniques. In addition, he established a systematic analytic approach to patients with mitral disease known as the "pathophysiologic triad of mitral valve regurgitation." The triad emphasized the importance of distinguishing between the medical condition causing the disease (etiology), the resulting lesions, and finally how these lesions affect leaflet motion (dysfunction).

Currently, mitral valve repair is the gold standard for patients with mitral valve disease, especially in the setting of degenerative disease. Recent data have demonstrated that it is possible to repair practically all prolapsing valves with a mortality risk of less than 1% in expert valve centers.

PRINCIPLES AND JUSTIFICATION

Mitral regurgitation (MR) predisposes the left ventricle to a volume overload in order to compensate for the volume lost to the regurgitant jet. While mild to moderate MR might be well tolerated for long periods of time, severe MR is fatal at a determined stage. At an early stage, the pure volume overload of MR is compensated for by eccentric left ventricular hypertrophy, which enables rapid left ventricular diastolic filling and an increase in stroke volume. However, this remodeling eventually encumbers systolic emptying. This maladaptive geometry together with the adrenergic overactivation results in decreased contractility. Severe MR is often divided into three clinical stages: acute, chronic compensated, and chronic decompensated, and each stage will have a different management as well as different surgical triggers. If MR is corrected in a timely fashion, this progression in stage can be reversed.

Severe MR is a mechanical problem with surgery as the only definitive solution, either by mitral valve repair or mitral valve replacement. Although the lack of randomized trials has led to controversy, especially in the setting of functional MR, repair is favored over replacement, particularly in patients with degenerative mitral valve disease, for multiple reasons including:

- a likely lower perioperative risk
- improved event-free survival
- freedom from the numerous complications of prosthetic heart valves
- better postoperative left ventricular function.

Despite the general consensus regarding the clinical superiority of mitral valve repair versus mitral valve replacement, it is sobering to note that many patients still undergo unnecessary valve replacement due to lack of surgical skill or experience. It is important to estimate the reparability of a valve based on the identified echocardiographic lesions in order to inform the patient about surgical expectations. Recent data from high-volume centers have shown a near 100% repair rate for degenerative mitral valve disease, with an operative risk of less than 1%. Matching surgical expertise and experience to the complexity of a specific valve morphology and patient is important in the modern era to assure high repair rates.

PREOPERATIVE ASSESSMENT AND PREPARATION

In general, transthoracic evaluation is adequate to assess mitral valve lesions and left ventricular function. A workup of coronary anatomy should generally be performed in patients over the age of 45 years, and a chest computed tomography (CT) scan done in elderly patients to rule out aortic or lung pathology. Otherwise, no other specific studies are mandatory in otherwise healthy patients.

ANESTHESIA

There are no specific changes to anesthetic management versus other open-heart procedures.

OPERATION

Classification of mitral valve disease

Structural lesions cause MR or MS by reducing leaflet coaptation or impairing leaflet opening respectively. An exhaustive interrogation (identification, localization, and magnitude) for mitral lesions is essential to determine the chances of successful valve repair and to proceed with a tailored therapeutic plan for each patient. As mentioned above, Carpentier described a systematic analytic approach to patients with MR known as the "pathophysiologic triad of mitral valve regurgitation." Besides emphasizing the importance of distinguishing

between etiology, lesions, and dysfunction, the triad also represents a very consistent way to elucidate which are the most appropriate techniques to achieve a successful repair. Given the very generic characteristics of mitral valve repair as an operative procedure, in part due to the vast armamentarium of techniques available, we use the classification of mitral valve disease based on the presence of abnormal leaflet motion (dysfunction) (**Figure 16.1**) in order to describe and analyze every technique in an organized fashion.

The differentiation of leaflet dysfunction is based on the position of the leaflet margins with respect to the mitral annular plane.

- *Type I dysfunction* implies normal leaflet motion, and the most common cause of significant MR is the perforation (e.g. endocarditis) of one of the leaflets or severe annular dilatation with a central regurgitant jet (e.g. long-standing atrial fibrillation).
- *Type II dysfunction* denotes excess leaflet motion generally secondary to chordal elongation or rupture (e.g. fibroelastic deficiency) or myxomatous degeneration (e.g. Barlow's disease) of the leaflets (regurgitant jet directed to the opposite site of the prolapsing leaflet).
- *Type III dysfunction* designates restricted leaflet motion and results typically from retraction of the subvalvular apparatus (IIIa, rheumatic valve disease or other inflammatory scenarios that lead to scarring and calcification) or papillary muscle displacement (leaflet tethering) from ventricular remodeling or dilatation (IIIb, ischemic or dilated cardiomyopathy).

Exposure of the mitral valve

Perfect exposure of the mitral valve is essential before any procedure is attempted and plays a key role in the success of the operation. Although multiple approaches have been described, including horizontal biatrial transseptal, superior biatrial transseptal, and interatrial approach through Sondergaard's groove, the latter remains the most efficient (better view and less tissue damage) when performing mitral valve repair.

DYSFUNCTION	FREQUENTLY ENCOUNTERED LESIONS

Type I

Normal leaflet motion

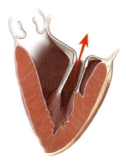 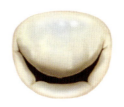 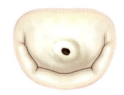

Type II

Increased leaflet motion
(leaflet prolapse)

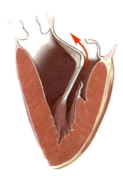 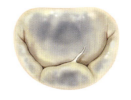 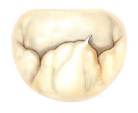

Type IIIa

Restricted leaflet motion
(restricted opening)

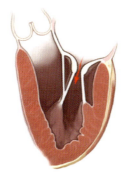 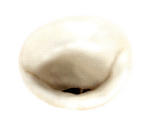 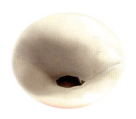

Type IIIb

Restricted leaflet motion
(restricted closure)

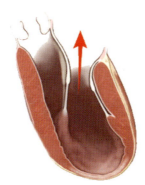 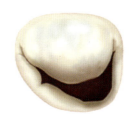 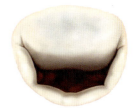

16.1

The interatrial groove is dissected and both atria are divided up to the fossa ovalis. The right atrium can be retracted medially and anteriorly. The right superior pulmonary vein at its junction to the left atrium is exposed (**Figure 16.2a**).

The dissection exposes the roof of the left atrium, which is opened at the midpoint between the right superior pulmonary vein insertion and the groove. During this maneuver, it is important not to inadvertently injure the posterior wall of the left atrium (**Figure 16.2b**).

The curvilinear incision is extended longitudinally both superiorly to 1 cm from the superior vena cava and inferiorly to the midpoint between the right inferior pulmonary vein and the inferior vena cava (**Figure 16.2c**).

If further exposure of the left atrium is required, the pericardial reflection on both vena cavae can be released and blunt dissection can be used to free the lateral aspects of both veins for about 2–3 cm (**Figure 16.2d**).

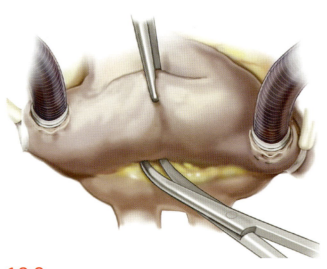

16.2a

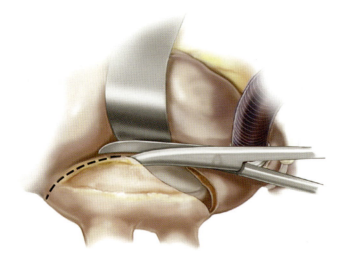

16.2c

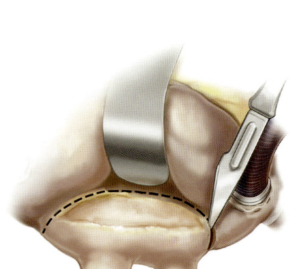

16.2b

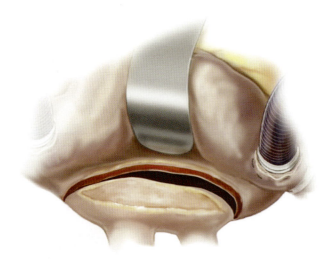

16.2d

Valve analysis

Valve analysis starts with the echocardiogram. Intraoperative valve inspection, performed in a systematic fashion (annulus, leaflets, chordae, and papillary muscles), confirms echocardiographic findings or further characterizes the existent lesions (**Figure 16.3**). This allows an accurate assessment of repair feasibility and helps to plan a surgical strategy and to choose the most appropriate techniques. Initially, the endocardium of the left atrium is carefully examined for jet lesions, thickening, thrombus, and areas of calcification. In the presence of large distended leaflets, placement of posterior annular sutures might be undertaken first to allow adequate exposure for valve analysis.

The mitral annulus is then evaluated first to assess shape, symmetry, and any degree of dilation, as well as areas of severe calcification that may require special consideration when placing annular sutures. The leaflets are examined with a nerve hook. We first identify and document the pathologic segments (A1-3; P1-3, anterior and posterior commissures).

Filling the ventricle with saline helps identify "functional" leaflet lesions. This may also identify migration of the leaflet hinges onto the left atrium. Subsequently, chordae tendinae are commonly interrogated for elongation, rupture, or a combination of both. Thickened, fibrotic, fused, or calcified chords should also be noted in patients with more complex scenarios. Finally, the papillary muscles are examined for calcification, fusion, and/or abnormal ventricular insertion.

Type I dysfunction – annular dilation

Every patient undergoing mitral valve repair requires a remodeling annuloplasty in order to restore the native annular size and shape allowing full leaflet motion, and preventing any risk of recurrence by stabilizing the annulus (especially the posterior aspect) with a prosthetic device. Those valves with type I dysfunction and isolated annular dilation can be successfully repaired with only a remodeling annuloplasty (**Figure 16.4a**).

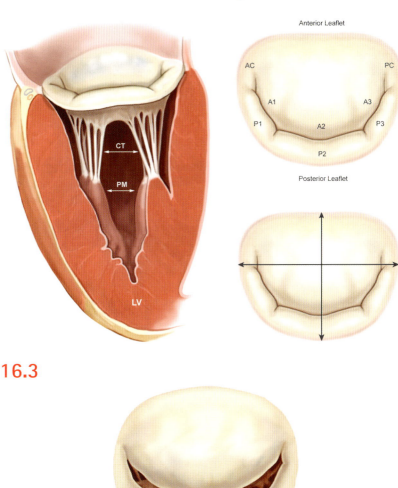

16.3

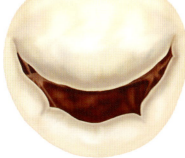

16.4a

Placement of the annular sutures (12–15 2-0 braided polyester mattress sutures) mandates complete visualization and identification of the mitral annulus (located approximately 2 mm away from the leaflet hinge). Grasping the leaflets transversally (as close to the annulus as possible) while applying traction towards the ventricle provides exposure and facilitates positioning of the sutures. Placing sutures along the anterior leaflet should be done using a backhand position with the needle tip oriented towards the ventricle (avoiding the aortic cusps). Sutures within the posterior annulus follow the same premises but require slightly deeper bites to reach the fibrous skeleton. For sutures along the posterior commissure, sutures are placed using a forehand position and oriented downwards. Finally, placing sutures within the anterior commissure requires a forehand position and the needle tip must be oriented towards the ventricle in order to avoid the circumflex artery (**Figure 16.4b**).

Selection of the ring size is based on the assessment of the base (intercommissural distance) and height of the anterior leaflet (**Figure 16.4c**).

After remodeling annuloplasty, saline testing should show a competent valve, with a symmetric and posterior line of coaptation (**Figure 16.4d**).

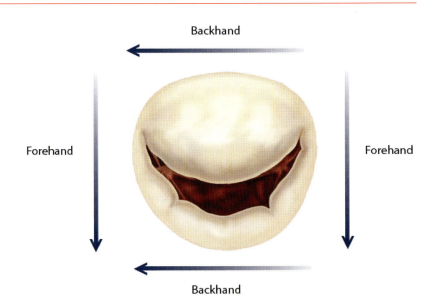

16.4b

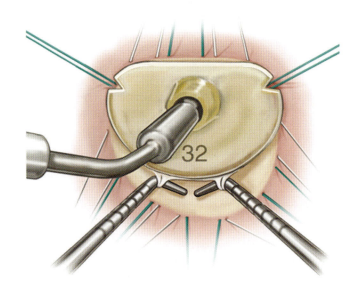

16.4c

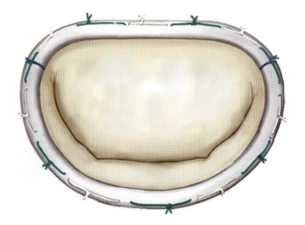

16.4d

Type I dysfunction – leaflet perforation

The second most common lesion leading to type I dysfunction is leaflet perforation, mostly due to bacterial endocarditis. The infection process usually leads to the formation of a vegetation-abscess on the body of the anterior leaflet (atrial side) that eventually becomes a true aneurysm, often with perforation (**Figure 16.5a**).

Early surgical intervention should be performed after isolation and identification of the organism and initiation of the appropriate antibiotic therapy. Debridement of the infected tissue mandates a minimum of 2 mm margins of macroscopically healthy tissue (**Figure 16.5b**).

A piece of autologous pericardium is immersed in 0.625% buffered glutaraldehyde solution (Poly Scientific, Bay Shore, NY) for 10 minutes. Afterwards, the patch is rinsed in saline solution. The patch is then tailored to match the shape of the leaflet defect (accounting for 2–3 mm of margin for the suturing) and then secured using a 5-0 continuous polypropylene suture (**Figure 16.5c**).

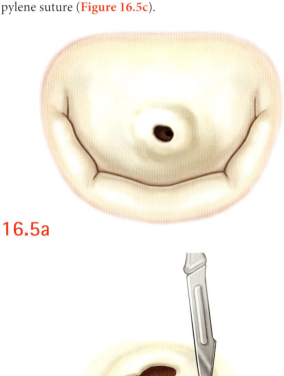

16.5a

16.5b

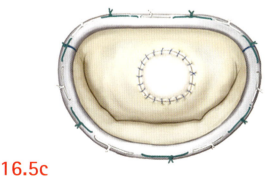

16.5c

Type II dysfunction – anterior leaflet prolapse

Due to its anatomy, the anterior leaflet does not allow aggressive margin resections. Every surgical strategy to address anterior leaflet prolapse therefore includes minimal or non-resection techniques. Non-resection techniques mainly comprise chordal transfer, chordal transposition, and polytetrafluoroethylene neochordoplasty (loop technique and its variants). If resection is necessary, a triangular resection limited to the rough area of the leaflet (so as not to compromise the leaflet body) should be carefully performed (**Figure 16.6a**).

Chordal transfer describes the mobilization of strong secondary chordae to the free margin of the prolapsed area (using a 5-0 polypropylene suture). Alternatively, *chordal transposition or posterior leaflet flip technique* involves the mobilization of an isolated chord or a segment of the posterior leaflet (usually the one opposed to the prolapsing area of the anterior leaflet in order to match the chordal length) with its marginal chordae. After complete mobilization and inspection of the chordae, the strip of posterior leaflet is attached to the free edge of the anterior leaflet using 5-0 polypropylene sutures (**Figure 16.6b**).

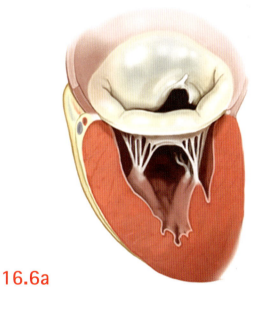

16.6a

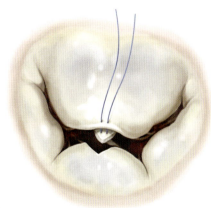

16.6b

Polytetrafluoroethylene neochordoplasty has been increasingly used in mitral valve repair. First, a CV-5 double-armed polytetrafluoroethylene suture is passed and looped through the fibrous tip of the papillary muscle. Next, the two ends of the artificial chord are passed through the leaflet margin (with a distance of approximately 3 mm between them) and two slip knots are tied (**Figure 16.6c**).

In the setting of isolated anterior leaflet prolapse, we generally proceed with a remodeling annuloplasty first. Functional (using saline testing) adjustment of the final length of the neochordae can then be performed always after remodeling annuloplasty. A catheter is attached to a bulb syringe and saline is pushed into the ventricle. A nerve hook is used to adjust the length of the artificial chord. A minimum of six knots are then completed to secure the chord (**Figure 16.6d**).

The loop technique was introduced to avoid problems of functional adjustment of the neochordae (inadvertent alteration of the chordal length during fixation). Three pre-measured CV-5 polytetrafluoroethylene loops are attached to the body of the papillary muscle (mandatory use of pledgets) and the free margin of the prolapsing leaflet (using 5-0 polypropylene sutures) (**Figure 16.6e**) to complete the repair (**Figure 16.6f**).

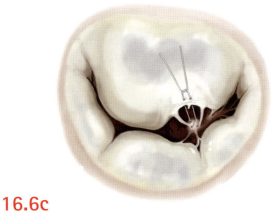

16.6c

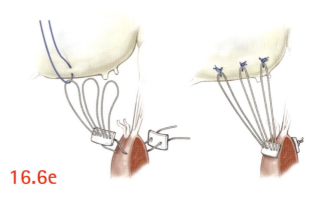

16.6e

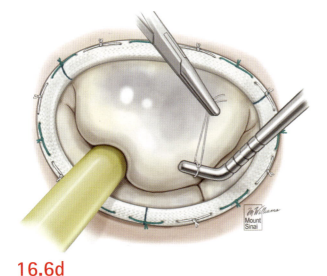

16.6d

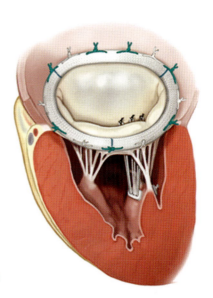

16.6f

Type II dysfunction – P2 prolapse

Posterior leaflet prolapse (particularly isolated P2 prolapse) is the most common cause of mitral valve regurgitation (**Figure 16.7a**).

Several approaches have been suggested including chordal techniques (see previous section), leaflet plication techniques (McGoon's), and resection techniques (triangular and quadrangular resection). McGoon's technique is used to repair very limited prolapses and involves the placement of two imbricated "magic" 5-0 polypropylene sutures to plicate the prolapsing leaflet segment (**Figure 16.7b and c**).

Triangular resection is a very useful technique. The resection is generally limited to within a few millimeters of good marginal chords, and extends to the midpoint of the belly of the leaflet (**Figure 16.8a**).

Leaflet continuity is restored using either interrupted or continuous 5-0 polypropylene sutures, depending on the pliability of the tissue (**Figure 16.8b**). A continuous suture technique is best avoided in the setting of leaflet calcification or retraction. After completion of the sutures, a nerve hook is utilized to assess leaflet continuity and to detect residual defects.

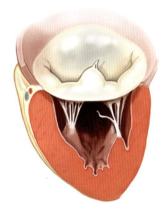

16.7a

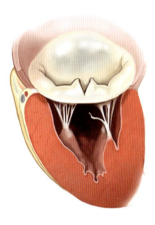

16.8a

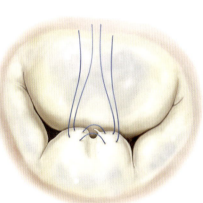
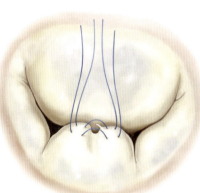

16.7b

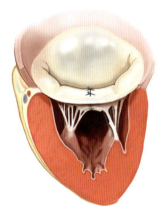

16.8b

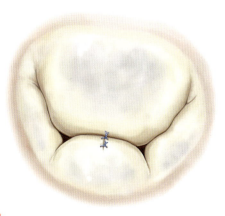

16.7c

Type II dysfunction – posterior leaflet prolapse

In the presence of a more extensive (excess tissue) posterior leaflet prolapse, more aggressive resection techniques are needed including quadrangular resection, annular plication, and sliding leaflet plasty. In this regard, quadrangular resection is the most frequently used technique in posterior leaflet prolapse. However, with the growing adoption of chordal techniques, many surgeons have decided to respect as much tissue as possible and abandon more complex techniques that involve large resections. After valve analysis, a quadrangular resection of the prolapsing area is carried out to the annulus (**Figure 16.9a**).

Generally, the tallest portion of the leaflet is excised, and well within the margin of normal chordae. Clefts or indentations are often targeted as one margin of the resection (**Figure 16.9b**).

If the residual leaflet defect is less than 2 cm, plication techniques are applied in order to avoid excess leaflet tension. Interrupted 2-0 braided polyester sutures are placed through the annulus at the limit of the resected area (**Figure 16.9c**).

The leaflet continuity is restored using 5-0 polypropylene sutures (**Figure 16.9d**).

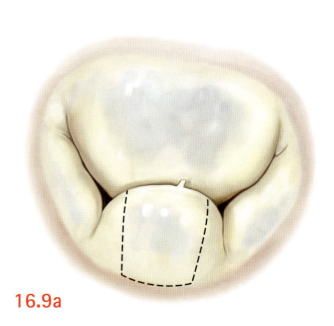

16.9a

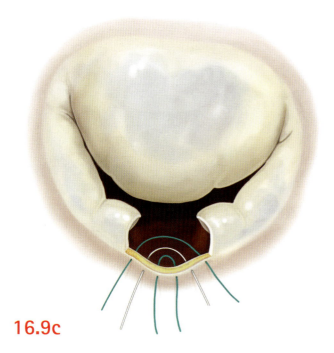

16.9c

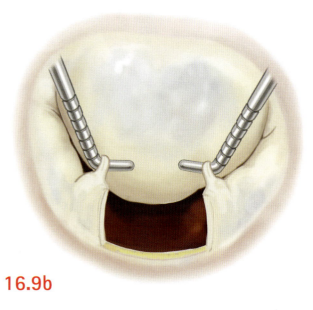

16.9b

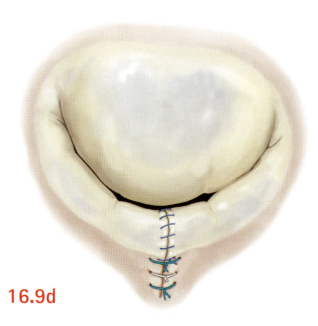

16.9d

Sliding leaflet plasty is a useful technique to avoid excess height and tension and is often employed in scenarios of more diffuse prolapse and leaflet myxomatous changes (**Figure 16.10a**).

A targeted (including deep indentations if present) leaflet quadrangular resection is usually performed where the prolapse is greatest or leaflet is tallest (**Figure 16.10b**). This resection is typically about 1 cm wide (additional excess tissue can be removed later). It is important not to remove all abnormal tissue. In the setting of additional deep indentations, we close these first with a figure-eight suture in order to treat the segments as one.

If the height is more than 15 mm in any residual leaflet segment, a sliding leaflet plasty (asymmetric in this case) to reduce the residual leaflet height to 12–15 mm needs to be performed. Specially angled scissors are used to detach the leaflet remnant, starting from the remaining left position of P2 and going to the anterior commissure (**Figure 16.10c**). At this point, the leaflet is suspended by the primary and secondary chordae with the basal chordae remaining on the annular side. Secondary chordae are detached to maintain free mobility of segments after advancement. This prevents secondary chords from restricting the leaflet after leaflet advancement. Additionally, at this stage, further resection of the base of P1–P2 may be considered in order to re-establish a uniform leaflet height.

A double layer of 4-0 polypropylene running suture is used to reattach the leaflet to the annulus, assuring no excess tension on either segment. Excess height is compensated for by taking sutures up to 5 mm deep into the leaflet; in areas of adequate height, sutures are taken just 1–2 mm from the leaflet edge. The two leaflet margins are then joined using a running 5-0 polypropylene suture (**Figure 16.10d**). The margins of the reconstructed posterior leaflet are examined to ensure that all segments are adequately supported. Any gaps in support, or areas supported by thinned out chordate (even in the absence of prolapse), are reinforced by transposition of previously detached secondary chordate, or now more commonly implantation of artificial neochordae.

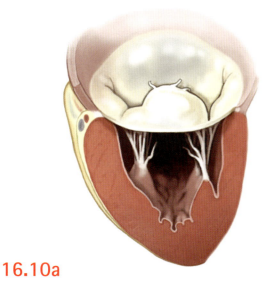

16.10a

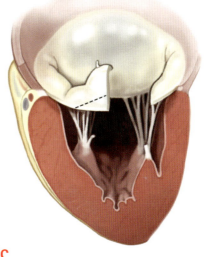

16.10c

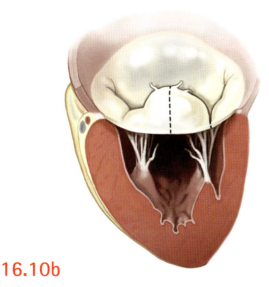

16.10b

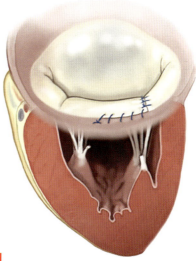

16.10d

Type IIIa dysfunction – commissural fusion

The majority of lesions leading to type IIIa (commissural fusion, leaflet thickening and retraction, and chordal thickening and shortening or fusion) have a rheumatic origin. The limitation of the leaflet excursion often results in combined valve stenosis and regurgitation. In this scenario, commissurotomy is the technique of choice. Traction of the commissure with a nerve hook helps to identify the commissural line (incision). An 11 blade is then used to make an incision about 5 mm from the annulus (**Figure 16.11a**).

The incision is completed leaving one chord on each side of the defect. The papillary muscle is then split in order to create a subcommissural orifice which will avoid future refusion (**Figure 16.11b**).

In cases of combined valve stenosis and regurgitation or pure stenosis and concomitant annular dilation, the commissures may need reconstruction (commissurotomy may contribute to further annular dilation and MR). In this scenario, also seen in diffuse leaflet prolapse or acute bacterial endocarditis, the optimal technique is the "magic suture" or commissuroplasty. This is performed using 5-0 polypropylene sutures (**Figure 16.11c**).

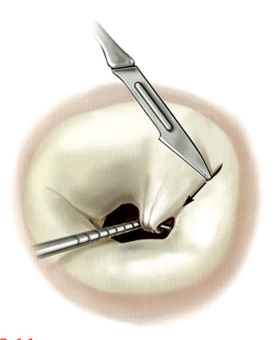

16.11a

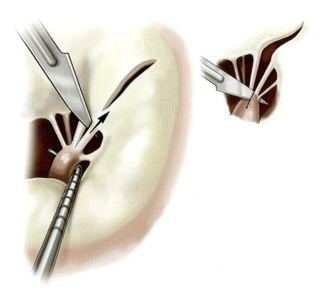

16.11b

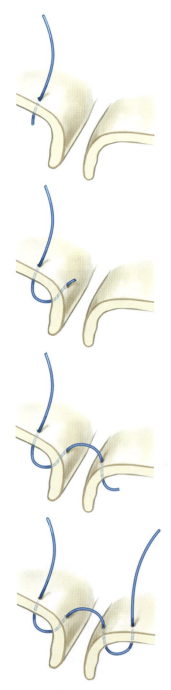

16.11c

Type IIIa dysfunction – severe leaflet restriction

Leaflet retraction in the context of type IIIa dysfunction is mainly due to abnormalities of the subvalvular apparatus (chordal thickening and shortening or fusion). In this case, leaflet mobilization should be achieved by resecting secondary chords, splitting fused hypertrophic chords and fenestrating isolated thickened chords (**Figure 16.12a**).

When leaflet mobilization cannot be achieved with subvalvular techniques, pericardial patch extension of the leaflet is indicated. Traction sutures (5-0 polypropylene) are placed in order to unfold the leaflet as much as possible and the incision is made about 5 mm from and parallel to the annulus (**Figure 16.12b**). The extent of the incision depends on the degree of leaflet retraction.

All secondary chordae are resected to free the leaflet and achieve adequate mobilization (**Figure 16.12c**).

A semilunar autologous pericardial patch (see previous section for further details) is tailored to the leaflet defect adding a 2 mm margin for suturing. The patch is then sutured using continuous 4-0 polypropylene sutures. Interlocked bites are used on the leaflet side to prevent a potential purse-string effect (**Figure 16.12d**).

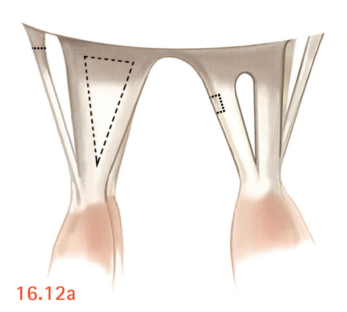

16.12a

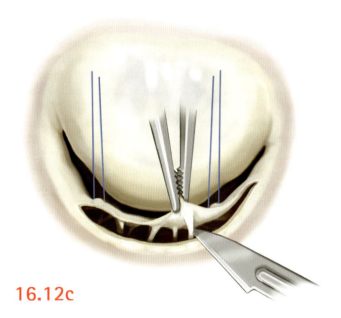

16.12c

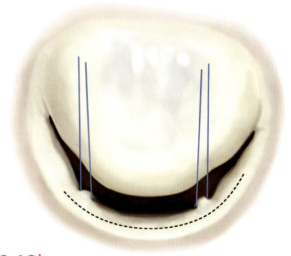

16.12b

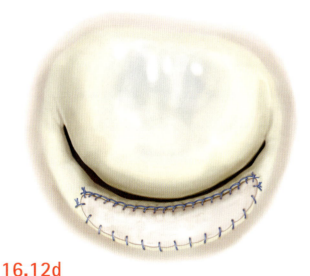

16.12d

Type IIIb dysfunction – posterior leaflet tethering

The primary ventricular alteration leading to ischemic MR is papillary muscle displacement. The papillary muscle tips are displaced away from the midseptal (anterior) annulus, i.e. posterolaterally, apically, and away from each other. Papillary muscle tethering leads to apical tenting of the leaflets (restriction of the motion of the free margins of the leaflets), which prevents them from rising to the plane of the annulus to provide good coaptation (**Figure 16.13a**).

Because leaflet restriction in ischemic MR results in less leaflet tissue available for coaptation, it is necessary to downsize a complete remodeling ring by one or two sizes or to use a true-sized asymmetric ring to ensure an adequate surface of coaptation following annuloplasty. The potential increased tension with associated annular dilation mandates placing the sutures very close together along the annulus, and suture crossover may be warranted, especially in the P3 area (**Figure 16.13b**).

The battery of adjunct techniques to downsized rigid ring annuloplasty include cutting of the secondary strut chord to the anterior leaflet in the setting of a "hockey-stick" deformity of the closure line, closure of all clefts and indentations in the posterior leaflet if severe leaflet tethering is present, and cutting restricted marginal chords if a residual leak is still present (replacing them with chordal transfer or artificial neochordae) (**Figure 16.13c**).

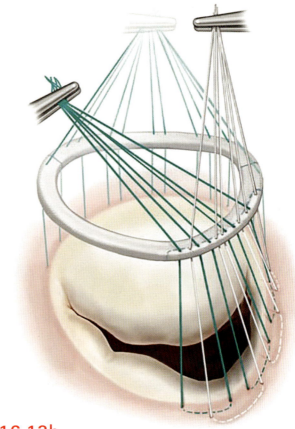

16.13b

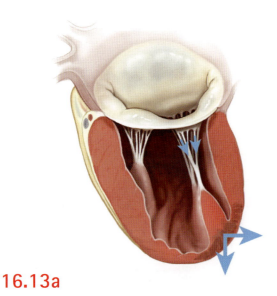

16.13a

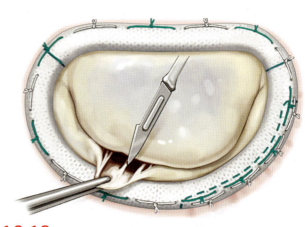

16.13c

Objectives of mitral valve repair

The most important goal for patients with MR is to achieve a competent and durable mitral valve repair. In this regard, the procedure should mainly restore the native annular shape meeting the following criteria:

- competent valve on saline and ink testing
- good surface of coaptation
- symmetric line of closure where the anterior leaflet occupies ≥80% of the valve area
- no residual areas of billowing
- no tendency to systolic anterior motion.

Evaluation for all these points may require two different intraoperative tests including the saline test and the ink test. The saline test is performed by filling the ventricle with saline and confirming all the aforementioned prerequisites. The ink test is performed by drawing a line on the valve closure line during maximum saline insufflations. The coaptation zone beyond the ink is examined with the help of nerve hooks and should be at least 6 mm in length (this will transform to approximately 8 mm on echocardiography as some of the ink is within the coaptation zone). Also, there should be no more than 10 mm of anterior leaflet beyond the ink line as this would signify a risk for systolic anterior motion.

POSTOPERATIVE CARE

The application of rigorous postoperative care following strict protocols is critical to ensure optimal success of mitral valve repair. Major physiological and mechanical derangements can occur in patients recovering from a cardiac operation as a consequence of pre-existing conditions or due to changes secondary to cardiopulmonary bypass and the surgical procedure. In this regard, a system-based approach is necessary to deal with problems in an organized fashion. The cardiovascular system frequently deranged and primary determinant of recovery will be the main focus of attention. If patients have preserved ventricular function and consequently good urine output, adequate oxygenation (optimal arterial blood gases) and preserved neurological status, they can be extubated fairly early, within hours following the procedure. In the presence of ventricular dysfunction, vasodilators for afterload reduction (ACE inhibitors preferentially) should be initiated in combination with inotropic agents. If pulmonary hypertension persists after surgery, the administration of nitric oxide has been demonstrated to be very effective. In addition, volume overload may require the administration of diuretics for a few weeks after hospital discharge.

Chronic or paroxysmal atrial fibrillation is common in patients with chronic MR due to increased left atrial pressure and progressive atrial stretch and dilation. It is present in 20–40% of patients undergoing mitral valve repair and current trials have reported the restoration of sinus rhythm postoperatively in up to 90% of patients undergoing adjunct ablation procedures. New onset of postoperative atrial fibrillation has been shown to be present in around 20% of patients. In this scenario, the rate control strategy should include the use of beta blockers or amiodarone and oral anticoagulation in refractory cases. Note that intravenous coagulation should be used with caution to avoid possible mediastinal bleeding. In patients with persisting atrial fibrillation up to 2–3 months after surgery, cardioversion might be indicated; transesophageal echocardiography must demonstrate the absence of atrial thrombus before any cardioversion attempt.

Anticoagulation is a very important aspect of the early postoperative care, although different centers have different treatment plans. We tend to use aspirin therapy alone in patients in normal sinus rhythm with no risk factors, and warfarin therapy in patients with preoperative or postoperative atrial fibrillation. Rhythm should be reassessed at 3 months to determine who should continue on warfarin therapy. Cardioversion should be coordinated with the patient's cardiologist.

OUTCOME

Contemporary data have shown a trend towards very low operative mortality rates after mitral valve repair regardless of the etiology. Preoperative factors that might significantly affect mid-and long-term survival in patients with MR include the presence of left ventricular dysfunction (left ventricular ejection fraction <60%), functional class III or IV, effective regurgitant orifice of ≥40 mm^2, a left ventricular end systolic dimension of >40 mm, a left atrial index of ≥60 mL/m^2, a left atrial dimension of >55 mm, pulmonary hypertension or exercise pulmonary hypertension, and the presence of atrial fibrillation. Patients with preoperative symptoms have increased postoperative mortality despite symptom relief (especially those with a left ventricular ejection fraction that is <50%), whereas in those with no or few symptoms, restoration of life expectancy can be potentially achieved. Durability of repair (assessed as freedom from moderate or greater MR) in patients with degenerative mitral valve has been reported to be between 90% and 95% at 5 years in high volume centers, with a recurrence rate of 1–1.5% a year. The failure to use an annuloplasty ring, chordal shortening techniques (which are now uncommon), the presence of anterior leaflet pathology, and, of course, the unavailability of pliable leaflet tissue (more often seen in patients with rheumatic disease) have been associated with higher repair failure rates.

ACKNOWLEDGEMENT

We would like to thank M. Williams for preparation of the images in this chapter.

FURTHER READING

Carpentier AC, Adams DH, Filsoufi F. *Carpentier's reconstructive valve surgery*. Maryland Heights: Saunders Elsevier; 2010.

Castillo JG, Anyanwu AC, Fuster V, et al. A near 100% repair rate for mitral valve prolapse is achievable in a reference center: implications for future guidelines. *J Thorac Cardiovasc Surg.* 2012; 144: 308–12.

Castillo JG, Anyanwu AC, El-Eshmawi A, et al. All anterior and bileaflet mitral valve prolapses are repairable in the modern era of reconstructive surgery. *Eur J Cardiothorac Surg.* 2014; 45(1): 139–45.

O'Gara PT, Grayburn PA, Badhwar V, et al. ACC Expert Consensus Decision Pathway on the Management of Mitral Regurgitation: a report of the American College of Cardiology Task Force on Expert Consensus Decision Pathways. *J Am Coll Cardiol.* 2017; 70: 2421–49.

Castillo JG, Adams DH, Carabello BA, et al. Degenerative mitral valve disease. In: Fuster V, Walsh RA, Harrington RA (eds). *Hurst's the heart.* 14th edn. London: McGraw-Hill Medical; 2017: pp. 1215–37.

El-Eshmawi A, Castillo JG, Tang GHL, et al. Developing a mitral valve center of excellence. *Curr Opin Cardiol.* 2018; 33: 155–61.

17

Minimal access mitral valve surgery

ARMAN KILIC, PAVAN ATLURI, AND W. CLARK HARGROVE III

HISTORY

The success and increasing utilization of laparoscopic approaches for general surgical procedures in the early 1990s fueled an interest in developing minimal access approaches to cardiac surgery. In the same decade, pioneering work from a number of surgeons led to the use of alternative incisions for heart surgery, including parasternal, partial sternotomy, and right thoracotomy or mini-thoracotomy approaches. The development of technology allowing for percutaneous cardiopulmonary bypass (CPB) and more recently aortic occlusion, cardioplegia administration, and venting have also facilitated refinements in minimal access cardiac surgical technique. In the realm of minimal access mitral valve surgery (MAMVS), our preference has been to use the Heartport platform utilizing a right mini-thoracotomy.

PRINCIPLES AND JUSTIFICATION

Patient selection and contraindications

Some of the relative contraindications for MAMVS are more applicable to surgeons with less experience with these techniques whereas others are relevant regardless of surgeon or institutional experience. For example, early in one's experience, isolated MAMVS should be performed prior to attempting mitral valve operations concomitant with tricuspid valve or atrial fibrillation procedures. Simple mitral valve repairs such as P2 triangular resections with annuloplasty should be performed initially prior to attempting complex mitral repairs using minimal access approaches. Patients who are morbidly obese can also present technical challenges and surgeons learning MAMVS should select thinner patients in their early experience.

Significant peripheral arterial disease that limits the ability to use femoral arterial cannulation is a contraindication to MAMVS. Patients with low ejection fractions (<25%), more than mild aortic insufficiency, severe right ventricular dysfunction, significant mitral annular calcification, or severe pulmonary hypertension are generally excluded from MAMVS. Significant pulmonary disease with the inability to tolerate single-lung ventilation as well as prior right thoracotomy are other contraindications to a right mini-thoracotomy approach for mitral valve surgery. Chest wall deformities such as pectus excavatum can hinder exposure. Large abdominal pannus, inguinal hernias, or prior groin incisions can also limit the ability to perform femoral cannulation.

PREOPERATIVE ASSESSMENT AND PREPARATION

Preoperative evaluation begins with a thorough history and physical examination to identify potential contraindications to MAMVS such as those listed above. Attention should be paid to body habitus and, in females, the presence of breast implants should be noted. Left heart catheterization should be performed in males over the age of 40 and postmenopausal women undergoing mitral valve surgery. Some surgeons will obtain preoperative catheterizations in all patients to assess coronary dominance, proximity of the circumflex artery relative to the mitral annulus, and the presence of severe mitral annular calcification. Right heart catheterization should be performed in patients with significant pulmonary hypertension or those with left or right heart failure.

Other important preoperative studies include a high-quality transthoracic or transesophageal echocardiogram. The preoperative echocardiogram is the cornerstone to mitral valve surgery planning and can help delineate several important points relative to surgical technique. The etiology and lesions of the mitral valve, mitral annulus size, presence of mitral annular calcification, leaflet thickening, elongated or flail chords, and risk factors for systolic anterior motion are some examples of pertinent information obtained by the echocardiogram. These findings should be confirmed with the findings of the intraoperative pre-incision transesophageal echocardiogram. Three-dimensional echocardiography is being used with increasing frequency for evaluation of the mitral valve as well.

Computed tomography (CT) of the chest, abdomen, and pelvis is important in delineating the suitability of the iliofemoral vessels for peripheral cannulation. Severe tortuosity, calcification, or small arterial diameter can preclude femoral cannulation. The thoracic aorta should also be evaluated for the presence of calcification, whether a Chitwood clamp or an endoballoon is used. It may not be possible to use the endoballoon in aortas with diameters greater than 4 cm, which can be sized preoperatively with CT. Carotid duplex scan and pulmonary function tests are also included in the preoperative evaluation in select patients.

ANESTHESIA

Double lumen endotracheal tubes are preferable as the right lung is deflated when entering the right chest and for exposure throughout the operation. Central venous access and invasive arterial monitoring are routinely established. We routinely have our anesthesia team place a 16–18 French cannula in the superior vena cava (SVC) via the right internal jugular vein with ultrasound guidance prior to positioning and draping the patient.

OPERATION

Positioning

The patient is positioned in a modified 30-degree left lateral decubitus position with the aid of a large bump tucked under the right torso. The patient should be shifted towards the right side of the operating room table to minimize the distance from the operating surgeon. Prior to draping the patient, we routinely mark with a sterile pen the suprasternal notch, the xiphoid process, the midline of the sternum, the inferior border of the right clavicle, the costal margins, the anterior axillary line, the border of the nipple circumferentially, and the femoral arterial pulse, preferably in the right groin (**Figure 17.1**).

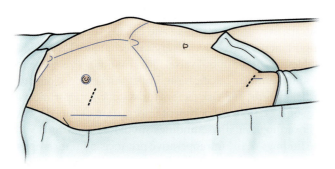

17.1

Incisions

An oblique right groin incision overlying the femoral vessels at the inguinal ligament is made and the femoral artery and vein are identified. We limit the amount of dissection we perform in the groin to avoid seromas, lymphatic leaks, nerve injury, and other complications related to more extensive dissection. Once the femoral vessels are identified, the wound is packed and attention is turned to the chest.

The right mini-thoracotomy is the initial incision that is made in the chest (**Figure 17.2**). In males, this is a 6 cm incision that is made under the nipple and extending laterally. In females, this is also a 6 cm incision but is made just superior to the inframammary crease. We have found that placing the incision just above the crease causes less discomfort as bras sit right in the crease and cause irritation if the incision is made there. After skin incision, the subcutaneous tissue is divided with electrocautery and the fourth interspace entered with the right lung deflated. A small thoracotomy is made first and the surgeon's index finger is inserted to palpate the proximity of the diaphragm. Occasionally, we will enter an interspace above if the incision is made too close to the diaphragm. After confirming that the interspace is suitable, the thoracotomy is extended medially and laterally.

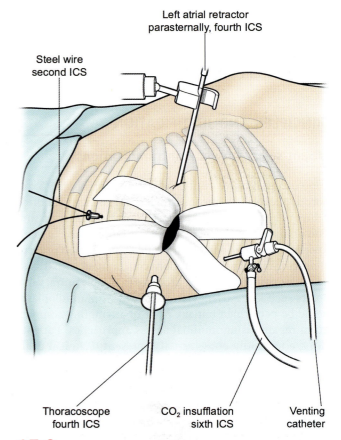

Left atrial retractor parasternally, fourth ICS

Steel wire second ICS

Thoracoscope fourth ICS

CO_2 insufflation sixth ICS

Venting catheter

17.2

Next, a stab wound is made two interspaces inferiorly from the mini-thoracotomy on the lateral edge with a #11 blade. A krile is then placed through the stab wound and into the chest, followed by a port that is connected to tubing for CO_2 insufflation. After this, a soft-tissue retractor is placed within the mini-thoracotomy. Another stab wound is made with a #11 blade in the same interspace as the mini-thoracotomy a few fingerbreadths lateral to the wound just outside of the soft-tissue retractor. A krile followed by camera port is then inserted. A 0-degree camera is then placed through the camera holder, which is secured on the operating room table on the right-sided rail, and then into the chest through the camera port. If the diaphragm is obscuring the view, a retraction suture may be necessary on the diaphragm with a #1 Vicryl suture in a figure-eight fashion. This suture is tied down to prevent bleeding when it is cut out at the end of the case before being passed through the chest wall with an endoclose and secured to the drape with a hemostat. A 16-gauge angiocath is then inserted into the chest superiorly and medially to the mini-thoracotomy wound and a 24-gauge wire is placed into the chest through the angiocath. A long krile is then used to grasp the wire through the thoracotomy and brought out through the wound. Suture guides are adhered to the chest wall and the wire is secured on the superior suture guide.

Cannulation

A Weitlaner retractor is placed in the right groin incision and a 4-0 Prolene pursestring is placed in the femoral vein and secured to a tourniquet. For the femoral artery, we use two 5-0 Gore-Tex sutures with micropledgets and run two U-stitches on either side of where the arterial puncture will be, with two bites per arm of each suture. The free ends of the suture for each Gore-Tex are then placed through another micropledget such that each of the two U-stitches has two pledgets for a total of four pledgets on the femoral artery. Each of these two U-stitches is then secured with a tourniquet. It is important to catch only adventitia with each bite to avoid hematomas. When pulling on the tourniquets, excessive force should be avoided as it can tear the femoral artery.

A needle with a syringe is then inserted into the femoral vein, a long wire is fed into the inferior vena cava and then right atrium under echocardiographic guidance, and the vein is dilated with a dilator. We typically use a 25-French venous cannula over the wire and position it under echocardiographic guidance. This cannula is then connected with the superior vena cava cannula via a Y-connector (**Figure 17.3**). We usually do not secure the femoral venous cannula with any stitches as repositioning is often necessary.

A needle is then inserted into the femoral artery between the two U-stitches. A wire is advanced into the descending thoracic aorta under echocardiographic guidance. If a Chitwood clamp is to be used, we would then dilate the femoral artery with a dilator and insert a 16 Fr or 18 Fr arterial cannula. However, if an endoballoon is used, the femoral

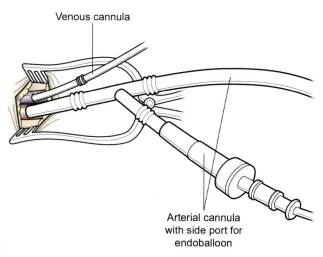

Venous cannula

Arterial cannula
with side port for
endoballoon

17.3

artery is dilated with a dilator followed by the venous cannula obturator or white inner cannula that is sheathed inside the venous cannula, which we trim with heavy scissors to use for the final arterial dilation. The Heartport arterial cannula is then advanced over the wire and into the femoral artery. If resistance is met at the entry of the artery, we typically make a small anterior nick in the artery with a #11 blade to facilitate passage. After the cannula is inserted, the side cannula is de-aired by turning the knob counterclockwise to backbleed it. The cannula is secured to the tourniquet as well as the skin with 2-0 silk stitches.

The endoballoon is prepared by de-airing the lines by flushing them and then inserting the endoballoon into the side port and advancing it to the 15 cm mark. We then obtain an echocardiographic view of the descending thoracic aorta and advance the wire through the endoballoon into view. Following this, an echocardiographic view of the ascending aorta is obtained and the wire is advanced to above the sinotubular junction (STJ). Care must be taken not to advance the wire through the aortic valve as leaflet perforation can occur. The endoballoon is advanced over the wire to a position above the STJ and the screw is turned clockwise to secure it in place.

Exposure

CPB is initiated and the heart drained out. This helps to drop the heart away from the pericardium and avoid inadvertent electrocautery injury to the heart. A stay suture may be used to help lift the pericardium away from the heart. An incision is made into the pericardium 2–3 cm anterior to the phrenic nerve with the electrocautery, and this is extended inferiorly to the diaphragm and superiorly such that the ascending aorta is in view. We extend even further superiorly if a Chitwood clamp is to be used.

A Ti-Cron suture is then placed in the middle of the upper part of the pericardial edge and secured to a suture guide.

Two Ti-Cron sutures are subsequently placed on the superior and inferior portions of the bottom part of the pericardial edge. A #11 blade is used to make a skin incision laterally and between the camera and CO_2 ports, and an endoclose is introduced through that incision to grasp these bottom pericardial stay sutures and bring them out through the lateral chest wall. These are secured to a Rummel and snared down. The handheld sucker is then used to bluntly dissect the space around the inferior vena cava. Electrocautery is used to develop Waterston's interatrial groove.

If a Chitwood clamp is used, a 2-0 pledgeted suture is placed in the ascending aorta and a cardioplegia line inserted and secured to a tourniquet. We use a 2-0 suture because typically we will use the Cor-Knot device to secure this pursestring at the end of the case when it is removed. The Chitwood clamp is inserted through a small skin incision in the chest wall just superior and lateral to the CO_2 port, with the curve of the clamp facing inferiorly and with the top clamp being the moving clamp and the bottom being stationary. The clamp is applied through the transverse sinus to limit injury to the pulmonary artery. Attention must also be paid to the left atrial appendage as it too can be injured by the clamp. After cross-clamping, antegrade cardioplegia is delivered.

If the endoballoon is used, the balloon is inflated via the blue port with a 30 mL syringe of heparinized saline under echocardiographic guidance. Adjustment of the balloon position may be necessary. A balloon pressure of around 300–400 mmHg is satisfactory. Adenosine is also given via a 10 mL syringe in the red port. Cardioplegia is then delivered through the endoballoon. Frequently, the balloon migrates with delivery of cardioplegia, so active readjustment of balloon position under real-time echocardiography of the ascending aorta is therefore essential.

After adequate cardioplegia has been delivered, a long handled #11 blade is used to incise the left atrium. A pump sucker is placed inside the left atrium and Potts scissors are used to extend the atriotomy cephalad towards the SVC and inferiorly between the right inferior pulmonary vein and the inferior vena cava. A Ti-Cron suture is placed on the upper lip of the atriotomy in the middle in a figure-eight fashion and then secured on a suture guide. The left hand of the surgeon is placed inside the chest to palpate the right internal mammary artery and the edge of the sternum and an incision is made with a #11 blade just on the right edge of the sternum. A krile is introduced into the chest via this incision. The metal obturator for the left atrial retractor is then placed in this incision and the retractor is introduced into the chest via the mini-thoracotomy on a long holder (**Figure 17.4**). The obturator is screwed onto the retractor and the retractor placed inside the left atrium, with retraction upwards to expose the mitral valve. The metal piece is then secured to an arm holder that is attached to the left-sided rail of the operating table to keep the retractor in place. A floppy sucker is placed through the CO_2 port and into the left inferior pulmonary vein. The 0-degree camera is exchanged for a 30-degree camera.

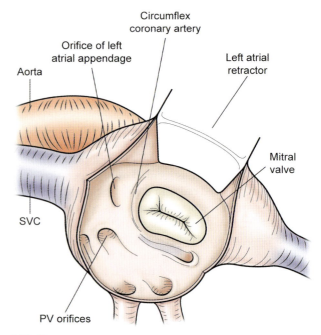

17.4

Mitral valve repair

Mitral valve repair is commenced in a similar fashion to when it is performed via sternotomy. A nerve hook is used to analyze the valve in a systematic fashion. We proceed with the annular stitches first and prefer to use an annuloplasty band in degenerative disease and a complete rigid ring in ischemic mitral disease. Unlike with the sternotomy approach, where the A1/P1 area of the annulus is most difficult to expose, the P3 area is most difficult to expose in a right mini-thoracotomy approach. We therefore start the annular stitches at the right fibrous trigone where visualization is easiest and proceed in a counterclockwise manner. These initial sutures are placed in the suture guide that is located inferiorly such that the sutures cross over the operative field. This helps to maintain a view of the annulus. After the first three or four annular stitches, the portion of the 24-gauge wire that is inside the chest is wrapped around these sutures and the other end of the wire is pulled out of the skin and a Kelly clamp placed at the skin level. This helps to move the sutures out of the way of the operative field and avoid crossing of sutures when the remaining annular sutures are placed. The remaining annular stitches are placed. At the P3 portion, the left atrium can often obscure the view making it necessary to use a Heartport forcep to retract the atrial tissue out of the way to visualize the annulus. Pulling on adjacent annular stitches can also help bring the annulus into view.

Leaflet repairs are similar to our sternotomy techniques and include anterior or posterior neochords, triangular or quadrangular resections, and cleft repairs, to name a few. Essentially, any repair technique that can be performed via sternotomy can be performed via right mini-thoracotomy in experienced hands. Early in a surgeon's MAMVS experience we would recommend starting with simple repairs such as annuloplasties only, or P2 prolapse with triangular resection and annuloplasty. As experience accumulates, more complex repairs can be performed. When performing neochords, we use 5-0 Gore-Tex sutures, place these as a U-stitch through the papillary muscle, and bring the arms up as a figure eight through the prolapsed leaflet edge. A long Heartport forcep can then be used to grasp the sutures at the intended length after pressurizing the valve with a tester and antegrade cardioplegia and then the sutures tied down with the knot on top of the forcep to maintain the desired length of neochord. Retesting the valve can then ensure an adequate neochord length.

The band is then sized. We typically tie a long silk suture on the sizers to help facilitate its retrieval from the chest, especially if the grasp on the sizer is inadvertently lost. The wire around the P1 sutures is removed and the P1 sutures are handed to the assistant in order and secured on a suture guide. The annular sutures are brought up through the band and the band seated. We have been using the Cor-Knot automated tying device to secure our knots as this can help expedite the suture tying and reduce cross-clamp time. If this device is not used, traditional extracorporeal tying with a knot pusher is performed.

The valve is tested with a long tester and, if a satisfactory result is achieved, the floppy suction is placed through the mitral valve to vent the left ventricle. The left atrium is closed with two running 3-0 Prolene sutures that are secured with a tourniquet in the middle of the atriotomy. The initial stitches in the corners are figure-eight stitches, after which the sutures are tied and then run to the middle of the atriotomy. Before snaring the tourniquet, the heart is filled and the left atrium de-aired through the atriotomy. Before the cross-clamp comes off, we place a bipolar ventricular pacing wire. The pacing wire is grabbed by the flaccid portion adjacent to the needle with an endoclose that is introduced through a small skin incision inferior to the mini-thoracotomy. After this, the cross-clamp is removed or the endoballoon deflated. The repair is evaluated with echocardiography, the heart is de-aired and CPB is weaned. Decannulation is performed in the usual fashion. It is important to evaluate for a distal femoral pulse after femoral arterial decannulation. If the distal femoral pulse is absent or weak, the artery can be clamped and an interrupted repair with 5-0 Prolene sutures can be performed. The arteriotomy may also be augmented with a bovine pericardial patch.

We place a Blake drain in the mediastinum through the left atrial retractor incision in males; in females, we make an additional incision inferior to the mini-thoracotomy and medial to the CO_2 port to place this Blake. An angled chest tube is placed in the right chest through the CO_2 port in both males and females. The pericardium is closed with two Ti-Cron sutures. The port sites including the mammary vessels are also checked with a dental mirror and the camera to ensure that they are not bleeding. Mammary vein bleeding can sometimes be controlled with an inflated Foley balloon. Significant vein bleeding or internal mammary artery bleeding is controlled with suture ligation. A long-acting intercostal block is performed before wound closure. A single #1 loop Maxon suture is used for pericostal closure to prevent lung herniation.

Mitral valve replacement and concomitant procedures

Mitral valve replacement with a bioprosthesis or mechanical prosthesis can be performed through MAMVS as well. This is performed in a similar manner to the mitral valve repair procedure described above. We tend to perform total chordal sparing replacement when possible. After incising the anterior leaflet in the A2 portion, we take scissors and bisect the leaflet and then tack the leaflets onto either side of the annulus around P1 and P3. Sutures are placed in either an everting or non-everting manner. The posterior sutures are brought through the edge of the posterior leaflet to help "tuck" the leaflet so that it does not hinder the valve. Although replacements are a good initial operation for the early MAMVS surgeon, cases of severe mitral annular calcification are viewed as a contraindication to a minimal access approach even in many experienced hands.

Concomitant procedures such as ablation procedures including left atrial appendage ligation and tricuspid valve procedures can be performed through the right mini-thoracotomy approach. Left atrial appendage ligation can be performed by lifting the aorta with suction and then grasping the left atrial appendage with a forcep through the transverse sinus and applying a large clip across the base of the appendage. It can also be performed by running a Prolene suture from inside the left atrium and closing the appendage from the inside in two layers. Tricuspid valve repairs or replacements can also be performed but require the placement of tourniquets around the superior and inferior vena cava for inflow occlusion. Surgeons early in their experience with MAMVS should start with isolated mitral valve surgery before proceeding to MAMVS with other concomitant procedures.

POSTOPERATIVE CARE

Most of the postoperative care in MAMVS patients is similar to that in all cardiac postsurgical patients. In appropriate candidates, early extubation within 6 hours is the goal. Pain control is facilitated in the usual manner although long-acting intercostal nerve blocks are an important intraoperative adjunct. Atrial fibrillation is common and treated in the usual manner. Pacing wires are removed on the first or second postoperative day. Chest tubes are removed when the output is less than 250 mL per day. Aggressive diuresis is important as pleural effusions and volume overload are common reasons for readmission. Sternal precautions are not needed in patients approached with a right mini-thoracotomy and physical restrictions are generally removed after the second postoperative week.

OUTCOME

Although there is undoubtedly a learning curve associated with MAMVS, reports from multiple institutions have established the safety and feasibility of this approach. A combined report from the East Carolina University and University of Pennsylvania groups demonstrated an operative mortality of 0.2% for isolated primary mitral valve repair. A meta-analysis of 10 papers publishing on 1358 MAMVS and 1469 sternotomy patients demonstrated that, although CPB and cross-clamp times were longer with MAMVS, there was no difference in mortality, stroke, atrial fibrillation, reoperation for bleeding, or length of intensive care unit or hospital stay between approaches. A report of over 28 000 mitral valve operations using the Society of Thoracic Surgeons National Database found that, despite longer CPB and cross-clamp times, there was similar adjusted operative mortality, fewer blood transfusions, and shorter hospital stay with MAMVS. However, stroke rates were higher with MAMVS and, in particular, with the beating or fibrillating heart approach. From a cost perspective, we have found that lower postoperative costs offset the higher operative costs with MAMVS therefore resulting in similar overall costs for MAMVS and traditional sternotomy. With further refinements in surgical technique and technology, outcomes with MAMVS will hopefully continue to improve in coming years.

FURTHER READING

Ailawadi G, Agnihotri AK, Mehall JR, et al. Minimally invasive mitral valve surgery I: Patient selection, evaluation, and planning. *Innovations (Phila)*. 2016; 11(4): 243–50.

Atluri P, et al. Port access cardiac operations can be safely performed with either endoaortic balloon or Chitwood clamp. *Ann Thorac Surg* 2014; 98: 1579–83.

Wolfe JA, Malaisrie SC, Farivar RS, et al. Minimally invasive mitral valve surgery II: Surgical technique and postoperative management. *Innovations (Phila)*. 2016; 11(4): 251–9.

18

Robot-assisted mitral valve surgery

KAUSHIK MANDAL AND W. RANDOLPH CHITWOOD JR.

INTRODUCTION

Robot-assisted minimally invasive cardiac surgery is facilitated by remote controlled telemanipulators that have 7 degrees of motion freedom and an operative console, which provides a high-definition three-dimensional magnified operative field view. Robotics introduced a paradigm shift in cardiac surgery with enhanced patient satisfaction. The advantages of operating through smaller incisions include reduced postoperative pain, quicker recovery, improved cosmesis, and earlier return to work.[1]

The transition from long-instrument, direct-vision minimally invasive surgery to robotics began in the early 2000s. This was spawned by advancements in endoscopic instruments, improved endoscopes, and modified cardiopulmonary bypass (CPB) perfusion systems using peripheral cannulation.[2–8] Approximately 20% of all mitral valve operations in the United States are currently performed using minimally invasive techniques, with half of them being robot-assisted.[9]

THE DA VINCI™ SURGICAL ROBOTIC SYSTEM

The mitral valve lies in an annular plane that approximates the thoracic sagittal axis. Hence, a 3–4 cm anterolateral thoracic incision (working port) is well suited for cardiac exposure. With the incision placed more laterally, the visual angle becomes even more direct. In this instance, long robotic instruments overcome the limitations imposed by the increased distance between the working port and the mitral valve. Today, the da Vinci SI™ surgical system (Intuitive Surgical, Mountain View, CA, USA) is the only robotic device that is FDA approved for cardiac surgery. The system comprises a surgeon operating console, a tableside instrument cart, and a video platform. Finger and wrist movements are registered through tiny sensors and are translated digitally into motion-scaled, tremor-free instrument tip movements. This device avoids the fulcrum effects and shaft shear forces present when working with long-shafted endoscopic instruments. Wrist-like end-effectors bring the pivoting action of the micro-instruments into the operative field, improving dexterity in confined spaces and allowing truly ambidextrous suture placement.

During robot-assisted procedures, the surgeon sits at the operating console and manipulates mechanical wrists which have 7 degrees of motion freedom. The tableside surgical assistant and scrub nurse exchange instruments and provide materials necessary for the mitral valve repair. The da Vinci system scales surgeon movements and corrects for human natural tremor before sending filtered information to the computer-driven robotic arms. Two parallel camera lenses provide high definition 3D visualization. A dynamic intra-atrial retractor enables rapid repositioning to optimize valve exposure, which is a significant advantage over a traditional fixed retractor used in non-robotic endoscopic mitral operations.[10]

The lack of tactile feedback in robotic procedures seemingly is a limitation; however, surgeons quickly learn to rely on visual cues to determine tissue deformation and suture strain when tying. Difficulties with robotic knot tying of annuloplasty band sutures have been overcome with the employment of the Cor-Knot™ device (LSI Solutions, Victor, NY). Pre-looped polytetrafluoroethylene (PTFE) (Leyla) sutures facilitate and speed left atrial closure.[11] These advances have significantly reduced all operative times. Between May 2000 and December 2012, 800 patients underwent robot-assisted mitral valve surgery at the East Carolina Heart Institute.

EARLY OUTCOMES

The first robot-assisted mitral valve surgery operation was performed by Carpentier and colleagues in 1997 using a prototype of the current da Vinci robotic system.[12] In 2000 the East Carolina University team performed the first complete robotic mitral valve repair in the United States using the first-generation da Vinci.[13] Following a pivotal investigational device exemption multicenter trial in 2002, the Food and Drug Administration (FDA) approved the da Vinci system for use in cardiac surgery.[14]

Mounting publications demonstrate improved recovery times and less pain associated with these procedures.[15–18]

Murphy and colleagues reported that over 60% of his robot-assisted mitral valve patients were discharged within 4 days after surgery.[19] A recent meta-analysis by Cheng and colleagues showed a significant reduction in bleeding, transfusions, incidence of atrial fibrillation, and time to resumption of normal activities, compared with conventional mitral valve surgery.[20] Optimal clinical outcomes and mitral valve repair durability remain sentinel goals regardless of the surgical approach. Two large single-center studies showed that perioperative and long-term mortality are equivalent to traditional operations as is long-term freedom from reoperation.[15, 20–21] Eight-year freedom from a reoperation was better than a traditional operation as were both short-term and 1-year survival.[22, 23] It is important to note that most of the robot-assisted patients have been pre-selected and generally do not include high-risk ones. Cheng showed that patients were younger and had a lower incidence of baseline renal failure and pulmonary disease.[20] The largest single-center report of robot-assisted mitral valve surgery comes from our group at the East Carolina Heart Institute.[24] In 540 consecutive patients with a 2.9% reoperation rate, we showed a low short- and long-term mortality of 0.4% and 1.7% respectively. These results compared favorably with the meta-analysis published by Cheng et al., in which 30-day mortality was 1.2% and reoperation rate was 2.3%.[20]

A significant learning curve exists for robotic-assisted procedures.[25] Both Cheng and our group have shown a decrease in mitral valve repair failure rate after 74 and 100 robot-assisted cases respectively.[26, 27] Compared with the sternotomy approach, operative times, including the cardiopulmonary and aortic cross-clamp times, have been shown to be longer with robot-assisted minimally invasive mitral valve procedures.[20]

PREOPERATIVE ASSESSMENT AND PREPARATION

Preoperative evaluation

The preoperative evaluation of patients for robot mitral valve surgery is similar to patients undergoing a traditional mitral valve operation with a few exceptions. Peripheral vascular cannulation for CPB is necessary. In patients with significant atherosclerosis, computed tomographic angiography (CTA) should be carried out. In a study of 141 patients, scheduled for minimally invasive cardiac surgery at the Cleveland Clinic, 20% of patients had the surgical approach changed to sternotomy because of CTA findings, which included

significant aortoiliac atherosclerosis and mitral annular calcification.[28] Previous right thoracotomy or adhesions and presence of breast implants are additional issues that could preclude a robot-assisted procedure. At East Carolina University, we carry out preoperative pulmonary function tests (PFTs) in patients with a significant pulmonary history. PFTs also indicate whether the patient can tolerate single-lung ventilation. Preoperative lung function abnormalities (FEV1 <40% predicted, DLCO <40% predicted) should alert the surgeon regarding potential problems with single-lung ventilation. Most patients undergo coronary angiography although in younger patients CT angiography is often selected. In patients where there is concern regarding pulmonary hypertension, we prefer to obtain right heart catheterization data. The combination of severe pulmonary hypertension, chronic obstructive pulmonary disease, and a dilated right ventricle generally lead us to opt for a sternotomy-based operation.

Echocardiographic operative planning

The importance of transesophageal echocardiography (TEE) guidance in making mitral valve repair decisions cannot be overemphasized and has been well established.[29–31] We use the Carpentier functional and topographic classifications to describe TEE evaluations. Pre-incision 2D (**Figures 18.1 and 18.2**) and 3D TEE (**Figure 18.3**) studies are essential to formulate a repair plan.[32] Also, quantitative mitral valve 3D echo modeling (**Figure 18.4**) has been a very useful adjunct.[33] **Figure 18.5** shows the 2D and 3D TEE measurements that we use to develop an intraoperative "blueprint" for every mitral repair. The direction of each jet (leak) is mapped, and both the mobility and the level of leaflet prolapse/restriction are determined. Each leaflet segment (P1–P3, A1–A3) is measured with specific attention to both the A2 length and P1–P3 heights (annulus to coapting edge). Adding 7 mm to the A2 length in the 120-degree midesophageal view guides us during annuloplasty band size selection (**Figure 18.1**). The planar angle between the aortic and mitral valve annulus is determined (**Figure 18.2**). Finally, the annular diameter, outflow tract septal thickness, and coaptation point to septal (C–sept) distances are measured. All TEE studies can be transmitted to the operating console Tile-Pro™ (Intuitive Surgical, Sunnyvale, CA) for intraoperative visualization during the repair. The TEE also alerts us to the presence of aortic regurgitation and left ventricular hypertrophy, both of which warrant adjustment in myocardial preservation strategy.

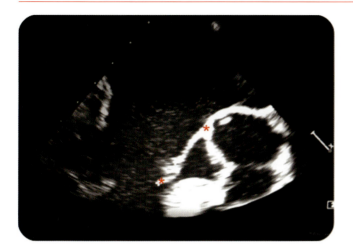

18.1 The 120° midesophageal TEE view for measuring the anterior mitral valve leaflet length.

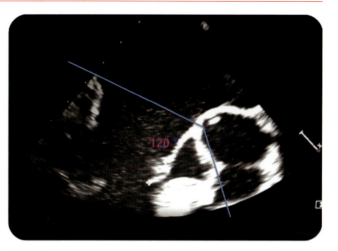

18.2 Measuring the aortomitral angle for assessing the risk of postoperative systolic anterior motion (SAM).

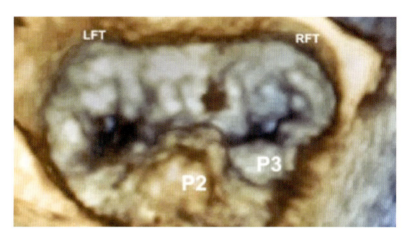

18.3 3D echo showing P2 prolapse.

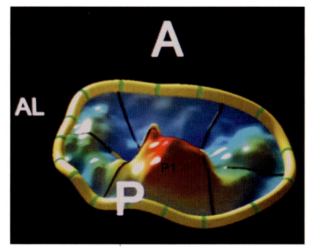

18.4 3D model of mitral valve generated using MVQ™ (Phillips) software.

120 ME long axis

	Reference
LVOT _____	<2.2 cm (divided by 0.8 = intertrigonal estimate)
A2 _____	2.5–3.0 cm, early diastole, leaflet extended
P2 _____	1.0–1.5 cm, early diastole, leaflet extended
Annulus (short/high) _____	<3.8 cm, early diastole, leaflets open
Annular calcium? _____	

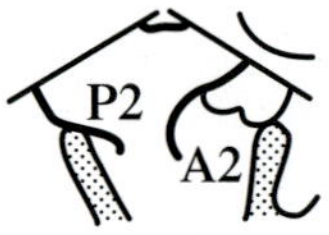

60 ME commissural

	Reference
P1 _____	1–1.5 cm, early diastole, leaflet extended
P3 _____	1–1.5 cm, early diastole, leaflet extended
Annulus (long/low) _____	< 4.0 cm
Annular calcium? _____	

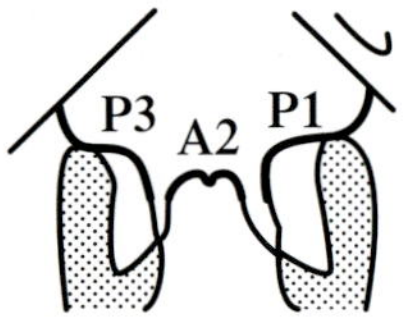

0 ME 4 chamber   Left atrium _____   <5.2 cm, end sys

3D Model

Annulus   long/low _____ (cm) (DAIPm)

Height _____ (mm)

short/high _____ (cm) (DAP)

Aortic–mitral angle _____ want > 120

Commissure length _____ (mm)

Leaflets   Total lengths = L3OT (mm)   Exposed lengths = L3OE (mm)

A2 _____   P1 _____

P2 _____   P3 _____

Max prolapse _____ (mm)

MR type   1 – central 2 – prolapse   3 – restricted (A - rheum, B - ischemic)

3D Live   Commissural leaflet? _____   Clefts? _____

Increased SAMS risk   AL>3.0   C–sept<2.5 cm   (septum to ant coapt LA side)
PL>1.6   MV/Ao<120
AL/PL<1.3

Estimates of ring/valve size = LVOT/0.8, commissural distance, short annular height, ant leaflet area

18.5 Mitral valve repair checklist for planning the repair.

ANESTHESIA

Patient positioning is typically supine with the right thorax elevated (**Figure 18.6**). To improve surgical exposure, the right arm is positioned by the side, allowing the shoulder to become displaced posteriorly. To avoid brachial plexus and neck stress, the right shoulder should be supported. External defibrillator pads should be applied, crossing the cardiac mass, and connected before starting the procedure. As a right anterolateral mini-thoracotomy working port is used, right lung isolation is essential. The most common techniques for achieving lung isolation are with either a double-lumen endotracheal tube (DLT) or a right-sided bronchial blocker. After separation from CPB, single-lung ventilation is often needed to check surgically for bleeding. **Figure 18.7** illustrates the anesthetic preparation that is typical for these and includes a DLT, a TEE probe, a Swan–Ganz pulmonary artery catheter, and the right internal jugular superior vena cava (SVC) cannula.

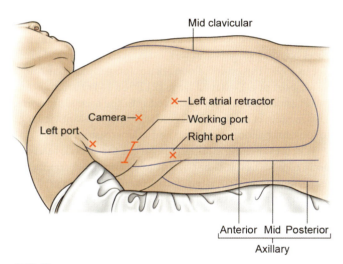

18.6 Patient positioning for right anterolateral thoracotomy approach with port and access sites marked.

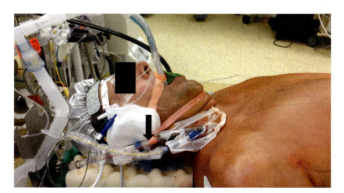

18.7 Anesthetic setup showing the double-lumen endotracheal tube, TEE probe, Swan–Ganz catheter and right internal jugular SVC cannula (arrow) in place.

OPERATION

Cardiopulmonary bypass

Venous return to the CPB circuit can be achieved in several ways. We establish inferior vena caval (IVC) drainage using either a 23 Fr or 25 Fr RAP™ femoral venous cannula (Estech, San Ramon, CA). After accessing the femoral vein, a guide-wire is advanced into the right atrium under TEE guidance, and the cannula is inserted over the wire using the Seldinger technique. Also, we prefer to place a thin-walled (15 Fr or 17 Fr) Bio-Medicus™ cannula (Medtronic, Minneapolis, MN) through the right internal jugular vein (double-puncture method) and position it in the distal SVC. **Figures 18.7** and **18.8** show the venous cannulae in place. Vacuum assistance is used to assist venous drainage.[34] Long percutaneous cannulae and vacuum assistance can increase venous return by 20–40%. In contradistinction, adequate total body venous drainage can be achieved with a single femoral venous cannula as long as the major side holes reside within the mid right atrium with the tip passed into the proximal SVC. The dynamic atrial retractor can impede venous drainage and repositioning will usually solve this problem. The placement of a large-bore drainage catheter in the neck is not without potential risks. Care must be taken when inserting this cannula to avoid the internal jugular vein (IJ) or SVC perforation. TEE guidance for both wire and cannula placement is essential for safety.[35] A small dose of heparin should be administered just before IJ cannulation. When the right atrium must be opened for a concomitant tricuspid valve repair, caval tapes are applied to prevent air entrainment.

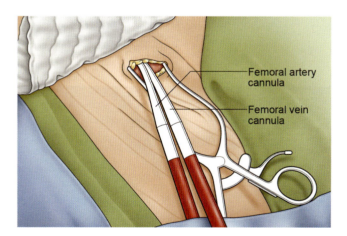

18.8 Right groin cannulae comprising the femoral arterial and the femoral venous cannulae. The femoral venous cannula is positioned in the right atrium using TEE guidance.

During femoral artery cannulation, the guidewire should be passed into the distal aorta and observed by TEE before beginning catheter insertion. Elevation of the arterial inflow-line pressure is often the first indicator of a possible retrograde aortic dissection. Thus, it is best to assess the aorta by TEE just after beginning CPB. Early recognition and conversion to antegrade central arterial flow may limit the damage of this potentially devastating complication.

When using peripheral arterial cannulation, we monitor oxygen saturation in both legs to decrease the risk of ischemia. By using the NIRS probe (INVOS® Cerebral/Somatic Oximeter, Medtronic, Minneapolis, MN) and a dual-chamber monitor to record simultaneously cerebral and leg arterial saturations (**Figure 18.9**), we are alerted to any significant drop in peripheral saturation (to less than 20% baseline). In this instance we shunt the affected leg by introducing a 5 Fr sheath into the distal femoral artery. This technique has prevented us from having any patients with devastating limb injury. Complications associated with vascular access and retrograde arterial perfusion using endoballoon aortic occlusion devices were reported by Mohr and colleagues.[36] New York University surgeons described a decrease in neurologic events from 4.7% to 1.2% by using central aortic cannulation during minimally invasive valve surgery.[37] Murphy and colleagues report the use of a screening protocol to identify and avoid femoral cannulation in patients considered at higher risk for retrograde embolization.[19]

Aortic occlusion

Our preferred method for cross-clamping the aorta is the Chitwood Transthoracic Aortic Cross-clamp (Scanlan International, Minneapolis, MN), which is inserted through the chest wall and guided toward the ascending aorta under either direct or endoscopic vision. We prefer the method to endoballoon aortic occlusion because of decreased infrastructure demands and costs, as well as shorter operative and cross-clamp times.[38] One disadvantage is the need to place a separate aortic root vent through the working port and into the ascending aorta for cardiac venting and antegrade cardioplegia administration.

The Port Access system (Edwards Lifesciences, Irvine, CA) with the EndoClamp was designed to facilitate minimal access cardiac surgery and was introduced into clinical practice in 1997. This endoballoon aortic clamp is placed through a side port of a Y-shaped large (21 Fr or 24 Fr) arterial cannula (EndoReturn) and advanced into the ascending aorta. This maneuver requires TEE guidance and constant vigilance to look for balloon migration and malperfusion.

When evaluating studies comparing the overall safety of both approaches, it is important to consider the significant learning curve associated with Port Access surgery. The learning curve was exemplified by results shown in the Port Access International Registry, in which the incidence of iatrogenic aortic dissection was 1.3% in the first half of the study followed by a decrease to 0.2% in the second half.[39]

Other alternatives to aortic cross-clamping exist, the simplest of which involves operating on a beating heart. The obvious advantage of this method is that it allows coronary flow to remain uninterrupted. The disadvantages of this approach include a wet surgical field and the possibility of systemic air embolization. In reoperative procedures or in the presence of mild–moderate aortic insufficiency, we have used cold fibrillatory arrest with excellent results without aortic cross-clamping. One has to be cognizant of the left atrial retractor position to avoid increased aortic regurgitation. Fibrillation can be achieved either by an electrical fibrillator or through rapid pacing with a special Swan–Ganz catheter.[40]

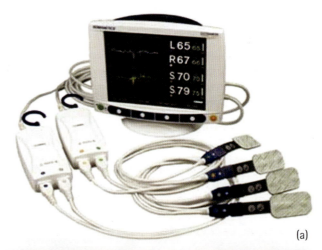

(a)

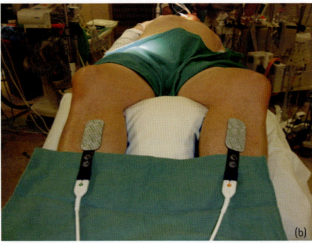

(b)

18.9a, b Setup for monitoring the peripheral leg saturations during the case.

Myocardial protection

We generally systemically cool patients to 26–28 °C. Warm CO_2 is insufflated continuously into the operative field to prevent camera fogging and to displace air from the hemithorax. For cardioplegia delivery, we use a long aortic root vent/cardioplegia cannula inserted through the working port incision through a 3-0 PTFE pursestring suture. Another option is to use a percutaneous coronary sinus catheter for retrograde cardioplegia delivery.[41, 42] The EndoPledge Coronary Sinus Catheter (Edwards Lifesciences, Irvine, CA) is advanced through an 11 Fr right IJ vein introducer sheath. This catheter has a triple lumen with a terminal balloon, which provides coronary sinus occlusion, distal pressure measurement, and infusion of cardioplegia. With this technique, retrograde cardioplegia can be administered while continuing with the robotic repair. The TEE is used most commonly to direct the cannula into the coronary sinus ostia. The generation of a "ventricularized" distal pressure waveform during inflation of the occlusion balloon suggests adequate sinus occlusion. Though appealing conceptually, the EndoPledge cannula has not been adopted widely because of concerns regarding the risk of a coronary sinus perforation, catheter placement difficulties, and a significant chance of intraoperative dislodgement. Many surgeons do not believe that retrograde cardioplegia is necessary for cardiac protection in the presence of normal coronary arteries.[43, 44]

Our preferred cardioplegia solution for robot-assisted mitral valve surgery is antegrade Custodiol® HTK. It is an intracellular solution, containing low concentrations of the electrolytes sodium, calcium, potassium, and magnesium. The normal osmolarity mix contains a high concentration of the amino acid buffering agent histidine/histidine hydrochloride, the amino acid tryptophan α-ketoglutarate, and an osmotic agent (mannitol). A single cold 2–2.5 L dose, administered slowly over 10–15 minutes, allows electromechanical silence for up to an hour and allows the surgeon to focus on uninterrupted surgery. Smaller infusions of 100–300 mL can be administered for any recurrent ECG activity. This large volume, low sodium infusate often drops the serum sodium and pH. Standard blood cardioplegia is still a viable alternative; however, surgery must be interrupted for frequent doses and this creates an increased chance of introducing coronary air. Data regarding the safety and efficacy of using Custodiol® HTK have been published.[45]

Robot-assisted mitral valve repair: technique

A 4 cm working port (mini-thoracotomy) is made in the right fourth interspace, lateral to the anterior axillary line. Instrument trocars (Figure 18.10) are positioned as follows:

1. *left robotic arm* – third interspace (anterior axillary line)
2. *right robotic arm* – fifth interspace (mid-axillary line)
3. *dynamic retractor arm* – fifth interspace (mid-clavicular line).

The da Vinci™ robotic instrument cart is docked at the left side of the table and instruments are passed through these trocars. The 30-degree 3D HD endoscopic camera is positioned looking up through either the working port or a separate fifth interspace port. We use the following

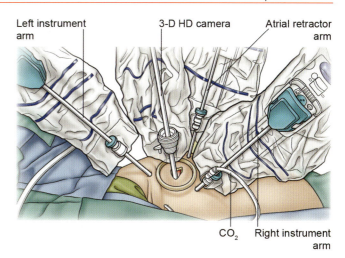

18.10 Typical setup for a robot-assisted mitral valve repair with the da Vinci system docked.

robotic instruments for mitral valve surgery: Resano (8 mm) Endowrist™ forceps, which are deployed through the left trocar, and either curved Endowrist™ scissors or Suture-cut™ needle holders, both of which are inserted through the right port. Lastly, the dynamic retractor is positioned in the chest before initiating cardiopulmonary perfusion.

After systemic perfusion (28 °C) has decompressed the heart, the pericardium is opened linearly 3 cm anterior to the phrenic nerve. To expose the aorta, the right superior pulmonary vein, and interatrial groove, three transthoracic 2-0 braided suture loops are placed along the posterior pericardial edge and passed through the chest wall to distract it laterally (Figure 18.11). For the cardioplegia vent catheter a 3-0 pledgeted H-shaped PTFE suture is placed robotically in the ascending aorta just proximal to the fatty fold of Rindfleisch. A long Medtronic catheter (Medtronic, Minneapolis, MN) is inserted through either the incision or a separate port and

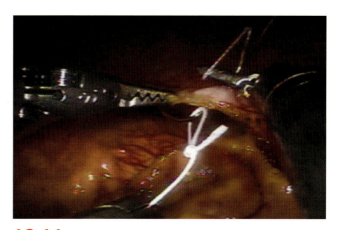

18.11 Pericardial retraction suture using Leyla loops.

secured (**Figure 18.12**). The tableside assistant then introduces the transthoracic aortic cross-clamp through the third interspace at the posterior axillary line, passing it across the SVC–pericardial junction. With robotic instruments lifting the aorta and under videoscopic guidance, the posterior clamp time is passed through the transverse sinus (**Figure 18.13**). The right pulmonary artery and left atrial appendage should be viewed at this time. After aortic clamping, 25 mL/kg of HTK Bretschneider solution is administered with an additional small dose of cardioplegia given after 1 hour.

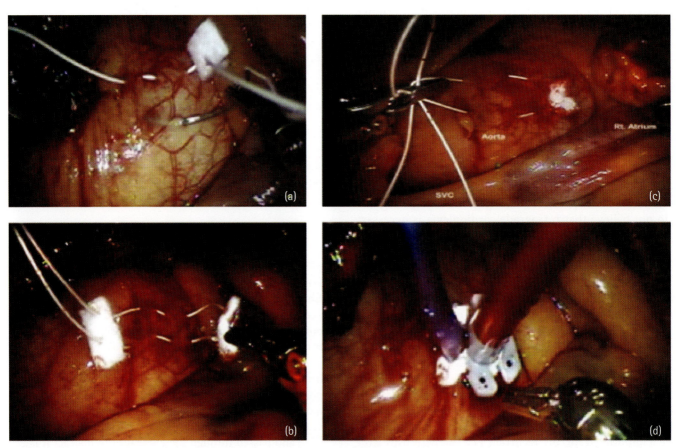

18.12a–d   A 3-0 Gor-Tex cardioplegia stitch and the antegrade cardioplegia cannula in situ.

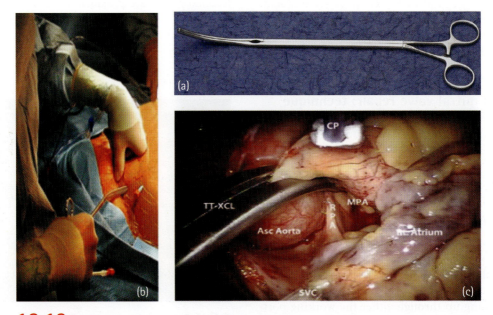

18.13a–c   Chitwood transthoracic clamp: insertion and placement.

Using the curved Endowrist™ scissors, minimal dissection is performed along the right superior pulmonary vein and toward the interatrial groove. The left atrium is opened radially, being careful not to damage either pulmonary vein. Thereafter, the dynamic retractor (**Figure 18.14**) is positioned

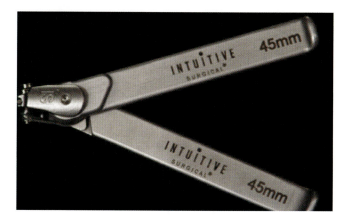

18.14   Dynamic left atrial retractor.

in the left atrium to expose the mitral apparatus, and a transthoracic sump sucker is placed in the left superior pulmonary vein. At the end of the repair the atriotomy is closed using 4-0 PTFE suture loops.[11]

POSTERIOR LEAFLET REPAIRS

All of our leaflet repairs are based on the preoperative TEE measurements shown in **Figure 18.5**. With degenerative mitral insufficiency, 80% of pathology relates to posterior leaflet defects. In many circumstances a simple triangular resection will correct isolated segmental prolapse (**Figure 18.15**).[46] We suggest using this method first to correct isolated scallops having mid-prolapse or ruptured chords, and then testing the repair early with ventricular saline filling. Leaflet segments that remain longer than 2 cm should be reduced in height using either a folding-plasty (**Figure 18.16**) or an additional triangular resection. Additional techniques can be used to provide a uniform coaptation line.

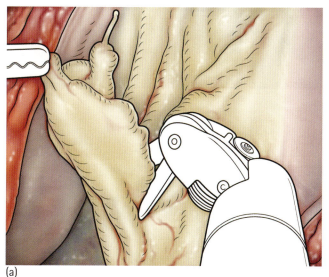

(a)

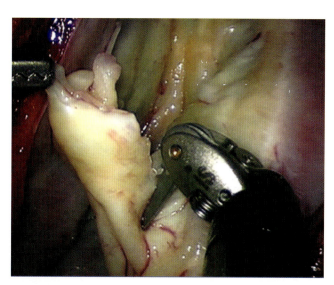

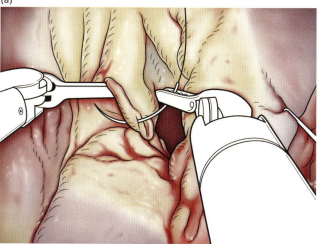

(b)

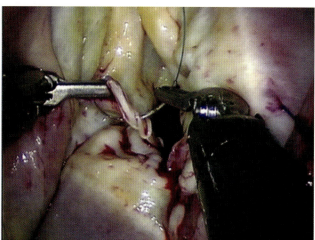

18.15a, b   Triangular leaflet resection and repair.

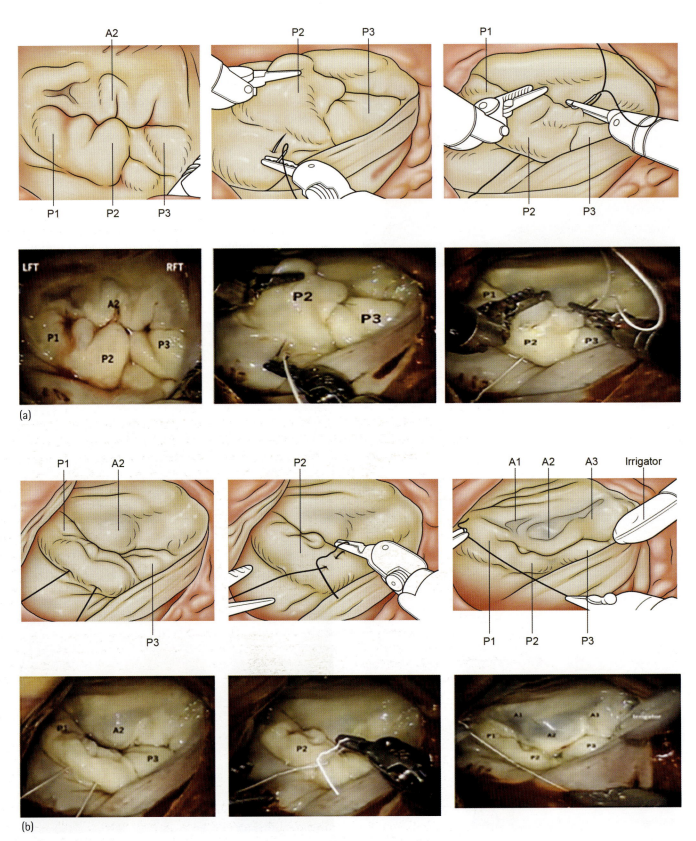

(a)

(b)

18.16   Posterior leaflet folding-plasty.

In the presence of diminutive P_1 and P_2 scallops and a very large P_2, one should consider either the "haircut" resection technique (**Figure 18.17**) or insertion of several PTFE neochords.[47–49] For multiple prolapsing scallops or those longer than 2 cm, several folding-plasties can be adjusted to create the best coaptation line. Final scallop height folding adjustments are made after the annuloplasty band has been implanted. An alternative to several triangular resections or folding-plasties is multiple PTFE neochord replacements, using the Frater–David technique (**Figure 18.18**).[48, 49] In severely prolapsing Barlow's valves with very elongated scallops, we still defer to a classic mid-scallop (P2) resection with a posterior leaflet annular sliding-plasty (**Figure 18.19**). However, multiple triangular resections, folding-plasties and/or multiple neochords can be used to repair moderately severe Barlow's valves.[50, 51]

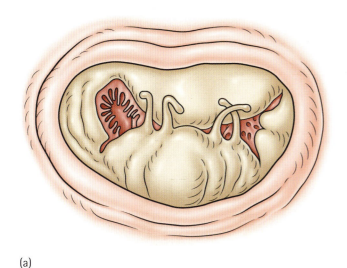

(a)

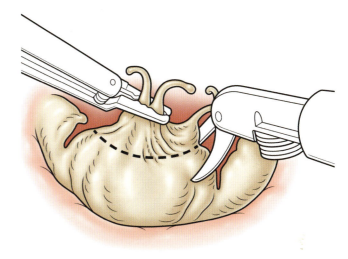

(b)

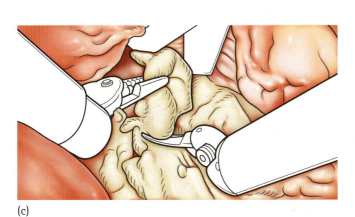

(c)

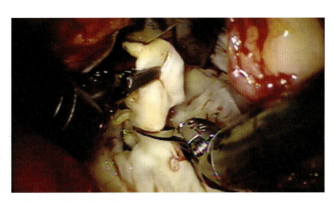

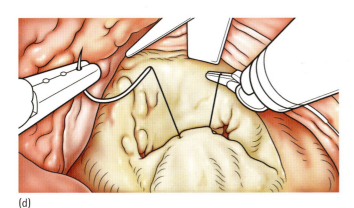

(d)

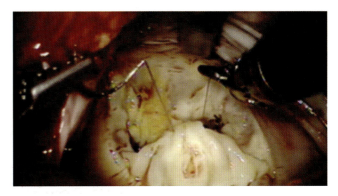

18.17a–d   "Haircut" P2 resection and repair for large prolapsing P2.

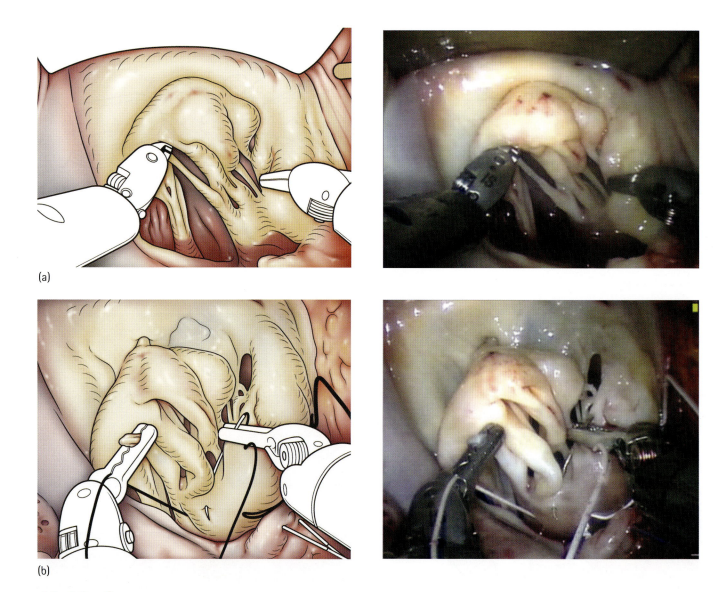

(a)

(b)

18.18a, b Robot-assisted neochord implantation.

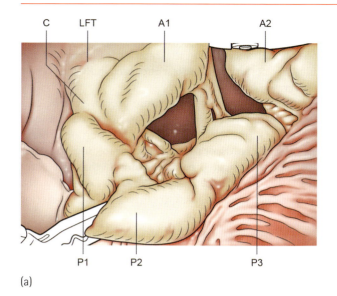

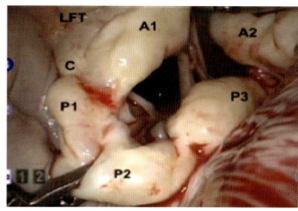

(a)

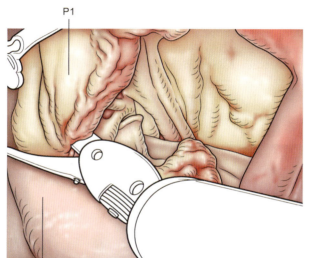

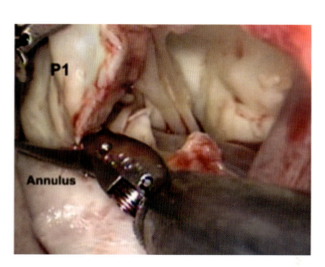

(b)

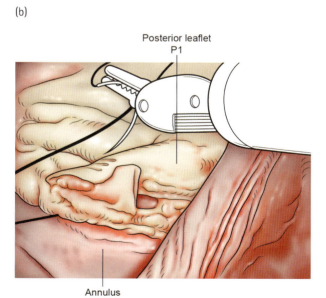

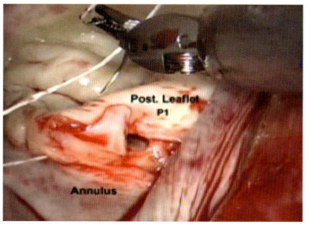

(c)

18.19a–c Posterior leaflet sliding-plasty.

Most of our mitral repairs have been supported by a trigone-to-trigone Cosgrove™ annuloplasty band (Edwards Lifesciences, Irvine, CA). We prefer to use multipoint band fixation, using deep braided sutures (2-0 Cardioflon, Peters, Paris, France) secured by Cor-Knot™ (LSI Solutions, Victor, NY) titanium clips (**Figures 18.20 and 18.21**). Some robotic surgeons prefer to use a running suture technique with extra-corporeal knot tying.[52]

ANTERIOR LEAFLET REPAIRS

With an isolated uniform anterior leaflet prolapse of less than 2–3 mm, we place the annuloplasty band first and then saline test to determine the level of coaptation. Most of these will be corrected by insertion of the band. When significant anterior prolapse exists, individual leaflet zones can be addressed by a local triangular resection, a secondary chord transfer, insertion of PTFE neochords, or a combination of these (**Figure 18.22**).[53] In elderly patients, especially with significant comorbid conditions, we may perform an ("Alfieri") edge-to-edge mid-leaflet repair combined with an annuloplasty. When a large anterior leaflet prolapsing segment is related to multiple chords from an elongated papillary muscle, correction can be accomplished either by muscle shortening (folding) (**Figure 18.23**) or by insertion

of several PTFE chords. For large areas of uniform anterior leaflet prolapse, a leading edge strip (rough zone) can be incised and advanced along the anterior leaflet toward the annulus. We perform a saline test after each individual repair maneuver.

In most circumstances commissure prolapse can be corrected by closure with a Carpentier "magic" stitch (Lembert edge-to-edge suture) (**Figure 18.24**) or by insertion of commissural PTFE chords, or papillary muscle folding. The latter can correct an elongated papillary muscle that originates chords to both anterior and posterior leaflet edges. Rarely, a leaflet sliding-plasty is used to correct a single posterior scallop commissure prolapse.

Robot-assisted mitral valve repair in reoperative surgery

In well-selected patients previous cardiac surgery does not preclude using robotic assistance and even provides significant advantages. Multiple studies have shown equal or better mortality when using a right thoracotomy for reoperative mitral valve surgery than after a second or third sternotomy.[54–56] Infections, transfusions, and length of hospital

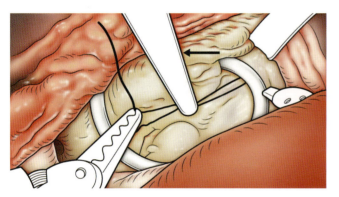
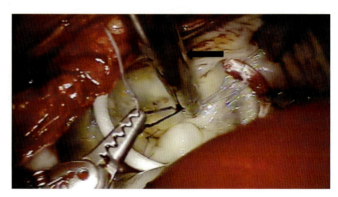

18.20 Intraoperative view showing annuloplasty ring being secured with Cor-Knot™ (arrow).

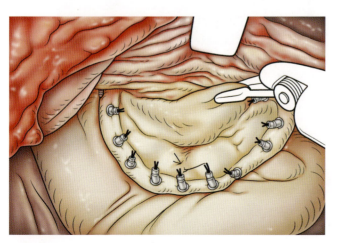
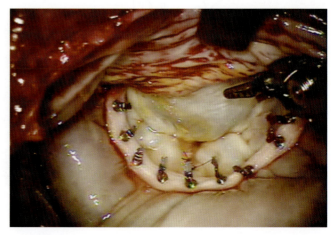

18.21 Intraoperative view of a completed annuloplasty, secured using Cor-Knot™.

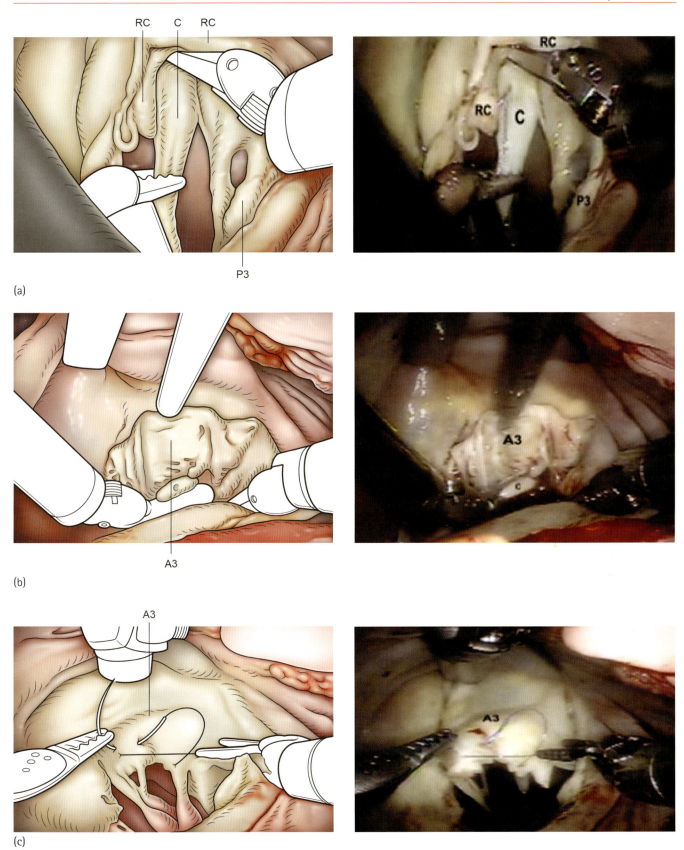

(a)

(b)

(c)

18.22a–c Anterior leaflet repair using triangular resection and secondary chord transfer.

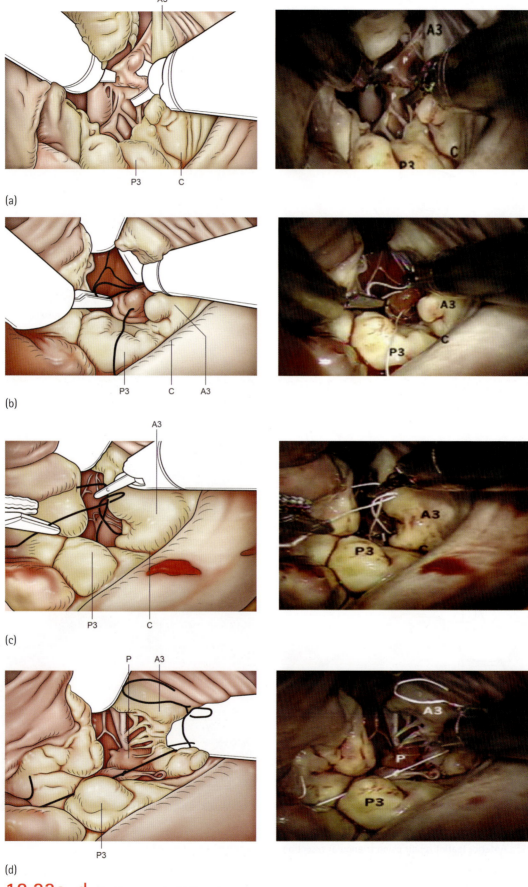

(a)

(b)

(c)

(d)

18.23a–d Papillary muscle folding-plasty.

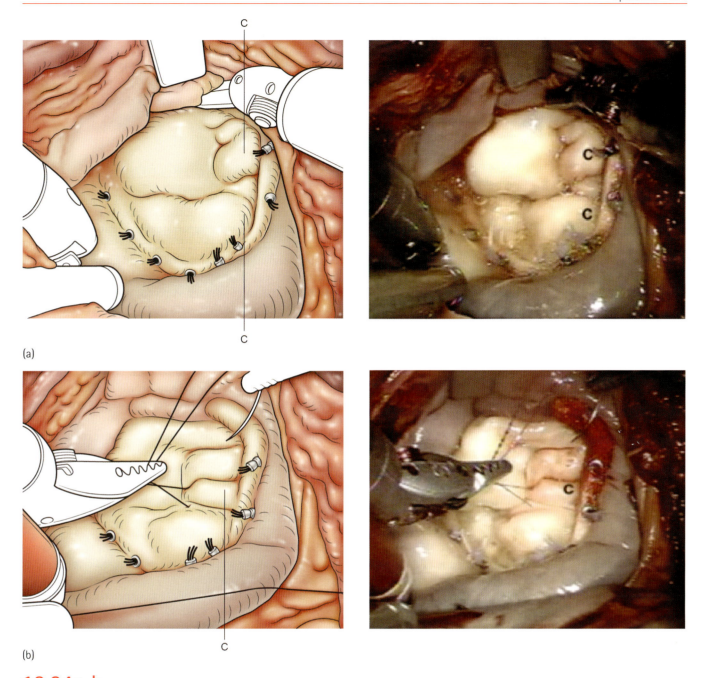

(a)

(b)

18.24a, b Commissural prolapse being corrected with a "magic" stitch.

stay were consistently reduced in these studies. Our group reported a 3.0% 30-day mortality in 167 patients who had had a previous sternotomy over a 15-year period, who underwent reoperation using a right anterolateral mini-thoracotomy.[57] Included in this were 19 robot-assisted cases. Over the last 5 years, we have had no 30-day deaths in 85 patients with a low stroke rate. It should be noted, however, that there was a significant increase in pulmonary complications compared with a reoperative sternotomy. Svensson et al. reported a higher incidence of repair failures and strokes in 80 patients undergoing mitral valve reoperations through a right thoracotomy[58] when compared to a 2444 patient cohort, who had a mitral repair performed via a reoperative sternotomy. Nevertheless, the operative mortality was similar between the two groups (6.7% and 6.3% respectively). Reoperative patients who have a patent left internal thoracic artery (LITA) coronary bypass graft require additional consideration. As the LITA cannot be clamped through a right mini-thoracotomy, either aggressive systemic cooling (26°C) or "beating-heart" strategies should be considered.[58, 59]

Anterior chest-wall adhesions from a previous sternotomy may limit right ventricular exposure and prevent insertion of temporary pacing wires. The preoperative placement of a pacing Swan–Ganz catheter will often alleviate this problem. Similarly, previous operations often create difficulties in achieving total vena caval occlusion. Placing bulldog clamps on both venae cavae during robotic surgery has been reported.[60] We have used a "no caval occlusion" method when entering the right atrium for a beating-heart tricuspid repair. Our perfusionists insert a hard shell venous reservoir in the CPB circuit to handle entrained air during aggressive assisted venous drainage. The IVC cannula is withdrawn to the mid-liver level and an additional right atrial sucker is added. The SVC can either be left open or occluded using a balloon catheter.

Separation from cardiopulmonary bypass

During separation from CPB, there are no dramatic differences from open operations. However, any increased cross-clamp and CPB times may need to be factored into decision making regarding post-CPB pharmacologic, ventilatory, fluid, and blood-product management. If a pacing Swan–Ganz catheter is being used, adjustments in position may be needed because, when the heart fills, the pacing electrode may migrate away from the ventricular wall. Ventilation of both lungs should be reinstituted as soon as possible. The ability to dislodge retained left atrial air is typically not hampered by the incision, but exposure to the left ventricular apex is not possible. In patients with pre-existing aortic regurgitation, a left ventricular vent should be placed across the mitral valve. This is especially important in patients with any degree of left ventricular impairment or hypertrophy.

As the aortic valve non-coronary leaflet is close to the left fibrous trigone, it is important to carry out TEE examination for any new aortic insufficiency. Similarly, as the circumflex coronary artery is close to the posterior and lateral annulus, ventricular wall motion assessment is important to rule out coronary injury. Right pulmonary vein patency and flow should be evaluated before separation from CPB.

During chest closure, single-lung ventilation is typically needed. This additional strain (hypoxemia and shunting) can lead to cardiac compensation in the presence of pre-existing right ventricular dysfunction or residual myocardial stunning. Continued positive end-expiratory pressure on the ventilated lung or intermittent collapsed lung recruitment may be necessary.

At the conclusion of surgery the DLT should be changed to a single-lumen tube. The use of an airway-exchange catheter may be helpful. Adequate hemostasis should be secured at the SVC cannulation site. Before moving the patient to the intensive care unit, peripheral pulses in the perfused leg should be evaluated. Many patients are excellent candidates for extubation on the operating table, but caution must be exercised because of the remote potential of postoperative chest wall bleeding.

POSTOPERATIVE PAIN MANAGEMENT

The simplest adjunctive pain management involves intercostal injections of a local anesthetic during closure. Longer-duration anesthetic catheters fed by an infusion pump may be left in the subcutaneous tissue or in the extrapleural space before closure.[61–63]

SUMMARY

Robot-assisted mitral valve surgery is rapidly becoming a "gold-standard," and the outcomes are now being use as the benchmark for valve repair quality.[64] Patients are experiencing faster recoveries with reduced pain and yet have a durable surgical repair. More importantly, these results can be achieved with morbidity and mortality equivalent to traditional mitral valve surgery. A recent publication from the Mayo Clinic suggests that, with system engineering, robot-assisted cardiac surgery can be cost-effective.[65]

Today, the majority of robotic cases are performed at a few centers. Advantages of robotic surgery are being shown, and expansion is inevitable. Technological advancements and patient demands will continue to promote this minimally invasive modality. Even in the presence of good results and device evolution, successful outcomes require an investment in training and greater experience for the entire robotic team. A well-organized and synchronous team has become the essence of success in these endeavors.

REFERENCES

1. Suri RM, Antiel RM, Burkhart HM, et al. Quality of life after early mitral valve repair using conventional and robotic approaches. *Ann Thorac Surg.* 2012; 93(3): 761–9.
2. Arom KV, Emery RW. Minimally invasive mitral operations. *Ann Thorac Surg.* 1997; 63(4): 1219–20.
3. Chitwood WR Jr, Wixon CL, Elbeery JR, et al. Video-assisted minimally invasive mitral valve surgery. *J Thorac Cardiovasc Surg.* 1997; 114(5): 773–80; discussion: 780–2.
4. Chitwood WR Jr, Elbeery JR, Moran JF. Minimally invasive mitral valve repair using transthoracic aortic occlusion. *Ann Thorac Surg.* 1997; 63(5): 1477–9.
5. Mohr FW, Falk V, Diegeler A, et al. Minimally invasive port-access mitral valve surgery. *J Thorac Cardiovasc Surg.* 1998; 115(3): 567–74; discussion: 574–6.
6. Navia JL, Cosgrove DM 3rd. Minimally invasive mitral valve operations. *Ann Thorac Surg.* 1996; 62(5): 1542–4.
7. Schwartz DS, Ribakove GH, Grossi EA, et al. Minimally invasive cardiopulmonary bypass with cardioplegic arrest: a closed chest technique with equivalent myocardial protection. *J Thorac Cardiovasc Surg.* 1996; 111(3): 556–66.
8. Glower DD, Siegel LC, Frischmeyer KJ, et al. Predictors of outcome in a multi-center port-access valve registry. *Ann Thorac Surg.* 2000; 70(3): 1054–9.
9. Gammie JS, Zhao Y, Peterson ED, et al. J. Maxwell Chamberlain

Memorial Paper for adult cardiac surgery. Less-invasive mitral valve operations: trends and outcomes from the Society of Thoracic Surgeons Adult Cardiac Surgery Database. *Ann Thorac Surg.* 2010; 90(5): 1401–8, 1410.e1; discussion: 1408–10.

10. Smith JM, Stein H, Engel AM, et al. Totally endoscopic mitral valve repair using a robotic-controlled atrial retractor. *Ann Thorac Surg.* 2007; 84(2): 633–7.

11. Kilic L, Sahin SA, Gullu U, et al. Leyla loop: a time-saving suture technique for robotic atrial closure. *Interact Cardiovasc Thorac Surg.* 2013; 17: 579–80.

12. Carpentier A, Loulmet D, Aupecle B, et al. Computer assisted open heart surgery: first case operated on with success. *C R Acad Sci III.* 1998; 321(5): 437–42 [in French].

13. Chitwood WR Jr, Nifong LW, Elbeery JE, et al. Robotic mitral valve repair: trapezoidal resection and prosthetic annuloplasty with the da Vinci surgical system. *J Thorac Cardiovasc Surg.* 2000; 120(6): 1171–2.

14. Nifong WL, Chitwood WR, Pappas PE, et al. Robotic Mitral Valve Surgery: a United States multicenter trial. *J Thorac Cardiovasc Surg.* 2005; 129(6): 1395–1404.

15. Modi P, Hassan A, Chitwood WR Jr. Minimally invasive mitral valve surgery: a systematic review and meta-analysis. *Eur J Cardiothorac Surg.* 2008; 34(5): 943–52.

16. Yamada T, Ochiai R, Takeda J, et al. Comparison of early postoperative quality of life in minimally invasive versus conventional valve surgery. *J Anesth.* 2003; 17(3): 171–6.

17. Walther T, Falk V, Metz S, et al. Pain and quality of life after minimally invasive versus conventional cardiac surgery. *Ann Thorac Surg.* 1999; 67(6): 1643–7.

18. Vleissis AA, Bolling SF. Mini-reoperative mitral valve surgery. *J Card Surg.* 1998; 13(6): 468–70.

19. Murphy DA, Miller JS, Langford DA. Endoscopic robotic mitral valve surgery. *J Thorac Cardiovasc Surg.* 2006; 132(4): 776–81.

20. Cheng DC, Martin J, Avtar L, et al. Minimally invasive versus conventional open mitral valve surgery: a meta-analysis and systematic review. *Innovations.* 2011; 6(2): 84–103.

21. Suri RM, Schaff HV, Dearani JA, et al. Survival advantage and improved durability of mitral repair for leaflet prolapse subsets in the current era. *Ann Thorac Surg.* 2006; 82(3): 819–26.

22. Galloway AC, Schwartz CF, Ribakove GH, et al. A decade of minimally invasive mitral repair: long-term outcomes. *Ann Thorac Surg.* 2009; 88(4): 1180–4.

23. Iribarne A, Karpenko A, Russo MJ, et al. Eight-year experience with minimally invasive cardiothoracic surgery. *World J Surg.* 2010; 34(4): 611–15.

24. Nifong WL, Rodriguez E, Chitwood WR. 540 consecutive mitral valve repairs including concomitant atrial fibrillation cryoablation. *Ann Thorac Surg.* 2012; 94: 38–43.

25. Charland PJ, Robbins T, Rodriguez E, et al. Learning curve analysis of mitral valve repair using telemanipulative technology. *J Thorac Cardiovasc Surg.* 2011; 142(2): 404–10.

26. Cheng W, Fontana GP, De Robertis MA, et al. Is robotic mitral valve repair a reproducible approach? *J Thorac Cardiovasc Surg.* 2010; 139(3): 628–33.

27. Chitwood WR Jr, Rodriguez E, Chu MW, et al. Robotic mitral valve repairs in 300 patients: a single-center experience. *J Thorac Cardiovasc Surg.* 2008; 136(2): 436–41.

28. Moodley S, Schoenhagen P, Gillinov AM, et al. Preoperative multidetector computed tomography angiography for planning of minimally invasive robotic mitral valve surgery: impact on decision making. *J Thorac Cardiovasc Surg.* 2013; 146(2): 262–8.

29. Eltzschig HK, Rossenberger P, Loffler M, et al. Impact of intraoperative transesophageal echocardiography on surgical decisions in 12 566 patients undergoing cardiac surgery. *Ann Thorac Surg.* 2008; 85(3): 845–52.

30. Minhaj M, Patel K, Muzic D, et al. The effect of routine intraoperative transesophageal echocardiography on surgical management. *J Cardiothorac Vasc Anesth.* 2007; 21(6): 800–4.

31. Freeman WK, Schaff HV, Khandheria BK, et al. Intraoperative evaluation of mitral valve regurgitation and repair by transesophageal echocardiography: incidence and significance of systolic anterior motion. *J Am Coll Cardiol.* 1992; 20(3): 599–609.

32. Wang Y, Gao CQ, Wang JL, et al. The role of intraoperative transesophageal echocardiography in robotic mitral valve repair. *Echocardiography.* 2011; 28(1): 85–91.

33. Jassar AS, Brinster CJ, Vergnat M, et al. Quantitative mitral valve modeling using real-time 3D echocardiography: technique and repeatability. *Ann Thorac Surg.* 2011; 91: 165–71.

34. Toomasian JM, McCarthy JP. Total extrathoracic cardiopulmonary support with kinetic assisted venous drainage: experience in 50 patients. *Perfusion.* 1998; 13(2): 137–43.

35. Chaney MA, Minhaj MM, Patel K, et al. Transoesophageal echocardiography and central line insertion. *Ann Card Anaesth.* 2007; 10(2): 127–31.

36. Mohr FW, Onnasch JF, Falk V, et al. The evolution of minimally invasive valve surgery: 2 year experience. *Eur J Cardiothorac Surg.* 1999; 15(3): 233–8; discussion: 238–9.

37. Grossi EA, Loulmet DF, Schwartz CF, et al. Evolution of operative techniques and perfusion strategies for minimally invasive mitral valve repair. *J Thorac Cardiovasc Surg.* 2012; 143(4 Suppl): S68–70.

38. Reichenspurner H, Detter C, Deuse T, et al. Video and robotic-assisted minimally invasive mitral valve surgery: a comparison of the Port-Access and transthoracic clamp techniques. *Ann Thorac Surg.* 2005; 79(2): 485–90; discussion: 490–1.

39. Galloway AC, Shemin RJ, Glower DD, et al. First report of the Port Access International Registry. *Ann Thorac Surg.* 1999; 67(1): 51–6; discussion: 57–8.

40. Levin R, Leacche M, Petracek MR, et al. Extending the use of the pacing pulmonary artery catheter for safe minimally invasive cardiac surgery. *J Cardiothorac Vasc Anesth.* 2010; 24(4): 568–73.

41. Siegel LC. Coronary sinus catheterization for minimally invasive cardiac surgery. *Anesthesiology.* 1999; 90(4): 1232–3.

42. Plotkin IM, Collard CD, Aranki SF, et al. Percutaneous coronary sinus cannulation guided by transesophageal echocardiography. *Ann Thorac Surg.* 1998; 66(6): 2085–7.

43. Lebon JS, Coutre P, Rochon AG, et al. The endovascular coronary sinus catheter in minimally invasive mitral and tricuspid valve surgery: a case series. *J Cardiothorac Vasc Anesth.* 2010; 24(5): 746–51.

44. Casselman FP, La Meir M, Jeanmart H, et al. Endoscopic mitral and tricuspid valve surgery after previous cardiac surgery. *Circulation.* 2007; 116(11 Suppl): I-270–5.

45. Viana FF, Shi WA, Hayward PA, et al. Custodial versus blood cardioplegia in complex cardiac operations: an Australian experience. *Eur J Cardiothorac Surg.* 2013; 43(3): 526–31.

46. Gazoni LM, Fedoruk LM, Kern JA, et al. A simplified approach to degenerative disease: triangular resections of the mitral valve. *Ann Thorac Surg.* 2007; 83: 1658–64.

47. Chu MWA, Gersch KA, Rodriguez E, et al. Robotic "haircut" mitral valve repair: posterior leaflet-plasty. *Ann Thorac Surg.* 2008; 85: 1460–2.

48. David TE, Armstrong S, Ivanov J. Chordal replacement with polytetrafluoroethylene sutures for mitral valve repair: a 25-year experience. *J Thorac Cardiovasc Surg.* 2013; 145: 1563–9.

49. Mihaljevic T, Pattakos G, Gillinov AM, et al. Robotic posterior mitral leaflet repair: neochordal versus resectional techniques. *Ann Thoracic Surg.* 2013; 95: 787–94.

50. Gregorini R, Chiappini B, De Remigis F, et al. Multiple triangular resection: a reliable technique for correction of multiple prolapse of the mitral valve. *J Cardiovasc Med.* 2009; 10: 804–5.

51. Mihaljevic T, Blackstone EH, Lytle BW. Folding valvuloplasty without leaflet resection: simplified method for mitral valve repair. *Ann Thorac Surg.* 2006; 82: 46–8.

52. Mihaljevic T, Jarrett CM, Gillinov AM, Blackstone EH. A novel running annuloplasty suture technique for robotically assisted mitral valve repair. *J Thorac Cardiovasc Surg.* 2010; 139: 1343–4.

53. Spencer FC, Galloway AC, Grossi EA, et al. Recent developments and evolving techniques of mitral valve reconstruction. *Ann Thoracic Surg.* 1998; 65: 307–13.

54. Sharony R, Grossi EA, Saunders PC, et al. Minimally invasive reoperative isolated valve surgery: early and mid-term results. *J Card Surg.* 2006; 21(3): 240–4.

55. Bolotin G, Kypson AP, Reade CC, et al. Should a video-assisted mini-thoracotomy be the approach of choice for reoperative mitral valve surgery? *J Heart Valve Dis.* 2004; 13(2): 155–8; discussion: 158.

56. Burfeind WR, Glower DD, Davis RD, et al. Mitral surgery after prior cardiac operation: port-access versus sternotomy or thoracotomy. *Ann Thorac Surg.* 2002; 74(4): S1323–5.

57. Arcidi JM Jr, Rodriguez E, Elbeery JR, et al. Fifteen-year experience with minimally invasive approach for reoperations involving the mitral valve. *J Thorac Cardiovasc Surg.* 2012; 143(5): 1062–8.

58. Svensson LG, Gillinov AM, Blackstone EH, et al. Does right thoracotomy increase the risk of mitral valve reoperation? *J Thorac Cardiovasc Surg.* 2007; 134(3): 677–82.

59. Umakanthan R, Petracek MR, Leacche M, et al. Minimally invasive right lateral thoracotomy without aortic cross-clamping: an attractive alternative to repeat sternotomy for reoperative mitral valve surgery. *J Heart Valve Dis.* 2010; 19(2): 236–43.

60. Gullu AU, Senay S, Kocyigit M, et al. A simple method for occlusion of both venae cavae in total cardiopulmonary bypass for robotic surgery. *Interact Cardiovasc Thorac Surg.* 2012; 14(2): 138–9.

61. Sostaric M, Gersak B, Novak-Jankovic V. The analgesic efficacy of local anesthetics for the incisional administration following port access heart surgery: bupivacaine versus ropivacaine. *Heart Surg Forum.* 2010; 13(2): E96–100.

62. Sostaric M. Incisional administration of local anesthetic provides satisfactory analgesia following port access heart surgery. *Heart Surg Forum.* 2005; 8(6): E406–8.

63. Ganapathy S. Anaesthesia for minimally invasive cardiac surgery. *Best Pract Res Clin Anaesthesiol.* 2002; 16(1): 63–80.

64. Suri RM, Burkhart HM, Daly RC, et al. Robotic mitral valve repair for all prolapse subsets using techniques identical to open valvuloplasty: establishing the benchmark against which percutaneous interventions should be judged. *J Thorac Cardiovasc Surg.* 2011; 142(5): 970–9.

65. Suri RM, Thompson JE, Burkhart HM, et al. Improving affordability through innovation in the surgical treatment of mitral valve disease. *Mayo Clin Proc.* 2013; 88(10): 1075–84.

19

Tricuspid valve surgery

TAKEYOSHI OTA AND VALLUVAN JEEVANANDAM

ANATOMY

The tricuspid valve structure consists of three leaflets, the fibrous tricuspid annulus, the subvalvular apparatus including the chordae tendineae and papillary muscles, the right atrium, and the right ventricle (**Figure 19.1**).

The septal leaflet is the smallest and semicircular in shape, and it is attached directly to the fibrous trigone of the heart above the interventricular septum. This attachment means that the septal leaflet is relatively spared from annular dilatation and it is therefore used as a benchmark for tricuspid annular sizing. The anterior leaflet is roughly quadrangular in shape and is the largest. The posterior is nearly triangular, is slightly smaller than the anterior leaflet, and is positioned rightward and lateral when the valve is viewed from the atrium.

While there are many variations, the papillary muscles are divided into three groups: anterior, posterior, and septal. The anterior papillary muscle(s) provide chordae to the anterior and posterior leaflets, and the posterior papillary muscle(s) provide to the posterior and septal leaflets. The septal papillary muscles or septal wall provide chordae to the anterior and septal leaflets. There are often accessory chordae attached to the right ventricular free wall and/or the moderator band.

The tricuspid valve annulus is not a planar configuration but a complex three-dimensional (3D) structure composed of intermixed fibroelastic fibers in continuity with the leaflets, the atrium, and the ventricle (**Figure 19.2**). The lowest portion of the annulus is the anteroseptal commissure, and the highest portion is around the middle of the annulus of the anterior leaflet which corresponds to the right ventricular outflow tract. During the cardiac cycle, the annular circumference and the annular area vary, with reductions of up to 20% and 30% respectively.[1–3]

Of particular surgical significance are two important anatomical structures close to the tricuspid valve annulus: the atrioventricular (AV) node and conduction bundle, and the aortic valve and sinuses. The AV node lies at

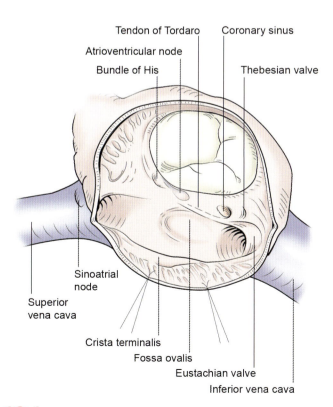

Tendon of Tordaro
Atrioventricular node
Bundle of His
Coronary sinus
Thebesian valve
Superior vena cava
Sinoatrial node
Crista terminalis
Fossa ovalis
Eustachian valve
Inferior vena cava

19.1

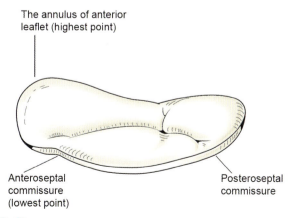

The annulus of anterior leaflet (highest point)
Anteroseptal commissure (lowest point)
Posteroseptal commissure

19.2

the apex of the triangle of Koch, which is bordered by the tendon of Todaro, the septal leaflet, and the coronary sinus. The AV conduction bundle (bundle of His) extends from the AV node toward the central fibrous body and the ventricles beneath the membranous septum (see **Figure 19.1**). These can be injured if sutures are placed in this area during valve annuloplasty or replacement or membranous ventricular septal defect closure, and this can result in rhythm disturbances. The aortic valve and sinuses (i.e. non-coronary sinus of Valsalva, non-coronary and right coronary leaflet and its commissure) are located in the vicinity of the portion of the annulus of the anterior leaflet. Care needs to be taken not to injure these structures during annuloplasty.

ETIOLOGY

Tricuspid regurgitation

As with the mitral valve, the Carpentier functional classification is frequently used to classify tricuspid regurgitation (**Figure 19.3**). It is classified in terms of leaflet motion:

- *Type I* – tricuspid regurgitation with normal leaflet motion
- *Type II* – tricuspid regurgitation with excess leaflet motion/prolapse
- *Type IIIa* – tricuspid regurgitation with restricted leaflet motion in diastole
- *Type IIIb* – tricuspid regurgitation with restricted leaflet motion in systole.

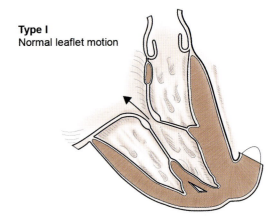

Type I
Normal leaflet motion

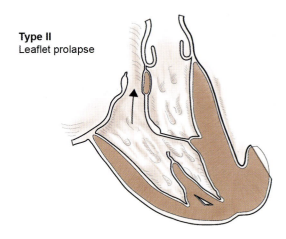

Type II
Leaflet prolapse

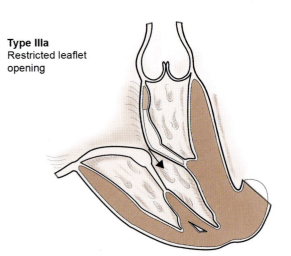

Type IIIa
Restricted leaflet opening

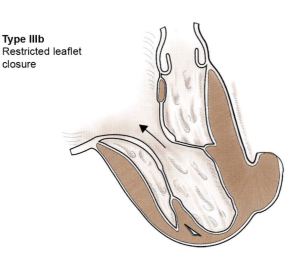

Type IIIb
Restricted leaflet closure

19.3

Functional tricuspid regurgitation is the most frequent cause of tricuspid valve dysfunction. The main pathology of functional tricuspid regurgitation is annular dilatation (Type I). Because the septal leaflet is directly attached to the fibrous trigone and therefore spared from annular dilatation, dilatation of the tricuspid annulus occurs only in the annulus of the anterior and posterior leaflet (Figure 19.4). The causes of functional tricuspid regurgitation include right ventricular dysfunction, pulmonary artery hypertension resulting from any cause, and left-sided valvular lesions. In addition, many other "reversible" factors contribute to the degree of functional tricuspid regurgitation including cardiac output, ventricular contractility, blood volume, and systemic afterload. This often makes it difficult to assess the indication of surgical interventions of the tricuspid valve.

Organic tricuspid regurgitation is caused by primary involvement of the tricuspid valve from a variety of conditions. Rheumatic tricuspid valve disease almost always accompanies mitral valve dysfunction and usually results in tricuspid regurgitation, which is typically Type IIIa, as well as stenosis. Marfan syndrome and other myxomatous diseases that could involve the tricuspid valve can also result in leaflet prolapse, elongated chordae, or chordal rupture, leading to tricuspid regurgitation. The endocardial right ventricular lead of a pacemaker/defibrillator can also cause tricuspid regurgitation by distorting the leaflets and interfering with leaflet coaptation. While it is recommended to avoid lead removal at the time of surgery in the setting of attempting to repair the tricuspid valve because of the risk of injury of the leaflet and sub-apparatus,[4] the surgeon needs to consider the high recurrence rate in 42% of patients who underwent successful tricuspid repair with the indwelling endocardial ventricular lead in place at 5 years from the initial surgery.[5] Organic tricuspid regurgitation can also be caused by blunt

chest trauma, carcinoid heart disease, chest irradiation, and certain drugs such as fenfluramine-phentermine.[6–9]

Tricuspid stenosis

The predominant cause of tricuspid stenosis is rheumatic disease. It is therefore commonly accompanied by mitral valve dysfunction, and much less frequently, by aortic valve lesion. The anatomical features include fused and shortened chordae, leaflet thickening, and, more rarely, calcification, leading to restricted leaflet motion. The diastolic mean gradient across the valve reaches more than 5 mmHg in severe tricuspid stenosis. Carcinoid heart disease and infectious endocarditis can also cause tricuspid stenosis.

Tricuspid valve endocarditis

Tricuspid valve endocarditis can result in tricuspid regurgitation and/or stenosis, and it is not uncommon and frequently associated with intravenous drug use. The tricuspid valve is involved in roughly 50% of patients, with endocarditis related to intravenous drug use, while the majority of patients with non-drug-related endocarditis have left-sided lesion(s).[10] The organism most commonly responsible is *Staphylococcus aureus*, followed by *Streptococcus viridians*.[11]

INDICATIONS FOR SURGERY

The appropriate timing of surgical interventions for tricuspid valve dysfunction is still not well established. In patients with tricuspid regurgitation, unless the tricuspid valve has intrinsic valve disease with severe regurgitation, medical therapy should be maximized before considering surgical interventions since many of the factors affecting tricuspid valve regurgitation are reversible. Surgical interventions should be considered in severe or moderate-to-severe tricuspid regurgitation refractory to maximum medical therapy. Surgical indications depend on whether surgery for other valve disease (i.e. mitral and/or aortic valve) is indicated because it is reasonable to assume that tricuspid regurgitation would decrease after correction of left-sided valve(s). In the setting of left-sided valve surgery, both the American College of Cardiology (ACC)/American Heart Association (AHA) guideline and the European Society of Cardiology (ESC) and the European Association for Cardio-Thoracic Surgery (EACTS) guideline recommend tricuspid valve surgery for severe tricuspid regurgitation (Class I, Level B).[12, 13] The ACC/AHA guideline also recommends concomitant tricuspid annuloplasty for mild/moderate tricuspid regurgitation with pulmonary hypertension and/or tricuspid annular dilatation in left-sided valve surgery (Class IIb, Level C). The size of the annular diameter is more than 40 mm in four-chamber view in transthoracic echocardiography, which roughly corresponds to the length from the

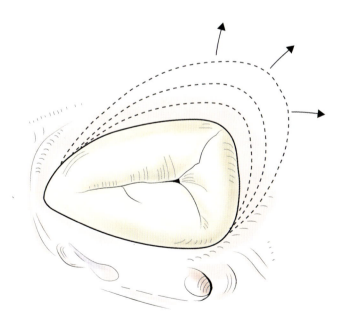

19.4

middle of the septal leaflet annulus to the anteroposterior commissure, or more than 70 mm in two-chamber view, which is from the middle of the anterior leaflet annulus to the posteroseptal commissure. Regarding primary tricuspid regurgitation, both guidelines noted that it is reasonable to perform tricuspid surgery in symptomatic patients with severe tricuspid regurgitation (Class IIa, Level C). Neither guideline supports tricuspid surgery for those who have no symptoms with less than 60 mmHg of pulmonary artery systolic pressure or for those who have mild tricuspid regurgitation (Class III, Level C). Of note, however, it is reported that moderate/severe tricuspid regurgitation is associated with increased mortality regardless of the presence of related symptoms.[14] In addition, significant tricuspid valve regurgitation contributes to a poor postoperative outcome even after successful mitral valve surgery and requires subsequent reoperation for tricuspid valve surgery.[15] It is critical to follow up closely and perform surgery in a timely manner before development of irreversible right ventricular failure and/or end-organ damage.

Tricuspid valve stenosis is usually due to rheumatic heart disease and most commonly involves mitral stenosis as well. Surgical intervention is indicated for symptomatic severe stenosis. Treatment is valve replacement.

The surgical indications in patients with tricuspid valve endocarditis and active intravenous drug users are generally the same as for others with endocarditis.[16] However, there are difficult ethical and practical problems when patients who are actively abusing injection drugs develop recurrent endocarditis and require surgery. Knowing there are many exceptions in the clinical practice, surgical intervention is not generally advisable in active intravenous drug users unless the patient agrees to enrol on a drug rehab program. Consultation with an ethics committee service is helpful in such a situation where the surgeon makes a decision not to offer surgery for non-compliant patients with recurrent endocarditis.

SURGICAL EXPOSURE AND CARDIOPULMONARY BYPASS TECHNIQUES

The surgical approach and exposure for tricuspid surgery is dependent upon the concomitant procedure and the preference of both patient and surgeon.

For patients undergoing concomitant coronary artery bypass grafting (CABG) and/or aortic valve surgery, median sternotomy, which allows full access to all cardiac structures, is usually the approach of choice. Minimally invasive approaches such as partial lower sternotomy and right thoracotomy are also possible surgical approaches, according to the preferences of the patient and surgeon and mainly in isolated tricuspid valve surgery or when combined with mitral valve procedures.[17] A minimally invasive right thoracotomy has the advantage of avoiding adhesions and preventing possible right ventricular injury during re-sternotomy in the setting of reoperations.

Median sternotomy

The traditional exposure of the tricuspid valve through median sternotomy includes central arterial aortic cannulation, bicaval venous cannulation with caval snares that are essential to isolate the right atrium. The left-sided valve repair or replacement is performed under cardiac arrest with antegrade and/or retrograde cardioplegia and moderate systemic hypothermia. The mitral valve can be exposed through an interatrial groove approach or through a transseptal approach. Similarly, the aortic valve can be exposed via a transverse aortotomy. After completing the left-sided valve procedures and/or CABG, the aortic clamp is released. The tricuspid valve can be exposed through an oblique right atriotomy from the atrial appendage toward the IVC cannula passing through approximately 2–3 cm posterior to the AV groove. Tricuspid surgery can be done while rewarming the heart and waiting for the return of cardiac rhythm. By performing tricuspid surgery on a beating heart, misplacement of a suture adversely affecting the conduction system can immediately be detected. It is also an option to perform tricuspid valve surgery while keeping the aortic cross-clamp in place. It gives better surgical exposure and adds only a little extra cross-clamp time. It would be the surgeon's preference/decision whether tricuspid valve procedure is performed on the beating heart or with cardioplegic arrest based on the patient's medical status and the complexity of procedures.

Right thoracotomy

The minimally invasive right anterior/lateral thoracotomy approach is widely used for mitral and tricuspid valve surgery, with direct vision, video-assisted, or robot-assisted surgery.[17, 18] Cannulation is usually through the femoral vessels, for both arterial and venous access. The venous cannulation should be with two separate cannulae, one from the groin to the inferior vena cava (IVC), and the second via the jugular vein or through the lateral thoracotomy directly to the superior vena cava (SVC). Isolation of the right atrium can be established by means of conventional snaring through the thoracotomy. Aortic cross-clamping is facilitated by using a single shaft instrument such as the Chitwood aortic clamp.

TRICUSPID ANNULOPLASTY

De Vega technique

De Vega annuloplasty can be used for mild to moderate tricuspid valve, especially when performed concomitantly with other cardiac procedures.[19, 20] It is a simple and cost-effective procedure and should be performed where it is anticipated that good long-term function does not depend on the integrity of the repair.

A double-armed 2-0 or 3-0 polyester suture with Teflon

felt pledget is used. The pursestring bites are placed at the junction of the annulus and right ventricular free wall (1–2 mm from the hinge of the leaflets), running around the anterior and posterior leaflets from the posteroseptal commissure to the anteroseptal commissure, avoiding the septal leaflet annulus (**Figure 19.5**). The second limb of the suture is placed through the pledget and runs parallel and 1–3 mm above the first suture line in the same counterclockwise direction in an alternative sequence (**Figure 19.6**). The suture depth should be 2–3 mm and 10–12 bites are typically needed for each limb. Both needles are then passed through a second pledget at the anteroseptal commissure for a buttress. The suture is tightened, producing a pursestring effect and reducing the length of the anterior and posterior annulus. The annular size should be reduced to the point at which two or three fingerbreadths fit snugly through the orifice. An annuloplasty sizer, Hegar sizer, or equivalent can be used as an alternative (**Figure 19.7**). Often a sufficient repair can be done applying the aforementioned stitch only in the lateral

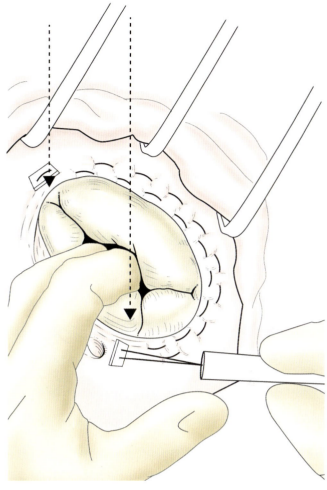

19.6

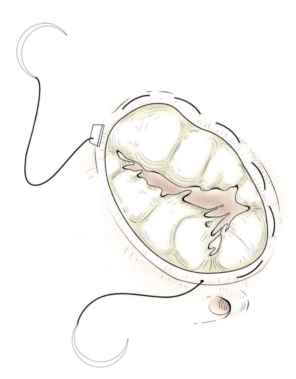

19.5

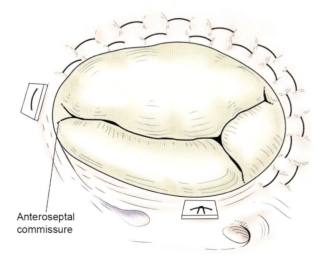

Anteroseptal commissure

19.7

half of the anterior leaflet and the base of the posterior leaflet (**Figure 19.8**). An autologous pericardium strip or a Teflon felt can also be utilized for reinforcement (**Figure 19.9**).

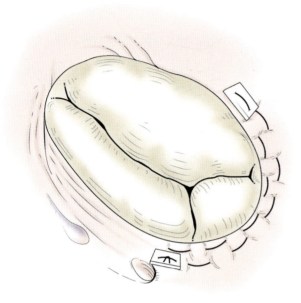

19.8

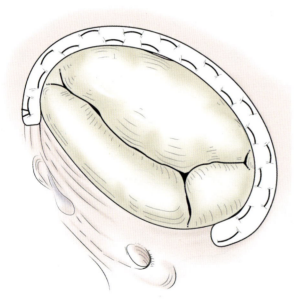

19.9

Ring and band annuloplasty

Ring or band annuloplasties are usually preferred for moderate or severe tricuspid regurgitation, especially if this is the main part of the operation. A ring or band allows significant degrees of annular reduction with long-term durability. Several devices are available including rigid rings (e.g. Edwards MC3 Tricuspid [Edwards Lifesciences, Irvine, CA], Medtronic Contour 3D [Medtronic, Minneapolis, MN), flexible rings (e.g. Medtronic Duran Ancore), flexible bands (e.g. Cosgrove–Edwards annuloplasty system [Edwards Lifesciences, Irvine, CA]), or semi-rigid rings (e.g. Medtronic Tri-Ad). These devices are designed to avoid suture placement in the region of the AV node to preserve the conduction system. The size of the ring or band is determined according to the length of the base of the septal leaflet or the surface area of the leaflet tissue attached to the chorea arising from the anterior papillary muscle, typically corresponding to a large portion of the anterior leaflet and a small portion of the posterior leaflet.

A series of horizontal mattress sutures is placed circumferentially using 3-0 Ticron sutures, with wider bites on the annulus and smaller corresponding bites through the ring or band, thus producing annular plication (**Figure 19.10**). Gentle tension by grasping the leaflet tissue transversely should be applied to identify the hinge. The depth of the bites should be substantial to avoid tearing. At the same time, care needs to be taken not to injure important surrounding structures (i.e. the aortic root, right coronary artery, AV conduction system). In order to avoid those injuries, it is helpful

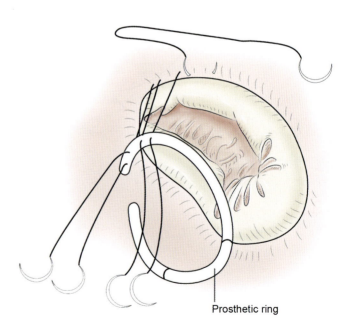

Prosthetic ring

19.10

to place sutures with the tip of needle oriented toward the direction to the right ventricular side. Then, the ring/band is lowered in place and the sutures tied (**Figure 19.11**). The reduction in the annular size is mainly along the annulus of the posterior leaflet. At the end of the procedure the tricuspid valve orifice is primarily occluded by the leaflet tissue of the anterior and septal leaflets.

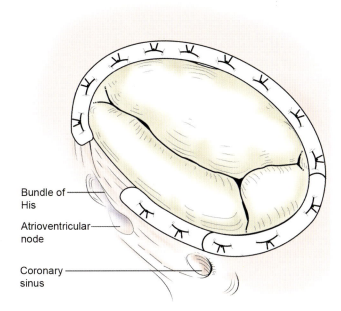

19.11

Bicuspidization

A third and less used option is bicuspidization of the tricuspid valve. By plicating the annulus over the posterior tricuspid valve leaflet, this leaflet is excluded, thus converting the tricuspid valve into a bicuspid valve. Technically, a 2-0 monofilament polypropylene suture with pledget is passed through the annulus at the anteroposterior commissure, through the annulus at the center of the posterior leaflet, and then through the annulus at the posteroseptal commissure (**Figure 19.12**). It is often necessary to place a second suture to reduce the annulus and reinforce it. It is also an option to simply place some figure-eight stitches to exclude the entire posterior annulus (Kay technique).[21] The repair is not at the area of the AV node, but care needs to be taken not to place sutures away from the coronary sinus. At the end of the repair the tricuspid valve should reach normal diameter.

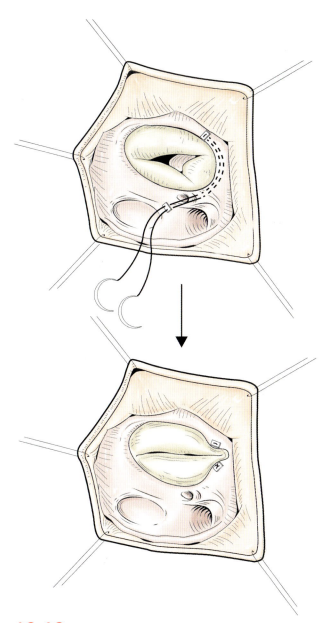

19.12

TRICUSPID VALVE REPLACEMENT

As a general and important principle, tricuspid valve repair is preferable to tricuspid valve replacement as long as valve repair is technically feasible, and surgery should be carried out early enough to avoid irreversible right ventricular dysfunction or end-organ failure (e.g. congestive liver cirrhosis). Surgical mortality for tricuspid valve replacement is significantly higher than for tricuspid valve repair.[22] Nevertheless, tricuspid valve replacement becomes mandatory when the native valve is too deformed and not suitable for repair. The prosthesis size is selected based on the diameter of the annulus. Whenever possible, the subvalvular apparatus should be preserved to maintain the postoperative right ventricular function, and the leaflet tissues should be incorporated in suturing to anchor the prosthetic valve. If there is a concern that the anterior leaflet tissue may obstruct the right ventricular outflow, the leaflet can be excised and only chordal attachments can be preserved. In cases where the tricuspid valve leaflets and/or subvalvular apparatus need to be resected due to a condition such as endocarditis, it is critical to leave a 2–3 mm fringe of leaflet tissue so that one can avoid injury to the conduction system by placing the sutures directly onto the fringe. The right ventricle of patients with chronic tricuspid valve disease is usually so dilated that it can easily accommodate the struts of a bioprosthetic valve. If not (e.g. in patients with acute valve failure due to endocarditis), the surgeon may need to consider using a mechanical valve. Care needs to be taken that the leaflet motion of the mechanical valve is not compromised by the preserved subvalvular apparatus when the mechanical valve is seated in the annulus.

Interrupted 2-0 polyester sutures with Teflon felt pledget are placed through the annulus with the exception of the area of the septal leaflet where sutures should be passed through the leaflet tissue to avoid damage to the conduction system. The sutures are then passed through the sewing ring of the prosthetic valve (**Figure 19.13**). The prosthetic valve is lowered onto the annulus and the sutures are tied. Care needs to be taken not to injure the interventricular septum with the struts if a bioprosthetic valve is chosen. It is also an option to place pledgeted mattress sutures only in the septal leaflet area, followed by continuous running sutures along the anterior and posterior annulus (**Figure 19.14**). As a less frequently utilized technique, the suture line can go around

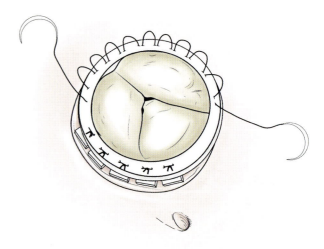

19.14

the atrial aspect of the coronary sinus to avoid the conduction system. The surgeon should consider placing permanent epicardial ventricular pacing leads at the time of tricuspid valve replacement because there is a persistent risk of late heart block, especially when concomitantly performed with mitral valve replacement.[23] The epicardial leads can be buried in a pocket in the left upper quadrant abdominal wall for later permanent pacemaker implant if indicated.

The choice of prosthetic valves in the tricuspid position is based on the same algorithm as in other valves. The considerations include, but are not limited to, age, anticoagulation, psychiatric issues, and social issues. Generally, mechanical prosthesis is recommended for younger patients unless there is a contraindication to anticoagulation.[24] It is interesting to note that it is generally accepted that patients with a bioprosthetic valve in the tricuspid position require no anticoagulation. However, 97% of living patients with tricuspid bioprostheses are on anticoagulant medication.[25] In terms of survival benefit from the choice of prosthetic valves, while it is reported that a bioprosthetic valve offers superior long-term survival over a mechanical valve,[26] the majority of studies which compare outcomes between bioprosthetic and mechanical valves in the tricuspid position showed no significant difference in survival.[25, 27–31] The durability of bioprosthetic valves in the tricuspid position is reasonable in the long-term follow-up. However, non-structural dysfunction due to pannus formation occurs frequently in bioprosthetic valves.[32] There is a greater chance of reoperation in bioprosthetic valves compared to mechanical valves.[30] It should also be noted that implantation of a mechanical valve will obviate any opportunity to place a transvenous right ventricular electrode if needed in the future. In addition, the use of mechanical valves in the tricuspid position could cause high occurrence of thromboemolic events even with adequately controlled anticoagulation. The choice of tricuspid prosthesis

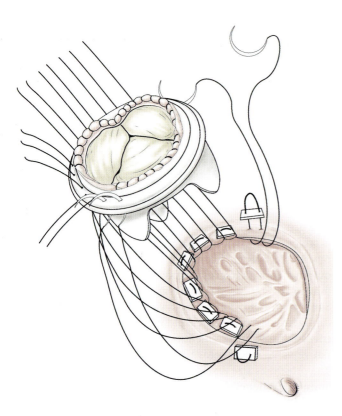

19.13

should be made on a case-by-case basis according to the surgeon's clinical judgment, and the age, heart disease, etiology, comorbidities, and background of the patient.

OTHER SURGICAL TECHNIQUES

Tricuspid resection

In the past surgical resection of the tricuspid valve was an acceptable treatment for tricuspid endocarditis, especially if there was the potential for continued intravenous drug abuse.[33, 34] Most patients tolerate the absence of the tricuspid valve well, at least for a while. However, 30% decompensate, especially with any increase in pulmonary vascular resistance or pulmonary valve insufficiency and develop subsequent right heart failure.[33, 35] Today, tricuspid vegetectomy, repair, or replacement are the surgical treatments of choice for tricuspid valve disease.[36]

Inflow occlusion technique

The inflow occlusion technique may be used for removal of vegetations/thrombus on the tricuspid valve and/or pacing leads. Tricuspid valve endocarditis is often treated surgically by preserving the tricuspid valve while removing infected material. Surgical intervention in the setting of sepsis carries a great risk of worsening pulmonary function with exposure to cardiopulmonary bypass. In addition, cardiopulmonary bypass causes an inflammatory response with activation of complement and a host of cytokines that can amplify a septic state.[37–39] For these reasons, the "off-pump" route employing vena caval inflow occlusion is suggested.

The chest is opened through a median sternotomy. The superior and inferior venae cavae are dissected free and slings are placed around them. The body of the right atrium is brought into view and four stay sutures are placed. Ten thousand units of heparin are administered systemically. The venae cavae are then snared and the body of the right atrium opened vertically between the stay sutures. The tricuspid valve is visualized and the vegetation excised. The right atrial cavity is washed out with antibiotic solution.

At the end of the "safe" 2-minute period a partial occluding clamp with a long, flat jaw is applied to the right atrium incorporating the edges and the stay sutures and the caval clamps are then released. If needed, a second opening of the atrium for 2 minutes can be applied. The edges of the atrial incision are approximated within the clamp with 4-0 monofilament polypropylene sutures. The pericardium is then closed.

This procedure removes the septic focus while preserving the valve and avoids the drawbacks of cardiopulmonary bypass. However, the technique is not useful if there is significant destruction of the tricuspid valve, a significant patent foramen ovale, or significant involvement of left-sided heart valves.[40, 41]

SURGICAL OUTCOME OF TRICUSPID VALVE SURGERY

Tricuspid valve annuloplasty

Since tricuspid valve annuloplasty is mostly performed concomitant with left-sided valve surgery, its isolated effect on survival is not simple to assess. The durability of De Vega annuloplasty has been reported acceptable when employed for mild to moderate tricuspid regurgitation. The long-term freedom from reoperation of the De Vega technique has been reported to be in the range of 75.7–91.6% with adequate long-term survival.[42–44] Chang and colleagues showed that recurrence-free survival was better with pericardial strip annuloplasty (86.8%) than with the De Vega technique (71.9%).[45] When comparing suture-based techniques (i.e. De Vega technique, bicupidization) and ring/band annuloplasty, there are a significant number of reports that support the superiority of ring annuloplasty over the suture-based techniques. McCarthy and colleagues reported a comparison between ring/band annuloplasty (Carpentier–Edwards ring, Cosgrove band) and suture-based techniques (De Vega technique, Peri-Guard annuloplasty) in long-term durability. Residual tricuspid regurgitation occurred in 14% of patients early after operation for all types of annuloplasty. While the severity of regurgitation was stable or slowly increased in the ring/band annuloplasty across time, it got worse more rapidly in the suture-based techniques, with statistically significant difference. Risk factors for worsening regurgitation included higher preoperative regurgitation grade, poor left ventricular function, permanent pacemaker, and repair type other than ring annuloplasty.[5] Generally, multiple factors such as right and left ventricular function, pulmonary hypertension, and end-organ dysfunctions are associated with long-term survival, and therefore it is difficult to link a history of tricuspid valve or the presence of tricuspid dysfunction and late mortality. However, some studies demonstrated the superiority of ring/band annuloplasty in long-term survival compared to De Vega annuloplasty.[46–48]

Tricuspid repair during heart transplant

Tricuspid regurgitation was reported often after orthotopic heart transplantation and the incidence varies from 36% to 98%.[49–53] The cause of tricuspid regurgitation is multifactorial and includes allograft dysfunction with right ventricular dilatation, pulmonary hypertension, severe donor–recipient size mismatch, and alteration in the geometry of the tricuspid valve and right atrium related to the technique of right atrial anastomosis.[54, 55] In several studies, moderate and greater levels of tricuspid regurgitation have been found to be associated with right-sided heart failure symptoms, renal and hepatic dysfunction, and decreased long-term survival.[53, 56] In a recent prospective randomized study a preventive tricuspid valve annuloplasty of the donor heart before bicaval orthotopic heart transplantation was found to improve immediate donor heart function as demonstrated by better right ventricular performance, lower perioperative mortality, and shorter reperfusion times. At 1 and 6 years after heart transplantation, there was less tricuspid valve regurgitation and less incidence of cardiac mortality in the patients with tricuspid annuloplasty.[57, 58] Prophylactic De Vega annuloplasty, which is a quick and cost-effective procedure, should be performed as a routine adjunct with bicaval orthotopic heart transplantation.

Tricuspid repair during left ventricular assist device implant

Patients with end-stage heart failure requiring a left ventricular assist device (LVAD) usually have dilated ventricles and frequently have significant secondary functional tricuspid regurgitation.[59] With LVAD support, global right ventricular function could be impaired due to a left-shifted septal wall. However, right ventricular myocardial efficiency is maintained by decreased afterload with a reduction in the secondarily elevated pulmonary artery pressures. Because of this mechanism, tricuspid regurgitation can be postoperatively reduced/resolved without surgical intervention to the tricuspid valve. On the other hand, it is also true that the improved cardiac output with LVAD support increases the venous return, augmenting right ventricular preload, and worsens tricuspid regurgitation. Right ventricular failure after the LVAD implantation remains a critical issue, and it has been reported that post-LVAD right ventricular failure occurred in 20–30%.[60, 61] Several investigators reported that tricuspid valve surgery concomitant with LVAD surgery did not increase surgical mortality,[62] reduced postoperative right ventricular failure,[63] and improved clinical outcomes.[64] Theoretically, the concomitant tricuspid procedure should benefit LVAD patients by improving survival, although no study has been reported to prove the long-term survival benefit.

Tricuspid valve replacement

Tricuspid valve replacement is an uncommon surgery since most tricuspid valve regurgitation is repairable with annuloplasty techniques and the incidence of tricuspid stenosis, which is likely to require valve replacement, is very low. Tricuspid valve replacement is traditionally associated with high mortality and morbidity, and today this problem has not been resolved despite recent medical advances in peri- and intraoperative care. A meta-analysis of 11 series of studies showed an early mortality of 19.2%.[24] The long-term survival at 10 years after surgery varies from 38% to 65%.[27, 28, 65] Chang and colleagues, however, reported respectable results that the long-term survival at 15 years after surgery was 73.8%, the incidence of valve thrombus was 1.28%/patient-year, and anticoagulation-related bleeding was 0.37%/patient-year. They did not mention the reason

for their better outcome, but their policy is to perform early surgical intervention for severe tricuspid regurgitation to prevent progressive right heart failure.[30]

REFERENCES

1. Tei C, Pilgrim JP, Shah PM, et al. The tricuspid valve annulus: study of size and motion in normal subjects and in patients with tricuspid regurgitation. *Circulation.* 1982; 66(3): 665–71.

2. Jouan J, Pagel MR, Hiro ME, et al. Further information from a sonometric study of the normal tricuspid valve annulus in sheep: geometric changes during the cardiac cycle. *J Heart Valve Dis.* 2007; 16(5): 511–18.

3. Fukuda S, Saracino G, Matsumura Y, et al. Three-dimensional geometry of the tricuspid annulus in healthy subjects and in patients with functional tricuspid regurgitation: a real-time, 3-dimensional echocardiographic study. *Circulation.* 2006; 114(1 Suppl): I492–8.

4. Love CJ, Wilkoff BL, Byrd CL, et al. Recommendations for extraction of chronically implanted transvenous pacing and defibrillator leads: indications, facilities, training. North American Society of Pacing and Electrophysiology Lead Extraction Conference Faculty. *Pacing Clin Electrophysiol.* 2000; 23(4 Pt 1): 544–51.

5. McCarthy PM, Bhudia SK, Rajeswaran J, et al. Tricuspid valve repair: durability and risk factors for failure. *J Thorac Cardiovasc Surg.* 2004; 127(3): 674–85.

6. Dounis G, Matsakas E, Poularas J, et al. Traumatic tricuspid insufficiency: a case report with a review of the literature. *Eur J Emerg Med.* 2002; 9(3): 258–61.

7. Palaniswamy C, Frishman WH, Aronow WS. Carcinoid heart disease. *Cardiol Rev.* 2012; 20(4): 167–76.

8. Knight CJ, Sutton GC. Complete heart block and severe tricuspid regurgitation after radiotherapy: case report and review of the literature. *Chest.* 1995; 108(6): 1748–51.

9. Connolly HM, Crary JL, McGoon MD, et al. Valvular heart disease associated with fenfluramine-phentermine. *N Engl J Med.* 1997; 337(9): 581–8.

10. Mathew J, Addai T, Anand A, et al. Clinical features, site of involvement, bacteriologic findings, and outcome of infective endocarditis in intravenous drug users. *Arch Intern Med.* 1995; 155(15): 1641–8.

11. Ota T, Gleason TG, Salizzoni S, et al. Midterm surgical outcomes of noncomplicated active native multivalve endocarditis: single-center experience. *Ann Thorac Surg.* 2011; 91(5): 1414–19.

12. Vahanian A, Alfieri O, Andreotti F, et al. Guidelines on the management of valvular heart disease (version 2012): the Joint Task Force on the Management of Valvular Heart Disease of the European Society of Cardiology (ESC) and the European Association for Cardio-Thoracic Surgery (EACTS). *Eur J Cardiothorac Surg.* 2012; 42(4): S1–44.

13. Bonow RO, Carabello BA, Chatterjee K, et al. 2008 Focused update incorporated into the ACC/AHA 2006 guidelines for the management of patients with valvular heart disease: a report of the American College of Cardiology/American

Heart Association Task Force on Practice Guidelines (Writing Committee to Revise the 1998 Guidelines for the Management of Patients With Valvular Heart Disease): endorsed by the Society of Cardiovascular Anesthesiologists, Society for Cardiovascular Angiography and Interventions, and Society of Thoracic Surgeons. *Circulation.* 2008; 118(15): e523–661.

14. Nath J, Foster E, Heidenreich PA. Impact of tricuspid regurgitation on long-term survival. *J Am Coll Cardiol.* 2004; 43(3): 405–9.

15. King RM, Schaff HV, Danielson GK, et al. Surgery for tricuspid regurgitation late after mitral valve replacement. *Circulation.* 1984; 70(3 Pt 2): I193–7.

16. Byrne JG, Rezai K, Sanchez JA, et al. Surgical management of endocarditis: the Society of Thoracic Surgeons clinical practice guideline. *Ann Thorac Surg.* 2011; 91(6): 2012–19.

17. Schmitto JD, Mokashi SA, Cohn LH. Minimally invasive valve surgery. *J Am Coll Cardiol.* 2010; 56(6): 455–62.

18. Modi P, Rodriguez E, Chitwood WR Jr. Robot-assisted cardiac surgery. *Interact Cardiovasc Thorac Surg.* 2009; 9(3): 500–5.

19. De Vega NG. Selective, adjustable and permanent annuloplasty. An original technic [sic] for the treatment of tricuspid insufficiency. *Rev Esp Cardiol.* 1972; 25(6): 555–6. [Article in Spanish]

20. Cohn LH. Tricuspid regurgitation secondary to mitral valve disease: when and how to repair. *J Card Surg.* 1994; 9(2 Suppl): 237–41.

21. Kay JH, Maselli-Campagna G, Tsuji KK. Surgical treatment of tricuspid insufficiency. *Ann Surg.* 1965; 162: 53–8.

22. Vassileva CM, Shabosky J, Boley T, et al. Tricuspid valve surgery: the past 10 years from the Nationwide Inpatient Sample (NIS) database. *J Thorac Cardiovasc Surg.* 2012; 143(5): 1043–9.

23. Barratt-Boyes BG, Rutherford JD, Whitlock RM, Pemberton JR. A review of surgery for acquired tricuspid valve disease, including an assessment of the stented semilunar homograft valve, and the results of operation for multivalvular heart disease. *Aust N Z J Surg.* 1988; 58(1): 23–34.

24. Carrier M, Hébert Y, Pellerin M, et al. Tricuspid valve replacement: an analysis of 25 years of experience at a single center. *Ann Thorac Surg.* 2003; 75(1): 47–50.

25. Rizzoli G, Vendramin I, Nesseris G, et al. Biological or mechanical prostheses in tricuspid position? A meta-analysis of intra-institutional results. *Ann Thorac Surg.* 2004; 77(5): 1607–14.

26. Brown ML, Dearani JA, Danielson GK, et al. Comparison of the outcome of porcine bioprosthetic versus mechanical prosthetic replacement of the tricuspid valve in the Ebstein anomaly. *Am J Cardiol.* 2009; 103(4): 555–61.

27. Kaplan M, Kut MS, Demirtas MM, et al. Prosthetic replacement of tricuspid valve: bioprosthetic or mechanical. *Ann Thorac Surg.* 2002; 73(2): 467–73.

28. Filsoufi F, Anyanwu AC, Salzberg SP, et al. Long-term outcomes of tricuspid valve replacement in the current era. *Ann Thorac Surg.* 2005; 80(3): 845–50.

29. Garatti A, Nano G, Bruschi G, et al. Twenty-five year outcomes of tricuspid valve replacement comparing mechanical and biologic prostheses. *Ann Thorac Surg.* 2012; 93(4): 1146–53.

30. Chang BC, Lim SH, Yi G, et al. Long-term clinical results of tricuspid valve replacement. *Ann Thorac Surg.* 2006; 81(4): 1317–24.

31. Solomon NA, Lim RC, Nand P, Graham KJ. Tricuspid valve replacement: bioprosthetic or mechanical valve? *Asian Cardiovasc Thorac Ann.* 2004; 12(2): 143–8.

32. Nakano K, Ishibashi-Ueda H, Kobayashi J, et al. Tricuspid valve replacement with bioprostheses: long-term results and causes of valve dysfunction. *Ann Thorac Surg.* 2001; 71(1): 105–9.

33. Wright JS, Glennie JS. Excision of tricuspid valve with later replacement in endocarditis of drug addiction. *Thorax.* 1978; 33(4): 518–19.

34. Arneborn P, Björk VO, Rodriguez L, Svanbom M. Two-stage replacement of tricuspid valve in active endocarditis. *Br Heart J.* 1977; 39(11): 1276–8.

35. Stern HJ, Sisto DA, Strom JA, et al. Immediate tricuspid valve replacement for endocarditis. Indications and results. *J Thorac Cardiovasc Surg.* 1986; 91(2): 163–7.

36. Lange R, De Simone R, Bauernschmitt R, et al. Tricuspid valve reconstruction, a treatment option in acute endocarditis. *Eur J Cardiothorac Surg.* 1996; 10(5): 320–6.

37. Kirklin JK, Westaby S, Blackstone EH, et al. Complement and the damaging effects of cardiopulmonary bypass. *J Thorac Cardiovasc Surg* 1983; 86: 845–57.

38. Asimakopoulos G. Systemic inflammation and cardiac surgery: an update. *Perfusion.* 2001; 16: 353–60.

39. Wan S, LeClerc JL, Vincent JL. Inflammatory response to cardiopulmonary bypass: mechanisms involved and possible therapeutic strategies. *Chest.* 1997; 112: 676–92.

40. Raman J, Bellomo R, Shah P. Avoiding the pump in tricuspid valve endocarditis: vegetectomy under inflow occlusion. *Ann Thorac Cardiovasc Surg.* 2002; 8(6): 350–3.

41. Gokalp O, Yurekli I, Yilik L, et al. Comparison of inflow occlusion on the beating heart with cardiopulmonary bypass in the extraction of a mass lesion or a foreign body from the right heart. *Eur J Cardiothorac Surg.* 2011; 39: 689–92.

42. Bernal JM, Gutiérrez-Morlote J, Llorca J, et al. Tricuspid valve repair: an old disease, a modern experience. *Ann Thorac Surg.* 2004; 78(6): 2069–74.

43. Morishita A, Kitamura M, Noji S, et al. Long-term results after De Vega's tricuspid annuloplasty. *J Cardiovasc Surg (Torino).* 2002; 43(6): 773–7.

44. Chidambaram M, Abdulali SA, Baliga BG, Ionescu MI. Long-term results of De Vega tricuspid annuloplasty. *Ann Thorac Surg.* 1987; 43(2): 185–8.

45. Chang BC, Song SW, Lee S, et al. Eight-year outcomes of tricuspid annuloplasty using autologous pericardial strip for functional tricuspid regurgitation. *Ann Thorac Surg.* 2008; 86(5): 1485–92.

46. Tang GH, David TE, Singh SK, et al. Tricuspid valve repair with an annuloplasty ring results in improved long-term outcomes. *Circulation.* 2006; 114(1 Suppl): I577–81.

47. Sarralde JA, Bernal JM, Llorca J, et al. Repair of rheumatic tricuspid valve disease: predictors of very long-term mortality and reoperation. *Ann Thorac Surg.* 2010; 90(2): 503–8.

48. Ghanta RK, Chen R, Narayanasamy N, et al. Suture bicuspidization of the tricuspid valve versus ring annuloplasty for repair of functional tricuspid regurgitation: midterm results

of 237 consecutive patients. *J Thorac Cardiovasc Surg.* 2007; 133(1): 117–26.

49. Lewen MK, Bryg RJ, Miller LW, et al. Tricuspid regurgitation by Doppler echocardiography after orthotopic cardiac transplantation. *Am J Cardiol.* 1987; 59: 1371–4.

50. Chan MC, Giannetti N, Kato T, et al. Severe tricuspid regurgitation after heart transplantation. *J Heart Lung Transplant.* 2001; 20: 709–17.

51. Marelli D, Esmailian F, Wong SY, et al. Tricuspid valve regurgitation after heart transplantation. *J Thorac Cardiovasc Surg.* 2009; 137(6): 1557–9.

52. Huddleston CB, Rosenbloom M, Goldstein JA, Pasque MK. Biopsy-induced tricuspid regurgitation after cardiac transplantation. *Ann Thorac Surg.* 1994; 57(4): 832–6.

53. Aziz TM, Saad RA, Burgess MI, et al. Clinical significance of tricuspid valve dysfunction after orthotopic heart transplantation. *J Heart Lung Transplant.* 2002; 21(10): 1101–8.

54. Sahar G, Stamler A, Erez E, et al. Etiological factors influencing the development of atrioventricular valve incompetence after heart transplantation. *Transplant Proc.* 1997; 29: 2675–6.

55. De Simone R, Lange R, Sack RU, et al. Atrioventricular valve insufficiency and atrial geometry after orthotopic heart transplantation. *Ann Thorac Surg.* 1995; 60: 1683–6.

56. Anderson CA, Shernan SK, Leacche M, et al. Severity of intraoperative tricuspid regurgitation predicts poor late survival following cardiac transplantation. *Ann Thorac Surg.* 2004; 78(5): 1635–42.

57. Jeevanandam V, Russell H, Mather P, et al. A one-year comparison of prophylactic donor tricuspid annuloplasty in heart transplantation. *Ann Thorac Surg.* 2004; 78(3): 759–66.

58. Jeevanandam V, Russell H, Mather P, et al. Donor tricuspid annuloplasty during orthotopic heart transplantation: long-term results of a prospective controlled study. *Ann Thorac Surg.* 2006; 82(6): 2089–95.

59. Piacentino V 3rd, Williams ML, Depp T, et al. Impact of tricuspid valve regurgitation in patients treated with implantable left ventricular assist devices. *Ann Thorac Surg.* 2011; 91(5): 1342–6.

60. Kormos RL, Teuteberg JJ, Pagani FD, et al. Right ventricular failure in patients with the HeartMate II continuous-flow left ventricular assist device: incidence, risk factors, and effect on outcomes. *J Thorac Cardiovasc Surg.* 2010; 139(5): 1316–24.

61. Kaul TK, Fields BL. Postoperative acute refractory right ventricular failure: incidence, pathogenesis, management and prognosis. *Cardiovasc Surg.* 2000; 8(1): 1–9.

62. Krishan K, Nair A, Pinney S, et al. Liberal use of tricuspid-valve annuloplasty during left-ventricular assist device implantation. *Eur J Cardiothorac Surg.* 2012; 41(1): 213–17.

63. Piacentino V 3rd, Ganapathi AM, Stafford-Smith M, et al. Utility of concomitant tricuspid valve procedures for patients undergoing implantation of a continuous-flow left ventricular device. *J Thorac Cardiovasc Surg.* 2012; 144(5): 1217–21.

64. Piacentino V 3rd, Troupes CD, Ganapathi AM, et al. Clinical impact of concomitant tricuspid valve procedures during left ventricular assist device implantation. *Ann Thorac Surg.* 2011; 92(4): 1414–18.

65. Rizzoli G, De Perini L, Bottio T, et al. Prosthetic replacement of the tricuspid valve: biological or mechanical? *Ann Thorac Surg.* 1998; 66(6 Suppl): S62–7.

20

The pulmonary autograft for aortic valve replacement

ZOHAIR Y. AL HALEES

HISTORY

Aortic valve replacement (AVR) has been shown to improve the natural history of patients with severe symptomatic aortic valve (AV) disease. Survival after surgery is often worse than in the general population. Often the degree of improvement depends on the valve substitute used. To date, there is no "ideal" valve substitute but the pulmonary autograft to replace the AV (the Ross procedure, first described by Ross in 1967) comes closest to the ideal. It is silent, non-thrombogenic, generally not requiring anticoagulation, gives best hemodynamics at rest and during exercise, and has the potential for growth.

When the procedure was initially reported, it was associated with excessive mortality and morbidity. In addition, the surgical technique described was subcoronary implantation of the autograft into the native aortic root, which is considered technically demanding. Some felt it was turning a single valve disease into a double valve disease in the same patient. Hence the adoption rate of the Ross procedure was very low. However, when excellent long-term outcomes were demonstrated, the operation was met with renewed enthusiasm. The introduction of the full aortic root replacement technique, which made early outcomes more predictable than when the subcoronary technique was used, resulted in widespread popularity of the Ross procedure. It was then offered, perhaps unwisely, for almost all types of AV pathology and for a wide age range.

With longer follow-up, it was found that patients developed progressive autograft root dilatation, which was often accompanied by aortic insufficiency (AI) and need for reoperation. It became obvious that the procedure is not suitable for all AV pathologies. Proper selection is now considered crucial for maintaining good long-term outcomes.

PRINCIPLES AND JUSTIFICATION

Multiple options are available for AVR. These include mechanical and biological options. There is no doubt that modern mechanical prostheses provide excellent hemodynamics and can be suitable for a wide range of patients, male or female, young or old. However, they need anticoagulation with its major drawbacks, particularly in the young and in females of child-bearing age. Biological valves, on the other hand, require no anticoagulation but generally deteriorate with time. The younger the patient, the faster the degeneration. Nevertheless, any choice can be associated with late complications, valve deterioration, or infection, which may need reoperation.

The Ross procedure emerged as a good alternative for AVR. It is the only surgical procedure that provides continued long-term viability of the valve tissue. The pulmonary autograft exhibits hemodynamic characteristics similar to the normal human AV, even under conditions of enhanced cardiac output. With its growth potential it is most suited for children with significant irreparable AV disease. The addition of Konno-type aortoventriculoplasty in conjunction with the Ross procedure (modified Ross–Konno; mini Ross–Konno) has further allowed the successful management of small children with AV disease associated with significant annular hypoplasia and complex left ventricular outflow tract obstruction (LVOTO). In the young, the Ross procedure conferred a survival advantage when compared to mechanical valve.

Early expectation was that autograft longevity would be superior to that of other valve substitutes. Unfortunately, longer follow-up demonstrated problems related to development of neoaortic root dilatation and AI after the technique of aortic root replacement. The techniques of subcoronary implantation and aortic root inclusion (pulmonary root inside the aortic root) prevented dilatation.

In our own experience, which includes more than 600 patients and expands over more than two decades, we utilized the procedure initially to replace the AV for almost any pathology which included rheumatic etiology in almost 85% of the patients. Most patients had AI with dilated annuli and left ventricle. In this initial cohort, we faced a high reoperation rate with most of the failures occurring in patients with rheumatic etiology and dilated aortic roots.

Rheumatic valvulitis was documented in some explanted autograft valves at reoperation indicating that the autograft can be sensitive to rheumatic fever. Because of this, we limited the use of the procedure in patients with rheumatic etiology. Other factors that were found to increase risk of autograft failure include pure AI, dilated aortic roots >27 mm (16 mm/m²) and concomitant severe rheumatic mitral valve regurgitation. We believe that dilated aortic roots continue to dilate because of intrinsic aortic root pathology. We do not recommend annular reduction. In our opinion patients with dilated aortic roots are not good candidates for the Ross procedure, particularly if they present with pure AI.

Patients with predominant aortic stenosis (AS), and particularly those with congenital etiology, had a much better long-term outcome with hardly any need for reoperation on the autograft. Based on this, congenital AV disease is currently our major indication for the Ross procedure. Ross procedure for a previous prosthetic valve failure is a reasonable option as previous surgery does stabilize the root and prevent progressive dilatation.

Progressive autograft dilatation with and without AI has been reported to occur in children and young adults and has emerged as a major concern after the Ross procedure. Because of this concern there has been a trend towards less utilization of the Ross procedure in young adults. A modification to the Ross procedure that may eliminate late autograft dilatation where the autograft is completely housed in a Dacron graft (size 28–32 mm, straight or Valsalva) prior to implantation has been suggested. In our cohort of patients, we demonstrated autograft growth that paralleled somatic growth as our neonates, infants, and children grew. We have not seen a disproportionate increase in the neoaortic root dimensions that led to progressive AI. We therefore believe that this problem is mostly related to selection and techniques of implantation.

From our experience and literature review there are good candidates, probably good candidates, and non-candidates for the procedure.

1. *Good candidates*
   - Congenital AV disease with and without LVOTO at any age. This may even be indicated in some neonates and infants.
   - Aortic valve stenosis as the predominant lesion with an annulus size less than 27 mm – (16 mm/m²) (even in those with a bicuspid AV).
   - Patients who started with AS and developed AI after balloon dilatation.
   - Redo AV surgery including a previous prosthesis provided that aortic annulus is less than 27 mm.
   - Patients with endocarditis of the AV as long as the aortic annulus is less than 27 mm. This is a good indication for the procedure as the autograft is viable and probably resists infection better than other valve substitutes.
2. *Probably good but not ideal candidates*
   - Patients with rheumatic AV disease with stenosis as the predominant lesion.
   - Patients with AI provided the annulus size is less than 27 mm. These patients should probably have root reinforcement ± sinotubular junction reinforcement.
3. *Non-candidates*
   - Patients with rheumatic AI, particularly if the annulus is dilated to more than 27 mm (16 mm/m²) with large left ventricle ± concomitant severe MR.
   - Patients with degenerated bicuspid AV with dilated annulus >27 mm.
   - Patients with connective tissue disorders such as Marfan syndrome, rheumatoid arthritis, and lupus erythematosus.

The procedure should be reserved for younger age groups <60 years of age as it probably loses a lot of its advantages beyond that age and the many biological options available will do as well. Some other relative contraindications include advanced three-vessel coronary artery disease, multiple valve replacements, severely depressed left ventricular function, and multisystem organ failure.

The major absolute contraindication to the Ross procedure is abnormal pulmonary valve anatomy. Quadricuspid pulmonary valve and a pulmonary valve with too many fenestrations or distortion of the commissural attachments should not be used. Though a bicuspid pulmonary valve has been used as an AV in repair of dextrotransposition of the great arteries with acceptable long-term outcome, we do not recommend the use of a bicuspid pulmonary valve in the context of a Ross procedure.

PREOPERATIVE ASSESSMENT

The indications for surgery are similar to those considered for any type of AV surgery. The patients should undergo a detailed transthoracic echocardiography study with all the necessary measurements. The pulmonary valve should be evaluated making sure that it is normal and suitable to use as an autograft. It should not have more than mild (1+) leakage. Hemodynamic evaluation is performed as necessary. Coronary angiography to rule out coronary artery disease should be carried out if indicated. If more information is needed, a transesophageal echocardiography study should be performed. Other diagnositic modalities like cardiac CT scan or MRI may be occasionally required.

ANESTHESIA

Anesthetic techniques for the Ross procedure are similar to those used for any major open heart operation for valve replacement.

A transesophageal echocardiography probe is inserted for further preoperative assessment if needed and to check on the immediate result of the operation after coming off cardiopulmonary bypass.

OPERATION

A standard median sternotomy incision is used. After suspension of the heart in a pericardial cradle and after full heparinization, aortic cannulation is done near the innominate artery origin followed by bicaval cannulation. The heart is usually vented through the left atrium. The systemic temperature can be lowered to 32–28 °C. Myocardial protection is provided by cardioplegic solution administered through an antegrade ± retrograde route. Either blood or crystalloid cardioplegia can be used.

There are three techniques for implanting the pulmonary autograft:

1. The *subcoronary position* using two suture lines (**Figure 20.1**).

   This technique has the advantage of retaining normal aortic wall around the autograft. This is believed to prevent progressive dilatation of the aortic root.

2. The *inclusion technique*, which theoretically keeps both autograft root and original aortic root intact. This technique is not suitable for the small aortic root (**Figure 20.2**).

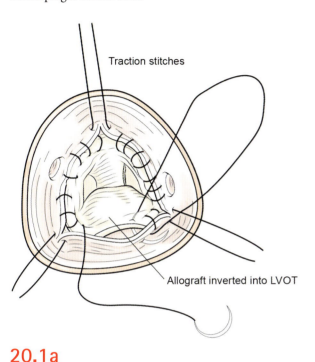

20.1a

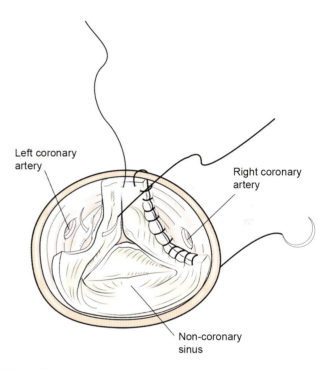

20.1b

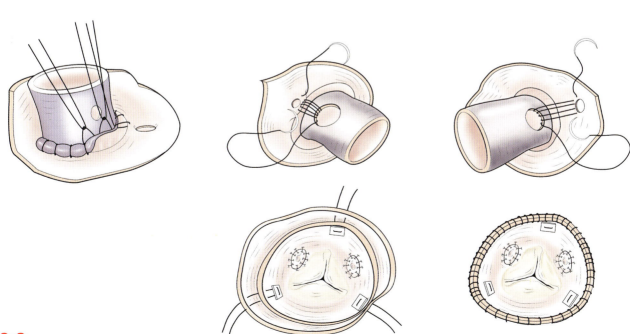

20.2

3. The technique of *full aortic root replacement*. This is our technique of choice and it will be described in detail .

Before arresting the heart, mobilization of the fat pad at the proximal aorta to identify the origin of the right coronary artery is advisable, and dissection of the pulmonary artery away from the ascending aorta with limited mobilization of the pulmonary artery branches is useful to facilitate reconstruction of the right ventricular outflow tract (RVOT) after the autograft has been harvested (**Figure 20.3**).

With the aorta cross-clamped and after cardioplegia administration, a transverse aortotomy is made approximately 1.5 cm distal to the origin of the right coronary artery and the aortic valve is examined. If the aortic valve is not repairable, the valve is excised and additional cardioplegia is injected antegrade into the coronary ostia as necessary (**Figure 20.4**).

PULMONARY VALVE HARVESTING

The pulmonary artery is incised and transected a few millimeters above the valve commissures. Careful examination is performed to ensure that the pulmonary valve is anatomically normal and therefore usable as an autograft valve replacement (**Figure 20.5a**). If the pulmonary valve is

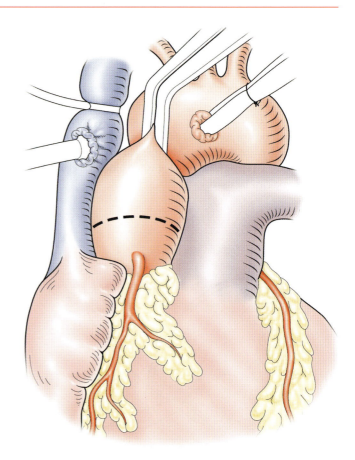

20.4

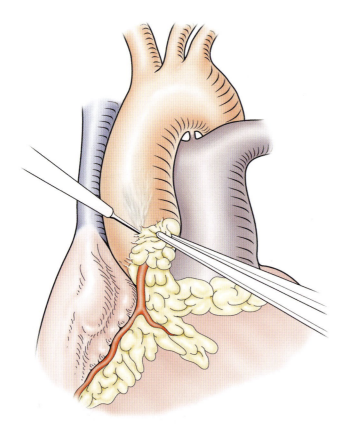

20.3

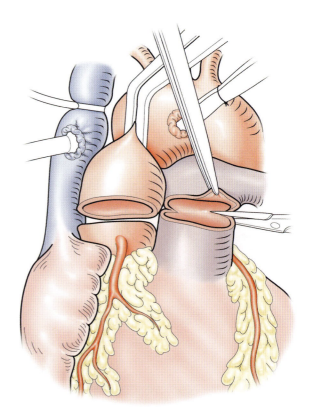

20.5a

bicuspid but otherwise anatomically suitable, and if the Ross procedure is definitely the preferred procedure, then use of the bicuspid pulmonary valve can be considered, but we do not recommend this, not least because the later results of the use of these valves are not known. More significant valvular abnormalities, such as abnormal commissural attachments or extra or diminutive cusps, have been associated with early failure, and the valve should not be used in this circumstance. If the pulmonary valve is abnormal, the pulmonary artery can be closed, and valve replacement of the aortic valve is performed with any of the numerous other potential prosthetic valve options.

If the autograft is usable, the pulmonary valve is retracted anteriorly, and initial dissection is begun on the posterior aspect of the proximal pulmonary artery adjacent to the pulmonary artery until septal myocardium is encountered. Staying close to the posterior aspect of the pulmonary valve

will avoid the left coronary artery. Use of electrocautery dissection in this area is advantageous to cauterize any small epicardial vessels that may cause troublesome postoperative bleeding (**Figure 20.5b**).

After mobilization of the posterior aspect of the pulmonary valve, a right-angle clamp is placed through the pulmonary valve approximately 4–5 mm below the pulmonary valve annulus where the anterior aspect of the right ventricular RVOT can be identified, and a small transverse incision is made below the pulmonary valve annulus in the outflow tract (**Figure 20.5c**).

Once the incision is made in the right ventricle (RV) and the pulmonary valve leaflets are readily visible, it is possible to extend the incision in the outflow tract anteriorly and posteriorly, staying approximately 4 mm from the pulmonary valve annulus and avoiding major epicardial coronary branches.

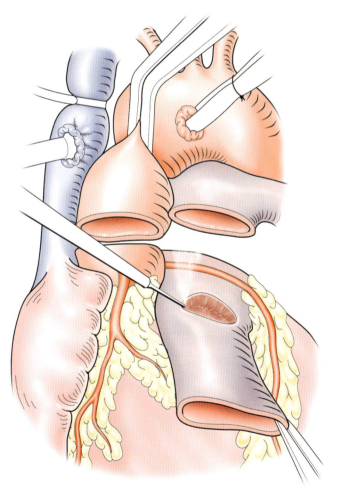

20.5b

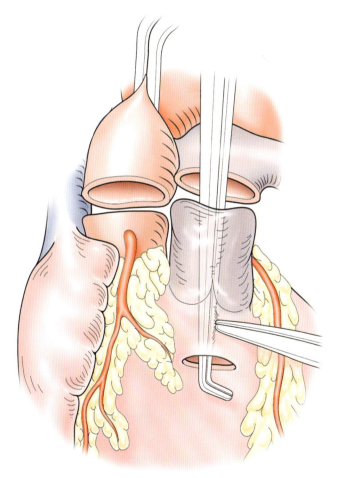

20.5c

Completion of the enucleation of the pulmonary autograft from the RVOT is performed by partially incising the posterior ventricular muscle of the septum. A fat pad and plane of dissection are usually present in the place of penetration of the first septal perforator off the anterior descending coronary artery, which traverses the septal musculature toward the conal papillary muscle of the tricuspid valve. Care must be taken to avoid interference with this vessel; if the dissection is carefully kept in the plane adjacent to the anterior muscle of the septum, it can be readily avoided. Often a fibrous tissue connection (i.e. the conus tendon) is present between the pulmonary artery and the aortic annulus, which may require sharp division to complete the enucleation of the autograft (**Figure 20.5d**).

After enucleation of the pulmonary valve and pulmonary artery, the muscle beneath the pulmonary valve should be trimmed 2–3 mm below the valve annulus. It is often advantageous to bevel the muscle to thin the muscular annulus, which will then be placed in the left ventricular outflow tract (LVOT) to avoid potential subaortic narrowing (**Figure 20.6a and b**).

The left and right coronary ostia are then mobilized and excised with a large button of aortic wall for reimplantation into the autograft. If feasible, the non-coronary sinus is kept intact as it can provide support for the autograft (**Figure 20.7**).

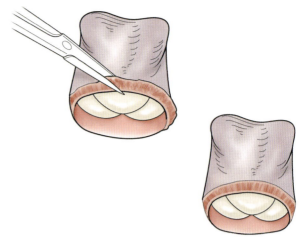

20.6a

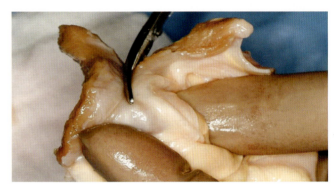

20.6b

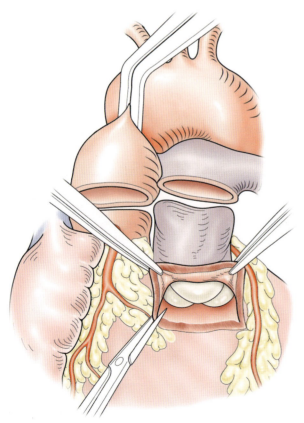

20.5d

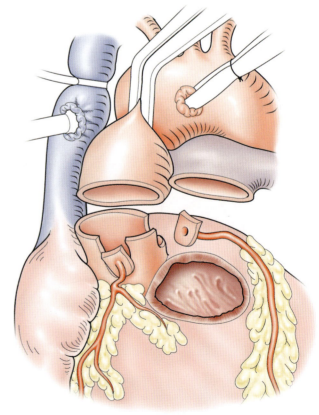

20.7

A major consideration for the pulmonary autograft implantation is the size-matching between the autograft valve and the aortic annulus. A maximum of 3–4 mm discrepancy is allowed. One should not try to compensate for an existing discrepancy between a large aortic annulus and a smaller pulmonary valve annulus by harvesting more RV muscle below the pulmonary valve. This may lead to progressive dilatation and autograft failure. The autograft should also be short and only a few millimeters above the commissures. (If the ascending aorta is dilated and needs replacement, an interposition graft should be used.) Although annular reduction is feasible and there are many ways to do it, we do not recommend it: basically, patients with a dilated aortic annulus to more than 27 mm are not good candidates for the Ross procedure.

If the pulmonary autograft is larger than the aortic annulus, which is often the case when doing the procedure for AS with a small aortic annulus, the excision of the aortic valve usually allows the annulus to dilate to match the autograft. Cutting the aortic annulus 5-6 mm to the left of the right coronary ostium will allow enlargement of the annulus to match the autograft in most cases. In patients with complex LVOTO associated with AS (**Figure 20.8a**) generous septal myomectomy should be performed. With both the aortic and pulmonary valves excised, the exposure is excellent. The resection can be guided by palpating the ventricular septum between the fingers to avoid creating a ventricular septal defect (mini Ross–Konno technique). Enlarging the LVOT just enough to match the pulmonary autograft is adequate as the autograft will grow, resulting in no recurrence of stenosis (**Figure 20.8b–d**).

Implantation of the autograft is performed by orienting

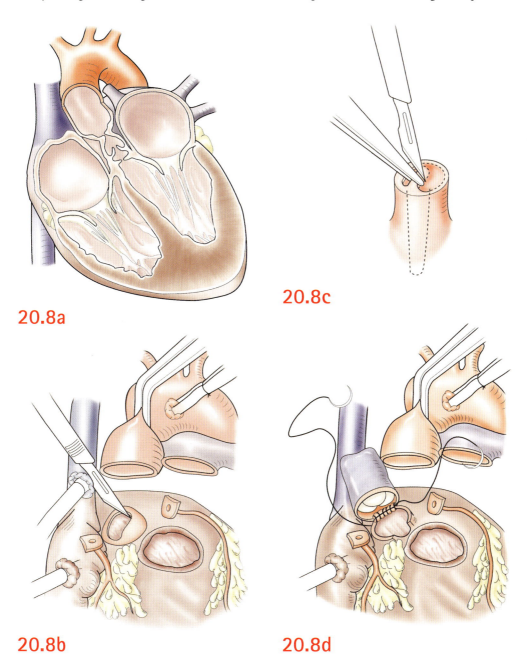

20.8a

20.8c

20.8b

20.8d

the autograft such that the pulmonary valve sinuses line up with the reimplantation sites for the coronary ostia. A suture is placed at the base of each commissure of the pulmonary autograft and positioned in the aortic annulus, trifurcated by the three sutures. Because the pulmonary valve sinuses are equal in size and the AV sinuses are rarely equal in AV pathology, adjustment of these sutures is necessary to align the autograft in the aortic annulus. Whether an interrupted or a continuous suturing is utilized, the suture should strictly follow the original level of the AV annulus (**Figure 20.9**).

While suturing the autograft, the needle is placed at the bottom of the sinus very close to the autograft leaflet insertion, ensuring that no RV muscle is incorporated in the suture line. This allows the hinge mechanism of the pulmonary autograft to be supported by the native aortic annulus (**Figure 20.10**).

If the annulus is to be fixed, as is recommended in virtually all patients with borderline dilated annulus undergoing the Ross procedure, the sutures should be replaced through a continuous strip of Dacron or Teflon felt; alternatively, with the interrupted technique, the sutures can be tied over a strip of Dacron graft material to fix the aortic annulus at a set size. Care is taken to inspect the AV leaflets all the time to ensure that no injury has occurred (**Figure 20.11**). Annular fixation is usually not done in young children.

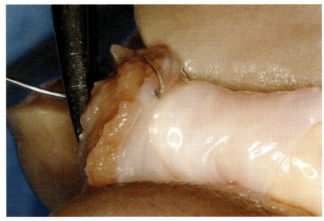

20.10a

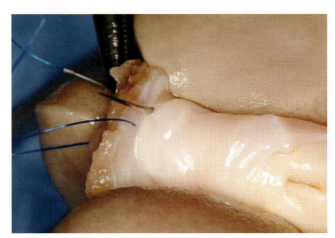

20.10b

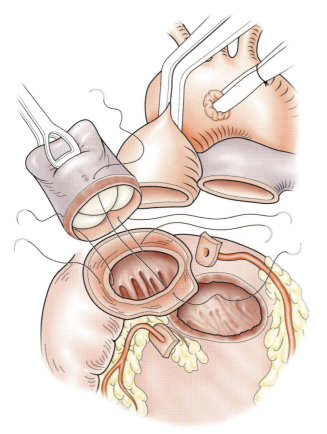

20.9

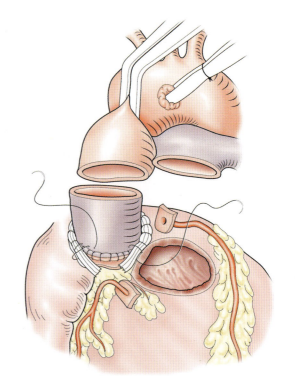

20.11

Both the right and left coronary arteries can be implanted at this time, or the left coronary can be initially implanted and the distal suture line created to allow the pulmonary autograft to distend to better judge the location for reimplantation of the right coronary, which can be higher than normal on the autograft wall (**Figure 20.12**).

After completion of the coronary implantation, the distal suture line to the ascending aorta is created. It may be necessary to tailor the distal aortic size to be equal to the autograft diameter by excision of a wedge of tissue anteriorly. It is also preferable to reinforce the aortic suture line using a strip of Teflon felt or Dacron graft material if there is any potential size discrepancy (sinotubular junction reinforcement, **Figure 20.13a–c**). This is usually not necessary in children. After completion of the reconstruction, cardioplegia can be injected through the aortic suture line just before tying to ensure dilation of the aortic root without autograft insufficiency and to check for any potential bleeding sites.

At this time, the aortic clamp can be released, if desired, to test the integrity of the suture lines and to ensure absence of AI. It may be necessary to manipulate the perfusion pressure if additional sutures are necessary in the autograft suture lines at this time. However, meticulous hemostasis should be secured before the RV outflow tract reconstruction is begun. The RVOT reconstruction can be done with the aortic cross-clamp on as well.

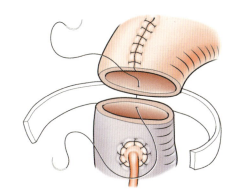

20.13a

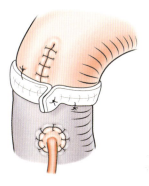

20.13b

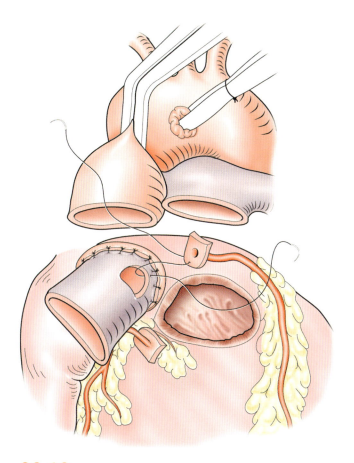

20.12

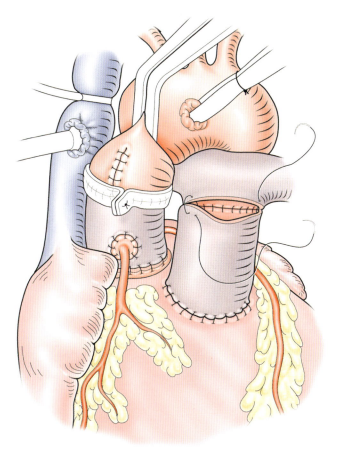

20.13c

The RV outflow tract is reconstructed with use of a pulmonary homograft (**Figure 20.14**). Recent modifications of cryopreservation have improved the lack of antigenicity of homografts, which may improve late results. A pulmonary homograft of a suitable adult size is selected, thawed, and then trimmed to match the length and width of the subpulmonary muscle tissue, the excised pulmonary autograft. After the aortic clamp is released, the distention of the autograft may actually make exposure to the pulmonary bifurcation more difficult for suturing of the pulmonary homograft; for this reason we prefer to do the entire procedure with the aorta cross-clamped. The distal anastomosis of the homograft is then created, and the proximal anastomosis of the homograft to the RVOT is created with a running polypropylene suture, with care being taken to place the posterior suture line superficially in the septal muscle to avoid interference with the septal perforators of the anterior descending coronary artery. If homograft is not available, other substitutes can be used, such as the Contegra® bovine jugular vein valved xenograft.

After completion of the pulmonary homograft insertion, the patient is rewarmed to normothermia, the vent is removed, and the patient is weaned off cardiopulmonary bypass. Transesophageal echocardiography is routinely performed in the operating room to assess the pulmonary autograft function; only trace insufficiency is generally seen. Moderate or greater insufficiency of the autograft is an indication for either revision or replacement with a different prosthesis.

POSTOPERATIVE CARE

Meticulous hemostasis is necessary in the operating room because extensive suture lines are present in this procedure. Use of topical hemostatic agents is helpful. Antithrombolytic agents can aid in achieving hemostasis. Postoperative management is similar to that of other valve procedures. Avoidance of hypertension is very important not only because it may exacerbate bleeding but also to avoid autograft dilatation. It is postulated that it may take several months for the autograft to adapt to the higher aortic pressure. Control of blood pressure is therefore important while this adaptation process takes place.

In the absence of significant chest tube drainage and with stable hemodynamics, early extubation is recommended. Early postoperative arrhythmias are common but they are generally minor and usually do not require more than short-term medical therapy.

20.14

OUTCOME IN CHILDREN

The Ross procedure in most series can be performed with an operative risk that is no higher than and possibly less than other types of AVR. The operative risk does not exceed 2.5% and some centers approached 0% mortality. However, the risk is higher in neonates and infants and is mostly related to the LV function and the status of the mitral valve. The need for concomitant mitral valve surgery significantly increases the risk. Postoperative complications are not different from those seen in a similar patient population undergoing other types of prosthetic AVR.

Anticoagulation is generally not required as the incidence of thromboembolism is exceedingly rare. Valve-related complications are also rare and survival has been excellent. In a propensity-adjusted comparison of long-term outcomes of mechanical valves versus the Ross procedure for AVR in children, we demonstrated that the Ross procedure confers a survival advantage over mechanical valves.

Frequent echocardiographic follow-up is necessary, probably every 3–6 months early on and yearly thereafter.

A major concern for the use of the Ross procedure is the potential development of late autograft root dilatation and autograft insufficiency requiring reoperation. This, however, was in most early series when there was probably an overenthusiasm for the procedure. With proper selection criteria and with proper surgical techniques paying attention to small details, this should no longer be a problem.

The major weakness of the Ross procedure is the fate of the pulmonary outflow tract. Progressive homograft degeneration does occur with time, resulting in homograft stenosis, regurgitation, or both. Homografts nevertheless have been lasting longer in Ross patients as they usually have a normal pulmonary vascular bed with normal vascular resistance and mostly normal right ventricle. Postoperatively, a gradient across the RVOT is frequently detected but this is usually insignificant. Only about 10% of the patients will have a Doppler gradient of more than 36 mmHg. Patients who need intervention usually belong to this group. It also appears that, after an initial increase in the gradient, progression slows down and the gradient stabilizes. Pulmonary regurgitation is usually well tolerated.

Balloon dilatation has generally been ineffective in relieving this obstruction. Surgical conduit replacement or patching of the narrowing has been required and has been accomplished with very minimal morbidity. The need for reoperation to deal with RVOT is low and, in our series, it was around 12% over a 10-year period.

Newer techniques are being developed to make homografts and xenografts last longer. Tissue-engineered valves may also become readily available. The prospect of percutaneous transcatheter pulmonary valve implantation should reduce the apprehension about this issue.

Patient satisfaction with the pulmonary autograft valve replacement has been excellent. Patients are able to resume a normal lifestyle with almost no restrictions. Exercise tolerance in athletes after the operation has been also excellent and essentially normal.

FURTHER READING

Al-Halees ZY, Pieters F, Qadoura F, et al. The Ross procedure is the procedure of choice for congenital aortic valve disease. *J Thorac Cardiovasc Surg.* 2002; 23: 437–42.

Al-Soufi B, Al-Halees ZY. Mechanical valves versus Ross procedure for aortic valve replacement in children. *J Thorac Cardiovasc Surg.* 2009; 137: 362–70.

Elkins RC, Knott-Craig CJ, Howell CE. Pulmonary autografts in patients with aortic annulus dysplasia. *Ann Thorac Surg.* 1996; 61: 1141–5.

Elkins RC, Lane MM, McCue C. Pulmonary autograft reoperation: incidence and management. *Ann Thorac Surg.* 1996; 62: 450–5.

Fadel BM, Al-Halees ZY. The fate of neoaortic valve and root after the modified Ross-Konno. *J Thorac Cardiovasc Surg.* 2013; 145: 430–7.

Kouchoukos NT, Davila-Roman VG, Spray TL, et al. Replacement of the aortic root with a pulmonary autograft for aortic valve disease in children and young adults. *N Engl J Med.* 1994; 330(1): 1–6.

Oury JH, Hiro SP, Maxwell JM, et al. The Ross procedure: current registry results. *Ann Thorac Surg.* 1998; 66(6 Suppl): S162–5.

Ross D, Jackson M, Davies J. The pulmonary autograft: a permanent aortic valve. *Eur J Cardiothorac Surg.* 1992; 6: 113–16.

Schmidtke C, Bechtel JF, Noetzold A, Sievers HH. Up to seven years of experience with the Ross procedure in patients >60 years of age. *J Am Coll Cardiol.* 2000; 36: 1173–7.

21

Valvular endocarditis

NISHANT SARAN AND ALBERTO POCHETTINO

PRINCIPLES AND JUSTIFICATION

Infective endocarditis (IE) is defined as the microbial invasion and the inflammatory reaction of the endocardium to a given organism. It mostly affects cardiac valves. The condition has an incidence ranging from 3 to 7 per 100 000 person-years, with a mortality approaching 30% at 1 year. Individuals with rheumatic heart disease, prosthetic valves, congenital heart disease, abnormal valves, and indwelling cardiovascular devices, and intravenous (IV) drug abusers are at higher risk for IE. Advanced age leads to both a higher incidence and higher mortality rate.

IE can affect either right- or left-sided valves, and involve native or prosthetic valves. An infection leading to symptoms within days is classified as acute, while a more indolent clinical course over several weeks is defined as subacute. Right-sided IE involving the tricuspid and/or pulmonary valve is more common among IV drug abusers or individuals with chronic indwelling intravenous lines. Among native valve endocarditis (NVE), 25–35% are nosocomial. Prosthetic valve endocarditis (PVE) comprises 16–30% of all IE. PVE risk is highest during the first 6–12 months after valve implantation and tends to stabilize thereafter, with portals of entry and responsible organisms similar to NVE once the early phase is past. PVE developing within the first 2 months post implant is mostly due to contamination during surgery and/or bacteremia in the immediate postoperative period.

Staphylococcus aureus is the most common organism responsible for nosocomial NVE and right-sided endocarditis in IV drug abusers, while coagulase-negative *Staphylococcus* is the most common organism responsible for PVE within 12 months of implant; 65–85% of these are methicillin resistant. Streptococci continue to be the most common organisms responsible for community-acquired NVE. Other organisms responsible include enterococci and HACEK group (*Haemophilus* species, *Aggregatibacter aphrophilus*, *A. actinomycetemcomitans*, *Cardiobacterium* species, *Eikenella* species, and *Kingella* species). Streptococci, *S. aureus*, and pneumococci typically result in an acute course, although *S. aureus* occasionally causes subacute disease.

Endocarditis caused by *Staphylococcus lugdunensis* (a coagulase-negative species) or by enterococci may also present acutely. Subacute endocarditis is typically caused by viridans streptococci, enterococci, coagulase-negative staphylococci, and the HACEK group.

IE lesions develop at sites of endothelial injury either by direct microbial invasion or by platelet–fibrin complex that becomes adherent to the injury site. This platelet–fibrin complex may grow to form a "vegetation." If it does not contain infectious agents, it is called non-bacterial thrombotic endocarditis (NBTE). These, however, can become sites for later organism invasion leading to IE. This process is most common in areas of pre-existing valvular lesions such as regions responsible for regurgitation and/or stenosis. Hypercoagulable states like malignancy and other chronic diseases may also lead to NBTE and are called marantic endocarditis. IE lesions in the form of vegetations are more commonly found on the atrial side of atrioventricular valves and ventricular surfaces of regurgitant semilunar valves. Low-pressure anatomic structures downstream to high-pressure zones also have a predilection for IE lesions (aorta distal to a coarctation, pulmonary arterial side of a patent ductus arterious, the lower pressure side of an intracardiac high-gradient left-to-right shunt). Vegetations typically have an infected core resistant to antimicrobials, or may have proliferating organisms at the surface being continuously shed into the bloodstream. Infectious organisms may further spread to form abscesses that can extend beyond the annulus of the affected valve into the myocardium, or lead to "kissing lesions" in the adjacent valve, such as across the aortomitral continuity. The most commonly affected valve is the aortic valve followed by the mitral, the tricuspid, and the pulmonary valves in that order.

Classically, patients present at first with unremitting fevers, chills, night sweats, and positive blood cultures, often followed by a new murmur and signs of heart failure. Echocardiography typically demonstrates valvular lesions with mobile echogenic densities. Occasionally, embolic episodes can lead to neurological deficits, renal dysfunction, and other peripheral signs. Classical "Oslerian" manifestations may be present too. Modified Duke's criteria are commonly invoked to arrive at a diagnosis of IE. Most of the patients who are not in heart failure and do not have large vegetations (>10 mm) are good candidates for medical management. Indications for surgery include:

- periannular extension with abscess or fistulous tract formation
- giant mobile vegetations (>10 mm) with high risk for embolic showers
- persistent sepsis
- severe heart failure due to significant structural valve destruction
- silent cerebral ischemic episodes
- PVE. Most PVE needs to be taken to surgery urgently, especially when *S. aureus* is the culprit organism, or when dehiscence is readily demonstrated.

Surgery can worsen an intracranial hemorrhage when carried out within 4–6 weeks of the event, hence close consultation between the surgical team and neurology/neurosurgery is important to make the best possible decision on timing of cardiac surgery.

PREOPERATIVE ASSESSMENT AND PREPARATION

Detailed transesophageal echocardiography (TEE) depicting all valvular lesions and vegetations is of paramount importance. Any suspicion of abscess should lead to a cardiac gated computed tomography (CT) scan. All patients who had undergone previous cardiac surgery should also get a gated CT angiogram scan. Details of prosthetic valve involvement, extension of lesions to other valves, and the presence of any pseudoaneurysms should be assessed. TEE may detect a rocking prosthetic valve as the infection spreads to the annulus and beyond. Coronary angiography should be sought in patients over 40 years of age if deemed safe based on the location of aortic vegetations. Coronary CT angiogram is a reasonable alternative.

Blood cultures must be sought and antibiotics started accordingly. It is desirable that any source of extracardiac infection, if identified, be eliminated prior to surgery. Some patients who present with negative cultures, possibly secondary to partly treated infection, may benefit from a leukocyte scan to localize an infectious focus. If the patient's clinical condition allows, achievement of negative blood cultures should be sought. However, persistent bacteremia resistant to appropriate antibiotics, the risk of embolic showers from mobile vegetations, and/or the presence of abscess, are all strong indications for urgent surgery. Postoperative continued treatment with appropriate antibiotics is an additional factor important to achieving a successful outcome.

Patients with PVE involving a left-sided mechanical valve may be at a greater risk for a cerebral hemorrhagic event if they are on oral anticoagulation. It is generally preferred to transition them to heparin while antibiotics are initiated and a decision for surgery is being made.

SURGERY

There are two cardinal rules in the management of any IE patient: debridement of all infected or devitalized tissue until healthy tissue margins are achieved, and removal of all prosthetic material including pledgets and suture remnants from previous surgery.

The mode of surgery, whether repair or replacement is carried out, and the choice of prosthesis should not have significant bearing on operative mortality as long as the basic principles are followed.

OPERATION

Approach

Most patients are approached via midline sternotomy as it allows the most flexibility in the conduct of the surgery. All patients who require redo sternotomy should be approached with appropriate precaution to insure safe re-entry. In particularly high-risk situations, femoral or axillary cannulation can be employed. The ascending aorta/proximal arch is typically the arterial cannulation site. While a two-stage right atrial cannula is typically sufficient for venous cannulation in most aortic valve endocarditis, bicaval cannulation should be considered if a large patent foramen ovale (PFO) is present, if mitral or tricuspid valve endocarditis is being treated, or if any fistula is present or suspected. Left ventricular venting is important, yet placement of an appropriate cannula may be delayed until after the aorta is cross-clamped to minimize the risk of distal embolism.

Myocardial protection

As many of these procedures can be complex and prolonged, it is important to keep the myocardium well protected. We typically use cold blood cardioplegia at a dose of 150 mL/m^2 at induction, roughly two-thirds of the dose given in an antegrade fashion often via ostial cannulae, and the remainder is given in a retrograde fashion. We repeat cardioplegia delivery every 20–25 minutes to maintain a quiet and cold myocardium. Moderate systemic hypothermia can be added, especially in the more complex reconstructions, to minimize myocardial rewarming between cardioplegia doses. Some surgeons have used Del Nido cardioplegia that may be repeated every 40–50 minutes. Its effectiveness in the setting of complex and prolonged operations has not been demonstrated, and we have continued to rely on cold blood cardioplegia for such situations.

Aortic root replacement

Earlier studies had suggested that homograft tissue has an increased resistance to recurrent infection in aortic IE, although it may lead to a higher late complication rate and challenging reoperations because of intense calcifications. More recent studies have shown that complication rates and late mortality in the treatment of aortic root abscess are comparable whether one uses a mechanical valved conduit, a non-homograft biologic valve conduit, or a homograft. Hence, it has become our practice in the treatment of complex aortic root infections to use either a porcine root if anticoagulation is undesirable, or a mechanical valved conduit. Homografts may be used selectively, when an abscess cavity extends well into the septum or across the aortomitral continuity with destruction of a significant portion of the anterior mitral leaflet. The homograft with its attached mitral leaflet can then be used in the reconstruction of the root to patch the septum or the partly destroyed mitral leaflet.

PROCEDURE

If a redo sternotomy is to be done, careful dissection is carried out, especially when pseudoaneurysms may be present.

The right atrium is usually completely dissected with exposure of the proximal superior vena cava (SVC) if feasible. Early visualization of the right superior pulmonary vein is useful for early venting in the setting of severe aortic insufficiency (AI).

The distal ascending aorta is completely dissected out. The arterial cannulation site is usually chosen distal to the origin of the innominate artery. Retrograde cardioplegia cannula is inserted into the coronary sinus. Cardiopulmonary bypass is initiated and a left ventricular vent is inserted through the right superior pulmonary vein. Cross-clamping is applied and retrograde cold blood cardioplegia is delivered while the ascending aorta is opened. Once the coronary ostia are visualized, cardioplegia delivery is switched to antegrade mode.

The aorta is transected completely if an aortic root replacement is planned (**Figure 21.1a**). The distal aorta is then dissected free of the posterior right pulmonary artery and retracted cranially. The next step is the complete mobilization of the root. The plane between the pulmonary artery and aortic root is developed carefully to avoid damaging the left coronary (**Figure 21.1b**).

The aortic valve is then inspected and the extent of infection is assessed. The anterior mitral leaflet is inspected to

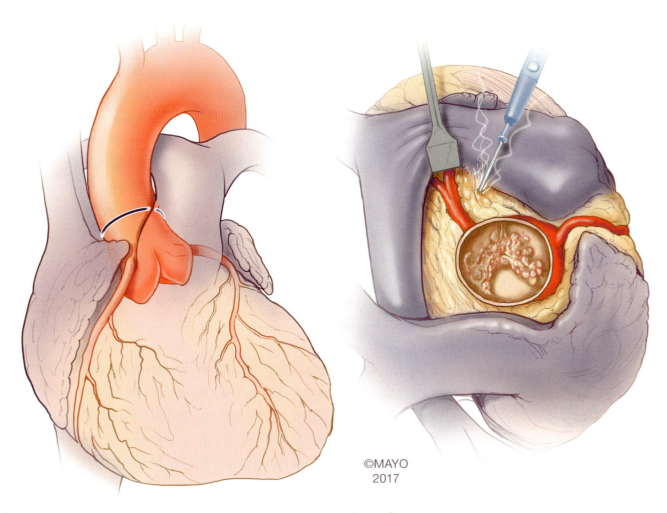

©MAYO
2017

21.1a   **21.1b**

assess for any infectious extension onto it. The coronary buttons are excised from the respective sinuses and mobilized sufficiently for a later tension-free anastomosis to the new root (**Figure 21.2a–c**).

The tissues may be fragile and friable. Radical debridement of all the infected tissue is of vital importance for a successful outcome. The valve leaflets are excised and the annulus is debrided until we reach healthy margins (**Figure 21.3a–c**). The residual left ventricular outflow tract (LVOT) is again completely examined for any residual tissue of questionable nature. A thorough irrigation with saline is then performed. If the tissue removed was grossly infected, we also use povidone iodine solution to thoroughly irrigate the field insuring that all pump suckers are turned off.

The aortic root is then sized for the appropriate root replacement. If significant missing tissue is noted, to allow a standard root replacement, bovine pericardium may be used as patch material to reconstruct the LVOT, the membranous septum, or the anterior leaflet of the mitral valve (**Figure 21.3d**).

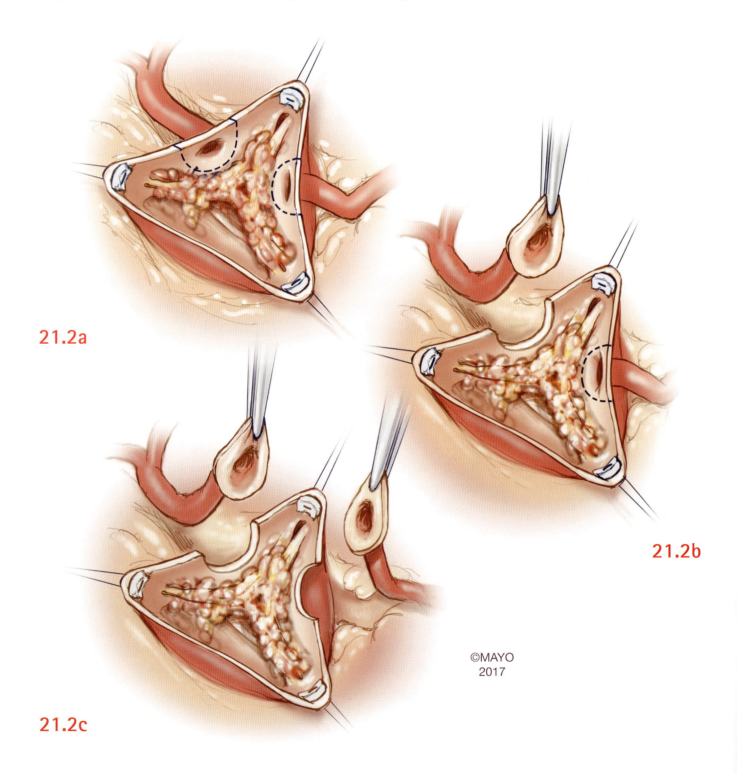

21.2a

21.2b

21.2c

©MAYO
2017

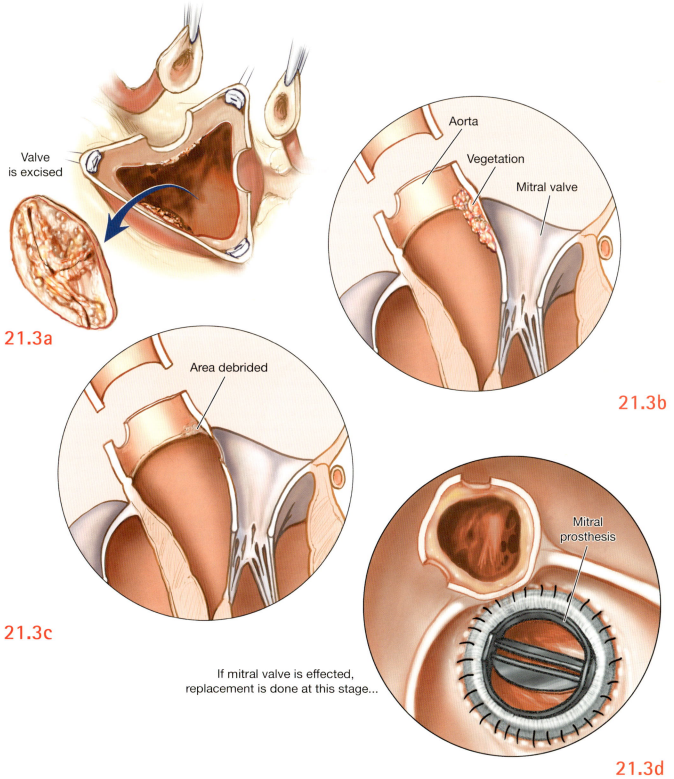

21.3a

Valve
is excised

Aorta

Vegetation

Mitral valve

21.3b

Area debrided

21.3c

If mitral valve is effected,
replacement is done at this stage...

Mitral
prosthesis

21.3d

Pledgeted 2-0 ethibond sutures are then passed through the LVOT, membranous septum, and anterior leaflet of the mitral valve in a circumferential intra-annular fashion. It is important that sutures be taken with adequate depth and optimum spacing as the tissue quality may be suboptimal. Between 15 and 18 mattress sutures are typically placed (**Figure 21.4a and b**).

Once all the sutures are in place, each suture is then passed through the sewing cuff of the chosen root. When implanting a porcine root, we would typically tie the sutures over a Hegar's dilator to avoid pursestringing or overtying the muscular tissue. The few sutures along the pulmonary artery are usually tied without the Hegar's dilator because of the awkward angle that the dilator causes with respect to the LVOT, which may lead to tissue tearing.

The left coronary button is then anastomosed with 5-0 prolene in a continuous fashion, followed by the right coronary button (**Figure 21.4c**). We generally avoid any glue or permanent hemostatic agents around the root as we believe these may cause a late pseudoaneurysm or potentially become a focus for persistent or future infection. It is therefore of extreme importance that each suture be placed with meticulous care to avoid deep root bleeding.

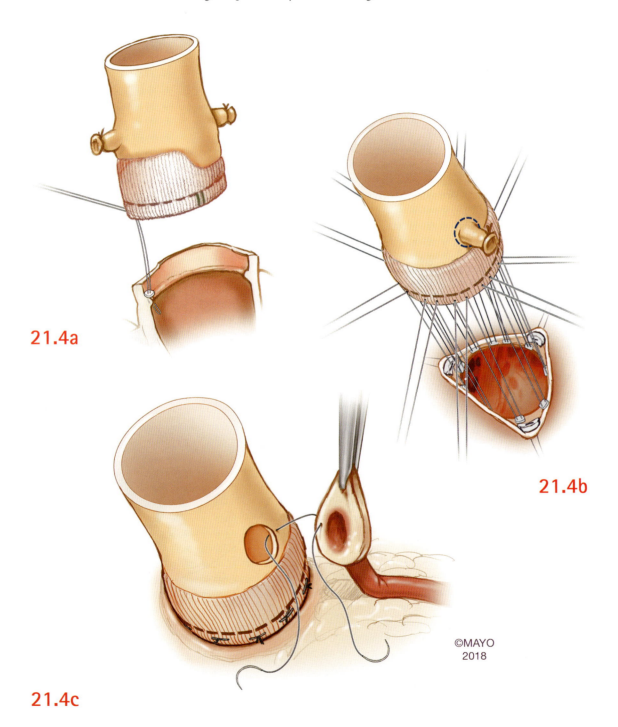

21.4a

21.4b

21.4c

©MAYO
2018

Once the buttons are in place, ascending aorta to the porcine root anastomsis is completed with a running Prolene 4-0 suture (**Figure 21.5a and b**).

Mitral valve surgery

If the IE lesion is localized to a particular leaflet or there is a small perforation that can be primarily repaired using a pericardial patch, one should opt for repair given the superior long-term results and increased resistance to recurrent IE. An infected prosthetic valve should be excised in its entirety including all pledget and suture material. Once excision is complete, the mitral annulus should be carefully assessed. It should be debrided until healthy margins are achieved. If need be, the annulus can be reconstructed using a pericardial (autologous or bovine) strip. The strip needs to be wide enough to cover the debrided annulus and also have a redundant margin that can be used as a sewing cuff for the prosthetic valve. 4-0 Prolene in a continuous fashion is used

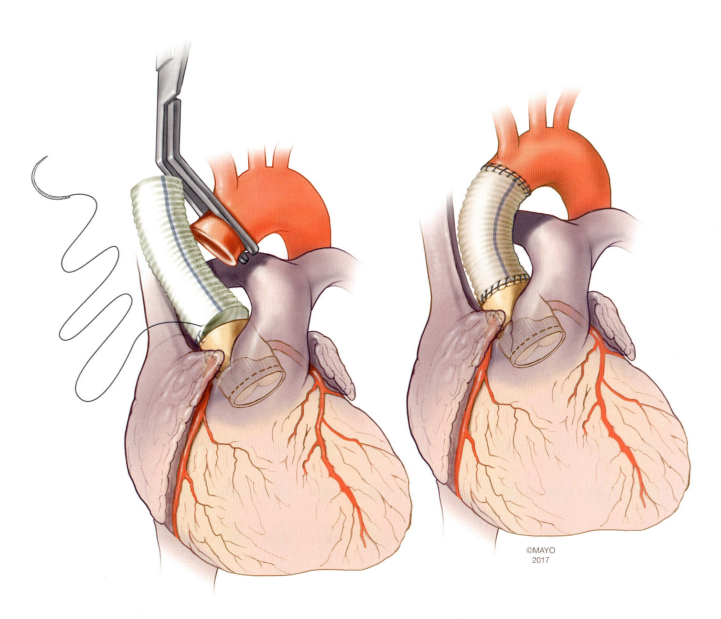

©MAYO
2017

21.5a

21.5b

to suture the pericardial strip to the atrial side superiorly and ventricular side inferiorly (**Figure 21.6a and b**). The valve is sized and the valve sutures are then placed using 2-0 ethibond sutures, following which the valve is seated.

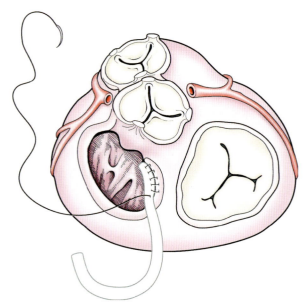

21.6a

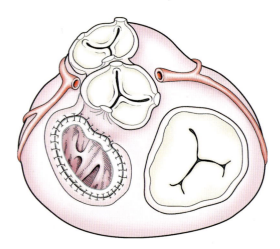

21.6b

Tricuspid valve surgery

This is the most common valve involved with IV drug abusers and infected pacemaker leads which, if present, must be removed completely. The results of tricuspid valve repair are superior to replacement and hence repair should be attempted whenever feasible. Tricuspid valve excision without replacement has been reported as an option in young

IV drug abusers. We have never favored such an approach and, when the valve cannot be repaired, we have used a tissue valve in this position. Relative undersize may be of value to allow for a gradient of at least 3–4 mmHg; a lower gradient can lead to inadequate opening of the leaflets with possible thrombus formation.

Pulmonary valve surgery

This is the valve least commonly affected by IE. A tissue valve is used most commonly which allows future transcatheter valve-in-valve implantation with ease. The tissue valve can be implanted beyond the pulmonary annulus in the pulmonary artery proper with a running 3-0 Prolene suture in a continous fashion. A bovine pericardial anterior patch allows ease of closure of the pulmonary artery.

OUTCOME

Overall surgical mortality in active IE is 6–25%, with long-term survival rates of approximately 70% in most series. Prognosis is better if surgery is undertaken early, before extensive abscess or intracardiac fistulae formation. Preoperative deterioration in the overall patient condition further increases the hazards of intervention. Final outcome has never been related to the duration and intensity of prior antibiotic treatment, and surgery should not be delayed when clearly indicated in the vain hope that a sterile operative field can be achieved.

FURTHER READING

Aksoy O, Sexton DJ, Wang A, et al. Early surgery in patients with infective endocarditis: a propensity score analysis. *Clin Infect Dis.* 2007; 44(3): 364–72.

Baddour LM, Wilson WR, Bayer AS, et al. Infective endocarditis in adults: diagnosis, antimicrobial therapy, and management of complications: a scientific statement for healthcare professionals from the American Heart Association. *Circulation.* 2015; 132: 1435.

Jassar AS, Bavaria JE, Szeto WY, et al. Graft selection for aortic root replacement in complex active endocarditis: does it matter? *Ann Thorac Surg.* 2012; 93: 480–7.

Musci M, Weng Y, Hübler M, et al. Homograft aortic root replacement in native or prosthetic active infective endocarditis: twenty-year single-center experience. *J Thorac Cardiovasc Surg.* 2010; 139: 665–73.

Prendergast BD, Tornos P. Surgery for infective endocarditis: who and when? *Circulation.* 2010; 121: 1141–52.

22

Valve-sparing aortic root replacement

IBRAHIM SULTAN AND THOMAS G. GLEASON

HISTORY, PRINCIPLES AND JUSTIFICATION

Valve-sparing aortic root replacement (VSRR) was described as a new surgical procedure in the 1980s by Sir Magdi Yacoub. He described a case series of 10 patients and introduced the concept of remodeling the aortic root. In the 1990s Christopher Feindel and Tirone David presented their technique of reimplantation of the aortic root in a polyester tube graft. This involved reimplantation of the aortic root while preserving the aortic valve in patients with aortic root aneurysm and aortic insufficiency. Subsequently, various modifications to the reimplantation and remodeling techniques have been performed and are now utilized by multiple cardiac surgical programs around the world. This is a very attractive operation in young patients with a life expectancy greater than 15 years where aortic valve repair can be a durable option.

PREOPERATIVE PLANNING AND PREPARATION

VSRR procedures are generally carried out in select patients but can have prolonged operative time, particularly in patients with leaflet pathology undergoing complex aortic valve repair at the time of reimplantation. Coagulation profile including platelet function should be normalized. Antiplatelets and anticoagulants should be held when appropriate prior to surgery. Dental hygiene should be assured prior to any valve surgery when possible. Patients with a family history of coronary artery disease or those over 40 years of age should have a preoperative coronary catheterization to rule out obstructive coronary disease. Three-dimensional computed tomography (CT) is used on all patients so orthogonal measurements of the aorta at various anatomic landmarks are performed. Echocardiography is critical in evaluating whether the aortic valve may be spared. Attention is directed to the aortic valve leaflets, sinus of Valsalva, annulus, and sinotubular junction. The coaptation height and zone of the aortic valve are carefully assessed. Aortic regurgitation is accounted for and the eccentricity of the aortic regurgitation jet is carefully examined. This enables a judgment to be made whether prolapse or restriction of one or more leaflets exists, thus causing the aortic regurgitation, or whether there is quite simply annular and sinus of Valsalva dilatation, which generally results in central aortic regurgitation.

OPERATION

Incision and cannulation

Our standard exposure for a VSRR is via a median sternotomy with a limited skin incision. The thymus is divided and the pericardium opened and suspended high on to the right chest. The patient is systemically heparinized and the lesser curvature of the aortic arch is utilized for aortic cannulation. If the arch is to be replaced at the time of the operation, the extrapericardial ascending aorta is cannulated. The right atrial appendage is used for venous cannulation with a dual-stage venous cannula. Cardiopulmonary bypass is commenced. We do not systemically cool the patient unless arch replacement is being performed at the time of surgery. We do not use a left ventricular vent as we have not noticed any benefit in doing so. Instead, a weighted cardiotomy sucker is placed across the aortic valve.

Myocardial protection is ensured with an induction dose of blood-based cardioplegia and additional direct ostial and retrograde cardioplegia every 20 minutes throughout the operation. A myocardial temperature probe can be utilized for monitoring myocardial cooling by placing it in the interventricular septum.

Mobilization of the aorta and excision of the aneurysm

Further dissection is carried out to create an aortopulmonary window and cross-clamping is applied. In the absence of aortic regurgitation, cardioplegia is given with a large-bored needle into the aortic root. If significant aortic regurgitation is present, induction retrograde cardioplegia is given followed by direct ostial cardioplegia into both coronary arteries. The aorta is then transected at the level of the sino-tubular junction. The distal aorta is then mobilized up to the cross-clamp. The aortic root is dissected carefully away from the right pulmonary artery, clearing the transverse sinus.

The left and the right coronary arteries are both excluded from the sinus of Valsalva by creating a 3–4 mm cuff of tissue. The left coronary button is best fashioned by mobilizing the soft tissue posterior to the main pulmonary artery and parallel to the left ventricular outflow tract (LVOT). Similarly, the right coronary button is fashioned by mobilizing the right ventricle (RV) off the proximal aorta. Aneurysmal tissue from all three sinus segments or two in the setting of a bicuspid aortic valve is resected in its entirety, leaving a 2 mm cuff of tissue attached to the aortic annulus. This is done from the commissure to the nadir of each sinus.

Valve analysis

The aortic valve is carefully analyzed at this stage for symmetry, prolapse, restriction, calcifications, and fenestrations. Once it is deemed that the valve is repairable, we proceed with the reimplantation procedure prior to attempting valve repair. Commissural fenestrations are typically not responsible for significant aortic regurgitation so they are deemed acceptable when small in size and number. Prolapse in one or more of the leaflets is typically easiest to repair because of the abundance of leaflet tissue.

Preparation of the aortic root and reimplantation

The aortic annulus is dissected 2 mm below the nadir of the ventriculoaortic junction (VAJ) circumferentially. This deep dissection is critical to establish a plane below the VAJ to perform appropriate annuloplasty by seating the tailored graft below the plane of the VAJ. This can be challenging around the RV and the membranous septum where the RV inserts onto the aorta.

We prefer the reimplantation method over the remodeling method as it allows the entire aortic root apparatus to be seated within a single graft. The length and the depth of each post-repair cusp determine the size of the graft and in turn the final internal annular diameter. This diameter is based on our reimplantation formula, adapted from seminal work performed by Milton Swanson and Richard Clarke, which revealed dimension relationships of the aortic root apparatus. The details of the formula and validation have been described previously. Simply, the constant measurement in the aortic root apparatus will be the height of the cusp. The simplified formula ensures that the graft size is approximately twice the size of the height of the cusp and 1–2 mm are added to round up to achieve the accurate graft size. A straight polyester woven graft is then chosen and neosinuses created after calculating the final annular diameter. This is done by dividing the cusp height by a constant of 0.7. Typical cusp heights of 13–18 mm will yield graft sizes of approximately 28–38 mm (**Figure 22.1**).

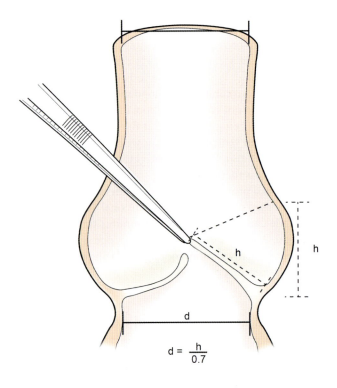

$$d = \frac{h}{0.7}$$

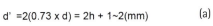

d' = 2(0.73 × d) = 2h + 1~2 (mm)   (a)

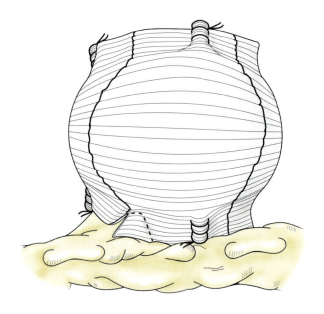

(b)

22.1a, b Formulation of a tailored graft with neosinuses for reimplantation.

Once the aortic root is appropriately dissected as described above, 21 non-pledged 2-0 Ti-Cron (Medtronic, Minneapolis, MN, USA) sutures are placed circumferentially 2 mm below the annulus in a coronet fashion. The graft is tailored after calculating the final internal annular diameter by placing pleats at the base of the graft and the neosinotubular junction to create distinct neosinuses. Three pleats and hence three neosinuses are created for trileaflet valves and two neosinuses in a setting of a true biscuspid valve. The two pleats in a true bicuspid valve are placed at two-fifths and three-fifths from each commissure.

The subannular sutures are then passed through the graft in a similar coronet fashion (**Figure 22.2a**). A groove is cut within the graft to accommodate insertion at the left–right commissure. The graft is then lowered down to the VAJ and secured by tying the knots in place (**Figure 22.2b**). This completes the annuloplasty. The commissures are then suspended high onto the graft at the sinotubular junction.

Valve analysis and repair

The valve is once again examined for any pathology. Aortic valve repair itself requires significant discussion and is beyond the scope of this chapter but we will briefly discuss our approach to valve repair in this section.

CUSP PERFORATIONS AND FENESTRATIONS

Cusp perforations are typically a result of infection. If this is invasive and caused by endocarditis, the aortic valve may not be able to be spared and a modified Bentall operation should be performed. Commissural fenestrations that are small in size and do not partake in the aortic regurgitant jet do not need to be surgically addressed. Relevant fenestrations that cause regurgitation can be addressed by surgical reinforcement by running fine (6-0) Gore-Tex (Gore, Flagstaff, AZ) sutures along the cusp. Larger fenestrations may preclude VSRR.

CUSP PROLAPSE

Prolapse of the aortic cusp can occur in one or all three cusps. A bicuspid aortic valve is easier to repair in this setting where the non-prolapsed cusp acts as a reference cusp and the prolapsed cusp can be tailored to achieve symmetry and coaptation. This can be done in the following ways:

- *Plication of the leaflet.* This can be accomplished by central plication or plication at the commissures with fine Gore-Tex suture. This is an easy technique to use when there is a small amount of prolapse/excess tissue. Central plication should be avoided when there is a prominent or calcified nodule of Arantius. The knots should be tied away from the leading edge on the aortic side in order to avoid any turbulent blood flow or hemolysis.

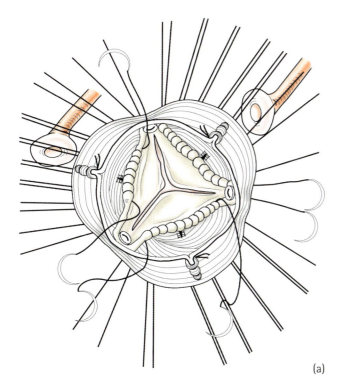

(a)

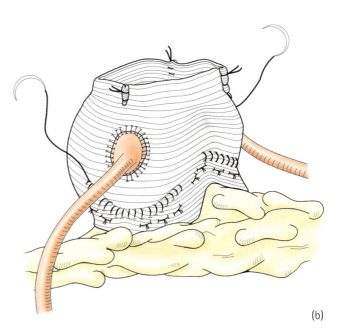

(b)

22.2a, b   Circumferential non-pledgeted sutures are passed through the graft (a), which is then lowered into the functional aortic annulus and secured by tying the knots in place (b).

- *Triangular resection,* similar to the classic teaching of posterior leaflet repair of the mitral valve. A small triangle of excess tissue is resected around the nodule of Arantius and the free edges sewn together with 6-0 Gore-Tex suture. This is generally used in a bicuspid aortic valve while using the non-prolapsed cusp as a reference cusp.
- *Free-margin reinforcement* can be performed by running 6-0 Gore-Tex suture from one commissure to the next and back. This is useful to shorten the leading edge of the cusp and may also help close any fenestrations that may be responsible for aortic regurgitation.

Secondary suture line

This is the hemostatic suture line and care must be taken to do it with precision. A 4-0 polypropylene suture is used to form the nadir of each neosinus to the commissure in a back and forth manner until the entire annulus is incorporated into the graft. We will occasionally place interrupted sutures if necessary to ensure hemostasis. Careful suturing is needed so as not to distort the annulus and hence the cusps after valve repair (**Figure 22.3a–c**).

Coronary reimplantation

The left main coronary is reimplanted first. A 2–3 mm cuff of the coronary artery is created and an appropriate spot is chosen on the graft. Ophthalmic cautery is used to create an orifice in the graft that is slightly larger than the ostium of the coronary. This is done while protecting the valve leaflets and the secondary suture line from cautery injury. The coronary is then reimplanted onto the graft using running 5-0 Prolene. The anastomosis is confirmed to be hemostatic by using a fine hook and ensuring that there are no loops before tying the knots in place. In a similar way, the right coronary is reimplanted high onto the graft. Care is taken to

ensure that the right coronary does not kink once the heart is full and ejecting.

Aortic anastomosis

If the arch is to be replaced during the operation, both the proximal and distal aortic grafts are left untrimmed, bevelled, and sewn to each other using a running 2-0 polypropylene suture. If the arch is not replaced, the aorta is trimmed up to the aortic cross-clamp. All aneurysmal aorta is removed. The graft is then bevelled appropriately and sewn to the aorta using running 4-0 polypropylene. This is done in an onlay intussuscepting fashion in order to ensure hemostasis.

De-airing

At the conclusion of the aortic anastomosis, the heart and the graft are carefully de-aired. This is done with the heart filled, retrograde cardioplegia, and some hand ventilation. Once the heart is de-aired, hot shot cardioplegia is given in a retrograde and antegrade fashion to de-air the coronary arteries. The cross-clamp is removed and the heart is allowed to reperfuse.

Weaning from cardiopulmonary bypass

While the heart is being reperfused, all visible suture lines are inspected carefully and any repair sutures placed at this time. After an adequate period of reperfusion, the heart is allowed to fill, eject, and wean off cardiopulmonary bypass. Occasionally, some inotropic support is required to wean off cardiopulmonary bypass. Any ventricular arrhythmias or depression of biventricular function should prompt one's attention to the possibility of kinking of the coronary buttons, and this should be addressed before weaning from

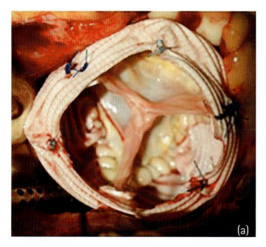
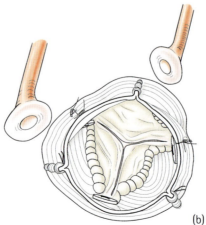
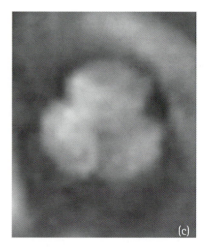

22.3a–c An intraoperative view (a), cartoon (b), and imaging view (c) of the finished secondary suture line and the representative view of the neosinuses with the tailored graft.

cardiopulmonary bypass. Two atrial and two ventricular wires are applied to the heart. Transesophageal echocardiography (TEE) of the valve is used to inspect the coaptation zone and height, and to ensure that there is no gradient or regurgitation across the aortic valve. Once satisfactory repair is confirmed, the heart is decannulated and protamine is administered.

We do not use any Teflon felt as part of our anastomoses as we do not feel it is necessary. Furthermore, reoperative surgery can be challenging when felt is used at the time of the index operation. The thymus and the pericardium are closed over the graft up to the RV in order to prevent any scarring of the graft to the chest wall.

POSTOPERATIVE CARE

The postoperative management for patients who have undergone VSRR is similar to that for those who have had any other proximal aortic surgery. Management of cardiac rhythm, output, and acid–base balance is important. It is uncommon for us to transfuse patients who have undergone VSRR. One Blake drain is placed at the time of surgery which is generally removed once the patient is ambulating and the output has decreased significantly. Atrial

fibrillation is managed aggressively with cardioversion prior to discharge.

Patients return 4 weeks after discharge with a high-quality transthoracic echocardiogram to ensure aortic valve competence. Periodic echocardiograms are performed to monitor valve repair. Long-term follow-up is critical in these patients. Any evidence of aortic regurgitation needs to be investigated and managed appropriately.

FURTHER READING

David TE, David CM, Feindel CM, Manlhiot C. Reimplantation of the aortic valve at 20 years. *J Thorac Cardiovasc Surg.* 2017; 153(2): 232–8.

Gleason TG. New graft formulation and modification of the David reimplantation technique. *J Thorac Cardiovasc Surg.* 2005; 130: 601–3.

Gleason TG. Current perspective on aortic valve repair and valve-sparing aortic root replacement. *Semin Thorac Cardiovasc Surg.* 2006; 18(2): 154–64.

Sarsam MAI, Yacoub M. Remodeling of the aortic valve annulus. *J Thorac Cardiovasc Surg.* 1993; 105: 435–8.

Sultan I, Comlo KM, Bavaria JE. How I teach a valve-sparing root replacement. *Ann Thorac Surg.* 2016; 101(2): 422–5.

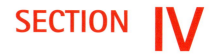

Surgery for heart failure

23

Heart transplantation

ARMAN KILIC AND PAVAN ATLURI

HISTORY

The first successful heart transplant was performed in 1967 by Dr Christiaan Barnard in Cape Town in South Africa. The 55-year-old recipient was transplanted with a heart from a 25-year-old donor who died in an automobile accident. The recipient survived 18 days. The initial enthusiasm in heart transplantation was met with the sobering reality of tissue rejection and associated poor survival. As a result, the number of heart transplants declined dramatically from 100 in 1968 to 18 in 1970. It was not until the advent and maturation of immunosuppressive therapy that transplantation volume began to rise globally. In recent years, approximately 5000 heart transplants have been performed annually throughout the world with 1-year survival rates of 85–90%.

Despite favorable post-transplant outcomes, there remain several limitations to this therapy for end-stage heart failure. Foremost, donor shortages continue to be the Achilles' heel of heart transplantation. Although 5000 heart transplants are performed throughout the world annually, approximately 50 000 patients are estimated to be candidates, highlighting the supply and demand mismatch that exists. Another area that requires further refinement is the optimization of bridging algorithms for high-risk patients. Moreover, it is unclear what support platforms such as extracorporeal membrane oxygenation or percutaneous or implantable ventricular assist devices should be utilized, particularly in patients presenting in cardiogenic shock with evidence of end-organ dysfunction who are otherwise suitable transplant candidates. The management and approach to these patients undoubtedly vary substantially between institutions and even providers within the same institution and are likely a reflection of the lack of trials and evidence-based guidelines. Despite these limitations, heart transplantation is a success story, offering the potential for long-term survival and improved quality of life in patients with end-stage heart failure.

PRINCIPLES AND JUSTIFICATION

Recipient selection

Potential candidates for heart transplantation should be reviewed by a multidisciplinary committee consisting of cardiac surgeons, cardiologists, nurse practitioners, coordinators, nurses, and social workers. In general, heart transplantation is considered in patients with end-stage heart failure with an expected survival of less than 1 year. More specifically, patients in cardiogenic shock requiring mechanical hemodynamic support and/or continuous intravenous inotropes, those with progressive, refractory, or stage D heart failure symptoms despite optimal therapy, those with recurrent and life-threatening arrhythmias despite optimal therapy including implantable defibrillators, and those with refractory angina without the possibility of further medical or surgical intervention may all be considered for heart transplantation. A limited exercise capacity as evaluated by peak oxygen consumption is frequently utilized in the evaluation of heart failure patients who are able to exercise. Peak oxygen consumption less than 12 mL/kg/min is indicative of poor prognosis with an estimated survival less than that of heart transplantation.

There are several contraindications to heart transplant therapy. Patients with advanced irreversible liver or renal disease are at high risk of post-transplant mortality following isolated heart transplantation. In these cases some centers will perform simultaneous heart and liver or heart and kidney transplantation. Similarly, advanced irreversible lung parenchymal disease is a contraindication and in select cases can be treated with a combined heart–lung transplant. Recent or active malignancy is also considered a contraindication given the higher risk of recurrence on immunosuppressive medications and shorter life expectancy.

An absolute contraindication is advanced irreversible pulmonary hypertension despite vasodilator therapy as the transplanted right heart is at increased risk for acute failure in the setting of high pulmonary vascular resistance.

Although the threshold for pulmonary vascular resistance above which heart transplantation is contraindicated can vary between institutions, greater than 3 Wood units is generally accepted as significantly elevated and associated with unacceptably high risk of post-transplant mortality. Heart–lung transplantation can be considered in some cases of irreversible pulmonary arterial hypertension.

Relative contraindications to heart transplantation include severe peripheral vascular disease, severe cerebrovascular disease, cachexia or morbid obesity, current or recent tobacco use, alcohol or illicit substance use, active pulmonary embolism, active or recent infection, diabetes mellitus that is poorly controlled or associated with end-organ damage, psychiatric disorders, poor compliance, or lack of social support. Patients with systemic illnesses such as acquired immunodeficiency syndrome (not necessarily human immunodeficiency virus infection that is well controlled) that portend a poor expected survival of less than 2 years are also generally not offered heart transplantation. Advanced age (>70 years) is also considered by some to be a contraindication although more recent data suggest that heart transplantation can be performed with acceptable outcomes in this higher-risk subset.

Donor selection

Donor selection is as important a contributor to overall outcomes as recipient selection. The quality of the donor heart should be evaluated not only in and of itself but also in relation to the recipient. Certain factors such as height and weight of the donor, ABO blood type, and positive serologic status including hepatitis B, C, and human immunodeficiency virus, may preclude a donor from being utilized. Size matching between an adult donor and recipient should generally be such that the donor weight is within 30% of the recipient weight. Other donor factors to consider include age, mechanism of death, gender, hospital course, inotropic support, and laboratory parameters. With regards to donor age, there is sufficient evidence to suggest that the older the donor, the worse the outcomes. However, similar to recipient age, the age threshold above which is considered a contraindication varies between institutions and providers. Donor age should be considered in the context of other donor risk factors, such as projected cold ischemic time, to provide a better sense of how marginal the donor organ truly is and to determine whether it should be used for that particular recipient. Many centers will employ a strategy of matching marginal donors with marginal recipients, particularly if the odds of finding another suitable donor organ for that recipient are estimated to be low given sensitization, blood type, and other factors that impact waiting list time.

PREOPERATIVE ASSESSMENT AND PREPARATION

Preoperative assessment of the recipient begins with a review of all aforementioned criteria to ensure that the recipient is indeed a suitable candidate for transplantation. Various risk models, such as the Index for Mortality Prediction After Cardiac Transplantation, or IMPACT score, have been developed that can be used for risk stratification and prognostication in heart transplantation. Evaluative tests for the recipient may include laboratory data with particular attention to end-organ function, serologic studies, chest X-ray, electrocardiogram, echocardiogram, and cardiac catheterization. Immunologic evaluation including blood typing, human leukocyte antigen typing, and panel-reactive antibody determination are performed. Virtual cross-matching is also frequently performed to identify antibody specificities. In patients bridged with a ventricular assist device, a computed tomography (CT) scan of the chest can help delineate the proximity of the outflow graft, aorta, and other structures to the sternum to aid in sternal re-entry.

Donor evaluative tests include a chest X-ray, arterial blood gas, and echocardiogram. Cardiac catheterization should be obtained in males over the age of 45 years or females over the age of 50 years, or in patients with risk factors for coronary artery disease. Although donors with mild coronary artery disease or mild reductions in left ventricular ejection fraction can be used, those with more significant coronary lesions or reduced function are typically not utilized for transplantation.

ANESTHESIA

Some patients undergoing heart transplantation are already mechanically ventilated but, for those who are not, endotracheal intubation is performed in the operating room. Radial arterial monitoring and central venous access are also established. A Swan–Ganz catheter is placed. In patients who have had a prior sternotomy, some surgeons will place a femoral arterial line with or without a femoral venous line for vascular access in case there is injury on sternal re-entry requiring emergent initiation of cardiopulmonary bypass (CPB). Other surgeons will perform a cutdown of the groin to expose the femoral vessels and potentially go on CPB prior to re-entry, particularly if the preoperative CT scan demonstrates structures that are in close proximity to the posterior table of the sternum. Many patients undergoing heart transplantation have implanted automated internal cardioverter defibrillators or permanent pacemakers. In patients who are pacemaker-dependent and have only a permanent pacemaker without defibrillating function, a magnet can be placed over the device to convert it to an asynchronous mode compatible with electrocautery use. In patients with devices that have both pacemaker and defibrillating function, a magnet will only deactivate the defibrillating function and therefore a member of the cardiac electrophysiology team should come to the operating room to program the device to an asynchronous mode.

OPERATION

Donor cardiectomy

The donor procurement process begins with a thorough review of all necessary documentation including establishment of demographics, brain death, blood typing, and consent by family members. Laboratory and imaging studies including echocardiography and cardiac catheterization are also reviewed. Communication with the recipient team is crucial throughout this process for coordination of operative timing.

A median sternotomy is performed and the bilateral pleural spaces are opened wide. The pericardium is then opened and tied off widely at the base near the diaphragm to maximize exposure, and pericardial 0-silk stay sutures are placed and secured to the drapes with hemostats. Manual inspection and palpation of the coronary arteries is performed and any anatomic abnormalities are noted. The superior vena cava (SVC) is mobilized medially and laterally and the azygous vein is identified and ligated with 0-silk sutures and divided. The pericardium is mobilized off the inferior vena cava (IVC). The aortopulmonary window is developed to allow placement of an aortic cross-clamp. An antegrade cardioplegia catheter is inserted into the ascending aorta and the cardioplegia circuit de-aired and connected (**Figure 23.1**).

In coordination with the abdominal procurement team, 30 000 units of intravenous heparin are administered. The SVC is then clamped or ligated. The IVC is incised midway between the junction with the right atrium and the

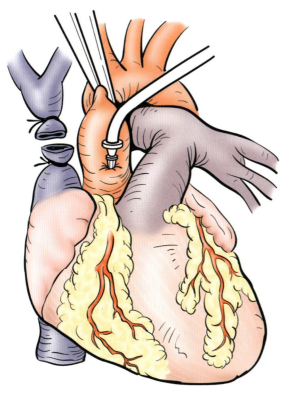

23.1

diaphragm. The left heart is vented either through incision of the pulmonary veins if the lungs are not being procured, or through the left atrial appendage if the lungs are being procured. In the latter case, the left atrial appendage can be clamped and then divided and venting can be accomplished by merely releasing the clamp once the IVC is incised. The distal ascending aorta is then cross-clamped and 2 liters of cardioplegia are delivered. Two pool-tip suctions are placed by the IVC to prevent warm blood from returning into the chest. Ice is dumped into the mediastinum and pleural spaces to keep the organs cold. The heart should be palpated occasionally to make sure it is not distending. If distension occurs, manual decompression of the heart and ensuring that the venting incisions are adequate is necessary to prevent injury to the donor heart.

After cardioplegia delivery, the ice is removed from the chest. The aortic cross-clamp and cardioplegia catheter are removed. If the SVC was not ligated before, it is ligated above the junction with the azygous vein. The IVC is completely transected making sure there is enough distance from the right atrium and the coronary sinus. The aorta is transected distally, either through the distal ascending aorta, the aortic arch, or in the proximal descending thoracic aorta with transection of each of the head vessels. The pulmonary artery is transected at the bifurcation. If the lungs are not being procured and the left-sided venting was done through the pulmonary veins, the pulmonary veins are completely transected bilaterally. If the lungs are being procured, then an incision is made in the left atrium from the right side after developing Sondergaard's groove. This incision is then carried inferiorly, keeping in view the IVC and ensuring that the right atrium is not inadvertently entered. The heart is retracted to the right and an incision is also made halfway between the reflection of the left pulmonary veins with the left atrium and the left atrial appendage. This incision is similarly carried inferiorly and joined with the incision from the right side. It is important to identify the pulmonary vein orifices while fashioning the left atrial cuff to ensure that the incisions are not made too close, which can result in pulmonary vein stenosis.

Recipient cardiectomy

The bicaval technique for heart transplantation is the most commonly utilized and our preference, and will be described here. In patients bridged with a ventricular assist device or with other prior open-heart surgery, a preoperative CT scan should be reviewed to evaluate the proximity of critical structures including the aorta, innominate vein, outflow graft, coronary bypass grafts, and right ventricle and atrium, to the posterior sternum. Percutaneous access to the femoral vein and femoral artery should be obtained at a minimum. In cases where critical structures are in close proximity, some surgeons will perform surgical exposure of the femoral vessels and obtain wire access and leave the wires in holders. This will minimize time to emergent CPB if there is inadvertent injury to the outflow graft or right ventricle, for instance. The outflow graft is ideally placed to the right of midline at the time of ventricular assist device implantation (**Figure 23.2**).

After sternotomy (and adhesiolysis in reoperative cases), intravenous heparin is administered and aortic and bicaval cannulation (or femoral cannulation) is performed. Rummel tourniquets are placed around the superior and inferior venae cavae (**Figure 23.3**). If groin cannulation is performed, we prefer to centrally cannulate the SVC and Y-connect this to the groin-cannulated IVC cannula. In reoperative cases, adhesiolysis around the apex of the heart is usually best tolerated on CPB.

CPB is initiated and, if there is a ventricular assist device, it is turned off and the outflow graft is clamped. An aortic cross-clamp is applied, and the Rummel tourniquets are snared around both cavae. The cardiectomy begins with an incision in the middle of the right atrium. This incision is carried to the right and posteriorly to the inferior edge of the right inferior pulmonary vein. It is also carried toward but not too close to the atrioventricular groove and then down onto the coronary sinus. Once the right atrium is open, the posterior IVC cuff is fashioned. The posterior incision should be made extending from the inferior edge of the right inferior pulmonary vein to the coronary sinus, keeping in mind that enough posterior cuff should be left to make suturing of this portion of the IVC anastomosis technically easier, as it is often the most difficult suture line in the operation.

The SVC is transected at its junction with the right atrium, and the posterior soft tissue mobilized. If an automated internal cardioverter defibrillator is in place, the wires are pulled down from the SVC and transected as proximally as possible with heavy Mayo scissors. The aorta is transected at the sinotubular junction or, if a ventricular assist device is in place, through the outflow graft where it is anastomosed to the aorta. The pulmonary artery is similarly transected just above the commissures. The fossa ovalis is then incised to enter the left atrium. The incision is carried up to the dome of the left atrium and toward the left atrial appendage. Once the left atrium is opened, the mitral annulus and orifices of the pulmonary veins should be noted. The left atrial cuff can be fashioned by making the incision approximately 1–2 cm superiorly to where the mitral annulus is, and aimed toward the superior edge of the left atrial appendage, again keeping in mind where the pulmonary vein orifices are located. It is helpful for the assistant to place their index and middle fingers in the orifices of the transected aorta and pulmonary artery and lift to retract the recipient heart up to help complete the cardiectomy. Once the recipient heart is removed, the edge of the left atrial cuff and surrounding fat are cauterized as this can lead to nuisance bleeding after implantation of the donor heart. A left ventricular vent catheter is placed

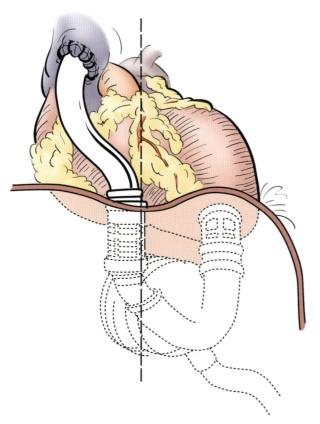

23.2

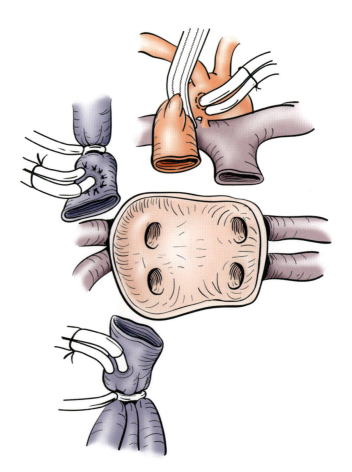

23.3

through the right superior pulmonary vein and the tip placed in the posterior atrial cuff to help keep the field dry during the left atrial anastomosis.

Implantation of the donor heart

The donor heart is removed from its packaging and placed in a bowl with ice. The heart is evaluated for damage. In particular, the IVC cuff should be evaluated and the coronary sinus identified. The SVC and suture-ligated azygous vein should be in view as well. The intervening soft tissue between the aorta and pulmonary artery is divided. The aorta is trimmed to exclude the aortic arch. The confluence of the right and left pulmonary artery is opened and the pulmonary artery is then transected to approximately 5 mm above each commissure (**Figure 23.4**). If left-sided venting was achieved through the pulmonary veins, then a forcep is placed through the orifice of one of the pulmonary veins to the orifice of another pulmonary vein, and the intervening tissue is divided with scissors. This is repeated until each of the pulmonary veins is opened to create the left atrial cuff,

which can then be trimmed as necessary. If venting was done through the left atrial appendage, it is closed in two layers with 4-0 polypropylene suture.

The donor heart is anatomically oriented. The left atrial anastomosis is started with a long 3-0 polypropylene suture and aligned such that the donor left atrial appendage matches with the recipient left superior pulmonary vein. The sutures in the posterior row should be imbricated so that there is endocardium-to-endocardium apposition. The left ventricular vent can be repositioned through the donor mitral valve and into the left ventricle then secured. After the left atrial anastomosis is completed, the IVC is anastomosed with 4-0 polypropylene suture. We typically place a stay suture on the right side at 9 o'clock to avoid kinking and to help with size matching. The suture line is started on the left side at 3 o'clock and the posterior suture line completed first (**Figure 23.5**). If there are concerns of a narrow anastomosis or substantial size mismatch, the donor IVC size can be increased by making a slit anteriorly into the right atrium. In cases where narrowing persists, the anastomosis can be augmented with a bovine pericardial patch.

The donor SVC is then stretched and transected after

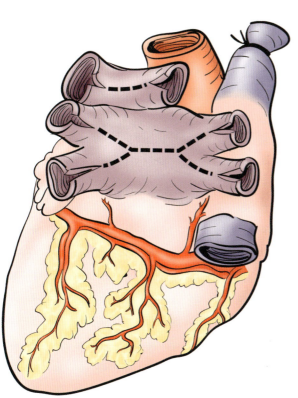

23.4

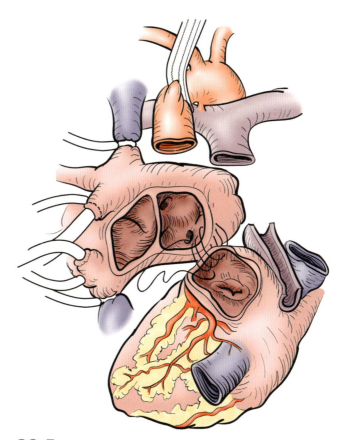

23.5

sizing, and the SVC anastomosis is performed with 5-0 polypropylene starting at 3 o'clock (**Figure 23.6**). A stay suture is similarly used on the right side at 9 o'clock to prevent a pursestring effect and to help in size matching. This anastomosis can also be performed as the last anastomosis after removing the aortic cross-clamp if there is concern for prolonged ischemic time.

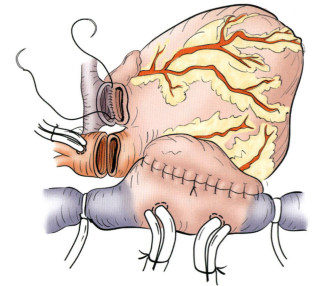

23.7a

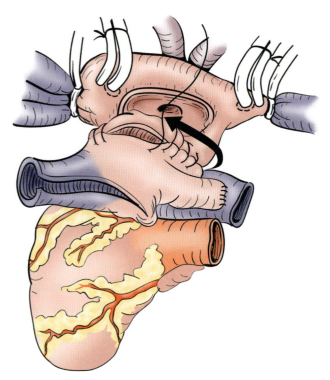

23.6

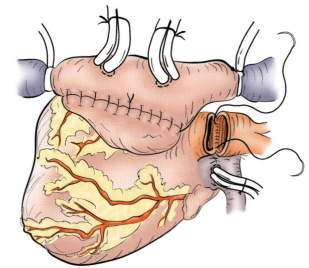

23.7b

The pulmonary artery anastomosis is completed with 4-0 polypropylene suture after placing a stay suture on the right side (**Figure 23.7a**). Excessive length of the anastomosed pulmonary artery should be avoided to prevent kinking. Systemic rewarming is initiated and the aortic anastomosis is performed with 4-0 polypropylene (**Figure 23.7b**). Some redundancy is acceptable with the aortic anastomosis because it will allow for access to the posterior suture line if repair sutures are needed for hemostasis.

After completion of the anastomoses, 500 mg of Solu-Medrol is given, an aortic root vent is placed, the aortic cross-clamp removed, and temporary atrial and ventricular pacing wires placed (**Figure 23.8**). After a period of adequate reperfusion, CPB is weaned and the patient is decannulated in standard fashion.

23.8

POSTOPERATIVE CARE

Primary graft dysfunction

An immediate concern following implantation of the donor heart is primary graft dysfunction. This is typically evidenced by impaired biventricular function after a period of adequate reperfusion with hemodynamic instability. An intra-aortic balloon pump can be used for left ventricular support and to facilitate weaning from CPB. In more severe cases, the recipient's chest may need to be left open and the patient converted to extracorporeal membrane oxygenation if unable to wean from bypass.

Right ventricular failure

In some cases, and particularly when there is elevated pulmonary vascular resistance, right heart failure ensues after implantation. Transesophageal echocardiography will demonstrate a depressed right ventricular contractility and an underfilled and vigorously contracting left ventricle. This will be accompanied by low cardiac output with rising central venous pressure. Right ventricular function typically improves over time, and aggressive hemodynamic support during the susceptible period is essential. Pharmacological support should ideally lower pulmonary vascular resistance and provide inotropic support to the right ventricle. Typical agents used for right ventricle support include dobutamine, milrinone, inhaled nitric oxide, and inhaled Flolan. Diuresis and avoiding volume overloading are important in managing the right heart. In more severe cases, temporary right ventricular assist device placement may be necessary.

Bleeding

Another concern particularly in the reoperative setting is bleeding. Many patients are coagulopathic at baseline and, after giving protamine and ruling out surgical sources, our preference is to proceed with synthetic factor VII or prothrombin complex concentrate. The advantage of these procoagulant products is that they limit the volume overloading that occurs with infusion of multiple blood products. When transfused, blood products should be leukocyte-depleted and cytomegalovirus negative if the donor and recipient are cytomegalovirus negative.

Arrhythmias

Pharmacologic chronotropic agents such as isoproterenol are used in the immediate post-transplant period to maintain a heart rate over 90 beats per minute. Temporary atrial and ventricular epicardial pacing wires should be placed during the operation even if the patient is in sinus rhythm. Persistent tachyarrhythmias should prompt an investigation of possible rejection.

Immunosuppression and rejection

Immunosuppression consists of glucocorticoids, antiproliferative agents, and calcineurin inhibitors. Nearly half of recipients also receive induction therapy, which improves immune tolerance and also avoids the use of nephrotoxic agents in the immediate postoperative period. The presence of hyperacute and acute rejection is monitored closely in the early postoperative period. Hyperacute rejection results from pre-existing antibodies to vascular endothelial cells of the donor heart, resulting in graft dysfunction within minutes to hours after implantation. Acute cellular rejection, which is more common and occurs in the first week to several years after implantation, is a mononuclear inflammatory response against the donor heart and can occur in up to 30% of patients in the first post-transplant year. Transjugular endomyocardial biopsies are the gold standard for diagnosing acute cellular rejection and are performed weekly and then every other week for several months. Acute antibody-mediated rejection occurs days to months after transplantation and is initiated by antibodies directed against donor endothelial cells or human leukocyte antigens.

Renal failure

Renal failure requiring hemodialysis occurs in 1–15% of heart transplant recipients and is associated with substantially higher mortality rates and an increased risk of chronic renal failure. The use of monoclonal or polyclonal antibodies can help in delaying the use of nephrotoxic immunosuppressive medications, and should be considered in high-risk patients or patients who develop worsening renal failure in the immediate post-transplant period. Diuretic therapy is generally initiated in the first few days after transplantation and the central venous pressure maintained at 5–12 mmHg. If the patient has low or no urine output, or has a steep increase in serum creatinine, hemodialysis should be considered early for volume management and renal replacement therapy.

OUTCOME

Approximately 85–90% of patients survive 1 year after heart transplantation, with a 3-year survival rate of 75%. Recipient risk factors for early death include older age, female sex, pre-existing liver or renal dysfunction, ischemic or congenital etiology of heart failure, mechanical ventilation, and intra-aortic balloon pump or extracorporeal membrane oxygenation as a bridging modality. Donor risk factors include donor age, ischemic time, left ventricular hypertrophy, and elevated troponin. The most common etiologies of early recipient mortality include graft failure, rejection, and infection. Late mortality is more commonly attributed to allograft vasculopathy, infection, and malignancy. Approximately 90% of surviving patients report no functional limitations at 1 year post-transplant, with 35% returning to work.

FURTHER READING

John R Liao K. Orthotopic heart transplantation. *Oper Tech Thorac Cardiovasc Surg.* 2010; 15: 138–46.

Kilic A, Allen JG, Weiss ES. Validation of the United States-derived Index for Mortality Prediction After Cardiac Transplantation (IMPACT) using international registry data. *J Heart Lung Transplant.* 2013; 32(5): 492–8.

Lund LH, Edwards LB, Kucheryavaya AY, et al. The Registry of the International Society for Heart and Lung Transplantation: Thirtieth Official Adult Heart Transplant Report – 2013; focus theme: age. *J Heart Lung Transplant.* 2013; 32(10): 951–64.

24

Heart–lung transplantation

CHRISTIAN A. BERMUDEZ

HISTORY

The surgical technique of heart and lung transplantation was initially developed by Demikhov and Lower between 1940 and 1960 using canine models, followed by Shumway, Reitz, and colleagues at Stanford University using a primate model that allowed a better understanding of the potential effects of heart–lung transplant surgery in humans. The anatomic and physiologic similarities, such as the absence of the suppression of the respiratory drive post-transplant that was seen in dogs due to ablation of the Hering–Breuer reflex, allowed longer survival and refinement of the surgical technique and postoperative management.

The first clinical heart–lung transplant was performed on August 31, 1968, by Denton Cooley on a 2-month-old patient with a congenital heart disease (CHD) and pulmonary hypertension. The patient survived only a few hours. Further attempts were made without success by Lillehei and Barnard in 1969 and 1971 respectively. It was not until a decade later that the first successful heart–lung transplant surgery was performed by Bruce Reitz and colleagues on March 8, 1981, in a patient suffering from end-stage pulmonary arterial hypertension (PAH). This case was followed by a second successful heart–lung transplant less than a month later by the same team, consolidating the heart–lung transplant procedure.

The first successful heart-lung transplant was the culmination of relentless experimental work by the Stanford group during the 1970s to overcome some of the technical challenges involving the vascular and airway anastomoses, and also immunological obstacles that were, in some way, surmounted by the addition of cyclosporine to improve the immunosuppression regime in 1981. Since then, important experience has been gained, and heart–lung transplant is used for patients with end-stage cardiac and pulmonary disease. More than 3800 patients have received heart–lung transplants worldwide, as reported recently by the International Society for Heart and Lung Transplantation (ISHLT).

Combined heart and lung transplantation was originally considered primarily for patients with advanced end-stage pulmonary vascular disease, which was seen in patients with primary pulmonary hypertension (now known as PAH), and patients with advanced CHD in the form of atrial or ventricular septal defects associated with Eisenmenger syndrome. Heart–lung transplant was also initially widely applied to patients with pulmonary diseases including cystic fibrosis (CF), chronic obstructive pulmonary disease (COPD), and idiopathic pulmonary fibrosis (IPF), because the technique of isolated lung transplantation lagged behind in its development. As lung transplantation techniques became more popular after the first successful series of single-lung transplants reported by Cooper in 1983 and the series of double-lung transplants reported by Patterson and colleagues in 1985, the lung transplant procedure became the preferred treatment for isolated, end-stage pulmonary parenchymal disease, limiting the considerations for heart–lung transplant.

A recent ISHLT report on heart–lung transplant indications, which examined all the heart–lung transplant cases in the ISHLT registry between January 1982 and June 2015 (3733 cases), demonstrated that CHD including Eisenmenger syndrome comprised 35.4%, PAH comprised 27.4%, CF 13.5%, cardiomyopathy 5.7%, COPD 4.2%, interstitial lung diseases 3.9%, and other diagnoses 10%. Most recently (2004–2015), close to 50% of the heart–lung transplants documented in the ISHLT registry were performed in patients with CHD and only 12–14% were in patients with PAH. Due to the increasing experience in lung transplantation and organ shortages, there has been a shift in favor of the use of double-lung transplant for patients with severe PAH who were historically considered candidates, limiting the indications for heart–lung transplant to patients with important anatomic distortion of the pulmonary vasculature or massive right ventricular (RV) dilatation and dysfunction.

A shift away from heart–lung transplantation in favor of lung transplantation has also occurred to a certain extent in patients with restrictive or obstructive lung disease with mild to moderate left ventricular (LV) dysfunction (ejection fraction, EF, over 40%) or with concomitant coronary artery disease (CAD). The ability to perform percutaneous interventions and stenting prior to transplant or concomitant revascularization at the time of lung transplant with bypass grafting has further limited the current indications for heart–lung transplant. These changes are reflected in a steep decrease in heart–lung transplant volumes, with 50 cases performed worldwide in 2014 and 2015 compared with 151 in 1997.

PRINCIPLES AND JUSTIFICATION

The current indications for heart–lung transplant include patients with advanced cardiac and lung diseases not amenable to either isolated heart or isolated lung transplant. Most commonly, patients with irreversible myocardial dysfunction or congenital abnormalities with irreparable defects of the valves or chambers of the heart in conjunction with intrinsic lung disease or severe pulmonary hypertension are considered for heart–lung transplantation. From a functional standpoint, patients considered for heart-lung transplant generally present with New York Heart Association (NYHA) functional class III–IV heart failure, have a life expectancy of less than 2 years, and have no contraindications for transplant.

Determining the timing of transplantation can be challenging, particularly in patients with PAH. However, signs of rapid and progressive clinical and functional deterioration, symptoms of atrial or ventricular arrhythmias, syncopal episodes and indices of RV failure, such as persistent NYHA functional class IV symptoms on maximal medical therapy especially in the presence of a decreased cardiac index of less than 2 liters/min/m^2 and right arterial pressure greater than 15 mmHg, are indications to proceed with transplant listing.

Some patients pose additional challenges when determining if a heart–lung transplant is appropriate. Patients with CHD pose unique challenges, especially patients with cyanotic diseases. The chronic cyanotic conditions seen in pulmonary atresia and other forms of advanced tetralogy of Fallot (TOF) can favor the development of large and diffuse aortopulmonary collaterals that frequently are considered a contraindication to heart–lung transplant due to high bleeding risk. Corrective cardiac surgery with concomitant lung transplant is frequently preferred to a heart–lung transplant in patients with intrinsic cardiac diseases, such as CAD, valvular heart disease, or septal defects without myocardial dysfunction, and with associated intrinsic parenchymal or vascular pulmonary disease requiring transplantation unless the cardiac disease is extensive and requires complex interventions (diffuse CAD or multi-valve disease).

In patients suffering chronic cardiomyopathies and elevated pulmonary vascular resistance (PVR), defined as PVR >5 Woods units, PVR index >6 or a transpulmonary pressure gradient (TPG) >16–20 mmHg, these hemodynamic parameters are considered contraindications to isolated cardiac transplantation, unless they can be reversed (PVR <2.5) with the use of pulmonary vasodilators. Heart–lung transplant is the procedure of choice in these patients.

Of note, and as a historical consideration, heart–lung transplant has also been used as part of the so-called domino procedure that involves implanting a heart–lung block into a patient with end-stage lung disease whose explanted normal heart is then given to an isolated heart transplant candidate. This technique was primarily performed in centers that advocated heart–lung transplantation as opposed to double-lung transplantation for CF and was applied mostly in some European centers. The proponents of this technique suggested that a heart with moderate RV hypertrophy has a better response to pulmonary hypertension and was ideal for a heart recipient with an increased TPG. This procedure has now been mostly abandoned.

PREOPERATIVE ASSESSMENT AND PREPARATION

Donor selection

The donor selection for heart–lung transplantation is based on ABO compatibility, functional characteristics of the donor's heart and lungs, donor size, and immunologic, human lymphocyte antigen (HLA) matching. For pulmonary evaluation, an appropriate X-ray, bronchoscopy, computed tomography (CT) scan, and oxygen challenge should be performed. The absence of major pulmonary infections, aspiration or contusion in the presence of adequate oxygenation (PaO$_2$ >300 mmHg), and lung compliance are the most relevant considerations at the time of donor lung assessment. The cardiac evaluation is based on an echocardiogram, a coronary angiogram in donors older than 45 years or with risk factors for CAD, and hemodynamic parameters of the donor. For heart–lung transplant, donor heart function should be ideally preserved (LV EF >50%), with the absence of significant valve abnormalities, coronary disease, or RV dysfunction and only modest doses of vasoconstrictors should be accepted to maintain donor hemodynamic stability.

The donor-size matching in heart–lung transplant has been less clearly defined than for isolated heart or lung transplant. Our strategy for donor selection in heart–lung transplant is based on matching appropriate lung donor and recipient size using transplantation criteria. We consider an assessment of the donor and recipient chest cavity size using standard measurement of the donor chest with vertical and transverse distances obtained from a recent X-ray that is matched to the recipient's measurements allowing a 10–20% difference depending on the chest wall characteristics. The presence of a severely enlarged heart in the recipient, which is seen in some patients with PAH, may allow oversized lungs in certain circumstances. On the other hand, the absence of chronic pulmonary vascular disease in the donor lungs allows less strict consideration of the standard 25–30% donor–recipient weight difference used to match donors for heart transplantation, allowing some significant cardiac undersizing between donor and recipient in heart–lung transplantation.

Regarding the immunological matching, the presence of donor-specific preformed antihuman lymphocyte antibodies (DSA) is confirmed preoperatively in the recipient. Using the HLA of the donor and history of DSA present in the recipient, a virtual cross-match is performed in case of sensitization, and occasionally a prospective cross-match using donor and recipient blood will be considered, especially in highly sensitized recipients.

ANESTHESIA AND MONITORING

Heart–lung transplantation is performed under general anesthesia. The patient is intubated using a single-lumen or double-lumen endotracheal tube depending on the technique utilized. Patients undergoing the heart–lung transplant through a sternotomy using a tracheal anastomosis require a single-lumen tube, while patients undergoing the procedure through a bilateral thoracosternotomy (clamshell incision) usually are intubated with a left-sided, double-lumen endotracheal tube. In patients with tracheal deformities and occasionally in other patients, a single-lumen tube with a selective endobronchial blocker can be utilized if single-lung ventilation is necessary.

Adequate monitoring is critical during heart–lung transplantation and, ideally, two arterial lines (radial and femoral) are utilized to provide accurate perioperative blood pressure assessment. A continuous output Swan–Ganz catheter is placed in the right internal jugular vein to be advanced following heart–lung block implantation. This catheter provides important information to facilitate postoperative management including pulmonary pressures, cardiac output, and central venous pressure. Transesophageal echocardiogram (TEE) is routinely used to assess postoperative allograft function and confirm adequate cardiac de-airing.

OPERATION

Incisions and surgical approach

MEDIAN STERNOTOMY

The median sternotomy is the original incision used for heart–lung transplant and continues to be used at many centers due to its technical simplicity and lower postoperative pain (**Figure 24.1a and b**). It provides good exposure of the cardiac structures and the pleural cavities in the primary chest cavity, although it can be associated with more difficult exposure of the posterior aspect of the pleural cavities in patients with previous thoracic or cardiac surgery, pleurodesis, or severe adhesions. Median sternotomy has been frequently used in combination with direct tracheal anastomosis to reconstruct the airway, although bilateral sequential bronchial anastomosis can eventually be accomplished with

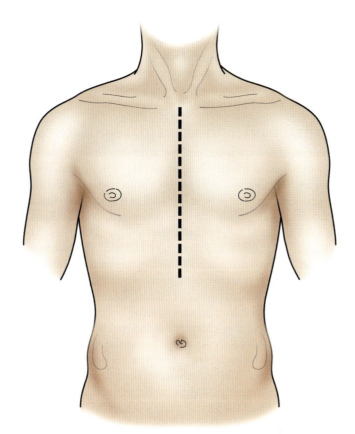

24.1a

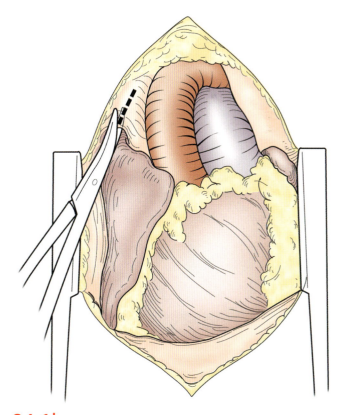

24.1b

the appropriate exposure while on cardiopulmonary bypass (CPB). The need to use a tracheal anastomosis could be considered the "Achilles' heel" of the medial sternotomy approach due to the potential risk of anastomotic complications including dehiscence, which may be present in 25–30% of patients and can be associated with high morbidity and a mortality rate of up to 25%.

BILATERAL THORACOSTERNOTOMY (CLAMSHELL INCISION)

Bilateral thoracosternotomy is currently our approach of choice to perform heart–lung transplant. This approach was adapted from extensive experience with its use in double-lung transplant. The patient is placed in the supine position; their arms can be kept by their sides or can be abducted to facilitate exposure of the posterior hilar structures. The incision includes a submammary bilateral thoracotomy with an axillary extension in the fourth or fifth intercostal spaces and a transverse sternotomy, usually at the level of the fourth intercostal space requiring ligation proximally and distally of both mammary arteries (**Figure 24.2a and b**). Once the chest is entered, the internal thoracotomy is completed posteriorly, sparing the latissimus dorsi and serratus anterior muscles. This incision provides excellent exposure and allows easier dissection of adhesions involving the posterior aspect of the thoracic cavities and reconstruction of the airway using a sequential bibronchial anastomosis. Anastomotic complications are less frequent using bronchial anastomoses (5–15%) than with tracheal anastomoses and can be managed conservatively with chest tubes and occasionally stenting with a lower risk of mortality. The negative aspects associated with the bilateral thoracosternotomy approach are the more frequent presence of acute and chronic postoperative pain complications and sternal malunion or dehiscence in up to 20% of patients and occasionally requiring reinterventions.

PLEURAL INSPECTION

After the chest cavity is entered, the anterior pericardium is opened longitudinally with an inverted-T incision and retracted with 3-0 silk sutures on each side of the pericardial edges. The pleural spaces are entered bilaterally, extending this opening from the innominate vein superiorly and to the pleurodiaphragmatic reflection inferiorly to allow adequate exposure of both pleural cavities and the pulmonary hilum. Mediastinal and pleural adhesions are dissected with an electrocautery. In some cases, pleural adhesion can be highly vascularized, especially in patients with cyanotic CHD or patients with previous pleurodesis, and generally the dissection should be performed as extensively as possible before heparin administration. In these patients, single-lung ventilation using a double-lumen endotracheal tube may facilitate exposure and dissection of the posterior aspect of the chest cavity that otherwise would require prolonged CPB. If a bilateral thoracosternotomy approach is used, we

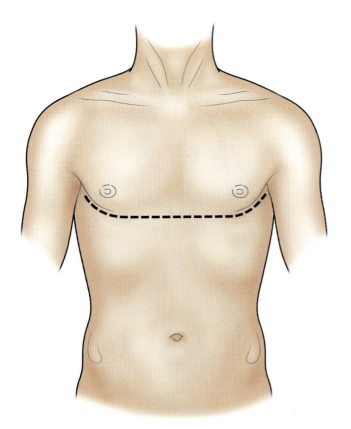

24.2a

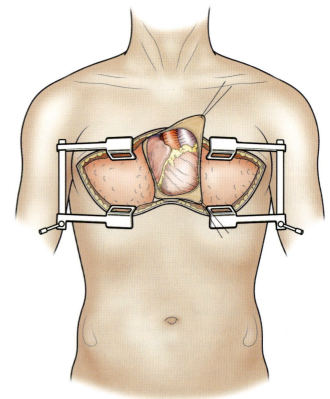

24.2b

would also perform hilar dissection, isolating the pulmonary artery and pulmonary veins individually with umbilical tapes, in preparation for the pneumonectomy as long as the patient tolerates single-lung ventilation. In patients where the sternotomy approach is used and in patients with severe pulmonary hypertension, we prefer to proceed immediately to cannulation and CPB as the exposure is more limited and the patient may not tolerate single-lung ventilation due to severe pulmonary hypertension.

Cannulation for cardiopulmonary bypass

After intravenous heparinization (300 units/kg), the distal aorta or preferably the proximal aortic arch is cannulated using a 20–22 Fr aortic cannula for arterial return. The superior vena cava (SVC) is freed from the pericardial reflection to allow distal cannulation close to the junction with the innominate vein. A 24 Fr venous cannula is inserted in adults. Occasionally, an innominate vein cannulation is necessary using a 20–22 Fr venous cannula when partial or complete obstruction makes SVC access impossible, which is often seen in the presence of chronic implanted cardioverter defibrillator (ICD) leads or multiple internal jugular vein accesses. The inferior vena cava (IVC) is cannulated in the IVC–right atrial (RA) junction using a 32 Fr cannula for venous return. We use this cannulation irrespective of the atrial anastomotic technique planned (biatrial or bicaval) (**Figure 24.3**). After cannulation is completed, the cannulae are secured. When the activated clotting time (ACT) is more than 450 seconds, we initiate CPB, cooling the patient to 30 °C, and ventilation is discontinued.

Recipient cardiectomy

Cardiectomy (removal of the heart) is performed after the initiation of CPB. In cases using the sternotomy approach, we perform cardiectomy first followed by bilateral pneumonectomy. During the dissection of the cardiac structures and pulmonary hilum, it is important to avoid damage to the nerves including the phrenic nerves and left recurrent laryngeal nerve of the recipient. To avoid nerve injury, we use a marker to delineate the positions of the phrenic nerves along the pericardium before we initiate the cardiectomy.

We surround the SVC and IVC with umbilical tapes, separate the aorta from the pulmonary artery, and clamp the distal ascending aorta, proximal to the cannulation site. After snaring the SVC and IVC, we perform a right atrial incision from the RA appendage down the IVC–RA junction and extend this incision into the coronary sinus leaving at least 1–2 cm of space away from the IVC cannula to facilitate the subsequent RA anastomosis. We then transect the ascending aorta at the level of the sinotubular junction and the pulmonary artery 1–2 cm above the pulmonary valve (**Figure 24.4**). After gentle retraction of the heart toward the

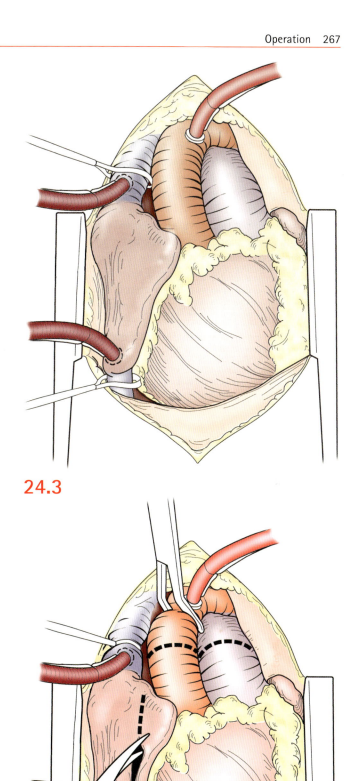

24.3

24.4

left, we open the roof of the left atrium (LA) and follow the posterior aspect annulus of the mitral valve (atrioventricular groove), connecting this incision to the incision originated previously on the coronary sinus (**Figure 24.5**). The heart is then removed from the pericardial cavity.

After completing the cardiectomy, we complete the dissection of the posterior pericardium and intrapericardial vascular structures. The posterior wall of the LA is divided medially and carefully dissected bilaterally to the posterior pericardial reflection (**Figure 24.6a**). It is important to maintain visualization of the previously marked phrenic nerve to avoid injury. The plane between the aorta and pulmonary artery is dissected superiorly allowing mobilization of these structures. The pulmonary artery is divided at its bifurcation, and a circular pulmonary artery patch is created at the level of the insertion of the ligamentum arteriosus (dimple) to avoid injury to the left recurrent laryngeal nerve that travels under the aortic arch in proximity to the ligamentum. A patch of at least 1 cm is created at the insertion of the ligamentum, avoiding use of the electrocautery (**Figure 24.6a, b and c**). At this point, we need to determine the method of anastomosis to reconstruct the RA during donor heart implantation.

In the case of biatrial anastomosis, the RA cuff is left intact and mobilized away from the LA to allow the mobilization and passage of the right lung through a posterior pericardial opening made later, after the right pneumonectomy is completed (**Figure 24.7a–c**). In our center, we prefer to perform bicaval venous anastomosis. In these cases, the SVC is transected with an electrocautery at the SVC–RA junction and mobilized superiorly. The IVC is transected 2 cm above the IVC cannulation site, usually at the IVC–RA junction, and then is mobilized away from the LA (**Figure 24.8**). The remnant of the RA cuff is dissected from the LA with an electrocautery and removed. A silk suture is placed at the 12 o'clock position on the SVC and IVC to guide the suture line during cardiac implantation. After completing the dissection of the cardiac and vascular structures that will be anastomosed during heart–lung block implantation (i.e. the aorta, SVC and IVC, or the RA cuff), we focus our attention to the right and left pulmonary hilar structures to complete the bilateral pneumonectomy and the dissection of the trachea in the posterior pericardium if a tracheal anastomosis is planned.

Bilateral pneumonectomy

Bilateral pneumonectomy is initiated by exposing the right hilum with gentle retraction of the pericardium using the traction sutures. The phrenic nerves have been previously marked bilaterally. Using blunt dissection and electrocautery at low energy, we dissect the pulmonary artery and pulmonary veins individually and mobilize them away from the pericardium. We then isolate the bronchus proximal to the bifurcation. Using blunt dissection with a peanut sponge, we mobilize the vagus nerve in the posterior aspect

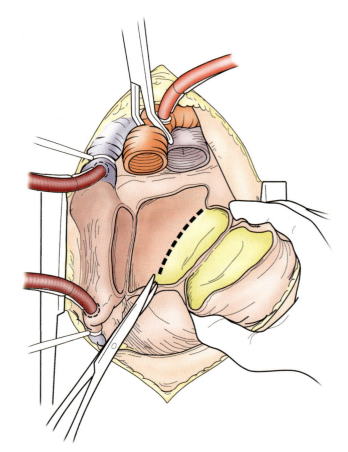

24.5

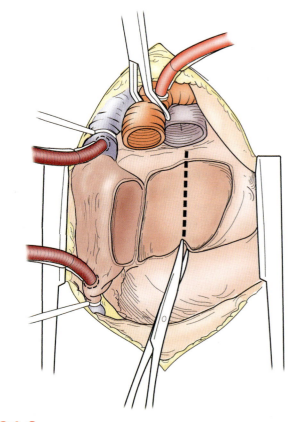

24.6a

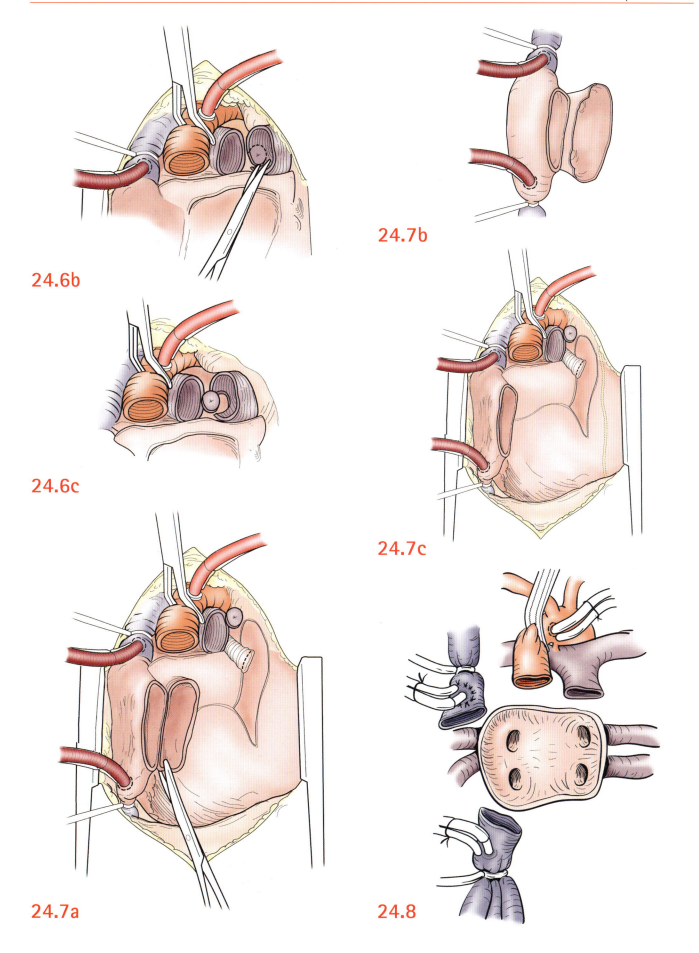

24.6b

24.6c

24.7a

24.7b

24.7c

24.8

of the hilum to avoid injury. At this point, we open a relatively wide incision in the pericardial reflection below the phrenic nerve. Careful attention is needed to perform this incision as the phrenic nerve on the right lies in close proximity to the hilum and follows a more posterior direction to the right diaphragm. We complete transection of the right bronchus using a TA30 stapler, cutting distal to it to avoid contamination of the field. We previously mobilized the pulmonary artery, pulmonary veins, and atrial cuff, and at this point we are able to complete the pneumonectomy (**Figure 24.9a**).

A similar technique is used on the left side. We place some traction on the pericardial sutures and complete the dissection of the left hilum using a combination of blunt dissection and low-energy electrocautery, always maintaining the phrenic nerve under direct visualization to avoid injury. In general, this nerve follows a higher course on the right side. We also open a moderate-size pericardial incision 2 cm below the phrenic nerve to allow the passage of the left donor lung into the left chest cavity. This pericardial opening on the left size should allow the mobilization and passage of the left donor lung but a large opening should be avoided or a partial closure after completing block implantation should be considered to avoid postoperative cardiac or pulmonary herniation. After isolating and transecting the bronchus using a TA30 stapler, we mobilize the remnant of the left pulmonary vein cuff and left pulmonary artery and complete the pneumonectomy (**Figure 24.9b**). Careful hemostasis should be performed in the posterior hilum and pulmonary ligaments bilaterally as these are common sources of postoperative bleeding and hemothorax.

After completing the pneumonectomy, we address the dissection and preparation of the trachea if tracheal anastomosis is considered. We open an incision of the posterior pericardium between the aorta and SVC. We use an electrocautery to make a transverse opening in the envelope of soft tissues surrounding the tracheal carina (**Figure 24.10**). This incision should be made as low as possible to maintain the blood supply to the distal trachea. The distal carina and the bronchial stumps are skeletonized by blunt dissection. The vagus nerves are close to the posterior wall of the trachea and its bifurcation, so only minor traction should be applied and electrocautery use should be minimized to avoid nerve injury. At this point, the dissection of the mediastinum is completed and careful hemostasis should be obtained.

In patients where a bibronchial anastomosis (our preferred approach) is planned, the mediastinum and trachea are left intact as the bronchial anastomosis will be performed outside the pericardial cavity, using the same technique used during double-lung transplant. After completing the pneumonectomy bilaterally, only the bronchus is left on the hilum. We avoid proximal dissection and manipulation and perform careful hemostasis, ligating the bronchial arteries

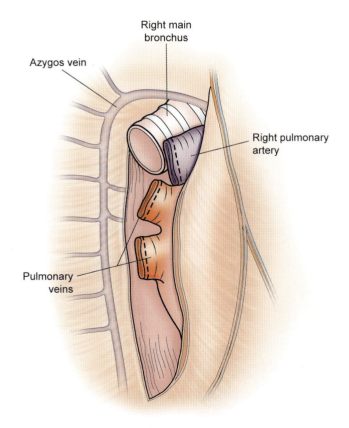

24.9a

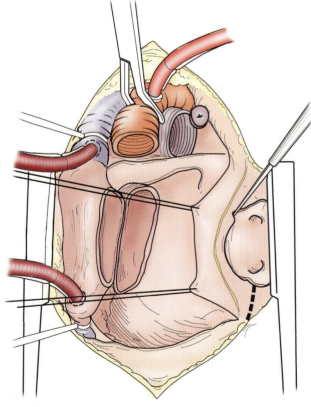

24.9b

SVC should be closed using 4-0 polypropylene continuous suture.

The only other structures requiring preparation are the trachea (in cases with tracheal anastomosis) and both bronchi in the cases with sequential bibronchial anastomosis. The trachea is transected 2 cm above the donor carina and, after careful suction of the donor airway and gentle lavage with saline solution, the trachea is finally trimmed leaving one or two cartilage rings (**Figure 24.11**). In the cases of bibronchial anastomosis, we remove the stapler suture line on the right and left donor bronchi and perform careful suction of secretions and lavage with 10 mL of saline solution. We then cut the donor bronchi leaving two rings above the lobar takeoff.

After completing preparation of the donor block, the organs are left in a container covered with ice. Attention is directed to the preparation of the recipient's trachea or bronchi that have been left, to this point, closed with staples to avoid mediastinal or chest contamination.

Preparation of the recipient trachea or bronchus for implantation

Once the heart–lung block is ready for implantation, the recipient's trachea is opened just above the carina using a 15 scalpel blade. The incision is continued with scissors in the cartilaginous segment. The membranous portion is

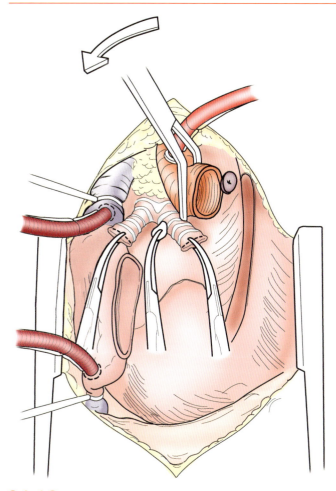

24.10

with hemoclips. The stapler suture lines in the bronchus are left until the heart–lung block has been positioned in the chest.

Preparation of the donor heart–lung block

Preparation of the heart–lung block is relatively simple as most structures are left intact during procurement. After a careful inspection to assess possible harvesting injuries, we remove the excess pericardium to facilitate visualization of the pulmonary hilum, especially when the bibronchial technique is considered. The donor's aorta is left long by transecting below the donor's innominate artery. Different from the preparation of donor hearts for isolated heart transplantation, the pulmonary artery is preserved during procurement for a heart–lung transplant as is the entire LA. No preparation of these structures is needed.

When bicaval anastomosis is planned, the donor IVC and SVC are left intact. Patent foramen ovale (PFO) should be identified and closed with 4-0 polypropylene suture. If a biatrial anastomosis is planned at the time of implant, an oblique incision going to the middle of the RA is performed originating from the IVC and directed to the edge of the RA appendage (**Figure 24.11**). In these cases, the

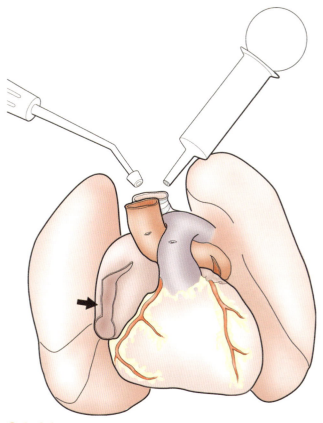

24.11

sectioned, avoiding traction on the stump that would lead to a retraction of this membranous segment. It is important to avoid the use of electrocautery and extensive manipulation of the stump to preserve the limited tracheal-stump blood supply. After the sectioning of the trachea is completed, the carina is excised (**Figure 24.12a and b**).

In cases where bibronchial anastomosis is performed, we have found that it is easier to prepare both bronchial stumps before placing the heart–lung block in the field due to the limited exposure. We cover one of them with gauze until the first anastomosis is completed. The bronchi are opened proximal to the stapler suture line using an angled scalpel at the desired length. On the right side, we prefer to cut two or three rings from the carina. During this preparation, the mediastinal lymph nodes are liberated such that a safe anastomosis may be performed. The bronchial arteries are ligated with cautery and clips to prevent significant bleeding. Denudation of the recipient bronchus should be avoided to prevent ischemic complications. Any secretions within the bronchus are suctioned liberally, and the double-lumen endotracheal tube is adjusted appropriately.

Implantation of the heart–lung block

With the cardiectomy and pneumonectomy completed and with an empty thorax (**Figure 24.13**), the donor heart–lung block is brought into the chest cavity. First, the right lung is passed under the right pericardial opening underneath the phrenic nerve. If the RA cuff has been maintained (**Figure 24.14a and b**), the right lung should gently be maneuvered to pass under it and through the pericardial opening. The surgeon sustains the heart with his/her left hand and then passes the left lung through the pericardial opening into the left chest cavity, while the assistant retracts the pericardial traction sutures. The orientation of the different pulmonary lobes should be checked carefully to avoid torsion. Partially closing the left pericardial opening should be considered at this point to avoid postoperative cardiac herniation. With the heart–lung block in position, we then cover the heart and lungs with ice slush.

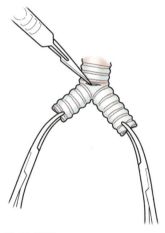

24.12a

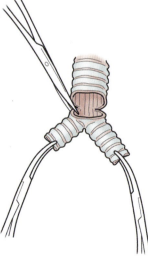

24.12b

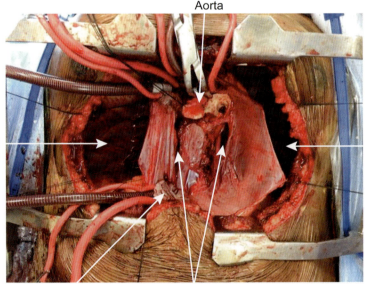

Aorta

Right chest cavity

Left chest cavity

Inferior vena cava   Pericardial openings

24.13

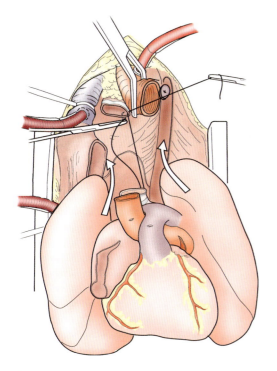

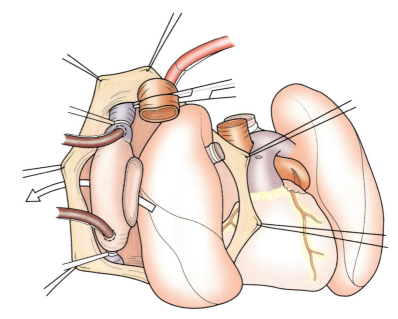

24.14a   **24.14b**

Airway anastomosis

TRACHEAL ANASTOMOSIS

A silk traction suture is placed in the donor aorta to move it downwards and provide exposure to complete the tracheal anastomosis (**Figure 24.15**). The tracheal anastomosis is performed using a 3-0 polypropylene suture starting from the left cartilage–membranous transition area. This running, posterior suture line continues throughout the membranous part of the trachea and follows the anterior cartilaginous suture line. Once the tracheal anastomosis is completed, the donor and recipient peritracheal soft tissue is approximated with a 3-0 polypropylene suture to cover the anastomosis. The anesthesiologist performs a bronchoscopy, aspirates residual blood and secretions, and performs an inspection of the anastomosis to confirm that it is free from defects. We usually do not ventilate to test the anastomosis as a significant gap should be easily observed by bronchoscopy. We would only use a ventilation test if any doubts persist.

BRONCHIAL ANASTOMOSIS

When a bronchial anastomosis is planned, the trachea is not manipulated, and the bronchial anastomoses are sequentially performed similar to a standard double-lung transplant protocol. The donor and recipient bronchi have been previously prepared. After placing the heart–lung block in the chest, the bronchial anastomoses are completed first using a running 3-0 polypropylene suture that begins with the membranous portion of the airway and ends anteriorly on the cartilaginous portion. Each anastomosis is performed in an end-to-end fashion taking great care to

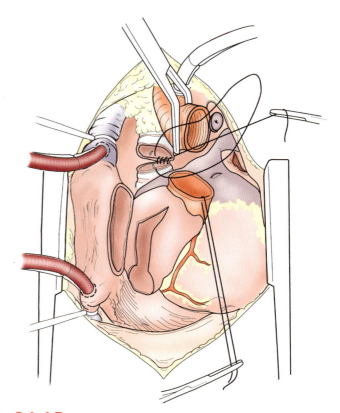

24.15

achieve membranous-to-membranous and cartilaginous-to-cartilaginous apposition (**Figure 24.16a and b**). After completing the anastomosis, we reinforce the suture line at the 10 o'clock and 2 o'clock positions with two additional 3-0 polypropylene sutures, which are also used to attach peribronchial tissue and pericardium to cover the anastomosis. The anastomoses are inspected using bronchoscopy to confirm indemnity of the suture line and proper orientation of the donor and recipient bronchi.

Right atrial reconstruction: biatrial and bicaval techniques

RIGHT ATRIAL ANASTOMOSIS (BIATRIAL TECHNIQUE)

For RA anastomosis using the biatrial technique, the donor SVC is closed with a 4-0 polypropylene suture. An RA opening, made during the block preparation from the lateral aspect of the IVC toward the RA appendage, is matched to the recipient RA cuff. The RA anastomosis is performed with a continuous 3-0 polypropylene suture line starting in the superior and posterior aspect of the anastomosis (**Figure 24.17**). This anastomosis should be performed with care taken to avoid significant stretch and deformation of the RA of the donor heart.

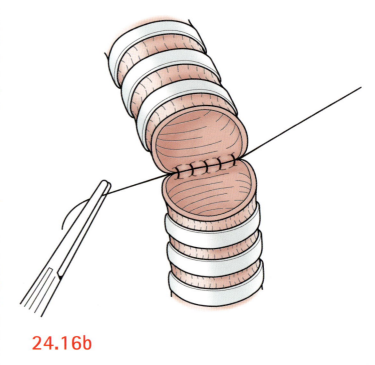

24.16b

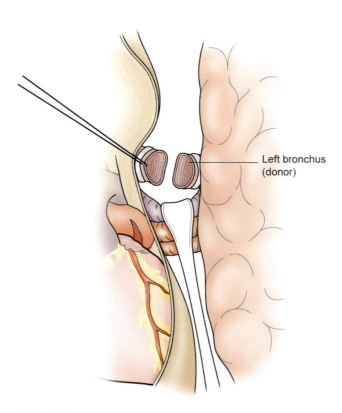

Left bronchus (donor)

24.16a

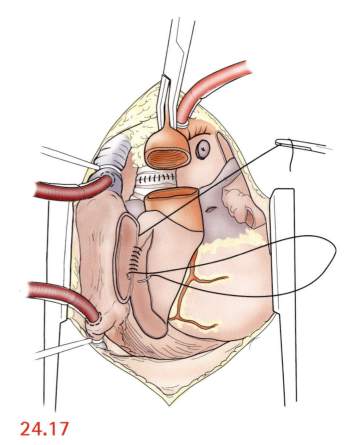

24.17

SVC-IVC ANASTOMOSIS (BICAVAL TECHNIQUE)

SVC–IVC anastomosis (the bicaval technique) is our preferred method of RA reconstruction and has been associated with decreases in recipient atrial arrhythmias, heart blockages, and tricuspid regurgitation and allows easier access to perform endomyocardial biopsies. When using the bicaval technique, it is important to preserve an adequate IVC cuff during the cardiectomy in the recipient and adequate SVC length. During the cardiectomy, we place a silk traction suture at the 12 o'clock position on the recipient's IVC. We start the anastomosis at the donor's 3 o'clock position, which usually corresponds to the coronary sinus, completing the posterior suture line first and anterior suture line afterwards. The SVC anastomosis requires adequate matching, length, and positioning to avoid torsion. We use a single continuous 4-0 or 5-0 polypropylene suture starting at the 3 o'clock position on the recipient side and create the posterior suture line first, completing the anterior suture line with the opposite suture, and intermittently locking this anastomosis to prevent a pursestring effect (**Figure 24.18**).

Aortic anastomosis

When creating the aortic anastomosis, the donor and recipient aortas are aligned, such that the neoaorta will be long enough to mobilize and repair posterior anastomotic bleeding sites.

We have learned that leaving this neoaorta longer decreases tension on the suture lines and the risk of postoperative bleeding. While we rewarm the patient to 37 °C, we perform the aortic anastomosis with a 4-0 polypropylene continuous suture. We start this suture line at the 5 o'clock position on the recipient's aorta, continue with the posterior suture line, and complete the anterior suture line with the opposite suture (**Figure 24.19**).

Reperfusion and de-airing

De-airing is an important step in the reperfusion process as massive amounts of air can produce not just systemic embolism but also coronary embolism after aortic clamp removal. After finishing the aortic anastomosis, we place an aortic root vent and a cardioplegia line. We place a vent in the right superior pulmonary vein into the LV. We give 1000 mL of warm-blood reperfusion through the ascending aorta and simultaneously place a vent in the proximal pulmonary artery, which will be used later to reperfuse the lungs while rewarming and reperfuse the patient before coming off CPB.

The patient is placed in the Trendelenburg position, and the IVC and SVC snares are removed, filling the heart. The Valsalva maneuver is performed, the aortic clamp is removed, and reperfusion is initiated. All vents are functionally maintained. Next, we connect the pulmonary vent

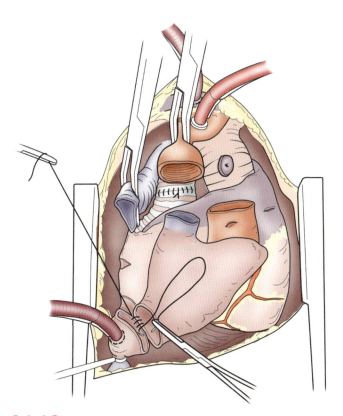

24.18

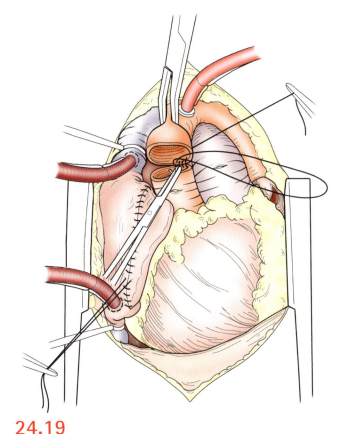

24.19

cannula (15–17 Fr) to the cardioplegia circuit to provide 500 mL/min of blood while we reperfuse the heart–lung block and rewarm the patient.

Temporary pacing wires are secured to the donor RA and inferior wall of the RV and brought out through the skin below the incision. The heart is paced to maintain a heart rate of 90–110 beats/min. Ventilation is initiated at a rate of 16–18 respirations/min using a tidal volume of 5–6 mL/kg of the donor weight and FiO_2 between 40% and 50%. Inotropic support is started with low to moderate doses of inotropes including epinephrine, milrinone, and isoproterenol or as per center protocol. We have also liberally used nitric oxide (NO), starting at 20–40 ppm, to improve the oxygenation–perfusion mismatch seen early after lung transplant.

After adequate organ reperfusion has been obtained and cardiac contractility is vigorous, we discontinue pulmonary artery perfusion and remove the cannula in preparation to wean off CPB. We fill the heart and assess residual cardiac air pockets using TEE. We then remove the right superior pulmonary vent and maintain the root vent. When the patient is normothermic, we remove the patient from CPB. Overdistension of the heart must be avoided at this stage.

After confirming adequate cardiac and pulmonary function by TEE and adequate arterial blood gases, we remove the venous cannulae and reverse the heparin using protamine sulfate (3 mg/kg). Blood products, including fresh frozen plasma, cryoprecipitate, and platelets, are transfused to revert the coagulopathy frequently seen after this extensive procedure. Finally, the aortic cannula is removed.

Chest closure

An adequate number and adequate positioning of chest tubes to enable detection of postoperative bleeding and prevent cardiac tamponade or hemothorax is crucial before chest closure. If the sternotomy approach was used, we place two chest tubes posteriorly and two mediastinal drains. The pleural tubes include a 32 Fr right-angle tube on the posterior costophrenic angle and a 24 Fr Blake drain following the paravertebral gutter to the apex of the pleural cavity. Mediastinal drainage includes a 32 Fr anterior drain toward the RA and a second drain posteriorly in the diaphragmatic surface of the pericardium toward the apex. If a bilateral thoracosternotomy and bibronchial anastomoses were performed, we add a 28 Fr chest tube that sits anterior to the pulmonary hilum on each side.

The longitudinal sternotomy is closed using standard techniques with 6–7 stainless steel wires, or the bilateral thoracosternotomy (clamshell incision) is closed using interrupted 5 poly-suture (ethylene, terephthalate) in a figure-eight fashion. The sternum is approximated using three 6 sternal wires. The pectoral fascial layer, the subcutaneous layer, the subdermal layer, and the skin are reapproximated with absorbable sutures and staples for skin closure. If the lungs are oversized or if there is significant primary graft dysfunction (PGD) or hemodynamic instability, we do not hesitate to the leave the chest open.

If a double-lumen endotracheal tube was used during the operation, this tube is exchanged for a single-lumen endotracheal tube. Bronchoscopy is performed for pulmonary toilet immediately post-procedure. A nasoenteric feeding tube is also placed at this time with the added benefit of placement with endoscopic control of the airway to avoid the inadvertent placement of the feeding tube within the airway.

POSTOPERATIVE CARE

Early postoperative care after a heart–lung transplant must focus on the maintenance of hemodynamic stability, adequate organ perfusion, and prevention of ischemia–reperfusion injury of the heart and lungs, which usually presents early post-transplant as cardiac dysfunction, pulmonary failure with hypoxemia, and pulmonary edema, or a combination of both. Patients are kept sedated and mechanically ventilated with close monitoring of all hemodynamic parameters for the first 6–12 hours post-transplant. Generally, a mean arterial pressure >65–70 mmHg is desirable, with a central venous pressure maintained between 8–15 mmHg. Low to moderate doses of epinephrine, isoproterenol, milrinone, and vasopressin are utilized in different combinations. In our center, a combination of epinephrine (0.03–0.1 mcg/kg/min) and milrinone (0.125–0.5 mcg/kg/min) is initiated intraoperatively for inotropic support, and low-dose isoproterenol (0.01–0.02 mcg/kg/min) is administered for its chronotropic effects. The goal cardiac index should be >2.2 L/min/m². A progressive deterioration in the cardiac index may be the first sign of early cardiac allograft dysfunction, intrathoracic bleeding, an undrained hemothorax, or tamponade and should be rapidly assessed with TEE and chest X-ray to define the etiology and manage accordingly.

Ventilation is performed using protective lung ventilation strategies with low tidal volume (5–6 mL/kg), a high respiration rate (16–20 respirations/min), positive end-expiratory pressure (PEEP) between 10–15 cm H_2O, and the lowest FiO_2 possible to maintain a PaO_2 of >80 mmHg. Ideally, we try to keep the FiO_2 between 40% and 50%, if tolerated. This theoretically avoids the risk of free-radical-induced oxygen toxicity. Increases in oxygen requirements to maintain target oxygenation with a PaO_2 above 70 mmHg and requiring FiO_2 greater than 80% in the presence of bilateral and increasing infiltrates on the X-ray may be signs of PGD. These changes require close observation as they may rapidly progress to the need for extracorporeal membrane oxygenation, which is our preferred method of postoperative allograft support for PGD.

There is a fine balance between adequate fluid resuscitation and fluid overload that may affect lung function, and this will depend on the clinical course of the patient. Although historically we have tried to keep patients who have undergone a lung transplant "dry," avoiding excessive fluid administration, it is not advisable to liberally increase inotropes and vasoconstrictors as this may affect end-organ function and increase the risk of renal failure and, most importantly, the risk of airway ischemia leading to the feared complication of tracheal necrosis and dehiscence, which carries an elevated morbidity and mortality. For this reason, we usually provide adequate fluid to maintain normal hemodynamics and avoid the liberal use of vasoconstrictors. If pulmonary allograft function is marginal, we do try to minimize fluid administration.

Weaning from mechanical ventilation occurs after hemodynamic stabilization has been obtained, usually 12–24 hours post-transplant in the absence of active bleeding, residual hemothorax, or signs of cardiac dysfunction or pulmonary hypertension. NO is discontinued in a slow and progressive fashion on postoperative day 2 as rebound pulmonary hypertension can occur and lead to RV dysfunction.

It is important to consider that allograft dysfunction can occur intraoperatively and also later (24–72 hours after the procedure), affecting the heart, the lungs, or both. In general, the progression of dysfunction of one organ will invariably affect the other organ to some extent, making it difficult at times to differentiate the culprit. The recommended mechanism to support the patient in the presence of severe allograft dysfunction is venoarterial extracorporeal membrane oxygenation allowing simultaneous cardiac and pulmonary support. Generally, this is performed centrally with cannulation in the RA and ascending aorta.

Immunosuppression

Our immunosuppression protocol is initiated in the operating room at the time of anesthesia induction with basiliximab, a chimeric mouse–human monoclonal antibody specific for the IL-2 receptor of the T cell (20 mg i.v.; with a second dose on postoperative day 4). Methylprednisolone (Solu-Medrol, 1000 mg i.v.) is given after reperfusion of the allograft.

Postoperative immunosuppression is initiated in the ICU and includes tacrolimus administered orally (0.1 mg/kg/day, divided in two doses) started within 24 hours to maintain serum levels of 12–15 mcg/L, accompanied by mycophenolate mofetil (1000 mg, orally, twice a day). Methylprednisolone (Solu-Medrol) is initiated after ICU admission in a dose of 125 mg i.v. three times a day and is then tapered and replaced by oral prednisone, which is also tapered over the next 2 weeks until a 20 mg dose is reached. Modifications to the standard immunosuppression regimen using lymphocytic induction with rabbit antithymocyte globulin (rATG) and plasmapheresis, intraoperatively and/or postoperatively, are used in highly sensitized patients.

OUTCOME

Outcomes after heart–lung transplant have improved over time and continue to have a close correlation with the transplant-center expertise and experience in the management of these complex patients. The ISHLT 33rd Adult Lung and Heart–Lung Transplant Report (2016) recently detailed the outcomes of 3775 primary heart–lung transplants performed between 1982 and 2014. The recipients had survival rates of 71% 3 months post-transplant, 63% 1 year post-transplant, 52% 3 years post-transplant, 45% 5 years post-transplant, and 32% 10 years post-transplant. Survival after heart–lung transplant has improved with transplant era, such that median survival for patients transplanted in the last decade has improved to 5.8 years with a median survival of more than 10 years conditional on survival 1 year after transplant. In comparison with lung-only transplantation, primary heart–lung transplantation has a more pronounced early mortality but better long-term survival. When survival after heart–lung transplant is stratified by diagnosis, younger patients transplanted for CF, PAH, or CHD have better survival as compared with those transplanted for COPD or cardiomyopathy.

For heart–lung transplant recipients who have the two most common diagnostic indications (CHD and PAH), the most common identifiable causes of death in the first 30 days post-transplant are graft failure (lung or heart) and technical complications. After the first year, obliterative bronchiolitis (OB)/bronchiolitis obliterans syndrome (BOS), late graft failure (lung or heart), and non-CMV (cytomegalovirus) infections are the most common causes of mortality. Cardiovascular causes of death account for a small but important proportion of deaths.

The Stanford group recently reviewed their experience with acute allograft rejection and reported that at 5 years post-transplant only 33.8% of the patients were still free from acute lung rejection, whereas 66.7% were free from acute heart rejection; both rejection curves plateaued after 5 years. In their experience, the number of rejection episodes within the first year was highly predictive of patient outcome. Median survival significantly decreased from 8.6 years with no rejection episodes to 7.2 years with one rejection episode, 3.1 years with two rejection episodes, 1.3 years after three rejection episodes, and 1.1 years after four rejection episodes.

The tools for diagnosing acute rejection have changed over the years. Initially, sequential endomyocardial biopsies of the transplanted heart were analyzed to monitor graft rejection, and rejection of the lung was assumed when cardiac rejection was diagnosed. Since the late 1990s, fiber-optic bronchoscopy with transbronchial lung biopsy has become the standard diagnostic tool to diagnose acute lung rejection, turning the focus to the more susceptible organ: the lung. Biased by this development, heart rejection was diagnosed in 45.7% of rejection episodes in the 1980s and in only 16.5% of rejection episodes in the 1990s. Overall, the heart seems to be protected by the lung grafts; pulmonary infiltration usually precedes or prevents myocardial infiltration.

Lung allograft dysfunction (e.g. OB/BOS) plays a significant role in the causes of late death, a unique feature of heart–lung transplant recipients as compared with heart transplant recipients. OB represents chronic rejection of the pulmonary allograft and has shown strong correlations with early CMV infection and clinical or subclinical episodes of cellular and antibody-mediated rejection. At earlier stages, OB may respond to augmentation of immunosuppression but, unfortunately, once OB is established, there is no effective treatment available and deterioration is progressive.

In contrast with heart transplantation, cardiac allograft vasculopathy is a less common problem after heart–lung transplant, accounting for 2–4% of late deaths. Vasculopathy invariably occurs in patients who have already developed advanced OB. In heart–lung transplant recipients, coronary artery vasculopathy (CAV) occurs less frequently than BOS. One year after heart–lung transplantation, 8% of recipients develop BOS in comparison with 3% who develop CAV. After 3 years, 27% of recipients develop BOS in comparison with 7% who develop CAV. After 5 years , 42% develop BOS and 9% develop CAV, and 10 years after heart–lung transplant 62% of patients have BOS and only 27% have developed CAV.

In summary, heart–lung transplantation is an established treatment option for patients suffering from cardiopulmonary disease who are not candidates for isolated heart or lung transplant. When performed at an experienced center, the outcomes in the most recent era have been associated with up to 40% survival 10 years post-transplant with excellent quality of life. Unfortunately, as the number of patients considered for thoracic organ transplant has increased and organ availability continues to be limited, the current allocation systems have favored single-organ transplantation, limiting the options for patients requiring a heart–lung transplant. As a consequence, we have seen a pronounced decline in the number of heart–lung transplants performed worldwide. A reassessment of the current allocation policies and a better understanding of techniques to improve organ utilization in marginal donors may allow transplantation to an increasing number of patients requiring both a heart and lungs.

FURTHER READING

Deuse T, Sista R, Weill D, et al. Review of heart-lung transplantation at Stanford. *Ann Thorac Surg.* 2010; 90(1): 329–37.

Griffith BP, Magliato KE. Heart-lung transplantation. *Oper Tech Thorac Cardiovasc Surg.* 1999; 4(2): 124–41.

Weill D, Benden C, Corris PA, et al. A consensus document for the selection of lung transplant candidates – 2014; an update from the Pulmonary Transplantation Council of the International Society for Heart and Lung Transplantation. *J Heart Lung Transplant.* 2015; 34(1): 1–15.

Yusen RD, Edwards LB, Dipchand AI, et al. The Registry of the International Society for Heart and Lung Transplantation: Thirty-third Adult Lung and Heart-Lung Transplant Report – 2016; Focus theme: Primary diagnostic indications for transplant. *J Heart Lung Transplant.* 2016; 35(10): 1170–84.

Yusen RD, Edwards LB, Kucheryavaya AY, et al. The Registry of the International Society for Heart and Lung Transplantation: Thirty-second Official Adult Lung and Heart-Lung Transplantation Report – 2015; Focus theme: Early graft failure. *J Heart Lung Transplant.* 2015; 34(10): 1264–77.

25

Lung transplantation

EDWARD CANTU

HISTORY

The first reported technical success in human lung transplantation occurred in 1963 by James Hardy at the University of Mississippi. Following this report, it was apparent that results were extremely limited, with significant perioperative mortality. This did not change until 1983 when Joel Cooper and his team at Toronto General Hospital performed the first clinically successful lung transplant. This clinical success established lung transplantation as an effective treatment for patients with end-stage lung disease. Since that time, there has been tremendous progress with surgical techniques, donor organ preservation, organ perfusion techniques, and peri- and postoperative care.

PRINCIPLES AND JUSTIFICATION

The decision to list a candidate for lung transplant is complex and takes into consideration not only clinical but psychosocial and programmatic factors. In general, lung transplant is considered in patients with end-stage lung disease who have a greater than 50% risk of death within 2 years of their lung disease and greater than 80% likelihood of surviving 3 months after transplant and 5 years from non-lung-related medical problems.

Absolute contraindications to candidacy include active or recent (<2–5 year interval) malignancy, multi-organ system dysfunction (unless planned combined transplant is planned), uncorrectable myocardial ischemia risk, uncorrectable bleeding diathesis, chronic infection with highly virulent organisms, psychosocial factors that limit adherence to complex medical regimen, BMI greater than 35, and severely limited functional status. Many other relative contraindications have been suggested and are further discussed in the International Society for Heart and Lung Transplantation (ISHLT) consensus guidelines; however, it must be understood that evidence for these contraindications is limited and guidelines are based on expert opinion. Centers can and do sometimes make exceptions to these guidelines depending on individual circumstances.

Decisions regarding type of transplant procedure (single versus bilateral) depend on patient characteristics. Although the majority of patients with non-infectious lung diseases and without pulmonary hypertension can safely receive a single lung transplant, bilateral lung transplantation is the preferred procedure for the majority of candidates. Single lung transplant is preferred when patient characteristics suggest perioperative mortality is too high for bilateral, survival advantage is not clear with bilateral, or the candidate's condition precludes further waiting.

Conversations with candidates should always include the risks involved from both lifelong immunosuppression and surgical complications. Although immunosuppressive regimens have improved, there remains the risk of diabetes, osteoporosis, hypertension, hyperlipidemia, renal injury and failure, gastrointestinal effects, infection, and malignancy. This is in addition to the risks of the procedure, which include hemorrhage, stroke, primary graft dysfunction, acute kidney injury, phrenic nerve injury, airway stricture/dehiscence, pneumonia, and death.

PREOPERATIVE ASSESSMENT AND PREPARATION

Transplant candidates are among the most diagnostically evaluated patients in all of cardiothoracic surgery. Though a comprehensive review of the diagnostic workup is beyond the scope of this chapter, there are a few critical diagnostic findings that would alter operative planning and should be considered.

Patients identified to have severe pulmonary hypertension are at exceedingly high risk of arrest at induction of anesthesia. In our practice, these patients are not induced until the surgeon is in the room and femoral arterial and venous catheters have been placed. Significant pleural calcification and scar suggest that pneumonectomy will be challenging. In these instances, we anticipate prolonged explant and commonly use the argon beam to control hemorrhage. Identification of a patent foramen ovale or less commonly atrial septal defect may require repair (significant shunt flow), which might require altering cannulation strategy. Additional findings of significantly calcified or diseased femoral vessels would preclude peripheral cannulation strategies for transplant.

ANESTHESIA

Anesthetic agents and techniques are similar to those typically used in open heart procedures. Required access includes large-bore intravenous access, a pulmonary artery (PA) catheter, and a radial arterial catheter. Decisions regarding site of placement should be made in the context of the transplant to be performed, donor lung quality, and predicted risk of required post-transplant mechanical support. For example, for a left single lung transplant the radial arterial catheter is placed on the right; in a recipient who will require extracorporeal membrane oxygenation (ECMO) post-transplant the PA catheter is placed on the left internal jugular vein.

Because the left bronchus is longer than the right and misplacement of endotracheal tubes is less frequent, our practice is to use left-sided double-lumen endotracheal tubes in all cases. Fiber-optic bronchoscopic confirmation of tube placement is required. In situations where tube placement is not possible, single-lumen tube placement with the use of bronchial blockers and tube repositioning can be used for lung isolation. However, in these circumstances the surgical team should be aware that isolation may not be ideal and ECMO/cardiopulmonary bypass may be needed.

Intraoperative management of lung transplant recipients is complex and requires continuous communication between surgeons and anesthesiologists. General principles during the procedure include minimization of crystalloids, liberal use of inotropes to maintain hemodynamics, and maintenance of appropriate red cell volume and clotting factors. Transesophageal echocardiography (TEE) is critical for evaluation of cardiac function and filling to guide decisions regarding use of volume or inotropes.

OPERATION

Positioning and preparation

Decisions for positioning are guided by patient and operative characteristics. Our practice has been to place all patients in a supine position with arm(s) abducted and flexed on a temperature-regulated pad. This allows for standardized bilateral and single lung transplant positioning and preparation that improves operative workflow (**Figure 25.1a and b**). The base of the neck, chest, abdomen, and bilateral groins are prepped and draped into the surgical field. A left femoral arterial line is placed for blood pressure monitoring given the variable reliability of upper extremity arterial monitoring (**Figure 25.1c**). In patients with tenuous cardiopulmonary status, a right femoral venous and left femoral arterial lines can also be placed prior to induction when necessary (**Figure 25.2**).

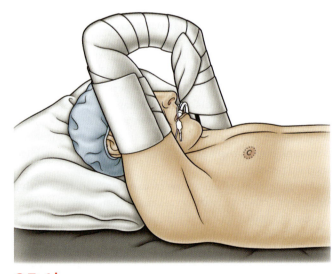

25.1b

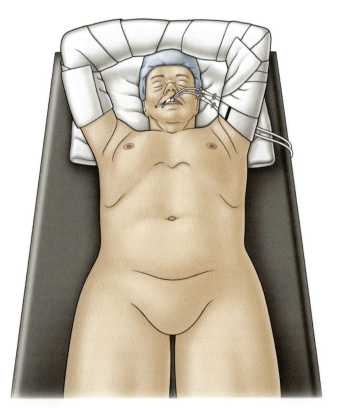

25.1a

Incision and exposure

For single lung transplants an anterior thoracotomy in the fourth or fifth intercostal space is made depending on positioning of the inferior pulmonary vein (typically fourth for restrictive and fifth for obstructive lung diseases). Bilateral lung transplants can be performed through sternal-sparing anterior thoracotomies (**Figure 25.3a**) or through a standard anterior trans-sternal thoracotomy (**Figure 25.3b**). Choice

25.1c

25.2

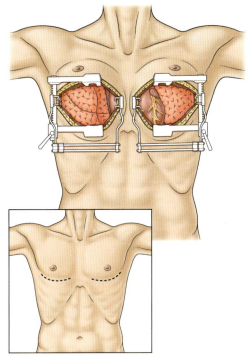

25.3a

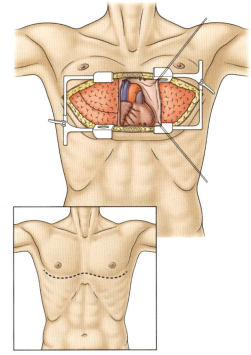

25.3b

of approach is dictated by anticipated need for support and exposure dictated by patient diagnosis. Most commonly, sternal-sparing anterior thoracotomies are used in patients with obstructive diseases and clamshell in patients with restrictive and pulmonary vascular diseases. In women there is a minor modification: the incision is made in the inframammary crease and a flap is raised similar to mastectomy, taking care to carefully control perforators.

Once the incisions are made and entry to the chest has been gained, the intercostal muscles are divided with cautery anteriorly and posteriorly to allow for the placement of retractors. Latissimus and serratus muscles can be spared laterally. If a clamshell is anticipated, the mammary arteries and veins are exposed, clipped, divided, and ligated. The anterior mediastinal pleura is then divided with cautery to the level of the anterior mammary veins. Retractors are placed and adhesions are taken down with cautery. Care should be taken when taking down mediastinal adhesions in close proximity to the phrenic nerve.

In circumstances where additional exposure is required, a figure-eight 0-silk retraction suture can be placed in the membranous dome of the diaphragm and passed through the chest in the most inferiorlateral intercostal space and secured with a small clamp (**Figure 25.4**).

Hilar dissection is begun with retraction from the surgical assistant and lung isolation (**Figure 25.5a and b**). Care is taken to identify and protect the phrenic nerve. Control of the pulmonary veins and PA is established using umbilical tapes. The inferior pulmonary ligament is taken down using cautery. A test occlusion of the PA is performed using a Rummel tourniquet fashioned from a red Robinson catheter

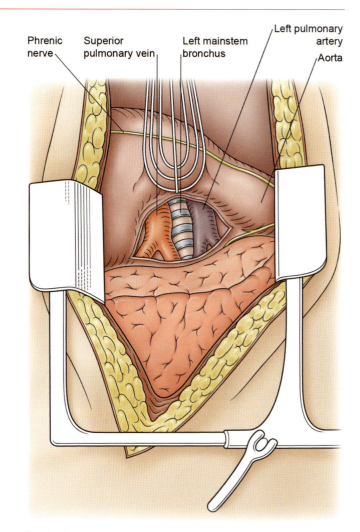

25.5a

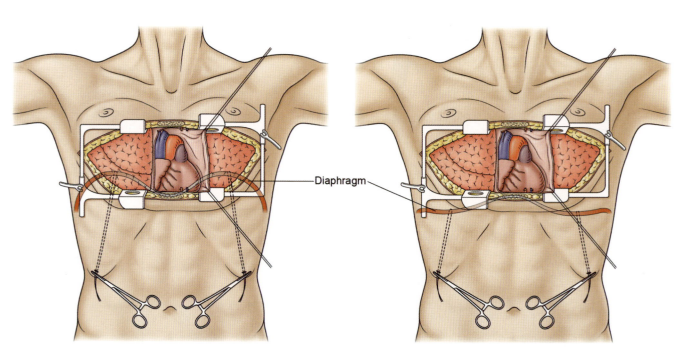

25.4

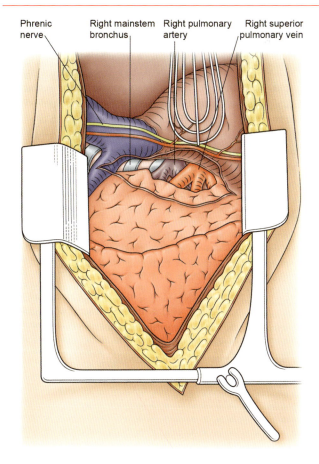

Phrenic nerve   Right mainstem bronchus   Right pulmonary artery   Right superior pulmonary vein

25.5b

to ensure cardiopulmonary stability (**Figure 25.6a and b**). If unstable, the tourniquet is released and the decision for proceeding with the contralateral lung, adding other adjuncts (nitric oxide, inotropes) or establishing mechanical support (ECMO/bypass) is considered. Ideally, once control of all vessels has been achieved, the donor organs should arrive in the operating room.

Pneumonectomy

Once the donor organs have arrived, ABO verification has been performed, and the organs are judged suitable for implantation, the recipient pneumonectomy is performed. For bilateral lung transplants the decision which side to perform first is based on individual patient lung function, donor lung quality, technical difficulty, and tolerance to test occlusion.

Division of the vessels is performed using an endo GIA stapler in such a way as to maximize vessel length. Once completed, the fraction of inspired oxygen is reduced and attention is focused on the bronchus, which is divided just after the takeoff of the upper lobe using cautery (**Figure 25.7a and b**). Division in such a way precludes injury to the bronchus by creating a handle that can be controlled with an Allis clamp for more precise sharp division (**Figure 25.7a inset**). The native lung is then removed, cultured, and sent for pathologic analysis. The chest is copiously irrigated with antibiotic saline.

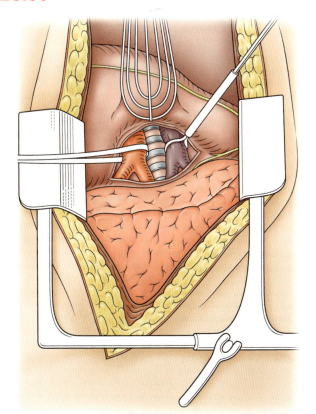

25.6a

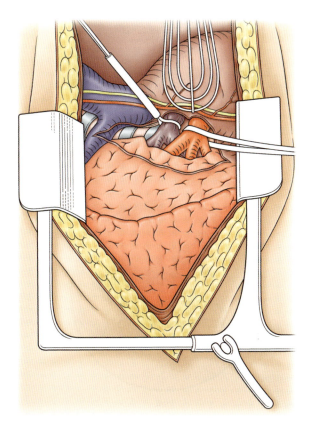

25.6b

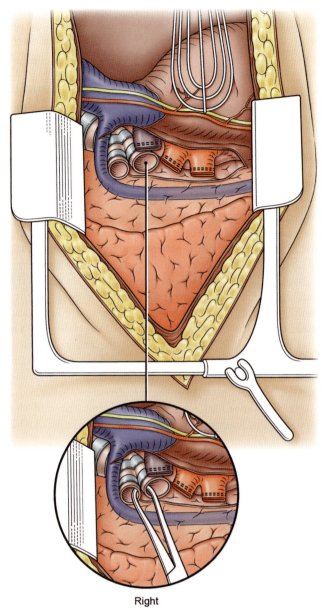

Right

25.7a

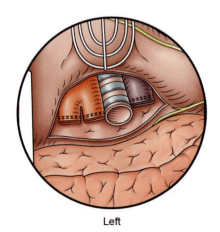

Left

25.7b

Attention is then turned to the pulmonary veins, which are circumferentially released from the pericardium providing sufficient length for control using a large Satinsky clamp. Silk stay sutures are placed in the veins to retract from the operative field. Next the PA is mobilized and similarly retracted. Last, the bronchus is divided sharply using a scalpel within one or two rings of the carina and a retraction stitch is placed anteriorly. The endotracheal tube positioning is confirmed and aspiration of any secretions is performed. Care is taken to identify and control any areas of hemorrhage.

Implantation

Similar techniques are used for left or right lung implantation. The left side is usually more difficult due to challenges of exposure caused by the heart and left atrial appendage. The bronchial anastomosis is performed using a 3-0 polypropylene suture beginning at the membranous/cartilaginous junction in an end-to-end continuous fashion (**Figure 25.8a and b**). Two simple interrupted 3-0 polypropylene sutures are used to reinforce and fix pericardium over the bronchus to facilitate potential future retransplants.

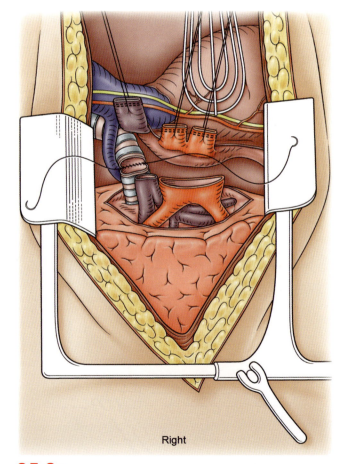

Right

25.8a

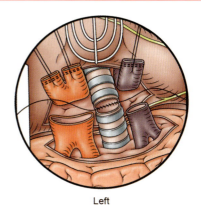

Left

25.8b

Cold supplemented blood (400 mL) is then delivered to the PA via a cardioplegia line to maintain hypothermia and clear debris from the left atrium (**Figure 25.9a and b**). A small or medium Satinsky clamp is placed on the recipient PA, placed on traction using an umbilical tape, and then opened. The donor PA is trimmed to an appropriate length taking care to avoid redundancy, which can result in obstruction. The anastomosis is performed using a continuous 5-0 polypropylene suture (**Figure 25.10a and b**). Once completed the suture is placed on a shod for later de-airing maneuvers.

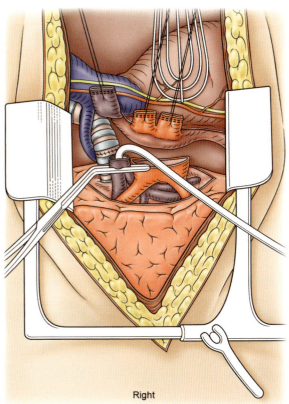

Right

25.9a

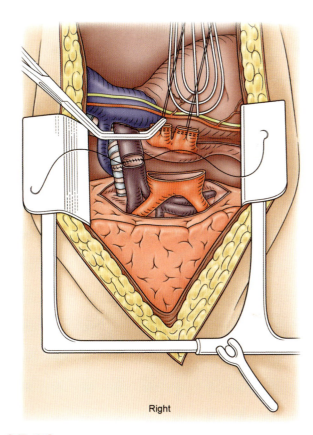

Right

25.10a

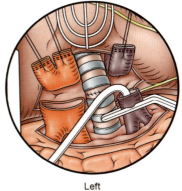

Left

25.9b

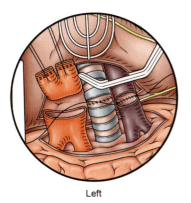

Left

25.10b

The left atrial anastomosis follows with control gained by lateral retraction on the pulmonary veins and placement of a large Satinsky clamp. Care must be taken to ensure that there is sufficient cuff distal to the clamp. The clamp is placed on traction using an umbilical tape to enhance exposure. The donor left atrium is appropriately sized and imbricated to facilitate endothelial intima-to-intima apposition using a running 4-0 polypropylene suture (**Figure 25.11a and b**). After the posterior suture line is completed, 500 mg methylprednisolone is administered.

The suture is shodded and de-airing through the PA is performed using normothermic supplemented blood delivered via a non-vented cardioplegia cannula in antegrade fashion through the PA staple line (**Figure 25.12a and b**). After all air and debris have been cleared from the left atrium, the left atrial anastomotic suture is tied and the clamp removed. De-airing continues through the PA until no air or debris is seen and the suture is tied. The PA clamp is slowly released over 5–10 minutes for controlled reperfusion. Ventilation is then resumed with gentle recruitment performed by hand

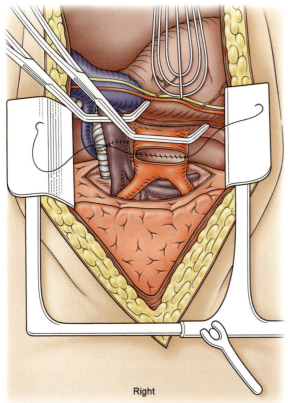

Right

25.11a

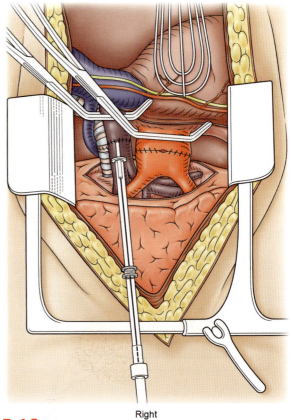

Right

25.12a

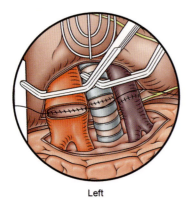

Left

25.11b

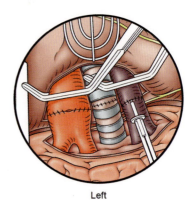

Left

25.12b

and lowest tolerable FiO_2. Mechanical ventilation is then resumed with positive end-expiratory pressure (PEEP) set at 5–10 cm H_2O and with tidal volumes approximately 5–7 mL/kg donor weight. Suture lines and pericardial edges are inspected to ensure adequate hemostasis while TEE confirms adequate heart function and flow across vessels.

For bilateral lung transplants, attention is focused on the contralateral lung after 10 minutes of stability. Isolation is initiated and the PA is controlled using a Rommel tourniquet to ensure cardiopulmonary stability. Once confirmed, pneumonectomy and implantation continue in a similar fashion to that previously described.

Closure

Upon completion of the implantation, the chest is copiously irrigated with antibiotic saline. Three chest tubes are routinely placed in each pleural cavity: a 28 Fr placed anteriorly in the apex, a 32 Fr right-angle tube placed posteriorly and a 24 Fr Blake tube placed along the diaphragm posteriorly that then reaches toward the apex in the chest. For bilateral lung transplants performed through a clamshell incision, three simple 6 wires are placed in the sternum to reapproximate the sternum. Several simple interrupted 5 braided polyester or 1 polyglyconate pericostal sutures are placed depending on the level of contamination. The pectoral fascial layer, the subcutaneous layer, and the subdermal layer are reapproximated with absorbable suture. The skin is closed with staples.

LUNG PROCUREMENT

Exposure

Exposure of the thoracic organs is performed via median sternotomy. The pericardium is opened anteriorly in an inverted Y with wide extension laterally to the diaphragm. Pericardial stay sutures are placed for exposure. Both pleural cavities are opened wide from the mammary pedicles superiorly to the diaphragm inferiorly. Manual examination of the lungs is performed sequentially to assess the general appearance and note any abnormalities (consolidation, infarct, nodules, edema, and compliance). Suspicious findings are sent for pathologic examination. Aggressive recruitment is performed to eliminate any atelectasis and differential gases are sent. We use a minimum PaO_2 of 300 mmHg on a 100% FiO_2 with 5 cm H_2O of PEEP to determine suitability.

Perfusion

Once the lungs are deemed suitable for transplant by the team, preparation for procurement will begin. Using cautery, mobilization of the aorta, PA, superior vena cava (SVC), and inferior vena cava (IVC) are performed with additional dissection along Waterston's groove (**Figure 25.13a**). These maneuvers decrease the risk for two common procurement injuries (right PA injury at the bifurcation and inadequate anterior atrial cuff). Once the assembled teams are ready for cannulation the donor is fully heparinized (250–300 units/kg), a standard cardioplegia cannula is placed, a 4-0 Prolene pursestring is placed, and cannulation of the PA positioned such that both pulmonary arteries are adequately perfused. Just prior to cross-clamp a 500 µg bolus of prostaglandin is administered directly into the PA, the SVC is ligated/clamped, the IVC is divided, the aorta cross-clamped, cardioplegia delivered, the left atrial appendage vented, and lung preservation solution administered (**Figure 25.13b**).

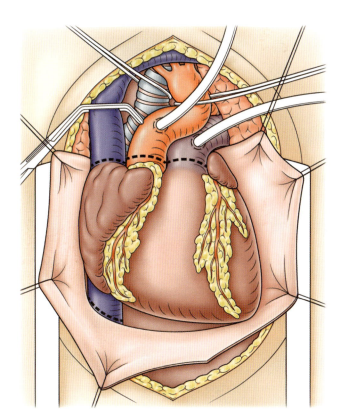

25.13a

Approximately 3 liters (35–50 mL/kg) of preservation fluid is administered through the PA as the chest cavity is covered in saline slush. Successful perfusion is indicated with clear effluent through the left atrium.

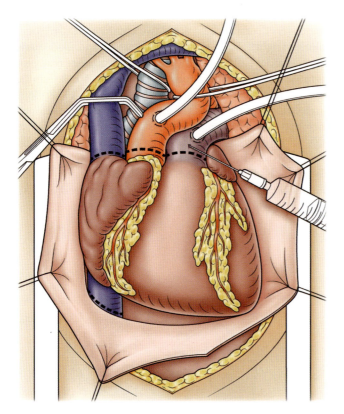

25.13b

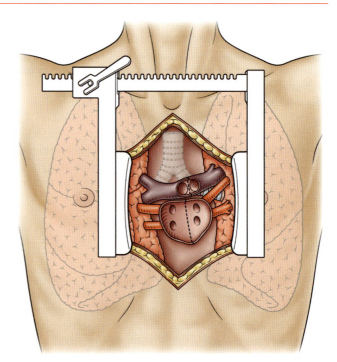

25.14a

Explant

After adequate perfusion of the heart and lungs with preservation solution, it is imperative that adequate tissue for implantation of both the heart and the lung allografts is achieved. Perfusion cannulae are removed. The SVC is divided proximal to the ligature/clamp as is the aorta. Next, the PA is divided at the bifurcation. The heart is retracted to the right and the left atrium is divided midway between the coronary sinus and the pulmonary veins which extend toward the right pulmonary veins. The heart is then retracted to the left and the atriotomy completed along Waterston's groove. The heart is removed from the field (**Figure 25.14a**).

Retrograde perfusion of the lung is performed through the pulmonary venous orifices (**Figure 25.14b**). Typically, 250–500 mL of preservation solution is needed to ensure clear effluent from the PA. Inspection of the PA, for pulmonary emboli is performed.

The trachea is exposed through the pericardium and is bluntly mobilized to expose at least three rings above the carina. The endotracheal tube is slowly withdrawn and

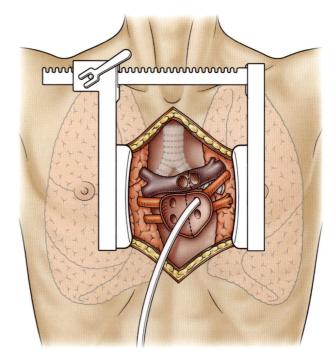

25.14b

a TA30 stapler is fired when the lung is at 70–80% vital capacity to prevent injury. An additional staple load is fired proximately and divided with a scalpel between staple lines to prevent contamination **Figure 25.14c**).

Removal of the lungs can proceed after division of the inferior pulmonary ligaments and remaining posterior

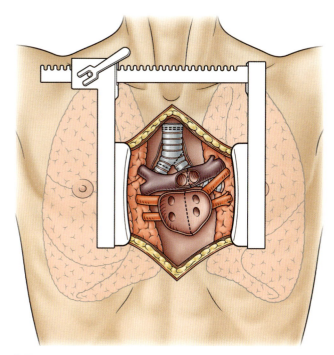

25.14c

mediastinal tissue anterior to the esophagus. The lungs are then triple bagged en bloc at 4 °C and brought back to the recipient hospital for back-table preparation and implant. If organs require separation at the donor hospital due to multiple recipients, preparation follows as described below.

Preparation of donor organ(s)

After arrival at the recipient hospital, ABO verification takes place and the donor lungs are sterilely passed to the back table. The posterior pericardium is divided in the midline, the left atrium midway between the pulmonary veins, and the PA at the raphe. The bronchus is divided using a TA30 stapling device placed just distal to the carina on the left bronchus (**Figure 24.14c**, dotted lines). If both lungs need to remain inflated (e.g. lungs divided at donor hospital for multiple recipients), an additional firing of the TA30 just distal to the original staple is performed and the bronchus is divided with a scalpel between the staple lines. Next, the vessels are inspected for injury and excess tissue is excised. The separated lungs are then covered with laparotomy pads and placed in saline slush to remain at 4 °C (or individually packaged for transport).

POSTOPERATIVE CARE

The postoperative care of transplant patients is complex and requires the expertise of several disciplines. While an extensive discussion is not the intent of this section, a few central principles should be considered.

Upon arrival in the intensive care unit, hemodynamic monitoring, baseline laboratory, and imaging exams are performed, and goal-directed resuscitation and weaning of hemodynamic and ventilator support are initiated. Most patients are liberated from mechanical ventilation in less than 24 hours. Just prior to extubation, fiber-optic bronchoscopy is performed to evacuate secretions and inspect the anastomosis. Adequate pain control is the cornerstone of postoperative care of the lung transplant patient. Patients with poor pain control cannot take deep breaths, control secretions, or participate in physical therapy. Promotility and stool softeners are required to mitigate the side effects of narcotics. Immunosuppressive regimens are standardized and tailored to local practice. Initiation of oral intake in our group is delayed until confirmation of safe deglutition thereby minimizing the risk of aspiration and preventing aspiration pneumonia. Patients with known or newly identified dysphagia or esophageal dysmotility receive nutritional support via enteral tubes until safe deglutition is achieved. Low thresholds for bronchoscopy are maintained until the recipient can adequately mobilize secretions. Deep-vein thrombosis (DVT) is common therefore all patients are placed on DVT prophylaxis. Patients are discharged to home when patients and care providers are able to manage their care at home.

OUTCOME

There has been significant improvement in lung transplant outcomes over the last 30 years. ISHLT Kaplan–Meier comparisons of survival by era (1990–1998, 1999–2008, and 2009–2014) have demonstrated increasing median survival from 4.2 to 6.1 years for primary lung transplants. Almost 80% of patients alive 3 years after transplant can carry out normal activity and 25% of those patients have returned to work. However, the continued limitation of available donors, the unpredictability of primary graft dysfunction, and the development of chronic lung allograft dysfunction continue to pose significant challenges which are the topics of significant research efforts. With better understanding of these challenges additional improvement in outcomes will be achievable.

FURTHER READING

Diamond JM, Lee JC, Kawut SM, et al. Clinical risk factors for primary graft dysfunction after lung transplantation. *Am J Respir Crit Care Med.* 2013; 187: 527–34.

Erasmus ME, van Raemdonck D, Akhtar MZ, et al. DCD lung donation: donor criteria, procedural criteria, pulmonary graft function validation, and preservation. *Transpl Int.* 2016; 29: 790–7.

Kotloff RM, Blosser S, Fulda GJ, et al. Management of the potential organ donor in the ICU: Society of Critical Care Medicine/ American College of Chest Physicians/Association of Organ

Procurement Organizations consensus statement. *Crit Care Med.* 2015; 43: 1291–325.

Orens JB, Boehler A, de Perrot M, et al. A review of lung transplant donor acceptability criteria. *J Heart Lung Transplant.* 2003; 22: 1183–200.

Pasque MK. Standardizing thoracic organ procurement for transplantation. *J Thorac Cardiovasc Surg.* 2010; 139: 13–17.

Weill D, Benden C, Corris PA, et al. A consensus document for the selection of lung transplant candidates: 2014 – an update from the Pulmonary Transplantation Council of the International Society for Heart and Lung Transplantation. *J Heart Lung Transplant.* 2015; 34: 1–15.

26

Permanent continuous-flow left ventricular assist devices

ERIN M. SCHUMER AND MARK S. SLAUGHTER

HISTORY

The first left ventricular assist device (LVAD) was implanted in 1963 by deBakey in a patient with postcardiotomy shock.[1] As the incidence of heart failure rose to epidemic proportions, LVADs emerged as a new solution to this devastating disease and superiority over medical treatment was demonstrated in the Randomized Evaluation of Mechanical Assistance for the Treatment of Congestive Heart Failure (REMATCH) trial.[2] The first-generation devices were pulsatile, in an attempt to replicate native cardiac physiology. When compared to medical management alone, therapy with these devices showed improved survival; however, their large size limited patient selection to mainly male patients, required large, pneumatic drivers, and decreased durability.

Thus, second- and third-generation devices were developed using continuous-flow pumps. These devices were smaller, allowing implantation in a broader population including women and children. The improved technology allowed for lengthened battery life, longer support times, and overall better quality of life for patients with advanced heart failure.[3] Continuous-flow devices have continued to dominate the market since their introduction and are implanted in more than 90% of patients with heart failure.[4]

PRINCIPLES AND DEVICE SELECTION

Chronic support of the left ventricle (LV) should entail long-term reliability, portability, and adequate cardiac flow for active patients. Two devices currently on the market are widely used: the HeartMate II™ (HMII) LVAS (Thoratec Corporation, Pleasanton, CA, USA) and the HeartWare HVAD™ (HeartWare Inc., Framingham, MA, USA), while the newly approved HeartMate III (HMIII) LVAS (Thoratec Corporation, Pleasanton, CA, USA) continues to gain popularity. All three pumps have inflow cannulae, which are placed in the LV apex. These cannulae are connected to a pump body, which then is connected to an outflow cannula and graft that

is subsequently sewn onto the ascending aorta. An electrical driveline from the pump exits the patient via a subcutaneous tunnel in the upper abdomen.

These pumps differ in several significant ways. The HMII, a second-generation device, uses an axial flow pump and, in general, requires a preperitoneal pocket for placement.[3] Both the HVAD and HMIII, third-generation devices, utilize centrifugal flow in a smaller configuration allowing for intrapericardial implantation.[5] While the survival outcomes are similar for the HMII and HVAD,[6] complication rates differ: the HVAD has a higher stroke rate while the HMII has a higher rate of driveline infection, both with significant clinical impact.[7] The smaller size of the HVAD is more conducive to a minimally invasive approach via thoracotomy either at the initial operation or if a redo operation is required. Additionally, biventricular configuration of the HVAD has been reported; however, the size of the HMII does not allow for biventricular support. Early results with the HMIII are promising, as this device appears to have a lower rate of thrombosis; however, survival and disabling stroke rates are similar when compared to the HMII.[8] Ultimately, it appears that device selection must be individualized for each patient, underscoring the importance of patient selection.[9]

PREOPERATIVE ASSESSMENT AND PREPARATION

Indication for LVAD placement varies by individual patient and is a current area of controversy. Historically, LVAD implantation has been indicated for patients with New York Heart Association Class IV heart failure and may include those patients with intractable arrhythmias and/or angina, end-organ dysfunction attributed to heart failure, or postcardiotomy shock.[10] Patients are classified by therapy goals into bridge-to-transplantation therapy (BTT), destination therapy (DT), bridge-to-recovery therapy, and bridge-to-decision therapy. The Interagency Registry for Mechanically Assisted Circulatory Support (INTERMACS) scoring system is useful to identify appropriate patients and timing of LVAD support.[4] Optimal patient selection is crucial for success in chronic LVAD implantation and it is achieved through an array of diagnostic studies.

Assessment considerations are divided into cardiac and non-cardiac considerations. Cardiac considerations include right ventricular function, valvular function and structure, intracardiac shunting, and arrhythmias. Transesophageal echocardiography (TEE) is an essential part of the pre-operative evaluation. Irreversible and severe right heart failure is a contraindication to placement of an LVAD, and these patients may be considered for biventricular VADs, total artificial heart placement, or heart transplantation. Non-cardiac considerations include end-organ function, particularly pulmonary, renal, and hepatic, nutrition and body habitus, and social and psychiatric issues. End-organ function must be optimized through the use of inotropes and potentially intra-aortic balloon pump and/or extracorporeal membrane oxygenation if shock is present.

OPERATION

Hemodynamic monitoring is performed using a pulmonary artery catheter, arterial line, and TEE. After induction and skin preparation, a midline sternotomy incision is performed. A preperitoneal pocket is made using sharp and blunt dissection in the case of HMII implantation (**Figure 26.1**). As VAD placements are most often repeat sternotomies, extra care must be taken during the dissection of the LV from the scar tissue. Following this dissection, the patient is systemically heparinized.

Aortic cannulation should be placed as high as possible, close to the arch (**Figure 26.2**). Single two-stage venous cannulation will suffice in the majority of cases, but bicaval cannulation may afford better drainage and, in the case of a right ventricular device, the appendage can be used for venous return with the VAD cannula. Cardiopulmonary bypass (CPB) is then initiated. If more dissection of the LV is needed, it is performed at this time with the heart beating but decompressed. At this point, the driveline is tunneled

percutaneously under the rectus muscle to exit usually over the left upper quadrant of the abdomen (**Figure 26.3**).

The heart is then elevated, bringing the LV to the midline of the wound. Pledgeted Ethibond® sutures are placed circumferentially around a chosen spot for the inflow cannula (**Figure 26.4**). Proper orientation of the inflow cannula is crucial to postoperative success: it must be pointed towards the left ventricular outflow tract for optimal flow and placed at the apex. Sutures are then placed through the sewing ring, which is then

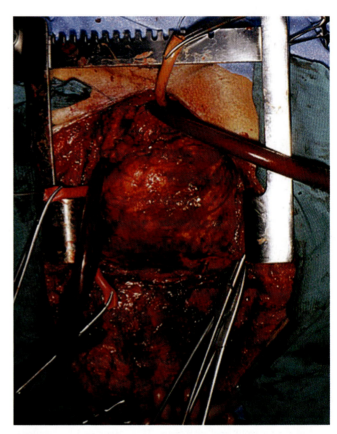

26.2   Cannulation strategy for cardiopulmonary bypass.

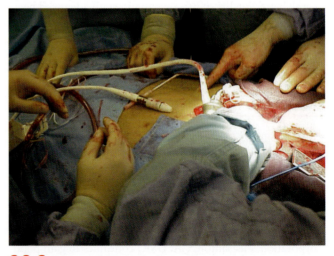

26.3   The driveline is tunneled out through the upper abdomen using the device tunneler far enough from the costal margin to prevent rubbing.

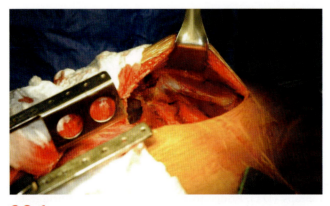

26.1   A preperitoneal pocket is created using sharp and blunt dissection for the HeartMate II implantation.

seated and tied down. In the case of HMII implantation, coring is performed prior to placement of the sewing ring.

At this point, the patient is placed in Trendelenberg position in preparation for coring. The heart is emptied and a cruciate incision is made at the apex. The coring tool is used to perform the left ventriculotomy (**Figure 26.5**). Following coring, the ventricle is inspected for crossing fibers, thrombus, or muscle, and any identified is resected. Once clear, the heart is de-aired and the inflow cannula of the pump is inserted (**Figure 26.6**). The pump is secured after proper

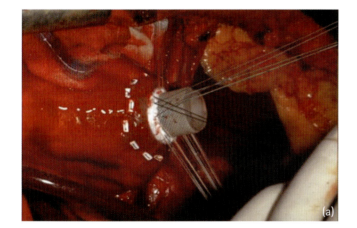

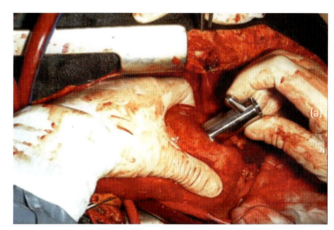

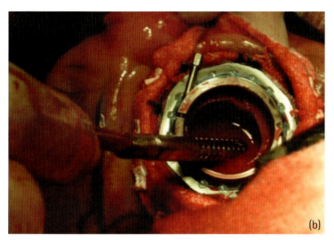

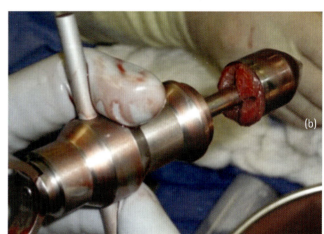

26.4a,b Sutures are placed circumferentially around the left ventricular apex for the sewing ring. The sutures are passed through the sewing ring, and the ring is seated after the sutures are tied down. (a) HeartMate II; (b) HVAD.

26.5a,b Coring is performed using the coring tool. (a) HeartMate II; (b) HVAD.

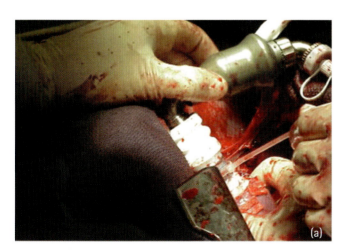

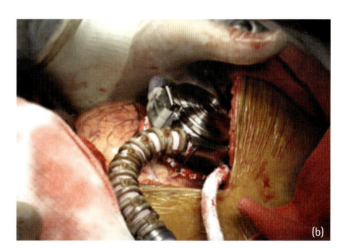

26.6a,b The inflow cannula of the pump is inserted into the ventriculotomy and secured within the sewing ring. (a) HeartMate II; (b) HVAD.

orientation is confirmed, and the heart is then placed back in its normal anatomic position in the chest.

Further de-airing is then performed through the outflow graft. The graft is then measured, clamped, and cut. A partial occluding clamp is placed on the greater curvature of the ascending aorta. After aortotomy, a running end-to-side anastomosis with 4-0 Prolene is performed (**Figure 26.7**).

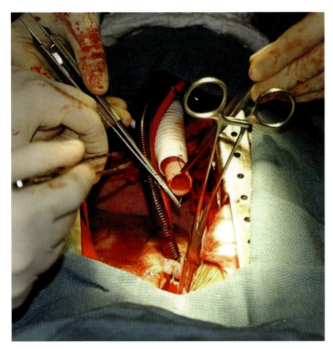

26.7 The aortic anastomosis is performed using a running Prolene suture in an end-to-side fashion.

Normal ventilation is resumed and inhaled prostaglandin and inotropes are started. The driveline is passed off the field and connected to the system controller. Following rewarming to normothermia, CPB is weaned while increasing the LVAD pump speed to achieve adequate flow.

After weaning from CPB, the right heart should be assessed for a short period before reversing anticoagulation. Pulmonary hypertension by itself is not a clear indication for RV support. Heavy bleeding, with resultant massive transfusion, will often lead to RV failure and should be corrected before weaning from bypass. Protamine infusion is administered, and the patient is decannulated. The bend relief and outflow graft are placed inside a 20 mm Gelweave graft. Left pleural, mediastinal, and right pleural drains are inserted. Once adequate hemostasis is achieved, the chest is closed.

POSTOPERATIVE CARE

Following implantation, hemodynamic monitoring in the cardiac intensive care unit is essential. This is accomplished by pulmonary artery catheter and echocardiography that guides titration of pump speed, parenteral fluids, inotropes, and vasopressor agents. Pump speed is optimized to several parameters including maintenance of septum location in the midline and reduction of mitral regurgitation while maintaining adequate flow to end organs. Average pump speeds are 8000–10 000 rpm, 2200–2800 rpm and 3000–9000 rpm for the HMII HVAD and HMIII respectively. If an intraaortic balloon pump is present, it must be placed on flutter and removed as soon as possible.

Additionally, right heart function is monitored by echocardiography. The incidence of right heart failure following LVAD implantation is 0.49/100 patient-months[4] and is often difficult to predict. Pulmonary vascular resistance (PVR) is minimized by careful ventilator management in addition to judicious fluid management. Agents such as inhaled nitric oxide or intravenous prostaglandins can help to lower PVR; however, if right heart failure is refractory to medical management, then right VAD support may be required. Currently, the HVAD is most commonly used as the configuration of the HMII does not allow for RVAD support.

Anticoagulation with heparin is started once postoperative bleeding is minimal, making meticulous intraoperative hemostasis crucial to this aspect of postoperative care. Transition to long-term anticoagulation with warfarin is not initiated until the patient is stable, usually 48–72 hours postimplantation. An INR of 2.5–3.5 is targeted. Antiplatelet therapy is additionally started at this point.

Other aspects of postoperative care include the use of perioperative antibiotics for a period of 72 hours in an effort to reduce infection aimed at coverage of both Gram-positive and Gram-negative organisms. The driveline dressing changes are performed daily under sterile conditions, and it is paramount that this technique is taught to the patient and their caregiver. Enteral nutrition should be initiated as soon as the patient's clinical condition warrants. Finally, a multidisciplinary team is crucial to the success of the patient both as an inpatient and after discharge.

OUTCOME

Outcomes for continuous-flow devices continue to improve, with a current expected 1-year survival rate of 80%, with BTT survival slightly better than DT survival.[4] Likewise, no survival difference post-transplantation exists between the HMII and HVAD or HMII and HMIII. Currently, there is no head-to-head comparison of survival between the HVAD and HMIII. Approximately 29.2% of patients experience adverse events within 1 year of implantation, the most significant of those including bleeding, infection, and cardiac arrhythmias.[4] However, this rate continues to decrease when compared to the earlier era of continuous-flow devices.[4]

Further investigation into LVAD implantation in patients with ambulatory heart failure is ongoing. The Risk Assessment and Comparative Effectiveness of Left Ventricular Assist Device and Medical Management in Ambulatory Heart Failure Patients (ROADMAP) trial demonstrated improved quality of life at the cost of increased adverse events with no survival benefit when comparing HMII implantation with optimal medical management in DT patients.[11] The ongoing Medical Arm of the Mechanically Associated Circulatory Support (MedaMACS) study aims to examine the results of patients on optimal medical support who have not yet received mechanical support and suggests a survival benefit for implantation in INTERMACS level 4 and 5 patients.[12] The data imply benefits for earlier implantation of patients with ambulatory heart failure; however, patient selection is crucial to clinical success.

In conclusion, LVAD therapy has improved quality of life and survival for many patients with advanced heart failure; however, the optimal device and patient for LVAD implantation is an ongoing debate. With improvement in technology, LVAD therapy will likely be an option for more patients with a reduced adverse event profile, which will translate to overall enhanced care for patients with heart failure.

REFERENCES

1. DeBakey ME. Development of mechanical heart devices. *Ann Thorac Surg*. 2005; 79: S2228–31.
2. Rose EA, Gelijns AC, Moskowitz AJ, et al. Long-term use of a left ventricular assist device for end-stage heart failure. *N Engl J Med*. 2001; 345: 1435–43.
3. Slaughter MS, Rogers JG, Milano CA, et al. Advanced heart failure treated with continuous-flow left ventricular assist device. *N Engl J Med*. 2009; 361: 2241–51.
4. Kirklin JK, Naftel DC, Pagani FD, et al. Seventh INTERMACS annual report: 15 000 patients and counting. *J Heart Lung Transplant*. 2015; 34: 1495–504.
5. Slaughter MS, Pagani FD, McGee EC, et al. HeartWare ventricular assist system for bridge to transplant: combined results of the bridge to transplant and continued access protocol trial. *J Heart Lung Transplant*. 2013; 32: 675–83.
6. Lalonde SD, Alba AC, Rigobon A, et al. Clinical differences between continuous flow ventricular assist devices: a comparison between HeartMate II and HeartWare HVAD. *J Card Surg*. 2013; 28: 604–10.
7. Stulak JM, Davis ME, Haglund N, et al. Adverse events in contemporary continuous-flow left ventricular assist devices: a multi-institutional comparison shows significant differences. *J Thorac Cardiovasc Surg*. 2016; 151: 177–89.
8. Mehra MR, Goldstein DJ, Uriel N, et al. Two-Year Outcomes with a Magnetically Levitated Cardiac Pump in Heart Failure. *N Engl J Med* 2018; 378: 1386–95.
9. Shah P, Birk S, Maltais S, et al. Left ventricular assist device outcomes based on flow configuration and pre-operative left ventricular dimension: an Interagency Registry for Mechanically Assisted Circulatory Support Analysis. *J Heart Lung Transplant*. 2017; 36(6): 640–9.
10. Go AS, Mozaffarian D, Roger VL, et al. Heart disease and stroke statistics – 2014 update: a report from the American Heart Association. *Circulation*. 2014; 129: e28–e292.
11. Estep JD, Starling RC, Horstmanshof DA, et al. Risk assessment and comparative effectiveness of left ventricular assist device and medical management in ambulatory heart failure patients: results from the ROADMAP study. *J Am Coll Cardiol*. 2015; 66: 1747–61.
12. Stewart GC, Kittleson MM, Cowger JA, et al. Who wants a left ventricular assist device for ambulatory heart failure? Early insights from the MEDAMACS screening pilot. *J Heart Lung Transplant*. 2015; 34: 1630–3.

27

ECMO and temporary mechanical circulatory assistance

CHRISTIAN A. BERMUDEZ AND JEFFREY POYNTER

INTRODUCTION AND HISTORY

The modern era of mechanical circulatory assistance (MCA) began in the early 1950s when cardiopulmonary bypass (CPB) was first used to support patients during open-heart operations for the repair of congenital heart defects. As the field of cardiac surgery evolved throughout the 1960s, the need for mechanical support able to provide short- and long-term assistance became evident. Different attempts to develop a durable ventricular-assist device and later a total artificial heart during that decade were conducted with only modest success, diverting efforts to the design of short-term temporary support devices with the intention to sustain patients with cardiogenic shock (CS), avoiding organ failure, and providing time for recovery of the myocardial function.

Counterpulsation with the intra-aortic balloon pump (IABP), the first temporary MCA device, was introduced in 1968 to augment cardiac function by improving cardiac output and decreasing myocardial work. With modifications in the 1980s, which led to its percutaneous implantation, IABP use rapidly increased; the IABP continues to be the most used mechanical support worldwide. At the same time, improvements were made in CPB oxygenator technology. The design of the membrane oxygenator in the early 1970s led to the development of a more portable CPB system – extracorporeal membrane oxygenation (ECMO) – allowing efficient bypass of the blood between the venous and arterial circulations while actively oxygenating the blood to provide cardiac and respiratory support. This technology was also adapted to be used in the intensive care unit (ICU) setting. The first report of a patient supported on ECMO in the ICU was in 1971, in a patient suffering severe pulmonary contusion. Initially used in patients with advanced respiratory failure, ECMO use was expanded during the 1970s to adult patients with acute CS refractory to medical therapy and was not infrequently used in patients unable to come off CPB after complex cardiac operations. Bleeding complications, due to the need for significant anticoagulation, and early oxygenator failures limited ECMO application for years. More recently, the use of the ECMO technology has expanded due to technological improvements in both the design and biocompatibility of cannulae, pumps, and oxygenators. ECMO has become an MCA workhorse and is the most frequently used MCA in patients in advanced cardiogenic and respiratory failure.

During the 1980s and 1990s, attention was focused on the development and clinical use of long-term or durable MCA. These efforts led to the development of left ventricular assist devices (LVADs) using pulsatile pumps for long-term support. The significant improvements in outcomes seen with these technologies, first with paracorporeal pulsatile pumps (Thoratec PVAD) followed by implantable intracorporeal pulsatile systems (HeartMate XE™ and HeartMate XVE™ [Thoratec Corporation, Pleasanton, CA], and NOVACOR), led to their approval by the United States Food and Drug Administration (USFDA) for use as a bridge to transplant therapy (BTT) and then as a destination therapy for permanent support in the case of the HeartMate XVE™ (REMATCH Trial). Durable LVAD technology for long-term support has continued to evolve with the incorporation of axial flow technology (HeartMate II™) and centrifugal flow technology (HeartWare®, [HeartWare Inc., Framingham, MA]) with excellent long-term survival.

Because durable VAD technology was not an option for many patients presenting with profound decompensation or who were not LVAD candidates, the need for temporary, less invasive temporary MCA became evident. In the early 2000s, conceptual technologies similar to those used in durable LVADs (axial and centrifugal flow pumps) were successfully applied to temporary MCA in the form of percutaneous support devices, such as the Impella Recover® (Abiomed Inc., Danvers, MA) and TandemHeart® (LivaNova) and other paracorporeal pumps including the Centrimag™ (Thoratec Corporation, Pleasanton, CA). These temporary devices and ECMO have come to play a major role in patients presenting in acutely decompensated states as an alternative to stabilize the patient and provide time to define the most appropriate treatment strategy.

Although patients requiring temporary MCA remain at high risk of morbidity and mortality, refinement in patient selection, improvements in medical and pharmacological support, a trend toward earlier intervention, and advancements in device design have reduced the complication rates of these life-saving procedures. Moreover, a paradigm shift toward earlier institution of MCA seems to be associated with improved outcomes and decreased costs. Progress in these areas has led to an explosive increase in the utilization of these life-saving technologies to bridge patients to recovery and occasionally to transplantation.

TEMPORARY MECHANICAL SUPPORT OPTIONS

Intra-aortic balloon pump

The IABP has two major components: a balloon catheter and a pump console to control the balloon. The IABP is a two-lumen catheter (7.5–8.0 Fr) with a polyethylene balloon attached at its distal end. The balloon is inflated with helium. Timing of balloon inflation and deflation is based on electrocardiogram (ECG) or pressure triggers. The balloon inflates with the onset of diastole, which corresponds with electrophysiologic repolarization. Following diastole, the balloon rapidly deflates at the onset of left ventricular (LV) systole, which is timed to the peak of the R-wave on the surface ECG. The hemodynamic effects of the IABP include an increase in diastolic blood pressure and coronary perfusion, a decrease in afterload and myocardial oxygen consumption, and a partial increase in the cardiac output. The IABP provides modest ventricular unloading but does increase mean arterial pressure and coronary blood flow. Patients must have some level of LV function and electrical stability for an IABP to be effective. The IABP is generally placed percutaneously in the femoral artery, but axillary and direct aortic cannulation are also used clinically, especially in the presence of peripheral vascular disease.

Extracorporeal membrane oxygenation

ECMO requires a circuit composed of a centrifugal, non-pulsatile pump for blood propulsion, and a membrane oxygenator for gas exchange. ECMO can be either veno-venous (VV) for oxygenation only or venoarterial (VA) for oxygenation and circulatory support. In cases of biventricular failure, VA ECMO is the MCA of choice for patients in CS and impaired oxygenation, as it provides full cardiopulmonary support. Modern pumps are generally well tolerated with excellent biocompatibility; there is no evidence to support superiority of one over the others. Significant improvements in the technology of ECMO oxygenators, mostly based on PMP (polymethylpentene) fibers that allow days to weeks of uninterrupted support, have drastically changed the field. Improvements in cannula design and quality have decreased cannula size, which has reduced vascular complications. In cases of CS, VA ECMO can be implemented peripherally in the femoral vessels or using subclavian/axillary cannulation in patients with peripheral vascular disease. A central open configuration (aorta and right atrium) is frequently used in patients with postcardiotomy failure. ECMO has been increasingly used in the emergency department to treat profound CS or cardiac arrest (CA) and can be done at the bedside using arterial cannulae ranging from 15 Fr to 19 Fr and venous cannulae of 22–25 Fr.

There are some limitations to ECMO MCA. The need for an oxygenator in addition to the pump requires a higher level of anticoagulation, especially in VA ECMO, with a partial thromboplastin time (PTT) of 50–70 seconds or an activated clotting time (ACT) of 180–220 seconds. For this reason, ECMO has been associated with an increased rate of bleeding and thromboembolic complication, and in the VA configuration has more limited support duration as compared with other temporary MCA systems. In cases of femoral peripheral cannulation, the retrograde flow provided by VA ECMO has been associated in certain patients with an increase in LV pressures and inadequate LV unloading as compared with other temporary MCA, especially in cases of very profound LV dysfunction or the absence of LV contractility. In such circumstances, ECMO support is combined with other devices (Impella®) or with directly unloading the LV using modified techniques such as direct apical cannulation or conversion to central cannulation.

Impella®

The Impella® is a catheter-mounted, small axial-flow blood pump that is positioned in the ascending aorta with the low-profile pump placed across the aortic valve and the tip in the LV cavity allowing antegrade flow to propel blood from the LV into the ascending aorta while unloading the LV (**Figure 27.1**). The Impella® device has been used for temporary hemodynamic support in patients with acute heart failure presenting with shock and to provide support to patients undergoing high-risk percutaneous coronary intervention (PCI) or other percutaneous interventions. This pump has three different options to support the LV including the Impella 2.5®, Impella 3.5 (CP)® and Impella 5.0® or 5.0 LD® (**Figure 27.1c**). The Impella 2.5® and Impella CP are implanted percutaneously in the arterial system, while the Impella 5.0® requires implantation via a surgical, open technique. The Impella RP® (22 Fr axial pump) became available more recently and can be placed through the femoral vein and positioned in the right ventricle (RV) and pulmonary artery. The Impella RP® is approved by the US FDA for right-sided hemodynamic support in patients suffering an acute myocardial infarction (AMI) or patients with RV failure after LVAD implantation (**Figure 27.1c**).

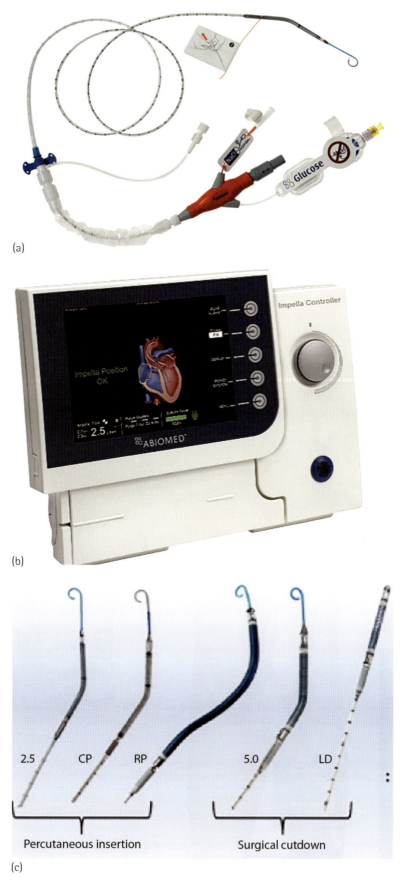

(a)

(b)

(c)

27.1a–c Impella® system. (a) Catheter-based axial flow pump; (b) pump controller; (c) pump options available. Used with permission from ABIOMED.

TANDEMHEART®

The TandemHeart® is a percutaneous temporary MCA device that functions as an LVAD, providing support by pumping blood from the left atrium to the femoral artery. Blood flow is provided by a paracorporeal, centrifugal-flow pump that has hydrodynamic bearings and uses a transseptal inflow cannula (21 Fr) and a femoral outflow cannula (17 Fr) providing up to 3.5 liters of retrograde aortic flow (**Figure 27.2a–c**). The TandemHeart® has been used mainly for temporary support in patients with CS and for brief support during high-risk PCI. More recently, a new dual-lumen cannula design, the Protek Duo catheter (TandemLife, Pittsburgh, PA) (29 Fr or 31 Fr), positioned from the right internal jugular vein (RIJV) into the proximal pulmonary artery, has allowed the use of the TandemHeart® pump as a right ventricular assist device (RVAD) providing up to 4–4.5 liters/min of support (**Figure 27.2d**).

Centrimag™

The Centrimag™ VAD is a versatile, magnetically levitated, paracorporeal centrifugal pump that requires surgical implantation and can be used to support both the LV and RV and was, up until recently, one of the few alternatives to provide temporary biventricular support (BiVAD). Due to its flow (up to 6 liters/min in standard clinical conditions) and biocompatibility characteristics, with decreased risk of pump thrombosis secondary to its bearing-free design, it has become one of the most frequently used surgically implanted MCA devices. The Centrimag™ device allows short- to mid-term stable support (weeks to months) and provides advantages over the other temporary MCAs in certain clinical conditions. This versatility allows this device to be used as a temporary LVAD, RVAD, and BiVAD and also as a centrifugal pump during ECMO support. The system is widely utilized worldwide.

PRINCIPLES AND JUSTIFICATION

Acute heart failure and CS can rapidly progress with end-organ dysfunction and a secondary systemic inflammatory response leading to irreversible organ damage and mortality. Historically, inotropes and vasopressors have been first-line therapy for hemodynamic instability and CS in its early stages. In patients in advanced CS, high doses of inotropes have not shown a benefit in outcomes with the potential for harm due to coronary and peripheral vasoconstriction. MCA has been increasingly considered in patients with severe hemodynamically unstable cardiovascular presentations.

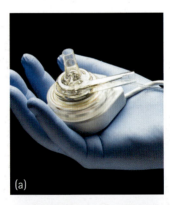

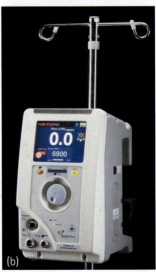

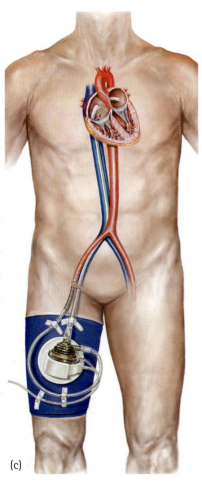

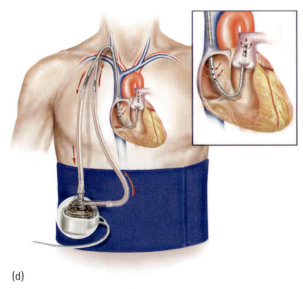

27.2a–d TandemHeart® system. (a) Centrifugal pump; (b) controller; (c) left atrium to femoral artery (transseptal approach, LVAD); (d) right atrium to pulmonary artery using the Protek Duo double–lumen catheter (RVAD). Copyright CardiacAssist Inc./TandemLife. Used with permission.

ECMO and other temporary MCA have been utilized to stabilize these patients and revert this physiological cascade. A safe and prompt MCA insertion allows the possibility of decompressing the heart, limiting the infarct size and risk of pulmonary congestion, maintaining end-organ perfusion, and eventually providing a stable physiological condition to allow myocardial recovery or to consider other advanced options including heart transplant or durable LVAD support.

Current indications for temporary MCA including ECMO

The different temporary MCA systems available have different capabilities and limitations that are important to consider depending on the clinical condition of the patient. Several specific patient populations are likely to benefit from temporary mechanical support. These include patients undergoing high-risk PCI, as a mechanism to prevent intraprocedural decompensation, and those presenting with acute decompensated heart failure associated with CS. Temporary MCA has also gained popularity for managing the advanced stages of shock with acute heart failure.

Temporary MCA is most frequently used in patients suffering from AMI and CS with LV dysfunction or mechanical complications (ventricular septal defect and acute mitral regurgitation). MCA is also used in patients with other forms of acute heart failure including decompensated non-ischemic cardiomyopathies, fulminant myocarditis, post-partum cardiomyopathy, life-threatening ventricular arrhythmic storm, severe cardiac dysfunction after drug intoxication, and massive pulmonary embolism. Other frequent indications include postcardiotomy shock or the inability to come off CPB following a cardiac operation and in heart transplant patients with primary graft dysfunction or ventricular dysfunction following rejection. Most recently, ECMO has been increasingly utilized as an alternative to extracorporeal cardiopulmonary resuscitation (ECPR) in patients who do not respond to conventional resuscitation maneuvers in the absence of contraindications.

The use of temporary MCA has been associated with some potential benefits. If properly selected, temporary MCA can provide a significant increase in cardiac output and unloading of the left cardiac structures. The clinical consequences include maintaining vital organ perfusion, preventing systemic shock syndrome, reducing intracardiac filling pressures and consequently decreasing pulmonary congestion, reducing LV volumes, wall stress, and myocardial oxygen consumption, and augmenting coronary perfusion eventually limiting the infarct size.

Despite their potential benefits, ECMO and other temporary MCA devices are not options for all patients. Their cost, potential complications, and lack of efficacy if chosen inadequately may lead to futile support impacting patient care. In general, the percutaneous devices, especially those requiring larger cannulae and arterial instrumentation (ECMO, Impella®, TandemHeart®), have been associated with a significant incidence of vascular and bleeding and thromboembolic complications. Systemic infections are frequent, especially in patients requiring prolonged support, and may be controlled only with device replacement in certain conditions. The balance between bleeding, secondary to heparinization, and thromboembolic and vascular complications continues to be a challenge despite improvements in the technology.

At our institution, we have emphasized the contraindications for MCA, including ECMO, as a mechanism to prevent futile support and improve patient outcomes. VA ECMO and the Impella® devices are the most frequently used MCA at our institution. Contraindications for VA ECMO include age over 75 years (except in cases of postcardiotomy failure), active malignancy with estimated survival of less than 1 year, severe pulmonary veno-occlusive disease, chronic respiratory failure, advanced chronic liver disease, acute aortic dissection, severe aortic insufficiency, current intracranial hemorrhage, witnessed cardiopulmonary resuscitation (CPR) greater than 60 min in the absence of return of spontaneous circulation, unwitnessed CA of longer than 5 min, end-stage renal disease on dialysis, and weight over 140 kg. Contraindications of MCA with Impella® devices include LV thrombus, mechanical aortic valve, severe peripheral vascular disease, tortuous iliac arteries, RV failure, morbid obesity, moderate-to-severe aortic insufficiency, aortic valve stenosis or calcification, and femoral or axillary vessels less than 7 mm in diameter (for Impella 5.0®).

PREOPERATIVE ASSESSMENT AND PREPARATION

Identifying patients with impending severe heart failure in advance is ideal. This permits an ordered, thorough review of the medical records and an assessment of the patient's likelihood of meaningful recovery and/or eligibility for future transplantation or LVAD support.

A detailed clinical history pertinent to previous cardiac or vascular interventions and heparin use or allergy (heparin-induced thrombocytopenia) is relevant. The presence of a mechanical aortic valve may preclude the use of Impella devices and a history of femoral stents or abdominal aortic aneurysm repair may preclude the use of the femoral approach for any of these devices.

Clinical examination to rule out the presence of peripheral vascular disease is critical for decision-making if percutaneous MCA is considered. In cases of profound hemodynamic decompensation or CA, the physical exam may evidence the presence of a significant neurologic complication (dilated, areflexic, and asymmetric pupils) that may preclude the use of temporary support. A recent echocardiogram is important to confirm the presence of severe LV dysfunction but also to rule out the presence of severe aortic insufficiency that may preclude the use of most percutaneous MCA options or to confirm the presence of LV thrombus, which may exclude the option of the Impella devices as support. The assessment of a recent X-ray is useful to define the degree of pulmonary involvement (congestion) that may direct the selection of MCA to be utilized. Occasionally, only limited information will be available, especially in patients with ongoing CA considered for ECMO support. A clear absence of the contraindications and the absence of peripheral vascular disease may be the most relevant information to obtain before initiation of support.

Device selection

Different factors must be considered when choosing the type of MCA. These include the hemodynamic condition of the patient, degree of support required (left, right, or biventricular), hemodynamic impact of the device based on the flow provided, need to provide oxygenation, duration of support, and technical considerations including ease and rapidity of insertion, and the ultimate goal of support (bridge to recovery or bridge to a more durable device).

A summary of the basic temporary MCA characteristics is provided in **Table 27.1**. In general, in patients presenting with acute heart failure in the presence on early stages of shock, an IABP is the most frequently utilized system to obtain hemodynamic stability, especially in the presence of an AMI where increased coronary perfusion may be desirable. The IABP has limitations with only modest increases in cardiac output and systemic perfusion, and the IABP requires maintenance of high doses of inotropic support, limiting its effect on outcomes in patients presenting with advanced stages of shock. It is in the more advanced stages of shock, with increasing doses of vasopressors and/or signs of organ malperfusion (increase in lactate, decrease in urine output) that temporary MCA and ECMO are considered.

In patients with only predominant LV dysfunction, the Impella® and TandemHeart® devices are considered as first-line MCA. Although the Impella 2.5® is an option for support in patients with CS, instead of an IABP, recent studies have demonstrated only limited hemodynamic improvement with the potential to increase vascular and bleeding complications. More recently, the Impella CP® (using the same percutaneous implantation delivery system as the Impella 2.5®) has been increasingly utilized in patients with CS, with some positive effect on LV unloading but without clear improvement in outcomes. It seems that, in very advanced stages of CS with predominantly LV dysfunction, the Impella 5.0®, using the femoral or subclavian cannulation, is the Impella® system that provides the best option to revert the physiologic derangement and improve ventricular unloading based on an increasing number of published series, but also without conclusive evidence to support it.

The TandemHeart® is also an appropriate alternative, and is probably comparable with the Impella 5.0®. It is important to note that, due to the need of transseptal cannulation for the inflow cannula, the placement of this device percutaneously requires the presence of an experienced interventional cardiologist, and the cardiologist may not always be available in emergent conditions. In an experienced center, a randomized study showed significant improvement in outcomes using this technology with limited vascular and bleeding complications.

ECMO has continued to be the most used temporary MCA for the advanced stages of CS including in patients with CA. Although generally ECMO has been considered for patients with CS and biventricular failure, especially in the presence of hypoxemia (frequently seen as a consequence of pulmonary congestion due to elevated LV filling pressures), ECMO is frequently utilized also in cases of isolated LV or RV dysfunction due to its implantation simplicity. ECMO can provide up to 6 L/min of flow and, due to its oxygenation capability, can rapidly revert advanced stages of shock. It is important to emphasize that ECMO using peripheral femoral cannulation and retrograde flow may be associated with an increase in left ventricular end-diastolic pressure (LVEDP) and insufficient LV unloading, which can worsen pre-existing mitral regurgitation and increase pulmonary congestion. In these patients, consideration to modify the peripheral approach to central (aortic) or axillary cannulation or even the addition of a second device (Impella®) or direct LV unloading cannula may be necessary to correct an unfavorable situation.

Although ECMO was, until recently, the only percutaneous biventricular support option, other options have become available. The Impella RP® (femoral vein cannulation) has been approved for RV support. This device can provide up to 4 L/min of support and, in combination with left-sided

Table 27.1 Characteristics of common MCA devices

	TandemHeart® LVAD	Impella 2.5–3.5 CP®	ECMO	Impella 5.0®	CentriMag™
Bedside implantation	No	No	Yes	No	No (surgical)
Flow (L/min)	3–3.5	2.5–3.5	3–6	4–5	4–6
LV unloading	Yes	Yes	Partial	Yes	Yes
RV support	No	No	Yes	No	Yes
Pulmonary support	No	No	Yes	No	No
Duration of support	Days–weeks	Days–weeks	<2 weeks	Weeks	Weeks–months
Insertion	Percutaneous	Percutaneous	Percutaneous/sternotomy	Graft	Sternotomy
Cannula size	17–21 Fr LVAD	9 Fr catheter	15–17 Fr artery	9 Fr catheter	
	29–31 Fr RVAD	12–14 Fr sheath	22–25 Fr vein	21 Fr sheath	

ECMO, extracorporeal membrane oxygenation; LV, left ventricular; LVAD, left ventricular assist device; RV, right ventricular; RVAD, right ventricular assist device.

Impella®, can provide biventricular support. A similar situation has occurred with the TandemHeart® pump, which can be used with a double-lumen Protek Duo cannula (placed in the internal jugular vein) and provide up to 4–5 L/min of RV support.

Finally, surgically implanted, temporary MCA, such as the Centrimag™, continues to be used in patients who require high levels of support (flow) due to profound ventricular dysfunction. These devices are approved for up to 14 days of support but have been used safely for periods that are more prolonged and they may be an excellent option in patients in whom slow recovery is suspected (myocarditis) or who require prolonged support directly as a bridge to heart transplant. If an adequate implantation technique is utilized for this device, it may allow mobilization and facilitate recovery. The apical LV cannulation provides excellent LV unloading and may be of use in patients with severely dilated ventricles and in patients with persistent pulmonary congestion with percutaneous support.

ANESTHESIA

Ideally, ECMO and other percutaneous MCA devices should be placed in the operating room or catheterization laboratory under general anesthesia or deep sedation depending on the clinical circumstances. We prefer general anesthesia for patients in profound shock when an emergent open vascular or sternotomy approach may be necessary. In cases where MCA is used as intraoperative support to PCI, sedation and local anesthesia may be used safely. In an emergency, during CA or in patients with impending arrest, only local anesthesia may be needed.

Monitoring of the arterial blood pressure should be obtained with an arterial line. In the case of peripheral femoral VA ECMO, right radial or brachial access is preferred to detect central hypoxemia and, in the case of right axillary access for VA ECMO or Impella®, a left radial or femoral arterial line should be considered.

OPERATIVE TECHNIQUES

Intra-aortic balloon pump insertion

Prior to percutaneous access to place an IABP, the catheter is prepared by flushing the central lumen and evacuating the balloon by applying and maintaining a vacuum and leaving the one-way valve in place until after the catheter is inserted. The femoral artery is accessed using the modified Seldinger technique. The guidewire (0.025 inch × 145–175 cm 3 mm) is inserted and advanced to the proximal descending aorta. Fluoroscopic or transesophageal echocardiographic guidance may be used, if available. There are different balloon sizes (7 Fr, 30 mL; 7.5 Fr, 30 mL and 40 mL; and 8 Fr, 50 mL). A 7.5 Fr or 8 Fr introducer sheath can be used for placement depending on IABP size. In large patients, a sheath may be

placed to facilitate passage of the balloon catheter through the soft tissue without kinking or damage to the catheter.

The intra-aortic balloon is passed over the guidewire to a position just distal to the origin of the left subclavian artery. The catheter is secured to the skin using the provided stabilizer. The pressure tubing is connected to the distal port on the catheter, and the balloon tubing to the controller. The ECG tracing lines are connected to the IABP controller, the balloon is activated on a 1:3 setting, and the arterial waveform observed. An augmented diastolic blood pressure exceeding the peak systolic blood pressure suggests good catheter positioning. Confirm the appropriate positioning of the balloon by chest X-ray or echocardiography. The ideal position for an IABP is approximately 2–4 cm distal to the left subclavian artery. Once positioning is confirmed, the controller may be turned up to 1:1 or 1:2, as needed. Heparin should be considered, in the absence of active bleeding, in cases of prolonged IABP use.

The IABP can also be placed in the axillary artery in cases where peripheral vascular disease is considered or in patients in whom prolonged support and ambulation is desirable. This technique requires open access, using a 5 cm subclavicular incision (right or left), suture of a 6–8 mm Dacron graft using a continuous 5-0 polypropylene suture, and advancement of the IABP over a wire under fluoroscopic guidance into the distal descending aorta (**Figure 27.3**).

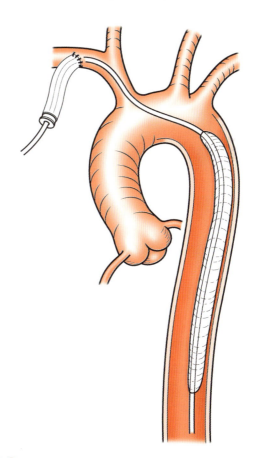

27.3 Intra-aortic balloon pump using subclavian cannulation (open technique).

Veno-arterial ECMO cannulation

Different cannulation techniques can be used for VA ECMO depending on the clinical condition of the patient and vascular access. In adult patients with non-operative CS (AMI, myocarditis, and other), percutaneous peripheral cannulation of the femoral vessels is the most frequently used technique (**Figure 27.4**). In the presence of peripheral vascular disease or inadequate peripheral access, peripheral open subclavian artery cannulation is a useful option and is utilized with the interposition of a Dacron graft to prevent subclavian arterial damage (**Figure 27.5**). In patients presenting with shock during or after cardiac surgery through a sternotomy, central cannulation is the method of choice and involves cannulation of the right atrium and aorta, although other variations can be used.

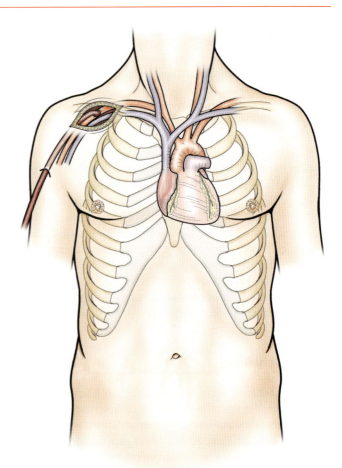

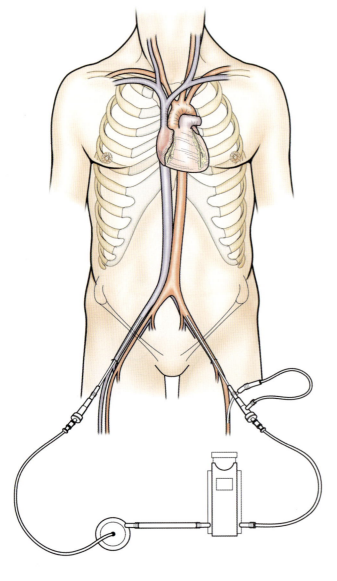

27.4 Femorofemoral peripheral venoarterial ECMO. Cannulation of the femoral artery and vein is usually percutaneous, but this can be done using an open technique if necessary.

27.5 Subclavian arterial cannulation. Cannulation of the subclavian artery using a Dacron graft (open technique) and percutaneous cannulation of the femoral or jugular vein.

PERCUTANEOUS PERIPHERAL FEMORAL CANNULATION

To place ECMO MCA with percutaneous peripheral femoral cannulation, the femoral artery is accessed using the modified Seldinger technique. Ultrasound guidance is helpful to identify the vascular structures, decreasing the risk of vascular complications and cannula malposition, and its use should be encouraged (**Figure 27.6**). A 16–18 gauge needle is inserted in the femoral artery (**Figure 27.7a**) and a guidewire (0.035 inch) is advanced into the femoral artery proximally (**Figure 27.7b**). Progressive arterial dilation is performed using tapered dilators (**Figure 27.7c**). After heparinization (10 000 U heparin to target an ACT of 180–250 seconds), the arterial cannula is inserted over the guidewire (**Figure 27.7d**) using rotational motion and keeping the guidewire under tension. We prefer 15 Fr or 16 Fr ECMO arterial cannulae for smaller patients (<60 kg) and 17–19 Fr for larger patients. After placement, the arterial cannula is secured to the skin. After removing the cannula introducer, a tubing clamp is used to prevent retrograde bleeding. Proper position is confirmed with fluoroscopy if available or by the presence of bright red blood and high blood return pressure in the emergent cannulation.

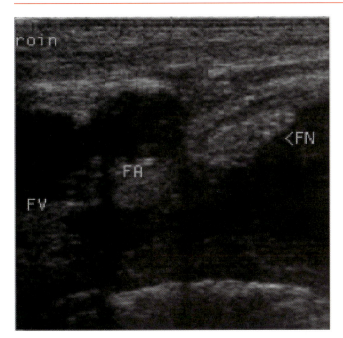

27.6 Femoral ultrasound depicting the femoral vein (FV) in proximity with the femoral artery (FA) and the femoral nerve (FN), which is more externally located.

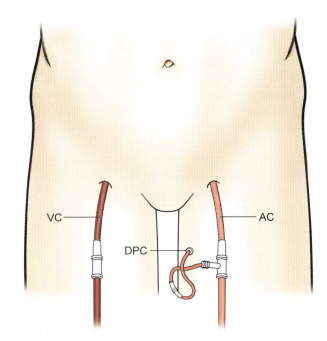

27.8 Contralateral venoarterial ECMO cannulation. AC, arterial cannula; DPC, distal perfusion cannula; VC, venous cannula.

The femoral vein is accessed using a similar technique as used for femoral artery cannulation. In emergent cannulation, we frequently consider ipsilateral arterial and venous cannulation, generally involving the right femoral vessels. In patients in more stable condition, we prefer to cannulate the right femoral vein and the contralateral (left) femoral artery (**Figure 27.8**) to facilitate venous return on the side with

arterial cannulation and decrease the risk of limb ischemia. A needle is introduced into the femoral vein and, using the modified Seldinger technique, a 0.035 inch guidewire is advanced through the femoral vein into the inferior vena cava up to the right atrium, watching the monitor for ventricular ectopy. Fluoroscopy or transesophageal guidance is recommended when available. In obese patients, a stiff guidewire

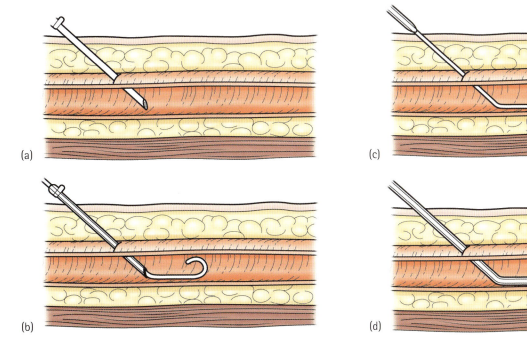

(a)

(b)

(c)

(d)

27.7a–d Seldinger technique. (a) The needle is introduced in the femoral vessel; (b) the guidewire is advanced proximally; (c) tapered dilators are used to dilate the vessel; (d) the cannula is advanced in its final position.

is preferable (0.035 inch Amplatz or Lunderquist guidewire) to prevent guidewire kinking during the introduction of the cannula. At our center, we would generally use a 22 Fr multifenestrated venous cannula in smaller patients (<60 kg) and a 25 Fr multifenestrated venous cannula in larger patients. After incising the skin, the venous cannula is inserted to a depth that delivers the tip of the cannula into the mid-right atrium. The guidewire and introducer are removed, and the cannula is clamped and secured to the skin. With both cannulae secure, we connect them to the ECMO circuit.

The ECMO circuit, including the pump and oxygenator, has been previously de-aired. The ECMO circuit tubing is clamped and divided. The arterial and venous cannulae are connected to the circuit tubing with care to avoid introduction of air into the circuit. Flow is initiated in a slow progression to avoid ventricular arrhythmia due to suction events.

Attention must be given to distal perfusion of the leg used for femoral arterial cannulation. We have modified our technique, and we use distal arterial perfusion in all patients undergoing peripheral VA ECMO support due to increasing evidence, including our own previously published experience, that distal arterial perfusion decreases the rate of serious vascular complications. In emergent cannulation, a distal perfusion cannula is inserted after placement of the arterial and venous cannula. In non-emergent cannulation, we prefer to access the distal superficial femoral artery first to facilitate the localization of the artery when it is completely filled. Using ultrasound, we identify the arterial vessel and using the modified Seldinger technique, we insert a 0.035 inch guidewire distally and place a 7–9 Fr sheath (**Figure 27.9**) or cannula (**Figure 27.10**). It is important to confirm the passage of the wire with ease into the distal part of the artery, because the guidewire and cannula can easily be positioned in the profunda femoris leading to subsequent ischemia of the lower extremity. It is our routine to confirm the proper position using angiography (**Figure 27.11**) if the procedure is performed in the operating room or if there is a concern regarding distal lower extremity perfusion. To minimize the risk of vascular

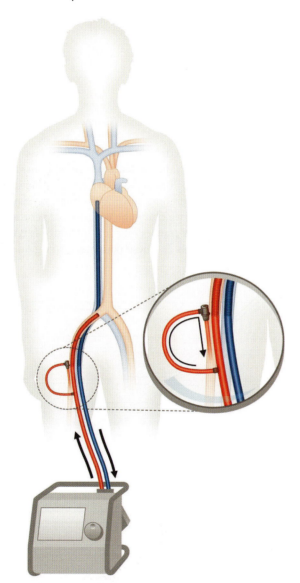

27.9 Distal perfusion using a 7–8 Fr sheath. Reprinted by permission from Springer Nature: *Clin Res Cardiol.* 105(4): 283–96. Cannulation strategies for percutaneous extracorporeal membrane oxygenation in adults. Napp LC, et al. Copyright 2016.

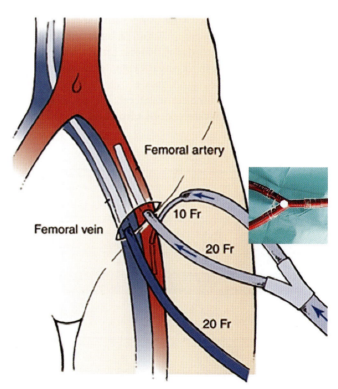

27.10 Distal femoral perfusion using a cannula. Reprinted from McGee JEC, Moazami N. Temporary Mechanical Circulatory Support. In *Cardiac Surgery in the Adult*, 5e, (2017) Cohn LH, Adams DH (eds). Used with permission of McGraw-Hill Education. Inset: Reprinted by permission from Springer Nature: *Clin Res Cardiol.* 105(4):283-96. Cannulation strategies for percutaneous extracorporeal membrane oxygenation in adults. Napp LC et al., Copyright 2016.

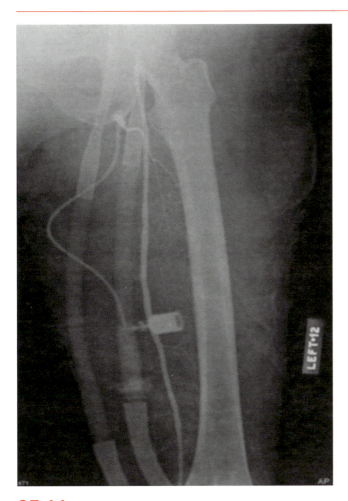

27.11 Angiograph verifying positioning in the artery.

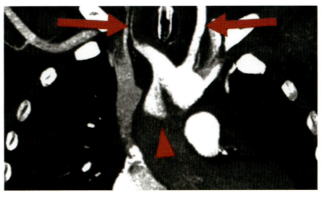

27.12 Central hypoxia (north-south syndrome) due to increased pulmonary shunting in the presence of primary or secondary lung injury in patients on peripheral VA ECMO. Reprinted by permission from Springer Nature: *Clin Res Cardiol.* 105(4): 283–96. Cannulation strategies for percutaneous extracorporeal membrane oxygenation in adults. Napp LC, et al. Copyright 2016.

complications, it is our practice to continuously monitor perfusion to both legs using near-infrared spectroscopy for the duration of ECMO support.

Primary lung injury or pulmonary injury secondary to cardiac dysfunction and severe pulmonary congestion or edema may lead to significant pulmonary shunting with poorly oxygenated blood filling the LV in patients who have been femorally cannulated for peripheral VA ECMO for CS. This poorly oxygenated blood is ejected on every cardiac cycle and could lead to hypoxic blood filling the root of the aorta and head vessels (**Figure 27.12**) with the potential of central hypoxia. A modification of femoral VA ECMO, called venoarterial–venous ECMO (VAV ECMO) (**Figure 27.13**) has been utilized to decrease the pulmonary shunting of deoxygenated blood. A second cannula (16–18 Fr) is placed in the RIJV and connected to the arterial limb of the ECMO circuit using a 0.375 inch Y connector. The inflow of oxygenated blood will then be through the femoral artery and RIJV. Flow through this RIJV cannula can be controlled and decreased as needed to maintain systemic blood pressure using a Hoffman clamp. The insertion of this internal jugular cannula is similar to femoral venous cannulation using the modified Seldinger technique.

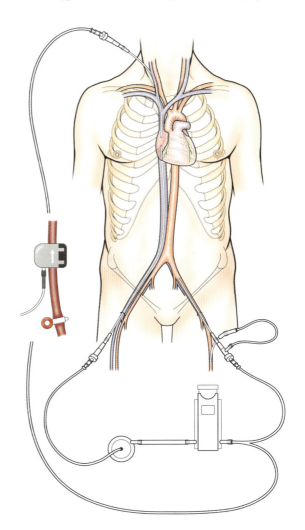

27.13 Venoarterial-venous (VAV) ECMO. Cannulation of the femoral artery and vein with the addition of a right internal jugular venous cannula providing arterial blood. This cannulation is usually percutaneous. Flow through the internal jugular cannula should be monitored with a flow probe and adjusted with a vascular clamp.

OPEN PERIPHERAL FEMORAL AND AXILLARY ARTERY CANNULATION

In case of concerns regarding femoral vessel size or an inability to localize the vascular structures, an open technique can be utilized to institute VA ECMO. The cannulation can be performed in several different ways, using open cutdown and direct vessel cannulation, open cutdown and the Seldinger technique ("semi-Seldinger"), or open cutdown with end-to-side graft (Dacron) to the artery.

In the case of open cannulation, a standard surgical cutdown is performed in a longitudinal or oblique fashion. After placing a soft-tissue retractor and using electrocautery and blunt dissection, the vascular structures, including the femoral artery and femoral veins, are identified. If a direct cutdown of the vessels is considered, proximal and distal control of the vessel is necessary using a vascular clamp or vessel loops. Once a longitudinal incision is performed in the vessel, the cannula is advanced, and then the vessel is snared proximally and distally with an umbilical tape or a heavy-silk tie. In these cases, distal perfusion of the femoral artery is necessary as the arterial flow is completely interrupted at the cannulation site (**Figure 27.14**).

The semi-Seldinger technique combines open access with the arterial cannulation using the Seldinger technique to cannulate the femoral artery and vein (**Figure 27.15a–d**).

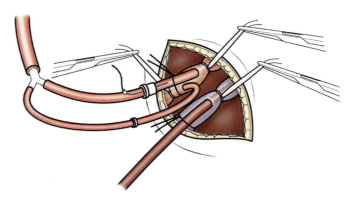

27.14 Distal femoral cannulation using the open femoral cannulation technique.

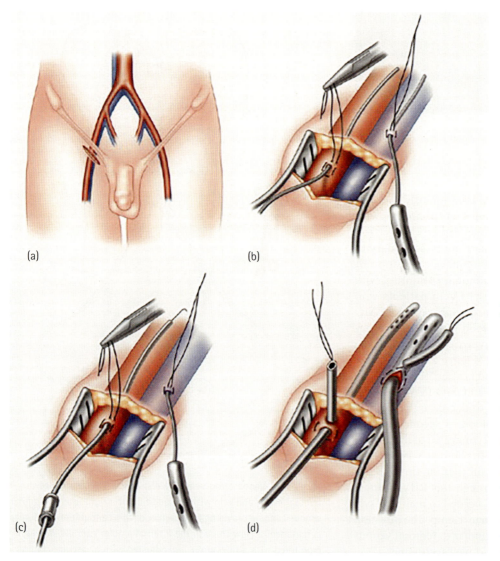

(a)

(b)

(c)

(d)

27.15a–d Arterial and venous cannulation using the semi-Seldinger technique. After direct exposure of the femoral vessels, the cannulae are advanced over the guidewire (similar to the percutaneous technique) and a pursestring suture using a 5-0 polypropylene suture is used to minimize bleeding. Reprinted by permission from Springer Nature: Cardiopulmonary perfusion during robotic cardiac surgery. Kypson AP, et al. In: Chitwood WR Jr (ed.). *Atlas of robotic cardiac surgery.* Copyright 2014.

The technique involves the insertion of a 16–18 gauge needle, advancement of a 0.035 inch guidewire, and insertion of the arterial and venous cannula after stepwise dilation. A 5-0 polypropylene pursestring suture can be used at the cannulation site to decrease bleeding and used later at the time of cannula removal. The cannulae are secured to the skin with multiple silk sutures to prevent cannula displacement.

In patients with small femoral arterial vessels, a Dacron graft, sutured in a terminolateral fashion to the femoral artery, can be utilized to insert the arterial cannula. Using a 5 cm groin incision (right or left) and after identifying the femoral artery, heparin is administered and, after clamping the artery proximally and distally, an 8–10 mm longitudinal arteriotomy is created. A 10 mm Dacron graft with a 70-degree angle bevel is sutured with a continuous 5-0 polypropylene suture to the femoral artery (**Figure 27.16**). After confirming absence of anastomotic bleeding, a 20 Fr arterial cannula is inserted and secured to the graft with multiple silk ties.

The right axillary artery can also be used for open arterial ECMO cannulation (**Figure 27.17**). A 3–5 cm longitudinal incision is performed to expose the axillary artery. By dividing the fibers of the pectoralis major, the subclavian vein and axillary artery beneath it are visualized. Upward traction on the clavicle may be required. Careful dissection is performed to expose the axillary artery. Inferior retraction of the subclavian vein is generally needed to expose the artery. Medial extension should be avoided to ensure preservation of the phrenic nerve on the anterior scalene muscle. This section should be free of significant branches, but you should avoid the thyrocervical

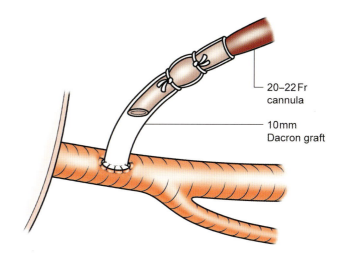

27.16 Open femoral cannulation using a 10 mm Dacron graft.

branch even though, if encountered, you should be able to take it without consequence. An 8–10 mm arteriotomy is created after heparinization and proximal and distal control of the vessel. A 10 mm Dacron graft is beveled in a 70-degree angle and is anastomosed in a terminolateral fashion using 5-0 polypropylene suture. After confirming the absence of anastomotic bleeding, a 20–22 Fr arterial cannula is inserted and secured to the graft with multiple silk ties. The graft is exteriorized through a separate incision. We routinely use a vessel loop to decrease the distal vessel lumen size by 50% to prevent right upper extremity hyperperfusion. We believe it is important

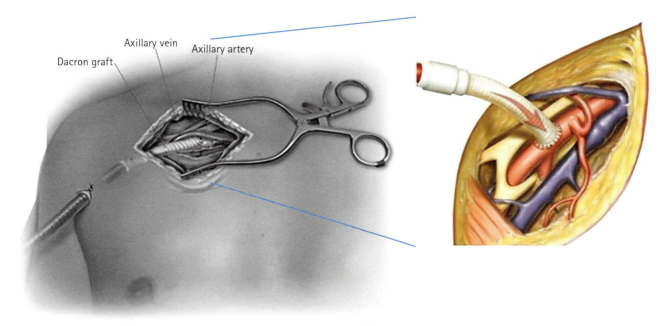

27.17 Open subclavian/axillary cannulation using a 10 mm Dacron graft. Left panel: © 2016 Chand Ramaiah and Ashok Babu. Adapted from: ECMO cannulation techniques; originally published by IntechOpen under the terms of the Creative Commons Attribution 3.0 License. Available from DOI: 10.5772/64338. https://www.intechopen.com/books/extracorporeal-membrane-oxygenation-advances-in-therapy/ecmo-cannulation-techniques. Right panel: From LeMaire SA, et al. Surgical adhesives. In: Coselli JS, LeMaire SA. *Aortic arch surgery: principles, strategies, and outcomes.* Chichester, UK: Wiley-Blackwell, 2008. Used with permission of John Wiley and Sons.

to leave a drain, because this anastomosis tends to bleed and could produce recurrent hematoma leading to vascular and nerve compression. The venous return to the ECMO circuit can be done through percutaneous femoral or right internal jugular cannulation.

CENTRAL CANNULATION FOR VA ECMO

VA ECMO using central cannulation is used frequently in patients presenting with CS after cardiac operations. Due to the antegrade direction of the flow in the aorta, it is generally associated with better unloading of the LV and RV than femoral ECMO.

After exposure of the heart via sternotomy, two concentric 4-0 polypropylene pursestring sutures are placed in the ascending aorta and captured with tourniquets. The aortic adventitia is dissected off the site selected for cannula insertion. Although standard surgical cannulae can be used for ECMO, we prefer ECMO with straight, tapered 18–22 Fr cannulae that allow exteriorization through the abdominal wall. After heparinization (10 000 U i.v.), a needle is inserted through the center of the pursestring sutures into the aortic lumen. A wire is gently advanced to the proximal descending thoracic aorta with confirmation of position by transesophageal echocardiography. Dilators from the PicA (Medtronic, Minneapolis, MN) cannula kit are sequentially inserted, maintaining control of the wire at all times. After dilation, the cannula is inserted into the aortic lumen. A central position, avoiding contact with the aortic wall or direction toward the head vessels, must be confirmed. The tourniquets are snared down, and two 0-silk ligatures are used to secure the cannula to the tourniquets. The tourniquets are secured using a sterile button or with four or five large vascular clips in their midsections, and the suture is folded over onto the tourniquet and secured with an additional large vascular clip.

For venous drainage, typically a large venous cannula is selected (28–32 Fr). A single 4-0 braided pursestring suture over pledgets is placed at the right atrial appendage or body and captured in a tourniquet. The right atrium is incised in the middle of the pursestring, and the venous cannula is inserted into the inferior vena cava. The cannula is secured to the tourniquet with two silk ligatures, and the ends of the tourniquet secured in the same manner as used for the arterial cannula. The cannulae are passed through the abdominal wall using a 26–40 Fr straight chest tube and then the cannulae are inserted as described above (**Figure 27.18**). The ECMO circuit is clamped, divided, and connected to the cannulae with care to remove any air; then ECMO flow is initiated.

In patients with persistent LV dilation despite adequate ECMO flows, a second drainage cannula can be added directly into the LV apex (**Figure 27.19**). Cannulation is performed using two or three polypropylene 4-0 sutures over pledgets and captured with tourniquets. At least two silk suture ties are used to secure the cannula to the tourniquets. The LV cannula is then connected to the right atrial return line. Other options to improve LV and RV decompression include a second pulmonary artery or right superior pulmonary vein cannula.

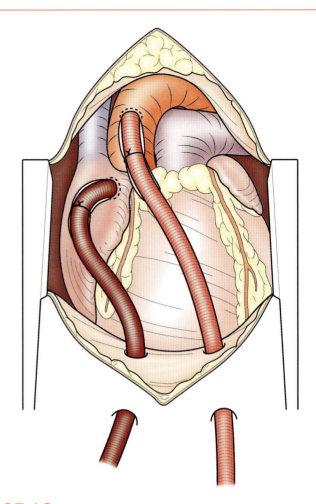

27.18 Final appearance of central VA ECMO using right atrial-to-aorta cannulation.

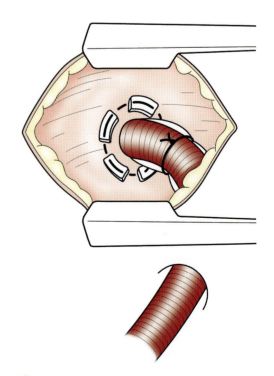

27.19 Left ventricular venting using a drainage cannula.

Usually, temporary closure of the sternotomy is achieved using an Esmarch patch. The patch is sutured to the skin with care to minimize any gaps around the cannulae as they exit the sternotomy from underneath the patch. Each cannula is firmly secured to the patient's skin using at least five 0-silk stitches. Alternatively, the surgeon may wish to bring the cannulae out of the body through separate skin sites. If this is desired, it is important for the surgeon to identify cannula sites before cannulation stitches are placed. The sternotomy may be left open with temporary patch closure, or the surgeon may wish to close the skin or close the sternotomy entirely. Before partial or complete chest closure at least three mediastinal chest tubes (inferior and anterior) should be placed to prevent early tamponade and decreased ECMO flows.

Insertion of Impella® devices

INSERTION OF THE IMPELLA 2.5® OR IMPELLA CP® DEVICE

The Impella® 2.5 and CP devices can be inserted via a standard catheterization procedure through the femoral artery, into the ascending aorta, across the valve, and into the LV. The Impella 2.5® and Impella CP® can also be placed through an open subclavian approach using a Dacron graft, as described for axillary cannulation for the Impella 5.0®.

To begin the catheterization procedure, obtain access to the femoral artery. Insert a 5–8 Fr introducer over a 0.035 inch guidewire to pre-dilate the vessel and then remove the introducer. Sequentially insert and remove 8 Fr, 10 Fr, and 12 Fr dilators and then insert a 13 Fr peel-away introducer with dilator. For the Impella CP® device, the introducer is 14 Fr. While inserting the introducer, hold the shaft of the introducer to slide it into the artery. Administer heparin, and remove the dilator when the ACT is greater than or equal to 250 seconds. Insert a diagnostic catheter (6 Fr AL1 or multipurpose without side holes or a 5 Fr pigtail without side holes) over a 0.035 inch diagnostic guidewire into the introducer and advance it into the left ventricle. Remove the 0.035 inch diagnostic guidewire, leaving the diagnostic catheter in the ventricle. Form a curve or bend on the end of a 0.018 inch placement guidewire and advance it into the apex of the left ventricle. Remove the diagnostic catheter. Insert the placement guidewire into the red EasyGuide lumen at the tip of the pigtail. Advance the guidewire until it exits the red lumen near the label. Remove the EasyGuide lumen by gently pulling the label in line with the catheter shaft while holding the Impella® catheter. Advance the catheter through the hemostatic valve into the femoral artery, along the placement guidewire, and across the aortic valve using a fixed-wire technique. Follow the catheter under fluoroscopy as it is advanced across the aortic valve, positioning the inlet area of the catheter 3.5 cm below the aortic valve annulus and in the middle of the ventricular chamber, free from the mitral valve chordae. Be careful not to coil the guidewire in the left ventricle. Remove the placement guidewire. Finally, confirm the position of the Impella® with fluoroscopy and confirm that an aortic waveform is displayed on the automated Impella® controller.

IMPELLA 5.0® INSERTION VIA FEMORAL ARTERY CUTDOWN

The Impella 5.0® can be placed with either a femoral artery cutdown or an axillary artery cutdown. After exposing the common femoral artery via a 3–5 cm incision, prepare the insertion site with a 5-0 polypropylene pursestring suture captured with a short tourniquet. Place vessel loops proximal and distal to the planned insertion site. Administer heparin to achieve an ACT of at least 250 seconds. Access the femoral artery in the middle of the pursestring with a needle and insert a 0.035 inch guidewire. Remove the needle. Insert a diagnostic pigtail catheter (6 Fr AL1 or multipurpose without side holes or 5 Fr pigtail without side holes) over the guide and advance the guidewire and diagnostic catheter into the LV. Exchange the guidewire for a 0.018 inch placement guidewire. Remove the diagnostic catheter. Backload the Impella 5.0® over the guidewire. Place the vessel loops on tension. Make a transverse arteriotomy at the arterial puncture site. Insert the device into the femoral artery as tension on the proximal vessel loop is released (**Figure 27.20a**). Advance the placement guidewire into the Impella 5.0® catheter and stabilize the cannula between the fingers. This prevents pinching of the inlet area. The placement guidewire must exit the outlet area on the inner radius of the cannula (**Figure 27.20b**), and align with the straight black line on the catheter. The catheter can be hyperextended as necessary to ensure the placement guidewire exits on the inner radius of the cannula. Guide the device into position within the LV using fluoroscopy. The inlet of the device should lie 3.5–4 cm below the aortic annulus. Remove the guidewire and start the device. Advance the repositioning sheath into position in the femoral artery and secure the pursestring suture and tourniquet as described previously. Close the incision and secure the repositioning device wings to the skin. Advance the sterile sleeve to the repositioning device and confirm the device position. Lock the device in position by tightening the repositioning device rings.

Rather than directly accessing the femoral artery, the Impella 5.0® may also be placed through a graft (**Figure 27.20c**). In this circumstance, the surgeon performs a femoral artery cutdown, obtains proximal and distal control, and anastomoses a beveled 10 mm × 20 cm Dacron graft in end-to-side fashion. A standard 6 Fr sheath is inserted through the graft into the femoral artery, and is used to control bleeding during manipulation of the 0.035 inch guidewire and 5 Fr pigtail catheter used to advance into the LV in the same manner as described above. After positioning the 0.018 inch guidewire in the LV, backload the device onto the guidewire and advance it through the graft and into the LV.

Regardless of the technique employed, obtain meticulous hemostasis and close the groin incision. If there is troublesome bleeding, you can leave a closed-suction drain in place.

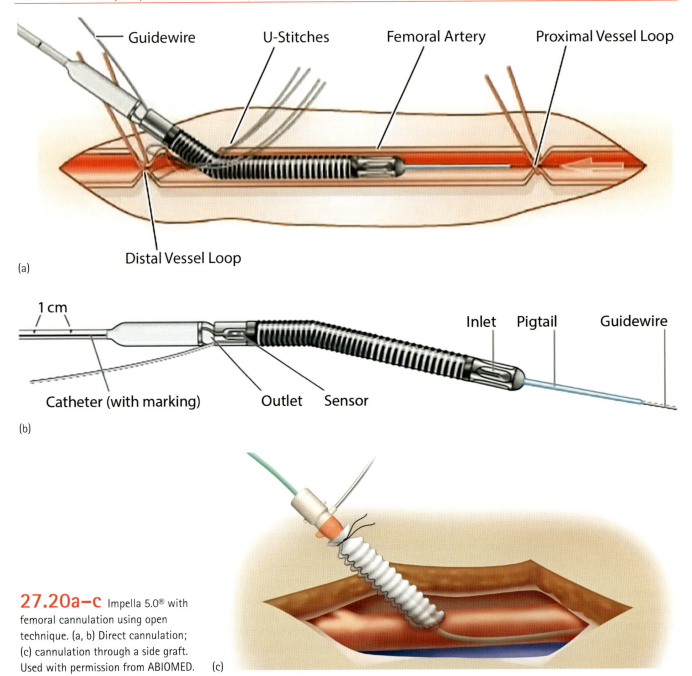

27.20a–c Impella 5.0® with femoral cannulation using open technique. (a, b) Direct cannulation; (c) cannulation through a side graft. Used with permission from ABIOMED.

IMPELLA 5.0® INSERTION VIA AXILLARY ARTERY CUTDOWN

After performing an axillary artery cutdown and obtaining proximal and distal control with vessel loops and/or vascular clamps, a longitudinal arteriotomy is made (**Figure 27.21a**) and a 20 cm × 10 cm Dacron graft is anastomosed to the axillary artery in end-to-side fashion (**Figure 27.21b**). Do not trim the graft. Apply a soft-jawed vascular clamp to the graft just distal to the anastomosis. Insert the 8 Fr peel-away sheath from the kit into the graft (**Figure 27.21b**). Secure the graft to the sheath with the graft blocks found in the kit, and release the clamp. Insert a 5 Fr diagnostic pigtail catheter with a 0.035 inch J-tipped guidewire through the sheath and advance across the aortic valve into the LV under fluoroscopic guidance. Exchange the 0.035 inch diagnostic guidewire for the 0.018 inch placement guidewire. Remove the pigtail catheter. Reapply the soft-jawed clamp to the graft. Advance the included 8 Fr silicone-coated dilator through the peel-away sheath into the graft. This lubricates the hemostatic valve with silicone, facilitating insertion of the device.

Backload the Impella 5.0® onto the guidewire, and advance it through the sheath. Keep the graft clamped until the device has passed all the way through the hemostatic valve to prevent bleeding through the device. Once the motor housing of the Impella® passes through the valve, the graft may be unclamped, and the device may be advanced over the wire into the LV under fluoroscopic guidance. Adjust the position such that the inlet of the device lies approximately 3.5 cm below the aortic annulus. The surgeon may then remove the guidewire and start the device. Reapply the soft-jawed clamp to the graft just above the anastomosis, and remove the graft blocks and the peel-away sheath (**Figure 27.21c**). Shorten the graft material such that the graft does not protrude above the level of the skin. Tighten the vessel loops, remove the clamp, and advance the repositioning sheath into the trimmed graft (**Figure 27.21d**). Secure the repositioning unit with 0-silk ligatures. Close the subcutaneous tissue and skin, and secure the wings of the repositioning device to the skin (**Figure 27.21e**). Confirm appropriate positioning of the device within the LV. Advance the sterile sleeve, and secure the catheter in position by tightening the repositioning device rings.

INSERTION OF THE IMPELLA RP® FOR RIGHT VENTRICULAR SUPPORT

Before beginning the implantation of the Impella RP® for RV support, confirm that purge fluid is exiting the Impella® catheter. Obtain access to the femoral vein. Insert a 5–8 Fr introducer over a 0.035 inch guidewire to pre-dilate the vessel, and then remove the introducer. Insert the 8 Fr, 12 Fr, 16 Fr, and 20 Fr dilators sequentially, as needed. After removing the 20 Fr dilator, insert the 23 Fr introducer with dilator. While inserting the 23 Fr introducer, hold the shaft of the introducer to advance it into the vein. Administer heparin. When ACT is at least 250 seconds, remove the 23 Fr dilator. Insert a flow-directed, balloon-tipped catheter into the 23 Fr introducer and advance it over a guidewire into the left (preferred) or right pulmonary artery. Remove the 0.035 inch diagnostic guidewire, leaving the diagnostic or balloon-tipped catheter in the pulmonary artery. Form a curve or bend on the 0.027 inch placement guidewire and then insert it. Advance the placement guidewire deep into the left pulmonary artery until the wire prolapses. Remove the diagnostic or balloon-tipped catheter. Wet the cannula with sterile water and backload the catheter onto the placement guidewire. One or two people can load the catheter on the guidewire. Advance the guidewire into the Impella RP® System catheter, and stabilize the cannula between the fingers. The scrub

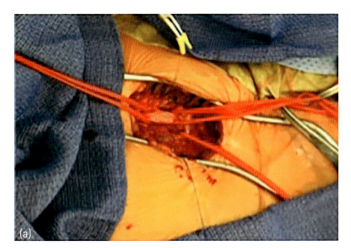

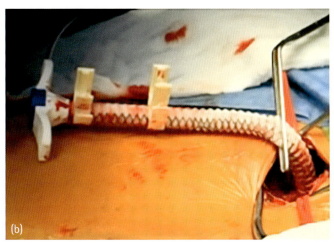

27.21a–e Impella 5.0® with axillary cannulation. Used with permission from ABIOMED.

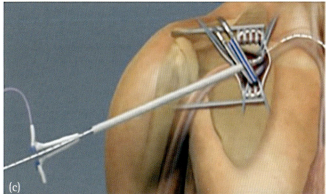

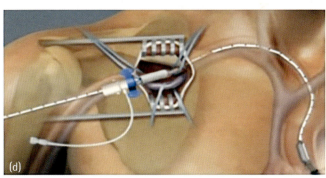

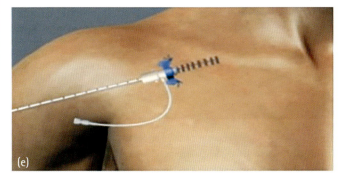

assistant can help stabilize the catheter by holding it proximal to the motor. The physician can focus on advancing the guidewire and, if the cannula needs to be hyperextended, the scrub assistant is available to assist. Advance the catheter through the hemostatic valve into the femoral vein and along the placement guidewire using a fixed-wire technique. Follow the catheter under fluoroscopy, and rotate the catheter as it enters the RV to direct the cannula tip upward and across the pulmonary valve. Position the outlet area of the cannula approximately 4 cm past the pulmonary valve annulus. While the entire pump is in the abdominal inferior vena cava, calibrate the sensor. Remove the placement guidewire, and confirm positioning with fluoroscopy.

Insertion of the TandemHeart® device

TANDEMHEART® INSERTION: LVAD CONFIGURATION

To begin insertion of the TandemHeart device for LVAD support, left femoral arterial access and right femoral venous access are obtained using the modified Seldinger technique. Ensure the patient is appropriately heparinized to an ACT above 400 seconds. Serially dilate the arteriotomy, then insert the cannula. Backbleed the cannula and clamp it. Access the femoral vein, and advance a guidewire under fluoroscopic guidance. Advance a Mullins guide catheter (Medtronic, Minneapolis, MN) and position it in the *fossa ovalis*. Create a transseptal puncture with a transseptal needle (Cook, Bloomington, IN) and dilator and introduce a guidewire into the left atrium, (via the left superior pulmonary vein). Then, remove the transseptal needle and Mullins sheath. Advance the two-stage dilator over the guidewire until the section with

the largest diameter enters the left atrium, then remove the dilator. Insert the introducer 21 Fr cannula over the guidewire into the left atrium. Confirm the position of the tip of the transseptal cannula in the left atrium using a combination of blood gas analysis, pressure measurement, fluoroscopy, and echocardiography. Confirm that adequate volume exists in the left atrium via pressure transduction. Next, remove the guidewire and introducer until they are beyond the clamp area of the cannula. Then, leaving the hemostatic valve in place to control blood loss, clamp the cannula in the clamping area and remove the obturator and wire. Once the cannula is fully clamped, remove the hemostatic valve.

After transseptal cannula placement, serially dilate the arteriotomy, then insert a 17 Fr arterial cannula. Backbleed the cannula, and clamp it. Ensure both cannulae are secured and connect them to the pump with a wet-to-wet connection with complete purge of any air. Turn on the pump, which will start at 5500 rpm. Check again for air bubbles. If the tubing and pump are air free, slowly release the clamp on the outflow cannula. Gradually increase the pump speed until the desired flow is achieved. Secure the pump and tubing.

TANDEMHEART INSERTION: RVAD CONFIGURATION USING PROTEK DUO CANNULA

To place the TandemHeart with the protek Duo cannula for RVAD support, use the modified Seldinger technique to introduce a 0.035 inch guidewire into the right internal jugular vein and advance it, under fluoroscopy, into the main pulmonary artery. Advance a 6 Fr multipurpose or a one-flow-directed Swan–Ganz catheter over the wire into the distal main pulmonary artery (**Figure 27.22a**). Remove the guidewire, and replace it with a stiff 0.035 inch Amplatz or

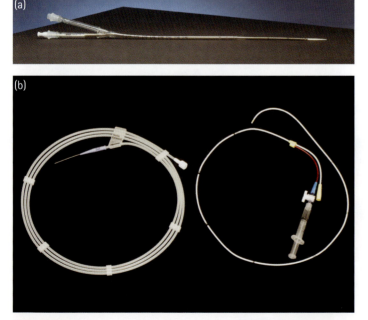

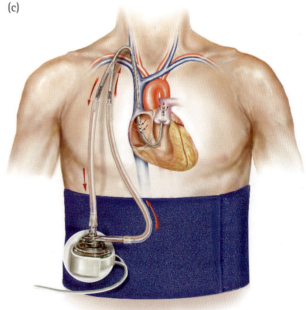

27.22a–c Placement of the TandemHeart® percutaneous RVAD. (a) Protek Duo: dual-lumen cannula; (b) flow-directed pulmonary artery catheter and COOK® 0.035 inch Lunderquist guidewire used to advance the cannula; (c) adequate position in the distal pulmonary artery. Copyright CardiacAssist Inc./TandemLife. Used with permission.

Lunderquist wire while keeping the catheter in place. Then, remove the catheter. Serially dilate the vein. Administer heparin to achieve an ACT above 400 seconds. Insert the Protek Duo cannula assembly over the guidewire, and advance it into the distal pulmonary artery under fluoroscopy guidance. A 29 Fr Protek Duo double-lumen cannula and a 31 Fr Protek Duo double-lumen cannula are available (**Figure 27.22b**). Confirm the appropriate position of the tip of the outflow lumen in the distal main pulmonary artery using pressure, echocardiography, or angiography (**Figure 27.22c**). Immediately secure the cannula at its insertion site. Remove the guidewire and introducer until they are beyond the clamp area of the cannula, leaving the hemostatic valve in place temporarily to control blood loss. Clamp the distal cannula port, and remove its hemostatic valve. You may then remove the hemostatic valve from the proximal port, backbleed it, and clamp the cannula. You can connect the inflow and outflow tubing to the ports. You may unclamp the inflow cannula, but leave the outflow cannula clamped. Turn on the pump, which starts at 5500 rpm. Check again for air. If no air is present, slowly release the outflow cannula clamp. You may then increase the pump speed until the desired flow rate is achieved. Secure the cannula, tubing, and pump.

Implantation of the CentriMag™ ventricular assist device

The CentriMag™ ventricular assist device requires surgical implantation, which is usually through sternotomy although minimally invasive approaches have recently been described. CPB is frequently needed, especially in cases of hemodynamic decompensation, but occasionally an off-pump technique is possible in cases of isolated RVAD or LVAD placement.

The Centrimag™ VAS has been used for left, right, and biventricular support in patients with different causes of primary CS or following cardiac operation. Different techniques of cannulation can be used. (**Figure 27.23a–c**). Cannulation is normally accomplished with standard CPB cannulae and techniques. There is no predetermined size of the cannulae, and their selection will be determined by the patient's characteristics and type of support required. For left ventricular support, we prefer a malleable, wire-reinforced inflow cannula and a large, low-resistance outflow cannula. For postcardiotomy failure, the existing CPB cannulae can be used if necessary. Otherwise, for left support, a 28 or 32 Fr inflow cannula is inserted into the left atrium at the level of the junction between the superior and inferior pulmonary veins (**Figure 27.23b**) or directly into the left ventricle (our preferred approach) (**Figure 27.23c**). A 20 Fr or 22 Fr elongated, one-piece outflow cannula is inserted preferably into the ascending aorta; when this site is unavailable, the cannula can be inserted via the femoral artery. In the case of RVAD, a 20 Fr arterial cannula is placed in the pulmonary artery. At each cannulation site, we use two 4-0 polypropylene or braided pursestring sutures secured with tourniquets, as described earlier in the chapter. If long-term

support is considered, a 10 mm Dacron graft can be sewn to the aorta and the pulmonary artery, and then the cannula can be secured to the proximal segment on the graft with silk sutures (**Figure 27.3b**). This technique may decrease the risk of bleeding with ambulation of the patient, because there is no direct contact between the cannula and the vessel wall. A similar technique has been described to insert the LV apical cannula where a Dacron skirt is sutured around the apical cannulation site to minimize postoperative bleeding. In general, we have used the apical LV apical cannulation with two 4-0 polypropylene U stitches over pledgets with no inconvenience and this is our preferred cannulation method.

After cannulation, the circuit and pumps are filled with saline solution. Then CPB flow is decreased to approximately 1–2 liters/min to allow for filling of the cardiac structures, and then the Centrimag™ system is started. Pump speed is gradually increased to achieve the desired level of cardiac output and to verify that suction has not occurred. When left atrial pressure is monitored, it should be maintained in the range of 10–15 mmHg. As the flow is increased, the operator should monitor the pump flow rate, the patient's blood pressure, and the circuit for signs of suction. The pump flow rate and the patient's total cardiac output, central venous pressure, pulmonary artery pressure, and arterial blood pressure should be monitored frequently, because hemodynamic conditions can change rapidly during the preoperative period. The cannulae are then secured with at least four or five silk sutures to the skin. Three or four chest tubes are placed in standard fashion (inferior, lateral, and anterior) to avoid postoperative fluid collection or tamponade.

POSTOPERATIVE CARE

Bleeding is of significant concern in patients with MCA. Strict hemostasis is essential, and extra time is spent in the operating room to ensure meticulous hemostasis. Occasionally, cutdown sites must be sterilely opened and repacked in the ICU, or the patient may need to return to the operating room to control bleeding at the device insertion site. We generally fully reverse heparin with protamine at the end of the procedure and initiate anticoagulation via a heparin infusion within 12–24 hours. Fibrin deposits and thrombi may form in oxygenators, pumps, tubing, or cannulae. Depending on the stability of the patient and the location of the debris, the affected portions of the circuit may be exchanged in the ICU or the operating room. Thromboembolic strokes are more common than hemorrhagic strokes, but either may occur. As mentioned previously, the presence of peripheral devices may compromise distal perfusion to the extremity. Extremity perfusion is routinely monitored with near-infrared spectroscopy, and antegrade superficial femoral artery perfusion cannulae are placed routinely unless difficult access raises concern for risk of vascular injury. The incidence of limb ischemia distal to the peripheral arterial cannula has been historically high, up to 30%, and approximately half of these patients require surgical intervention. However, more

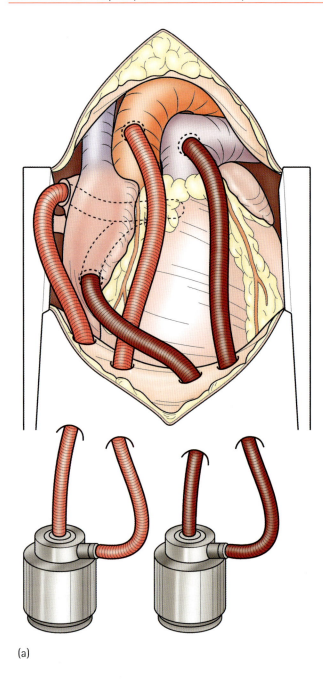

(a)

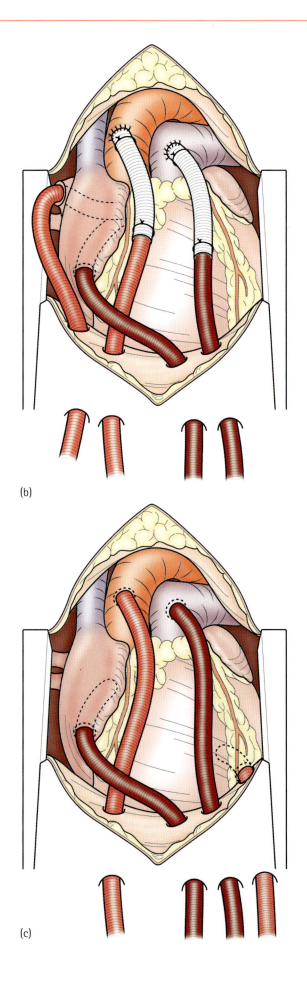

(b)

(c)

27.23a–c Cannulation techniques for the CentriMag™ device.

recently, with the use of these techniques, limb ischemia has decreased to less than 10%.

Intracardiac thrombus formation may be prevented by maintaining contractility and adequate anticoagulation. Typically, we try to maintain the PTT at 50–60 seconds or ACT above 250 seconds if there is no concern for bleeding. Good drainage of the left atrium and LV is also important to avoid thrombus formation. Drainage of the left-sided chambers may be increased by insertion of intra-aortic balloon pump or Impella® or by conversion to central cannulation with additional drainage via the pulmonary artery, a pulmonary vein, or direct apical cannulation of the LV. Judicious volume administration may avoid right-sided heart failure. Inotropes, diuretics, dialysis, and pulmonary vasodilators may also be useful to prevent this complication.

Infectious complications are less frequent in percutaneous device insertion sites with infection control techniques including impregnated dressings. Femoral cutdown sites are more prone to wound infection after device removal and skin closure.

After stabilizing the patient on temporary MCA, it is important to take active steps to prevent complications related to MCA to increase destination options. Final destination options should be expedited whenever possible. Myocardial recovery is most desirable, and should be pursued aggressively with use of revascularization, active unloading, and the potential use of long-acting inotropes although not infrequently these patients may become candidates for other long-term device options or heart transplant.

OUTCOME

The mortality rate for patients presenting in advanced CS requiring ECMO or other temporary mechanical circulatory support varies and depends on the clinical conditions at presentation, patient age and comorbidities, timing and quality of support provided, and the ability to prevent complications and rapidly transition the patient to recovery, LVAD support, or transplant. Although historical series have shown overall survival rates of 30–40%, more recently a better understanding of the potential and limitations of MCA devices and

improvements in perioperative care have positively impacted outcomes with survival rates of 50–60% in experienced centers.

The most common causes of death in this patient population include multisystem organ failure, life-threatening hemorrhage, and late infection with sepsis. More recently, active strategies to provide adequate resuscitation and flow and prevent vascular complications, broad antibiotic use to minimize infection complications, and a team-based approach to define an early transition to more permanent support or transplant, with the increasing ability to wean these patients safely, have made a significant impact on the overall outcomes. The increasing expertise and dedication of the teams providing care for these patients and the ability to recognize futile support are key factors when considering the use of ECMO and other temporary support devices.

FURTHER READING

Abrams D, Combes A, Brodie D. Extracorporeal membrane oxygenation in cardiopulmonary disease in adults. *J Am Coll Cardiol.* 2014; 63(25 Pt A): 2769–78.

Cheng JM, den Uil CA, Hoeks SE, et al. Percutaneous left ventricular assist devices vs. intra-aortic balloon pump counterpulsation for treatment of cardiogenic shock: a meta-analysis of controlled trials. *Eur Heart J.* 2009; 30(17): 2102–8.

Doersch KM, Tong CW, Gongora E, et al. Temporary left ventricular assist device through an axillary access is a promising approach to improve outcomes in refractory cardiogenic shock patients. *ASAIO J.* 2015; 61(3): 253–8.

Napp LC, Kühn C, Hoeper MM, et al. Cannulation strategies for percutaneous extracorporeal membrane oxygenation in adults. *Clin Res Cardiol.* 2016; 105(4): 283–96.

Rihal CS, Naidu SS, Givertz MM, et al. 2015 SCAI/ACC/HFSA/STS Clinical expert consensus statement on the use of percutaneous mechanical circulatory support devices in cardiovascular care (endorsed by the American Heart Association, the Cardiological Society of India, and Sociedad Latino Americana de Cardiologia Intervencion; affirmation of value by the Canadian Association of Interventional Cardiology–Association Canadienne de Cardiologie d'intervention). *J Card Fail.* 2015; 21(6): 499–518.

28

Left ventricular reconstruction

EDWIN C. MCGEE JR. AND PATRICK M. MCCARTHY

HISTORY

Denton Cooley reconstructed the first left ventricle (LV) when he repaired a left ventricular aneurysm by linear closure on cardiopulmonary bypass in 1958.[1] The surgical technique of aneurysm repair remained largely unchanged until 1985 when Jatene and Dor separately described repairs which included reconstruction of the aneurysmal portion of the septum as well as free wall.

PRINCIPLES AND JUSTIFICATION

Heart failure is increasing in prevalence as the population ages. Close to six million Americans are affected by heart failure.[2]

Medical therapy with neurohormonal antagonists is the cornerstone of care and guideline-based therapies should be applied to all patients with heart failure. Coronary artery disease is a leading cause of heart failure and is the second most common cause of heart failure of patients listed for transplant. Heart transplantation is the gold standard treatment in terms of length and quality life for patients with advanced (stage D) heart failure; however, heart transplantation is limited by both donor availability and the morbidity of lifelong immunosuppression. Left ventricular assist devices (LVADs) have been miniaturized and enhanced in terms of biocompatibility and complication profiles, but they remain costly and require specialized care. Coronary artery bypass is the most commonly applied surgical therapy for the patient with heart failure. In patients with ischemic cardiomyopathy, revascularization of ischemic but viable myocardium increases survival[3] by recruiting hibernating myocardium and thus alleviating heart failure and/or malignant ventricular arrhythmias.

However, not all patients with ischemic cardiomyopathy manifest viability. Transmural infarction of the left anterior descending (LAD) territory can lead to the development of a true left ventricular aneurysm. Such aneurysms occurred more commonly before prompt interventional revascularization became the standard of care for ST elevation myocardial infarction (MI). However, LV aneurysms still occur in patients sustaining an ST elevation MI who either present late or are misdiagnosed. Revascularization alone does not lead to reverse remodeling of these transmural infarcts or aneurysms. Left ventricular reconstruction (LVR) is a surgical procedure designed to actively remodel the dyskinetic aneurysmal myocardial segment that forms after a transmural infarct.

The law of Laplace states that the tension exerted on the wall of a sphere is proportional to the cube of its radius. The theory behind LVR relates directly to the law of Laplace. By excluding the aneurysmal segment and thereby reducing the size of the LV, wall stress is reduced, which counteracts further dilatation. Additionally, systolic function is further enhanced by the exclusion of the dyskinetic segment, which, left untreated, robs cardiac output by elastic expansion with every ventricular contraction. In this chapter we outline our thought process in terms of candidacy, preoperative workup, surgical procedure, and perioperative care of patients undergoing LVR.

PREOPERATIVE ASSESSMENT AND PREPARATION

Patients being prepared for LVR undergo the same preoperative battery of tests as any patient undergoing any type of cardiac surgical procedure. A complete history and physical, standard laboratory examinations, chest X-ray, cardiac angiogram, echocardiogram, and typically carotid Dopplers are obtained. Right heart catheterization is mandatory. Our group does not offer LVR to patients who are in decompensated heart failure or who are dependent on inotropic support to maintain a cardiac index of >2 L/min/m² or normal end-organ perfusion. Furthermore, myocardial viability must be present in the lateral and inferior territories.

ANESTHESIA

LVR is performed under general anesthesia with full hemo-dynamic monitoring, which includes an arterial line and an oximetry pulmonary artery catheter. Additionally, we typically place a femoral arterial line both to confirm the arterial blood pressure in these patients who usually are on numerous vasodilators and who are at risk for vasoplegia syndrome post cardiopulmonary bypass. We hold angio-tensin-converting-enzyme inhibitor (ACEI) for 48 hours pre-surgery to mitigate vasoplegia. A femoral arterial line serves as access for an intra-aortic balloon pump (IABP) should one be needed to support the ventricle post bypass. We typically separate from bypass on a low dose epinephrine infusion supplemented with milrinone if needed. An intra-operative transesophageal echocardiogram (TEE) is standard of care and assists both in indentifying concomitant valvular pathology and also helps identify the presence or absence of laminated ventricular thrombus and intracardiac shunts. Post bypass TEE helps confirm the adequacy of valvular repairs and replacements and revascularization as well as assisting with air evacuation.

OPERATION

A standard median sternotomy is performed and conduit is harvested. The patient is dosed with heparin for cardio-pulmonary bypass (CPB) (300 U/kg of heparin). Typically, a standard three-stage cannula introduced through the right atrial appendage is utilized for venous drainage. Chronic ischemic mitral regurgitation (Carpentier Type IIIb) and functional tricuspid regurgitation are frequently encoun-tered in patients with ischemic cardiomyopathy. In patients with 2+ or greater valvular regurgitation we carry out bicaval venous cannulation in anticipation of addressing the valvular pathology. A retrograde cardioplegia cannula is introduced via the right atrium and an aortic root vent/antegrade cardio-plegia catheter is introduced into the distal ascending aorta. A weighted flexible suction catheter assists with valvular surgery as well as the LVR.

Cardiopulmonary bypass is initiated when the activated clotting time (ACT) is greater than 480 seconds. Systemic normothermia is typically maintained. The heart is arrested with both antegrade and retrograde cold blood cardioplegia. Supplemental doses are given every 15 minutes. Coronary vein distal anastomoses are performed first and are con-nected to a cardioplegia manifold if mitral pathology exists. If not, proximal anastomoses are performed next. In patients undergoing LVR we typically use the left internal mammary artery to graft the best vessel on the lateral wall, which is usually the largest obtuse marginal (OM) branch. The LAD is typically grafted with reverse saphenous vein.

With the heart arrested and the aortic root vent on suction, the location for the initial ventriculotomy becomes appar-ent. This area is marked with a surgical pen (**Figure 28.1**). The heart is filled and Valsalva maneuvers are performed as the aortic root vent is placed on high suction. Manual

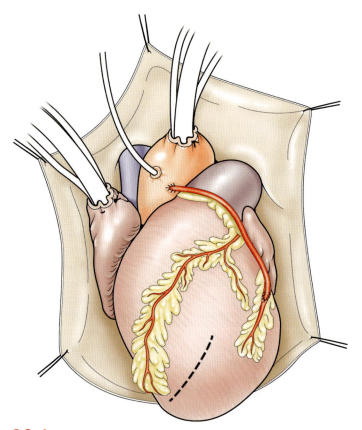

28.1

compression of the LV is performed to assist in air removal and a terminal dose of warm substrate-enhanced cardioplegia is administered by retrograde and then antegrade routes. The patient is placed in the Trendelenburg position and the aortic cross-clamp is removed. If the heart fibrillates, cardioversion is performed.

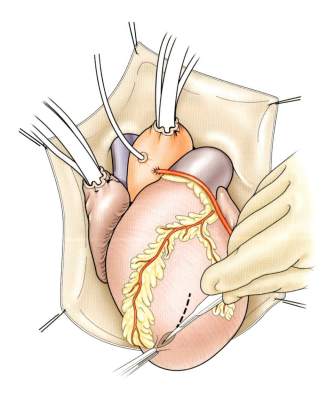

28.2

The LV apex is then elevated on laparotomy pads or by traction sutures placed in the pericardial well. The ventricle is incised sharply in the middle aspect of the zone of infarct, which is usually a few centimeters lateral to the LAD (**Figure 28.2**). The ventriculotomy is extended with scissors to define the transition zone between infarct and viable muscle. Our preference is to perform LVR with the heart beating as the delineation of the infarct and viable contracting muscle is clearly evident. It is easy to distinguish viable muscle, both visibly and tactilely, in the beating heart. During this portion of the case, the heart is also being reperfused, which we feel mitigates postcardiotomy low cardiac output states.

Blood is evacuated from the open LV with a flexible weighted suction catheter. As long as the aortic root is pressurized the risk of air embolism from the empty beating ventricle is very low. We take care not to lower our systemic perfusion while the ventricle is open because, if the aortic valve is not pressurized, air may enter the aortic root and subsequently embolize.

The edges of the ventriculotomy are retracted with 2-0 traction sutures (**Figure 28.3a**). Any thrombus that is present is carefully removed. The first of two cerclage sutures is begun at the 12 o'clock position. We use a 0-0 polypropylene suture on a small circumference, heavy-cutting needle and place the stitches deep into the tissue of the junction between scar and muscle (**Figure 28.3b**). Deep bites of 1 cm depth and breadth are taken. The scarred myocardium is extremely strong and large, deep bites are encouraged. The first cerclage suture is completed and the tag ends are held with a hemostat. A second cerclage suture is placed about 1 cm above the last stitch and similarly retracted. The first stitch is securely tied followed by the second (**Figure 28.3c**). Typically, the two cerclage stitches tighten down leaving a ventricular defect

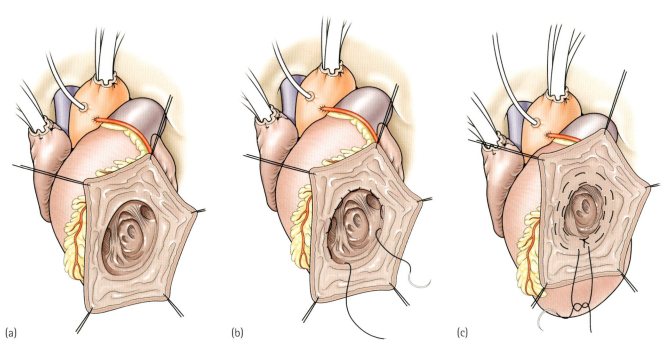

(a)   (b)   (c)

28.3a–c

less than a centimeter. If done correctly, all of the infracted non-viable tissue is excluded from the circulation.

Next, two strips of Teflon felt are fashioned, 1 cm wide and slightly longer than the ventriculotomy. Horizontal mattress sutures of 2-0 polypropylene suture are than placed entering and exiting the felt strips at the level of the first pursestring (**Figure 28.4a**). Five or six mattress sutures are generally required. The sutures placed at either end of the ventriculotomy are angled in to the ventriculotomy at 45 degrees whereas those placed in the mid portion are place at 90 degrees (**Figure 28.4b**). Lastly, a 2-0 stitch is placed in a running double-layer fashion through the felt and muscle. Additional hemostatic sutures are placed as needed (**Figure 28.4c**).

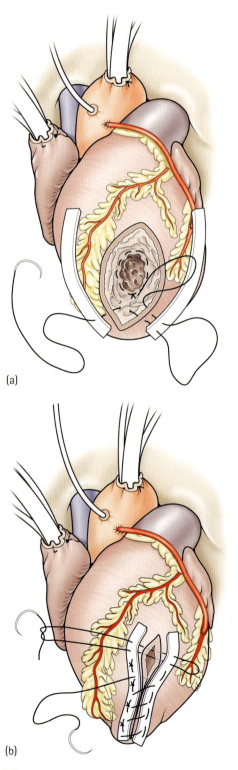

(a)

(b)

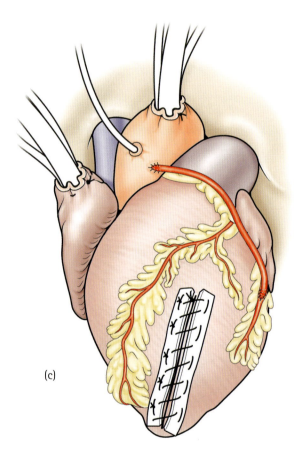

(c)

28.4a–c

If needed, tricuspid procedures are completed and the patient is weaned from bypass after additional dearing maneuvers. We liberally use low-dose epinephrine infusions and milrinone. We feel that prevention is the best treatment for low cardiac output. Prior to separation from bypass, additional alpha agents are utilized to ensure an adequate perfusion pressure.

If a heavily calcified aneurysm is encountered, debridement of the calcium is required to achieve adequate downsizing and closure. We generally use electrocautery on a low setting to accomplish the decalcification. Care must be taken especially on the septum as a ventricular septal defect can be created. For extensive aneurysms or those with heavy calcification, we occasionally use a patch fashioned from Gelweave Vascutek™ (Vascutek Ltd, a Terumo company, Scotland, UK). It is secured after the second pursestring suture is tied, typically with a running 2-0 suture (**Figures 28.5a and b**). The mattress closure is then placed above the patch as previously described. We have not found the use of commercially available mannequins to be helpful for performing LVR.[4]

POSTOPERATIVE CARE

The judicious use of inotropes to maintain vigorous hemodynamics is encouraged and helps prevent over-resuscitation with volume should cardiac index or mean arterial pressure sag at chest closure or in the immediate postoperative period. Postcardiotomy low cardiac output syndrome is a rare occurrence. Should it occur, we rule out a technical problem with a graft by graft inspection and flow measurement. We aggressively treat low cardiac output that is unresponsive to standard doses of milrinone and epinephrine initially with an IABP. We rarely need to utilize an IABP for support of cardiac output but readily use them if the patient develops vasoplegia syndrome. If hemodynamics and pressure are still compromised or labile, we move quickly to a temporary ventricular assist device. Temporary VADs can usually be weaned over a few days but, if chronic support is needed, we transition to a continuous-flow implantable LVAD. Reports in the past have described taking down the LV reconstruction in order

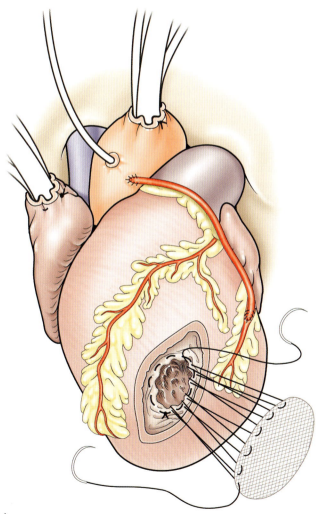

(a)

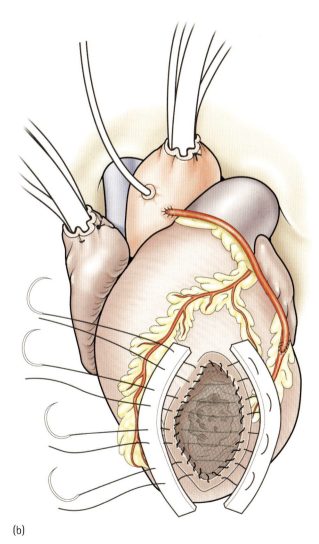

(b)

28.5a–b

to accomplish optimal placement of the inlet cannula; currently, in patients who have had prior LVR, we prefer to place the inlet cannula on the diaphragmatic surface of the LV as described by Frazier and colleagues.[5]

Meticulous attention is paid to hemostasis as tamponade can develop subtly and sets off a vicious cycle of hemodynamic compromise which can lead to the development of a shock state. The pulmonary artery catheter is removed once hemodynamics are stable on low-dose inotropes and the patient has normal end-organ function. It is common to wean intravenous milrinone clinically slowly over a few days after the PA catheter has been removed. A brisk diuresis is achieved with intravenous loop diuretics to return the patient to or below their preoperative weight. Guideline-based medical therapy, including beta blockade and an ACEI, is introduced as milrinone is tapered. The patient is discharged to home or outpatient rehab once a stable medical regimen is received. Although some groups have advocated routine AICD placement in those rare LVR patients who do not already have an AICD, we defer such decisions to our electrophysiology colleagues.

OUTCOME

Retrospective studies have shown LVR to be beneficial. The RESTORE (Reconstructive Endoventricular Surgery Returning Original Radius Elliptical Shape to the LV) was a multicenter international registry that reported on 1198 patients with ischemic cardiomyopathy who underwent LVR between 1998 and 2003.[6] CABG was performed in 95% and mitral valve surgery in 23%. Thirty-day mortality was 5.3%. Ejection fraction increased from $29.6 \pm 11\%$ to $39.5 \pm 12.3\%$ ($p < 0.001$). Left ventricular end-systolic volume index (LVESVI) decreased (29%) from $80.4 \pm 51.4 \, \text{mL/m}^2$ to $56.6 \pm 34.3 \, \text{mL/m}^2$ ($p < 0.001$). Improvement of NYHA functional class occurred (preop 67% NYHA class III and IV; postop 85% Class II). Five-year survival was $68.6 \pm 2.8\%$. Patients with dyskinetic aneurysms showed more improvement after LVR than those with akinetic segments.

Mickleborough reported on 285 patients with ischemic cardiomyopathy who underwent LVR at the University of Toronto. CABG was performed in 92% and mitral valve procedure in 2%. Operative mortality was 2.8% and 5-year survival was 82%. Sixty-seven per cent of patients experienced symptomatic improvement with a mean improvement in NYHA class of 1.3 ± 1.1. The average increase in ejection fraction was $10\% \pm 9\%$.[7]

Similarly, O'Neil and colleagues studied 220 patients from the Cleveland Clinic who underwent LVR from 1997 to 2003. Thirty-day mortality was 1% and 5-year survival was 80%. Eighty-six per cent underwent concomitant CABG and 49% underwent mitral surgery. Ejection fraction increased from $21.5 \pm 7.3\%$ to $24.7 \pm 8.86\%$ ($p < 0.01$). Preoperatively 66% of patients were NYHA class III or IV; postoperatively 85% were NYHA class I or II.[8]

The group from Johns Hopkins reported similar intermediate outcomes to heart transplant for patients undergoing LVR with much less cost associated.[9]

The recently completed STICH (Surgical Treatment of Ischemic Congestive Heart failure) trial was a randomized international multicenter trial sponsored by the National Heart Lung and Blood Institute (NHLBI) that was designed to ascertain the optimal treatment of patients with ischemic cardiomyopathy. Patients without left main disease or disabling angina were randomized to medical therapy or medical therapy plus coronary artery bypass grafting.[10] Hypothesis 1 of the trial was that the addition of coronary artery bypass would decrease overall mortality and the incidence of hospitalizations from cardiovascular causes.[10] Patients that randomized to surgery who had significant anterior wall akinesia or dyskinesia were further randomized to undergo LVR or just CABG alone. Hypothesis 2 surmised that the addition of LVR to CABG alone for patients with significant anterior wall akinesia or dyskinesia would have improved survival and fewer hospitalizations due to cardiovascular causes.[10] While overall survival was no better in patients who underwent coronary artery bypass as compared to medical therapy, those patients undergoing CABG had fewer hospitalizations and fewer deaths from cardiovascular causes than those patients treated only with medical therapy. When compared to CABG alone, the addition of LVR did not decrease rates of death or hospitalization due to cardiovascular cause. Left ventricular volumes were decreased by 19% for patients undergoing LVR as compared to 6% for those undergoing CABG alone.[11] The apparent negative outcome of STICH in terms of LVR has cast a cloud upon LVR as a beneficial surgical therapy.

There were several problems with STICH. In an effort to enhance patient accrual, which was initially slow, viability testing was made optional. As a result only 601 patients out of a total of 1212 in the trial underwent viability testing with single-photon-emission computed tomography (SPECT). As such the lack of benefit associated with LVR in the STICH trial may have been due to the fact that patients with viable anterior walls underwent LVR.[12] Furthermore, from the RESTORE and other groups we know that LVR for patients with primarily akinetic anterior walls is less beneficial than it is for those with dyskinetic anterior walls. If the majority of the patients in STICH underwent LVR for akinetic anterior walls, the overall improvements seen would likely be less.

A survival advantage for LVR as compared to CABG alone was demonstrated in those patients who achieved a postoperative end-systolic volume index of $70 \, \text{mL/m}^2$ or less.[13] Certainly, there are some patients with severely remodeled LVs who are past the point of no return and would be better served by LVAD and/or heart transplantation.

SUMMARY

LVR is a useful therapy for select patients with ischemic cardiomyopathy. We reserve this operation for those patients with non-viable dyskinetic anterior walls, with viable lateral and inferior walls, who do not have decompensated or inotropic-dependent heart failure.

ACKNOWLEDGMENT

We would like to thank Ms Patricia Alvarez for her editorial assistance with this manuscript.

REFERENCES

1. Cooley DA, Collins HA, Morris GC, et al. Ventricular aneurysm after myocardial infarction: surgical excision with the use of temporary cardiopulmonary bypass. *J Am Med Assoc.* 1958; 167: 557–60.

2. Lloyd-Jones D, Adams RJ, Brown TM, et al. Heart disease and stroke statistics: 2010 update – a report from the American Heart Association. *Circulation.* 2010; 121: e46–e215.

3. Velazquez EJ, Lee KL, Deja MA, et al. Coronary-artery bypass surgery in patients with left ventricular dysfunction. *N Engl J Med.* 2011; 364(17): 1607–16.

4. Caldeira C, McCarthy PM. A simple method of left ventricular reconstruction without patch for ischemic cardiomyopathy. *Ann Thorac Surg.* 2001; 72(6): 2148–9.

5. Gregoric ID, Cohn WE, Frazier OH. Diaphragmatic implantation of the HeartWare ventricular assist device. *J Heart Lung Transplant.* 2011; 30(4): 467–70.

6. Athanasuleas CL, Buckberg GD, Stanley AW, et al. Surgical ventricular restoration in the treatment of congestive heart failure due to post-infarction ventricular dilation. *J Am Coll Cardiol.* 2004; 44(7): 1439–45.

7. Mickleborough LL, Merchant N, Ivanov J, et al. Left ventricular reconstruction: early and late results. *J Thorac Cardiovasc Surg.* 2004; 128(1): 27–37.

8. O'Neill JO, Starling RC, McCarthy PM, et al. The impact of left ventricular reconstruction on survival in patients with ischemic cardiomyopathy. *Eur J Cardiothoracic Surg.* 2006; 30(5): 753–9.

9. Williams JA, Weiss ES, Patel ND, et al. Surgical ventricular restoration versus cardiac transplantation: a comparison of cost, outcomes, and survival. *J Card Fail.* 2008; 14(7): 547–54.

10. Velazquez EJ, Lee KL, O'Connor CM, et al. The rationale and design of the Surgical Treatment for Ischemic Heart Failure (STICH) trial. *J Thorac Cardiovasc Surg.* 2007; 134(6): 1540–7.

11. Jones RH, Velazquez EJ, Michler RE, et al. Coronary bypass surgery with or without surgical ventricular reconstruction. *N Engl J Med.* 2009; 360(127): 1705–17.

12. Bonow RO, Maurer G, Lee KL, et al. Myocardial viability and survival in ischemic left ventricular dysfunction. *N Engl J Med.* 2011; 364(17): 1617–25.

13. Michler RE, Rouleau JL, Al-Khalidi HR, et al. Insights from the STICH trial: change in left ventricular size after coronary artery bypass grafting with and without surgical ventricular reconstruction. *J Thorac Cardiovasc Surg.* 2013; 146(5): 1139–45.

29

Surgery for hypertrophic cardiomyopathy

ROBERT J. STEFFEN AND NICHOLAS G. SMEDIRA

INTRODUCTION

Hypertrophic cardiomyopathy is a genetic condition with an incidence of 1 in 500 characterized by excessive left ventricular hypertrophy and associated systolic anterior motion (SAM) of the mitral valve. Hypertrophic obstructive cardiomyopathy (HOCM) occurs when hypertrophy of the septum and SAM lead to an elevated pressure gradient across the left ventricular outflow tract (LVOT). This causes heart failure symptoms of varying severity. The goal of surgery is to eliminate the elevated pressure gradient, and thus the symptoms, by resecting a portion of the hypertrophied septum.

PREOPERATIVE ASSESSMENT

Patients with HOCM are diagnosed on echocardiogram as part of a general workup for shortness of breath. On taking the history, patients often complain of exertional dyspnea made worse by the initiation of antihypertensive medications and may have a murmur made worse with performing the Valsalva maneuver.

Transthoracic echocardiogram is imperative in making the diagnosis of HOCM. Key measurements to note are the width of the interventricular septum, the gradient across the LVOT, presence of SAM of the mitral valve, severity of mitral regurgitation (MR), along with any papillary muscle abnormalities.

The upper limit of normal for interventricular septal width is about 1.3 cm. Hypertrophy may be focal and isolated to a single segment of the septum or may be diffuse throughout the entire ventricle. The width of the septum at a given depth often changes from base to apex and from anterior to inferior. Understanding the patient's unique septal geometry using the intraoperative transesophageal echocardiogram (TEE) is key to the safe conduct of the operation and will be discussed later.

Patients with HOCM have an elevated gradient across their LVOT either at rest or with exertion. Patients who are able to exercise undergo a treadmill stress echo. Those unable to exercise can perform a Valsalva maneuver or receive a dose of amyl nitrate. The key is to measure the gradient while the heart is hyperdynamic by decreasing preload, increasing the heart rate, and reducing afterload.

High-velocity flow through the LVOT pulls the anterior mitral leaflet into the outflow tract. In addition to narrowing the LVOT further, the SAM prevents the anterior leaflet from coapting with the posterior leaflet, leading to a posteriorly directed jet of MR.

Papillary muscle abnormalities are present in approximately 10% of patients with hypertrophic cardiomyopathy. The muscles can be bifid, hypermobile, and displaced apically. Aberrant and abnormal papillary muscles as well as their chordae can lead to LVOT obstruction independent of septal hypertrophy.

OPERATION

In the operative series from the Cleveland Clinic, there was a slight male predominance with the average age at the time of operation being 50 years ± 14 years. Most patients had either New York Heart Association (NYHA) class II (54%), or III (35%) heart failure symptoms. The mean peak gradient across the LVOT was 68 mmHg ± 43 mmHg. The mean septal thickness was 2.3 cm ± 0.5 cm. Almost all patients had resting SAM and 80–90% had at least mild MR.

Most patients having surgery for HOCM underwent isolated septal myectomy. Between 10% and 20% of patients required a concomitant operation on their mitral valve. Patients requiring a mitral valve procedure were about 10 years older than the overall cohort and more likely to have a septal thickness of <2.0 cm. The most common lesions requiring mitral valve surgery were restricted or elongated leaflets, likely from long-standing SAM–septal contact. The majority of these valves could be repaired.

Surgery for HOCM significantly improved heart failure symptoms, decreased the gradient across the LVOT, and reduced MR. The mean postoperative septal thickness was 1.6 cm ± 0.3 cm; the mean residual gradient was 17 mmHg ± 11 mmHg; 80–90% of patients had NYHA class I or II symptoms. The percentage of patients free of MR increased from 20% to 45% after surgery and the majority of those with residual MR had only mild or mild–moderate in severity.

Over time, the peak LVOT gradient and interventricular septal thickness continued to decrease. At 5 years postoperative, 80% of patients still had NYHA class I or II symptoms and 96% of patients were free from reoperation. Patients with residual atrial fibrillation had worse outcomes than those in a sinus rhythm. Overall survival was similar to age-matched controls.

Surgery decreased the cardiac workload, provided immediate, durable improvement in symptoms, and provided a normal life expectancy.

The intraoperative TEE dictates the conduct of the myectomy. Key measurements are the thickness of the interventricular septum, how the thickness changes as you move horizontally through the septum and vertically towards the apex, and the depth below the nadir of the right coronary cusp (RCC) that SAM–septal contact occurs.

It is important to view both the anteroseptum seen in the 135-degree view (**Figure 29.1a**) and the inferoseptum seen with the four-chamber or 0-degree view (**Figure 29.1b**). As the septum moves from the anteroseptum (underneath the right ventricular outflow tract) to the inferoseptum (underneath the membranous septum), the thickness thins out by

around 3–4 mm. Additionally, this area near the inferoseptum is easier for the surgeon to see than the anteroseptum. Because of these factors, iatrogenic ventricular septal defects are most likely to occur in this area. As such, the resection is mainly focused on the anteroseptum and the resection specimen is not as thick as it moves towards the inferoseptum.

The operation is performed through a sternotomy with standard aortic and venous cannulation. Cardiopulmonary bypass (CPB) is initiated and the heart is arrested. A left atrial vent is placed through the right superior pulmonary vein to optimize visualization in the left ventricle. A transverse aortotomy is performed 1.5 cm above the right coronary ostia and the aortic walls are retracted. A malleable is used by the assistant to retract the RCC for visualization of the septum (**Figure 29.2**).

The septum is resected in three stages, starting with a piece from the middle and then taking one on either side (**Figure 29.2**). The resection is started 1.5–2.0 cm below the nadir of the RCC. In Morrow's original description of the operation, the myectomy was started 3 mm below the nadir of the RCC. Starting the resection that high risks both destabilizing the aortic valve, specifically the right cusp, as well as injury to the bundle of His. The point of SAM–septal contact typically occurs around 1.5–2.0 cm below the RCC. The myectomy is thus started just above this point, somewhere around 1.5 cm below the nadir of the RCC.

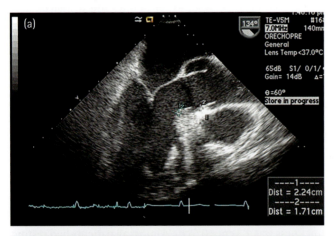

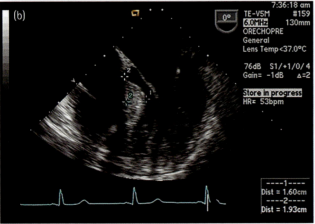

29.1a–b

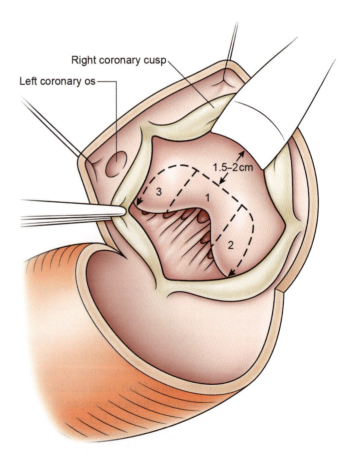

29.2

The initial myectomy incision is made using a 10 blade with the cutting end pointed towards the left ventricular cavity (**Figure 29.3**). The width of the blade at its thickest is 8 mm, so the width of the blade buried in the LV muscle gives the surgeon a sense of the thickness of specimen being resected (**Figure 29.4**).

Septal hypertrophy occurs in many forms. Patients can have an isolated proximal bulge at the base of the septum, mid-cavitary hypertrophy, apical hypertrophy, or diffuse hypertrophy that extends throughout the ventricle. The hypertrophy pattern must be determined using the preoperative echo as the geometry is not clear intraoperatively.

Once the middle resection slice is taken to the desired depth on either side, a 15 blade knife and long-toothed forceps are used to excise the muscle (**Figure 29.5**).

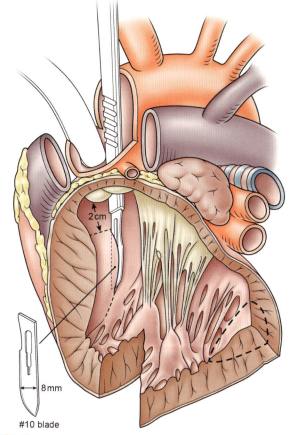

#10 blade

29.4

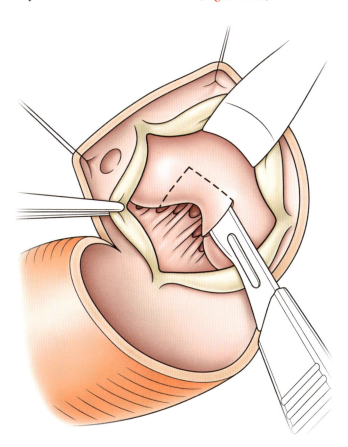

29.3

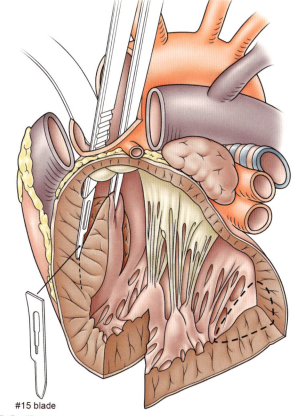

#15 blade

29.5

The middle specimen is now resected and you are left with septum on each side going towards the fibrous trigones (**Figure 29.6**). The resection must take place from trigone to trigone. Leaving residual septum on either side of a middle transection specimen is a common mode of residual outflow tract obstruction.

The myectomy is then taken from the edge of the middle resection towards the inferoseptum (**Figure 29.7**). As noted previously, the width of the septum in this area is 3–4 mm thinner than at the anteroseptum.

The myectomy is then completed by finishing the resection to the left trigone (**Figure 29.8**). For patients with diffuse, mid-cavitary, and apical hypertrophy, the myectomy must be taken well into the LV, at least to the mid-papillary muscle level. The mid-papillary muscle depth of an empty, decompressed heart translates to the tip of the papillary muscle in a full, dilated left ventricle. Residual mid-cavity hypertrophy can leave a persistent LV outflow tract gradient if not resected. As the middle and apex of the left ventricle can be difficult to see, a ring-forceps with a sponge on the end or similar instrument can be used to push the apex towards the aortic valve so the resection can be taken deeper.

Once the myectomy is complete the mitral valve is assessed. There are frequently aberrant chordae from the papillary muscles to the septum that can be resected. Secondary chordae to the body of the anterior mitral leaflet are also seen. These can lead to leaflet tethering across the LVOT and are resected as well.

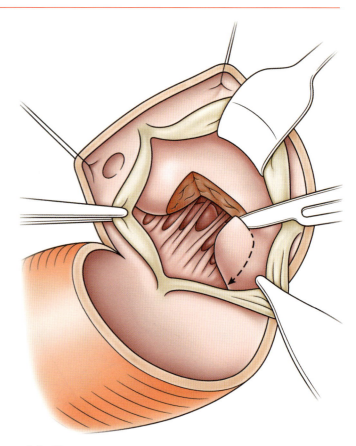

29.7

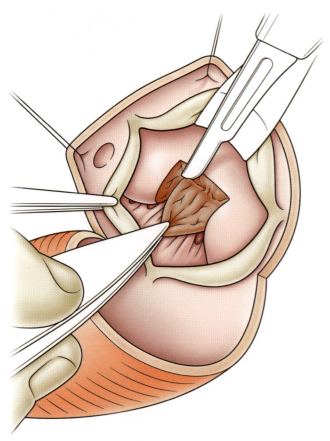

29.6

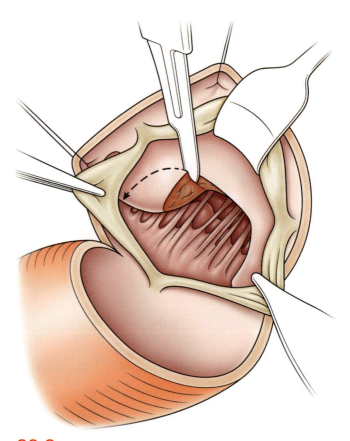

29.8

MR is seen in the majority of patients with HOCM, mostly due to SAM of the mitral valve. Septal myectomy cures the MR in half of the patients with preoperative MR. Residual postoperative MR is usually mild in degree. In our series, patients with postoperative MR tended to have a stable degree on follow-up, with no improvement or worsening.

In patients with 3–4+ MR postoperatively, the mitral valve is repaired using standard techniques. An oversized annuloplasty band is used, or none is used at all, as it puts the patient at risk for SAM. If the valve is unable to be repaired, then the valve is replaced.

The aortotomy is closed, the cross-clamp is removed, and the patient is weaned from CPB. Before removing the cannulae, the LVOT is assessed for persistent obstruction. The gradient is first measured at rest, then under stress. In order to induce a hyperdynamic state, the patient is given dobutamine at 20 mcg/kg/min and nitroglycerin to induce mild hypotension. If the gradient is normal, the patient is decannulated. If a gradient persists, the mode of obstruction must be identified. The septum is analyzed for residual hypertrophy that can be resected (**Figure 29.9**). Residual SAM leaving an elevated gradient may require valve replacement.

The postoperative specimen is weighed and measured at the end of the case (**Figure 29.10**). Myectomy specimens can weigh 4–24 g, averaging 7–8 g.

FURTHER READING

Desai MY, Bhonasle A, Smedira NG, et al. Predictors of long-term outcomes in symptomatic hypertrophic obstructive cardiomyopathy patients undergoing surgical relief of left ventricular outflow tract obstruction. *Circulation.* 2013; 128: 209–16.

Kaple RK, Murphy RT, DiPaola LM, et al. Mitral valve abnormalities in hypertrophic cardiomyopathy: echocardiographic features and surgical outcomes. *Ann Thorac Surg.* 2008; 85: 1527–36.

Kwon DH, Setser RM, Thamilarasan M, et al. Abnormal papillary muscle morphology is independently associated with increased left ventricular outflow tract obstruction in hypertrophic cardiomyopathy. *Heart.* 2008; 94: 1295–301.

Kwon DH, Smedira NG, Thamilarasan M, et al. Characteristics and surgical outcomes of symptomatic patients with hypertrophic cardiomyopathy with abnormal papillary muscle morphology undergoing papillary muscle reorientation. *J Thorac Cardiovasc Surg.* 2010; 140(2): 317–24.

Maron BJ, Gardin JM, Flack JM, et al. Prevalence of hypertrophic cardiomyopathy in a general population of young adults. *Circulation.* 1995; 92: 785–9.

Smedira NG, Lytle BW, Lever HM, et al. Current effectiveness and risks of isolated septal myectomy for hypertrophic obstructive cardiomyopathy. *Ann Thorac Surg.* 2008; 85: 127–34.

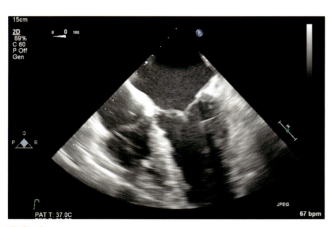

29.9

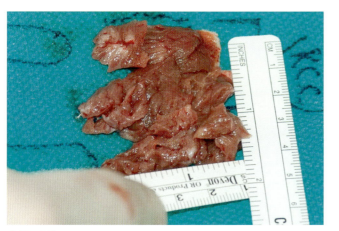

29.10

30

Congestive heart failure: surgical techniques for functional mitral regurgitation

SARAH T. WARD, ALEXANDER A. BRESCIA, MATTHEW A. ROMANO, AND STEVEN F. BOLLING

HISTORY

It has been well documented that even small amounts of functional mitral regurgitation (FMR) are harmful in patients with congestive heart failure (CHF). Several studies demonstrate that FMR is not just a sign of advanced CHF, but an independent determinant of CHF death. The severity of mitral regurgitation (MR) impacts quality of life, as well as survival. Furthermore, there is a strong association between the presence of ischemic FMR severity and heart failure hospitalizations. However, while the presence of FMR predicts a poor prognosis in patients with left ventricular (LV) dysfunction and heart failure, "proof" that correction of FMR improves prognosis unfortunately remains elusive.

Historically, the surgical approach to FMR was non valve-sparing mitral valve (MV) replacement, at a time when little was understood of the interdependence of ventricular function and the annular–papillary muscle continuity. Consequently, patients with low ejection fraction (EF) who underwent MV replacement with removal of the subvalvular apparatus had prohibitively high mortality rates. To explain this, the erroneous concept of a beneficial "pop-off" effect of FMR was conceived. This idea erroneously proposed that mitral incompetence provided low-pressure relief during systolic ejection for the failing ventricle, and that removal of this effect through mitral replacement was responsible for the perioperative deterioration of ventricular function. Consequently, MV replacement in patients with heart failure and FMR was discouraged.

PRINCIPLES AND JUSTIFICATION

The indications for surgery for FMR are more cautious than those for primary, degenerative MR due to the recognition that surgical outcomes are linked to underlying LV remodeling. Secondary FMR can acutely be corrected by MV surgery; however, it has never clearly been demonstrated that reducing or eliminating FMR alters the natural history or improves survival. Moreover, whether the response to surgery is different in secondary MR due to ischemic versus non-ischemic cardiomyopathy has also not been established. One-year mortality after MV surgery for severe ischemic MR (with or without coronary artery bypass graft, CABG) is up to 17%.[1] Therefore, the benefit of MV repair in patients with FMR and heart failure is unclear. Wu and colleagues showed no mortality benefit in FMR patients treated with MV repair, although they did not examine the effect of recurrent MR.[2] In ischemic cardiomyopathy patients, several non-randomized studies showed that MV repair in addition to CABG for FMR did not alter long-term functional status or survival when compared to CABG alone, while others did show a survival benefit when compared with medical therapy or CABG alone. Trichon demonstrated a survival advantage in ischemic cardiomyopathy patients who underwent CABG plus MV repair only compared with medical management, as there was no difference between CABG plus MV repair versus CABG alone.[3] Randomized trials have been performed but are not definitive. Fattouch[4] found no significant benefit to adding mitral repair to CABG in a single-center, underpowered trial with 102 patients. A substudy of the STICH trial by Deja[5] concluded a superior survival for CABG with mitral repair compared to CABG alone, but the decision to treat the mitral was left to the discretion of the surgeon rather than randomized. The randomized RIME trial of 73 patients showed better LV remodeling, MR severity, and functional class with CABG plus mitral repair versus CABG alone, but the trial was not powered for mortality.[6] The Cardiothoracic Surgical Trials Network Investigators concluded in an analysis of 301 patients that the additional of mitral repair to CABG did not result in a higher degree of LV reverse remodeling or improvement in survival and had more untoward events, though did reduce the prevalence of moderate or severe regurgitation and reported outcomes at only 1 year after surgery.[7]

The present AHA/ACC Valve Guidelines (2014)[8] and the European Society of Cardiology (ESC)/ European Association for Cardio-thoracic Surgery (EACTS) guidelines[9] have separate recommendations for functional or secondary ischemic mitral regurgitation. As noted, these guidelines state that treating ischemia with CABG or percutaneous methods should be primarily undertaken for FMR. Additionally, all FMR patients should have guideline-directed medical heart failure therapy (GDMT), with consideration for cardiac resynchronization therapy (CRT), if they have a QRS greater than 150 ms.[10] However, if the patients remain symptomatic with severe MR or stage D disease, they may be considered for "mitral valve surgery" as a IIb indication. Yet, from the surgeon's perspective, while it is recommended that surgical correction of FMR should be considered, exactly how to successfully correct FMR remains unclear.

PREOPERATIVE ASSESSMENT AND PREPARATION

It is important to note that the decision to operate for FMR should be made a priori and not based on intraoperative echocardiography. The decision should be made based on preoperative echocardiography, on guideline-directed medical therapy, and while the patient is euvolemic.

OPERATION

Currently, the most common technique to restore valve competence is placing an undersized or restrictive annuloplasty ring to reduce mitral annulus size and increase leaflet coaptation. Unfortunately, ischemic FMR may persist or recur after restrictive MV annuloplasty. Persistent or recurrent FMR in postoperative patients is understandably associated with unabated ventricular dilatation, an escalation of CHF symptomatology, and possible reduction in long-term survival.

Surgical mitral annuloplasty improves symptoms in patients with CHF and mitral repair is feasible with a low mortality. Several authors have demonstrated 30-day mortality rates as low as 1–5 % for mitral repair for MR in CHF. Recently, Geidel reported that the late results of restrictive annuloplasty in patients with FMR and advanced cardiomyopathy demonstrated a 3% 30-day mortality and 91% 12-month survival with little postoperative recurrence of significant MR.[11] Perhaps the most compelling data for the safety and efficacy of MV repair for FMR come from the MV surgery alone arm of the prospective Acorn trial (CorCap Cardiac Support Device, a prospective, randomized multicenter trial). The Acorn trial showed a 98% 30-day survival rate, 2% repeat reoperation, and 85% 24-month survival and significant improvements in quality of life, exercise performance, and New York Heart Association (NYHA) class. Furthermore, in the MV surgery arm, improvement in LV volumes, mass, and shape was sustained out to 5 years with little recurrence of significant MR.[12]

The "Achilles' heel" of MV repair in many series of FMR, however, is persistent, residual, or recurrent MR. It was learned that the intertrigonal distance is not stable in FMR, with dilatation occurring along not only the insertion of the posterior leaflet, but also in the anterior portion. This intertrigonal portion dilates and, although once considered to be a "measurable" standard by which to size annuloplasty rings, it is now known from a landmark paper of Hueb that this is not the case.[13] Previous methods of FMR sizing were therefore incorrect, and "undersizing" rings has become the standard for these functional MR patients. This may partly explain the operation "failing" and recurrence of mitral regurgitation in functional MR patients when using too large "classic-sized" rings or when using partial or flexible rings.

Despite undersizing rings, there is significant disparity in recurrence rates among FMR series. The lack of a mortality benefit may be partially explained by the absence of a durable repair. When McGee and Gillinov showed no mortality benefit in FMR after mitral repair, they also noticed the rate of recurrent significant MR to be 30–40% at 1 year.[14] Others have shown even higher rates of return of FMR, up to 80%.[15] This has led to an attempt to identify surgical predictors of recurrent MR and for improved surgical techniques that result in a more permanent repair. In order to observe a survival benefit in these patients after mitral repair, FMR must be fixed permanently, as residual and recurrent MR may obscure or obliterate any possible survival benefit.

There are some FMR patients who should be approached with clinical caution. Silberman showed the larger the ventricle, the worst the outcome for FMR patients.[16] This was also shown in a study from Braun and colleagues, which demonstrated that LV end-diastolic dimensions (LVEDDs) over 65 mm had a much poorer outcome than those starting at a smaller LV size.[17] There are probably some ventricles that are "too far gone" and mitral repair will not be beneficial in these patients. Furthermore, patients with poor RV function and very high PA pressures should be carefully evaluated and perhaps avoided.

Techniques of mitral surgery for FMR

For FMR operations, meticulous attention should be paid to myocardial preservation and cardiopulmonary perfusion. At the time of exposure of the MV, it can be noted that the MV appears "normal," while the pathology in FMR is created from a diseased ventricle (**Figure 30.1**). Asymmetric FMR may result from asymmetric ischemic changes within the LV (**Figure 30.2**). The reduction in AP diameter and orifice area of the MV is an overcorrection and overcompensation for a disease of the ventricle. This "undersizing" of the mitral ring was first proposed by Bolling in 1995 and has become a standard technical approach for FMR repair.[18] When undersizing a mitral ring, it is recommended that one use numerous annular sutures, as compared to degenerative MR repairs, to distribute the workload of annular reductive force. These sutures may be put very closely together, or even on a diagonal. Some

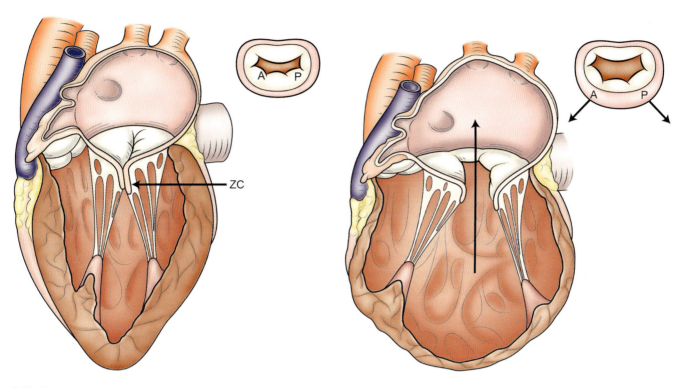

30.1   LV geometric distortion in FMR.

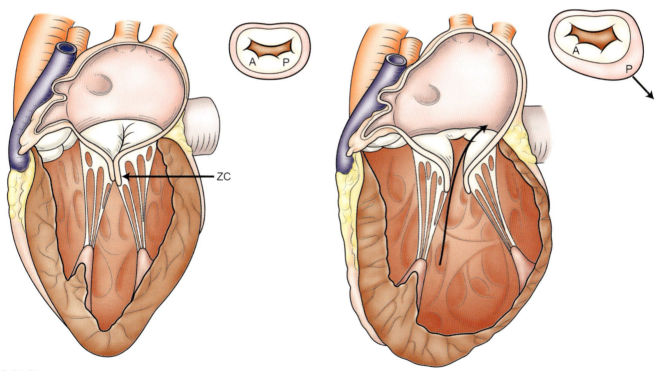

30.2   Asymmetric FMR noted with ischemic-related LV changes.

advocate the use of pledgeted sutures, or the use of an extra row or a few pledgeted reinforcement sutures posteriorly, once the ring is tied in place.

In terms of FMR ring sizing, the normal mitral annulus is roughly proportional to a patient's thumb and forefinger in a circle. One must "downsize" from there. There are some who have advocated double downsizing, meaning two sizes below that measured at the time of operation, but the vast majority of patients may be well served with a "small" 26 mm or 28 mm ring. Although initially in FMR patients there was concern for both systolic anterior motion (SAM) of the anterior leaflet and/or mitral stenosis from such downsizing, these have not resulted in significant clinical sequelae in long-term FMR follow-up series.[19] However, it must be noted that some investigators have reported "functional" mitral stenosis with provocative (dobutamine) testing with undersized rings.[20–25]

The type of ring utilized for FMR repairs is an important technical consideration. As noted, in a landmark paper by Hueb, the fibrous portion of the mitral annulus anteriorly between the two mitral trigones dilated proportionally and as much as the posterior muscular annulus.[13] Magne reported extraordinarily high failure rates with large flexible and/or partial bands for FMR patients in his meta-analysis.[15] Silberman reported on predictors of residual and recurrent mitral regurgitation in FMR and the two largest multivariate predictors were LV size and the type of ring. In fact, the type of ring was a better predictor than LV size, and small, rigid, and complete rings were found to be best for FMR.[16] In the specific disease of FMR, large partial or incomplete rings probably do not result in a durable repair and are not favored technically. Presently, there are numerous specific small rigid and complete FMR rings with a disproportionate AP diameter dimension reduction. While these rings have shown no clinical outcome differences between them, they are probably most favored for the repair of FMR.

When coming off cardiopulmonary bypass, there should be no mitral regurgitation seen on intraoperative postoperative transesophageal echocardiography (TEE). Furthermore, the zone of coaptation should be measured and should be at least 8–10 mm long. If this is not the case, then the patient certainly has a higher incidence of recurrence of MR when they are awake and removed from the unloading effects of general anesthesia.

There are other adjunct therapies that have been used for the FMR repair. In the dilated FMR mitral valve, there are often deep clefts between P1/P2 and P2/P3 which should be closed. Borger has advocated the use of lysis of secondary chords to both the anterior and posterior leaflets to allow for a longer zone of coaptation.[26] While this method has been technically successful, there is no long-term follow-up and the effect of disrupting any chordal structures on LV function is unknown.

FMR is a ventricular disease and surgeons have tried to add adjunctive and inventive "ventricular" therapies to an undersized mitral ring, thereby directing operative therapy to the ventricle itself. Kron has advocated the use of "ring and string" by placing a Gore-Tex traction suture in the posterior papillary muscle and bringing it up towards the annular plane.[27] Hvass has demonstrated the use a double annular ring, placing a standard annular ring at the annulus level and then a second one of Gore-Tex, woven around the papillary muscles to recreate the normal cylinder of closure.[28] Many authors have reported moving papillary muscles or even sewing them together. None of these operations has had long-term follow-up. Some surgeons have advocated augmenting the anterior or the posterior leaflet with bovine pericardium to improve the length of the zone of coaptation. While these approaches increase the technical difficulty of the operation, they are certainly appealing on the basis of altering the underlying problem. Other types of ventricular therapies which have been utilized include the ACORN restriction jacket, the Coapsys ventricular tether, and a silicon lifting pad behind the posterior inferior ventricular wall, amongst others. None of these therapies has had long-term follow-up.

Mitral valve replacement in FMR

Which FMR valves to replace primarily remains controversial. In a summary paper by Lancellotti,[29] the identified predictors of failed FMR repair are mild annular dilatation, coaptation depth more than 1 cm, reverse angulation of the posterior leaflet or LV remodeling end-diastolic diameter greater than 65 mm, or a LVEDV greater than 100 mm indexed. Kron has also shown in the follow-up paper to Acker (*NEJM*) that posterior-basilar dyskinesia or akinesia is associated with a high rate of MR recurrence, even with an undersized repair.[27]

While deciding which patient to replace in FMR remains controversial, there is a consensus on the technical aspects of MV replacement for FMR. MV replacement should be a total valve-sparing replacement. Yun demonstrated in a randomized trial comparing partial versus complete chordal-sparing MV replacement that the effects on LV volume and function were much better preserved with complete versus posterior leaflet sparing.[30] Non valve-sparing mitral replacement should be abandoned. There are numerous techniques for total valve-sparing MV replacement in FMR including anterior flip-over, in which a C-shaped incision is placed in the anterior leaflet and the entire anterior apparatus is moved posteriorly. Following appropriate valve sizing, pledgeted stitches are placed through the posterior annulus, the edge of the posterior leaflet, and the "flipped" anterior leaflet, placing both chordal apparatus and leaflets behind the MV prosthesis (**Figure 30.3a–d**).

A second method of achieving total valve sparing is to remove the center of the anterior leaflet then rotate the remaining portions of the anterior leaflet to the left and right. Valve sizing for FMR should be prudent and not oversized. With modern MV prostheses there should not be undue worry of stenosis and overly large bulky valves may impair LV dynamics in these already poor LVs. Acker showed in

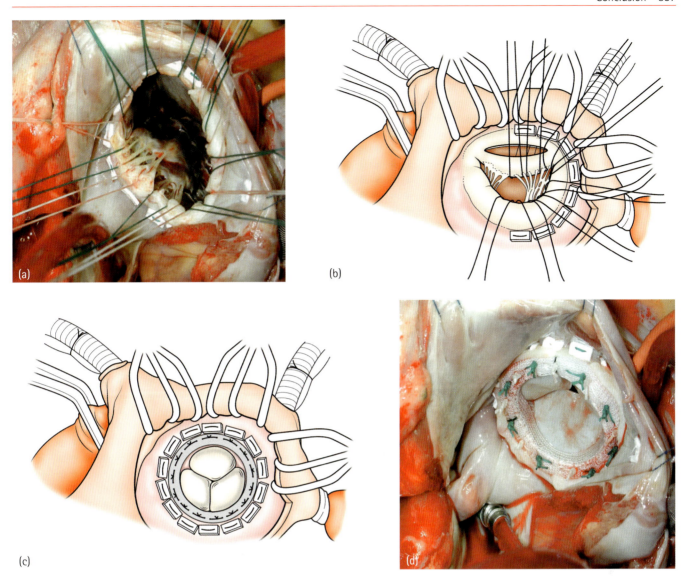

30.3a–d Valve-sparing MV replacement technique: anterior leaflet "flip-over."

severe FMR patients a total valve-sparing operative mortality of 4.2%, which was only slightly higher than the operative mortality of 1.6% mitral repair for FMR patients.[1]

POSTOPERATIVE CARE

Following repair or replacement for FMR, these patients may be managed largely the same as degenerative MR patients. However, we have found that this population tends to have significant down-regulation of beta receptors and we frequently utilize milrinone in the immediate postoperative setting.

CONCLUSION

FMR is a complex issue that occurs as a disease of the ventricle through disordered LV geometry and contractile function or via annular dilation from left atrial enlargement. Treatment should utilize guideline-directed medical therapy to address underlying LV dysfunction, in addition to CRT and/or coronary revascularization, when indicated. MV surgery should be considered when patients are undergoing concomitant cardiac surgery or when FMR symptoms persist despite medical therapy. MV repair should be preferred over replacement in most situations and undersizing the mitral ring remains paramount to achieving optimal results.

REFERENCES

1. Acker MA, Parides MK, Perrault LP, et al. for the CTSN. Mitral valve repair versus replacement for severe ischemic mitral regurgitation. *N Engl J Med.* 2014; 370(1): 23–32.

2. Wu AH, Aaronson KD, Bolling SF, et al. Impact of mitral valve annuloplasty on mortality risk in patients with mitral regurgitation and left ventricular systolic dysfunction. *J Am Coll Cardiol.* 2005; 45(3): 381–7.

3. Trichon BH, Glower DD, Shaw LK et al. Survival after coronary revascularization, with and without mitral valve surgery, in patients with ischemic mitral regurgitation. *Circulation.* 2003;108 Suppl 1: II103–10.

4. Fattouch K, Guccione F, Sampognaro R, et al. POINT: Efficacy of adding mitral valve restrictive annuloplasty to coronary artery bypass grafting in patients with moderate ischemic mitral valve regurgitation: a randomized trial. *J Thorac Cardiovasc Surg.* 2009; 138: 278–85.

5. Deja MA, Grayburn PA, Sun B, et al. Influence of mitral regurgitation repair on survival in the surgical treatment for ischemic heart failure trial. *Circulation.* 2012; 125(21): 2639–48.

6. Chan KM, Punjabi PP, Flather M, et al. Coronary artery bypass with or without mitral annuloplasty in moderate functional ischemic mitral regurgitation: final results of the Randomized Ischemic Mitral Evaluation (RIME) trial. *Circulation.* 2012; 126: 2502–10.

7. Smith PK, Puskas JD, Ascheim DD, et al. Surgical treatment of moderate ischemic mitral regurgitation. *N Engl J Med.* 2014; 371(23): 2178–88.

8. Nishimura RA, Otto CM, Bonow RO, et al. 2014 AHA/ACC guideline for the management of patients with valvular heart disease: a report of the American College of Cardiology/American Heart Association Task Force on Practice Guidelines. *J Am Coll Cardiol.* 2014; 63(22): e57–185.

9. Vahanian A, Alfieri O, Andreotti F, et al. Joint Task Force on the Management of Valvular Heart Disease of the European Society of Cardiology (ESC) and the European Association for Cardio-Thoracic Surgery (EACTS). Guidelines on the management of valvular heart disease (version 2012). *Eur J Cardiothorac Surg.* 2012; 42(4): S1–44.

10. Yancy CW, Jessup M, Bozkurt B, et al. 2013 ACCF/AHA guideline for the management of heart failure: a report of the American College of Cardiology Foundation/American Heart Association Task Force on Practice Guidelines. *J Am Coll Cardiol.* 2013; 62: e147–239.

11. Geidel S, Lass M, Schneider C, et al. Early and late results of restrictive mitral valve annuloplasty in 121 patients with cardiomyopathy and chronic mitral regurgitation. *Thorac Cardiovasc Surg.* 2008; 56(5): 262–8.

12. Acker MA, Jessup M, Bolling SF, et al. Mitral valve repair in heart failure: five-year follow-up from the mitral valve replacement stratum of the Acorn randomized trial. *J Thorac Cardiovasc Surg.* 2011; 142(3): 569–74.

13. Hueb AC, Jatene FB, Moreira LFP, et al. Ventricular remodeling and mitral valve modifications in dilated cardiomyopathy: new insights from anatomic study. *J Thorac Cardiovasc Surg.* 2002; 124: 1216–24.

14. McGee EC, Gillinov AM, Blackstone EH, et al. Recurrent mitral regurgitation after annuloplasty for functional ischemic mitral regurgitation. *J Thorac Cardiovasc Surg.* 2004; 128(6): 916–24.

15. Magne J, Senechal M, Dumesnil JG, Pibarot P. Ischemic mitral regurgitation: a complex multifaceted disease. *Cardiology.* 2009; 112: 244–59.

16. Silberman S, Klutstein MW, Sabag T, et al. Repair of ischemic mitral regurgitation: comparison between flexible and rigid annuloplasty rings. *Ann Thorac Surg.* 2009; 87(6): 1721–7.

17. Braun J, Bax JJ, Versteegh MI, et al. Preoperative left ventricular dimensions predict reverse remodeling following restrictive mitral annuloplasty in ischemic mitral regurgitation. *Eur J Cardiothorac Surg.* 2005; 27(5): 847–53.

18. Bolling SF, Deeb GM, Brunsting LA, Bach DS. Early outcome of mitral valve reconstruction in patients with end-stage cardiomyopathy. *J Thorac Cardiovasc Surg.* 1995; 4: 676–83.

19. Spoor MT, Geltz A, Bolling SF. Flexible versus nonflexible mitral valve rings for congestive heart failure: differential durability of repair. *Circulation.* 2006; 114(1 Suppl): I67–71.

20. Magne J, Sénéchal M, Mathieu P, et al. Restrictive annuloplasty for ischemic mitral regurgitation may induce functional mitral stenosis. *J Am Coll Cardiol.* 2008; 51: 1692–701.

21. Kubota K, Otsuji Y, Ueno T, et al. Functional mitral stenosis after surgical annuloplasty for ischemic mitral regurgitation: importance of subvalvular tethering in the mechanism and dynamic deterioration during exertion. *J Thorac Cardiovasc Surg.* 2010; 140: 617–23.

22. Kainuma S, Taniguchi K, Daimon T, et al. Does stringent restrictive annuloplasty for functional mitral regurgitation cause functional mitral stenosis and pulmonary hypertension? *Circulation.* 2011; 124(11 Suppl): S97–106.

23. Rubino AS, Onorati F, Santarpia G, et al. Impact of increased transmitral gradients after undersized annuloplasty for chronic ischemic mitral regurgitation. *Int J Cardiol.* 2012; 158: 71–7.

24. Nishida H, Takahara Y, Takeuchi S, Mogi K. Mitral stenosis after mitral valve repair using the duran flexible annuloplasty ring for degenerative mitral regurgitation. *J Heart Valve Dis.* 2005; 14: 563–4.

25. Lancellotti P, Pellikka PA, Budts W, et al. The clinical use of stress echocardiography in non-ischaemic heart disease: recommendations from the European Association of Cardiovascular Imaging and the American Society of Echocardiography. *Eur Heart J Cardiovasc Imaging.* 2016; 17(11): 1191–229.

26. Borger MA, Murphy PM, Alam A, et al. Initial results of the chordal-cutting operation for ischemic mitral regurgitation. *J Thorac Cardiovasc Surg.* 2007; 133: 1483–92.

27. Kron IL, Hung J, Overby JR, et al. Predicting recurrent mitral regurgitation after mitral valve repair for severe ischemic mitral regurgitation. *J Thorac Cardiovasc Surg.* 2015; 149(3): 752–61.

28. Hvass U, Joudinaud T. The papillary muscle sling for ischemic mitral regurgitation. *J Thorac Cardiovasc Surg.* 2010; 139(2): 418–23.

29. Lancellotti P, Moura L, Pierard LA, et al. European Association of Echocardiography recommendations for the assessment of valvular regurgitation. Part 2: Mitral and tricuspid regurgitation (native valve disease). *Eur J Echocardiogr.* 2010; 11: 307–32.

30. Yun KL, Sintek CF, Miller DC, et al. Randomized trial of partial versus complete chordal preservation methods of mitral valve replacement: a preliminary report. *Circulation.* 1999; 100(19 Suppl): II90–4.

Thoracic aortic disease

31

Ascending aortic aneurysm

RYAN P. PLICHTA AND G. CHAD HUGHES

HISTORY

Advances in surgical technique, cardiovascular anesthesia, mechanical circulatory support, and selective cerebral perfusion, as well as postoperative intensive care, have resulted in safe and effective surgical strategies for approaching aneurysms of the ascending aorta and root. Over the past 50 years, mortality rates for replacement of the proximal aorta have dropped from above 50% to well below 10% at high volume centers of excellence.

PRINCIPLES AND JUSTIFICATION

Aortic aneurysms represent a spectrum of typically asymptomatic disease with potentially devastating consequences. Aneurysmal disease of the ascending aorta often has an indolent course. In fact, the vast majority of these aneurysms are asymptomatic up until the time of an acute event. As an aortic root or ascending aortic aneurysm increases in diameter, the risk of dissection also increases. This relationship is not linear, however, and other less well-defined factors, such as wall tension or stress, likely contribute to dissection risk as well. Overall, the aortic root tends to exhibit the slowest growth of all aortic segments, at approximately 0.4 mm annually. Comparatively, the ascending aorta grows at approximately 1 mm per year.

In an era of improving and ubiquitous imaging, ascending aneurysms are increasingly identified, usually as incidental findings on studies performed for other indications. The decision to intervene is based upon absolute size criteria, rate of growth, family history, the presence or absence of a connective tissue disorder, and medical comorbidities. Patients with a history of aortic aneurysm are followed over their lifetime with serial imaging and medical therapy with blood pressure control, lipid control, and smoking cessation. The ultimate goal is to surgically repair an aneurysmal aorta when the risk of dissection or rupture exceeds the relatively low risk of surgical intervention. The rates of morbidity and mortality with elective proximal aortic surgery range from 2–5% with regards to risk of death or stroke. The morbidity and mortality risks of emergent surgery after an acute event are much higher.

Our algorithm regarding operative intervention for aortic root and ascending aneurysms is generally in accordance with current published guidelines, with surgery recommended at an outer-wall to outer-wall aortic diameter by computed tomography angiography (CTA) or magnetic resonance imaging (MRI) of 5.5 cm in patients with no other indication for surgery. Additionally, we intervene at 5.0 cm in patients with a congenital bicuspid aortic valve or associated moderate or worse stenosis or insufficiency of a trileaflet valve, although controversy exists regarding appropriate diameter thresholds for elective surgery in the bicuspid population. Finally, we operate at 4.5 cm in patients with a connective tissue disorder, or a family or personal history of aortic dissection. We also believe that modest dilation of the aortic root carries a greater risk of dissection than a similar degree of dilation of the supracoronary ascending aorta, and therefore will recommend aortic root replacement in non-syndromic trileaflet patients who are otherwise good surgical candidates at a diameter of 5.0 cm. Our practice is to remove all dilated aorta, and we therefore have a low threshold to perform concomitant hemi-arch repair when the aorta is 4.0 cm or greater at the level of the innominate artery, as current data and our own experience would suggest the addition of hemi-arch adds little to no additional operative risk. The treatment of aortic aneurysms associated with connective tissue disorders and procedures involving valve-sparing root remodeling and reimplantation will be covered in subsequent chapters (Chapters 33 and 34).

PREOPERATIVE ASSESSMENT AND PREPARATION

Preoperative evaluation of patients with ascending aortic aneurysms includes thin-cut (≤1 mm) CTA of the chest, abdomen, and pelvis to evaluate the entire aorta and first-degree branch vessels. Alternatively, magnetic resonance angiography (MRA) may be used in select patients, although we favor thin-cut CTA as our baseline procedure of choice.

Patients with an aneurysm of the ascending aorta are at an increased risk of harboring concomitant aneurysmal disease in other aortic segments. Additionally, these patients undergo transthoracic echocardiography to assess for ventricular function and valvular pathology. Each patient also undergoes an electrocardiogram (ECG) as well as left and right heart catheterization. Other studies such as arterial blood gas, pulmonary function testing, and carotid duplex may be obtained as indicated, depending on patient history and physical exam findings. Additional indications for surgery are addressed concomitantly at the time of ascending aortic repair.

ANESTHESIA

Cardiovascular anesthetic care of patients undergoing replacement of the ascending aorta is of critical importance. It is vital that the anesthesia and surgical teams work in close coordination to ensure a successful outcome. Good communication is needed, and a thorough preoperative briefing is key to confirming that everyone has a clear understanding of the operative plan.

The anesthesia team places bilateral radial arterial lines, central venous access in the right internal jugular vein, with or without a pulmonary artery catheter depending on patient comorbidities, a nasopharyngeal temperature probe, and a transesophageal echocardiography (TEE) probe. Warming pads are placed under the patient's legs and torso for the rewarming portion of the operation. Electroencephalographic (EEG) monitoring is performed routinely when hypothermic circulatory arrest (HCA) is utilized and therefore volatile agents only are used.

When separating from cardiopulmonary bypass (CPB), we anticipate some degree of coagulopathy due to the routine use of HCA for hemi-arch repair. As such, blood and blood products are available and administered as needed after protamine sulfate administration following separation from CPB. This includes packed red cells, fresh frozen plasma, platelets, cryo-precipitate, Desmopression (DDAVP), low dose recombinant activated Factor VII (rFVIIa), and pro-thrombin complex concentrate, all of which should be in the room and immediately available at the time of CPB separation. In our experience, administration of low dose rFVIIa (1 mg initial dose with additional 1 mg dosing 10–15 minutes later if coagulopathy persists) is a safe and effective way to improve hemostasis and correct coagulopathy early in the course of refractory blood loss without adverse effects given the very low dose administered. Additionally, mean arterial pressure goals while weaning from bypass are typically 60–70 mmHg to minimize bleeding. In the setting of more severe coagulopathy, as may be seen in complex redo operations and acute dissections, especially in elderly, frail, or medically compromised patients, low dose 3-factor prothrombin complex concentrate (initial dose 10 U/kg with an additional 10 U/kg given 10–15 minutes later if coagulopathy persists) may be required as well as higher doses of rFVIIa (up to 90 μg/kg total dose).

OPERATION

Aneurysms of the ascending aorta are typically approached via a median sternotomy. The majority of these aneurysms include a dilated proximal transverse aortic arch. As mentioned, we perform an aggressive hemi-arch repair when the aorta measures ≥ 4.0 cm at the level of the innominate artery. Although controversy currently exists regarding optimal temperature and adjunctive perfusion strategy for circulatory arrest, at our institution open arch repair is most often performed using moderate HCA with unilateral antegrade cerebral perfusion (ACP). Goal systemic temperature is 22–26 °C. Our preference for arterial cannulation is through the right axillary artery as this allows for easy administration of ACP and keeps the aortic and ACP cannulae out of the operative field. In our experience, this is a safe, quick, and reproducible method of arterial cannulation for the majority of our proximal aortic operations. Central cannulation of the distal ascending aorta/proximal arch, as well as femoral arterial cannulation, are also reasonable options but lack the benefit of providing ACP via the same access as for arterial inflow from the CPB circuit and therefore require additional cannulae inserted directly into the origins of the head vessels via the open arch. In instances where ACP is not used, an additional venous cannula (26–Fr angled) is placed in the SVC and utilized for retrograde cerebral perfusion (RCP) during the period of HCA.

All proximal aortic repairs are done under continuous TEE monitoring; EEG is added in the case of concomitant arch repair. The patient is placed in the supine position on the operating room table. Prophylactic antibiotics are administered perioperatively. Neuroprotective agents are also administered and include 1000 mg of methylprednisolone on the morning of surgery, as well as 2–4 mg magnesium and 200 mg of lidocaine while on CPB, although we recognize only low-level evidence supports the use of these neuroprotective agents. Invasive monitoring lines are placed by the cardiac anesthesia team as above. The bilateral radial arterial lines aid in monitoring during ACP. The neck, chest, abdomen, and legs, to just below the knees, are prepped and draped in the usual sterile manner. A surgical time out is then performed with the entire operating room team present and any concerns are addressed.

Right axillary cannulation

The procedure to obtain right axillary access is simple and easily reproducible (**Figure 31.1**). A 5–6 cm incision is made 1–2 finger-breadths below the lateral two-thirds of the right clavicle. The dissection is carried down to the pectoralis major fascia with the use of electrocautery. The deltopectoral groove is entered and the clavipectoral fascia is divided. The pectoralis minor muscle is partially divided with cautery. This affords excellent exposure of the axillary artery. Care is taken to avoid disturbing the brachial plexus. Then, 4–5000 units of IV heparin are administered

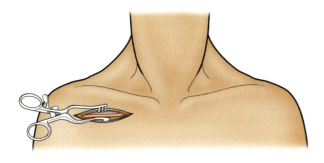

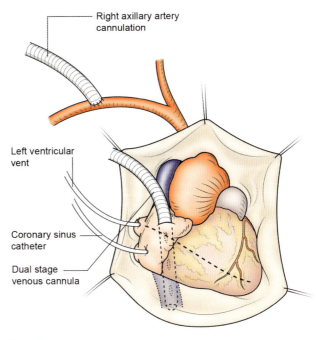

Right axillary artery cannulation

Left ventricular vent

Coronary sinus catheter

Dual stage venous cannula

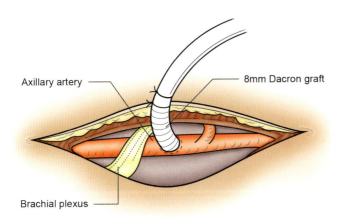

Axillary artery

8mm Dacron graft

Brachial plexus

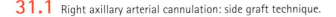

31.2

31.1 Right axillary arterial cannulation: side graft technique.

and the axillary artery is clamped and opened. Typically, an 8 mm knitted Dacron graft is then anastomosed to the axillary artery in an end-to-side manner using 5-0 Prolene suture (side-graft technique). To ensure excellent hemostasis throughout the case, several small pledgeted 5-0 Prolene sutures are placed in a horizontal mattress fashion around the completed anastomosis to reinforce it. The graft is then de-aired and a three-eighth-inch connector is placed inside the distal portion of the graft and secured with a zip tie or several heavy silk ties and connected to the arterial inflow line of the CPB circuit.

Cardiopulmonary bypass

A median sternotomy is then performed (**Figure 31.2**). The heart is suspended in a pericardial cradle and the patient is fully systemically heparinized. Using digital palpation and TEE guidance, the ascending aorta is carefully evaluated for any contraindications to ascending aortic cross-clamp; epiaortic ultrasound may also be used, although we rarely find this to be necessary given the excellent evaluation of the aorta provided by the combination of preoperative thin cut CTA imaging, manual palpation, and TEE. Venous cannulation is through the right atrium with a dual-stage venous cannula unless concomitant procedures such as mitral or tricuspid surgery or atrial septal defect closure requiring bicaval cannulation are planned. Systemic cooling is then

initiated, although cooling should be delayed until the left ventricular vent is in place and the aorta nearly ready to be cross-clamped in the setting of significant aortic insufficiency so as to avoid left ventricular distension following onset of ventricular fibrillation with cooling. As mentioned, moderate systemic hypothermia is used with neurocerebral monitoring with intraoperative EEG. The goal temperature is approximately 20–24 °C in the nasopharyngeal cavity, which typically correlates to a bladder temperature of approximately 24–26 °C. The heart is vented via the right superior pulmonary vein with an aortic root vent placed at the completion of the repair to assist with de-airing prior to removal of the aortic cross-clamp. If right axillary artery cannulation is contraindicated, or if there is no plan for arch repair, central aortic cannulation is performed, with the femoral artery rarely utilized. As above, an additional SVC venous cannula is utilized when RCP is planned.

Myocardial protection

Reliable and effective myocardial protection is a critical part of proximal aortic surgery, as these operations are complex and frequently involve prolonged aortic cross-clamp times. Our preference is to continuously monitor myocardial temperature with a septal temperature probe. Aortic occlusion is performed using a single clamp and cardioplegia is administered both antegrade and retrograde through the aortic root and the coronary sinus. If there is significant aortic insufficiency, antegrade cardioplegia can be given directly into the ostia of the coronary arteries after induction cardioplegia is begun via a retrograde route. Induction is performed using a cold blood/crystalloid solution and high potassium. Maintenance cardioplegia is performed with a cold blood/crystalloid solution and low potassium. Buckberg cardioplegia is typically utilized and re-administered via the retrograde route at 20-minute intervals. Retrograde cold blood may be given between cardioplegia doses as needed to maintain septal temperature < 14 °C.

Technical details of ascending aortic aneurysm repair

After the ascending aorta is clamped and induction cardioplegia administration completed, the ascending aorta is opened and divided down to the right pulmonary artery. The entire ascending aorta is removed from just above the sinotubular junction and sent to pathology for microscopic

examination. The aortic root is then mobilized off of the right and main pulmonary arteries posteriorly and medially, respectively, and off of the right ventricular outflow tract (RVOT) and right and left atria anteriorly and laterally, respectively.

With the aorta open and the root mobilized, the aortic valve and root are carefully examined. The status of these components dictates the particular technique for proximal reconstruction. If the aortic valve leaflets and the sinuses are normal (**Figure 31.3a**), reconstruction of the sinotubular junction and ascending aorta alone is required. In the scenario of central insufficiency of a trileaflet aortic valve, typically moderate or less in severity, due to isolated dilation of the sinotubular junction, replacement of the ascending aorta with an appropriately sized Dacron graft (as assessed based upon the aortic annular diameter as discussed below) restores the normal sinotubular junction anatomy

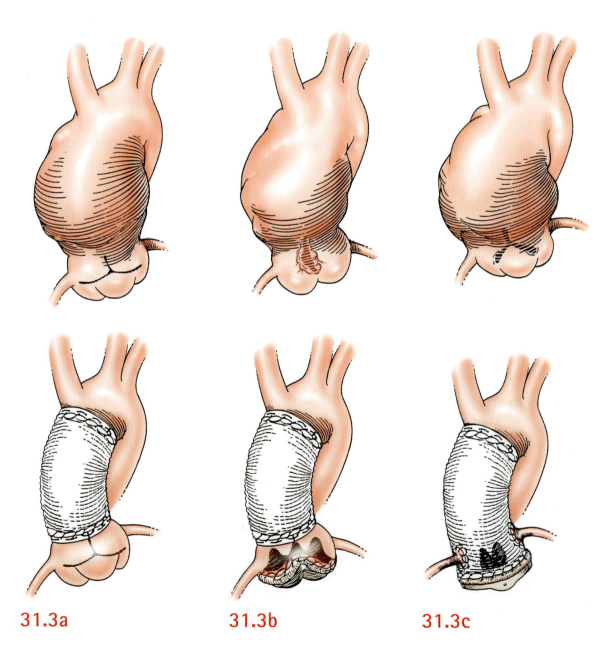

31.3a   31.3b   31.3c

and corrects any valve insufficiency that may be present. When the aortic valve leaflets themselves are abnormal yet the aortic root is of normal caliber, aortic valve replacement and separate placement of a supracoronary graft (Wheat procedure) is an excellent strategy (**Figure 31.3b**). Of note, the presence of a congenital bicuspid aortic valve alone does not mandate aortic valve replacement. If the bicuspid valve is non-calcified and normally functioning, it may be left in situ as described for a trileaflet valve and the supracoronary ascending aorta alone replaced if the root is normal. If both the aortic valve leaflets and aortic root are abnormal (**Figure 31.3c**), replacement of the aortic root with a valved conduit is indicated (modified Bentall procedure). Finally, if the aortic valve leaflets are relatively normal yet the root is abnormal, a valve sparing root replacement procedure should be considered, especially in the younger patient. This operation, which may be performed in the setting of both congenital bicuspid and trileaflet aortic valves, has proven to result in a safe and durable repair when performed by experienced surgeons at high volume centers and is covered in Chapter 22.

With a normal aortic valve and root, and mild-moderate central AI due to isolated dilation of the sinotubular junction, replacing the ascending aorta eliminates the aneurysm and restores the normal anatomy of the sinotubular junction, thereby correcting any potential valvular insufficiency. Sizing the aortic annulus with aortic valve sizers aids in approximating the ideal size of the sinotubular junction and the ascending graft. For example, for an aortic annulus that measures 25 mm, a 26 mm or 28 mm Dacron graft is selected. One must be careful not to excessively downsize the sinotubular junction as this will create cusp prolapse and subsequent AI. The proximal end of the graft is then anastomosed to the sinotubular junction using running 4-0 Prolene suture on a BB needle. A thin strip of Teflon felt, placed outside of the aorta, is incorporated into this anastomosis, and the graft is intussuscepted several millimeters down into the lumen of the aorta as it is sewn into place. This completes the proximal aortic reconstruction and re-establishes normal sinotubular junction anatomy. This proximal graft is then clamped and pressurized with antegrade cardioplegia, and valve competency and hemostasis are checked simultaneously. For patients with abnormal aortic valves and normal root anatomy, an aortic valve replacement is added to the above procedure in the usual manner (Wheat procedure) (**Figure 31.3b**).

BUTTON BENTALL PROCEDURE WITH AND WITHOUT "LEGS" TECHNIQUE

If the aortic root and aortic valve are both abnormal, a root replacement is performed. The aortic annulus is sized with a commercial valve sizer corresponding to the valve type to be implanted and the appropriate valved conduit is selected. For mechanical valved conduits, the composite valve and graft come attached out of the box. If the decision is made to utilize a bioprosthetic valve, typically the aortic graft chosen for attachment to the bioprosthetic valve is approximately 5 mm larger than the aortic valve size selected. For example, a 25 mm aortic valve will be paired with a 30 mm Dacron graft. We prefer to use the commercially available Gelweave Valsalva™ graft with premade sinuses of Valsalva (Vascutek; Terumo Cardiovascular Systems, Ann Arbor, Michigan), as the additional width of the sinus portion of the graft facilitates attachment of the coronary buttons requiring less mobilization. The valve is placed in the proximal portion of the graft and secured with a running 4-0 Prolene suture. Another option is a commercially available graft that can be utilized with the Sorin Mitroflow valve (Sorin Group Inc., Arvada CO), which allows the graft to be quickly coupled to the bioprosthetic valve by tying a single suture. The entire ascending aorta and non-coronary sinus are excised leaving a generous rim of native aorta around the annulus to allow quality bites with the valve sutures. The native valve tissue is removed and the annulus is debrided of any calcified deposits. The aortic root and left ventricular outflow tract are then copiously irrigated to remove any remaining debris that has the potential to embolize. The left and right main coronary artery buttons are dissected free from their respective sinus segments leaving a large cuff of tissue that can be trimmed to size later. Pledgeted valve sutures are placed around the circumference of the aortic annulus in a supra-annular position using 2-0 Ethibond horizontal mattress sutures. It should be noted that if the annulus is markedly dilated (> 33 mm in diameter), as can occasionally be encountered in cases of marked annuloaortic ectasia, a 2-0 Prolene pursestring suture is run around the base of the annulus just below the annular ridge and then tied down over a 31 mm Hegar dilator to downsize the annulus for an appropriate valve implant prior to placing the supra-annular pledgeted valve sutures. The valve sutures are then passed through the sewing ring of the aortic valve and the proximal cuff of the graft (**Figure 31.4a**). The aortic valved-conduit is then seated into the annulus and the sutures are secured with either manually tied knots or a knot-tying device.

Next, the left and right coronary buttons are sewn onto the composite graft in an orthotopic position using running 5-0 Prolene suture (**Figure 31.4b**). The left coronary button is sewn first, followed by the right. Of note, it is important to carefully assess the location of the graft where the coronaries will be re-implanted to minimize the risk of coronary kinking after button implant. For the right coronary button, this typically involves placing the button as high and anteriorly as possible. For the left coronary, one should attempt to assess the planned lie of the button to ensure that the coronary will not be kinked or twisted once the heart is full after weaning from CPB. A coronary probe can be helpful to assess this by having the assistant hold the button in the planned location and then gently probing the coronary artery to ensure that the probe passes easily without distal obstruction. The graft aortotomy is then made with a graft-cutting cautery at the estimated anatomic level on the root graft. In the redo-setting, adequate mobilization of the coronary buttons can be challenging and our practice has been to sew a short interposition 8 mm woven Dacron graft to the coronary button and

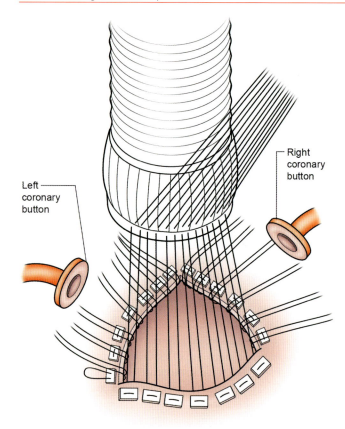

31.4a

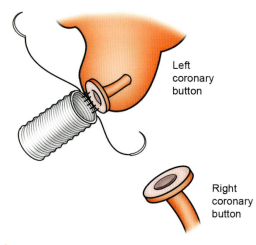

31.4c

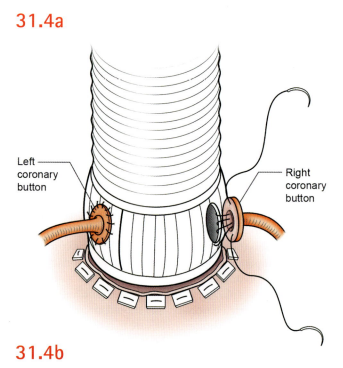

31.4b

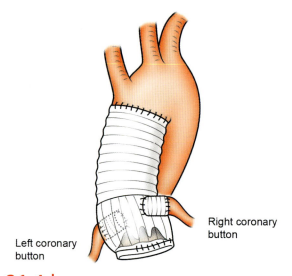

31.4d

then directly attach this "leg" to the ascending graft ("Legs" technique). The 8 mm graft is first sewn to the button and left long, such that it may be pressurized with antegrade cardioplegia; hemostasis is then ensured by reinforcing the anastomosis with interrupted 5-0 Prolene sutures as needed (**Figure 31.4c**). Once this has been completed and hemostasis

of the graft-to-button anastomosis confirmed, the 8 mm graft is cut to a short (2–3 mm) length as appropriate to reach the root graft without tension (**Figure 31.4d**). This technique may also be useful in the case of markedly dilated aortic roots whereby the ostia of the coronary arteries can be markedly displaced from the aortic annulus. The surgeon must be very wary of ventricular dysfunction or dysrhythmias coming off of bypass. This can frequently be the result of air embolizing into the coronary arteries. However, if the findings of coronary ischemia persist, the surgeon must suspect kinking of a coronary button until proven otherwise. The intraoperative TEE can be helpful in this scenario to assess which coronary distribution appears affected as adjunctive coronary bypass may be required.

Technical details of transverse aortic arch graft (hemi-arch)

After completion of cooling to the target temperature for HCA depending on institutional preference (NP temperature 20–24°C with use of ACP at our institution), the proximal aortic work is suspended and attention is turned the hemi-arch repair. The patient is placed in slight Trendelenburg position, the circulation is stopped, and the aortic clamp is removed. The aortic arch is then mobilized and the base of the innominate and left common carotid artery are completely exposed during a brief period of circulatory arrest. This dissection and mobilization can be started during cooling, prior to removal of the crossclamp, as this helps to reduce circulatory arrest time. The base of these arteries are then clamped and ACP initiated via the right axillary graft to a target right radial arterial line pressure of approximately 50–70 mmHg at an inflow temperature of 12°C (**Figure 31.5a**). This allows for a flow rate of approximately 5–15 cc/kg/min. The field is insufflated with CO_2 at 6 L/min during the entire open portion of the case to displace intracardiac/vascular air. Bright red blood will be seen emanating from the orifice of the left subclavian artery indicating an intact Circle of Willis and adequate left cerebral hemisphere perfusion. If this is not the case, a separate selective antegrade catheter can be placed in the left carotid artery while the distal anastomosis is performed (although this is rarely necessary in our experience) with the carotid ACP cannula removed just prior to anastomosis completion.

If RCP is employed, we prefer to utilize deeper hypothermia (< 20 NP) given the lack of cerebral nutrient flow with RCP. To initiate RCP, the SVC is snared and RCP provided via the SVC cannula to a target central venous pressure of approximately 25 mmHg at an inflow temperature of 12°C in a slight Trendelenburg position. This allows for a goal flow rate of approximately 150–450 cc/min. Dark red blood will be seen emanating from the orifices of the arch vessels indicating adequate RCP.

The entire underside of the aortic arch is resected as distally as possible (peninsula technique) so as to remove all diseased aorta. A separate straight woven Dacron graft is then used to reconstruct the aortic arch in an aggressive "Hemi-Arch" fashion. Utilizing a 4-0 BB Prolene running continuous suture, the arch reconstruction is performed. In the case of aneurysmal disease, we typically do not use Teflon felt reinforcement of the distal anastomosis as we have not found this to be necessary. At completion of both the posterior and anterior suture lines, the aorta and graft are allowed to fill via the right axillary artery, after removal of the clamps on the proximal innominate and left common carotid arteries, to completely de-air the cerebral vessels and cardiovascular system. The aortic cross-clamp is then placed on the graft just proximal to the arch anastomosis (**Figure 31.5b**). When RCP is utilized without axillary cannulation, the arch graft is re-cannulated with the aortic cannula just proximal to the arch suture line, and the graft carefully de-aired and then pressurized via the aortic cannula. Full flow CPB at 12°C (cold reperfusion) is then performed for approximately 5 minutes to allow free

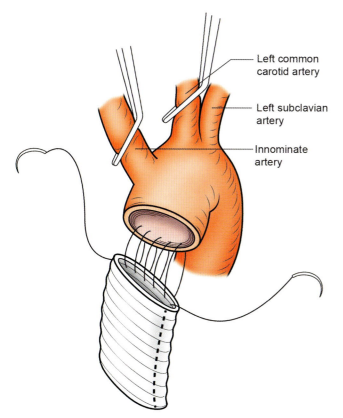
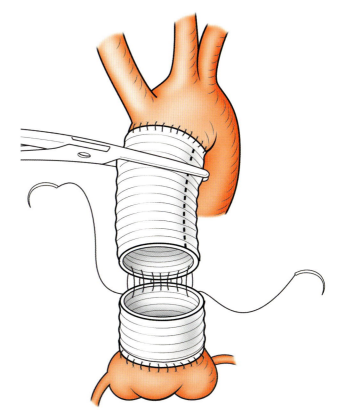

Left common carotid artery

Left subclavian artery

Innominate artery

31.5a–b Hemi-arch repair, distal and graft-to-graft anastomoses.

radical washout and minimize reperfusion injury. The pressurized aortic arch anastomosis is then checked for hemostasis. Pledgeted 4-0 Prolene sutures are placed along the posterior wall to address any bleeding. Attention is then again turned to the ascending aorta and root.

TOTAL AORTIC ARCH REPLACEMENT

Patients with aneurysms extending from the ascending aorta through the aortic arch may require total aortic arch replacement. The use of a branched graft allows for complete replacement of the ascending aorta and the aortic arch while simultaneously creating a proximal landing zone (PLZ) for future endograft placement. Total arch replacement may be performed either with or without creating an elephant trunk. In the case of a planned second stage endovascular repair, total arch replacement without creating an elephant trunk is easier as the distal anastomosis is quick and very similar to a hemi-arch anastomosis. Our practice is to use a branched Bavaria graft (Vascutek; Terumo Cardiovascular Systems, Ann Arbor, Michigan) for total arch replacements without elephant trunk. For elephant trunk procedures, we utilize a multibranch collared elephant trunk Gelweave TM Siena Plexus 4 branch graft (Vascutek; Terumo Cardiovascular Systems, Ann Arbor, Michigan). We create a 10 cm elephant trunk that will reach into the proximal descending thoracic aorta for easy access during a second stage repair. Frequently, the left subclavian artery (LSCA) arises distally from the arch and is left intact at the first stage total arch replacement with the left common carotid and the innominate arteries being reimplanted into the corresponding integral limbs of the arch graft.

As described above for hemi-arch replacement, after completion of cooling to the desired temperature for HCA, the circulation is stopped, the aortic clamp removed, and the distal ascending aorta opened. Dissection and mobilization of the distal ascending aorta and transverse arch is then fully completed during a brief period of circulatory arrest. Next, the base of the innominate artery, left common carotid artery, and the LSCA, if LSCA reimplantation is planned, are clamped and divided from the arch and ACP is then initiated as above. The entire proximal-mid aortic arch is resected, and the aorta is typically divided proximal to the LSCA so as to allow the distal arch anastomosis to be performed more anteriorly within the chest. This is technically easier and also helps avoid the risk of recurrent laryngeal or phrenic nerve injury, which can occur with a more distal anastomosis. Next, the arch graft of desired size is chosen and then anastomosed end-to-end to the divided arch with a 4-0 Prolene continuous running suture on a BB needle in the case of total arch without elephant trunk (**Figure 31.6a**). When an elephant trunk is created, a 3-0 Prolene on a larger SH needle is utilized, given the greater thickness of tissue (aorta plus graft), which must be incorporated into the distal anastomosis (**Figure 31.6b**).

Sizing of the arch graft bears considerable importance with regard to planning for a second stage endovascular operation.

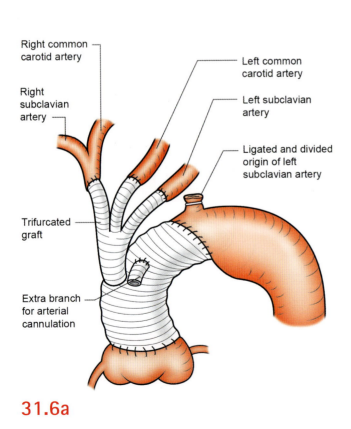

Right common carotid artery

Right subclavian artery

Left common carotid artery

Left subclavian artery

Ligated and divided origin of left subclavian artery

Trifurcated graft

Extra branch for arterial cannulation

31.6a

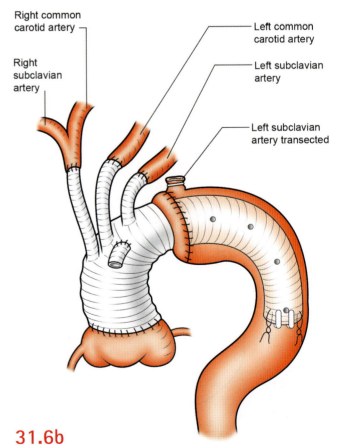

Right common carotid artery

Right subclavian artery

Left common carotid artery

Left subclavian artery

Left subclavian artery transected

31.6b

Our practice is to choose a graft size at least 4 mm smaller than the size of the distal landing zone, to allow for the dilation of the Dacron that occurs after implantation. Using a smaller arch graft size allows for the use of a single endograft for completion of the second stage repair in some cases, or allows for the endografts to be deployed from proximal to distal if multiple devices are required. When an elephant trunk has been created, we also place four large hemoclips on the distal end of the elephant trunk graft to aid in fluoroscopic identification for wire cannulation from the groin, as well as two 0 pacing wires that allow the graft to be snared for counter tension during endograft positioning and deployment (**Figure 31.6b**). This avoids the occasional tendency of the Dacron graft to fold on itself when cannulated with an endograft.

At the completion of the arch suture line, the prefabricated 10 mm perfusion sidearm of the branch graft is connected to a "Y" segment of the CPB arterial inflow circuit and full flow to the lower body (and left brain in the case where the LSCA is not reimplanted) is resumed after careful de-airing. Flow to the right brain continues via the right axillary graft. Rewarming is then initiated. The arch anastomosis is checked for bleeding as above.

Next, the distal 8 mm limb of the arch graft is either clipped and oversewn, if the LSCA is not reimplanted, or cut to length and anastomosed end-to-end to the LSCA using running 5-0 Prolene. If the LSCA is reimplanted, this limb must be carefully de-aired to avoid posterior circulation air emboli prior to re-establishing antegrade LSCA flow via the graft. Next, the proximal 8 mm graft limb is cut to length and anastomosed, end-to-end, to the left common carotid artery using running 5-0 Prolene. The graft limb is again carefully de-aired, and then flow to the anterior left brain is resumed via the perfusion side arm of the main graft. At this point, our preference is to complete the proximal aortic work and then anastomose the arch graft to the ascending or root graft, de-air the heart, and release the aortic cross-clamp with flow to the right brain during this entire period continuing to be provided via the right axillary graft into the innominate artery. This sequence of leaving the innominate artery reimplantation until last shortens the aortic cross-clamp time. Finally, once the aortic cross-clamp has been removed, the 12 mm integral limb of the arch graft is cut to length and anastomosed end-to-end to the innominate artery using running 5-0 Prolene. The innominate limb is then carefully de-aired, and flow to the entire body is then switched to be via the right axillary graft. This will minimize the risk of cerebral embolization as the flow pattern is away from the aortic arch. The patient is then weaned from CPB in the usual manner as described below. **Figure 31.6c** demonstrates a total arch replacement without elephant trunk and completed second stage with endograft PLZ just distal to the branched portion of the Bavaria graft.

When performing a total arch replacement with reimplantation of the LSCA, special consideration must be given to arterial pressure monitoring. In these cases, we place bilateral radial arterial lines as well as a left femoral arterial line. During the initial portions of the procedure prior to HCA,

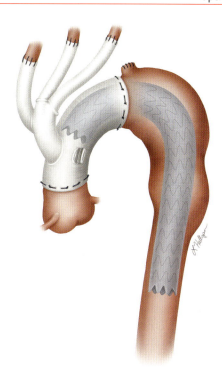

31.6c Total arch replacement and completion second stage endograft. The proximal landing zone is just distal to the branched portion of the Bavaria graft.

the left radial and left femoral arterial lines are displayed on the monitors and used to monitor systemic pressure. The right radial arterial line is not displayed at this point (the left and right radial arterial lines are attached to a single transducer that allows the anesthesia team to toggle between them depending on which is being monitored at any given point in the case) as the right radial arterial line will read falsely elevated pressures during the provision of systemic flow from the right axillary artery while on CPB. However, during the ACP portion of the procedure, the right radial arterial line is monitored to guide flow provided to the brain as described above. When flow is restored to the lower body following completion of the arch distal anastomosis, the left femoral arterial line is monitored in addition to the right radial a-line. After LSCA reimplantation is complete, we switch back to the left radial arterial line for monitoring of upper and lower body perfusion.

Redo operations

It is not uncommon to encounter a patient with a history of previous open heart surgery, frequently prior acute type A dissection repair. In all instances of previous median sternotomy or mini-thoracotomy, a preoperative CT scan should be thoroughly reviewed with regard to operative planning. The proximity of an aneurysmal aorta to the posterior sternal table, the presence of patent venous grafts, and the course of a patent mammary graft need to be noted, and care is taken when opening a redo-sternotomy to avoid injury to these structures. Right axillary artery cannulation with a side graft and central venous cannulation is a reasonable strategy in these cases. Alternatively, femoral venous cannulation is also an option, depending on surgeon preference and likelihood of injury upon opening the redo sternotomy. Given the frequent need for femoral venous cannulation in redo cases, a right femoral venous line should be placed at the beginning of the case to ensure venous access to facilitate rapid femoral venous cannulation should this become necessary during the procedure. Our practice is to obtain percutaneous access of the femoral vein with a micro puncture needle and 5F sheath prior to sternotomy. Further, for cases where injury to underlying structures is highly likely during sternal re-entry, as in the case of the aorta or other structure abutting the posterior sternal table, we recommend performing femoral venous cannulation after axillary cannulation and prior to sternal re-entry. The femoral venous cannula can be flushed/filled with heparinized saline and clamped such that additional heparinization beyond the small dose given for axillary cannulation is not required and thus lessening bone bleeding during redo sternotomy.

An oscillating saw is then used to divide the anterior table of the sternum along its entire length. To aid in lifting the sternum up and away from the contents of the mediastinum, two penetrating towel clips can be used by the first assistant and applied at the level of the sternal angle and the distal sternum. Alternatively, bone hooks can be used in a similar manner. After dividing the anterior table, heavy scissors are then used to divide the posterior table under direct vision. Care is taken to avoid excess upward tension on the sternum with the towel clips or retractors as the thin walled right ventricle is at risk for tearing when adherent to the posterior table.

With the sternum now open, the heart is dissected free of the pericardial space as needed and the operation continues as usual. It is advisable to limit the dissection to only what is necessary to carry out the operation, in order to limit bleeding from adhesions at the close of the case.

Completion

Finally, the graft-to-graft anastomosis of the proximal ascending/root graft to the distal arch graft is performed using running 3-0 Prolene suture (**Figure 31.7a and b**). The grafts should be cut to length while being held on tension to avoid excessive length and to ensure the final reconstruction nicely simulates the normal curvature of the ascending aorta. After this graft-to-graft anastomosis is completed, a root vent is placed and the patient is placed into a steep Trendelenburg position for standard de-airing maneuvers. Then the cross clamp is removed, the heart is defibrillated if needed and ventricular and atrial pacing wires are placed and pacing initiated. After a period of reperfusion and rewarming, the left ventricular vent and retrograde cardioplegia catheters are removed. The patient is then weaned from CPB.

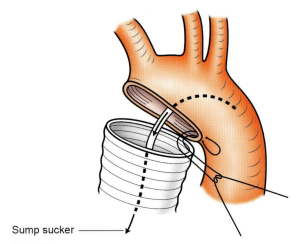

Sump sucker ⟶

31.7a   Ready for graft-to-graft anastomosis.

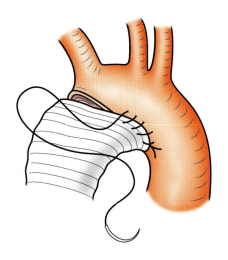

31.7b

POSTOPERATIVE CARE

Standard postoperative care is undertaken with the patient transported to the cardiovascular surgical intensive care unit. Inotropes are used to support the patient's ventricular function, mediastinal drains are monitored for excessive bleeding that may result in cardiac tamponade, and blood pressure is supported with vasoconstrictors as needed. The patient is extubated when they meet criteria and there is no concern for postoperative complication requiring a return to the operating room.

Postoperative imaging is obtained using CTA or MRI at 9 months post-discharge in most patients, although earlier imaging may be required in scenarios where a second stage procedure is planned or other concerns about the distal aorta exist. A follow-up CT or MRI scan is then obtained at 18 months after the initial postoperative scan and then every 24 months thereafter assuming stable findings on prior scans.

OUTCOME

Current outcomes for elective repairs of the ascending aorta/root and transverse arch are excellent. Outcomes for urgent or emergent repairs are less favorable and underscore the need for serial surveillance of known aneurysms and appropriate intervention when the aneurysms meet indication for repair. Operative mortality for these operations in the Society of Thoracic Surgeons Adult Cardiac Surgery Database was 3.4% in the elective setting and 15.4% for non-elective cases. Additionally, adding hemi-arch repair to replacement of the ascending aorta and root has been shown to be a safe strategy that does not increase the morbidity or mortality of the operation in experienced centers. However, failure to address a dilated proximal transverse arch can result in progressive arch dilatation, potential dissection or rupture, and need for reoperation.

FURTHER READING

Chau KH, Elefteriades JA. Natural history of thoracic aortic aneurysms: size matters, plus moving beyond size. *Prog Cardiovasc Dis.* 2013; 56(1): 74–80. doi:10.1016/j.pcad.2013.05.007

Hiratzka LF, Bakris GL, Beckman JA, et al. ACCF/AHA/AATS/ACR/ASA/SCA/SCAI/SIR/STS/SVM guidelines for the diagnosis and management of patients with thoracic aortic disease. *Circulation.* 2010; 121(13): e266–369.

Iribarne A, Keenan J, Benrashid E, et al. Imaging surveillance after proximal aortic operations: is it necessary? *Ann Thorac Surg.* 2017; 103(3): 734–41.

Malaisrie SC, Duncan BF, Mehta CK, et al. The addition of hemiarch replacement to aortic root surgery does not affect safety. *J Thorac Cardiovasc Surg.* 2015; 150(1): 118–24.

Peterss S, Bhandari R, Rizzo JA, et al. The aortic root: natural history after root-sparing ascending replacement in nonsyndromic aneurysmal patients. *Ann Thorac Surg.* 2017; 103(3): 828–33.

Williams JB, Peterson ED, Zhao Y, et al. Contemporary results for proximal aortic replacement in North America. *J Am Coll Cardiol.* 2012; 60(13): 1156–62.

32

Hybrid aortic arch repair

DANIEL-SEBASTIAN DOHLE AND NIMESH D. DESAI

HISTORY

The fast-developing era of aortic arch surgery began with the first report of Borst et al.[1] in 1964 about hypothermic circulatory arrest (HCA) for surgical aortic arch repair. Griepp et al.[2] reported a successful series of patients operated on with HCA in 1975 and this new technique was increasingly used for different aortic pathologies like aneurysms and acute and chronic aortic dissections of the arch. With this new tool for brain protection, surgical techniques like the open distal anastomosis developed, resulting in large series published by Svensson et al. in 1993[3] or Ergin et al. in 1994.[4] Nevertheless, the time frame for advanced surgical techniques under HCA was limited by the risk for stroke and mortality. The combination of HCA with RCP improved the results and the applicability worldwide. Even larger time frames of HCA could be tolerated with the introduction of unilateral and bilateral ACP. These perfusion techniques enabled further advancements of surgical techniques like the "elephant trunk procedure" and simultaneous brachiocephalic vessel reconstruction. Simultaneously another treatment option using endovascular stent grafts for thoracic aortic diseases (TEVAR) was developed in the late 1990s. The "frozen elephant technique" combined both principles, the antegrade implantation of a stent graft with regular arch surgery in a commercially available "hybrid-prosthesis."[5] Despite favorable results and further strategic developments resulting in reduction of HCA and CPB times, aortic arch surgery remains invasive major surgery with accordingly mortality and morbidity, especially in high-risk patients with prohibitive significant comorbidities or unfavorable anatomy. Further developments aimed at less invasive approaches combining endovascular aortic repair with surgical repair. The earliest "hybrid arch procedures" were therefore the extension of the proximal landing zone up to the LCA after carotid-subclavian bypass, followed by TEVAR. After overcoming several challenges regarding the proximal landing zone, debranching and reconstructive procedures of the ascending aorta and the aortic arch in combination with TEVAR resulted in today's hybrid arch surgery.

PRINCIPLES AND JUSTIFICATION

The hybrid arch repair has basically two components, the surgical aortic arch reconstruction with or without repair of the ascending aorta and the endovascular thoracic aortic repair (TEVAR), with different proportions of each component according to the extent of the underlying disease. As for any endovascular stent graft procedure, the proximal and distal landing zone are crucial. Therefore, the main focus of the open surgical component is always a favorable proximal landing zone > 3 cm for the endovascular component of the procedure. With the early hybrid procedures, a classification system for the proximal landing zone was established by Criado et al. in 2002 (**Figure 32.1**).[6] According to underlying aortic disease and its extent, different proximal landing zones for TEVAR can be prepared by intra- or extrathoracic

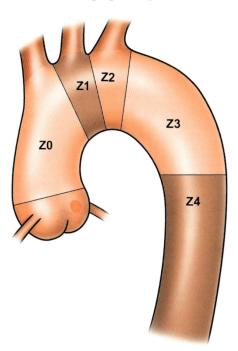

32.1

debranching and varying extent of aortic repair, which is the basis of the hybrid repair classification (**Figure 32.2**):

- **Type I hybrid repair:** The type I hybrid repair (**Figure 32.2a**) basically represents an aortic arch debranching with a proximal anastomosed multi-branch graft, resulting in a native zone 0 landing zone for subsequent TEVAR. Both the proximal and distal landing zones are favorable for TEVAR. In order to avoid retrograde dissection, a healthy ascending aorta with a diameter < 37 mm is a presumption. The TEVAR component can be performed at the same time, ante- or retrograde, as well as staged.
- **Type II hybrid repair:** In the type II hybrid repair (**Figure 32.2b**), only the distal landing zone is favorable. Therefore it includes a proximal repair to achieve a synthetic Dacron zone 0 landing zone for the TEVAR. It is indicated for aortic pathologies including the ascending and the aortic arch. As in type I hybrid repair, the TEVAR can be performed at the same time, ante- or retrograde, as well as staged.
- **Type III hybrid repair:** The type III hybrid repair (**Figure**

32.2c) is for extensive aortic disease involving the ascending aorta, arch and descending aorta. It is a two-staged approach including a type II repair or a complete arch repair with elephant trunk, completed by an staged retrograde TEVAR. In contrast to type I and II repairs, neither the proximal, nor the distal landing zone are favorable. It is less invasive compared to the conventional single or two-staged approach. This reduces the risk for complications between the intervals, and increases the compliance for completion of the second stage.

The main goal of the hybrid arch approach is reduction of morbidity and mortality. It is a therapeutic option for frail elderly individuals with significant comorbidities like renal failure, chronic obstructive disease and previous neurological events and patients with extensive atherosclerotic and thrombotic burden in the aortic arch, a subgroup that was identified to have mortality and stroke rates up to 20% in classic arch surgery.

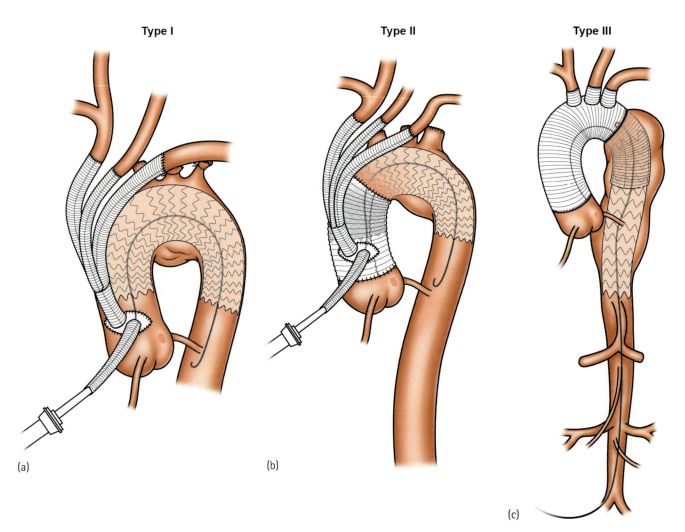

Type I   Type II   Type III

(a)   (b)   (c)

32.2a–c

The indications are aneurysmal diseases and aortic dissections. Aneurysms of the aortic arch can present variously and are usually diagnosed by computed tomography angiography (CTA). Typical clinical signs include back or chest pain. Hoarseness can result from stretching of the recurrent laryngeal nerve. Most aneuryms and penetrating ulcera result from excessive atherosclerotic disease. False lumen aneurysms occur after isolated proximal DeBakey type I dissection repair, or in chronic DeBakey type III dissections. No specific guidelines exist for the aortic arch. Generally accepted indications for surgery are aortic diameters over 6 cm or growth over 0.5 cm per year. Aortic size should be indexed to the patient's body surface area (BSA). Positive family history for aortic diseases should be considered. The use of TEVAR and hybrid surgical approaches remains controversial in patients with known or suspected connective tissue diseases like Marfan's, Loeys–Dietz or Turner syndrome. The risk for proximal or distal dissection induced by an oversized stent graft is high in these patients. Nevertheless, good results have been reported for the use of frozen elephant trunk, avoiding oversizing in these patients.

PREOPERATIVE ASSESSMENT AND PREPARATION

Imaging

As selection of the landing zones and planning is the key in hybrid arch surgery, the aortic anatomy has to be studied before incision extensively and thoughtful. The key imaging modality is therefore contrast enhanced ECG-triggered high resolution computed tomography (CT) with an early and late phase. The aortic arch is a complex 3D structure and advanced imaging software enabling at least 3D multiplanar reconstruction (3D MPR) and centerline reconstruction should be used. Comparing serial studies illustrates changes in specific areas and the dynamic of the pathology relevant for the indication of surgery. The exact longitudinal extent of the disease and the diameters of the proximal and distal landing zone, measured along the centerline, have to be known in order to prepare an appropriate combination of stent grafts. Atherosclerotic calcifications or debris in the arch vessels and anomalies like a bovine arch or vertebral arteries directly originating from the arch should be studied because they have huge impact on the cannulation and revascularization strategy. Also, the curvature of the arch should be considered to avoid "bird beak" at the proximal landing zone and high forces in the distal landing zone in severely curved "gothic arch". The distal extent of the aortic disease, additional abdominal or infrarenal aneurysms, and atherosclerotic or thrombotic burden have to be considered. False lumen perfusion of visceral organs, re-entries, true lumen size, and the stiffness of the dissection membrane itself have to be considered in dissection patients. These details are relevant for definition of the distal landing zone, and determine the strategy regarding an antegrade or retrograde TEVAR deployment.

Comorbid workup

Because hybrid aortic arch procedures often represent an alternative for frail, multimorbid, and old patients, a rigorous comorbid workup is essential. This includes echocardiography with evaluation of the cardiac and valve function, as well as cardiac catheterization to exclude or address an accessory coronary artery disease. Carotid and vertebral arteries should be evaluated by carotid ultrasound. The integrity of the Circle of Willis should be assessed, particularly in patients with a history of stroke. Pulmonary function should be tested for any obstructive or restrictive lung disease, medication optimized and patients educated and trained preoperatively. Peripheral arteries disease is not only relevant for the TEVAR approach but should also be addressed prior to aortic surgery to avoid critical limb ischemia early postoperatively. After completion of all preoperative studies a detailed plan should be made for the surgical access, perfusion, protection, monitoring and revascularization strategies, landing zones, needed grafts and stent grafts, materials, and alternative plans. These, and the potential risks and strategies to minimize them, should be discussed in detail with the patient and the family in order to achieve truly informed consent.

Hybrid operating room

A hybrid operating room is mandatory for hybrid aortic arch procedures and a one-stage approach. A hybrid operating room is a surgical theatre equipped with fixed C-Arm fluoroscopy, enabling open surgical repair and endovascular therapy on the same table within the same operation. Modern hybrid rooms integrate different imaging modalities like CTA, fluoroscopy, intravascular ultrasound (IVUS) and echocardiography with integrated post-processing.

ANESTHESIA

Hybrid arch procedures require standard cardiac anesthesia with experience in transesophageal echocardiogram (TEE), neuromonitoring, and neuroprotection. Arterial lines in both radial arteries as well as one femoral line are recommended for continuous blood pressure monitoring during debranching and HCA. Near infrared spectroscopy (NIRS) facilitates real-time information about the cerebral oxygenation, thus enabling the surgeon to test-clamp during debranching procedures and change or modify the cerebral perfusion strategies, and is therefore essential. Electroencephalography (EEG) and sensory-evoked potentials (SEP) augment the neuromonitoring. Hypothermia is crucial for neuroprotection. Nasopharyngeal temperature tracks the brain temperature most accurately, but bladder and rectal temperature monitoring are still widely used. Barbiturates and steroids are widely and variously used as neuroprotective agents, without evidence. Spinal fluid drainage for spinal cord protection should be considered in extended repairs. Blood products should be available for prompt bleeding control.

OPERATION

Cannulation, perfusion, and temperature management

Depending on the type of hybrid repair, cardiopulmonary bypass (CPB) is needed. CPB and HCA can be avoided most of the time in type I hybrid repair. Nevertheless, short CPB and cardiac arrest might be helpful. A short CPB run in type I hybrid repair allows mild cooling to 32 °C for further neuroprotection during the debranching procedure.

CPB is always needed in type II and III hybrid repair. Most proximal repairs require HCA for an open distal anastomosis. In conventional arch surgery, a paradigm shift from deep hypothermic circulatory arrest (DHCA 14.1–20 °C) to moderate hypothermic circulatory arrest (MHCA 20.1–28 °C) occurred, avoiding the hazards of prolonged CPB times due to rewarming and the risk for coagulopathy. MHCA without additional cerebral perfusion is only safe for 10 minutes. Therefore, either MHCA with antegrade cerebral perfusion (ACP), or DHCA with retrograde cerebral perfusion (RCP) is necessary.

DHCA with RCP is a good strategy for patients with an anticipated HCA time < 20 minutes. RCP is delivered via a snared superior vena cava cannula with internal jugular pressure 20–22 mmHg, flow rate of 150–300 cc / min and an inflow temperature of 10–12 °C (**Figure 32.3a**). Technical advantages of RCP are the elimination of arterial debris and excellent de-airing by back-bleeding.

In patients with anticipated HCA times > 20 minutes, MHCA with ACP is preferred (**Figure 32.3b**). Cannulation of the right axillary is preferred because it is rarely

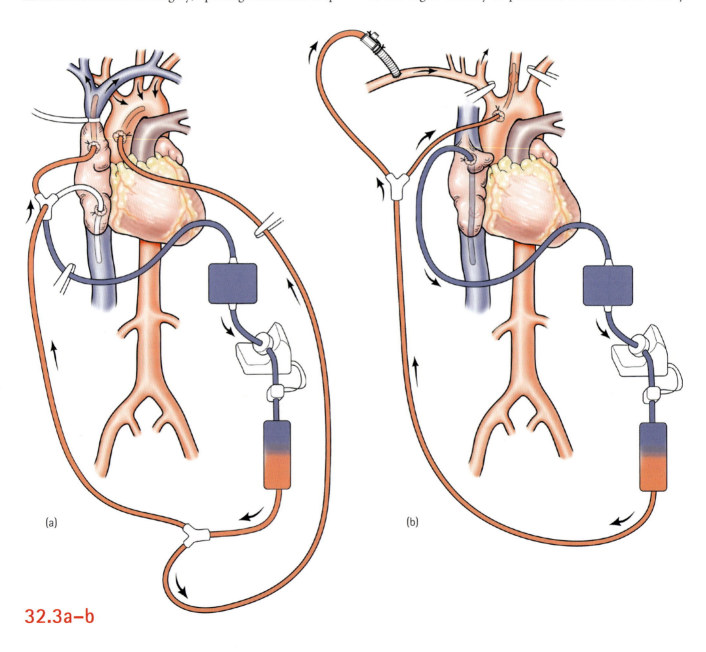

(a)

(b)

32.3a–b

atherosclerotic diseased, it has a low risk for retrograde aortic dissection, and it is easy to switch to unilateral ACP by clamping the innominate artery. Axillary cannulation can be performed by direct cannulation or with an end-to-side sewed 8 mm prosthesis (**Figure 32.4**). During unilateral ACP the left carotid artery (LCA) should also be clamped or occluded with a balloon-tipped catheter to avoid a steal phenomenon by excessive back-bleeding.

For longer HCA times, bilateral ACP can be easily established by inserting an additional cannula into the LCA connected via a Y adapter to the main pump-line. Generally, a flow rate of 10 cc / kg / min at 20 °C and a pressure of at least 40 mmHg in the radial artery is recommended.

Type I hybrid repair

Depending on the proximal landing zone, different surgical strategies are possible. Before the classic type I hybrid repair with landing zone 0 is described, variants with landing zone 2 and 1 are summarized, as these techniques are relevant for an endovascular zone 0 hybrid arch repair and used in different combinations for numerous variants.

LANDING ZONE 2

If coverage of the left subclavian artery (LSA) by TEVAR is necessary, recent Society for Vascular Surgery guidelines recommend prior subclavian revascularization. Sacrificing the LSA results in increased risk for paraplegia, arm and cerebral ischemia. Especially in patients with patent coronary, LIMA grafts, or dominant left vertebral artery, preoperative LSA revascularization is important.

By a supraclavicular incision, both the LSA and the LCA can be exposed. Revascularization of the LSA can be realized by a bypass or transposition to the LCA. The lateral insertion of the sternocleidomastoid muscle to the clavicle is mobilized for exposition of the LCA. If possible, the lymphatic duct should be identified and either preserved or ligated. By generous circumferential mobilization and lateral reflection of the jugular vein, the LCA and the vagus nerve can be exposed. The subclavian artery has to be mobilized extensively for transposition to avoid any tension on the anastomosis. After heparinization with 70 IU / kg, isolation and controlling the vertebral and internal thoracic artery with vessel loops, the subclavian artery can be clamped distally. Thereafter LSA can be ligated and transected proximal of the vertebral and thoracic artery. During clamping of

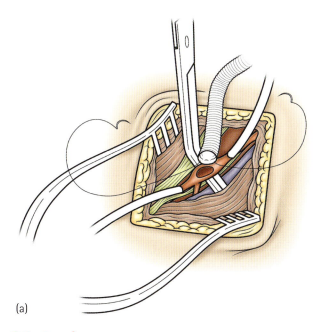

(a)

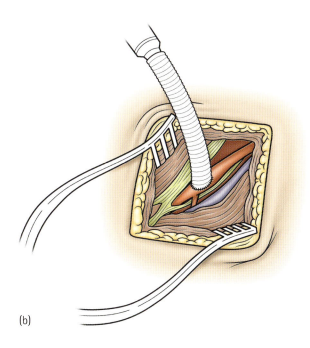

(b)

32.4a–b

the carotid artery, the vagus nerve has to be preserved. The mobilized LSA is sewn end-to-side to the carotid artery using a 5-0 Prolene running suture (**Figure 32.5**).

Alternatively, a short 8 mm Dacron graft can be used with the same exposition. This approach needs less extensive LSA dissection and mobilization, and might be necessary if the vertebral artery is very proximal or the thoracic artery used was previously used as a coronary bypass graft. The anastomosis to the subclavian anastomosis is usually performed more lateral behind the anterior scalene muscle and care has to be taken with the phrenic nerve (**Figure 32.6**). To avoid any type II endoleak the LSA has to be ligated or

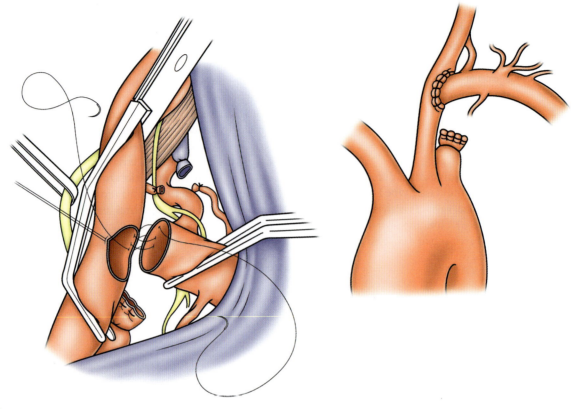

32.5

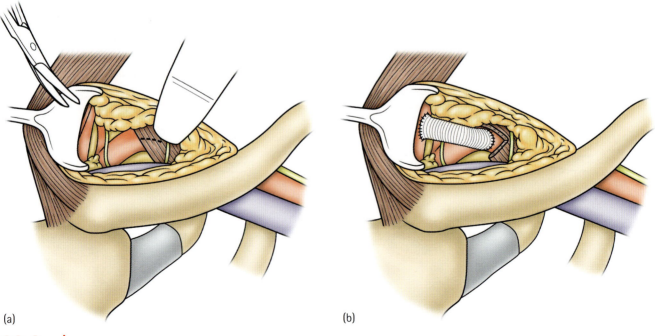

(a)

(b)

32.6a–b

clipped proximally of the vertebral and thoracic artery. If the origin of the LSA is very deep or the risk for aortic complications due to mobilization and manipulation is high, closure of the LSA can also be achieved endovascular using coils (**Figure 32.7**).

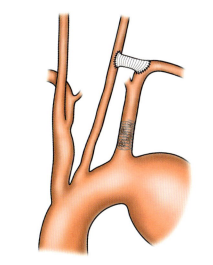

32.7

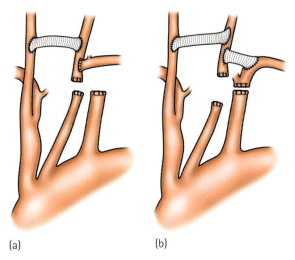

(a) (b)

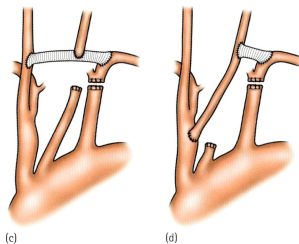

(c) (d)

32.8a–d

LANDING ZONE 1

For landing zone 1 the carotid artery has to be revascularized. Landing zone 1 is rarely used because the distance between the LCA and innominate artery is usually small and the additional landing zone compared to zone 2 therefore insufficient. Nevertheless, some of the various techniques will be described as they are valuable in combination with branched endoprothesis. Carotid to carotid bypass can be added after LSA transposition (**Figure 32.8a**) or bypass (**Figure 32.8b**), or with one cross-graft between right carotid artery and LSA with end-to-side LCA reimplantation (**Figure 32.8c**). The carotid–carotid bypass can be tunneled retropharyngeal.

The LCA can also be transpositioned to the innominate artery via mini-sternotomy, which is our preferred approach (**Figure 32.8d**). Adequate exposure is important for this procedure to allow tension-free anastomoses. Innominate and LCA should therefore be circumferentially mobilized cranial of the innominate vein to ensure tension-free anastomoses. After test-clamping of the LCA without significant drop in left NIRS, the LCA can be clamped proximal and distal, transected and proximal oversewn. A tangential clamp is placed on the innominate artery without restricting the cerebral perfusion, monitored by the right radial artery and NIRS. Hereupon the innominate artery can be opened longitudinally and the LCA anastomosed end-to-side using a 5-0 Prolene running suture. After careful flushing and de-airing maneuvers, full cerebral perfusion is restored.

LANDING ZONE 0

Branched endoprithesis

In combination with a Carotid-subclavian bypass and a LCA transposition a zone 0 repair can be achieved using a branched graft. For the US market, a novel trial device is currently available and favored in our practice (**Figure 32.9**). The basic principle of this device is a side branch delivered over a pre-cannulated side-branch-wire, after delivering the aortic component over the main wire.

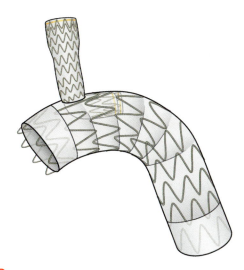

32.9

A long hydrophilic glide-wire is advanced into the descending aorta from the right radial or brachial artery over a 6F sheath. Percutaneous femoral artery access is a 20–26F Gore DrySeal sheath (**Figure 32.10a**). A contralateral 6F sheath is placed for diagnostic angiography. The glide-wire is snared in the descending aorta with a snare and carefully externalized for a through and through access (**Figure 32.10b**). The through and through glide-wire is exchanged with a guidewire and loaded to the side port of the TBE graft. The stiff guide wire in the ascending aorta is loaded to the central

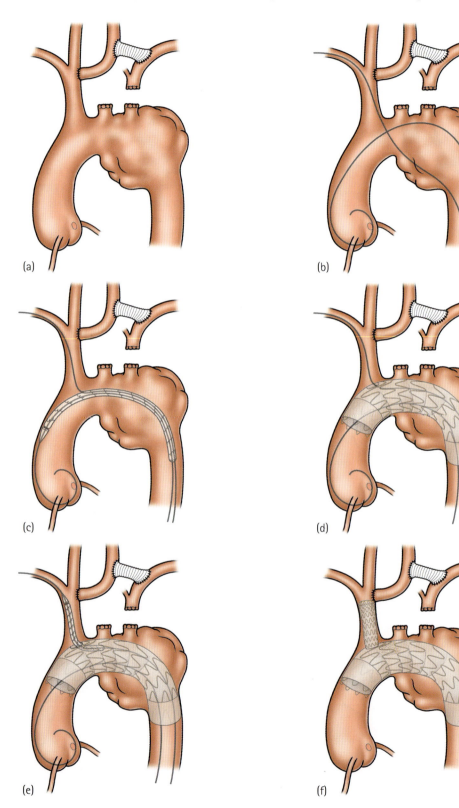

(a)

(b)

(c)

(d)

(e)

(f)

32.10a–f

port of the TBE graft. Avoiding any wire wrap by twisting the delivery catheter, the graft is advanced. Guided by the through and through wire the graft is positioned with the marked side-port facing the innominate artery at the outer curvature and deployed (**Figure 32.10c**). After deployment of the main body (**Figure 32.10d**) the delivery system is withdrawn and the side branch is introduced from the femoral over the through and through wire supported by a 14F sheath (**Figure 32.10e**). Advancing the delivery sheath through the portal can sometimes be difficult but reached by gentle push-push as well as push-pull maneuvers on the through and through wire. After careful branch positioning without compromising the origin if LCC off the innominate artery, the branch-graft can be deployed and carefully ballooned (**Figure 32.10f**). For perfect sealing of the main-body multilobed flow highly conformable balloon catheters can be used proximal and distal of the side-branch.

Intrathoracic arch debranching

The pericardium is opened after hemi- or total median sternotomy. After heparinization with 70 IU/kg and with strict pressure control, the ascending aorta can be tangentially clamped considering a proximal landing zone for TEVAR

>3 cm. The clamping site should be on the lateral site at 10 o'clock of the ascending aorta to avoid compression of the graft after chest closure (**Figure 32.11**).

If the ascending aorta is short or calcified, or the patient unstable, the use of CPB and cardiac arrest might be beneficial. Cannulation and clamping site can be the ascending aorta and right atrium in standard fashion, followed by cardioplegia, which enables a comfortable open proximal anastomosis (**Figure 32.12**).

After longitudinal opening of the ascending aorta the proximal end of a multibranched graft is sewed end-to-side on the ascending aorta with a running 4-0 Prolene suture. We prefer the use of a prefabricated prosthesis with four sides, whose fourth branch with a 45-degree angulation can be used for antegrade stent graft deployment (**Figure 32.13**). Subsequently the LSA is clamped, transected, the proximal stump oversewn and the LSA anastomosed with the third branch end-to-end. If the LSA cannot be exposed intrathoracic due to the large arch aneurysm or risk for rupture, the

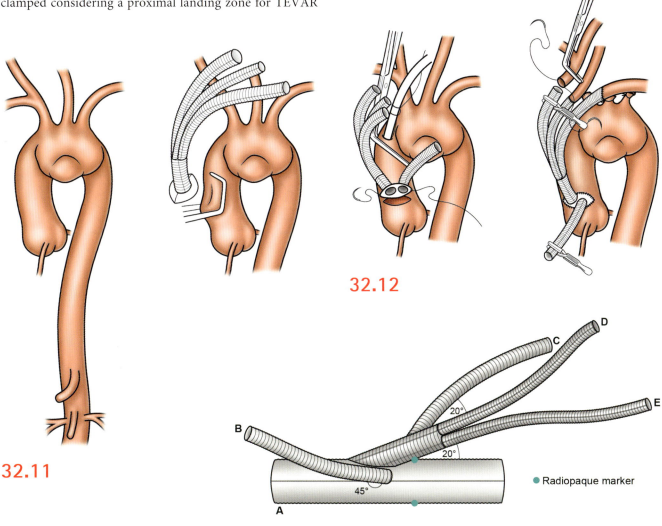

32.11

32.12

32.13

Radiopaque marker

LSA can also be revascularized extrathoracic by tunneling the third limb trough the second intercostal space. The LSA can be coiled proximally to avoid endoleaks. Usually problems with LSA exposure can be anticipated from CTA and carotid-subclavian bypass or subclavian transposition as described earlier can be performed 2–4 days earlier. With alert NIRS monitoring the LCA is clamped proximal and distal, transected and oversewn proximally. The second branch (the largest is for the innominate artery) is shortened appropriately, tunneled behind the innominate vein, and anastomosed end-to-end to the LCA with a 5-0 Prolene suture. After careful de-airing of the anastomosis LCA perfusion is restored. The innominate artery is debranched in the same way. If grafts without radiopaque markers and an extra limp are used, the proximal anastomosis should be marked with clips or pacing wires.

Antegrade stent graft deployment avoids further iliofemoral vascular complications and enables precision at the proximal landing zone. Over a sheath in the fourth branch, a pigtail-catheter is placed in the descending aorta and exchanged for a guidewire. In dissection, wire localization in the true lumen using angiography, TEE, or IVUS is essential. Thereafter the stent graft can be advanced and deployed straight behind the proximal anastomosis. Alternatively, the stent graft can be deployed retrograde with the guidewire in the left ventricle and rapid pacing to ensure precision during deployment. Either way, a control angiography should be performed to exclude endoleaks, which could be addressed by ballooning.

Type II hybrid repair

For type II hybrid repair the ascending aorta is replaced by a Dacron graft, but otherwise it is very similar to the type I hybrid repair and redundant steps are not repeated. Most type II hybrid repairs require an open distal anastomosis. Different cannulation and perfusion strategies have been discussed previously. Independently of the cannulation strategy, after dissection of the arch vessels and cannulation the distal ascending aorta is cross-clamped and the heart is arrested. The proximal ascending aorta is resected and any additional repair necessary on the root or aortic valve done during cooling. The main body of the branched graft has to be shortened appropriately before sewing it with a 4-0 Prolene suture to the ascending aorta right above the sinutubular junction, orienting the branches towards 10 o'clock. When reaching the target temperature, the patient is positioned in the Trendelenburg position and HCA is initiated by opening the aortic clamp and either snaring SVC and redirecting the flow into the venous cannula for RCP, or clamping the innominate artery and redirecting the flow into the right carotid artery for ACP. The length of the grafts main-body has to be adapted and sewed to the open arch with a 4-0 Prolene suture in a hemiarch fashion (**Figure 32.14a**). After careful de-airing of all branches in Trendelenburg position the fourth branch can be utilized as a cannulation site for whole body perfusion. During rewarming the arch anastomoses are performed in the same fashion as described for type I hybrid

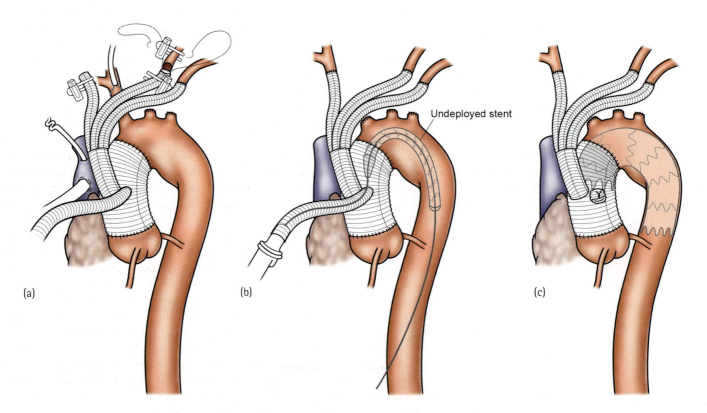

Undeployed stent

(a) (b) (c)

32.14a–c

repair. Alternatively, LSA and LCA can be anastomosed during HCA. The stent graft deployment is analogous to type I hybrid repair (**Figure 32.14b and c**).

Type III hybrid repair

Because the surgical techniques used for the type III hybrid repair include a broad spectrum including classic arch repair techniques described in other chapters, these techniques will be covered briefly only.

EXTENDED TYPE II REPAIR

After preparing a Dacron zone 0 according to hybrid type II repair, the entire distal aorta could be stented antegrade with multiple stent grafts down to the celiac artery. Nevertheless, a staged approach is preferred in order to reduce stress for the patient due to operation and ventilation time and contrast media exposition. Most important: a two-staged approach allows the spinal collateral network to adapt and reduces the risk of paraplegia. The second stage is minimally invasive and can be performed retrograde within weeks.

CLASSIC ELEPHANT TRUNK (ET)

For the classic elephant trunk, axillary cannulation and MHCA with ACP are described. The ascending aorta is clamped and the heart arrested. After proximal replacement of the ascending aorta with a straight Dacron prosthesis during cooling, HCA is initiated when reaching target temperature and unilateral ACP via the right carotid artery started by clamping the innominate artery. The aortic clamp is removed and the arch inspected. Bilateral ACP can be established with a second cannula in the LCA. The arch is opened and resected leaving a Carrel patch including innominate, LCA, and LSA. The aorta is resected to the level of the anticipated distal anastomosis, which is usually zone 3. After previous LSA revascularization, the distal can be performed comfortably and with reduced risk of recurrent nerve injury in zone 2.

The distal end of the prosthesis is marked circumferentially with pacing wires or clips for later radiographic use. The prosthesis is invaginated and plugged into the arch, the inner proximal and outer distal end of the prosthesis in the descending aorta and the double-layered edge proximally aligned to the open edge of the distal arch. This positioning of the graft allows a straightforward running suture with a 3-0 MH Prolene taking one layer aorta and two layers graft with every stitch. After finishing the distal anastomosis, the inner part of the prosthesis is pulled out.

Distal perfusion can now be achieved by cannulating the graft with a straight cannula close to the distal anastomosis at the inner curvature, secured by two pledgeted 3-0 Prolene U-stitches. The sidearm of branched prosthesis can be used alternatively, or a 24 F Foley catheter tied to a quarter-inch adapter can be used to establish early distal perfusion. After establishing distal perfusion, an appropriate orifice is burned into the arch prosthesis and the Carrel patch

anastomosed with 4-0 Prolene. After careful de-airing in the Trendelenburg position the innominate is unclamped and whole body perfusion established by clamping the graft close to the patch. Rewarming can be started. The proximal and distal grafts are anastomosed with appropriate shortening without kinking or tension.

FROZEN ELEPHANT TRUNK (FET)

Except for product specific details, the operative conduct of the classic and frozen elephant trunk procedure is identical. These are advanced into the open descending aorta over a previously ante- or retrograde placed guidewire. In both devices, the arch graft is already invaginated and a Dacron collar facilitates the distal anastomosis. Arch vessels are implanted into the Evita prosthesis as described for the elephant trunk, whereas the Thoraflex prosthesis has branches that are sewed to the arch vessels as described for the zone 2 repair.

POSTOPERATIVE CARE

Hemodynamic stability with high mean arterial pressures is important to ensure adequate organ perfusion after generalized ischemia reperfusion. Due to the coverage of segmental arteries the spinal perfusion is affected and has to be maintained via collaterals. Therefore, a high mean arterial pressure and continuous neurological assessment are important. If motoric or sensitive neurological deficits occur, blood pressure should even be increased urgently using vasopressors, and spinal drainage (10–12 mmHg) should be considered, if not already placed preoperatively. Frail and comorbid patients commonly get pneumonia after hybrid arch surgery. Early extubation and mobilization are crucial to avoid this life-threatening complication.

OUTCOME

Within the last years, technological innovations, growing experience, and spreading of the hybrid arch repair have led to very many heterogeneous publications. Most are retrospective single-center studies or registry studies, mixing a diversity of approaches.

Results published by our own group, comparing elective hybrid arch and conventional open arch surgery, demonstrated a stroke rate of 4% in the hybrid and 9% in the conventional group. In hospital, mortality was 11% in the hybrid and 16% in the conventional group. In patients older than 75 years it was 8% and 36%, respectively. This finding emphasizes the patient group that profits from hybrid arch surgery.[7]

The results of many excellent groups have been concluded in different meta-analyses: Antoniou et al. summarized 18 non-comparative studies with a total of 195 patients who had hybrid arch.[8] Overall they found 9% mortality, 7% stroke, and 9% endoleak. Morbidity, including cardiac and pulmonary complications, renal failure, infection, and dissection, was nevertheless 21%.

A large meta-analysis summarizing 46 studies with 2272 patients compared conventional and hybrid arch repair.[9] In hospital, mortality rates for conventional (9.5%) and hybrid arch repair (11.9%) were comparable; and also stroke rates (6.2% vs 7.6%) were similar. Nevertheless, in hybrid arch repair the new type A dissection rate was 4.5% and the endoleak rate was 16%, emphasizing the two major risks of type I hybrid repair that can be avoided by type II repair.

Another large meta-analysis, which included 53 studies and 1886 patients compared ET + TEVAR versus FET versus type I + II hybrid repair.[10] They found the lowest mortality rate (11.9% vs 9.8% vs 13.2%) and stroke rate (7.3 vs 6.2% vs 10.9%) in the FET group, and the lowest spinal cord ischemia incidence (4.3% vs 7.9% vs 7.2%) in the type I +II hybrid repair group. The subgroup analysis demonstrated a learning curve and better results in high volume centers. Due to the novelty of the hybrid approach, no solid long-term data are known yet. Despite high endoleak and re-intervention rates reported in some series, five-year survival rates of 72% are reported from a transcontinental registry.[11] Considering that patients treated with a hybrid approach were older and could not have withstood a conventional repair, these results are encouraging.

In conclusion, hybrid arch repair is a less invasive alternative to conventional surgical arch repair in old and multimorbid patients, and an advancement towards complete endovascular arch surgery. With further innovations in the future the armamentarium of the cardio-aortic surgeon will become even broader, increasing the variability of combinable surgical strategies toward a highly individual patient-tailored approach.

REFERENCES

1. Borst HG, Schaudig A, Rudolph W. Arteriovenous fistula of the aortic arch: repair during deep hypothermia and circulatory arrest. *J Thorac Cardiovasc Surg.* 1964; 48: 443.

2. Griepp RB, Stinson EB, Hollingsworth JF, Buehler D. Prosthetic replacement of the aortic arch. *J Thorac Cardiovasc Surg.* 1975; 70: 1051–63.

3. Svensson LG, Crawford ES, Hess KR, et al. Deep hypothermia with circulatory arrest: determinants of stroke and early mortality in 656 patients. *J Thorac Cardiovasc Surg.* 1993; 106: 19–28, discussion 28–31.

4. Ergin MA, Galla JD, Lansman SL, et al. Hypothermic circulatory arrest in operations on the thoracic arrest: determinants of operative mortality and neurologic outcome. *J Thorac Cardiovasc Surg.* 1994; 107: 788–97, discussion 797–9.

5. Jakob H, Tsagakis K, Leyh R, et al. Development of an integrated stent graft-dacron prosthesis for intended one-stage repair in complex thoracic aortic disease. *Herz.* 2005; 30: 766–8.

6. Criado FJ, Clark NS, Barnatan MF. Stent graft repair in the aortic arch and descending thoracic aorta: a 4-year experience. *YMVA.* 2002; 36: 1121–8.

7. Milewski RK, Szeto WY, Pochettino A, et al. Have hybrid procedures replaced open aortic arch reconstruction in high-risk patients? A comparative study of elective open arch debranching with endovascular stent graft placement and conventional elective open total and distal aortic arch reconstruction. *J Thorac Cardiovasc Surg.* 2010; 140: 590–7.

8. Antoniou GA, Mireskandari M, Bicknell CD, et al. Hybrid repair of the aortic arch in patients with extensive aortic disease. *Eur J Vasc Endovasc Surg.* 2010; 40: 715–21.

9. Moulakakis KG, Mylonas SN, Markatis F, et al. A systematic review and meta-analysis of hybrid aortic arch replacement. *Ann Cardiothorac Surg.* 2013; 2: 247–60.

10. Cao P, De Rango P, Czerny M, et al. Systematic review of clinical outcomes in hybrid procedures for aortic arch dissections and other arch diseases. *J Thorac Cardiovasc Surg.* 2012; 144: 1286–300, 1300.e1–2.

11. Czerny M, Weigang E, Sodeck G, et al. Targeting landing zone 0 by total arch rerouting and TEVAR: midterm results of a transcontinental registry. *Ann Thorac Surg.* 2012; 94: 84–9.

FURTHER READING

Bavaria J, Milewski RK, Baker J, et al. Classic hybrid evolving approach to distal arch aneurysms: toward the zone zero solution. *J Thorac Cardiovasc Surg.* 2010; 140: S77–80, discussion S86–91.

Bavaria J, Vallabhajosyula P, Moeller P, et al. Hybrid approaches in the treatment of aortic arch aneurysms: postoperative and midterm outcomes. *J Thorac Cardiovasc Surg.* 2013; 145: S85–S90.

Czerny M, Schmidli J, Carrel T, Grimm M. Hybrid aortic arch repair. *Ann Cardiothorac Surg.* 2013; 2: 372–7.

Szeto WY, Bavaria JE. Hybrid repair of aortic arch aneurysms: combined open arch reconstruction and endovascular repair. *Semin Thorac Cardiovasc Surg.* 2009; 21: 347–54.

Vallabhajosyula P, Szeto WY, Desai N, et al. Type II arch hybrid debranching procedure. *Ann Cardiothorac Surg.* 2013; 2: 378–86.

33

Thoracoabdominal aortic aneurysms

SHINICHI FUKUHARA AND NIMESH D. DESAI

INTRODUCTION

Thoracoabdominal aortic aneurysms (TAAAs) by definition traverse the diaphragm and involve portions of both the thoracic and the abdominal aorta. Therefore, thoracic aortic control is required for repair. These aneurysms can extend proximally to the transverse aortic arch and distally to the abdominal aortic bifurcation.

The Crawford classification of TAAAs (**Figure 33.1**) is based on the extent of aortic involvement. Accurate classification of TAAAs is important because the operative strategy, risks, and results vary based upon the extent of aortic replacement. Extent V, which was introduced in the last two decades, is from T6 to just above the renal arteries. Despite recent refinements and advances in endovascular approaches to aortic aneurysms, open repair remains the procedure of choice for successful management of these extensive TAAAs. While improvement in anesthesia, surgical technique, and critical care has allowed these operations to be performed successfully, they remain a formidable technical challenge. A variety of pathologies, extensive aortic involvement, and frequent medical comorbidities in these patients have contributed to this challenge. As this disease entity becomes more common in the ageing population, the need for therapeutic intervention will continue to increase.

HISTORY

TAAA repair was first performed in the 1950s. One of the first successful repairs was reported in 1955 by Etheredge[1]. A large aneurysm of the upper abdominal aorta involving the celiac and superior mesenteric arteries was replaced utilizing an aortic homograft and temporary aortic bypass with a 5 mm polyethylene tube. That same year, Rob also reported on his experience of six TAAA repairs that required lower thoracic aortic clamping via a thoracoabdominal incision.[2] These initial reports involved aneurysmectomy, which prolonged operative times and led to significant morbidity, and Crawford revolutionized TAAA repair by introducing the graft inclusion technique.[3] Along with the utilization of

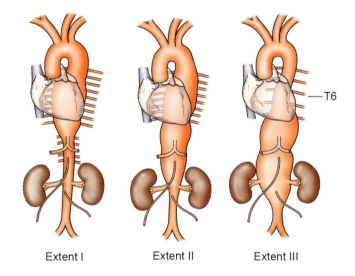

Extent I   Extent II   Extent III

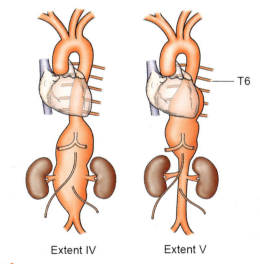

Extent IV   Extent V

33.1

cardiopulmonary bypass, hypothermic circulatory arrest, and cerebrospinal fluid (CSF) drainage, Crawford's approach most resembles contemporary techniques performed at major centers today.

PRINCIPLES AND JUSTIFICATION

The two most common disease processes that affect the thoracoabdominal aorta are medial degeneration and aortic dissection. Each of these mechanisms produces weakness and dilatation of the aortic wall, ultimately resulting in rupture. While both processes may exist separately, they serve as risk factors for one another, and thus often coexist. Dissection of the thoracoabdominal aorta can occur with/without involvement of the ascending and transverse arch aorta, with up to 40% of patients with chronic dissection eventually requiring repair.[4]

PREOPERATIVE ASSESSMENT AND PREPARATION

Presentation

Patients with TAAAs often remain asymptomatic until the aneurysm becomes large enough to compress surrounding structures or weak enough to dissect or rupture. Therefore, TAAAs are commonly found incidentally during imaging studies obtained for unrelated medical problems. Additionally, the onset of symptoms is generally considered an indication of imminent rupture. Unfortunately, very few patients present with symptoms prior to an acute aortic event, with up to 95% of the events occurring in the absence of any heralding symptoms.[5] The most common symptom is pain located in the chest, abdomen, or back, due to pressure from the aneurysm on adjacent structures, or the initiation of dissection or rupture. Wheezing, coughing, and pneumonitis may result from compression of the trachea or a segmental bronchus. Erosion of the aneurysm into the airway or pulmonary parenchyma may lead to hemoptysis, while similar compression or erosion of the esophagus may lead to dysphagia or hematemesis. Impingement of the left recurrent laryngeal nerve causes vocal cord paralysis and hoarseness.

Diagnosis

The diagnosis of thoracoabdominal aortic pathology is heavily dependent upon radiographic imaging.

Today, computed tomographic angiography (CTA) of the aorta with 3D reconstruction has become the gold standard for preoperative imaging, while contrast aortography is rarely required. CTA is critical to determining appropriate repair strategies, especially when considering endovascular/hybrid repairs. The ability to manipulate the 3D image while simultaneously viewing the axial slice is a helpful tool to assess aneurysmal anatomy. **Figure 33.2** depicts a 3D reconstructed CTA image with perpendicular axial slice designation of a TAAA with chronic dissection.

Indications for repair

Indications for surgical repair are primarily based upon the presence of symptoms and the size of the aneurysm. The development of any symptom is carefully evaluated and attributed to the aneurysm until proven otherwise. Signs of impending rupture, such as acute pain or hypotension, are clear indications for immediate surgical repair. For asymptomatic

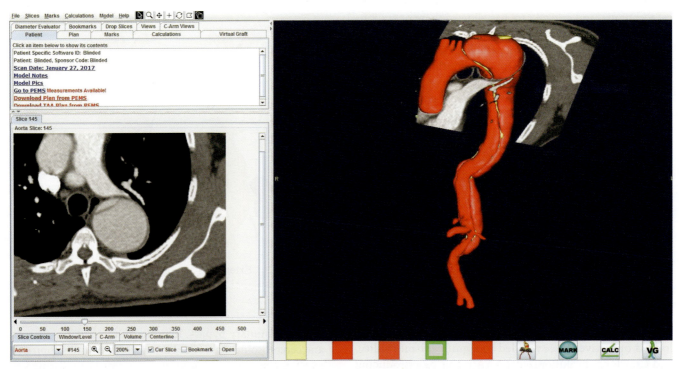

33.2

patients, elective repair is recommended when the aneurysm diameter exceeds 6.0 cm or when the rate of expansion exceeds 1 cm per year unless medical comorbidities prohibit this. Smaller than 60 mm size criteria can be applied to patients with connective tissue disorders such as Marfan and Loeys–Dietz syndromes. Absolute size criteria must be adjusted in patients of extreme size, and interventions are considered based on an aortic size index, which takes into account both aneurysm size and the patient's body surface area.

Preoperative evaluation

Regardless of the extent of repair, an extensive preoperative workup is the key to successful repair. Aside from stratifying routine cardiovascular risk factors, careful attention must be paid to pulmonary and renal function to ascertain the patient's potential operative risk and to determine their surgical candidacy.

Preoperative transthoracic echocardiography is a satisfactory non-invasive screening method that evaluates both valvular and biventricular function. Additional testing is obtained in patients with a left ventricular ejection fraction of less than 30% or other evidence of myocardial ischemia. Patients with significant coronary artery disease should undergo an appropriate coronary revascularization procedure prior to TAAA repair. Computed tomographic coronary angiography has recently emerged as a less invasive method to visualize the coronary arterial anatomy and has been utilized as a coronary screening in many centers. Importantly, patients with previous coronary artery bypass grafting using the left internal mammary artery may require left carotid-subclavian bypass before extent I or II TAAA repair to avoid cardiac ischemia if the aortic clamp is placed proximal to the left subclavian artery.

The most frequent cause of postoperative complications in patients undergoing TAAA repair is respiratory failure. Evaluation of pulmonary function with arterial blood gas and spirometry must be carefully evaluated because most repairs require single lung ventilation. Patients with a diminished forced expiratory volume-one second (FEV1) or a blood carbon dioxide partial pressure greater than 45 mmHg should undergo preoperative optimization of respiratory function including smoking cessation, an exercise regimen and bronchodilators. Patients with poor diffusing capacity or severe chronic obstructive pulmonary disease (COPD) may require the use of cardiopulmonary bypass for TAAA repair because they may not tolerate one-lung ventilation. Additionally, preoperative evaluation of right recurrent laryngeal nerve is important because it is not uncommon for the left recurrent laryngeal nerve to be damaged during extent I/II TAAA repair, which could lead to respiratory compromise upon extubation.

Assessment of preoperative renal function is important because preoperative renal insufficiency is strongly associated with early postoperative mortality. The National Kidney Foundation currently recommends the use of estimated glomerular filtration rate (GFR) to assess renal function in order to avoid the misclassification of patients on the basis of serum creatinine levels alone. Renal artery anatomy is determined from imaging studies. Occlusive disease of the renal arteries should be treated prior to, or during, TAAA repair.

ANESTHESIA

After induction of anesthesia and insertion of a double-lumen endotracheal tube, central venous access is obtained and a pulmonary artery catheter is inserted for hemodynamic monitoring. A Foley catheter is placed, and arterial lines are inserted in both the upper and lower extremities to monitor both proximal and distal perfusion during aortic clamping in cases where cardiopulmonary/left heart bypass is used. Arterial blood gas and serum electrolyte measurements are monitored closely and appropriate adjustments are made as needed. CSF drains are used routinely, maintaining the intrathecal pressure at 10 mmHg or less. Cranial and peripheral electrodes are placed for monitoring of somatosensory or motor evoked potentials to assess intraoperative spinal cord protection and perfusion. In the case of motor evoked potentials, special anesthetic considerations are required because the use of neuromuscular blocking agents can confound monitoring. Preoperative antibiotics are given prior to incision and a gram of Solu-Medrol and 12.5 grams of mannitol are given prior to the onset of left heart/cardiopulmonary bypass. Acidosis during aortic clamping is prevented with a continuous intravenous sodium bicarbonate infusion. The use of routine autotransfusion of washed red cells has led to a significant reduction in banked blood transfusion requirements. As some large aneurysms may contain up to 2000 mL of blood within them, autotransfusion during surgical repair is of paramount importance.

SPINAL CORD PROTECTION

Spinal cord protection during TAAA repair continues to be a major focus of investigation despite the refinements in operative technique. Risk factors for spinal cord ischemia are aneurysm extent, open repair, prior proximal/distal aortic operations, and perioperative hypotension. Early detection of spinal cord ischemia by intraoperative neurophysiologic monitoring and postoperative neurological examination is crucial to enable immediate treatment to prevent permanent paraplegia.

Vigilant attention to volume status is imperative during TAAA repair to avoid wide fluctuations in blood pressure. Crystalloid administration begins prior to the operation. Central venous and pulmonary arterial pressures are maintained at normal or pre-anesthetic levels. Maintaining spinal cord perfusion by augmenting arterial blood pressure and augmenting cardiac output, together with preventing hypotension, reducing CSF pressure, and reducing central venous pressure is the cornerstone for the prevention and treatment of spinal cord ischemia. Our approach to spinal cord protection is based on the extent of the aneurysm being repaired. In most TAAA repairs, mild permissive hypothermia (32–34°C) is employed by allowing the bladder temperature to decrease gradually from exposure after the induction of general anesthesia. In addition to routine use of CSF drainage and left heart bypass, sequential aortic clamping and aggressive reattachment of patent segmental intercostal and lumbar arteries when possible, particularly those between T8 and L1, are advocated. As for blood pressure maintenance, mean proximal pressure should be maintained around 80–100 mmHg and pressure distal to the clamp to be 60–80 mmHg. If proximal pressures are too high and distal pressures are too low, the arterial flow of the left heart bypass is increased. If both proximal and distal pressures are too high, volume is taken off to maintain optimal pressure. If both proximal and distal pressures are too low, volume is to be given. If proximal pressures are too low and distal pressures are too high, the flow is to be decreased. Rewarming after reperfusion can be accomplished with warmed saline and forced air warming blanket.

OPERATION

Operative strategies and techniques vary considerably depending upon the extent and characteristics of the aneurysm.

Preparation and exposure

Using a deflatable beanbag, the patient is positioned in a right lateral decubitus with the shoulders at 60 degrees and the hips at 30 degrees (**Figure 33.3**). The left arm is placed on an armrest. Pressure points are padded with foam. A shoulder roll is placed under the chest so that the right shoulder is free from pressure. The operating table is hyperextended to open the space between iliac crest and costal margin. Draping allows access to the entire left chest, abdomen, and both groins.

The level of the incision is based upon the proximal extent of the aneurysm in the thoracic aorta (**Figure 33.4**). In general, two surgeons are able to begin the thoracoabdominal exposure concurrently. A curvilinear thoracoabdominal incision is made from just posterior to the inferior aspect of the left scapula, curving along the 7th rib and across the costal margin toward a point about 3–4 cm to the left of the umbilicus. When a repair involves the iliac arteries, the incision may be extended inferiorly around the umbilicus and into the midline to just above the pubic symphysis. Aneurysms beginning near the diaphragm (extent IV) are exposed through the eighth interspace, while those extending more proximally (extents I, II, III and V) are usually approached through the sixth interspace. Proximal exposure may require division or resection of the sixth rib. The fifth space may be appropriate when improved exposure of the distal arch and left subclavian is required. Prior to entering the chest, the

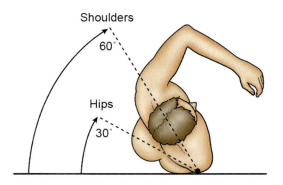

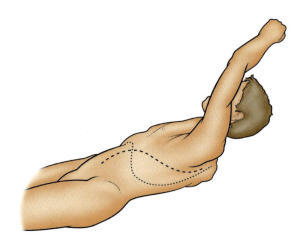

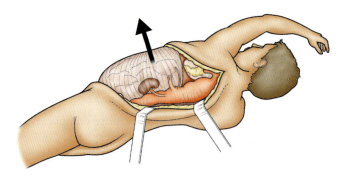

33.3

left lung is deflated and single lung ventilation is initiated.

Care must be taken not to injure the left phrenic nerve when the costal margin and diaphragm are divided. The retroperitoneal plane is accessed by splitting the transversalis muscle fibers, which are oriented transversely across the top of the peritoneal sac. The peritoneal sac and its contents are then bluntly dissected and moved medially from the left retroperitoneal space, developing the avascular plane anterior to the psoas muscle and posterior to the left kidney. The diaphragm is divided in a circumferential fashion to protect the phrenic nerve. A 2–3 cm cuff of diaphragmatic tissue is left on the chest wall, preserving the bulk of central musculature and allowing secure closure upon completion of the procedure (**Figure 33.5**). The diaphragmatic crus is divided. The left renal artery is identified and exposed. The superior

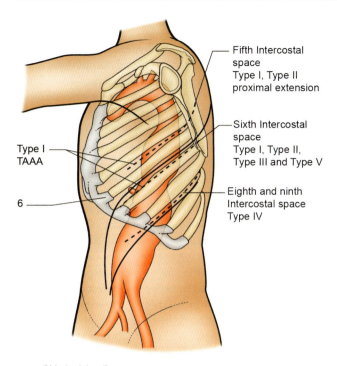

Fifth Intercostal
space
Type I, Type II
proximal extension

Sixth Intercostal
space
Type I, Type II,
Type III and Type V

Eighth and ninth
Intercostal space
Type IV

Type I
TAAA

6

—— Skin incision line

--- Interspace

33.4

mesenteric, celiac, and right renal arteries are not usually identified externally. The lumbar vein, which rises from the psoas groove to enter the renal vein, taking a course around the left side of the aorta, is often encountered nearby the left renal artery origin. At this point, self-retaining retractors are set up to provide and maintain stable exposure.

In preparation for placement of the proximal aortic clamp, the distal aortic arch is gently mobilized by dividing the remnant of the ductus arteriosus. Circumferential dissection of the distal transverse aortic arch allows its separation from the adjacent esophagus and pulmonary artery. The left vagus and recurrent laryngeal nerves are identified and protected. The vagus nerve may be divided distal to the takeoff of the recurrent laryngeal nerve if additional mobilization is required. The left subclavian artery is also mobilized circumferentially if proximal clamping between the left common carotid and left subclavian arteries is needed. The left superior intercostal vein may be ligated for exposure of the distal aortic arch (**Figure 33.6**). The distal clamp site for proximal anastomosis is also prepared at the level of the left pulmonary hilum. It is important to stay anterior to the hemiazygos vein and intercostal veins. Intercostal arteries around clamp sites are clipped or ligated. The adjacent esophagus is identified and dissected away from the aortic clamp site. Heparin is administered intravenously for left heart/cardiopulmonary bypass once the exposure is complete.

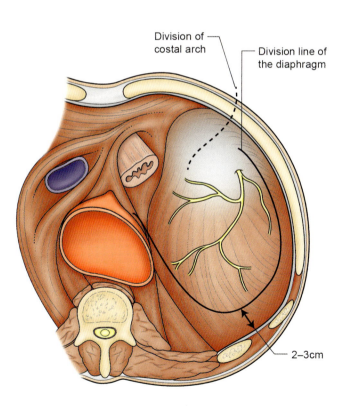

Division of
costal arch

Division line of
the diaphragm

2–3cm

33.5

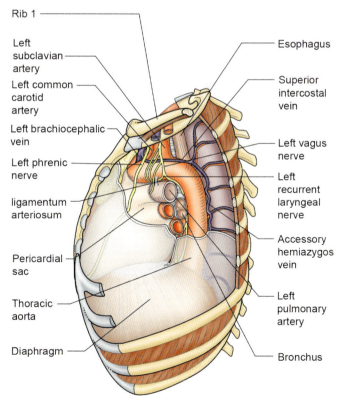

Rib 1

Left
subclavian
artery

Left common
carotid
artery

Left brachiocephalic
vein

Left phrenic
nerve

ligamentum
arteriosum

Pericardial
sac

Thoracic
aorta

Diaphragm

Esophagus

Superior
intercostal
vein

Left vagus
nerve

Left
recurrent
laryngeal
nerve

Accessory
hemiazygos
vein

Left
pulmonary
artery

Bronchus

33.6

Left heart bypass and preparation of the proximal aorta

Regarding circulatory support during TAAA repair, a variety of strategies have been described. However, it is fundamentally determined by the extent of repair. Most groups utilize left heart bypass at a minimum, and it is generally accepted that decompression of the proximal circulation in conjunction with distal perfusion of the abdominal viscera, spinal cord, and lower extremities ameliorates complications associated with ischemia. Our preferred method is left heart bypass with a closed circuit in-line centrifugal pump that comprises left atrial drainage via the left inferior pulmonary vein and arterial inflow by cannulation of the iliac system or distal abdominal aorta depending on the extent of repair (**Figure 33.7**). This configuration provides adequate retrograde flow to the visceral segment and the spinal cord via the internal iliac system and antegrade flow to the bilateral lower extremities. In patients with inadequate pulmonary reserve who may not tolerate single lung ventilation, partial cardiopulmonary bypass may be chosen, electing to cannulate the left femoral vein with an extended venous cannula that is advanced to the level of the right atrium and arterial inflow as described above. Selective visceral/renal perfusion is also routinely performed. This is accomplished by utilizing balloon-tipped catheters and a separate arterial inflow circuit from the bypass pump to perfuse the visceral/renal arteries with oxygenated blood.

In cases where proximal aortic clamping is not possible or extensive reconstruction of the aortic arch is inevitable, we utilize deep systemic hypothermia (18°C to 22°C) with temporary circulatory arrest with total body retrograde perfusion. Cardiopulmonary bypass is typically accomplished by cannulation of the right atrium via the femoral vein and direct cannulation of the aorta or femoral artery. Optimal hypothermic conditions for deep hypothermic circulatory arrest include electrocortical silence by electroencephalography, or at least 45 minutes of cooling on cardiopulmonary bypass. A left ventricular vent via the left upper pulmonary vein is placed using a standard left ventricular vent cannula, particularly in patients with aortic insufficiency.

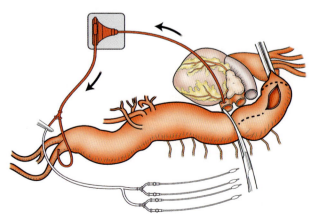

33.7

Sequential clamping strategy

Following institution of left heart bypass, the proximal portion of the aneurysm is isolated by placing clamps distal to the left subclavian artery and across the upper/mid-descending thoracic aorta (**Figure 33.7**). If the aneurysm extends more proximally, the aorta is clamped between the left common carotid and left subclavian arteries and a separate clamp is placed on the left subclavian artery. Left heart bypass flow is increased toward a target between 1.5 and 2.5 L/min to keep the patient's blood pressure appropriate as described above.

The aorta is transected at least 2 cm distal to the proximal clamp and separated from the esophagus to allow for full-thickness suturing of the aortic wall. This maneuver minimizes the risk of esophageal injury. In cases of aortic dissection, the dissecting membrane is usually excised. Intimal calcifications at the site of the anastomosis should be appropriately debrided in order to create a pliable aortic wall. Back-bleeding from intercostal arteries are ligated using 2-0 silk in a figure-eight fashion. A properly sized gelatin-impregnated woven Dacron graft is selected. We routinely use a commercially available prefabricated aortic graft with four side branches designed for reattaching the celiac, superior mesenteric, and both renal arteries. It is important to set up the proper orientation, as the graft will shift when the viscera are rotated back to the anatomic position. The proximal anastomosis is carried out using running 3-0 polypropylene suture. Alternatively, in patients with fragile aortic tissue, such as those with Marfan syndrome, 4-0 polypropylene suture is utilized. Teflon strips may be used to reinforce the anastomosis but are generally not necessary. In cases of aortic dissection, the false lumen is obliterated within the suture line. Similar principles are employed for the remaining anastomoses. Once the proximal anastomosis is complete, the proximal aortic cross-clamp is removed and the hemostasis is meticulously checked with reinforced with pledgeted mattress sutures as needed.

Distal anastomosis and viscera/renal vessel attachment

Before starting left heart bypass, selective visceral perfusion catheters are prepared for use. The size of the catheters varies in each vessel in each individual (6Fr–13Fr). These are attached to a line off of the arterial return tubing allowing continued delivery of oxygenated blood from the pump circuit to the abdominal viscera, usually at a flow rate of 200–400 mL/min when all four vessels are perfused. The flow rate is reduced as each vessel anastomosis is complete. Ideally, these selective cannulae are kept in place during anastomosis until reattachment is nearly complete. Prior to opening the remaining aorta, the aortic graft is placed under appropriate tension and trimmed to the appropriate length. One or more oval openings are made on the graft for reattachment of selected patent intercostal arteries from T8 to L1. Alternatively, a U-shaped 8 mm graft may be sewn proximally and distally to the main aortic graft and sewn side-to-side to the intercostals. The abdominal segment is clamped 2–3 cm below the proposed distal anastomotic site.

The remaining aorta is opened longitudinally down to the aortic bifurcation; care is taken to cut posterior to the origin of the left renal artery. The aortic edges are retracted laterally with stay sutures as needed. The origins of the visceral and renal arteries are identified and endarterectomized if necessary. Each visceral vessel and renal arteries are cannulated with an appropriate size cannula. Brisk intercostal/lumber artery back-bleeding is controlled with 2-0 silk figure-eight sutures in order to minimize blood loss, improve visualization, and prevent shunting of blood away from the spinal circulation. Large segmental arteries with little or no back-bleeding may be particularly important for spinal cord perfusion and reimplantation is strongly considered. After the patch reimplantation of the intercostal arteries is completed, the proximal aortic cross-clamp is moved down the aortic graft to a position immediately distal to the intercostal patch. This allows for reperfusion of the reimplanted intercostal arteries as part of the spinal protection strategy known as sequential cross-clamping (**Figure 33.8**).

The distal anastomosis is performed in an end-to-end configuration with a continuous 3-0 or 4-0 polypropylene suture depending on the aortic disease and reinforced with pledgeted 4-0 polypropylene sutures as needed. The aortic graft and its four branches are filled with blood from the distal anastomosis. Vascular clamps are placed across each branch of the graft and the aortic cross-clamp on the main body of the graft is slowly removed to re-establish pulsatile

blood flow to the pelvis and both lower extremities. At this point the patient is weaned from left heart bypass and the pump is used for selective visceral perfusion and return of suctioned blood from the operative field.

The sequence of visceral/renal vessel anastomosis varies depending on the anatomy. We usually perform celiac artery anastomosis first followed by superior mesenteric artery. While the celiac artery perfusion catheter is in place, the superior 10 mm branch, which is located anteriorly, is trimmed to the appropriate length and anastomosed in an end-to-end configuration with a continuous 5-0 polypropylene suture. The perfusion catheter is removed prior to completion of anastomosis. After the graft is de-aired, the anastomosis is finished and the graft clamp removed. The superior mesenteric artery is anastomosed to the other 10 mm branch in the same fashion. As for renal arteries, the right renal artery anastomosis is usually done first because of its medial location. The right-sided 8 mm side branch is trimmed to the appropriate length and anastomosed in the same fashion with a continuous 5-0 polypropylene suture. Often, the origin of the left renal artery is separated from the aortic wall as a button, and its proximal portion is mobilized. The remaining 8 mm side-branch graft is trimmed to the appropriate length and anastomosed to the left renal artery. Care is taken to ensure that the artery and the branch graft are not kinked when the peritoneal sac is returned to its anatomic position (**Figure 33.9**). Alternatively, a visceral patch including the celiac, superior mesenteric, and right renal arteries is fashioned and sewn to the graft in the same fashion; however, this should be avoided in patients with connective tissue disorders due to the possibility of developing visceral patch aneurysmal dilatation. The left renal artery mostly requires a separate branch graft anastomosis as well.

Following aortic reconstruction, heparin is reversed with protamine sulfate. Meticulous hemostasis must be achieved and secured at all suture lines and cannulation sites. The native aortic wall edge is cauterized as needed. Visceral, renal, and peripheral perfusion are thoroughly assessed. The remaining aneurysm wall is then wrapped around the

Superior mesenteric artery

Celiac artery

Left renal artery

Right renal artery

33.8

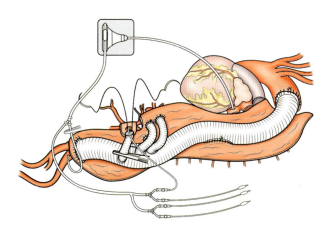

33.9

aortic graft and secured with a running suture. Two thoracic drainage tubes are positioned in the posterior pleural cavity. The diaphragm is re-approximated with a running #1 polypropylene suture. The thoracotomy is closed using heavy braided polyester suture. Stainless steel wires or rib plating system may be used around the costal margin if necessary.

POSTOPERATIVE CARE

Meticulous control of blood pressure is imperative during the initial 48 hours postoperatively, as even brief periods of hypertension may disrupt fresh suture lines, while maintaining adequate spinal cord and visceral perfusion. The mean arterial pressure during the early postoperative period is maintained between 80 and 100 mmHg. A lower blood pressure target may be selected in patients with particularly fragile tissue such as Marfan syndrome and acute aortic dissection. During augmentation of the arterial pressure, it is also important to assure that cardiac output is satisfactory and that the patient is not anemic in an effort to optimize oxygen delivery. The CSF drain is drained as needed to maintain CSF pressure between 10–12 mmHg. The CSF drain is usually removed in 48 hours if the patient is neurologically intact. In most cases, the ventilator is weaned and the patient is able to be extubated within 24 hours. Thoracic drainage tubes are removed once drainage is less 300 mL/day, commonly within 48–72 hours. Ambulation is initiated on the second or third postoperative day after CSF drain removal and aggressive physical rehabilitation is emphasized early in the postoperative course.

OUTCOMES

At experienced surgical centers, morbidity and mortality rates have greatly improved during the past 40 years, even in patients with extensive repairs or chronic aortic dissection. **Table 33.1** summarizes the contemporary outcomes from the largest series between 1986 and 2014,[6] excluding non-elective repair cases. Approximately two-thirds of repairs were performed to treat degenerative aneurysms without dissection (64.2%); the other one-third were performed to treat aortic dissection (35.8%).

REFERENCES

1. Etheredge SN, Yee J, Smith JV, et al. Successful resection of a large aneurysm of the upper abdominal aorta and replacement with homograft. *Surgery*. 1955; 38: 1071–81.
2. Rob C. The surgery of the abdominal aorta and its major branches. *Ann R Coll Surgeons Engl*. 1955; 17: 307–17.
3. Crawford ES. Thoraco-abdominal and abdominal aortic aneurysms involving renal, superior mesenteric, celiac arteries. *Ann Surg*. 1974; 179: 763–72.
4. Escobar GA, Upchurch GR Jr. Management of thoracoabdominal aortic aneurysms. *Curr Probl Surg*. 2011; 48: 70–133.
5. Elefteriades JA, Farkas EA. Thoracic aortic aneurysm clinically pertinent controversies and uncertainties. *J Am Coll Cardiol*. 2010; 55: 841–57.
6. Coselli JS, LeMaire SA, Preventza O, et al. Outcomes of 3309 thoracoabdominal aortic aneurysm repairs. *J Thorac Cardiovasc Surg*. 2016; 151(5): 1323–37.

FURTHER READING

Coselli JS, LeMaire SA, Köksoy C, et al. Cerebrospinal fluid drainage reduces paraplegia after thoracoabdominal aortic aneurysm repair: results of a randomized clinical trial. *J Vasc Surg*. 2002; 35: 631–9.

Estrera AL, Sandhu HK, Charlton-Ouw KM, et al. A quarter century of organ protection in open thoracoabdominal repair. *Ann Surg*. 2015; 262: 660–8.

Girardi LN, Lau C, Munjal M, et al. Impact of preoperative pulmonary function on outcomes after open repair of descending and thoracoabdominal aortic aneurysms. *J Thorac Cardiovasc Surg*. 2017; 153: S22–9.

Table 33.1 Results of thoracoabdominal aortic aneurysm repair in 2586 patients in the elective setting.[6]

	Extent I N = 700	Extent II N = 866	Extent III N = 504	Extent IV N = 516
Operative mortality	32 (4.6%)	72 (8.3%)	41 (8.1%)	16 (3.1%)
Paraplegia	8 (1.1%)	37 (4.3%)	18 (3.6%)	3 (0.6%)
Paraparesis	14 (2.0%)	25 (2.9%)	10 (2.0%)	8 (1.6%)
Stroke	17 (2.4%)	31 (3.6%)	5 (1.0%)	7 (1.4%)

34

Thoracic endovascular aortic repair

GEORGE J. ARNAOUTAKIS AND WILSON Y. SZETO

HISTORY

Open surgical repair of thoracic aortic aneurysms (TAA) was first performed in the 1950s. There have been significant advances in surgical techniques, anesthetic regimens, and perioperative care; however, the morbidity and mortality of these open procedures remains significant. In addition, the patient population presenting with thoracic aortic disease has become increasingly older and harbors more concomitant comorbidities. Thoracic endovascular aortic repair (TEVAR) emerged as a complementary treatment paradigm to minimize the morbidity and mortality associated with open repair for aneurysms of the thoracic aorta. Several non-randomized studies have documented improved mortality and morbidity (shorter length of stay, improved paraplegia rates, less bleeding complications) for the TEVAR approach. The US Food and Drug Administration (FDA) granted initial endograft approval for treatment of TAA in 2005, and presently four companies manufacture FDA-approved devices. Since then, indications for use have expanded with broader FDA approval for all lesions of the descending thoracic aorta. Furthermore, the myriad advancements in endovascular technology continue to expand the pool of patients who may be amenable to undergoing TEVAR for increasingly complex thoracic aortic pathology, especially involving the aortic arch.

PRINCIPLES AND JUSTIFICATION

Degenerative aneurysm, characterized by abnormal aortic dilation and medial degeneration of the aortic wall, is the most common disease process to require TEVAR. Symptomatic TAA are typically considered for urgent surgical repair. In asymptomatic TAA, surgical intervention is typically recommended at aortic diameter of 5.5–6 cm,

because the annual risk of rupture, dissection, or death exceeds 15% for aneurysms greater than 6 cm in maximal diameter. Patients with saccular aneurysms, rapid aneurysm growth rate, a connective tissue disorder, or family history of aortic-related complications should be considered for earlier intervention. The ultimate decision to operate on TAA must respect the surgical principle that peri-procedural risk should not exceed the risk of rupture.

In September 2013, the W.L. Gore & Associates (Flagstaff, AZ, USA) C-TAG device was granted FDA approval for all lesions of the descending thoracic aorta, followed in January 2014 by Medtronic, Inc. (Minneapolis, MN, USA) Valiant device receiving the same approval. This broad approval was granted with the provision that the efficacy of TEVAR be more completely analyzed, and has expanded indications for treatment to both acute and chronic Type B dissection, traumatic transections, penetrating ulcer, and intramural hematoma. Studies are ongoing to more fully elucidate those patients with Type B dissection who stand to benefit most from TEVAR therapy.

Surgical anatomy

The descending thoracic aorta begins just distal to the left subclavian artery, and is direct extension from the distal aortic arch. At the twelfth vertebral level, the descending aorta traverses the aortic hiatus in the diaphragm to become the abdominal aorta. There are branches emanating from the anterior surface of the thoracic aorta that consist of bronchial and esophageal branches. The intercostal segmental arteries originate from the posterior surface of the descending aorta, and supply segmental arterial blood flow to the spinal cord. In many patients, a dominant anterior medullary artery, the artery of Adamkiewicz, originates between T7 and L1, and comprises most of the blood supply to the anterior two-thirds of the spinal cord (**Figure 34.1**). The first major branch of the descending aorta is the celiac artery, thus permitting treatment of the entire descending thoracic aorta with TEVAR, albeit at increased risk of stroke and spinal cord ischemia.

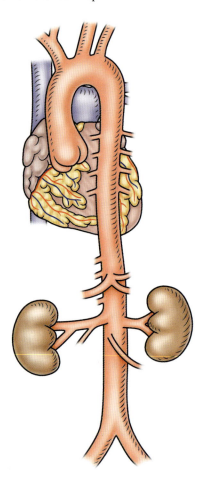

34.1

PREOPERATIVE ASSESSMENT AND PREPARATION

A thorough history and physical examination should be performed in all TEVAR candidates, with emphasis on cardiorespiratory comorbid conditions that increase the risk of perioperative complications. A detailed neurologic and cardiovascular examination is key, with attention to distal vascular pulses and any neurologic deficits. Cardiovascular evaluation with EKG, 2D transthoracic echocardiography, and carotid duplex ultrasound should be performed as indicated. Preoperative imaging with thin-slice helical computed tomography is necessary, with 3D aortic reconstructions whenever possible. The preoperative imaging will determine the anatomic suitability for a TEVAR approach.

Anatomic requirements

Satisfactory proximal and distal landing zones are the key determinants in whether a patient's thoracic aortic disease is amenable to TEVAR. The proximal and distal region of the endoprosthesis must be deployed in suitable caliber aorta to exclude the thoracic aneurysm properly without endoleak. For purposes of standardization, the proximal aorta is divided into landing zones (**Figure 34.2**). Unless great vessel revascularization is performed, deployment in zone 0 or zone 1 will cause occlusion of the innominate artery or left common carotid artery, respectively. Zone 2 deployment is routinely performed, and results in occlusion of the left subclavian artery. In zone 3, there may be steep angulation of the endograft that results in endoleak. Zone 4 proximal landing is typically straightforward due to lack of angulation in this region of the aorta.

The length of the landing zone and the diameter must both be considered. For most devices, the landing zone requirement is 2 cm without significant tapering of the aorta. When selecting device measurements for aneurysmal disease, upsizing of 10–20% is recommended. In the setting of dissection or traumatic transection, a more conservative approach is advocated with less than 10% oversizing. Exaggerated tapering, mural thrombus, calcification, and excessive tortuosity or angulation are additional anatomic factors that warrant consideration.

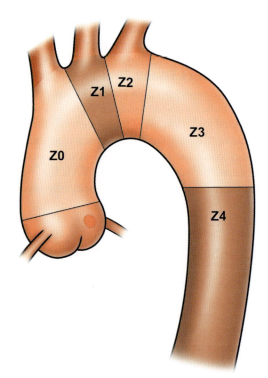

34.2

Vascular access

Adequate iliofemoral access is a prerequisite to safely performing TEVAR procedures. Complications related to vascular access are a major contributor to morbidity following TEVAR procedures. Current delivery systems range in size from 20F to 26F, and the iliac and femoral vessels must be assessed for diameter, degree of calcification, tortuosity, and angulation. A prior history of aortoiliac surgery may preclude safe delivery of the TEVAR device. For patients without acceptable femoral arterial access, retroperitoneal exposure may be used to gain direct iliac artery access.

ANESTHESIA

TEVAR procedures are performed using general anesthesia in most instances. This anesthetic technique permits respiratory control and enables more precise imaging during device deployment. Arterial line placement is routine, whereas central line placement and intraoperative transesophageal echocardiography are performed as needed. In addition, a lumbar drain is placed preoperatively when extensive coverage of the thoracic aorta is anticipated. Furthermore, patients with prior abdominal aortic repair should undergo preoperative lumbar drainage. Cerebrospinal fluid drainage augments spinal cord perfusion and is associated with lower paraplegia risk.

Neuromonitoring

Due to the risk of stroke and spinal cord ischemia, intraoperative neuromonitoring with somatosensory-evoked potentials and electroencephalography should be routine. These modalities of neuromonitoring may identify early signs of spinal cord ischemia before reliable neurologic examination can be performed. Clinical interventions such as increased lumbar drainage, volume expansion, and vasopressor use may potentially reverse spinal cord ischemia and prevent permanent paralysis.

OPERATION

Imaging

Intraoperative imaging for TEVAR relies principally on fluoroscopy. Fixed systems in hybrid operating rooms facilitate imaging, though the procedure can be accomplished with a portable C-arm. Real-time imaging is essential for proper endograft deployment. Digital subtraction angiography enables removal of background bony structures and enhances visualization of the descending thoracic aorta when injected with contrast. Road mapping permits transfer of a given reference image onto a live image for guidance during endograft deployment. Both are additional useful imaging features. Intravascular ultrasound (IVUS) is another imaging modality that is valuable in patients with renal insufficiency to minimize contrast exposure. IVUS offers intraluminal imaging. This modality can distinguish true from false lumen in dissection, and can be used to evaluate the suitability of proximal and distal landing zones.

Access

In most patients, vascular access for TEVAR can safely be performed via the femoral artery. With use of Perclose (Abbott, Santa Clara, CA) arterial closure devices, the procedure can be performed totally percutaneously. Alternatively, an open approach can be performed with a transverse incision at the level of the inguinal ligament. A retroperitoneal exposure can be used if the femoral vessel caliber is too small to accommodate the device. After access is achieved, a stable 5F sheath is inserted and a flexible guidewire is delivered retrograde to the aortic arch with the aid of fluoroscopy. Systemic heparin should be administered prior to wire manipulation. A super-stiff guidewire is required to deliver the endograft due to the natural angulation of the aortic arch. A wire exchange is needed, because the super-stiff guidewire should always be advanced to the arch over a catheter to minimize risk of dissection or rupture. A long guide catheter with a multipurpose angle (MPA) is suggested for performing this wire exchange. The super-stiff wire is then brought up the MPA catheter into the ascending aorta and is ready to accommodate the endograft. Through the contralateral artery, a diagnostic catheter (5F pigtail; Cordis) with several sideholes and radiographic markers is brought up into the aortic arch. Brachial access is occasionally needed for coil embolization of the left subclavian artery if a carotid-subclavian bypass has been performed.

Carotid–subclavian bypass

Proximal deployment in Z2 is often required to achieve a satisfactory length of normal caliber aorta for landing zone. In non-emergency situations, subclavian revascularization should be performed in advance, either subclavian-carotid transposition or with a bypass. Transposition entails more proximal exposure of the subclavian artery, and in the setting of a large TAA the anatomy can be distorted. When a carotid-subclavian bypass is performed, it is necessary to embolize the proximal left subclavian artery with coils to prevent type II endoleak. This may be performed via brachial artery access at time of the TEVAR, or can be performed directly through the subclavian vessel at the time of revascularization. Carotid-subclavian bypass is performed via a supraclavicular incision, and the sternocleidomastoid and omohyoid muscles are divided after division of the platysma. After the anterior scalene muscle is encountered, the phrenic nerve and thoracic duct are identified and protected from inadvertent traction or injury. The subclavian artery is identified deep to the anterior scalene muscle. Proximal and distal control are established for both the subclavian and carotid arteries (**Figure 34.3**). The synthetic graft used (expanded polytetrafluoroethylene or Dacron) must be measured properly to avoid undue tension or kinking. Running 5-0 or 6-0 Prolene sutures are used to complete both vascular anastomoses.

Device deployment

Proper preoperative imaging facilitates planning of the number, size, and sequence of endograft deployment. The projected coverage length of the thoracic aorta dictates the number and length of endografts. Due to angulation and tortuosity of the thoracic aorta in many patients, an aortic centerline measurement is useful to determine the length of endografts most suitable to use. Three-dimensional vascular reconstruction software is useful for these measurements. Proximal and distal

landing zone diameters determine the appropriate diameter of the endograft to use. To achieve a proper seal, the device should be selected to achieve a 15–20% oversize of the landing zone. However, in the setting of acute pathologies such as dissection or traumatic transection, a more conservative approach of 5–10% oversizing is preferred to avoid aortic rupture. Endografts are most often deployed beginning in the most proximal location first. However, in instances where the proximal endograft is larger than the distal device, or if precise deployment is required at the level of the celiac axis, the endografts may be deployed in distal to proximal sequence.

With the aid of fluoroscopy, the endograft is advanced over the Lunderquist wire to the proximal landing zone (**Figure 34.4**). For the Gore TAG endograft, an introducer sheath is available that permits hemostasis if multiple devices will be deployed. Other devices are advanced directly into the access artery without an introducer sheath. The C-arm is positioned in left anterior oblique view of approximately 45–50 degrees. A diagnostic angiogram is performed with temporary cessation of ventilation to achieve the best imaging. This confirms the anatomy and allows proper positioning of the endograft with respect to the landing zone. The road mapping functionality is useful during this stage of the procedure. The pigtail catheter is often withdrawn prior to deployment though this is not always necessary. Each available device has a specific deployment mechanism that should be reviewed prior to actual deployment, with relative advantages and disadvantages to each system. When exact landing at the level of the celiac artery is necessary, the C-arm is rotated to full lateral position for ideal imaging during diagnostic angiography.

For deployment of additional devices, the first device is exchanged over a stiff Lunderquist guidewire. When multiple

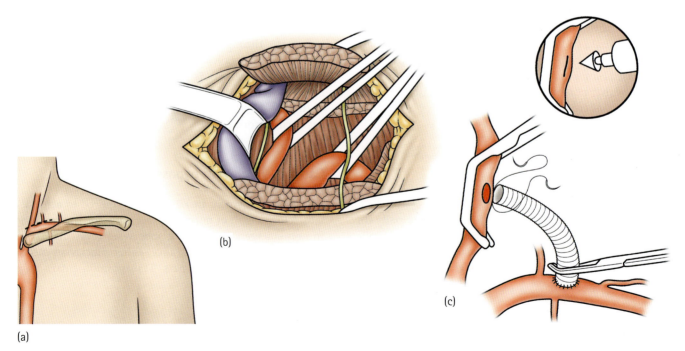

(a)

(b)

(c)

34.3

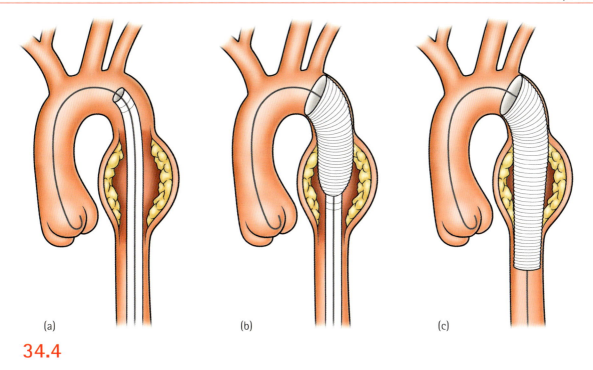

(a)   (b)   (c)

34.4

devices must be deployed, it is important to have satisfactory overlap distance to avoid inter-device, or type III, endoleaks. A minimum overlap of 5 cm is preferred. Additionally, ballooning of junctions between endograft devices is usually recommended to achieve ideal apposition and avoid endoleak. Ballooning of proximal and distal landing zones is usually performed to minimize type Ia or Ib endoleak, respectively. Caution while ballooning under fluoroscopic guidance is important to minimize risk of stent fracture or aortic dissection, as can occur with overly aggressive balloon dilation. A compliant tri-lobed balloon is used, with the sequence occurring proximal to distal, with the endograft junctions performed last. A final diagnostic angiogram is performed by advancing the pigtail catheter within the stent graft devices up into the aortic arch under fluoroscopic visualization. On this completion angiogram, one should carefully inspect for endograft position and endoleak. Additional devices or further ballooning are performed as necessary to treat endoleak. The delivery system is then withdrawn from the access vessel, keeping the guidewire in place. This serves as a precautionary measure by which an occlusive balloon can be advanced for temporary hemostasis in the event of a vascular injury. If a percutaneous approach was performed, the Perclose sytem is cinched down. After documentation of intact vascular integrity and confirmation of distal pulses, the guidewire can be removed and the Perclose sutures cut.

Special circumstances

AORTIC DISSECTION

Historically, acute type B aortic dissection was treated with aggressive medical management to control blood pressure and decrease shear forces on the aorta. However, a large percentage of patients who undergo optimal medical management develop complications related to their dissection that later require intervention. Surgical management for acute type B dissection has traditionally been reserved for patients with dissection-related complications such as malperfusion syndromes, impending or contained rupture, persistent pain, or degenerative aneurysm formation. Because conventional open operations are associated with significant morbidity and mortality, there has been recent enthusiasm in applying endovascular technology to the treatment of acute type B aortic dissection, both in the complicated and uncomplicated setting. For acute complicated type B aortic dissection, TEVAR is recommended when anatomically possible, due to an early mortality benefit compared to open surgery. In uncomplicated acute type B aortic dissection, recent data from the INSTEAD-XL randomized trial comparing early TEVAR plus optimal medical therapy to optimal medical therapy alone showed an aorta-specific survival benefit at five years. These encouraging results with TEVAR for type B dissection have led to recent FDA approval for treatment of all lesions of the descending thoracic aorta.

The optimal surgical management of degenerative aneurysm in the setting of chronic type B aortic dissection is not well defined. There are many documented reports of successful approaches with TEVAR. However, there can be difficulty achieving complete expansion of the endograft due to a thickened septum and thus difficulty achieving false lumen thrombosis. In addition, thoraco-abdominal involvement of the dissection with downstream abdominal fenestrations and branch vessel involvement of the dissection flap or false lumen complicates the endovascular approach. The emergence of fenestrated stent grafts may overcome some of these anatomic challenges. Nevertheless, the difficulty in managing chronic Type B aortic dissection with aneurysmal degeneration reinforces the need to identify patients in the acute setting with risk factors for aneurysmal degeneration. These are the patients who most stand to benefit from early TEVAR intervention.

The underlying principles that guide an endovascular approach to aortic dissection differ from those that apply to aneurysmal disease. The key objective in treatment of acute type B aortic dissection is coverage of the primary entry tear site, typically located distal to the left subclavian artery (**Figure 34.5**). The goal is to re-expand the true lumen and exclude false lumen flow, thereby leading to false lumen thrombosis and correction of malperfusion. It is imperative to confirm wire access in the true lumen throughout its course to the ascending aorta. For this purpose, IVUS is very useful. Depending on the anatomic location of the dissection, intraoperative transesophageal echocardiography can be a useful adjunct to IVUS in confirming true lumen wire placement. Sizing of devices for dissection should be more conservative than for aneurysmal disease, generally 10% oversized relative to the diameter of the dissected aorta. IVUS can be useful for appropriate aortic measurements as well. Aggressive ballooning should not be performed except in extreme circumstances due to risk of aortic rupture and retrograde type A aortic dissection. If important visceral or lower extremity vessels remain malperfused after proximal TEVAR deployment, treatment with bare metal or uncovered stents more distally may be necessary.

TRAUMATIC AORTIC INJURY

Traumatic aortic injury typically occurs just distal to the ligamentum arteriosum, where the aorta is relatively fixed. In high-energy deceleration injuries, this region of the aorta is particularly vulnerable to traumatic injury. In those patients who do not die immediately from free rupture, TEVAR offers significant improvement in morbidity and mortality compared to open repair.

Injuries classified as Grade 1 with intimal tear alone may be managed with heart rate and blood pressure control alone. However, more extensive injuries (Grade 2: intramural hematoma; Grade 3: pseudoaneurysm; Grade 4: rupture or transection) require operative repair. In patients who exhibit hemodynamic stability, repair can be deferred until other life threatening traumatic injuries have been treated. As the proximal and distal landing zones are generally healthy aorta and these patients tend to be younger in age, 5–10% oversizing is satisfactory.

HYBRID ARCH REPAIR

Management of aortic arch aneurysms is challenging, with complex procedures requiring circulatory arrest and complex cerebral protection strategies. The concept of hybrid aortic arch repair involves great vessel revascularization to establish a suitable proximal landing zone in Z0. This hybrid approach offers the advantage of avoiding circulatory arrest and possibly even use of cardiopulmonary bypass in those patients with suitable anatomy. The hybrid arch repair can be accomplished as a staged repair with initial revascularization followed by retrograde TEVAR with deployment in Z0 (**Figures 34.6 and 34.7**). Or, antegrade delivery can be performed simultaneously with the great vessel revascularization procedure. In those patients who have a dilated ascending aorta that is not suitable for proximal landing zone, the ascending aorta requires replacement. During the debranching procedure, neuromonitoring with continuous electroencephalography is recommended for detection of neurologic events that could influence the conduct of operation. The development of multiple branched arch endografts may replace the hybrid arch concept in the future. In properly selected patients who may be too high risk for conventional open arch surgery, at present the hybrid approach is an attractive surgical option.

POSTOPERATIVE CARE

Invasive hemodynamic monitoring in an intensive care unit setting is recommended following a TEVAR procedure. An arterial line is preferred for accurate blood pressure control, and a Swan-Ganz catheter is selectively used in those patients with known depressed cardiac function. Patients who have undergone TEVAR procedures require standard resuscitation that mirrors the usual resuscitation following any major cardiac operation. Higher blood pressure is acceptable because of the absence of an open aortic suture line, which promotes spinal cord perfusion. Expeditious

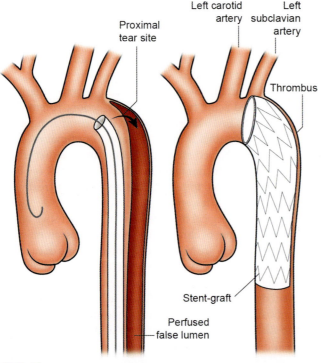

34.5

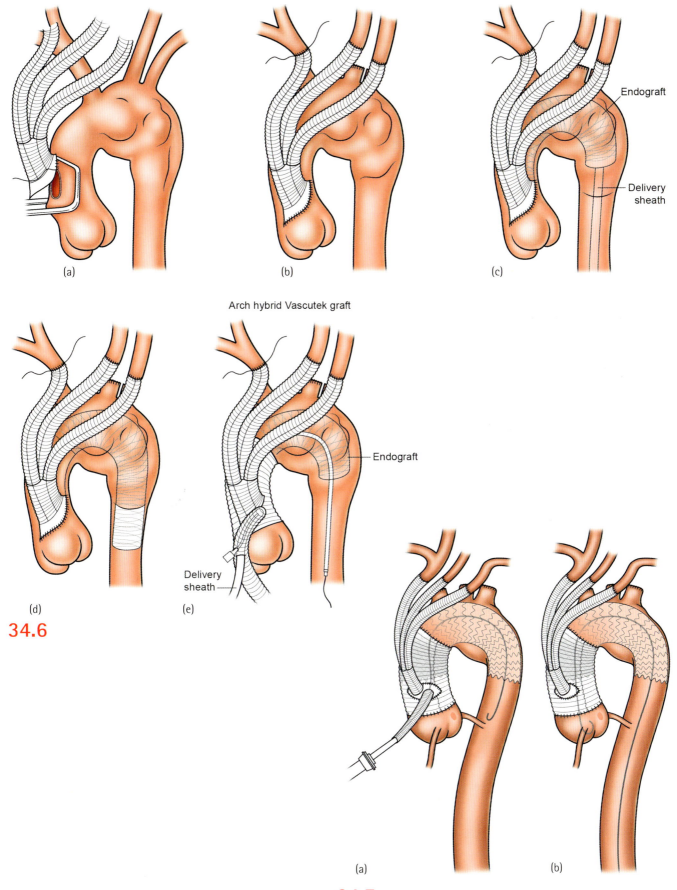

(a)

(b)

(c)
Endograft
Delivery sheath

Arch hybrid Vascutek graft

(d)

(e)
Endograft
Delivery sheath

34.6

(a)

(b)

34.7

neurologic assessment is crucial. In those cases where spinal cord ischemia is apparent or suspected, spinal drainage, volume expansion, and permissive hypertension, even with the use of added pressor agents, should be performed promptly. Atrial tachyarrhythmias should be treated aggressively, with electrical defibrillation if needed, as these rhythm disturbances often lead to abrupt hypotension. In patients who are completely neurologically intact, the spinal drain can usually be capped at 24 hours with removal at 48 hours.

OUTCOME

TEVAR has technical success rates exceeding 95%. Compared with open surgical repair, perioperative mortality for uncomplicated type B dissection is favorable, approximately 2%. Perioperative stroke occurs in 1–4% of patients and spinal cord ischemia occurs in approximately 5% of patients. Retrograde type A aortic dissection occurs in 5% of patients. For patients with acute complicated type B aortic dissection, perioperative mortality ranges between 5–8%, and compares favorably to open surgical repair with mortality rates between 15% and 20%, albeit no randomized data exist.

Ongoing surveillance is critical to identify endoleak, which occurs in 5–10% of patients. Approximately 5% of endografts will require secondary intervention in the future. CTA is the ideal imaging modality to identify endoleak. Type I and III endoleak can be treated with additional device deployment. Type II endoleak with progressively enlarging aneurysm sac can often be treated with embolization procedures.

FUTURE DIRECTIONS

There are several published reports of centers employing TEVAR technology to treat pathology of the ascending aorta, such as acute aortic dissection or pseudoaneurysm in patients who are too high risk for conventional surgery. Most of these reports involve use of devices not designed for the ascending aorta. Thus, at present there are limitations in the applicability of this technology to the ascending aorta. However, the Cook Medical (Bloomington, IN, USA) Zenith ascending dissection device is specifically designed for the ascending aorta, and there are likely to be additional devices in the future. Furthermore, development of branched endografts will facilitate treatment of aortic arch disease.

FURTHER READING

Czerny M, Roedler S, Fakhimi S, et al. Midterm results of thoracic endovascular aortic repair in patients with aneurysms involving the descending aorta originating from chronic type B dissections. *Ann Thorac Surg.* 2010; 90(1): 90–4.

Fattori R, Cao P, De Rango P, et al. Interdisciplinary expert consensus document on management of type B aortic dissection. *J Am Coll Cardiol.* 2013; 61(16): 1661–78.

Makaroun MS, Dillavou ED, Wheatley GH, et al. Five-year results of endovascular treatment with the Gore TAG device compared with open repair of thoracic aortic aneurysms. *J Vasc Surg.* 2008; 47(5): 912–8.

Nation DA, Wang GJ. TEVAR: Endovascular repair of the thoracic aorta. *Semin Intervent Radiol.* 2015; 32(3): 265–71.

Nienaber CA, Kische S, Rousseau H, et al. INSTEAD-XL trial. Endovascular repair of type B aortic dissection: long-term results of the randomized investigation of stent grafts in aortic dissection trial. *Circ Cardiovasc Interv.* 2013; 6(4): 407–16.

Szeto WY, Bavaria JE. Hybrid repair of aortic arch aneurysms: combined open arch reconstruction and endovascular repair. *Semin Thorac Cardiovasc Surg.* 2009; 21(4): 347–54.

Szeto WY, McGarvey M, Pochettino A, et al. Results of a new surgical paradigm: endovascular repair for acute complicated type B aortic dissection. *Ann Thorac Surg.* 2008; 86(1): 87–93.

35

Aortic dissection: type A and B

ARMAN KILIC AND PRASHANTH VALLABHAJOSYULA

HISTORY

Historical descriptions of aortic dissection date back several centuries. The death of the British King George II in 1760 from cardiac tamponade in the setting of a type A aortic dissection (TAAD) was documented in detail by his personal physician, Frank Nicholls. Rene Laennec, the inventor of the stethoscope, first used the term "dissecting aneurysm" in 1819. The first successful surgical repair of a dissecting thoracic aortic aneurysm was performed by DeBakey, Cooley, and Creech more than a century later, in 1954. This chapter provides an overview of the approach to patient management for both TAAD and uncomplicated and complicated type B aortic dissection (TBAD), with particular attention to technical details of surgical therapy.

PRINCIPLES AND JUSTIFICATION

Classification

Aortic dissections are classified according to the time from onset of symptoms to presentation, and anatomically according to the extent of the dissection. Acute aortic dissection corresponds to symptoms that have been present for 2 weeks or less. Traditionally, chronic dissection referred to symptoms lasting more than 2 weeks although further subdivisions are being considered to include such time classifications as hyperacute and subacute, the exact definitions of which are debated. Anatomic classification is based on either the Stanford or DeBakey classification (**Figure 35.1**). Stanford type A dissections involve the ascending aorta whereas Stanford type B aortic dissections do not involve the ascending aorta. DeBakey type I aortic dissection originates but is not confined to the ascending aorta. DeBakey type II aortic dissection originates and is confined to the ascending aorta, whereas DeBakey type III aortic dissection originates in the descending aorta. TBADs are further classified into uncomplicated versus complicated, the latter being defined as the presence of aortic rupture, malperfusion, refractory pain, or rapid expansion.

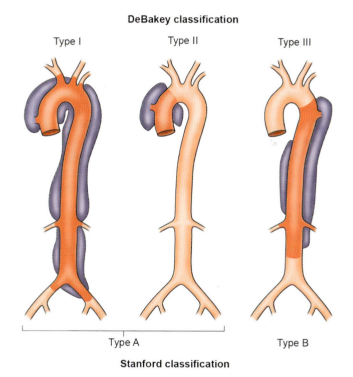

DeBakey classification

Type I   Type II   Type III

Type A   Type B

Stanford classification

35.1

Risk factors, presentation, and diagnosis

Predisposing risk factors for aortic dissection include a history of hypertension, aneurysmal disease of the aorta, and connective tissue disorders. Abrupt onset of chest pain is typical for acute TAAD whereas back pain or abdominal pain is more common in TBAD. Tachycardia and hypertension are usually presenting signs due to anxiety, pain, and baseline hypertension. Some patients will present with hypotension in the setting of aortic rupture, pericardial tamponade, myocardial ischemia from involvement of the coronary ostia, or acute aortic valve regurgitation. Diminished or absent pulses in the femoral arteries signify limb ischemia. Syncope, stroke, or other neurologic manifestations of cerebral malperfusion may be present as well. Renal malperfusion may present as rising creatinine or declining urine output.

In patients presenting with symptoms or signs concerning for an acute TAAD, expeditious diagnosis by imaging is essential. At some centers, patients with suspected TAAD who are being transferred are brought directly to the operating room for confirmation of the diagnosis. The most common imaging modalities for TAAD are computed tomography angiography and echocardiography. In hemodynamically unstable patients with suspected acute TAAD, transesophageal echocardiography in the operating room can be used for diagnosis in order to minimize time to emergent surgical repair. For patients with TBAD, computed tomography angiography of the chest, abdomen, and pelvis is important to delineate the entire extent of the dissection. Magnetic resonance imaging can also be used for both TAAD and TBAD although it is much less commonly utilized.

Indications for surgical repair of acute type A aortic dissection

Without treatment, acute TAAD has a mortality rate of approximately 1% per hour. Moreover, 50% of patients with untreated acute TAAD are dead by the third day and almost 80% are dead by the end of the second week. This high mortality rate has led to an aggressive surgical approach to acute TAAD, with the diagnosis itself being an indication for surgical repair. Although each case is evaluated in an individualized manner, relative contraindications to operative repair include age greater than 80 years, although this threshold is debated and differs between providers and between institutions, and severe comorbidities such as dialysis-dependent renal failure or advanced liver cirrhosis. Devastating neurologic injury is also viewed as a contraindication, although typically imaging evidence of neurologic injury is necessary to deem TAAD repair futile. Moreover, some patients who present with neurologic symptoms in the setting of TAAD will resolve these symptoms postoperatively, particularly when there are no intracranial abnormalities on imaging studies.

Indications for surgical repair of acute type B aortic dissection

In acute TBAD, it is important to distinguish whether it is uncomplicated or complicated. Approximately 70–80% of TBADs are uncomplicated and have traditionally been managed medically with anti-impulse and anti-hypertensive medications. In-hospital mortality with medical management in uncomplicated TBAD is less than 10%. Despite low rates of early mortality, emerging evidence suggests a 3-year survival of only 75–80% with a 25–50% rate of late aortic-related complications in medically managed patients. In patients with uncomplicated TBAD with high risk features, which include an initial aortic diameter of at least 4 cm or greater with a patent false lumen, intramural hematoma with a penetrating aortic ulcer in the proximal descending

thoracic aorta, initial false lumen diameter of 22 mm or greater in the proximal descending thoracic aorta, or recurrent or refractory pain or hypertension, there is now an increasing body of evidence to support thoracic endovascular repair (TEVAR) to help promote aortic remodeling and false lumen thrombosis and thereby prevent late aortic-related complications.

Repair is warranted in patients with complicated TBAD. This includes cases of end-organ malperfusion, refractory pain, rapidly expanding false lumen, impending or frank rupture, and chronic aneurysmal dilatation. Traditionally this has been done through an open repair; however, perioperative mortality with this approach has been high, ranging from 15% to 50%. Surgical therapy usually consists of graft replacement of the descending thoracic aorta or thoracoabdominal aorta, with hypothermic circulatory arrest used in approximately half of cases in multicenter registries. Remaining patients were treated with surgical fenestration. TEVAR has been used increasingly for complicated TBAD given the significant morbidity and mortality rates associated with open repair. In cases of dynamic malperfusion, placement of a stent graft reliably leads to reperfusion whereas in cases of a combination of dynamic and static malperfusion the rate of reperfusion is lower with stent placement alone. Multiple studies, including those from the International Registry of Acute Aortic Dissection, have demonstrated lower operative mortality and morbidity with TEVAR as compared to open surgical repair.

Indications for surgical repair of chronic aortic dissection

Chronic TAAD patients more frequently have undergone prior cardiac surgery. Indications for surgical repair include moderate or severe aortic insufficiency with left ventricular dilatation or heart failure symptoms, rapid aortic diameter increase of at least 0.5 cm per year, large dissecting aneurysm, hemodynamic instability, or onset of new chest pain or neurologic symptoms. In chronic TBAD, the most common indications for repair are aneurysmal dilatation of the dissected aorta greater than 5.0-6.0 cm, or rapid expansion greater than 1.0 cm per year.

PREOPERATIVE ASSESSMENT AND PREPARATION

Performing a thorough assessment, particularly in emergent cases such as TAAD or complicated TBAD, can be challenging given the ultimate goal of minimizing time to surgical repair. A quick assessment, sometimes even on the operating room table, of mental status and neurologic function, femoral pulses, abdominal pain, and hemodynamics is essential. This helps quickly establish a baseline assessment of the patient including presence of malperfusion. A review of the electrocardiogram and echocardiogram specifically for evidence of coronary ischemia and aortic regurgitation, pericardial effusion, and the extent of dissection are important. In cases of rupture and hemodynamic instability, permissive hypotension with avoidance of excessive fluid administration is acceptable as long as the patient is mentating. In the stable patient, aortic wall stress should be minimized such that the heart rate is less than 60 beats per minute and the systolic blood pressure is less than 120 mmHg. Intravenous beta-blockers are typically used to achieve these hemodynamic goals with the addition of vasodilators should the blood pressure remain elevated after heart rate control. Adequate pain control is also important.

Another critical component of preoperative assessment is a review of the imaging studies. The location of the primary tear, extent of dissection, presence of intramural hematoma or penetrating aortic ulcer, aneurysmal dilatation, and involvement of branch vessels can be delineated from computed tomography scans. In TAAD, this is important for operative planning as the right axillary artery should not be dissected if planning on axillary cannulation, and in addition, involvement of the root or tear in the aortic arch may necessitate more extensive surgery, which will be discussed in further detail later in this chapter. The preoperative computed tomography scan is equally important in TBAD in planning the surgical approach, including suitability for TEVAR based on access vessel diameter, tortuosity, and calcification and suitable landing zones. The proximal extent dictates whether the left subclavian artery will be covered with the need for potential revascularization. Distally, thoracoabdominal extension will also dictate the need for mesenteric debranching and revascularization. These details will also be discussed in further detail in the Operation section of this chapter.

ANESTHESIA

In open surgical repairs done through median sternotomy, standard anesthetic monitoring including non-invasive blood pressure monitoring, pulse oximetry, electrocardiogram, invasive arterial blood pressure monitoring, central venous access, Swan-Ganz catheter, temperature probe and temperature-sensing urinary catheter are utilized. In cases of TAAD, near infrared spectroscopy and electroencephalogram can be employed. Red blood cells for possible transfusion should be made available in an expeditious manner. Vasoactive agents such as nitroglycerin and phenylephrine should also be available as the patient can have labile hemodynamics. Moreover, patients with TAAD tend to develop hypertension upon opening the pericardium that untreated can lead to potential rupture in unruptured or contained rupture cases. Standard endotracheal tubes can be used but a double lumen endotracheal tube should be utilized in cases where the left chest will be entered such as TBAD given the need for single lung ventilation. TEVAR can be performed under general or local anesthesia. Some centers will use cerebrospinal fluid drainage to reduce the

risk of paraplegia following descending thoracic or thoracoabdominal repair although preoperative placement is not always possible especially in emergent cases.

OPERATION

Type A aortic dissection – cannulation and cerebral protection strategy

The cannulation and cerebral protection strategy for TAAD varies between centers and surgeons. Options for arterial cannulation include the right axillary artery provided it is not dissected, the ascending aorta via Seldinger technique with transesophageal echocardiography guidance, and the femoral artery. Right axillary cannulation is performed before sternotomy by making a 2 cm incision parallel and inferior to the lateral clavicle (**Figure 35.2**). The pectoralis major can be separated and the pectoralis minor identified and divided with electrocautery. The axillary artery can then be palpated inferior to the clavicle. The axillary vein is superficial to the artery and can be mobilized and retracted to provide optimal exposure to the artery. The nerves of the

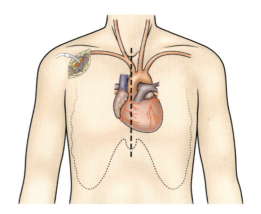

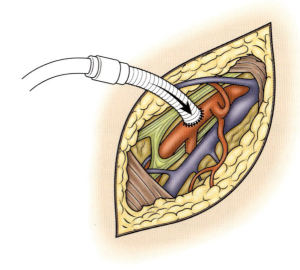

35.2

brachial plexus should not be handled and sharp dissection should be used near them to avoid electrocautery injury to the nerves. Small arterial branches can be ligated and vessels loops can be placed around larger branches. Once adequately exposed, 5000 units of intravenous heparin is administered and a side-biting clamp is placed on the axillary artery. An arteriotomy is made with an 11-blade and opened with Potts scissors. An 8 mm or 10 mm Dacron graft is then sewed end-to-side to the axillary artery and the arterial cannula placed within the graft and secured with silk ties.

For direct ascending aortic cannulation, a median sternotomy is performed, and the pericardium is opened and secured to the skin with silk sutures. A single pursestring is then placed in the distal ascending aorta on the lesser curve. A needle is then inserted inside the pursestring at a steep angle and aimed towards the left, a wire passed, and confirmation of the wire inside the true lumen should be done by transesophageal echocardiography (**Figure 35.3**). Once confirmed, the aortotomy is then serially dilated over the wire and the aortic cannula is inserted, again with confirmation of true lumen placement in the distal arch by echocardiography.

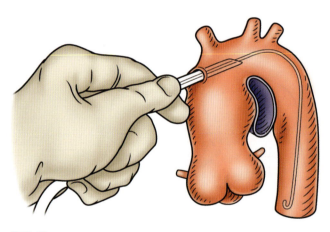

35.3

With respect to venous cannulation, the right atrium (with or without superior vena cava cannulation) or femoral venous cannulation is performed. The advantages and disadvantages of moderate versus deep hypothermic circulatory arrest (MHCA and DHCA, respectively) and antegrade versus retrograde cerebral perfusion (ACP and RCP, respectively) have been extensively debated. Options for ACP include delivery via the right axillary artery if cannulated in that manner with clamping of the innominate artery, direct ostial ACP (either unilateral via the innominate artery or bilateral via the innominate and left common carotid arteries), or direct innominate cannulation. RCP is typically delivered via a superior vena cava cannula that is connected via a y-connector to a right atrial cannula with snaring of the superior vena cana. In cases using ACP, flows are maintained between 10 and 12 mL / kg / min with right radial arterial pressures of 50–60 mmHg. RCP flow is regulated to maintain

a central venous pressure of 20–25 mmHg. A retrograde cardioplegia and left ventricular vent via the right superior pulmonary vein are also inserted.

Type A aortic dissection – proximal reconstruction

Cardiopulmonary bypass is instituted. Once the left ventricular vent is successfully inserted, the patient is cooled to the desired hypothermic temperature over a period of 45 minutes. During this time, proximal evaluation and reconstruction can be performed. Once the desired temperature is reached we typically proceed to the hypothermic circulatory arrest and distal reconstruction portion of the operation therefore allowing for rewarming during proximal reconstruction to help improve operative efficiency.

While the patient is being cooled, the aorta is cross-clamped, the proximal ascending aorta is opened with Metzenbaum scissors and the true and false lumens identified. Direct antegrade ostial cardioplegia is carefully given as the ostia are often friable and may be involved in the dissection. The ascending aorta is transected and a segment extending to 1–2 cm above the sinotubular junction removed after mobilization. The root is then inspected for evidence of intimal tear. Tears that extend to the sinotubular junction but do not involve the coronary ostia or significantly destruct the sinuses can be repaired with primary pledgeted 4-0 polypropylene sutures. If the tear is extensive or extends into the root, a root replacement is performed. Involvement of coronary ostia may necessitate coronary ligation and bypass with a vein graft.

Valve resuspension is performed by placing 4-0 pledgeted polypropylene sutures in a horizontal mattress 5 mm above each commissure, with pledgets on both the inside and outside of the aorta, and tying each of these sutures down (**Figure 35.4a–d**). The extent of the dissection is also evaluated and hematoma is removed carefully from between the intimal and adventitial layers. We use a neomedia technique whereby felt is trimmed to fit into semicircular spaces created by the dissection, and the felt is then secured by running a 5-0 polypropylene suture that goes through adventitia, the felt, and intima. This buttresses the friable dissected tissue. Some surgeons secure neomedia felt with bioglue although our preference is to suture the felt in place as described above. Cardioplegia can be run antegrade through the graft with clamping near the transected end to evaluate for any bleeding in the anastomosis and also to test for valve competency.

Type A aortic dissection – hemi-arch repair

Once the patient is sufficiently cooled, hypothermic circulatory arrest with ACP or RCP is initiated. The aortic cross-clamp is removed, and the aortic arch is inspected for evidence of tear. In the absence of an intimal tear in the arch, extensive dissection involving the arch branch vessels, or a

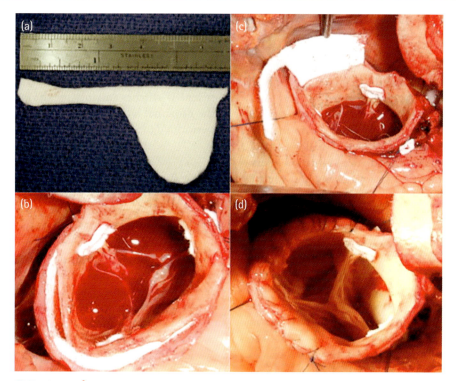

35.4a–d

pre-existing arch aneurysm, it is reasonable to proceed with a hemi-arch repair. We perform an aggressive hemi-arch with resection of most of the lesser curve of the arch. Similar to the proximal reconstruction, we utilize a neomedia technique to place felt in between dissected intimal and adventitial layers if the dissection extends to the arch. This helps reinforce the anastomosis that would otherwise involve friable tissue.

The hemi-arch anastomosis is performed by suturing an appropriately sized Dacron graft to the transected distal aorta using 4-0 SH polypropylene suture (**Figure 35.5**). The graft should be telescoped into the aorta for better hemostasis. This can be achieved by pulling the aorta down and the graft up and into the aorta while pulling up on the suture after each bite. Stitches on the aorta should be deep as the tissue is often friable and will tear if it is too shallow of a bite. Once this anastomosis is completed, circulatory arrest is stopped, the patient is rewarmed, and cardiopulmonary bypass restarted either using the axillary cannula if it was cannulated or by cannulating the distal graft after placing two polypropylene U stitches in the graft. Some surgeons prefer a graft with a side branch that can be cannulated as well. In addition, a graft-to-graft anastomosis is performed using 3-0 polypropylene suture, although some surgeons will use one graft particularly if there no significant discrepancy in diameter between the proximal and distal aortic diameters.

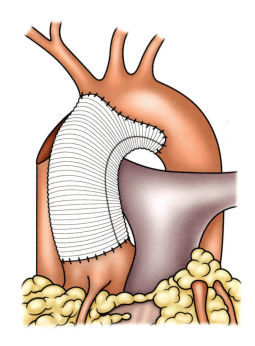

35.5

Type A aortic dissection – total arch replacement

In cases of a pre-existing arch aneurysm, tear in the arch, or extensive dissection involving the arch branch vessels, a total arch replacement should be performed (**Figure 35.6**). Total arch replacement is performed under hypothermic circulatory arrest with either axillary cannulation that can be used for ACP or direct ostial ACP with balloon-tipped catheters, or with RCP. After cannulation, initiation of cardiopulmonary bypass, aortic cross-clamping and varying degree of proximal reconstruction, attention is turned to the circulatory arrest portion of the operation when the desired hypothermic temperature is reached. The patient is placed in the Trendelenburg position. Hypothermic circulatory arrest is initiated and ACP, RCP, or both are delivered and the aortic cross-clamp is removed. In our practice, RCP alone is not utilized for arch repairs, but instead combined ACP and RCP or ACP alone. The arch and branch vessels are inspected for evidence of intimal tear and extent of dissection. The soft tissue around the arch is mobilized, as are the branch vessels. The distal arch is transected distal to the left subclavian artery. The three branch vessels are also transected near their origin from the arch. An appropriately sized trifurcated graft with or without a side branch for re-cannulation is then anastomosed. The distal graft is sewn to the transected distal arch using a 4-0 polypropylene suture. The left subclavian and left carotid anastomoses are sewn using 5-0 polypropylene.

After the left carotid anastomosis is completed, hypothermic circulatory arrest can be stopped and the patient transitioned back to cardiopulmonary bypass. The proximal graft should be clamped as well as the side branch graft for the innominate artery. If axillary cannulation and ACP is used, the native innominate artery is already clamped and the arterial tubing is already Y-ed. Cannulation of the distal graft via a side branch graft with partial clamping of the arterial tubing for the axillary cannula can then be performed. The innominate artery anastomosis can be performed off

of circulatory arrest with the innominate graft and native artery clamped. The innominate graft is then backbled and de-aired prior to releasing the clamp on the innominate graft. If direct ascending arterial cannulation was used, the graft is re-cannulated after placing two perpendicular 2-0 polypropylene U-stitches and incising the middle. After completing the proximal reconstruction, a graft-to-graft anastomosis is performed in standard fashion.

Type A aortic dissection – other distal reconstructive surgical options

Other distal reconstructive surgical options include performing a zone 2 arch repair and subsequent interval TEVAR via the groin. A zone 2 arch repair is similar to a total arch repair except that the left subclavian artery is left intact and the distal transection of the aorta occurs in between the left carotid artery and the left subclavian artery as opposed to distal to the left subclavian artery. This strategy can be employed if an arch tear is located in the more proximal arch with sparing of the left subclavian artery. The primary benefits are reducing circulatory arrest time and positive remodeling of the distal aorta with reduction in false lumen diameter and higher rates of complete false lumen thrombosis.

In the setting of a DeBakey type I aortic dissection, some groups have advocated for a total arch replacement with antegrade descending thoracic aortic stenting, otherwise known as a frozen elephant trunk (**Figure 35.7**). This is done to improve distal aortic remodeling and reduce rates of subsequent distal aortic interventions.

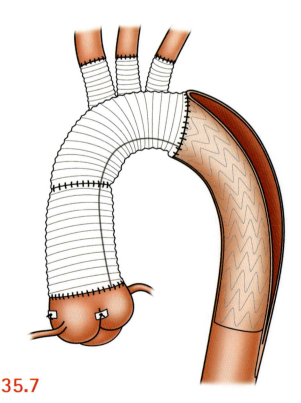

35.6

35.7

Another option we have utilized in select DeBakey type I malperfusion cases is primary arch tear repair with aggressive hemi-arch reconstruction and antegrade TEVAR (**Figure 35.8**). This is a technically easier operation, avoids manipulation of the arch vessels, and reduces circulatory arrest time. This is especially true in obese patients or those with large arch aneurysms where exposure of the distal arch and arch vessels can be difficult. The dissection flap is repaired with the neomedia felt technique described previously, with primary repair of the arch tear using interrupted pledgeted sutures. A GoreTAG stent graft that is 150 mm in length and ranges typically from 31 mm to 37 mm is then deployed in an antegrade fashion into the true lumen and the proximal end is secured with polypropylene sutures to include the repaired aorta and the stent.

Type B aortic dissection – open surgical repair

The patient is positioned in right lateral decubitus position with the pelvis tilted posteriorly to allow access to the femoral vessels (**Figure 35.9**). On single lung ventilation, a posterolateral thoracotomy is made in the fourth or fifth intercostal space. This can be extended into a thoracoabdominal incision if the abdominal aorta is to be included in the repair. The abdominal aorta can be accessed either through a transperitoneal or retroperitoneal approach. The diaphragm is divided in these cases. We typically disarticulate the thoracic cartilage using electrocautery and a rib cutter to help improve exposure. A Bookwalter retractor is then placed with the post connected to the left side of the operating table.

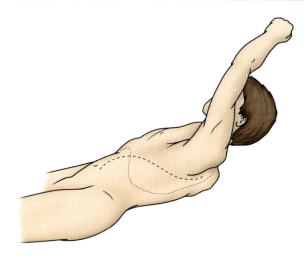

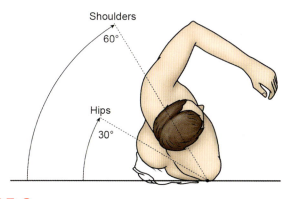

35.9

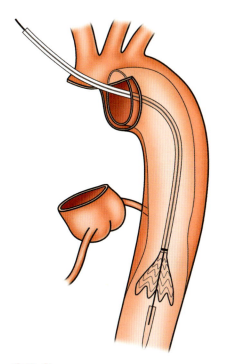
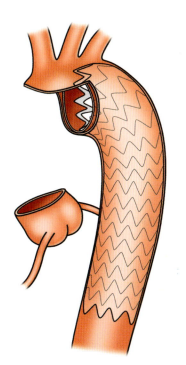
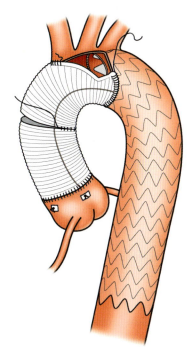

35.8

The proximal extent of the repair is determined with preoperative imaging. Circulatory management consists of either hypothermic circulatory arrest, which avoids clamping the dissected aorta, or left atrial to femoral artery bypass. Adhesiolysis is performed to mobilize the lung off of the aorta. The mediastinal pleura between the left subclavian and left common carotid arteries is opened and the left vagus and recurrent laryngeal nerve is identified. The inferior pulmonary ligament is taken down, and the soft tissue around the thoracic aorta is mobilized.

If hypothermic circulatory arrest is utilized, heparin is given and the distal aorta is cannulated with the tip pointed inferiorly if the repair is limited to the descending thoracic aorta. The femoral artery can be used for more extensive thoracoabdominal dissections. A long venous cannula is placed via the left femoral vein. Cardiopulmonary bypass is initiated and the patient is cooled. A left ventricular vent is placed through the left inferior pulmonary vein. The bypass tubing is arranged to allow for cross circulation. Once the desired hypothermic temperature is reached, the arterial tubing is clamped by the cannula and venous tubing is clamped by the portion that returns to the pump to allow for total body retrograde perfusion through the arterial tubing, across extension tubing connecting the arterial and venous side, and then via the venous cannula into the femoral vein. Once on circulatory arrest, the aortic cannula is removed and the operation proceeds.

If partial left heart bypass is utilized, the distal thoracic aorta or femoral artery is cannulated. It is important to ensure that the true lumen is being perfused. The left inferior pulmonary vein is used for venous cannulation. In cases involving the proximal descending thoracic aorta, the left subclavian artery can be encircled with an umbilical tape and a Rummel tourniquet applied. After snaring of the left subclavian artery, vascular clamps can be applied on the aortic arch in between the left common carotid and subclavian arteries, and distally on the descending thoracic aorta.

The aorta is opened longitudinally and bleeding from intercostal arteries controlled with suture ligation (**Figure 35.10**). The aorta is then transected. The diameter of the proximal aorta is sized and a Dacron graft is sewn using a 3-0 polypropylene suture. The proximal clamp is then removed and placed on the graft and the anastomosis is evaluated for hemostasis. If the repair is limited to the descending thoracic aorta, the distal diameter is sized as well and a Dacron graft similarly anastomosed in an end-to-end fashion using a 3-0 polypropylene suture. A graft-to-graft anastomosis is then performed. Cardiopulmonary bypass is weaned and the patient decannulated in standard fashion.

Treatment of the proximal dissection can often improve visceral or lower extremity malperfusion. If malperfusion persists, percutaneous or surgical fenestration may be necessary to create a communication between the false and true lumens and improve blood flow. Femoral–femoral bypass or axillo–femoral and femoral–femoral bypass can also be utilized in cases of unilateral or bilateral lower extremity malperfusion, respectively.

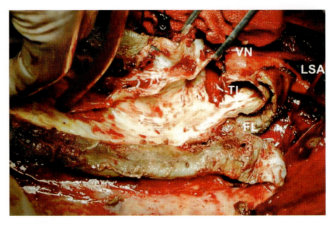

35.10

Type B aortic dissection – endovascular surgical repair

TEVAR has become the preferred treatment modality for aneurysmal disease, and more recent evidence has expanded its use in the setting of TBAD. A primary goal in TEVAR is to restore true lumen blood flow by covering the primary intimal tear. Radial pressure from the stent can also help in aortic remodeling by decreasing the diameter of the false lumen, helping promote false lumen thrombosis, and expanding the true lumen.

Preoperative computed tomography angiography is evaluated to assess the bilateral iliofemoral vessels. The femoral artery that will be used for delivery of the device should be the larger vessel with less calcification and tortuosity. If there are concerns for calcification or narrowing where the access will be achieved, surgical cutdown of the femoral artery is performed. In 10–20% of cases alternate access is established for device delivery. Most commonly this is achieved via a 10 mm conduit sewn to the common iliac artery through a retroperitoneal exposure.

A percutaneous 5 or 6 French sheath is placed in the contralateral femoral artery (**Figure 35.11**). If the contralateral femoral artery is not suitable, this can be performed through the brachial artery. A pigtail catheter is inserted and advanced to the aortic arch. Aortography or intravascular ultrasound is then used to confirm true lumen placement and to create an operative roadmap. The proximal landing zone is best visualized with a 45–75-degree left anterior oblique angle fluoroscopically. A super-stiff wire is inserted through the delivery sheath and advanced into the aortic arch under fluoroscopic guidance. The patient is heparinized. The sheath is advanced into the abdominal aorta and the device is advanced to the targeted area. In the setting of dissection, the stent graft should not be oversized more than 10% to mitigate the risk of retrograde dissection. The systolic blood pressure should be brought to 100 mmHg prior to deployment. The stent is deployed and the position confirmed by angiography

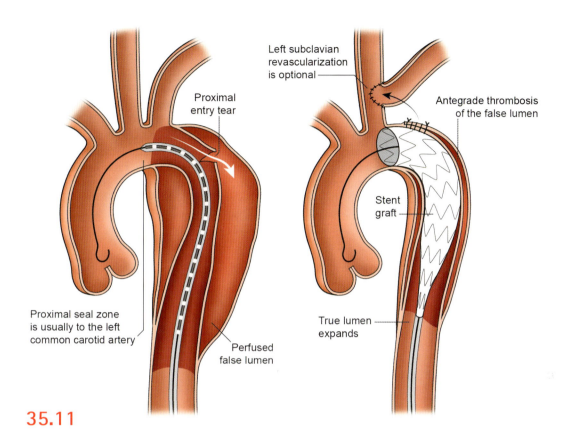

35.11

or intravascular ultrasound. Completion angiography through the pigtail catheter will help evaluate for the presence of endoleaks and blood flow to the branch vessels. Type I endoleaks can be treated with extension grafts or ballooning although the latter should be done carefully to minimize retrograde dissection or rupture risk. Persistent malperfusion can be treated with fenestration or branch vessel stenting.

POSTOPERATIVE CARE

Patients are brought to the intensive care unit. Invasive hemodynamic monitoring and vasoactive agents are used to keep the systolic blood pressure between 90 and 110 mmHg. Assuming the patient has stable hemodynamics and bleeding is not substantial, sedation should be weaned and a neurological exam obtained. In patients who fail to follow commands, computed tomography scans of the head are usually obtained in the first few postoperative days. In patients undergoing descending thoracic aortic repair, paraplegia should be treated aggressively as it can potentially be reversed using high mean arterial pressure goals of 85 to 95 mmHg, cerebrospinal fluid drainage at 10 cm H20, volume expansion, correction of anemia and hypoxia, and immediate neurology consultation.

Bleeding is an immediate concern in both type A and B dissection open repairs. We have used factor 7 or prothrombin complex concentrate intraoperatively in coagulopathic patients with significant bleeding after ruling out surgical sources, with good success. These agents are also advantageous as they avoid significant volume overloading that accompanies massive blood product transfusions.

Long-term management entails antihypertensive medication regimens to maintain systolic blood pressure less than 120 mmHg. Follow-up imaging is indicated initially prior to hospital discharge and at 6-month intervals for at least the first year. Computed tomography scans or magnetic resonance imaging for those with renal insufficiency can help evaluate the distal aorta true and false lumen diameters and false lumen thrombosis, particularly after type I TAAD repair when the distal aorta is left untreated. Imaging can also evaluate for endoleaks and enlargement of untreated but dissected aorta. Follow-up echocardiography should also be obtained following TAAD repair to evaluate for aortic valve insufficiency.

OUTCOME

According to the International Registry of Acute Aortic Dissections, the in-hospital mortality following TAAD repair remains high at 17–26%. Early survival seems to be affected more by patient characteristics and presentation than by surgical technique. Nonetheless, these rates are significantly lower than those in patients treated with medical management alone. Major postoperative complications include reoperation for bleeding (5–20%), acute renal failure (10–25%), limb ischemia (5–15%), myocardial ischemia (0–15%), stroke (5–15%), and prolonged mechanical ventilation (20–50%). Long-term survival after TAAD repair is approximately 70–90% at 5 years and 55–65% at 10 years, with survival of those discharged from the index admission being 96% at 1 year and 91% at 3 years. Long-term freedom from aortic reoperation is approximately 80–90% at 10 years.

In-hospital mortality following open surgical repair of acute complicated TBAD is 20–30%, with stroke rates of 5–10%, paraplegia rates of 5–10%, and acute renal failure rates of 5–20%. Large series of TEVAR for TBAD have demonstrated technical success rates of over 95%. Operative mortality rates are 0–15% with many series reporting less than 5%. Paraplegia rates are 0–5%, and long-term survival 65–100% with median follow-up ranging up to 40 months. The rates of endoleak are 2–40%. False lumen thrombosis is achieved in 60–100%. These mortality and morbidity rates compare favorably to open repair, which has supported the use of TEVAR for TBAD when technically feasible.

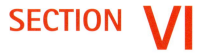

Surgery for cardiac rhythm disorders and tumors

36

The cut-and-sew Maze-III procedure for the treatment of atrial fibrillation

JAMES L. COX

INTRODUCTION

The first Maze procedure (now referred to as the "Maze-I" procedure) was performed on September 25, 1987.[1] There were two problems with the pattern of the Maze-I procedure:

1. One of the roof lesions crossed the "sinus tachycardia region" of the sino-atrial (SA) node where all sinus tachycardia originates. This region of the "atrial pacemaker complex"[2] lies immediately anterior to the junction of the SVC with the right atrium. Obliterating it with a surgical lesion led to the inability of several patients to generate an appropriate chronotropic response to exercise postoperatively as they usually could generate a heart rate of no more than 110 beats per minute.
2. The combination of interrupting Bachmann's bundle on the roof of the left atrium with the anterior approach to the left atrium and creating a conduction block in the posterior-inferior left atrial isthmus caused an intra-atrial conduction delay between the right atrium and left atrium. The delay was so long that the left atrium frequently activated (and contracted) simultaneously with the left ventricle while the mitral valve was closed, leading to an apparent loss of left atrial contractile function.

These two problems with the Maze-I procedure were the stimulus for the development of the Maze-II procedure in which the lesion through the sinus tachycardia region of the SA node was eliminated and the left atrial roof lesion was moved more posterior to preserve normal, rapid conduction of activation from the right atrium to the left atrium across Bachmann's bundle. Unfortunately, the Maze-II procedure was extremely difficult technically, stemming from the need to transect the SVC for exposure. There were two lesions in the Maze-II procedure itself that ended in the SVC at the level of its transection, resulting in the necessity of patching the SVC in every patient. Because of the technical difficulty of the Maze-II procedure, the lesions were further

modified, resulting in the Maze-III procedure described in this chapter, first introduced clinically in April 1992.[3] Prior to that time, we had performed 35 Maze-I procedures and 14 Maze-II procedures. Thereafter, only Maze-III procedures were performed.

The most common misunderstanding of the Maze-III procedure is that the term "Maze-III" is thought to be synonymous with the term "Cut-and-sew Maze". It is true that the first 200–250 Maze-I, II, and III procedures were performed via a median sternotomy with the cut-and-sew technique described herein. However, after mid-1997, all Maze-III procedures were performed via a 6 cm right antero-lateral thoracotomy and every lesion except the left atriotomy was performed with a cryoprobe. We considered calling this modification the "Maze-IV" procedure but decided against it because the lesion pattern was exactly the same as the cut-and-sew Maze-III pattern. Instead, we elected to call it the minimally-invasive cryosurgical Maze-III procedure.[4]

The Maze-IV procedure, introduced by Damiano and Gaynor in 2004, described a method for creating the same lesion pattern using a combination of radiofrequency clamps and cryosurgery, which was much quicker and easier to perform than the cut-and-sew Maze-III procedure.[5] The lesion patterns of the Maze-III and Maze-IV procedures are identical from an electrophysiologic standpoint except for the deletion of the septal lesion in the latter. Many authors now refer to the "Maze-III/IV" procedure, indicating that while the surgical techniques and energy sources are different, the patterns and electrophysiologic consequences are essentially the same. The major advantage of the Maze-IV procedure over the Maze-III procedure is that the Maze-IV lesions can be performed much more quickly while maintaining the same efficacy in treating AF.

There have been several modifications of the right atrial lesion pattern of the Maze-III and Maze-IV procedures but only the original cut-and-sew Maze-III technique will be described in this chapter. The description and illustrations are modified from a chapter on the same topic published in 1995.[6]

THE MAZE-III PROCEDURE

After total cardiopulmonary bypass is established and the caval tapes are secured, the right atrial appendage is excised (**Figure 36.1**). At least 2 cm of visible atrial muscle should be preserved between the superior end of the excised appendage (dashed line) and the orifice of the superior vena cava (SVC). Note that the SVC is cannulated directly approximately 2 cm above the right atrium and that the inferior vena cava (IVC) also is cannulated low. A pulmonary artery vent is shown in position, as is the combined cardioplegia infusion-aortic vent in the ascending aorta.

The lesion into the SVC has frequently been accused by others of causing damage to the SA node resulting in an increased need for postoperative pacemakers. However, we routinely performed extensive preoperative testing of SA node function prior to surgery except in those patients with long-standing or permanent AF. More than 100 patients were found to have normal SA node function preoperatively and only one of them had to have a postoperative pacemaker. This was in a patient who had undergone previous atrial surgery and the addition of the lesion into the SVC in his case resulted in complete isolation of the SA node. These findings effectively refute the notion that the SVC lesion causes postoperative SA node dysfunction.

A lateral incision, parallel to the right AV groove, is placed from the base of the excised atrial appendage toward the IVC, leaving 5–6 cm of right atrial free wall between the lower end of the incision and the IVC cannula (**Figure 36.2**). A posterior longitudinal incision is then placed from well into the SVC (dashed line) to well into the IVC. It is helpful to place a cardiotomy sucker into the opening of the coronary sinus via the atrial appendage during placement of the posterior longitudinal incision.

The lower portion of the posterior longitudinal incision is closed immediately to prevent inadvertent tearing and extension of the incision into the IVC during later retraction. The incision usually is closed to the level of the top of the IVC

cannula. A T incision is then made from this point across the lower right atrial free wall approximately 1 cm above the IVC cannula. The T incision is extended to the top of the right atrioventricular (AV) groove (**Figure 36.3**, dashed line). The remainder of the incision, extending to the tricuspid valve annulus, must be made from the inside the right atrium.

The right atrial free wall is retracted anteriorly and superiorly. The dashed line shows the planned extension of the T incision to the tricuspid annulus (**Figure 36.4**). This continues

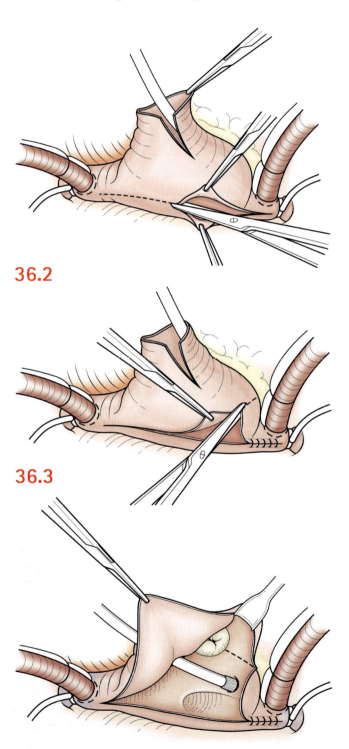

36.2

36.3

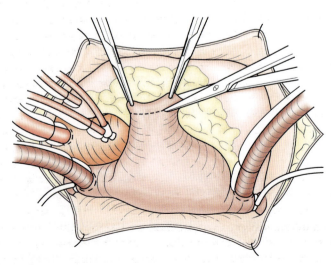

36.1

36.4

to be a transmural atriotomy, but underlying this portion of the incision is the fat pad of the right AV groove that harbors the right coronary artery. Therefore, this portion of the incision must be made with care. Once the atrial wall has been divided transmurally, the fat in the AV groove is visible.

Even when surgeons perform the classic cut-and-sew Maze-III procedure, most use a linear cryoprobe to complete this extension of the T incision.

It is essential to divide all atrial myocardial fibers traversing this portion of the T incision using either a knife or a nerve hook (**Figure 36.5**).

If a linear cryoprobe has been used to extend the T incision, it is not necessary to place a separate focal cryolesion at the tricuspid annulus.

A cryolesion is placed at the tricuspid end of the T incision to be certain that no remaining fibers traverse the incision at the level of the tricuspid valve annulus (**Figure 36.6**). A 3 mm cryoprobe is applied for 2 minutes at −60 °C.

The tricuspid end of the T incision is closed to the level of the top of the AV groove (**Figure 36.7**). The remainder of the incision is left unclosed in order to attain better surgical exposure during the remainder of the procedure.

Once the lower ends of the posterior longitudinal incision and the T incision have been closed, the anterior right atrial counter incision is performed beginning at the anteromedial border of the excised right atrial appendage (dashed line) (**Figure 36.8**). This incision extends to the anteromedial tricuspid valve annulus, and once begun

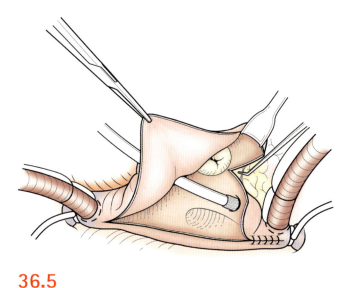

36.5

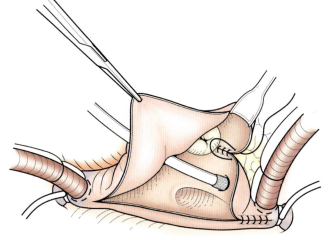

36.7

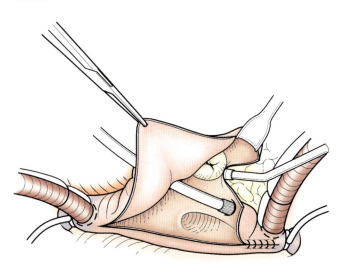

36.6

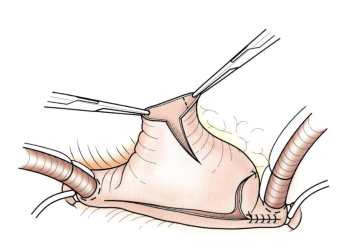

36.8

it is easier to complete from within the right atrium (**Figure 36.9**).

The right atrial free wall is retracted anteriorly and superiorly to expose the anteromedial portion of the tricuspid valve annulus and the upper portion of the counter incision that has been started from outside the right atrium. The dashed line shows the planned extension of this counter incision to the tricuspid valve annulus.

Again, this counterlesion is often performed today using a linear cryoprobe, as first suggested by Dr. Hartzell Schaff of the Mayo Clinic, Rochester, MN. When it is performed with a linear cryoprobe there is no need to add this separate focal cryolesion at the tricuspid annulus.

The counter incision is transmural, but care must be taken in dividing the final myocardial fibers because the right AV groove fat pad lies immediately beneath the incision. This portion of the right AV groove corresponds to the anterior septal space. In this case, the incision is approximately 2–3 cm anterior to the AV node–His bundle complex (**Figure 36.10**). The right coronary artery usually has not

joined the right AV groove at this point, although anatomic variations exist. A 3 mm cryolesion is also placed at the tricuspid end of this incision to ensure its completion. This is the final right atrial incision.

The entire counter incision is closed to the base of the excised atrial appendage (**Figure 36.11**).

Once the anteromedial counter incision has been closed, the remaining right atrial incisions are left unclosed until the left atrial procedure has been completed (**Figure 36.12**).

A standard left atriotomy is performed in the interatrial groove, its lower being extended around the lower lip of the orifice of the right inferior pulmonary vein. The atrial septum is then divided beginning 2–3 cm below the orifice of the SVC, traversing the anterior limbus of the fossa ovalis, and then traversing the fossa ovalis itself (dashed line) (**Figure 36.13**). This septal incision should be slanted in the general direction of the opening of the coronary sinus, but it is absolutely essential to terminate it at the bottom of the thin portion of the fossa ovalis.

The distal end of this incision terminates at the level of

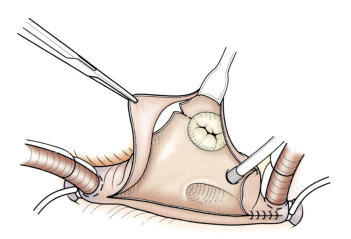

36.9

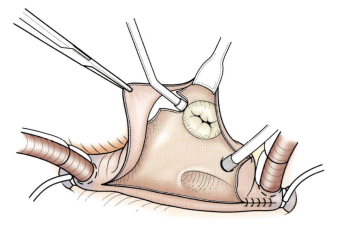

36.10

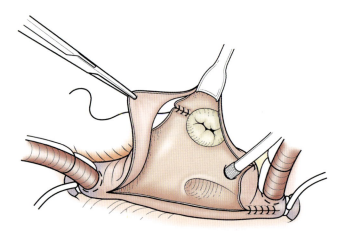

36.11

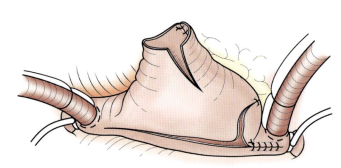

36.12

the Tendon of Todaro, which is the roof of the Triangle of Koch. The AV node always resides within the Triangle of Koch and therefore, cannot be injured by this septal incision without crossing the Tendon of Todaro. This is why heart block is not a complication of a correctly performed Maze procedure per se. However, heart block can occur following combined AF and valve surgery either due to valve sutures or prolonged cardioplegic arrest. As a safety precaution, it is helpful to place a pledgeted suture at the base of this incision to prevent its tearing and extending across the Tendon of Todaro during later retraction and exposure of the left atrium.

The atrial septum is retracted for optimal exposure of the left atrium, mitral valve, left pulmonary veins, and orifice of the left atrial appendage (**Figure 36.14**). The standard left atriotomy is extended *inferiorly* across the posterior left atrial free wall between the mitral valve and the orifices of the inferior pulmonary veins. Likewise, the *superior* portion

of the standard left atriotomy is extended around the lip of the left superior pulmonary vein orifice. Before the two ends of the pulmonary vein isolation incision are joined, the left atrial appendage is excised.

The left atrial appendage is inverted and amputated at its base (**Figure 36.15**). The base of the appendage to the right, as viewed by the surgeon in this orientation, must be approached with special care because the circumflex coronary artery may course very near to this portion of the incision. Once the appendage is excised, a small bridge of tissue remains between the appendage amputation site and the two ends of the pulmonary vein encircling incision (inset). This bridge of tissue can be divided and closed with sutures, or it can be left intact and cryoablated.

A 1.5 cm cryoprobe is applied to the bridge of tissue for 2 minutes at −60 °C (**Figure 36.16**). The isolation incision of the pulmonary vein is much easier to close if this tissue bridge is left intact rather than surgically divided.

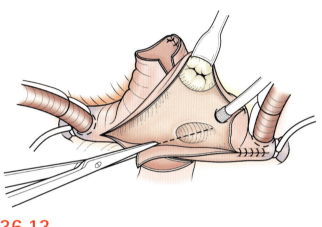

36.13

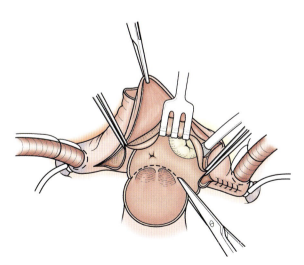

36.14

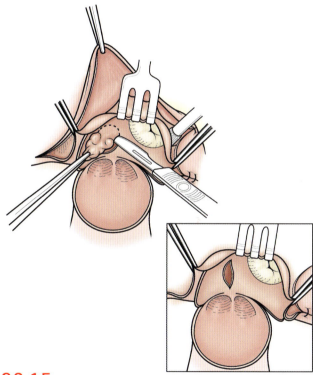

36.15

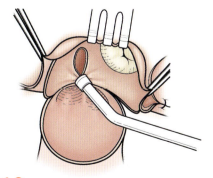

36.16

After the cryolesion is completed (dotted circle), the site of the appendage amputation is closed (**Figure 36.17**). The dashed line represents the site of the final incision, a posterior vertical left atriotomy that extends from the pulmonary vein isolation incision to the mitral valve annulus.

Once the posterior vertical incision is made and all visible atrial myocardial fibers spanning the fat pad of the underlying AV groove have been divided, the coronary sinus is subjected to transmural cryothermia at −60°C for 3 minutes (**Figure 36.18**). Care is taken to avoid applying cryosurgery to the circumflex coronary artery. In addition, if retrograde cardioplegia is used, the cannula should be removed during this portion of the procedure.

A 3 mm cryolesion is placed at the lower end of the incision adjacent to the mitral valve annulus (**Figure 36.19**). The posterior vertical left atriotomy is closed (**Figure 36.20**). The lower portion of the pulmonary vein isolation incision is closed across the posteroinferior free wall of the left atrium (**Figure 36.21**).

Once the lower portion of the pulmonary vein isolation incision has been closed to the level of the atrial septum, the incision again resembles a standard atriotomy in the interatrial groove (**Figure 36.22**). At this point, the septal incision

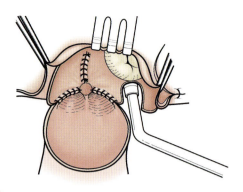

36.19

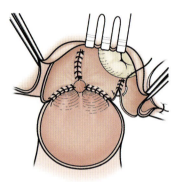

36.20

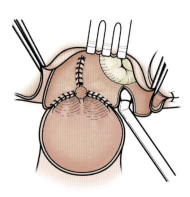

36.17

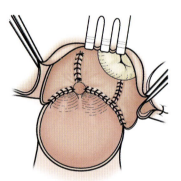

36.21

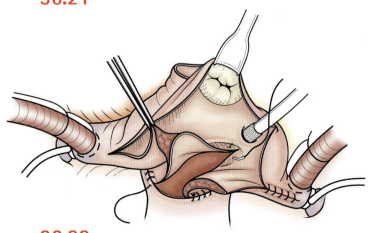

36.18

36.22

is closed beginning at its lower end. The thin portion of the fossa ovalis is closed up to the inferior margin of the anterior limbus (**Figure 36.23**). The left atrial side of the limbus of the fossa ovalis is closed in continuity with the remainder of the superior left atriotomy (**Figure 36.24**). The right side of the limbus of the fossa ovalis is closed in continuity with the portion of the posterior right atrial free wall that is medial

to the posterior longitudinal right atriotomy (**Figure 36.25**). The remainder of the right atrial T incision is closed (**Figure 36.26**). The remainder of the posterior longitudinal right atriotomy is closed (**Figure 36.27**). The lateral right atriotomy and the site of the amputated right atrial appendage are closed in continuity from a lateral to a medial direction (**Figure 36.28**).

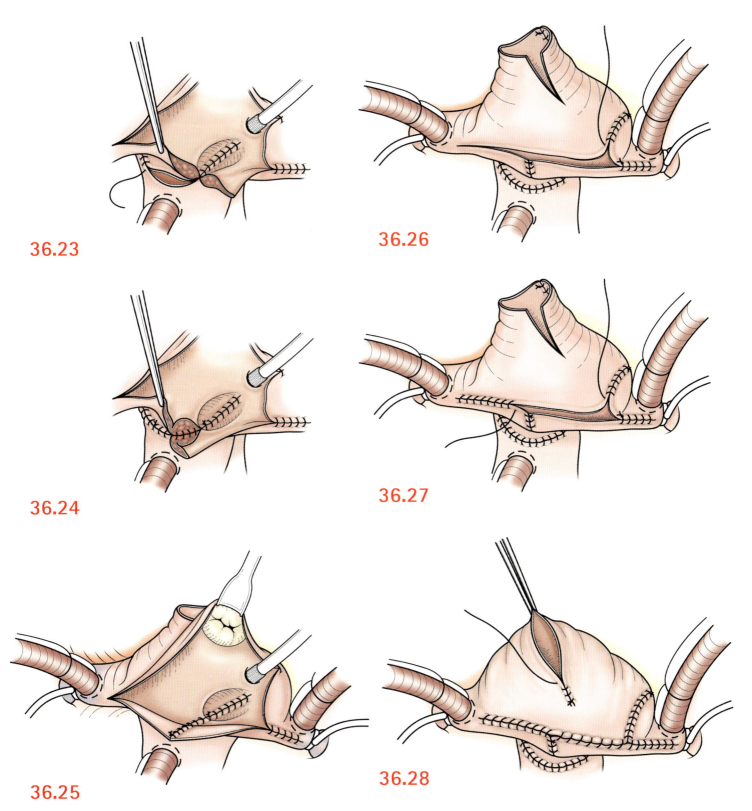

36.23

36.24

36.25

36.26

36.27

36.28

Figure 36.29 shows the appearance of the completed Maze-III procedure.

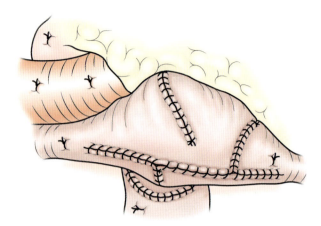

36.29

CLOSING COMMENTS

The Maze-I, II, III, and IV procedures have all had equivalent results on long-term follow-up. The 15-year results for the original cut-and-sew Maze procedures reported by Damiano et al. in 2003 documented an overall success rate of over 90%.[7] That report has been criticized because at the time there were no long-term monitoring devices available for follow-up, and the success rate would undoubtedly have been somewhat lower had those patients been monitored with some of the newer devices. However, the first 69 of those patients returned to Barnes Hospital (now Barnes-Jewish Hospital) 6 months after surgery on no anti-arrhythmic drugs and underwent a full formal electrophysiology study by Dr. Bruce Lindsay, the electrophysiologist who followed them. Dr. Lindsay subjected every patient to the same programed electrical stimulation protocol and burst-pacing protocol that they had been subjected to preoperatively. When atrial fibrillation could not be induced in a single patient, a continuous isoproterenol infusion was initiated and they were again put through the same pacing protocols. Still, not a single patient was inducible into atrial fibrillation. We stopped that practice after 69 patients because Dr. Lindsay said, "I'm wasting my time and the patients' time". At 15 years follow-up, there was no difference in the success rate between those 69 patients and the remainder of the patients who did not have this severe test of procedure efficacy.[7]

An additional, unexpected benefit of the Maze procedure was that the perioperative stroke rate was 0.7% and only one ischemic stroke occurred in the patient cohort on 15 years follow-up. The long-term freedom from stroke could be attributed to the fact that the vast majority of the patients were free of atrial fibrillation or to the absence of the left atrial appendage. However, the only explanation for the excessively low perioperative stroke rate in patients undergoing combined Maze surgery plus multi-valve surgery, CABG, or repair of adult congenital defects, 100 of whom had suffered preoperative strokes, was the absence of the left atrial appendage.

Numerous "Maze modifications" have been championed over the past three decades but none has matched the results of procedures that adhere to the concept of a Maze procedure (Maze-I, II, III, or IV). Unfortunately, the term "Maze procedure" has become generic for almost any surgical procedure that is used to treat AF and this has led many cardiologists, patients, and others to believe that true Maze procedures are not as successful as they actually are. Thus, it is important to understand that all so-called "Maze procedures" are not the same.

REFERENCES

1. Cox JL. The first Maze procedure. *J Thorac Cardiovasc Surg.* 2011; 141(5): 1093–7.
2. Boineau JP, Schuessler RB, Canavan TE, et al. The human atrial pacemaker complex. *J Electrocardiol* (Suppl). 1989; 22: 189–97.
3. Cox JL, Jaquiss RD, Schuessler RB, Boineau JP. Modification of the Maze procedure for atrial flutter and atrial fibrillation. II. Surgical technique of the Maze-III procedure. *J Thorac and Cardiovasc Surg.* 1995; 110(2): 485–95.
4. Cox JL. The minimally invasive Maze-III procedure. *Oper Tech Thorac Cardiovasc Surg.* 2000; 5: 79–92.
5. Gaynor SL, Diodato MD, Prasad SM, et al. A prospective, single-center clinical trial of a modified Cox Maze procedure with bipolar radiofrequency ablation. *J Thorac Cardiovasc Surg.* 2004; 128(4): 535–42.
6. Cox JL. The Maze-III procedure for treatment of atrial fibrillation. In: Sabiston DC (ed). *Atlas of Cardiothoracic Surgery.* Philadelphia: W.B. Saunders Co; 1995, pp. 460–75.
7. Prasad SM, Maniar HS, Camillo CJ, et al. The Cox Maze-III procedure for atrial fibrillation: long-term efficacy in patients undergoing lone versus concomitant procedures. *J Thorac Cardiovasc Surg.* 2003; 126: 1822–8.

37

Cardiac tumors

GABRIEL S. ALDEA AND EDWARD D. VERRIER

PRINCIPLES AND JUSTIFICATION

Primary tumors of the heart are infrequent, often asymptomatic, and much less common than metastatic tumors (20–50-fold less common), with an incidence of less than 0.03% in large autopsy series.[1] Over 75% of cardiac tumors are benign and present with a variety of non-specific clinical signs and symptoms that overlap with many other cardiovascular and systemic disorders. Symptoms are associated with size, location, mobility, propensity to cause intracardiac obstruction or valve incompetence, precipitate arrhythmias or conduction abnormalities, embolize (tumor fragments or clot on its surface) or cause constitutional symptoms. They remain an important consideration in the differential diagnosis of embolism (systemic or pulmonic), congestive heart failure, arrhythmias or conduction defects and syncope. The most common presenting complaints at presentation are: dyspnea (42%); acute embolic event (25%); and chest pain (22%). Notably 64% of patients presented with New York Heart Association (NYHA) class III/IV.[2]

The types and distribution of benign and malignant tumors of the heart are strikingly different in adults and children (Tables 37.1 and 37.2) and vary widely between autopsy studies and series of surgical resections.

Of all primary cardiac tumors, approximately 25% are malignant. In adults, most malignant cardiac tumors are sarcomas, commonly angiosarcoma as shown in Table 37.2. The right atrium is most commonly involved. Patients present with congestive heart failure, hemopericardium with or without tamponade, myocardial ischemia, or arrhythmias. In children and infants, the most common primary malignancy is a rhabdomyosarcoma. Children are more likely to present with complications related to intracavitary extension. The role of surgery in the management of primary cardiac malignancy is generally to establish a definitive diagnosis and guide multi-modality adjunctive therapy. Clinically, patients with sarcomas display a rapid downhill course and most patients die within a year of diagnosis, despite adjunctive multi-modality chemotherapy, radiation therapy, and resection of hematogenous spread. Rare long-term survival has been reported in patients with primary cardiac lymphomas.

Neoplasia of the heart and pericardium are much more likely to be secondary or metastatic, rather than primary. Reports of prevalence derived from large autopsy studies of patients with known malignancy demonstrate cardiac and/or pericardial involvement in up to one in five patients. Metastases may be seen as a result of either direct invasion or extension (such as lung cancer or mesothelioma), through lymphatic channels (such as Hodgkin's or large cell lymphoma) or via hematogenous routes (such as breast, melanoma, pancreas, gastric, and renal malignancies).

Table 37.1 Incidence of benign cardiac tumors

Tumor type	Adults (n = 241)	Children (n = 78)
Myxoma	49%	15.5%
Lipoma	19%	–
Papillary fibroelastoma	17%	–
Hemangioma	5%	5%
Rhabdomyoma	< 1%	45%
Teratoma	1%	14%
Fibroma	2%	15.5%
AV node mesothelioma	4%	4%
Other		

Modified from McAllister & Fegnolio, 1978.[3]

Table 37.2 Incidence of primary malignant cardiac tumors

Tumor type	Adults (n = 117)	Children (n = 9)
Angiosarcoma	33%	–
Rhabdomyosarcoma	21%	33%
Mesothelioma	16%	–
Fibrosarcoma	11%	11%
Malignant lymphoma	6%	–
Osteosarcoma	4%	–
Thymoma	3%	–
Neurogenic sarcoma	3%	11%
Other	3%	44%

Modified from Allard et al., 1996.[4]

Diagnostic evaluation

Transthoracic echocardiography (TTE), with its markedly improved resolution and quality, remains the procedure of choice for screening and initial assessment of intracardiac tumors. TTE has superb resolution of endocardial and intracavitary lesions and can demonstrate tissue characteristics including size, mobility, attachment, relation, and involvement of adjacent valve and chamber pressures. Transesophageal echocardiography (TEE) and 3D imaging further improves sensitivity, specificity, and spacial resolution.[4] Ultra-fast gated CT and cardiac MRI are complementary modalities. These modalities are better at defining tissue characteristics, assessing more fully thoracic, paracardiac mediastinal structures and pathology, and pericardial involvement, and are also better at differentiating thrombus from tumor. Positron emission tomography (PET) is also useful in identifying patients with metastatic tumors.[5,6]

PRIMARY BENIGN TUMORS OF THE HEART

Myxomas

Myxomas are the most common primary tumors of the heart and represent 80–90% of all primary cardiac tumors in adults.[2] Cardiac tumors, particularly myxomas, have a propensity to present with systemic manifestations that are often confused with collagen vascular diseases. These include fever, cachexia, malaise, arthralgias, rash, clubbings, Raynauld's, and atrial fibrillation. Laboratory evaluations may show elevated sedimentation rate, thrombocytopenia, and circulation antimyocardial antibodies. The systemic constitutional symptoms are thought to be due to secretion by the tumor cells of Interleukin-6,[7] a cytokine known to be a major promoter of acute phase response that leads to the activation and amplification of the inflammatory, complement, and clotting cascades. Although originally thought to represent myxomatous degeneration of organized thrombi, most experts recognize atrial myxoams as true neoplasms. Neuroendocrine markers have been identified in over 60% of these tumors, suggesting an endocardial nerve tissue origin.[8]

Myxomatous tumors arise from the endocardium and are often pedunculated, gelatinous, occasionally villous and friable, extending into the cardiac chamber. Embolization of tumor fragments and thrombi from the tumor surface is frequent. Over 80% of myxomas arise from the left atrium and over 90% are solitary.[9] Systemic embolization can result in infarction and hemorrhage of viscera, heart, brain, and extremities. These peripheral emboli can sometimes mimic and be confused with the presentation of infectious endocarditis and vasculitis. A biopsy of the skin can sometimes demonstrate intravascular tumor emboli. Right-sides tumors can also result in tumor emboli with secondary pulmonary hypertension and rarely in Cor Pulmonale. Pedunculated left atrial myxomas are mobile, with stalk often originating near the limbus of the fossa ovale. These tumors often prolapse across the orifice of the mitral valve and by obstructing flow across the valve orifice present with signs and symptoms of mitral stenosis or insufficiency.

Patients with myxomas often present with symptoms including dyspnea, orthopnea, paroxysmal nocturneal dyspnea, pulmonary edema, cough, hemoptysis, and fatigue.[3] Typically, symptoms are intermittent in nature and are characteristically elicited or accentuated by change in body position. On physical examination, a loud S1 is noted, with S4 (denoting congestive heart failure), and a systolic or diastolic murmur heard best at the apex consistent with mitral (or tricuspid with right-sided tumors) stenosis or regurgitation. Right atrial tumors frequently present with signs of right heart failure including peripheral edema, ascites, hepatomegaly, and prominent jugular venous pulse a-waves, and with murmurs consistent with obstruction to tricuspid valve flow. Familial cardiac myxomas constitute 10% of all myxomas and have an autosomal dominant transmission. The familial myxoma pattern is referred to as Carney's syndrome and consists of a cluster of symptoms including multiple spotty pigmentation, peripheral myxomas (breast and skin), and endocrine hyperactivity (pigmented adrenocortical disease with Cushing's syndrome, testicular Sertoli cell tumors or pituitary adenomas).[10, 11]

Lipomas

Lipomas are the second most common primary cardiac tumor occurring in adults. These tumors are often encapsulated, and occur in the subendocardium or subepicardium. Subendocardial tumors are frequently located in the interatrial septum. Symptoms result from the specific tumor size that can cause intracavitary obstruction or rhythm disturbance. Lipomatous hypertrophy of the atrial septum may be confused with cardiac tumors. It is commonly located in the limbus of the fossa ovalis and is associated with advanced age, obesity, and occasionally supraventricular tachycardia.

Papillary fibroelastomas

Papillary fibroelastomas are smaller pedunculated tumors with frond-like projections emanating from a short stalk, which share with myxomas a high incidence (> 30%) of systemic embolization, thought to be a consequence of thrombus formation on the tumor surface.[12, 13] They frequently arise from valves (75% of all valvular tumors, invariably left-sided valves, and 90% involve the aortic valve but are rarely any associated valve dysfunction), and more rarely involve papillary muscles, chords, or the endocardium. They are usually solitary. These tumors are increasingly recognized, perhaps because of improvements in imaging technologies (especially TEE), and in many series now surpass lipomas in incidence. Pathologically, tumors have a short pedicle and a "sea anemone-like" appearance.

Rhabdomyomas

Rhabdomyomas are the most common primary cardiac tumors in children and infants. They occur in equal frequency in the right ventricular, left ventricular, and septal myocardium, and nearly always occur as multiple lesions. Tumors are frequently intracavitary, result in obstructive symptoms, and are associated with a high incidence of ventricular pre-excitation and Wolff-Parkinson-White syndrome. These tumors are frequently associated with tuberous sclerosis, a familial syndrome presenting with diffuse hematomas, epilepsy, mental retardation, and adenoma sebaceum.[13] Spontaneous regression in size and number are commonly seen in patients under 4 years of age.

Fibromas

Fibromas are the second most common primary cardiac tumor seen in children. The tumors are characteristically solitary, are well circumscribed with central calcification, frequently involve the anterior free wall of the left ventricle, and have a biological behavior similar to fibromatous tumors at other sites.

PREOPERATIVE ASSESSMENT

The complementary modalities of TTE, TEE, CT, and MRI not only demonstrate the specific lesion, its appearance, size, and location (chamber, relation to valves, septum, stalk etc.) but also give very important anatomical information to plan appropriate surgical approaches, when indicated. Spiral ultra-fast CT or MRI is helpful to delineate other associated mediastinal pathology. Lipomas can be further identified by their characteristic density (Hodenshield units) on MRI.

Pathologically, the diagnosis of myxoma is made by identifying patterns of "lipidic" cells embedded in myxoid stroma rich in glycoseaminoglycans. The histological appearance of fibroelastomas demonstrate multiple papillary with a collagen core surrounded by elastic fibers and endocardial endothelium. Rhabdomyomas are grossly yellow-gray, are well circumscribed, and microscopically differ from normal myocardium by clusters of abnormal cells – "spider cells", large cells with a central cytoplasmic cell, suspended in fine fibrillar processes radiating to the periphery. The cytoplasm is rich in glycogen. These tumors are myocardial hamartomatous malformations rather than true neoplasms. Fibromas are typically encapsulated with a whorled appearance and microscopically demonstrate fibroblasts admixed with fibrous tissue and collagen. Lipomas are encapsulated as well and microscopically are composed of mature fat cells admixed with connective tissue and occasionally muscle.

OPERATION

Although histologically benign, most cardiac tumors are potentially lethal as a result of intracavitary and valvular obstruction, embolization, and rhythm disturbances. Complete operative excision is the treatment of choice for most cardiac tumors. Although some rare epicardial tumors can be excised without extracorporeal circulation, the removal of most tumors is done using the heart-lung machine. The major surgical consideration is avoiding manipulation and embolization, complete excision while trying to preserve adequate ventricular myocardium, conduction system, and valve function. Atrial myxomas are resected with their stalk and with at least a 1 cm portion of surrounding fossa ovale, to minimize risk of recurrence.[14, 15] Recurrence and the appearance of a second metachronous tumor is rare (less than 7%) except in patients with familial myxomas, Carney's syndrome, and synchronous tumors in which the incidence of tumor can reach 20%. Resection of papillary fibroelastomas typically requires shaving off its base or a localized valve resection with valve preservation. Recurrence after localized resection is extremely rare.

Left atrial myxoma

A myxoma should be resected with its stalk and with at least a 1 cm portion of surrounding fossa ovale or atrial wall to minimize risk of recurrence from a pretumorous focus (**Figures 37.1** and **37.2**). With the patient on full

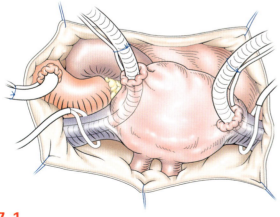

37.1

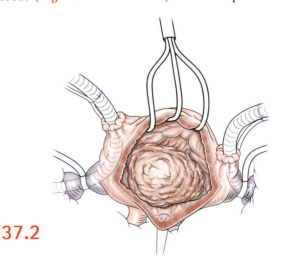

37.2

cardiopulmonary bypass using bicaval cannulation, and with the aorta cross-clamped, the left atrium is opened just anterior to the right pulmonary veins. The myxoma is carefully visualized and partially retracted through the atriotomy, exposing its base or stalk, which is resected with a small margin of normal atrial septal tissue or atrial wall. Especially in the case of a myxoma with a broad, sessile base, partial-thickness excision of the septum may be adequate. After excision of the myxoma and repair of the atrial septum or wall is completed, the atrial and ventricular cavities are irrigated to ensure that no residual tumor fragments remain in the heart. The left atriotomy is then closed in the usual fashion, with left-heart de-airing maneuvers undertaken as the aortic cross-clamp is removed.

Alternate exposure for a particularly large left atrial myxoma can be achieved via a right atrial approach (**Figures 37.3**

and **37.4**). Although this approach facilitates examination of the left atrium for residual tumor fragments and multicentric tumors, the transatrial septal incision may increase the occurrence of postoperative atrial arrhythmias. After establishing full cardiopulmonary bypass, the right atrium is opened and the right atrial cavity carefully examined for tumor involvement. A septal incision is made anterior to the fossa ovalis, and the left atrium is entered. Myxoma excision then proceeds as described previously.

Papillary fibroelastoma

A papillary fibroelastoma arising on the anterior leaflet of the mitral valve is shown in **Figures 37.5** and **37.6**. This tumor resembles a sea anemone with multiple papillary fronds. As

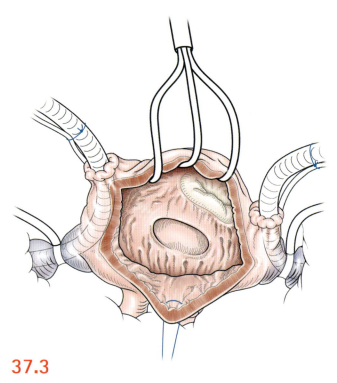

37.3

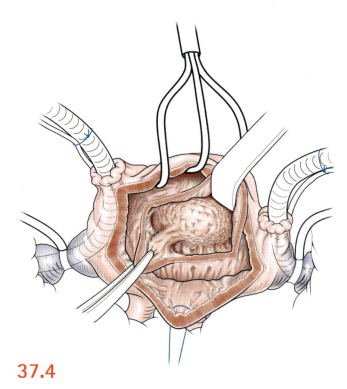

37.4

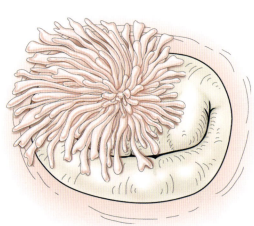

37.5

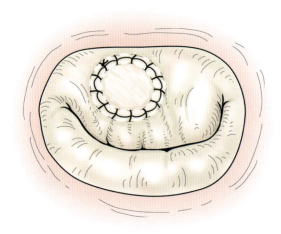

37.6

shown, the tumor is attached to the anterior mitral valve leaflet by a relatively short pedicle. After resection of the tumor with a portion of the leaflet, autologous or bovine pericardial patch repair is performed to reconstruct the anterior mitral leaflet.

Primary malignant cardiac tumors

Of all primary cardiac tumors 25% are malignant. In adults, almost all malignant cardiac tumors are sarcomas, most commonly angiosarcomas (Table 37.2). Malignant tumors occur in adults most commonly in the fourth decade of life and have a similar incidence in men and women. The right atrium is most commonly involved. Patients present with symptoms of congestive heart failure, hemopericardium with or without tamponade, and, rarely, myocardial ischemia from local coronary artery involvement or arrhythmias. In children and infants the most common primary cardiac malignancy is a rhabdomyosarcoma. Clinical presentation more commonly presents in children with complications resulting from intracavitary extension with obstructive symptoms. Clinically, patients with sarcomas display a rapid downhill course and most patients die within the first year of diagnosis despite adjunctive chemotherapy and radiation therapy because of the tumor's propensity for hematogenous spread. The role of surgery is generally to establish a definitive diagnosis and guide multi-modality adjunctive therapy.[17,18] Rare longer term survivals have been reported in patients with primary cardiac lymphomas.

Management of metastatic cardiac tumors

Most metastatic cardiac lesions are clinically silent and found only at autopsy. Pericardial and cardiac metastasis should be suspected whenever a patient with known malignancy develops new murmurs, electrocardiographic conduction delays, arrhythmias, congestive heart failure, or pericardial effusions. Metastatic disease has to be differentiated from the effects of concomitant cardiac toxicity from mediastinal radiation and chemotherapeutic agents such as the antracycline family, and those of infectious endocarditis that can occur in these immunosuppressed patients with indwelling central intravenous lines.

Cardiac compromise can arise from:

1. Direct tumor extension from the lung and mediastinum into the pericardium leading to pericardial effusion, tamponade or regional extra cardiac compression of cardiac chambers or coronary vessels. Depending on the degree of pericardial involvement (regional or diffuse), myocardial compression, and size rapidity of pericardial effusion, this can lead to either a restrictive or constrictive presentation, with exertional dyspnea, tachycardia, cough, and chest pain, with or without evidence of pulsus paradoxus and clinical signs of tamponade.

2. Direct intramyocardial involvement (either focal or diffuse) resulting in arrhythmia or conduction abnormalities.
3. Tumor growth into the cardiac chambers, resulting in obstructive phenomena and embolization such as congestive heart failure or vena caval obstruction with its associated facial edema, headaches, prominent collateral circulation, hepatic congestion, and peripheral edema.
4. Complications related to circulating tumor mediators leading to hypercoagulable states, which can present with non-bacterial thrombotic endocarditis manifesting with embolization in the absence of fever and leukocytosis.

Diagnostic evaluation of metastatic cardiac involvement

Most patients with thoracic and other malignancies can be evaluated by spiral, ultra-fast CT, MRI, and PET scans, which can demonstrate associate pulmonary and mediastinal pathologies. The diagnosis of secondary cardiac involvement, however, is most definitively confirmed by echocardiography, either transthoracic or transesophageal. This modality not only demonstrates the degree of pericardial and myocardial involvement but also allows physiological assessment. The definitive confirmation of metastatic cardiac disease or pericardial involvement frequently requires acquisition of tissue for diagnosis (biopsy or cytology) when appropriate.

Management of metastatic cardiac involvement

Initial treatment of malignant pericardial disease addresses the hemodynamic significance and hemodynamic consequences of the pericardial effusion with either open surgical or percutaneous echocardiographic guided drainage. Whereas pericardial effusions from lymphomas respond frequently to chemotherapy, those caused by lung cancer usually requires surgical drainage by either a subxyphoid or video-assisted thoracoscopic surgery (VATS) (anterior thoracotomy or thoracoscopy) approaches. Although surgical resection of a solitary cardiac metastasis may prolong survival, the main goal of surgical intervention is to establish a definitive diagnosis or palliate complications of an advanced systemic disease.

OUTCOME

As previously noted, benign primary cardiac tumors rarely recur. Only rarely are myxomas multicentric. Malignant degeneration of primary benign tumors is very unlikely. Because of progressive enlargement with obstruction and risk of embolization, complete excision of intracardiac tumors is recommended.

Primary malignant and metastatic tumors are associated with poor prognosis. Therapy directed at such malignancies should be diagnostic and palliative in nature.

REFERENCES

1. Lam KY, Dickens P, Chan AC. Tumors of the heart: a 20 year experience and review of over 12485 consecutive autopsies. *Arch Pathol Lab Med.* 1993; 117(10): 1027–31.
2. El Bardissi AW, Dearini JA, Mullany RC, et al. Survival after resection of primary cardiac tumors: a 48 year experience. *Circulation.* 2008; 118: S7–S15.
3. McAllister HA, Jr, Fegnolio JJ, Jr. Tumors of the cardiovascular system. In Hartman WH, Cowan W (eds.). *Atlas of tumor pathology.* Sec. Series, Fasc. 15, Washington, DC: Armed Forces Institute of Pathology; 1978.
4. Allard MF, Taylor GP, Wilson JE, et al. Primary cardiac tumors. In Goldhaber S, Braunwald E (eds.). *Atlas of heart diseases.* Philadelphia: Current Medicine; 1996: pp. 15.1–15.22.
5. Gulati G, Sharma S, Kothari SS, et al. Comparison of echo and MRI in imaging and evaluation of intracardiac masses. *Cardiovasc Intevent Radiol.* 2004; 27: 459–67.
6. Aaroz PA, Mulvagh SL, Tazelaart HD, et al. CT and MR of benign cardiac neoplasms with echocardiographic correlation. *Radiographics.* 2000; 20: 1303–19.
7. Jourdan, M. Bataille R, Sequin, J, et al. Constitutive production of IL-6 and immunologic features in cardiac myxomas. *Arthritis Reum.* 1990; 33: 398.
8. Kriekler DM, Rhode J, Davis MJ, et al. Atrial myxoma: a tumor in search of its origins. *Br Heart J.* 1992; 99: 1203.
9. Sabiston DC, Jr, Hattler BG, Jr. Tumors of the heart. In Sabiston DC, Jr, Spencer FC (eds.). *Gibbon's surgery of the chest.* 4th edn. Philadelphia: WB Saunders Company; 1983.
10. McCarthy PM, Piehler JM, Schaff HV, et al. The significance of multiple, recurrent and "complex" cardiac myxomas. *Thorac Cardiovasc Surg,* 1986; 91: 389.
11. Carney JA. Differences between nonfamilial and familial cardiac myxomas. *Am J Surg Path.* 1985; 9: 53.
12. McFadden PM, Lacy JR. Intracardial papillary fibroelastoma: an occult cause of embolic neurologic deficit. *Ann Thorac Surg.* 1987; 43: 667.l
13. Howard RA, Aldea GS, Shapira OM, et al. Papillary fibroelastoma: increasing recognition of a surgical disease. *Ann Thorac Surg.* 1999; 65: 1881–5.
14. Burke AP, Virmani R. Cardiac rhabdomyoma: a clinicopathologic study. *Mod Pathol.* 1991; 4: 70.
15. Castaneda AR, Varco RL. Tumors of the heart: surgical considerations. *Am J Cardiol.* 1968; 21: 357.
16. Chitwood WR, Jr. Cardiac neoplasms: current diagnosis, pathology and therapy. *J Card Surg.* 1988; 3: 119.
17. Bear PA, Moodie DS. Malignant primary cardiac tumors: the Cleveland Clinic experience, 1956–1986. *Chest.* 1987; 92: 860.
18. Murphy MC, Sweeney MS, Putram JB, et al. Surgical treatment of cardiac tumors: a 25 year experience. *Ann Thorac Surg.* 1990; 49: 612.

38

Pacers–BV pacers

MICHAEL J. GRUSHKO, ANDREW KRUMERMAN, AND JOSEPH J. DEROSE JR.

HISTORY

Congestive heart failure (CHF) results from a variety of different diseases affecting the ventricular myocardium. Left ventricular (LV) remodeling occurs, and ultimately, systolic dysfunction ensues with symptoms relating to elevated LV diastolic filling pressures and diminished cardiac output. Despite decongestive therapy and neuro-hormonal modification, morbidity and mortality remain high. Heart failure hospitalizations make up approximately 20% of all hospitalizations of people over the age of 65. Moreover, CHF patients are at a higher risk of malignant arrhythmias and sudden cardiac death. Several randomized controlled trials have demonstrated that ICDs reduce mortality related to the decreased risk of sustained ventricular arrhythmia. However, ICDs do not prevent CHF exacerbations, and nor do they improve symptoms independent of medical therapy.

The conduction system is often affected by the myopathic process as well. One-third of CHF patients develop a left bundle branch block (LBBB) resulting in abnormal intraventricular depolarization and ventricular electromechanical delay or dyssynchrony. Mechanically inefficient contraction within the LV results in reduced systolic function, decreased cardiac output and blood pressure, ventricular dilatation, and functional mitral regurgitation.[1]

Cardiac resynchronization therapy (CRT) allows for simultaneous pacing of both the left and right ventricles resulting in more efficient LV contraction. Multiple randomized controlled trials have demonstrated that CRT can improve LV systolic function, functional capacity, and quality of life. Moreover, CRT therapy has been shown to reduce CHF hospitalization as well as mortality.

In more than 90% of cases, transvenous biventricular pacing can be achieved. Standard endocardial right atrial (RA) and ventricular (RV) leads are placed. The LV lead is placed in a postero-lateral or lateral coronary sinus (CS) tributary, achieving biventricular pacing with simultaneous contraction of the septal and lateral LV walls. However, technical limitations owing to individual CS and coronary venous anatomy may require a surgical epicardial approach.

Historically this was done via an anterolateral thoracotomy, which is limited by its morbidity in these frail CHF patients and its limited access to the postero-lateral surface of the LV. Our group and others developed the robotic, totally endoscopic approach as a minimally invasive option for posterolateral lead placement in patients with a failure of transvenous CS cannulation.

PRINCIPLES AND JUSTIFICATION

The goal of CRT (biventricular) pacing is to restore mechanical LV synchrony for more efficient ventricular contraction. The transvenous procedure requires placement of RA and RV leads using standard technique followed by CS cannulation. Coronary venous anatomy is studied using retrograde venography and a suitable lateral (or postero-lateral, free wall) branch is selected for LV lead insertion. The operator must choose a venous branch while considering pacing threshold, diaphragmatic stimulation, and lead stability. If performed surgically, the goal is to obtain access to the postero-lateral LV epicardium.

Appropriate patient selection is essential for achieving optimal benefit and minimizing risk, and is based primarily on the joint ACC/AHA device implantation guidelines, which have recently been updated.[2] CRT is clearly indicated (Class I recommendation) in patients with a left ventricular ejection fraction (LVEF) < 35%, in sinus rhythm, with an LBBB and QRS > 150 ms, who are New York Heart Association (NYHA) Class II, III, or ambulatory Class IV despite being on optimal medical therapy. It is also indicated with the above prerequisites and a LBBB with QRS 120–149, or a non-LBBB pattern with a QRS of > 150 ms and Class III symptoms (Class IIa). CRT is *not recommended* for patients with EF > 35%, or in patients with EF < 35 but with NYHA Class I, II symptoms, with a non-LBBB ECG pattern, and a QRS duration < 150 ms. In addition, CRT is not indicated in those patients whose comorbidities and/or frailty limit survival with good functional capacity to less than 1 year.

Complications related to transvenous device implantation

Complications related to transvenous device implantation in general include pneumothorax and/or hemothorax relating to access site puncture, cardiac perforation during lead placement, pocket hematoma, and/or infection. Myocardial infarction, stroke, death, and complications due to anesthesia are rare but must be discussed when obtaining informed consent. Complications specific to endocardial LV lead placement include CS dissection or perforation, extra-cardiac stimulation by the LV lead such as diaphragmatic pacing, and acute heart failure. A small risk of renal injury or allergic reaction due to IV contrast injection must also be disclosed. Overall complications rate is approximately 2–4%, and major complication rate 1–2%.

Complications related to robotic LV lead placement

Complications related to robotic LV lead placement include a 1–2% risk of bleeding and/or infection. General anesthesia can precipitate a CHF exacerbation in patients with a very low LVEF. Finally, intercostal neuropathy can be seen in up to 5% of patients undergoing thoracoscopy.

PREOPERATIVE ASSESSMENT AND PREPARATION

The preoperative patient evaluation should substantiate the indications for CRT implantation above. Baseline 12-lead ECG and routine blood testing including type and screen, CBC, chemistry, and coagulation panel must be obtained. Medications should be reviewed in detail as well as allergies and contraindications to IV contrast injection. Recent or acute febrile illness should be explored, and it is prudent to postpone the procedure until afebrile and aseptic. Current volume status and ability to tolerate supine positioning for an extended period of time should be ascertained.

Transvenous approach

Patients should be fasting for at least 6–8 hours pre-procedure. Based on operator preference, a 20 gauge peripheral IV line should be placed *on the side* of implantation to facilitate possible venography with contrast to facilitate localization of the axillary and subclavian veins, and/or to confirm a cephalic vein.

Patients on anticoagulation or on antiplatelet therapy have a higher risk of pocket hematoma formation. In our laboratory aspirin and plavix therapies are continued peri-operatively. Warfarin or thrombin inhibitors are discontinued several days prior to implantation. In patients with moderate to high risk of thrombosis (e.g. mechanical

heart valves) warfarin therapy may be continued to avoid interruption in anticoagulation. Implantation may be performed safely if the international normalized ratio (INR) is maintained in low therapeutic range (2–2.5). The utility of pre-implantation prophylactic IV antibiotics covering skin flora is well established.

Surgical approach

Robotic LV lead insertion for biventricular pacing should be viewed as an elective procedure that is performed under general anesthesia with single lung ventilation. It is imperative to obtain a careful history regarding any prior cardiac or left chest surgery. Multiple prior pericardial entries are not a contraindication to robotic LV lead insertion given its posterior approach. It is important to know the location and patency of any coronary bypass grafts. Previous left chest surgery may require conversion to a mini-posterior thoracotomy. Prior left lung resection, however, is an absolute contraindication to a robotic approach.

A PA and lateral chest X-ray is necessary to evaluate the cardiac/pulmonary ratio and the posterior operating space. To allow for identification of the latest point of mechanical LV activation as the target zone for LV lead placement, we obtain a transthoracic echocardiogram with tissue synchronization imaging (TSI) in all patients preoperatively. This allows the surgeon to tailor his/her approach to the most ideal LV epicardial lead placement.

Finally, in patients with underlying pulmonary disease, an assessment of the patient's ability to tolerate single lung ventilation is critical. Therefore, a room air blood gas and pulmonary function tests can be helpful in determining a patient's candidacy for robotic LV lead insertion.

ANESTHESIA

Transvenous approach

CRT device implantation may be performed using conscious sedation. A combination of midazolam and fentanyl is generally used, in addition to liberal local anesthetic. Our group uses bupivacaine for local anesthesia given its longer half-life. Care must be taken to allow the medications to take effect prior to starting the procedure, and to tailor dosages on an individual basis. Standard precautions for administering conscious sedation should be followed. High-risk patients such as those with sleep apnea may require positive pressure ventilation to allow adequate and safe sedation.

Surgical approach

General anesthesia induction in patients with poor cardiac reserve, with or without underlying coronary artery disease, can potentially be complicated. Large bore IVs and a right radial arterial line (as the patient is in the right lateral decubitus position) are useful for hemodynamic monitoring and maintenance. Central access is reserved for those patients who may need inotropic support during the procedure.

Left lung isolation is achieved with a bronchoscopically placed double-lumen endotracheal tube. If this is difficult, owing to the relative large size and non-compliance of the tube, alternatives such as the Univent (Fuji Systems Corporation, Tokyo, Japan) or a bronchial blocker can be utilized to achieve single lung ventilation. The patient is then placed in the right lateral decubitus position. The procedure is done with the help of transesophageal echocardiography to monitor volume status, to assist in identifying the optimal location for the LV lead, and to assess the atrial appendage for clot prior to testing the defibrillation threshold of the ICD if placed. The majority of patients are extubated in the operating room and transferred to a monitored setting for observation.

In both the transvenous and surgical approaches, patients with a pre-existing ICD must have tachycardia detection and therapy deactivated prior to the procedure.

OPERATION

Transvenous approach

The operative procedure can be broadly divided into four parts:

1. venous access;
2. CS and branch vein cannulation;
3. LV lead placement; and
4. pocket management.

Following routine sterile preparation, draping, and institution of conscious sedation and local anesthesia, access to the venous system is obtained. We generally perform cephalic vein cut-down for insertion of the RA and RV leads. The axillary or subclavian vein is used for LV lead insertion. There is wide variability in the approach to access. Having a separate insertion site for the LV lead reduces the chance of displacement during manipulation of the RA or RV leads. Many operators inject 10–15 ml of intravenous contrast via a peripheral vein on the ipsilateral arm to visualize the cephalic and axillary veins prior to obtaining access (**Figure 38.1a**).

An incision approximately 3 fingerbreadths long is made over the delto-pectoral (DP) groove, with a medial slant of the cephalad incision to allow for easier axillary vein access. Blunt dissection is performed down to the DP groove, usually noticeable with a stripe of fatty tissue between the deltoid and the pectoralis major muscles (**Figure 38.1b and c**). The cephalic vein is identified and cleaned. Using a right angle clamp, two 0-ethibond ligatures are placed along the distal aspect of the vein and tied to occlude flow. These ties will also serve as anchoring ties for the future RA and RV leads should the vein remain intact. A hemostatic tie is placed over the proximal portion of the vein in anticipation of backbleeding post lead insertion, and at this point is clamped without

tension on the proximal vein. Partial venotomy is performed using iris scissors or a number 11 scalpel blade, held open by forceps, vein pick, or mosquito clamp. Two guidewires are inserted through the vein and advanced until the distal portion is visualized in the SVC on flouroscopy. Peel-away sheaths can then be placed over each guidewire to allow for the RA and RV lead insertion sequentially.

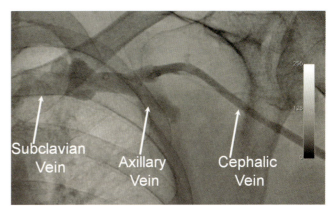

38.1a

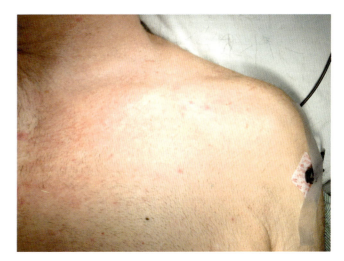

38.1b

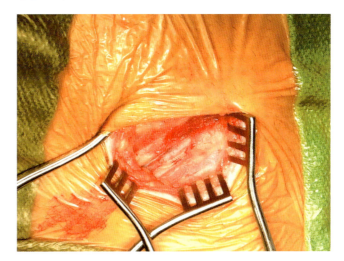

38.1c

Prior to placing the RV or RA leads, access for LV lead insertion is obtained. Using the method of Belott[3] for axillary venous access, a micropuncture needle is advanced under fluoroscopy to the confluence of the clavicle and the first rib, using the wires placed via the cephalic vein. Using this method, the needle should not be advanced beyond the medial border of the first rib for risk of pneumothorax. One can also use a peripheral upper extremity venogram or US guidance for axillary access, or, alternatively, use the seldinger technique for subclavian access. Following venous access, a long guide-wire (180 cm) is inserted and advanced to the IVC (to ensure venous vs arterial cannulation) in preparation for CS guide insertion. A figure-eight stitch is often placed around the wire insertion site to ensure hemostasis following guide catheter removal. Two non-absorbable sutures are tied to the pectoralis muscle near the insertion site and a few millimeters distally, which are used to anchor the LV lead.

After the RV and RA leads are placed and temporarily affixed in place, attention is now turned to the CS and branch vein access. There are multiple delivery systems for CS leads. Guide catheters are designed specifically to cannulate the CS and provide support for delivery of a LV lead to the target branch vein. A complete review of the various guide catheters used for CS and branch vein cannulation is not within the scope of this chapter and may be found elsewhere.[4] At our center, most operators use a CS guide catheter along with a Terumo wire to cannulate the CS. The guide catheter is positioned near the CS os and gentle counterclockwise rotation allows CS cannulation. Once engaged, the wire is advanced to the anterior portion or a branch vessel (**Figure 38.2**). Prior to advancing the guide catheter or guide wire into the CS the operator should ensure that the tip of the catheter is posteriorly positioned in the RAO projection and laterally positioned in the LAO projection. Some operators find it helpful to inject

contrast through the guide catheter to localize the CS os and assist with cannulation.

With the long terumo wire in the anterior portion of the CS or a branch vessel, the outer sheath is gently positioned securely in the body of the CS (**Figure 38.3a**). Retrograde venography of the CS is then performed via a balloon tipped catheter. Depending on the delivery system used, the guide-wire may need to be removed for this step. The balloon catheter is positioned at the tip of the outer sheath, which is then retracted until the balloon tip is out of the distal os of the sheath. With the balloon inflated, approximately 15 cc of contrast is used for retrograde venography in both the RAO and LAO views (**Figure 38.3b and c**). It is important

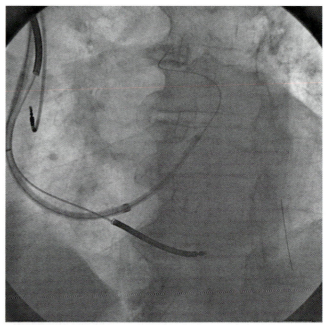

38.3a

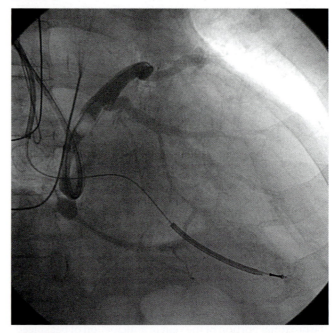

38.2

38.3b

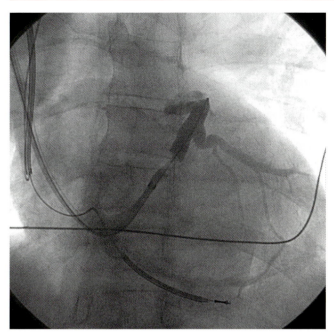

38.3c

to deflate the balloon in between and after the injections. A target vein ideally is one that is posterolateral to lateral (free wall), large enough to accommodate a lead, but small enough for the lead to be able to be securely anchored. The type of LV lead is chosen based on the target vein.

With the target vein selected, LV lead placement can be attempted directly using a variety of lead stylets and/or angioplasty wires. A second or inner guide catheter with different angulations may be necessary to help sub-select a particular venous branch based on the anatomical take-off of the branch os.[4] Once sub-selected with the lead or an inner sheath in the

target vein, the wire is advanced to a relatively secure position and the LV lead is pushed out of the sheath. In **Figure 38.4a**, an inner sheath with a 90-degree angulation is used to direct a guidewire and pacing lead into the target vein. Often, telescoping over the wire (pulling wire back while advancing the lead) is necessary to move distally in the target vein. Once in place, lead threshold is tested and phrenic nerve stimulation or direct diaphragmatic stimulation is evaluated with high output pacing. Bipolar and quadripolar leads may be used to overcome diaphragmatic stimulation by changing the vector of depolarization. This is sometimes referred to as virtual lead repositioning and may be accomplished postoperatively using a programmer without physically moving the lead to another location. With the LV lead in place and testing satisfactory, a straight stylet is placed in the lead to provide stability for removal of the outer and/or the inner sheaths without displacing the LV lead (**Figure 38.4b**). Guide catheter removal is performed using a peel-away or slitting technique. Careful attention to the LV lead while removing the sheath is essential to avoid displacement.

After confirmation that the LV lead has remained in place, the stylet is removed carefully, and the lead is tied down via previously placed anchoring sutures. A second pair of anchoring ties is placed either around an intact cephalic vein or via muscle tie for the RA and RV leads. A subcutaneous pocket is created inferomedial to the incision site, approximately 8 cm deep and 6 cm wide. The pocket is flushed with sterile saline or antibiotic solution and checked for bleeding. The pulse generator is placed onto the sterile field and all leads verified and connected to the pulse generator. The pulse generator is placed into the subcutaneous pocket and device interrogation is performed to ensure satisfactory sensing and pacing from all leads. Patients receiving CRT ICDs then undergo defibrillation threshold testing.

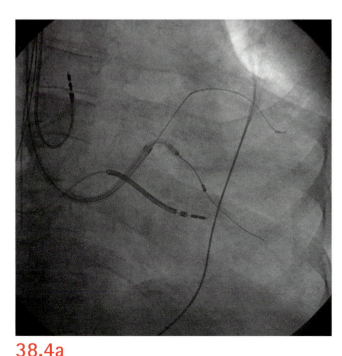

38.4a

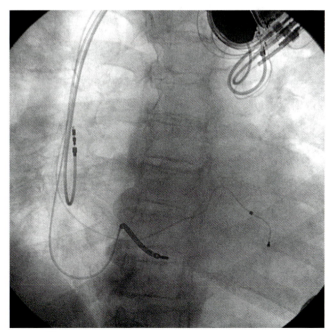

38.4b

The wound is closed in three layers. A 2.0 vicryl with interrupted sutures for the deep layer is important in preventing the device from angling upwards and causing tension on the skin, with erosion a possible future complication. A middle layer, using 3-0 vicryl, is next used for optimal skin opposition. Many operators will use a continuous stitch as opposed to interrupted in this layer. Finally, the subcuticular layer is performed with a continuous stitch using 3-0 or 4-0 vicryl, or 3-0 monocryl. Steri-strips aid in keeping the wound edges opposed.

Surgical epicardial approach

The patient is placed in the full posterolateral thoracotomy position such that the patient's back is aligned with the left side of the operating table with the help of a sand bag. The camera port is placed in the seventh intercostal space (ICS) in the posterior axillary line. Next, an anterior working port is made and an 11 mm soft port is inserted. This port is created under direct vision using the robotic camera in a hand-held, thoracosopic fashion. The port is placed in the anterior axillary line and is used to create a subcutaneous pocket for storage and later retrieval of the LV leads. Two Medtronic 5571 51-inch screw-on leads are then inserted through this port and the tips are left close to the lateral pericardium for robotic insertion. The left and right arms are then positioned in the eighth and fifth ICS respectively along a straight line with the tip of the scapula (**Figure 38.5**).

Left chest insufflation is not necessary. An 8–10 mm working soft port is inserted posterior to the camera port and is used by the assistant for lung retraction, introduction of sutures, and suture and needle retrieval. The pericardium is then opened posterior to the phrenic nerve, and extended inferiorly and superiorly as to visualize the obtuse marginal vessels. In the setting of prior cardiac surgery, the posterior entry into the pericardium allows for easier dissection of the posterior wall. The pericardium is then retracted posteriorly and anteriorly with sutures that are brought out through the working ports, and placed on tension with clamps for maximal exposure. Through the posterior working port, a peanut is used to reflect the left lung posteriorly away from the working field. The target zone is identified and a suitable area of bare myocardium is located (**Figure 38.6**).

The robotic arms are then used to fix the two LV leads to the myocardium at a level below the circumflex artery and between the first and second obtuse marginal arteries (with the second lead approximately 2.5 cm distal to the first lead). The screw-in leads are secured with 2.5 to 3 clockwise turns of the helix. It is helpful to use the right hand to screw in the lead and the left hand to stabilize the lead when "re-cocking" the right hand for further rotational torque. Round tooth or long tipped forceps provide the most secure grasp for this maneuver. Care needs to be taken to hold the lead only on the header or the fabric cuff and not to grasp the body of the lead itself as this can cause perforation of the lead insulation. In order to maximize working space, ventilation can be held during lead implantation.

Once both leads are secured, they are each tested by pacing above the native rate with one lead and grounding to the other lead. During this testing procedure, lead thresholds below 2.5 V are typically satisfactory and will show steady improvement once the lung is re-inflated. Prior to closure of the pericardium both pacemaker leads are made to lie in

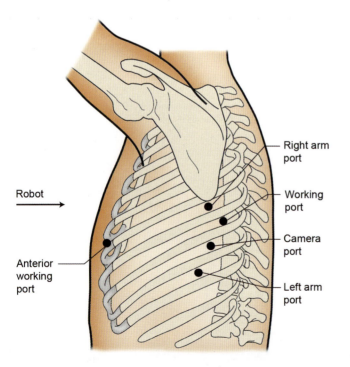

38.5

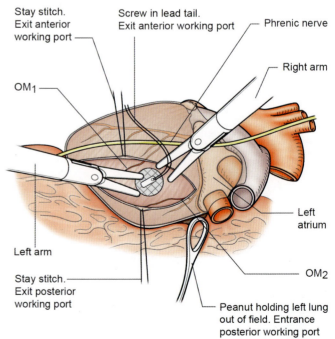

38.6

the superior direction, parallel to the pericardotomy. The pericardium is then closed over the leads in all cases with 3-0 silk sutures. The knots can be tied with the robotic arms or by the table surgeon using a knot tier. The closure of the pericardium aids in both lead thresholds and permanent distal fixation (**Figure 38.7**).

The robot is removed (and moved away from the table) and the camera is inserted through the anterior working port in a hand held fashion. A 24-French channel drain is then inserted through the left arm port and is positioned under direct vision. An intercostal nerve block is then performed with Marcaine (0.25%) by injecting along the chest wall from spaces 3 through 9 and observing the creation of a subpleural wheal with the thoracoscope. The scope is also used at this point to confirm that all port sites are hemostatic. The camera is removed and the leads are capped. A pocket is made in the anterior working port and the leads are left in this subcutaneous pocket for retrieval following repositioning. The port sites are then closed and the patient is repositioned in the supine position, with the left arm abducted to about 60 degrees.

If a device has previously been placed, this pocket is opened and the device is retrieved. The anterior working port pocket is opened and the LV leads are delivered into the field. A tunneling clamp is then placed into the device pocket and directed towards the anterior working port. One by one the leads are placed into the tip of the clamp and tunneled through the subcutaneous tissue into the device pocket. The leads are then once again tested (**Figure 38.8**). A "y" adaptor is used to connect the LV leads into the LV port on the device in a bipolar arrangement. This allows the device to be set with either lead as the active lead and multiple possibilities for a ground (the other LV lead, the can of the device, etc.). As such, should the thresholds on one lead increase, different

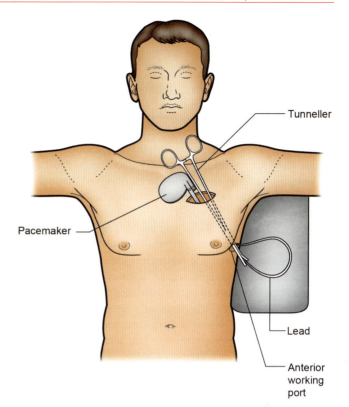

38.8

grounding arrangements can be set or a switch to the other LV lead can be made in order to maintain effective LV pacing. If a right-sided pacing or defibrillating lead is required, it is inserted at this time under fluoroscopy.

POSTOPERATIVE CARE

Transvenous approach

Monitoring post-procedure varies between centers. All patients should be on a unit with continuous cardiac rhythm monitoring. The activity level of the patient should be tempered. Bedrest should be avoided and the arm on the side of the implant *should not* be placed in a sling, as mild activity and arm motion can reveal a precariously placed electrode and prevent a "frozen shoulder". PA and lateral chest X-rays are obtained soon after the procedure to rule out pneumothorax and evaluate baseline radiographic lead placement. 12-lead ECG is performed post-procedure with and without pacing to document initial appropriate sensing and capture. Heparin subcutaneously or intravenously is avoided in the immediate postoperative period for fear of pocket/surgical site bleeding. Coumadin, as discussed above, can either be started the postoperative night, or can be continued if the procedure was done on therapeutic anticoagulation.

Patients are monitored overnight, and if on repeat interrogation of the device all parameters are satisfactory, they are discharged home that following day. Care is taken to keep the surgical site dry for 3–5 days post-procedure. Heavy lifting

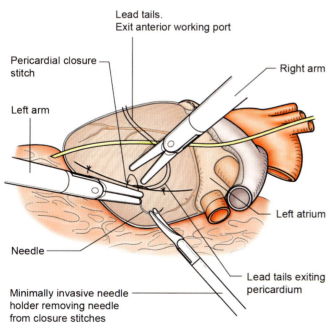

38.7

(greater than 25 pounds) is prohibited on the side of implantation for 1 month, but regular arm motion and activity are encouraged. Patients are seen 1 month post-procedure for wound and device check.

Surgical epicardial approach

All patients are observed in the intensive care unit overnight where they are monitored for CHF decompensation and/or arrhythmias. The chest tube can be removed the night of surgery or the following morning. Most patients can be discharged within 24–48 hours of the procedure. It is imperative to ensure patients are discharged on their prior heart failure regimen. Most patients require minimal pain medicine upon discharge and the narcotic regimen is identical to standard pacemaker placement. However, approximately 2–3% of patients can develop an intercostal neuropathy from the thoracoscopic ports. This can manifest as a burning pain radiating along a T-6 to T-8 dermatome and accompanied by severe skin hypersensitivity. The syndrome is nearly always self-limited but the use of Neurontin can be helpful in symptom control.

OUTCOME

In a relatively recent systematic review, the rate of transvenous LV lead implantation failure was approximately 5–7%, with an in-hospital mortality of <1%. Lead failure occurred in 5% of patients over 1 year. Response to biventricular pacing, defined as improved quality of life, improved symptomatology, decreased hospitalization, and reverse remodeling with increased EF, is seen in approximately two-thirds of patients, and benefit can occur as early as 1 month post-implantation, with a sustained effect >6 months to 1 year. However, the absolute benefit is variable and is not generally predictable. However, it has been shown that LV lead placement at the site of maximal dyssynchrony (latest LV activation) carries a much higher chance of success. Given transvenous limitations of delivering the LV lead into that area based on CS anatomy, other technical challenges, and a failure rate of >5%, minimally invasive epicardial LV lead placement may carry benefits over endocardial placement. Such an approach permits a greater freedom

of optimal lead placement and, in an initial report of 41 patients, there were no in-hospital deaths, intraoperative complications, or failures to implant the LV lead. Despite this, there are no randomized studies to show significant clinical benefit of this approach over transvenous placement. Our group has performed robotic LV lead insertion in more than 110 patients to date. Conversion to a mini-posterior thoracotomy has been rare (2%) with the major indication being a fused pleural space from prior pulmonary infection. Preoperative mapping studies have become routine and all patients have received leads in their target zones. Lead survival has been excellent with only two patients requiring lead revision over a 9-year period. Response rates and dyssynchrony measurements have improved when compared to conventional CS lead placement. Ongoing randomized studies comparing percutaneous to robotic biventricular pacing will not only delineate the role of robotics in primary implantations but will continue to expand our knowledge regarding the evolution resynchronization therapies for heart failure.

REFERENCES

1. Jarcho JA. Biventricular pacing. *N Engl J Med.* 2006; 355(3): 288–94.
2. Tracy CM, Epstein AE, Darbar D, et al. 2012 ACCF/AHA/HRS focused update of the 2008 guidelines for device-based therapy of cardiac rhythm abnormalities. *J Am Coll Cardiol.* 2012; 60(14): 1297–313.
3. Belott P. How to access the axillary vein. *Heart Rhythm.* 2006; 3(3): 366–9.
4. Ellenbogen KA, Wilkoff BL, Kay GN, et al. *Clinical cardiac pacing, defibrillation, and resynchronization therapy.* 4th ed. Philadelphia: Elsevier Saunders; 2011.

FURTHER READING

DeRose JJ, Belsley S, Swistel DG, et al. Robotically-assisted left ventricular epicardial lead implantation for biventricular pacing: The posterior approach. *Ann Thorac Surg.* 2004; 77: 1472–4.
Joshi S, Steinberg JS, Ashton RC, et al. Follow-up of robotically assisted left ventricular epicardial leads for cardiac resynchronization therapy. *J Am Coll Cardiol.* 2005; 46: 2358–9.

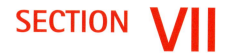

Surgery for congenital heart disease

39

The anatomy of congenital cardiac malformations

ROBERT H. ANDERSON AND DIANE E. SPICER

INTRODUCTION

Knowledge of detailed cardiac anatomy is a prerequisite for successful surgery. Nowhere is this more important than in the setting of congenital cardiac malformations. Although the anatomy displayed in these anomalies is often complex, it is not necessarily difficult to understand. In this chapter, we describe the basic rules of cardiac anatomy, which permit the surgeon, working in the operating room, to diagnose and recognize the arrangement of the cardiac chambers. As we will show, this knowledge, at the same time, will provide guidelines to the position of the vital conduction tissues. The basic layout of the heart should, of course, be established prior to commencement of intracardiac procedures. The diagnosis of even the most complex cases demands, in the first instance, no more than the distinction, in terms of morphology, of a right atrium from a left atrium, a right ventricle from a left ventricle, and an aorta from a pulmonary trunk. Distinction of these various chambers and vessels then provides the basis of the approach for simple sequential segmental analysis. The anatomy of "holes" and "stenoses" and so on are of equal, or even greater, significance. This morphology will be described in the appropriate chapters. Here we are concerned specifically with setting the ground rules for a systematic approach to cardiac anatomy.

APPROACHES TO THE HEART

When usually arranged, the heart lies in the mediastinum, with its apex pointing to the left and two-thirds of its bulk to the left of the midline. An unusual location of the heart should alert the surgeon to the possibility of complex malformations, although these are not always present when the heart is abnormally located. If abnormally positioned, we find it best to describe this finding in simple terms, such as heart mostly in the right chest with the apex pointing to the left, or as appropriate. Whatever its position, the heart and its great vessels can be approached either through the midline anteriorly or via the thoracic cavities.

A median sternotomy is used most frequently. The anterior mediastinum immediately behind the sternum is devoid of vital structures. This tissue plane is reached through separate incisions in the suprasternal notch and beneath the xiphoid process, the two being joined by blunt dissection.

Splitting the sternum will expose the pericardial sac, seen between the pleural cavities (**Figure 39.1**). In the infant, an important structure in this region is the thymus gland, which wraps itself over the anterolateral aspects of the pericardium in the area of the arterial pole. The gland itself is made up of two lateral lobes joined by a midline isthmus, which sometimes must be divided or partially excised to provide adequate exposure. Care must be taken with its arterial supply from the internal thoracic and inferior thyroid arteries. If divided, these arteries may retract beneath the sternum and produce troublesome bleeding. The thymic veins are also a potential problem, being fragile structures which often empty via a common trunk to the left brachiocephalic vein. This vein may be inadvertently damaged by undue traction.

Once the pericardium is exposed via a median sternotomy, access to the heart poses few problems. The vagus and phrenic nerves traverse the length of the pericardium well clear of the operative field, with the phrenic nerves anterior, and the vagus nerves posterior, to the lung hilums. The phrenic nerves may be vulnerable when the pericardium is harvested for use as an intracardiac patch or baffle. Excessive

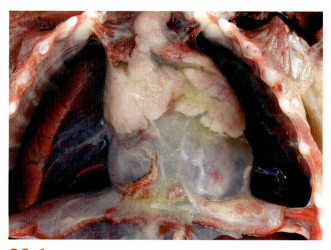

39.1

traction on the fibrous pericardium should be avoided, since this can avulse the origin of the pericardiacophrenic arteries, which accompany the phrenic nerves. The internal thoracic arteries themselves should not be at risk during exposure of the heart via a median sternotomy, but they may be damaged when the incision is closed.

Lateral thoracotomies provide exposure either to the heart or to the great vessels via the pleural spaces. Most frequently, these incisions are made in the fourth intercostal space, using the posterior bloodless triangle between the edges of the latissimus dorsi, trapezius, and the teres major muscles. The floor of this triangle is the sixth space, but division of the latissimus posteriorly, together with serratus anteriorly, frees the scapula and provides access to the fourth space, which is identified by counting from above. An incision midway between the ribs avoids the intercostal neurovascular bundle, which is protected beneath the lower margin of the fourth rib. Having entered the pleural space on the left side, retraction of the lung posteriorly exposes the middle mediastinum, with the left thymic lobe overlying the pericardium and the aortic arch with its associated nerves and vessels. If access is needed to the heart, this is usually achieved anterior to the phrenic nerve. More frequently, the aortic isthmus and descending aorta are approached and then the lung is retracted anteriorly, the parietal pleura being divided on its medial aspect posterior to the vagus nerve.

An important structure in this area is the left recurrent laryngeal nerve (**Figure 39.2**). This nerve takes origin from the vagus and curves round the inferior border of the arterial ligament, or duct if still patent. Excessive traction to the vagus can cause injury to this structure just as readily as direct trauma in the environs of the ligament. The thoracic duct ascends through this area to drain into the left jugular vein at its junction with the internal jugular vein. Accessory lymph channels draining into the duct can be troublesome when dissecting the origin of the left subclavian artery.

A right thoracotomy is performed in similar fashion, reaching the heart via the fifth interspace or the right-sided great vessels through the fourth interspace. When approaching the right pulmonary artery, it is sometimes useful to divide the azygos vein near its junction with the superior caval vein. On the right side, the recurrent laryngeal nerve passes round the subclavian artery as it courses medially from the vagus towards the larynx. Also encircling the artery on this side is the subclavian loop from the sympathetic trunk. Damage to this structure can result in Horner's syndrome.

Surface anatomy of the heart

Opening the pericardial cavity reveals the surface of the heart, which almost always is mostly in the left hemithorax with its apex pointing to the left. Important and readily recognizable landmarks enable the nature of the cardiac chambers to be determined with considerable accuracy by external inspection (**Figure 39.3**). Attention should first be directed to the atrial appendages. These anterolateral

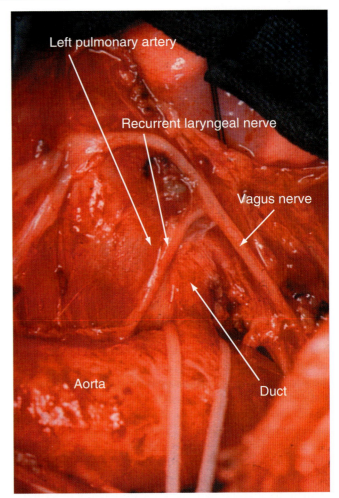

39.2

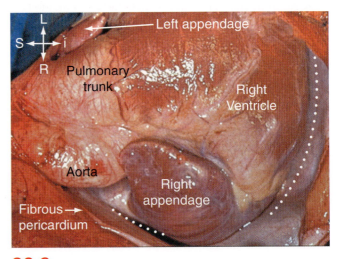

39.3

outpouchings from the atrial chambers usually clasp the arterial pedicle. The finding of both appendages on the same side of the pedicle is itself an anomaly – so-called juxtaposition of the atrial appendages. Left-sided juxtaposition is almost always associated with abnormal connections of the cardiac segments, but right-sided juxtaposition, whilst much rarer, tends to be found with relatively simple malformations such as atrial septal defect. Juxtaposition in itself is a nuisance to the surgeon, since it will necessitate alterations in planning

the cannulation, and so on. Juxtaposition can also markedly distort the architecture of atrial anatomy, and can produce problems unless properly recognized. Once recognized, nonetheless, the problems are readily surmountable.

Having established the position of the appendages, the next step is to establish their morphological nature. When the terms "right" and "left" are used in this chapter, they are used to indicate morphology rather than position. Where position is also abnormal, this situation will be indicated separately. Differences in the shape of the appendage are usually sufficient to permit the surgeon to distinguish the morphologically right from the morphologically left atrium, with the pectinate right appendage having a triangular shape (**Figure 39.4**) in contrast to the tubular left appendage (**Figure 39.4c**). The most reliable means of distinguishing between the appendages, however, is to examine the nature of their junctions with the remainder of the atrial chambers. It is often not appreciated that the entire anterior wall of the right atrium, as seen by the surgeon, is made up of the pectinate wall of the appendage. Thus, the pectinate muscles in the triangular morphologically right appendage extend to the crux of the heart, encircling the vestibule of the tricuspid valve. In contrast, the morphologically left atrioventricular junction is smooth, containing as it does the coronary sinus, and with the pectinate muscles confined within the antero-superiorly located tubular appendage. These differences are best appreciated by inspection of the isolated heart, as shown in **Figure 39.4a and b**, but can easily be seen at straightforward surgical inspection. In most instances, the triangular

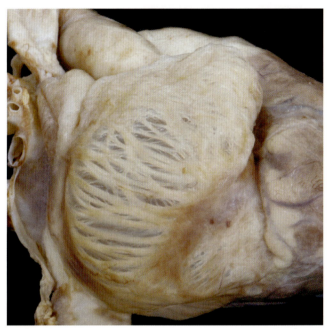

39.4a

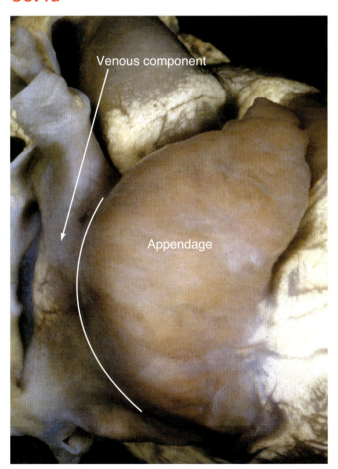

Venous component

Appendage

39.4b

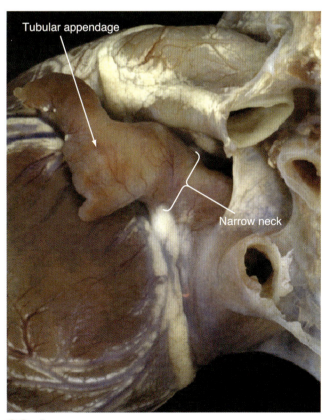

Tubular appendage

Narrow neck

39.4c

appendage is right-sided, and the narrow, tubular, append-age is left-sided. This usual arrangement is also called "situs solitus." Rarely, the tubular appendage is right-sided, and the triangular one is left-sided. This situation is the mirror-image or "inverted" arrangement. It is better to describe mirror-imagery than "inversus," since the appendages themselves are not turned upside down. More frequently, when the heart is complexly malformed, an arrangement will be found in which the appendages have comparable morphology.

In this latter situation, both appendages will be broad and triangular, with pectinate muscles extending all round the atrioventricular vestibules, or else tubular and narrow, with bilaterally smooth vestibules. The syndromes associated with this arrangement, which is one of isomerism, are also known as the "splenic syndromes" or visceral heterotaxy. Interest in these constellations has usually been the province of the pathologist. By the simple expedient of inspecting the appendages, nonetheless, the surgeon has the means of diagnosing these entities during life. This permits drawing all the inferences that go with the recognition of right isomerism ("asplenia"), or left isomerism ("polysplenia"), including the drawing of important information concerning the arrangement of the conduction tissues (**Figure 39.5**).

While inspecting the appendages, the surgeon should also examine their junctions with the venous components of the atriums. Here again, a vital difference exists between morphologically right and left sides. The right junction is the extensive terminal groove (or sulcus terminalis), marking the site internally of the terminal crest (or crista terminalis). Lying in the terminal groove, in an immediately subendo-cardial position, and usually lateral to the crest of the atrial appendage, is the sinus node (**Figure 39.6**). The left junc-tion is not marked by any such prominent groove, and no conduction tissue is present at this junction. These findings complement the information gained from the location of the appendages. With the usual arrangement, the sinus node

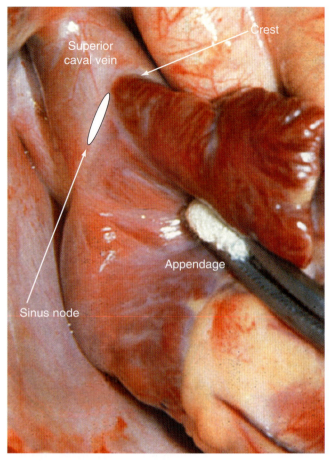

39.6

is right-sided, whereas in the setting of mirror-imagery, the node is a left-sided structure. In right isomerism, sinus nodes are present bilaterally, but in left isomerism the sinus node is hypoplastic and abnormally positioned, being vari-ously located in the atrial wall close to the atrioventricular junction.

Inspection of the appendages should lead attention directly to the venoatrial connections. Here, the important features to note are abnormal connections of either the pulmonary or the caval veins. A search should be made between the left appendage and the left pulmonary veins for a persistent left SCV, while the finding of left isomerism should always alert the surgeon to the likelihood that the inferior caval vein is interrupted, being continued via the azygos or hemiazygos veins, which would be correspondingly enlarged.

Considerable information concerning the ventricular arrangement can also be derived from external inspection. Here, it is the descending branches of the coronary arter-ies that are the guide. In the usual situation, the anterior interventricular coronary artery, a superior as well as an anterior structure, arises from the main stem of the left coronary artery. It descends close to the obtuse margin of the ventricular mass. When this anterior interventricular artery arises from the right-sided coronary artery, there is

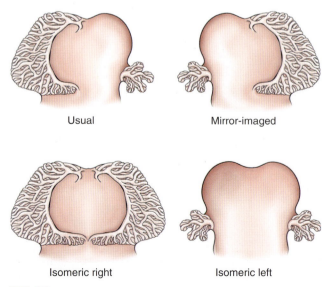

Usual　　　　　　　Mirror-imaged

Isomeric right　　　　Isomeric left

39.5

almost always a mirror-imaged ventricular arrangement, with the left ventricle found on the right side. The precise connections between the atriums and ventricles will depend on the arrangement of the atrial appendages, but this coronary arterial pattern should alert the surgeon to the potential presence of congenitally corrected transposition (see below). The other abnormal arrangement of the coronary arteries to be sought by inspection is the presence of two "delimiting" arteries on the anterior surface of the ventricular mass, rather than prominent interventricular arteries on the obtuse and diaphragmatic surfaces. This situation indicates a disproportion between the sizes of the ventricles. This finding suggests the presence of a dominant left ventricle and a small and incomplete right ventricle, such as is found in double-inlet left ventricle or tricuspid atresia. Alternatively, the absence of prominent interventricular arteries on the anterior ventricular surface should raise the suspicion of a solitary indeterminate ventricular chamber, or else a dominant right ventricle with a posteroinferior incomplete left ventricle. The latter will be revealed by inspection of the diaphragmatic surface.

The final feature to be inspected, which will usually be studied at the same time as the ventricular mass, is the relationship of the arterial trunks. The first step is to confirm the presence of separate aortic and pulmonary trunks, as opposed to a common trunk. When separate trunks are found, the aortic trunk is almost always posterior and right-sided, with the pulmonary trunk spiralling around the aorta as it divides into the right and left pulmonary arteries. Abnormal relationships of the great arterial trunks almost always indicate intracardiac malformations, but the connections of the cardiac chambers cannot be inferred from these abnormal relationships. At best, the anomalous arterial positions raise the suspicion of a given lesion. Most frequently, an anterior and right-sided aorta is found with discordant ventriculoarterial connections, usually described as transposition, but it can also be found with double-outlet right ventricle. An anterior and left-sided aorta suggests congenitally corrected transposition, but it, too, can be found with double-outlet right ventricle or, rarely, with concordant atrioventricular and ventriculoarterial connections – so-called "anatomically corrected malposition." In similar fashion, it cannot be presumed that the ventriculoarterial connections are normal simply because the arterial trunks are "normally related." Often there are "normal" spiralling arterial relationships in the presence of double outlet right ventricle. This spiralling arrangement can be found on very rare occasions when the arterial trunks are discordantly connected.

ANATOMY OF THE CARDIAC CHAMBERS

In the previous section, we placed emphasis on the recognition of the morphology of the different chambers, specifically the atriums, while stressing also that these chambers are not always in their usual position, nor connected to their anticipated neighbors. Each chamber, nonetheless, has a relatively constant anatomy irrespective of its position or its connections, although subtle changes in morphology are found when the chambers are connected together in abnormal fashion. In this section, we focus on the anticipated normal morphology, with additional remarks concerning abnormal structure made when pertinent.

The right atrium

The right atrium has its extensive triangular appendage separated from the systemic venous sinus by the terminal groove (shown by a white line in **Figure 39.4b**). As usually seen by the surgeon, the superior caval vein enters the left-hand side and the inferior caval vein the right-hand side of the sleeve-like sinus, which is separated inferiorly by the interatrial groove from the right pulmonary veins. This groove, known also as Waterston's or Sondergaard's groove, is the extensive interatrial gulley produced by the deep infolding of the right and left atrial walls. As discussed above, the terminal groove is a vital surgical landmark, since immediately beneath its epicardial surface lies the sinus node.

Opening the right atrium with the freedom permitted the morphologist reveals the extensive terminal crest which underlies the groove (**Figure 39.7** – anatomical position). This muscular crest swings round the orifices of both the superior and inferior caval veins. An extension from the inferior end of the terminal crest runs anteriorly towards the atrial septum, striking towards the vestibule of the tricuspid valve. This muscular ridge separates the orifice of the inferior caval vein from the mouth of the coronary sinus. Extending from it, as opposing sickle-shaped folds of varying dimensions, are the remnants of the Eustachian and Thebesian valves, which guard the venous orifices. The valves themselves are of varying dimensions in different hearts. Of more surgical significance is the fibrous commissure of these two valves, which buries itself in the musculature between

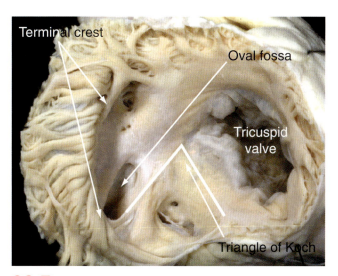

39.7

the coronary sinus and the oval fossa, and runs towards the left-hand margin of the tricuspid vestibule. This important structure is the tendon of Todaro, which forms one boundary of the triangle of Koch (see below).

As seen by the surgeon, an extensive pouch is present above the orifice of the coronary sinus, located between the sinus, the hinge of the tricuspid valve, and the inferoanterior extension of the terminal crest (**Figure 39.8**). This sinus is the so-called sub-Eustachian pouch. In reality, it is sub-Thebesian with the heart viewed anatomically. A triangular area is then formed, with the sub-Eustachian sinus as its base. Its inferior border, as viewed in the operating room, is the site of the tendon of Todaro, and its superior border is the site of annular attachment of the septal leaflet of the tricuspid valve. This vital area is the triangle of Koch. The atrioventricular node is entirely contained within its confines, and the atrioventricular bundle penetrates towards the left ventricular outflow tract at its apex.

Between the triangle of Koch and the orifice of the superior caval vein is the right atrial surface of the oval fossa. At first sight, this entire surface gives the impression of being interposed between the right and left atriums (**Figure 39.9a**). Sectioning another heart shows that this is not the case (**Figure 39.9b**). The true septal area is confined to the floor of the fossa and its anteroinferior margin. The extensive mound to the left-hand side of the fossa as viewed by the surgeon is the atrial wall overlying the aortic root. The rim between the fossa and the superior caval orifice, seen in inferior position by the surgeon, is no more than the infolded walls of the interatrial groove. The right-hand margin is the wall of the inferior caval vein. The inferior margin, seen superiorly by the surgeon, is the tissue separating the fossa from the coronary sinus, which becomes continuous with the floor of the triangle of Koch.

The left atrium

The proportions of the left atrium formed by the appendage and venous component are reversed compared to the right atrium, and overall the left atrium has a much simpler structure (**Figure 39.10**). The venous component, located posteriorly, receives the four pulmonary veins, one at each

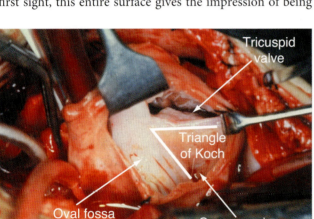

39.8

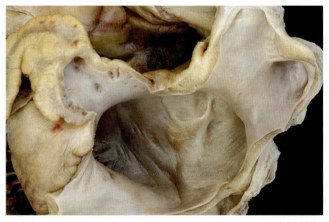

39.10

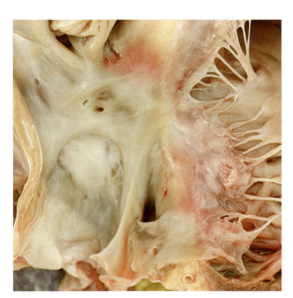

39.9a

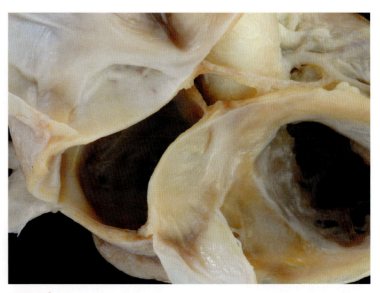

39.9b

corner. This component leads directly into the anteriorly positioned mitral vestibule. As seen by the surgeon entering through the atrial roof, the narrow opening of the tubular appendage is to the left hand, while the septal surface is to the right. The sweep of muscular tissue above the mitral vestibule is the extensive anterior atrial wall related to the aortic root. The smooth inferior and posterior margin of the mitral vestibule overlies the coronary sinus as it runs round from the obtuse margin of the ventricular mass. The septal surface of the left atrium is much simpler than the right, being formed by the flap valve of the oval fossa. The left atrium also has a body of significant size, a fact that can be deduced from examination of hearts from patients having totally anomalous pulmonary venous connection. In these hearts, in which the left atrium lacks its pulmonary venous component, a substantial part of the chamber still cannot be accounted for in terms of the appendage, the vestibule, and the septum. This part is the atrial body.

The atrioventricular junctions

The surgeon will never see the entirety of the atrioventricular junctions, although at different times he or she will be concerned with their various parts. Knowledge of the junctions in their entirety is, nonetheless, fundamental to the proper understanding of several congenital anomalies, particularly atrioventricular septal defects in the setting of common atrioventricular junctions.

In this section we will therefore discuss the detailed anatomy of the entire junctions. This anatomy is best appreciated by removing the atrial chambers and great arteries from the ventricular base, and viewing the heart from the superior aspect as in **Figure 39.11**. The dominant feature is the "wedged" position of the aortic valve. Equally significant is the oblique orientation of the mitral and tricuspid valvar orifices relative to the aortic root. Although we usually speak of the valvar annuli, none of the four cardiac valves has a true

and complete fibrous ring which supports its leaflets. The mitral annulus approximates most closely to the concept of a ring, although it is ovoid rather than circular. In its parietal component, nonetheless, it is often the case that very little collagenous tissue supports the mural leaflet of the valve and, at the same time, separates the atrial and ventricular myocardial masses. In the tricuspid orifice, it is rare to find a collagenous annulus. Instead, it is the fibrofatty tissues of the atrioventricular groove which usually separate the right atrial muscle from the ventricular mass. When considering the arterial valves, the concept of a "ring" becomes totally deficient. Rather, each of the semilunar valvar leaflets is attached in part to the arterial sinuses, and in part to the underlying ventricular structures. The subarterial roots, therefore, take the shape of coronets, tenting up in the areas of attachment to the sinotubular junction, and sweeping down to the nadir of the attachments to the ventricular bases. These attachments in the pulmonary "ring" are exclusively to right ventricular muscle – the free-standing subpulmonary infundibulum. In the case of the aortic valve, a good half of the circumference of the leaflets is supported by, and attached to, fibrous and collagenous tissues.

As a consequence of its wedged position, the aortic valve is in extensive fibrous continuity with the leaflets of both the mitral and tricuspid valves. The entirety of the aortic (or anterior) leaflet of the mitral valve is in fibrous continuity with two of the leaflets of the aortic valve (**Figure 39.12**). For this reason alone, this leaflet of the mitral valve is best termed, in the otherwise normal heart, the aortic leaflet, differentiating it in this way from the mural leaflet. The two ends of the region of aortic–mitral valve continuity are thickened to form the right and left fibrous trigones, respectively.

The right fibrous trigone is itself an integral part of the fibrous mass where the aortic root is continuous with the leaflets of the tricuspid valve. This whole area is usually called the central fibrous body. The part between the aortic root and the right side of the heart is the so-called membranous septum. This septum forms the medial wall of the subaortic

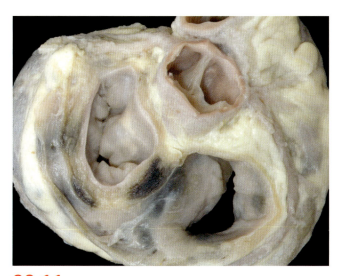

39.11

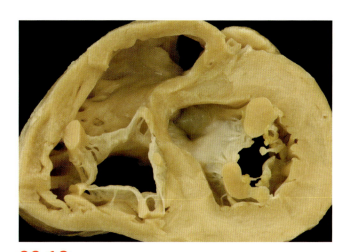

39.12

outflow tract, being positioned immediately beneath the zone of apposition between the right coronary and non-coronary leaflets of the aortic valve. Examination of long-axis sections taken at right angles to the septum through this region show that the leaflet of the tricuspid valve is attached to the right-sided aspect of this area. This attachment of the tricuspid valve divides the membranous septum into its atrioventricular and interventricular components, as shown by taking sections through the different components (**Figure 39.13a and b**). The arrangement is shown in a different plane by the arrows in **Figure 39.15**.

The obliquity of the mitral and tricuspid valvar orifices relative to each other is responsible for the unusual morphology of the muscular area immediately behind the central fibrous body. This area is the floor of the triangle of Koch (see above). Careful dissection of the region shows how the wedged aortic outflow tract "lifts" the aortic leaflet of the mitral valve away from the muscular ventricular septum (see **Figure 39.13b**). Because of this, it is only over a very short distance that the two atrioventricular valves are attached to opposite sides of the septum, or "facing" each other. In this short "facing" area, the tricuspid valve is attached to the septum more towards the ventricular apex than is the mitral valve. By virtue of these differential levels of attachment (indicated by the arrows in **Figure 39.14**), part of the ventricular septum interposes between the left ventricle and the right atrium, albeit with right atrial musculature on its atrial face. This area has previously been termed the "atrioventricular muscular septum." In reality, an extension of the fibrofatty inferior atrioventricular groove separates the atrial and ventricular musculatures between the valvar hinges, so that the area is better likened to a sandwich than a septum. Irrespective of such niceties, the area is short and shallow, because almost immediately inferior to the aortic root the two atrioventricular orifices diverge from each other, the inferior "swing" of the tricuspid orifice being more marked than that of the mitral valve. In this inferior bay, the coronary sinus opens to the right atrium, having traversed the posterior and inferior aspect of the left atrioventricular junction.

The atrioventricular muscular sandwich is of particular importance to the surgeon because its atrial component contains the atrioventricular node. The cross-sectional cut (**Figure 39.14**) shows the oblique nature of the atrioventricular junction at this site. The atrioventricular node lies on the sloping atrial aspect of this junction. As seen from the left atrial aspect, this point is marked by the inferomedial

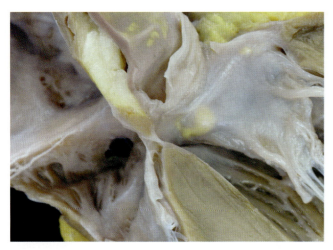

39.13a

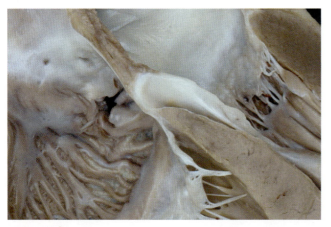

39.13b

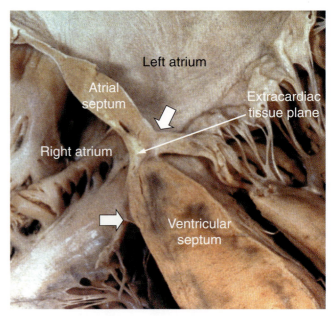

39.14

attachment of the zone of apposition of the leaflets of the mitral valve. By virtue of the extensive posteroinferior diverticulum of the aortic root, the atrioventricular bundle, having penetrated through the central fibrous body, passes directly into the left ventricular outflow tract. From the standpoint of the subaortic root, the landmark to the point of penetration is the zone of apposition between the right and non-coronary aortic valvar leaflets. As seen from the right atrium, therefore, it is the landmarks of the triangle of Koch that delineate the site of the specialized atrioventricular junction. Seen from the left atrium, it is the posteromedial attachment of the leaflets of the mitral valve which points to the danger area.

As seen from the aorta, it is the junction of the non-coronary and right coronary valvar leaflets which indicates the danger area. When seen from the right ventricle, it is the area immediately adjacent to the medial papillary muscle and the zone of apposition between the septal and antero-superior leaflets of the tricuspid valve that must be avoided (**Figure 39.15**).

Examination of the dissected atrioventricular junctions

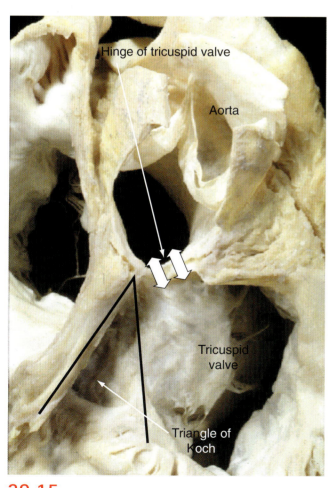

Hinge of tricuspid valve

Aorta

Tricuspid valve

Triangle of Koch

39.15

reveals other features of note. The encircling branches of the coronary arteries are an integral part of the junctions. The right coronary artery has an extensive junctional course. In its first few centimeters or so, it lies directly within the inner curvature of the heart. The right margin of this ventriculo-infundibular fold, when viewed from the right ventricle, is seen as the supraventricular crest. The left coronary artery emerges into the inner curvature, and then immediately branches into its anterior interventricular and circumflex branches. The anterior branch immediately moves out of the junction to become interventricular. The circumflex artery, in contrast, becomes an integral part of the left atrio-ventricular junction. The extent of its intimate relationship to the junction varies markedly from heart to heart. Most frequently, it fades out at the obtuse margin, and the right coronary artery extends across the crux to supply the diaphragmatic surface of the left ventricle. In other cases, the right coronary turns down at the crux to become the inferior, interventricular artery, usually described incorrectly as the posterior descending artery, while the circumflex artery supplies the diaphragmatic surface of the left ventricle. Least frequently, the circumflex artery supplies the diaphragmatic region, and continues to become the inferior interventricular artery. This highly significant variability cannot be expressed simply in terms of right and left "dominance" of the coronary arteries. Instead, it is necessary to specify separately the origins of the inferior interventricular coronary artery, and the nature of the arteries that supply the diaphragmatic surface of the left ventricle.

The right ventricle

Before going into specifics of ventricular morphology, it is appropriate to offer a few remarks concerning ventricular division and valvar morphology. Traditionally, ventricles have been divided simply into inlet and outlet parts, or sinus and conus. For the normal heart, this convention is adequate, although less than ideal. When abnormal hearts are considered, its deficiencies are soon evident. The incomplete right ventricle seen in tricuspid atresia, for example, lacks an inlet component. Nevertheless, it is unequivocally recognized as a right ventricle, because of the presence of the so-called "sinus" component. In tricuspid atresia, therefore, according to those still using the notion of "sinus" and "conus," the "sinus" is not the same thing as the ventricular inlet.

This potential controversy can be circumvented by assessing the ventricle from a different viewpoint. In terms of descriptive morphology, each ventricle can be considered to possess three rather than two components, namely the inlet, apical trabecular, and outlet portions. All ventricles, no matter how deformed, are readily described using this tripartite convention. **Figure 39.16a** shows these three components in the right ventricle; the three components in the left ventricle are shown in **Figure 39.16b**. For instance, the problematic incomplete right ventricle in tricuspid atresia possesses outlet and apical trabecular components. It lacks its inlet portion.

When considering valvar morphology, it is important to have a convention which enables leaflets to be distinguished one from another, and from so-called "scallops." The best way of distinguishing between the leaflets is to view the valve in its closed position. This orientation permits recognition of the zones of apposition between adjacent leaflets. Such an approach is much better than taking as the criterion of division between leaflets the presence of a commissural cord arising from a prominent and easily recognized papillary muscle. It can be impossible to distinguish morphologically such "commissural" cords from so-called "cleft'" cords – hence the problem of determining whether the mitral valve has two, four, or more leaflets. When viewed from the stance

of the closed valve, it is obvious that the mitral valve possesses two leaflets, with a solitary zone of apposition between them. In similar fashion, the tricuspid valve closes in trifoliate fashion and therefore possesses three leaflets. The leaflets within the orifice of the tricuspid valve are located septally, anterosuperiorly, and inferiorly.

Returning now to the right ventricle, this chamber, when normally constituted, possesses the tricuspid valve in its inlet portion. Its three leaflets are readily seen by the surgeon from the right atrium, although **Figure 39.17** shows the valve as seen from its ventricular aspect, revealing that the leaflets occupy anterosuperior, septal, and inferior positions. It is a mistake to describe the inferior leaflet as being posterior. The septal leaflet is the most posterior of the three. The peripheral attachment of the zone of apposition between the septal and anterosuperior leaflets, supported by the medial papillary muscle, is "round the corner" from the area of the membranous septum. Often the septal leaflet is itself cloven to the level of the membranous septum. This area is intimately related to the site of penetration of the atrioventricular bundle.

The apical trabecular component of the right ventricle has typically coarse trabeculations (see **Figure 39.16a**). It is on the basis of the nature of the apical trabeculations that the ventricle is most reliably differentiated from a left ventricle. Extending upwards and leftwards from the apical trabecular component is the outlet portion, supporting the leaflets of the pulmonary valve. In the normal right ventricle, this outlet component is a free-standing muscular

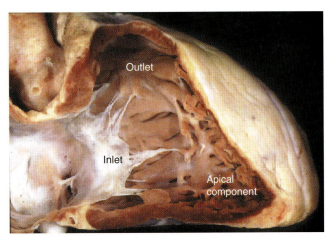

39.16a

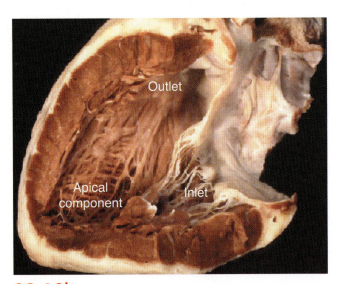

39.16b

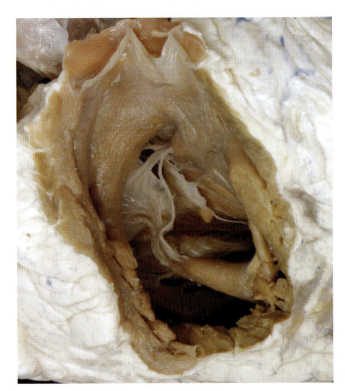

39.17

sleeve (**Figure 39.18**). (The black line indicates the junction between the infundibular musculature of the right ventricle and the wall of the pulmonary trunk.) The presence of this infundibulum provides another very characteristic feature of the right ventricle, namely the muscular supraventricular crest which separates the attachments of the leaflets of the tricuspid and pulmonary valves. As can be appreciated from study of the atrioventricular junctions (see **Figure 39.11**), this apparently extensive muscle bundle as seen from inside the ventricle is no more than the inner aspect of the parietal ventricular wall. In other words, it is the ventriculoinfundibular fold.

This observation is readily confirmed by dissection, which shows the extent of the free-standing subpulmonary muscular infundibulum. A very characteristic anatomical feature of the right ventricle is the extensive septal muscle bundle that runs down into the apical trabecular component, then splitting into its various trabeculations, including the moderator band, the anterior papillary muscle, and various septoparietal trabeculations (**Figure 39.19**). The basal part of this prominent bundle itself divides into two limbs which embrace the supraventricular crest. The posterior of these two limbs gives rise to the medial papillary muscle, while the anterior limb runs up to the pulmonary valve.

The extensive bundle is sometimes considered inappropriately to be part of the supraventricular crest. In North America, it is usually called the "septal band." This is an appropriate description, but even the most cursory examination shows that this structure, being septal, cannot also be part of the supraventricular crest. We distinguish this important structure as the septomarginal trabeculation, recognizing its relations to both the ventriculoinfundibular fold, which forms the supraventricular crest, and the free-standing muscular subpulmonary infundibulum (**Figure 39.20**). At the junction of the fold with the septomarginal trabeculation, we used to think that a small part of the muscular ventricular septum was interposed between the ventricular outflow tracts. We now know that this is not the case, and that the free-standing infundibular sleeve is separated from

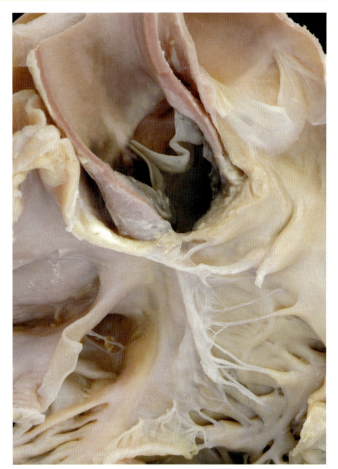

39.19

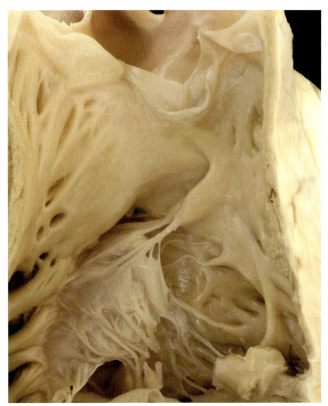

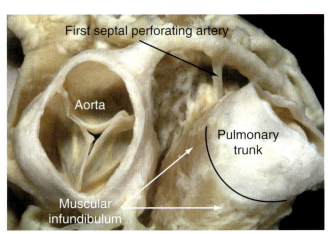

39.18

39.20

the aortic root through its entirety by an area of extracavitary space filled with fibrous, adipose tissue. This space is shown in the dissection made to produce **Figure 39.18**. The atrioventricular conduction axis branches in relation to the posterior limb of the septomarginal trabeculation, but on the left ventricular aspect of the septum. The right bundle branch then penetrates through the septum, and surfaces beneath the medial papillary muscle. It then runs down towards the apex either on the surface of, or embedded within, the body of the septomarginal trabeculation.

The left ventricle

As with the right ventricle, the left ventricle can readily be divided into inlet, apical trabecular, and outlet components (see **Figure 39.16b**). The inlet component contains the mitral valve. When viewed from the atrial aspect (**Figure 39.21a**), the ends of the solitary zone of apposition between the aortic and mural leaflets are in superolateral and inferomedial position, although usually described incorrectly as being posteromedial and anterolateral. By virtue of their position, the two leaflets themselves have grossly dissimilar annular attachments. The aortic leaflet has a relatively short attachment, guarding only about one-third of the circumference. As seen in the open valve, this leaflet has considerable depth, and is a well-defined sail-like structure (**Figure 39.21b**). In contrast, the mural leaflet, although having a much more extensive annular attachment, has much less depth, and is more curtain-like. In most hearts, this mural leaflet is further divided into a series of "scallops." Three such scallops are usually present, but five, or even six, may be seen on occasion, as in the specimen shown in **Figure 39.21a**. The overall result of these dissimilar arrangements, nonetheless, is that the two leaflets have more or less equal surface area. As discussed in the section on the atrioventricular junctions, it is the area around the inferomedial end of the zone of apposition which is related to the site of penetration of the atrioventricular bundle.

The apical trabecular component of the left ventricle is characterized by particularly fine trabeculations. The apex of the ventricle itself is remarkably thin, with often no more than 1 mm of myocardium between the epicardial and endocardial surfaces at this point. Unlike the right ventricle, the trabecular component of the left ventricle has a smooth septal surface, down which cascades the fan-like left bundle branch. The initial portion of the fan is an undivided fascicle; but having descended about one-third of the septum, the bundle divides into its interconnected anterior, septal, and posterior divisions.

Although not a completely muscular structure as in the right ventricle, the outlet portion is well formed in the left ventricle. It has a particularly prominent deep inferoposterior diverticulum (**Figure 39.22a**). Because of the fibrous continuity between the aortic and mitral valves, the outlet

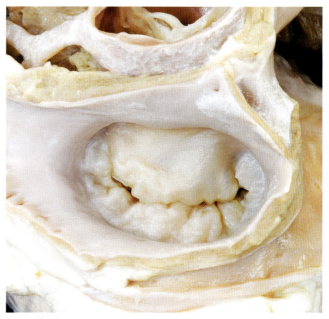

39.21a

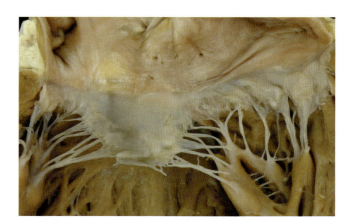

39.21b

does not have completely muscular walls, the ventriculo-infundibular fold usually being eradicated in this area. The significant surgical feature of this area, in addition to the fact that the inferoposterior diverticulum is related to a considerable area of the right atrium, is the coronet-like attachment of the aortic valve leaflets (**Figure 39.22b**: RC, right coronary; LC, left coronary; NC, non-coronary). At the apexes of the zones of apposition between the leaflets, the aortic outflow tract is directly related to such structures as the anterior wall of the left atrium and the transverse sinus. Further important features are the descent over the midseptal surface of the outflow tract of the left bundle branch (arrow in **Figure 39.22b**), and the origin of the coronary arteries from two of the aortic sinuses. All of these features are highly significant when planning operations to enlarge the aortic root.

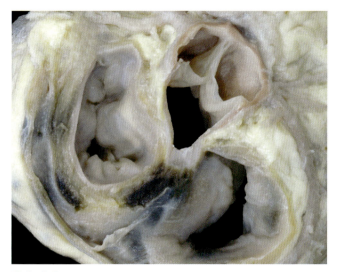

39.22a

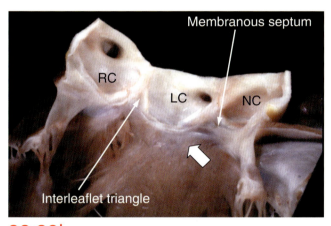

Membranous septum

RC

LC　　NC

Interleaflet triangle

39.22b

SEQUENTIAL SEGMENTAL ANALYSIS OF CONGENITALLY MALFORMED HEARTS

In the preceding paragraphs, we have described the basic morphology of the cardiac chambers, indicating how the key features may be recognized by the surgeon. At the same time, we have emphasized how the basic disposition of the conduction tissues is dictated by this morphology. Thus far, anatomy has been considered mostly in the setting of the normal heart. Almost all patients with congenital cardiac lesions undergoing surgery will have these malformations in the setting of the normal heart. For example, persistent patency of the arterial duct, or a simple aortic coarctation, in no way alters the basic cardiac morphology. Similarly, the presence of simple atrial or ventricular septal defects, or even an atrioventricular septal defect with common atrioventricular junction, does not distort the basic arrangement to such an extent that the heart is not readily recognized as being normal. In a few cases, nonetheless, the anatomy can be exceedingly bizarre, often with the heart itself being

abnormally positioned. Even in these complex cases, understanding can be simply achieved if attention is paid to the principles established in the previous paragraphs. The ways in which the atrial chambers themselves can be arranged are strictly limited, as are the ways in which the atrial chambers can connect to the ventricles, and the ventricles in turn connect to the great arteries. We conclude our discussion of surgical cardiac anatomy, therefore, with a brief description of the principles and philosophy of sequential segmental analysis, concentrating once more on the vital information provided by these principles concerning the distribution of the atrioventricular conduction tissues.

Philosophy of sequential segmental analysis

When describing any given congenital cardiac malformation, it is necessary to account separately for the features of the morphology of the individual cardiac segments, the connections of the segments to each other, and the interrelationships of the chambers within each segment. It does not particularly matter how each of these features is described, provided that each is accounted for using mutually exclusive terms. A variety of terms has been used for this purpose, but the value of using simple everyday words in description has become increasingly apparent, rather than having a vocabulary deeply rooted in classical etymology.

We have already described the essential morphological features of each of the cardiac chambers, but it is now necessary to decide which of these features is taken as the final arbiter for identification of a given chamber. In this respect, it is best to follow the so-called "morphological method." This states that chambers, however deformed or abnormal, should always be identifiable in terms of their own intrinisic characteristics. This system means, for example, that venous connections cannot be used to identify an atrium, since the veins themselves may connect anomalously. An atrioventricular valve cannot be used as the final arbiter of the nature of a ventricle because some ventricles do not possess atrioventricular valves. It is the morphology of the atrial appendages that turns out to be the most reliable feature for atrial recognition. For the ventricles, it is the nature of the apical trabeculations which is most useful. The great arteries have no intrinsic features which permit their recognition, but almost always their patterns of branching are sufficiently discrete to permit distinction of an aorta from a pulmonary trunk, and a common trunk from a solitary arterial trunk. For full description, it is necessary to account separately for connections and relations. Ideally, each element should have equal weight in description. Practically, the surgeon is most concerned with the way the cardiac components are joined together. In this account, therefore, it is the connections between the parts that are given the pre-eminent position, with relationships relegated to a secondary role.

Atrial arrangement

The importance of inspecting the morphology of the atrial appendages has already been stressed, and the possible variations have received attention. Recognition of the arrangement of the appendages is doubly important in sequential analysis, since the remainder of the heart cannot be described adequately without knowledge of the morphology of the atrial segment. There are only four ways in which the atrial appendages can be arranged (see **Figure 39.5**). In the first two patterns, morphologically right and morphologically left appendages are both present. These two arrangements are lateralized. When the right appendage is right-sided, this usual arrangement is often called "solitus," but this word means no more than usual! When the right appendage is left-sided, then a mirror-image arrangement is frequently called "inversus," despite the fact that the atriums are not upside down. The other two patterns are found when each appendage has comparable morphology, or in other words the two appendages are isomeric. Right isomerism then describes the existence of two appendages each having right morphology, while left isomerism exists when each appendage has left morphology. As discussed above, the disposition of the sinus node is dictated by the morphology of the atrial appendages, hence the importance of the surgeon recognizing the isomeric arrangements.

The atrioventricular junctions

Analysis of the atrioventricular junctions demands knowledge of the nature of both the atrial appendages and the ventricular chambers (**Figure 39.23**). It is necessary to determine first how the atriums are connected to the ventricles and, second, the morphology of the atrioventricular valves which guard the atrioventricular junctions. When each atrium connects to its own separate ventricle, there are biventricular atrioventricular connections. This situation can occur with either lateralized or isomeric atrial appendages. With lateralized appendages, there are then two possibilities, which can exist when the appendages themselves are either usually arranged or mirror-imaged. The first is when the right atrium connects to the right ventricle, and the left atrium to the left ventricle. This gives concordant atrioventricular connections. The second is when the right atrium connects to the left ventricle, and the left atrium to the right ventricle. This situation produces discordant connections.

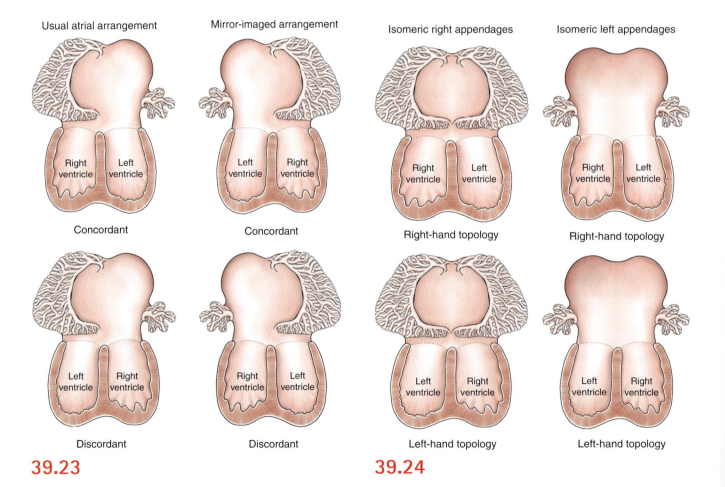

39.23

39.24

When the appendages are isomeric, whatever the arrangement of the ventricles, the atrioventricular connections must inevitably be mixed and biventricular (**Figure 39.24**). In this situation, it is crucial to recognize the topological arrangement of the ventricular mass.

There are only two basic patterns of ventricular topological architecture. The usual pattern is seen in the normal heart with usual atrial arrangement and concordant atrioventricular connections. The right ventricle more or less wraps itself round the left ventricle in such a way that, figuratively speaking, it is the palmar surface of only the observer's right hand that can be placed on the septal surface such that the thumb is in the inlet, the wrist in the apex, and the fingers in the outlet. This arrangement, therefore, can be described as right-handed topology (**Figure 39.25a**). The second basic pattern is typically seen in the heart with usually arranged atrial appendages, but with discordant atrioventricular connections. It is also seen in the situation of mirror-imaged atrial arrangement and concordant atrioventricular connections (**Figure 39.23**). With this topological arrangement, only the left hand can be placed upon the right ventricular septal surface, hence left-handed topology (**Figure 39.25b**).

Either of these two topological arrangements can exist with either right or left isomerism (see **Figure 39.24**), and they must be described so as to provide full categorization.

This knowledge is important, because the topological arrangement dictates the disposition of the conduction tissues when biventricular atrioventricular connections are mixed (see below). Almost without exception, in patients with lateralized atrial appendages the ventricular topology is harmonious with the atrioventricular connections. Usually, the ventricular relationships are also as expected, with the right ventricle to the right with right-handed topology, and right ventricle to the left with left-handed topology. Sometimes, however, the ventricular relationships may be unexpected, either because of rotation, or tilting of the ventricular mass around its long axis. Such rotation or tilting produces the so-called "criss-cross" or "upstairs-downstairs" hearts. Providing that relations are described, and identified separately from connections and topology, these hearts should not give problems in either diagnosis or description.

A second group of hearts is different from those with biventricular connections. In this group, the atriums connect to only one ventricle, or in other words the hearts have a univentricular atrioventricular connection. These hearts can exist with either lateralized or isomeric atrial appendages. The specific connections to be found in the hearts making up this group are double-inlet ventricle, and absence of either the right or the left atrioventricular

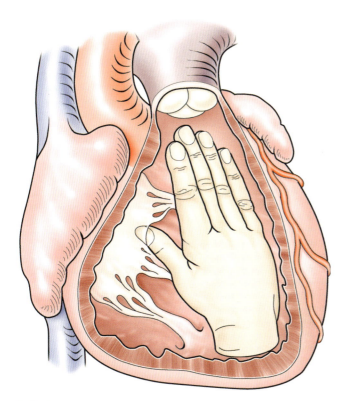

39.25a

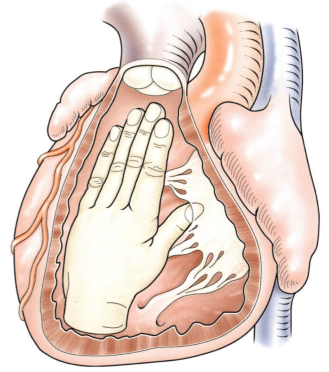

39.25b

connection (**Figure 39.26**). These univentricular connections can be found when the atriums are connected to a dominant left ventricle, to a dominant right ventricle, or to a solitary and indeterminate ventricle. Almost always when a univentricular connection to either a dominant left or a right ventricle exists, the complementary ventricle is present in hypoplastic and incomplete form because it lacks at least its inlet portion. Incomplete right ventricles, found with univentricular connection to a dominant left ventricle, are always in anterosuperior position, although they may be either right-sided or left-sided. Incomplete left ventricles, found with univentricular connection to a dominant right ventricle, are always posteroinferior, but again may be either right- or left-sided. By arguing from developmental principles, it is possible to account for the position of incomplete ventricles in terms of right-hand and left-hand topologic patterns. It is much simpler just to describe the position of the incomplete ventricle using anterior/posterior, superior/inferior, and right/left coordinates. Solitary and indeterminate ventricles do not possess second ventricles. Self-evidently, only these solitary ventricles, in morphological terms, are "single ventricles" or "univentricular hearts."

The so-called mode of atrioventricular connection describes the arrangement of the atrioventricular valves. When concordant, discordant, mixed, and double-inlet connections exist, both atriums are connected with the ventricular mass. The dual atrioventricular junctions can be guarded by two separate valves, or by a common atrioventricular valve. One of two valves, or rarely both, may straddle the ventricular septum when the tension apparatus is attached on both sides of the septum. When a valve straddles, its junction usually also overrides the septum. The degree of this override determines the commitment of the valve to the two ventricles. It is well known that spectrums of degrees of override exist with different segmental combinations. These extend from the hearts having effectively biventricular to effectively double-inlet atrioventricular connections. For the purposes of categorization of the precise connection in such hearts, in other words double-inlet versus biventricular connections, the overriding valve is assigned to the ventricle connected to its greater part, the so-called "50% law." Common valves usually straddle, but not always. For instance, a common valve in the presence of a double-inlet connection can be exclusively connected to one ventricle. A common valve, nonetheless, always guards two atrioventricular junctions, the right and the left, so this fact must be taken into account when assessing the degree of override. A further mode of connection when two valves exist is for one of the valves to be imperforate. This situation is different from absence of one atrioventricular connection, but both arrangements produce atrioventricular valvar atresia. Absence of one connection is the commonest cause of atrioventricular valvar atresia. When one atrioventricular

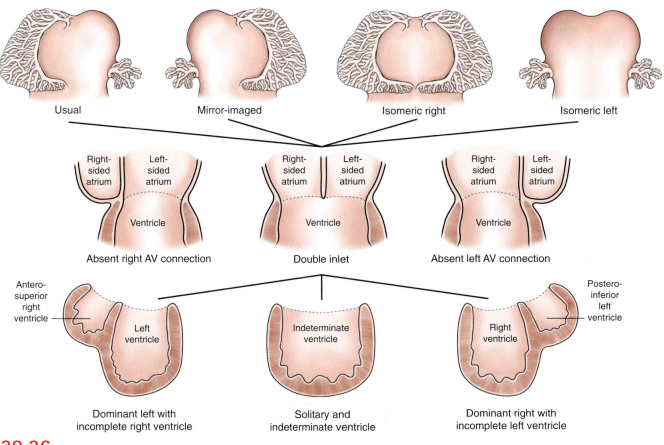

Usual   Mirror-imaged   Isomeric right   Isomeric left

Right-sided atrium | Left-sided atrium   Right-sided atrium | Left-sided atrium   Right-sided atrium | Left-sided atrium

Ventricle   Ventricle   Ventricle

Absent right AV connection   Double inlet   Absent left AV connection

Antero-superior right ventricle   Left ventricle   Indeterminate ventricle   Right ventricle   Postero-inferior left ventricle

Dominant left with incomplete right ventricle   Solitary and indeterminate ventricle   Dominant right with incomplete left ventricle

39.26

connection is absent, the modes of connection of the persisting junction are strictly limited. The atrioventricular valve may either be exclusively connected to one ventricle, or alternatively straddle or override. The latter arrangement gives a connection which is uniatrial but biventricular.

Influence of ventricular topology on conduction tissues

In the section on the normal atrioventricular junctions, we described how the triangle of Koch provides the landmarks to the atrioventricular junctional area. In hearts with abnormal atrioventricular connections, however, the regular atrioventricular node is not always the one which gives rise to the penetrating atrioventricular bundle. During fetal life, a complete ring of potential conduction tissue surrounds the atrioventricular junction. Remnants of this ring often persist into adult life, but then they are sequestered on the atrial aspect of the fibrous plane of insulation, and they do not give rise to atrioventricular conduction bundles. In the presence of abnormal connections between the atriums and ventricles, however, parts of this atrioventricular ring tissue can take over the role of the atrioventricular node. The rules which determine whether a regular or an anomalous node exists, or rarely both, are governed by several factors. The most important is whether good alignment exists between the atrial septum and the muscular ventricular septum. Almost always in hearts with concordant atrioventricular connections, there is good alignment, and hence a regular conduction system. The exception is found in the setting of straddling and overriding of the tricuspid valve, when an anomalous node is formed at the point at which the muscular ventricular septum makes contact with the atrioventricular junction. The normal septal alignment is lacking in hearts with usual atrial arrangement and discordant atrioventricular connections, and in hearts with univentricular connection to dominant left and indeterminate ventricles. In these hearts, therefore, there is usually an anomalous anterior atrioventricular node. In those with dominant left ventricles, the anterosuperior position of the muscular ventricular septum dictates that there cannot be alignment with the atrial septum, so that an anterior node is the rule. With univentricular connection to a dominant right ventricle, in contrast, septal alignment is maintained when the rudimentary left ventricle is left-sided, so that regular conduction systems are found. Similarly, when discordant atrioventricular connections are found with mirror-imaged atrial chambers, there is often good septal alignment because of associated pulmonary stenosis or atresia, and hence a regular conduction system. Ventricular topology, nonetheless, is also significant. Thus, abnormal systems are found most frequently in the presence of left-handed ventricular topology. This rule holds good also when a univentricular connection is made to a dominant right ventricle, and when biventricular atrioventricular connections are mixed in the setting of isomeric atrial appendages. The exception is found when left-handed topology coexists with

mirror-imaged atrial chambers, because almost always this situation means that the atrioventricular connections will be concordant. Thus, the atrioventricular connections are the best guide to disposition of the atrioventricular conduction axis, but the topological arrangement of the ventricular mass is also highly significant.

The ventriculoarterial junctions

At the ventriculoarterial junctions, it is again necessary to take account of the type and mode of connections. Additionally, attention should be paid to arterial relationships. The morphology of the ventricular outflow tracts, so-called infundibular or conal anatomy, is also variable but is rarely of surgical significance.

The ventriculoarterial connections are said to be concordant when the aorta is connected to the left ventricle, and the pulmonary trunk to the right ventricle. An aorta connected to a right ventricle, and a pulmonary trunk to a left ventricle, produces discordant connections. Both arteries connected to the same ventricle are described as double outlet, whereas single outlet of the heart is used to describe the situation in which only one patent arterial trunk can be traced to make contact with the ventricular mass. The latter may be a common trunk, or alternatively an aortic trunk with pulmonary atresia, a pulmonary trunk with aortic atresia, or a solitary arterial trunk when the intrapericardial pulmonary arteries are lacking. The modes of connection are more limited at the ventriculoarterial junctions. A common valve only exists with a common trunk. When two valves are present, both may be patent. One or both may then override the septum. As with overriding atrioventricular valves, the precise connection is determined by using the 50% law. One arterial valve may also be imperforate. In this situation, either the imperforate valve or the patent valve may override.

All of the above connections are determined irrespective of the arterial interrelationships. It is not possible to infer with complete accuracy the ventricular origin of the great arteries from their external relationships. In making this statement, we do not imply that relationships give no help in diagnosing connections. Certain basic arrangements are seen more frequently with one given connection, for example a right-sided and anterior aorta with concordant atrioventricular and discordant ventriculoarterial connections. Immutable laws, however, do not exist, and trends should be treated only as a guide to the possibility of abnormal connections. When describing the abnormal relationships, it is necessary to account for both the positions of the arterial valves and the orientation of the ascending portions of the arterial trunks. Valvar relationships are best described by accounting for the position of the aortic valve in comparison to the pulmonary valve in right/left and anterior/posterior coordinates. When describing the orientation of the arterial trunks, there are two basic patterns: either the pulmonary trunk spirals round the aorta towards its bifurcation or the trunks ascend in parallel fashion. By combining these two variables, it is an easy matter to describe all anticipated patterns of arterial interrelationships.

Although the morphology of the outflow tracts in itself is rarely of surgical significance, great emphasis has been placed in the past on the role of the bilateral conus or bilateral infundibulum. Each arterial valve is potentially capable of being supported by a complete muscular infundibulum in the setting of any ventriculoarterial connection. These infundibula have three basic components. One component separates the arterial valves, along with their subvalvar outflow tracts, from each other. This component is the muscular outlet, infundibular, or conal septum. The second part is the free parietal ventricular wall. The third part has given most problems in comprehension. This part represents the inner heart curvature between the anterosuperior wall of the atriums, and the posteroinferior wall of the great arterial trunks. This curvature separates the arterial valves from the atrioventricular valves and is called the ventriculoinfundibular fold. The variability in morphology of the outflow tracts usually depends on the integrity of this fold. When it is intact, there is discontinuity between the leaflets of the atrioventricular and arterial valves, and a complete muscular infundibulum is usually present. When the fold is deficient, continuity exists between the leaflets of the atrioventricular and arterial valves, and part of the infundibulum is deficient. The term "usually" is used above purposely, since it is possible for the ventriculoinfundibular fold to be intact, producing arterial–atrioventricular discontinuity, and yet for the outlet septum to be deficient, thus permitting valvar continuity between the leaflets of the aortic and pulmonary valves. In this setting, the muscular infundibula would be incomplete. Obviously, therefore, the integrity of the ventricular outflow tracts depends on the morphology of both the ventriculoinfundibular fold and the outlet septum. It should also be noted that this discussion has made no mention of the septomarginal trabeculation. This latter muscular structure is an integral part of the right ventricle and is not part of the subvalvar outflow tracts.

Subsequent steps in sequential analysis

The analysis described thus far accounts only for the segmental combination of the heart. In most instances, this will be normal. But it will have cost the surgeon nothing to prove this normality. Indeed, it is essential so to do. Having established the segmental pattern, analysis is concluded by assessing all the associated defects present. This assessment is also best done in segmental fashion, commencing by confirming the normality of the venoatrial connections. Attention can then be directed in turn to the atrial segment, the ventricular

segment, and the arterial segment, at the same time looking for any junctional malformations that may not have been accounted for during the analysis of the connections. Then, the anatomy of the aortic and pulmonary pathways is assessed. In this way, any congenital cardiac lesion, or combination of lesions, however simple or complex, is accounted for and understood in the segmental setting of the heart itself. Separate description is then provided for the location of the heart, the direction of its apex, and the arrangement of the thoracic and abdominal organs, taking care to describe each system separately when discrepancies are encountered from the anticipated patterns.

ACKNOWLEDGMENTS

It would not have been possible to prepare all the illustrations, or to write the surgical aspects of this chapter, without the considerable help of and intellectual input from Dr Benson Wilcox, from the University of North Carolina, Chapel Hill. Sadly, Ben passed away during the spring of 2010. We dedicate this revised chapter to his eternal memory. One of us (RHA) was indebted to him throughout his studies, and we remember fondly his freely given support and collaboration. **Figures 39.2, 39.3, 39.6** and **39.8** were photographed by him, and were reproduced with his permission. Some of the other illustrations were also prepared with the help of Siew Yen Ho, Andrew Cook, and Gemma Price. We thank them for their contributions.

FURTHER READING

Anderson RH. How should we optimally describe complex congenitally malformed hearts? *Ann Thorac Surg.* 1996; 62: 710–16.

Anderson RH, Ho SY. Sequential segmental analysis – description and categorisation for the millennium. *Cardiol Young.* 1997; 7: 98–116.

Anderson RH, Ho SY, Becker AE. Anatomy of the human atrioventricular junctions revisited. *Anat Rec.* 2000; 260: 81–91.

Anderson RH, Webb S, Brown NA. Clinical anatomy of the atrial septum with reference to its development components. *Clin Anat.* 1999; 12: 362–74.

Sutton JP 3rd, Ho SY, Anderson RH. The forgotten interleaflet triangles: a review of the surgical anatomy of the aortic valve. *Ann Thorac Surg.* 1995; 59: 419–27.

Uemura H, Ho SY, Devine WA, et al. Atrial appendages and venoatrial connections in hearts with patients with visceral heterotaxy. *Ann Thorac Surg.* 1995; 60: 561–9.

40

Palliative procedures: shunts and pulmonary artery banding

DAVID P. BICHELL

MODIFIED BLALOCK–TAUSSIG SHUNT

HISTORY

Introduced in 1945, the Blalock–Taussig shunt in its modified form has become a standard part of palliation for cyanotic heart defects. As neonatal and infant open-heart procedures have been refined, the use of the Blalock–Taussig shunt or other interim systemic-to-pulmonary shunts for many defects has given way to early complete anatomical repair. The role for the modified Blalock–Taussig shunt has become limited largely to short-term palliation in staged univentricular pathways.

PRINCIPLES AND JUSTIFICATION

In its current use, the modified Blalock–Taussig shunt is applied as a means of maintaining predictable pulmonary blood flow for defects of pulmonary hypoperfusion, or, most commonly, in univentricular palliations where the patent ductus arteriosus is typically divided, and the Blalock–Taussig shunt provides the exclusive source of pulmonary blood flow for 3–6 months. At the second stage, pulmonary vascular resistance has fallen sufficiently to accept passive venous flow by direct cavopulmonary anastomosis.

A successful shunt must be planned to conduct a narrow range of appropriate flow, providing pulmonary blood flow that is sufficient but not excessive, so as to avoid low cardiac output, pulmonary vascular damage, and excessive ventricular volume overload.

Some principles of hydrodynamics are integral to the planning and construction of the successful shunt. Assuming laminar flow, the volumetric flow rate through a regular cylindrical conduit is governed by the Hagen–Poiseuille equation:

$$Q = \Delta p \pi d^4 / 128 L \mu$$

in which Q = volumetric flow rate, Δp = pressure drop, d = diameter, L = length, and μ = fluid viscosity. This relationship illustrates the concept that a small change in shunt diameter results in a large change in flow, relating to the diameter raised to the fourth power. For a great majority of newborns, a 3.0–3.5 mm polytetrafluoroethylene (PTFE) conduit provides an appropriate balance of systemic-to-pulmonary blood flow. Overly bulky anastomotic suture lines can diminish the effective diameter of the shunt, with accordingly amplified effects on flow. Shunt length has a much weaker influence on flow. Placing the origin of a Blalock–Taussig shunt anastomosis more distal or proximal along the innominate or subclavian artery may modulate shunt flow, owing to the diameter of the vessel of origin, but the resulting small changes in shunt length with these maneuvers are of minor influence. Shunt length and angle of anastomosis are best planned to preserve, undistorted, the geometry of the innominate and pulmonary arteries. A shunt that is only millimeters too long can compress its own inflow or outflow; millimeters too short can place distorting tension on the pulmonary artery.

The modified Blalock–Taussig shunt can be constructed through a thoracotomy or a sternotomy. In recent years, the sternotomy approach has gained favor at most institutions for a variety of reasons, particularly because the shunt is used usually as an interim palliation that will be followed by a subsequent sternotomy-requiring procedure. Other advantages of the sternotomy approach include technical ease, better shunt patency, more even distribution of flow bilaterally, less pulmonary artery distortion, and better access to ligate the ductus arteriosus or perform other concomitant procedures.

PREOPERATIVE ASSESSMENT AND PREPARATION

Although a majority of newborns are appropriately served by a 3.5 mm PTFE shunt, smaller shunt diameters may better suit the infant weighing less than 2.5 kg. An arterial monitoring line, preferably not in the limb affected by the shunt, and venous access, are imperative before starting the procedure. Pulse oximetry and near-infrared spectroscopy aid in assessing the balance between pulmonary and systemic circulations, and the patient's tolerance for partial pulmonary artery clamping.

OPERATION

Modified Blalock–Taussig shunt

A standard median sternotomy is performed (**Figure 40.1**). The upper pericardium is incised, and pericardial suspension sutures assist in exposure of the upper mediastinal structures. The innominate artery is mobilized circumferentially beyond its bifurcation into subclavian and common carotid arteries. The innominate vein can be gently retracted with Silastic vessel loops. Between the aorta and superior vena cava (SVC), the right pulmonary artery is identified and mobilized circumferentially from its origin at the main pulmonary artery to beyond the origin of the upper lobe branch.

Before the placement of any clamp, a PTFE conduit is cut on an angle with a gentle S shape, corresponding to the angle of the innominate artery as it relates to the aorta (**Figure 40.2**).

A forcep is used to grasp the point of intended anastomosis to the innominate artery (**Figure 40.3**). Caudad traction on this point during the application of a C-clamp centers the point of anastomosis within the jaws of the clamp.

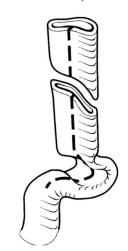

40.2

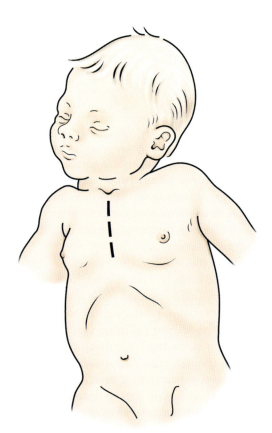

40.1

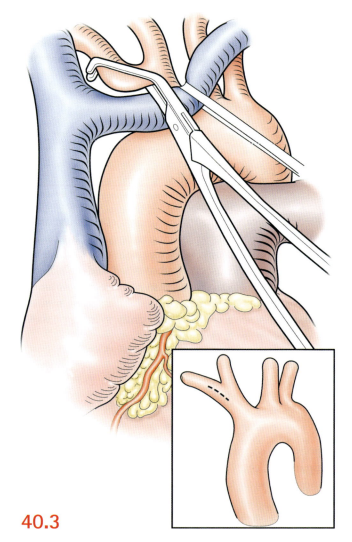

40.3

A 7-0 or 8-0 polypropylene suture is used to form the proximal anastomosis, with caution so as not to create a bulky, inverting, or distorted suture line (**Figure 40.4**). At the completion of the proximal anastomosis, the PTFE graft is clamped distally after passing it posterior to the innominate vein on its course toward the pulmonary artery.

As the graft is distended with blood, a point is chosen at which to divide it at a length and angle corresponding to the point of distal anastomosis to the right pulmonary artery. A vascular clamp is placed proximally on the graft to block flow without compromising exposure for the distal anastomosis (**Figure 40.5**). Traction sutures on the ascending aorta can aid in exposure for this anastomosis. The center point of the intended distal anastomosis on the right pulmonary artery is grasped and tented cephalad, to center it within a C-clamp. The patient's saturation and hemodynamics are observed during a trial pulmonary artery clamping before making the pulmonary arteriotomy. Care is taken to ensure that the clamp does not exert compression on the coronary arteries or aorta. A longitudinal pulmonary arteriotomy is made, and a 7-0 or 8-0 polypropylene suture is used to complete the distal anastomosis.

If the shunt is being created as an isolated procedure, the patent ductus is ligated and divided as the shunt is opened (**Figure 40.6**). Mobilization of a patent ductus before the

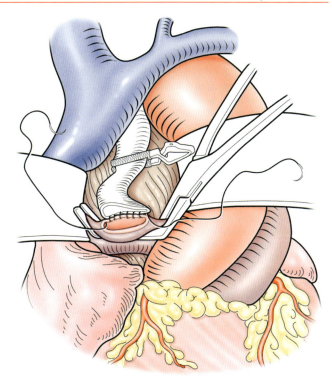

40.5

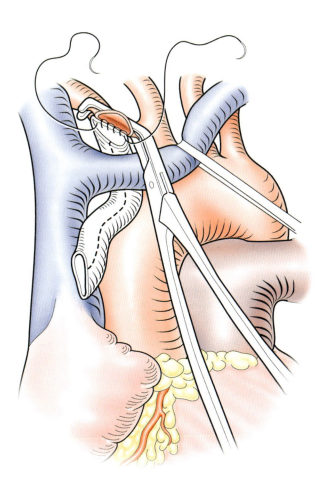

40.4

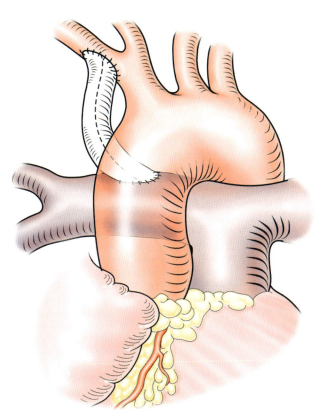

40.6

shunt construction in ductal-dependent lesions is ill-advised, as ductal spasm induced by the dissection can render the patient unstable before the establishment of an alternative source of pulmonary blood flow. Briefly test-clamping the shunt demonstrates patency and runoff, and careful hemodynamic monitoring ensures the appropriate balance of pulmonary and systemic circulations. Rarely, pulmonary overcirculation requires tailoring the shunt before closure.

Central aortopulmonary shunt

When the brachiocephalic vasculature is insufficient in caliber, condition, or geometry to support a modified Blalock–Taussig shunt, a central aortopulmonary shunt is an alternative approach.

Through a median sternotomy, the ascending aorta is exposed. Marking sutures are placed to delimit a diagonal course for a conduit that will direct flow toward the targeted distal anastomosis site on the pulmonary artery (**Figure 40.7a**). With retraction on the marking sutures, a straight or gently curved vascular clamp is placed so as to isolate the area delimited by the marking sutures, without compromising flow to the distal aorta. An aortotomy is made (**Figure 40.7b**).

A PTFE conduit is cut in a recurved bevel (**Figure 40.8a**), which, when positioned onto the curved aortotomy, will produce a uniform conduit shape, with inflow compromised neither by a restrictive edge at the heel of the graft nor by flattening along the greater curve of the graft (**Figure 40.8b**).

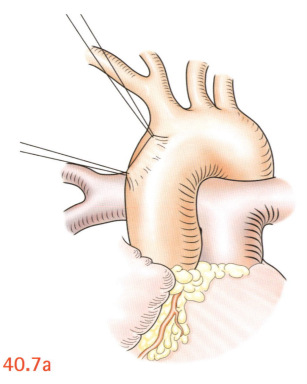

40.7a

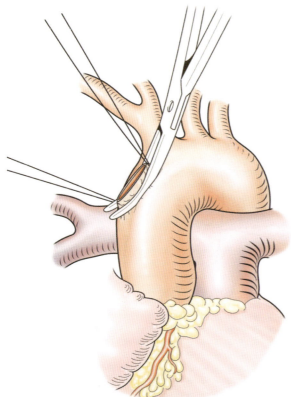

40.7b

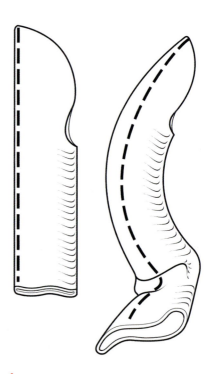

40.8a–b

The graft anastomosis is formed (**Figure 40.9a**), the partial occlusion clamp on the aorta is released, and the graft is allowed to fill (**Figure 40.9b**). The distal end of the graft is cut at an appropriate bevel for its anastomosis onto the pulmonary artery, which is carried out as for the modified Blalock–Taussig shunt.

POSTOPERATIVE CARE

Pulmonary overcirculation from an inappropriately large systemic-to-pulmonary shunt, high systemic vascular resistance, or low pulmonary vascular resistance can result in systemic hypoperfusion, excessive ventricular volume overload, acidosis, and arrest. Shunt thrombosis results in pulmonary hypoperfusion and cyanosis. Meticulous monitoring of hemodynamic data and arterial blood gas data must continue postoperatively, with a high index of suspicion and a low threshold for intervention to revise the shunt. In the presence of postcardiopulmonary bypass pulmonary edema or other comorbidities resulting in parenchymal lung disease or intrapulmonary shunting, gas exchange may be inefficient, resulting in the phenomenon of low arterial oxygen saturation despite pulmonary overcirculation. Venous O_2 saturation, near-infrared spectroscopy, and systemic acidosis are sensitive indicators of the adequacy of systemic perfusion, and a proactive treatment of these findings with a low threshold for reoperating must be pursued. Residual arch obstruction is important to rule out as an indirect etiology for pulmonary overcirculation.

When postoperative bleeding is not a concern, a continuous heparin infusion may prevent early thrombosis. Many centers maintain shunted patients on daily aspirin.

OUTCOME

Perioperative complications after the construction of a modified Blalock–Taussig shunt include phrenic nerve injury, Horner's syndrome, shunt thrombosis, pericardial effusion, and chylothorax.

Hospital mortality for the isolated construction of a palliative modified Blalock–Taussig shunt is reported as 8–11%. Shunt failure was a more prominent contributing factor to mortality in the thoracotomy group than in the sternotomy group, owing to pulmonary artery distortion. The majority of modified Blalock–Taussig shunts are created in conjunction with additional procedures, such as the Norwood stage I palliation, and outcomes depend on a variety of factors associated with the principle procedure. The parallel circulation imparted by the systemic-to-pulmonary shunt causes systemic ventricular volume overload and labile shifts in circulation from pulmonary to systemic circulations. The morbidity and mortality associated with these factors reinforces the principle that the modified Blalock–Taussig shunt should be left in place for only the shortest possible period before the subsequent repair or palliation is performed.

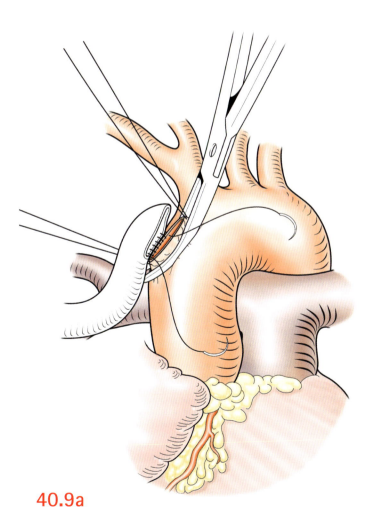

40.9a

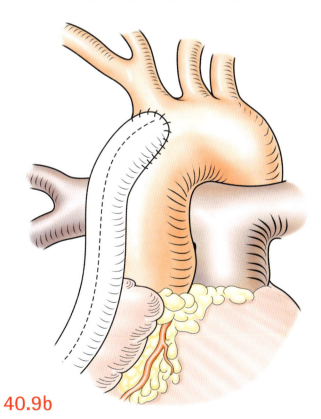

40.9b

BIDIRECTIONAL CAVOPULMONARY ANASTOMOSIS (BIDIRECTIONAL GLENN SHUNT)

HISTORY

Experimentally induced severe right ventricular damage in a dog model, performed in the 1940s, demonstrated only a minimal resultant increase in systemic venous pressure and no demonstrable reduction in pulmonary blood flow. These experiments established the scientific substrate for the development of right heart bypass procedures commonly in use today to palliate the univentricular heart. Carlton, Mondini, and de Marchi first described the cavopulmonary anastomosis in cadaveric and animal feasibility studies in 1950. The first clinical application of the cavopulmonary shunt was reported by Shumacher, and the first clinically successful reported cavopulmonary anastomosis was performed in 1956 by Meshalkin et al. After several years of detailed animal studies of right heart bypass physiology, William Glenn, for whom the superior cavopulmonary anastomosis is most commonly named, reported its use in a 7-year-old progressively cyanotic boy with single ventricle physiology and pulmonary stenosis. The classic Glenn shunt, diverting SVC flow exclusively to the right lung, resulted in an uneven distribution of pulmonary blood flow and pulmonary artery distortion complicating a subsequent Fontan and contributed to the formation of pulmonary arteriovenous malformations. Experimentally developed by Haller et al., the first clinical application of the end-to-side bidirectional cavopulmonary anastomosis was reported by Azzolina et al. in 1972. The bidirectional cavopulmonary anastomosis is the only form in common clinical use today, mostly as a second stage in the three-staged palliation of the univentricular heart.

PRINCIPLES AND JUSTIFICATION

The prolonged volume load burdening the single ventricle with parallel circulation contributes to ventricular dilatation, atrioventricular valve regurgitation, ventricular dysfunction, and the resultant risk of a suboptimal Fontan outcome. The bidirectional cavopulmonary anastomosis augments pulmonary blood flow while reducing ventricular work. For infants, the SVC contributes 50% of the total cardiac output, and so the bidirectional cavopulmonary anastomosis diverts a significant amount of volume load away from the ventricle. An early bidirectional cavopulmonary anastomosis in the univentricular heart may reduce the deleterious effects of prolonged hypoxia and volume overload. Early volume unloading has been shown to result in improved late exercise performance in Fontan patients when compared with those whose unloading procedures were performed later. Since the late 1980s, the bidirectional cavopulmonary anastomosis has become a routine interim stage for a majority of Fontan pathway patients.

Additionally, the bidirectional cavopulmonary anastomosis is used as an adjunct to 1.5 ventricle palliations for lesions such as pulmonary atresia with intact ventricular septum or Ebstein's anomaly and unbalanced atrioventricular septal defect, where a diminutive right ventricle or tricuspid valve may be capable of conducting inferior vena caval flow but not capable of conducting an entire cardiac output.

PREOPERATIVE ASSESSMENT AND PREPARATION

Age

Systemic venous-to-pulmonary artery blood flow without ventricular propulsion depends on a sufficiently low pulmonary vascular resistance to permit the passive transit of blood across the pulmonary circulation, and sufficiently low pulmonary artery pressures to avoid systemic venous hypertension. The newborn's pulmonary vascular resistance is too high to satisfy these criteria but falls in the first weeks or months of life, as the cross-sectional area of the pulmonary microvascular bed expands. A cavopulmonary anastomosis performed in the first weeks of life invariably results in prohibitive cyanosis and SVC hypertension. Although successful cavopulmonary shunts have been performed at 4 weeks of age, a majority are performed at or beyond 4 months. Within these constraints, several theoretical and practical advantages exist to performing the cavopulmonary anastomosis as early as reasonably possible.

Anatomical considerations

Every candidate for cavopulmonary anastomosis undergoes a preoperative diagnostic echocardiogram and often also a cardiac catheterization. Anatomical details must be clarified to plan modifications of the procedure to accommodate such findings as left SVC, or interrupted inferior vena cava with azygos continuation. Although some atrioventricular valve regurgitation may resolve with ventricular volume load reduction, important structural atrioventricular valve regurgitation can complicate the postoperative course and deserves attention. This situation should prompt the consideration of a concomitant valvuloplasty. Pulmonary artery stenosis or distortion is mapped for concomitant repair. Present or incipient ventricular outflow obstruction might require a Damus–Kaye–Stansel anastomosis or an intracardiac procedure concomitantly with the cavopulmonary anastomosis. Important venous collateral vessels to the lower compartment can be identified and coil-occluded preoperatively. Pulmonary vein obstruction is ruled out.

Hemodynamic criteria

Pulmonary artery pressure determinations and/or pulmonary venous wedge pressure data, ventricular end-diastolic pressure data, and saturation data are useful to assess the appropriateness of constructing the bidirectional cavopulmonary anastomosis. The omission of these determinations can result in postoperative cyanosis, systemic venous hypertension, poor cardiac output, and the need to disassemble the shunt. In general, though subject to exceptions, an indexed pulmonary vascular resistance greater than 2 U/m², a mean pulmonary artery pressure greater than 18 mmHg, a transpulmonary gradient greater than 10 mmHg, or ventricular end-diastolic pressure greater than 12 mmHg are catheterization values above which the cavopulmonary anastomosis may fail. A reversible etiology should be sought for any of these findings to improve a patient's likelihood of sufficient pulmonary blood flow without systemic venous hypertension.

Monitoring

A peripheral arterial monitoring line and venous access are important at the outset of the operation. Central venous access can be placed preoperatively or intraoperatively. A transduced upper-compartment (SVC) line and lower-compartment (atrial) line is a useful intraoperative determinant of the transpulmonary gradient. Although preoperative upper-compartment percutaneous venous lines are routine in some institutions, an indwelling line left in a low-flow system carries the risk of SVC thrombosis.

OPERATION

The SVC is mobilized circumferentially from its atrial attachment and cephalad onto the innominate vein (**Figure 40.10**). The azygos vein is ligated and divided. The ipsilateral pulmonary artery is mobilized fully, beyond the origin of the upper lobe branch. Cardiopulmonary bypass is initiated with bicaval venous cannulation.

A polypropylene pursestring is placed around the SVC just cephalad to the atriocaval junction (**Figure 40.11**). The SVC is divided and the atrial pursestring secured. A pursestring ligation of the SVC is preferred over a clamp at the SVC, so as to minimize tissue damage in the area of the sinoatrial node. The orientation of the SVC is carefully preserved. A spatulation of the lateral aspect of the SVC is performed (**Figure 40.12**).

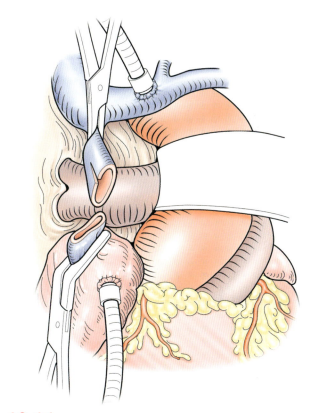

40.11

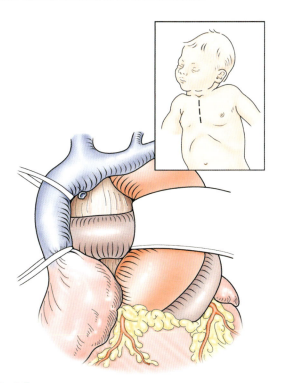

40.10

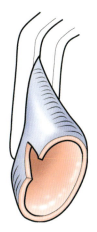

40.12

The mobilized pulmonary artery is grasped at a center point for the planned anastomosis, and a curved clamp is applied, taking care to not compress the coronary artery as it emerges from the adjacent aortic root (**Figure 40.13**). A longitudinal pulmonary arteriotomy is made, and the anastomosis is carried out with a 7-0 or 8-0 polypropylene suture (**Figure 40.14**).

The completed anastomosis should result in a smooth transition from SVC to pulmonary artery, without creasing, distortion, or stenosis (**Figure 40.15**).

When necessary to ameliorate pulmonary artery stenosis, to augment the cavopulmonary anastomosis to ensure no distortion, a patch augmentation of the branch pulmonary artery is made before the completion of the SVC–pulmonary artery anastomosis (**Figure 40.16**).

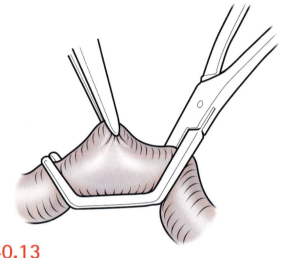

40.13

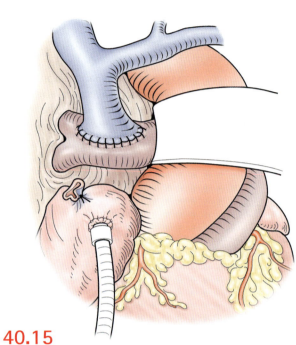

40.15

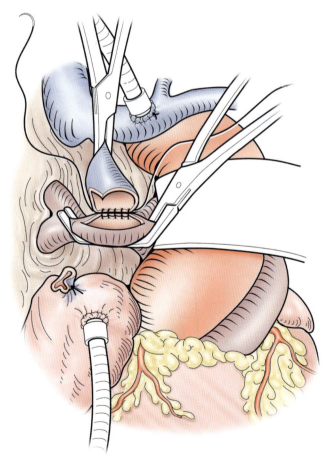

40.14

40.16

Fresh, autologous vein is an excellent, endothelialized material for use as a patch, fortuitously available at the time of cavopulmonary anastomosis. The azygos vein, routinely separated from the SVC to prevent upper-to-lower venous compartment decompression, can be harvested as a segment several centimeters in length (**Figure 40.17**).

The azygos vein segment is opened longitudinally to create a rectangular patch. Care must be taken to orient the patch such that any venous valve is oriented properly, with the direction of flow through the pulmonary artery (**Figure 40.18**).

The pulmonary artery is isolated from hilum to hilum with elastic vessel loops around upper and ongoing pulmonary artery branches. A broad pulmonary arteriotomy is made to encompass the segment to be augmented and the anastomotic site for the cavopulmonary anastomosis (**Figure 40.19**).

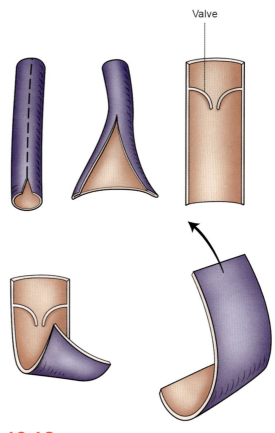

Valve

40.18

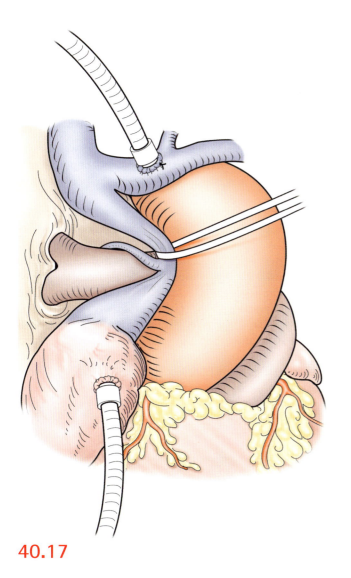

40.17

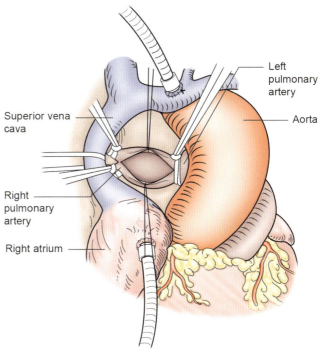

Left pulmonary artery

Superior vena cava

Aorta

Right pulmonary artery

Right atrium

40.19

The azygos vein onlay patch is applied to the pulmonary arteriotomy, tailoring its rightward aspect so as to accommodate the SVC anastomosis site (**Figure 40.20a–d**). The cavopulmonary anastomosis is formed, with the azygos vein patch tailored appropriately, to avoid distortion at the toe of the anastomosis (**Figure 40. 21**).

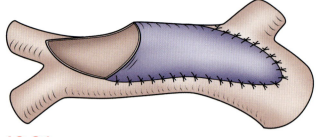

40.21

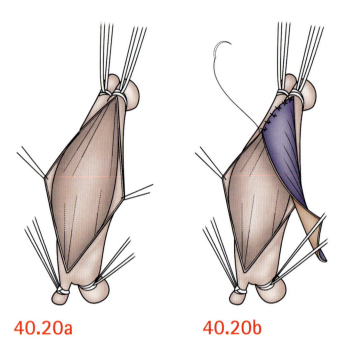

40.20a

40.20b

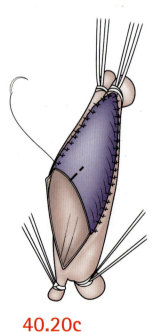

40.20c

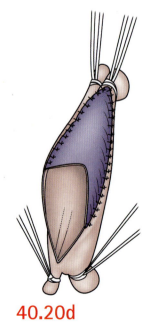

40.20d

POSTOPERATIVE CARE

The perioperative management of patients after bidirectional cavopulmonary anastomosis requires a concerted effort to promote the transit of blood through the pulmonary circulation. Positive pressure ventilation may itself impede pulmonary blood flow. This effect is minimized if strategies of low inspiratory-to-expiratory ratio and early extubation are pursued. Hyperventilation impairs oxygenation even as it lowers pulmonary vascular resistance, possibly as a result of cerebrovascular resistance increasing in response to a decreasing PCO_2. An elevation of the patient's head may help minimize upper body edema.

Pharmacological maneuvers to optimize pulmonary blood flow include the routine use of phosphodiesterase inhibitors such as milrinone, which affects pulmonary as well as systemic vasodilatation. Nitric oxide may augment pulmonary blood flow, but it is seldom necessary in the postoperative period.

Postoperative hypoxia, despite the previously described maneuvers, prompts an aggressive investigation of possible etiologies. A high level of suspicion is maintained for pulmonary artery or pre-pulmonary stenosis that could require surgical revision. Venovenous collaterals from the upper to lower compartment should be ruled out and can be the cause of early or late postoperative cyanosis. Atrioventricular valve regurgitation or poor ventricular function results in elevated atrial and ventricular end-diastolic pressures, and these problems are addressed with appropriate inotropic support or surgical intervention. In rare instances of hypoxia, it may be necessary to construct a second source of pulmonary blood flow in the form of a systemic-to-pulmonary shunt, although this strategy produces a volume load to the ventricle, and can exacerbate upper-compartment venous hypertension.

Other considerations in investigating an unstable postoperative course include acute geometric changes in the heart imparted by the acute reduction in volume load. A bulboventricular foramen, on which ventricular outflow depends, can become restrictive after ventricular unloading.

OUTCOME

Perioperative and late mortality from the construction of a bidirectional cavopulmonary anastomosis in the present era is less than 2%. Fontan morbidity may be reduced when the interim cavopulmonary anastomosis is used. Late sequelae include progressive cyanosis secondary to growth, venovenous collateral formation, and the development of pulmonary arteriovenous malformations. The late

development of pulmonary arteriovenous malformations has been reported to occur in 25–50% of patients with bidirectional cavopulmonary shunts, especially in heterotaxy patients. Fontan completion to incorporate hepatic venous effluent into the pulmonary vascular circulation contributes to their resolution. Aortopulmonary collateral formation may occur in two-thirds of patients, requiring coil embolization where possible.

THE PULMONARY ARTERY BAND

HISTORY

The pulmonary artery band, originating as an animal model for the study of hypertrophy, was introduced as palliation for excessive pulmonary blood flow by Muller and Dammann in 1952. Pulmonary artery banding gained popularity for many years for the palliation of large ventricular septal defects (VSDs) and a variety of other defects associated with pulmonary overcirculation, permitting an infant to gain sufficient size for a safe anatomical correction or additional palliation. Advances in cardiac surgery for infants and newborns have resulted in the early anatomical correction of a majority of defects that constituted former indications for pulmonary artery banding, and the procedure is currently uncommon. The pulmonary artery band is presently reserved for the short-term palliation of infants with excessive pulmonary blood flow, such as that associated with tricuspid atresia, double-inlet left ventricle, double-outlet single ventricle, multiple VSDs, or large VSDs requiring interim palliation owing to comorbidities that prohibit cardiopulmonary bypass. The pulmonary artery band is also used for the short-term conditioning of the left ventricle in preparation for the arterial switch procedure in patients not corrected as newborns.

PRINCIPLES AND JUSTIFICATION

In accordance with Poiseuille's equation, flow through a cylindrical constriction is proportional to its diameter raised to the fourth power. The diameter is such a powerful determinant of flow that a 1 mm change in band diameter can effect a threefold change in flow. Plotting band circumference and weight, Trusler and Mustard examined the adequacy of empirically placed pulmonary artery bands for patients with VSD, based on the absence or persistence of congestive symptoms. A formula was devised predicting the optimal band circumference to be 20 mm plus 1 mm for each kilogram of the patient's weight. Further analysis of survival data and anatomical features led to the following revised formulae of band circumference:

- 20 mm + 1 mm/kg for simple defects without intracardiac bidirectional mixing
- 24 mm + 1 mm/kg for mixing lesions, with loosening only if cyanosis or bradycardia occurs.

Infants weighing less than 2 kg were recommended to have bands measuring 1.0–1.5 mm smaller in circumference than Trusler's formula predicts. Taking into account the nonlinear growth of the pulmonary valve in infants, Kawahira et al. have derived a formula for determining the optimal pulmonary artery band circumference as 87% of the normal (angiographically derived) pulmonary artery circumference ($51.81 \times$ [BSA]0.45), which applies more consistently to infants of any weight and correlates with Trusler's rule when applied to larger children. Using Trusler's rule as a starting point, most centers add pre- and post-band direct pressure measurement and peripheral O_2 saturation measurement to fine-adjust the band. The objective is to reduce the systolic pulmonary artery pressure to as close as possible to 30 mmHg or half of the systemic pressure, without causing bradycardia or systemic desaturation below 80%.

PREOPERATIVE ASSESSMENT AND PREPARATION

Careful consideration of the patient's cardiac anatomy must be made to select appropriate candidates for a palliative pulmonary artery band. Hazardous sequelae result from its inappropriate application.

Subaortic or aortic obstruction presents a relative contraindication to the placement of a pulmonary artery band, as a band creates physiological biventricular outflow obstruction, promoting myocardial hypertrophy and ischemia-fibrosis. A bulboventricular foramen area index less than $2 \, cm^2/m^2$ predicts an obstructive outflow unless bypassed as an initial palliation. This anatomy should prompt the consideration of a Damus–Kaye–Stansel construction with shunt as the initial palliation rather than a pulmonary artery band.

OPERATION

Sternotomy approach

The sternotomy approach is used when concomitant thoracotomy-requiring procedures, such as coarctation repair, are not indicated. The median sternotomy provides a safe, precise exposure of the main pulmonary artery and its branches for positioning of the band. The median sternotomy is often needed for future staged palliations or anatomical repair, so this approach has the additional advantage of leaving the patient with only one scar. The main pulmonary artery is mobilized circumferentially (**Figure 40.22**) and the pulmonary artery band material, pre-marked at a circumference estimated by Trusler's formula, is passed around the mobilized segment (**Figure 40.23**). A polypropylene suture is passed through the band at the pre-marked endpoints and tied (**Figure 40.24**).

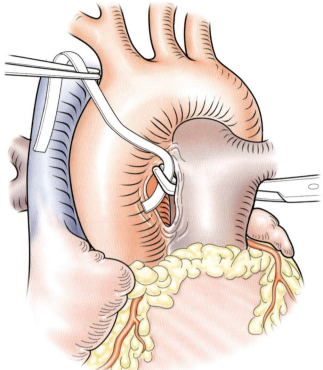

40.23

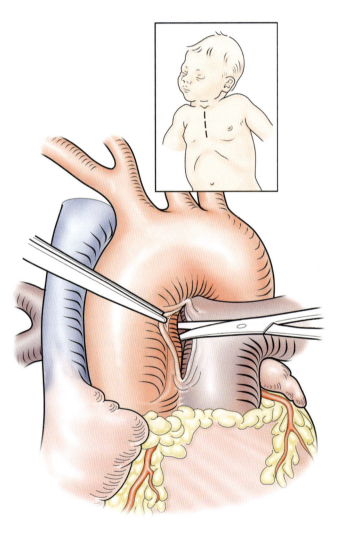

40.22

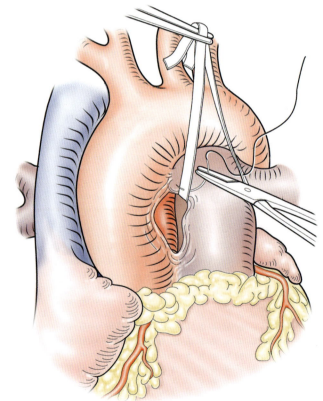

40.24

Direct pre- and post-band pressure measurements are made, and peripheral arterial line tracings and pulse oximetric determinations are observed. Additional mattress sutures are placed through the band to adjust its tightness to the goal of post-band pulmonary artery pressure equal to half the systemic pressure, while preserving O_2 saturations greater than 80% (**Figure 40.25**). Cyanosis or bradycardia suggests that the band should be loosened.

The band is positioned at a point sufficiently proximal to not impinge on the origin of the branch pulmonary arteries, approximately at the level of the sinotubular junction of the main pulmonary artery. Adventitial sutures secure this position and prevent band migration (**Figure 40.26**). The left main coronary artery is often in close proximity to the posterior aspect of the main pulmonary aretry, and caution is advised to assure no impingement on its course by the band.

The right branch pulmonary artery typically originates proximal to, and at a more acute angle than, the left branch pulmonary artery (**Figure 40.27**). Even a slight migration of the band can result in a partial or complete occlusion of the right branch pulmonary artery and insufficient limitation of flow to the left (**Figure 40.28**).

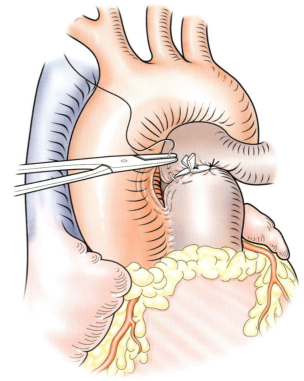

40.26

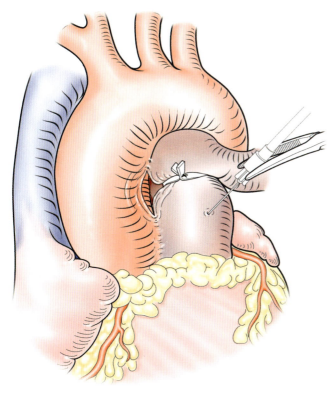

40.25

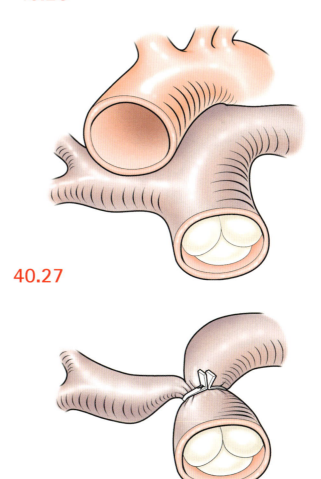

40.27

40.28

Pulmonary artery banding, thoracotomy

A left posterolateral thoracotomy is made in the fourth intercostal space to expose the juxtaductal aorta. A ductal ligation and/or concomitant aortic procedure is performed (**Figure 40.29**).

The pulmonary artery is exposed through an incision in the pericardium anterior to the phrenic nerve. Retraction sutures placed in the pericardium assist exposure of the main pulmonary artery and ascending aorta (**Figure 40.30**). A curved clamp is passed through the transverse sinus, and a tape, pre-marked at the appropriate band circumference as estimated by Trusler's formula, is passed to encircle the aorta and the pulmonary arteries together (**Figure 40.31**).

A plane is carefully dissected between the aorta and the main pulmonary artery, entering the transverse sinus under direct visualization (**Figure 40.32**). The dissection is carried out in a plane close to the back wall of the aorta, minimizing the chances of injuring the thin-walled right pulmonary artery as it passes in proximity to the posterior aorta. The clamp is then insinuated around the aorta to grasp the tape

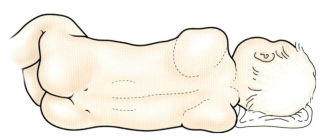

40.29

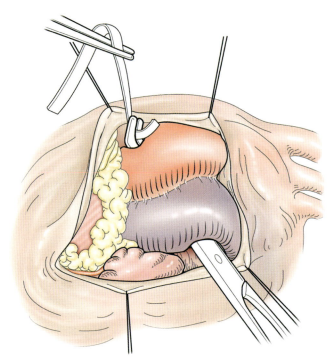

40.31

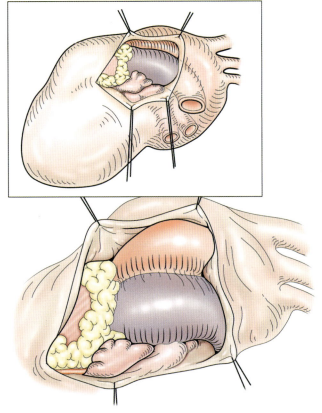

40.30

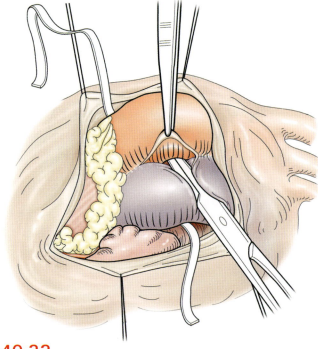

40.32

and exclude the aorta (**Figure 40.33**). This technique results in an encirclement of the main pulmonary artery without passing the clamp blindly around the thin-walled pulmonary artery itself (**Figure 40.34**).

A polypropylene suture is then placed through the band material at the marked endpoints to draw the band tight (**Figure 40.35**). Direct pre- and post-band pressure measurements are made, and peripheral arterial line tracings and pulse oximetric determinations are observed. Additional mattress sutures are placed through the band to adjust its tightness to the goal of post-band pulmonary artery pressure equal to half the systemic pressure, while preserving O_2 saturations greater than 80%. Cyanosis or bradycardia suggests that the band should be loosened.

After a satisfactory adjustment, the band is fixed to the adventitia of the pulmonary artery with several sutures to prevent its migration (**Figure 40.36**). The pericardium is reapproximated, and the thoracotomy is closed.

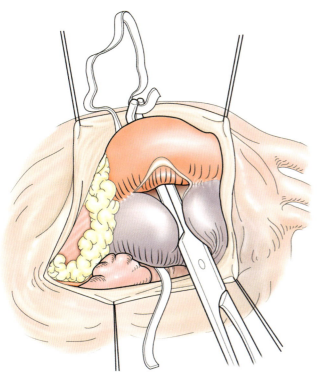

40.33

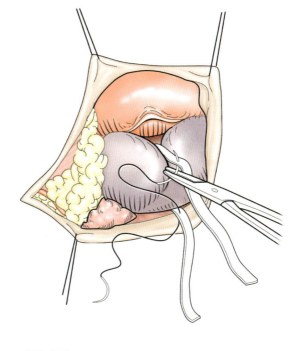

40.35

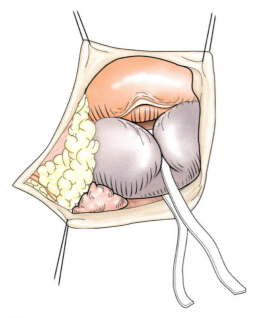

40.34

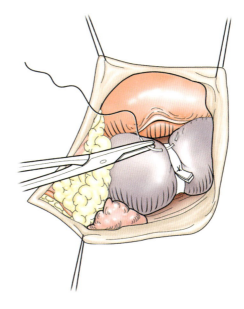

40.36

Pulmonary artery de-banding and reconstruction

The pulmonary artery is exposed through reoperative sternotomy, and main and branch pulmonary arteries are mobilized. Cicatricial tissue around the pulmonary artery band site results in a circumferential intimal ridge, and a simple anterior patch plasty of the band site results in residual obstruction from the retained posterior ridge. The pulmonary artery band and a segment of affected main pulmonary artery must be segmentally resected for a complete relief of obstruction (**Figure 40.37**).

As a segmental resection of the main pulmonary artery is carried out (**Figure 40.38**), particular caution is exercised at its posterior wall, as the left main coronary artery usually lies immediately subjacent. Along the posterior wall, the pulmonary artery is only resected as the structures deep to it are clearly visualized, and safety sometimes dictates that a portion of back wall be left intact. The pulmonary valve is inspected and repaired if necessary.

Further mobilization of the confluence and branch pulmonary arteries is carried out to minimize any distortion or tension on the planned anastomosis (**Figure 40.39**). A

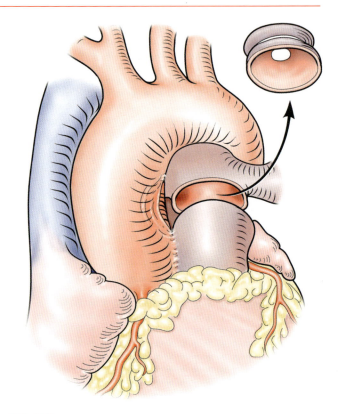

40.38

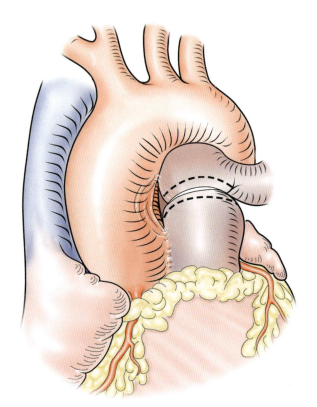

40.37

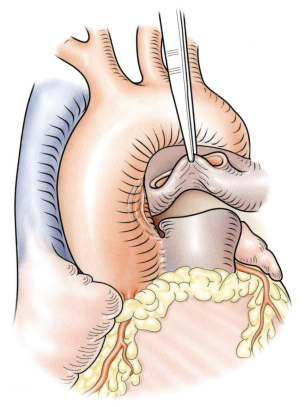

40.39

circumferential native pulmonary artery–to–pulmonary artery anastomosis is carried out with a continuous polypropylene suture technique (**Figure 40.40**). Where tissue is deficient, a pericardial patch augmentation is indicated.

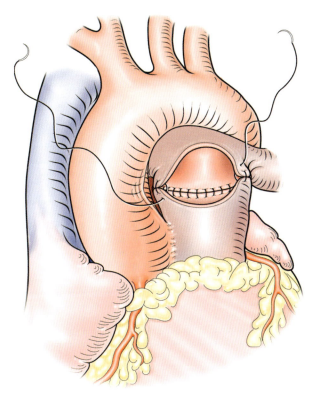

40.40

POSTOPERATIVE CARE

Early complications include phrenic or recurrent laryngeal nerve palsies, chylothorax, and coronary artery compromise. A loose band with ongoing congestive heart failure carries a significant associated mortality, and attention must be paid to the possibility of an inadequately protected pulmonary vascular bed, with a low threshold for returning to the operating room for band revision.

Late complications include congestive failure owing to an inadequate band, band migration resulting in right or bilateral branch pulmonary artery distortion, band erosion into the infundibulum, and pulmonary artery aneurysm or pulmonary valve distortion. Hypertrophy with exacerbation of subaortic obstruction from pulmonary artery banding is discussed above (see Preoperative assessment and preparation).

OUTCOME

A recent retrospective study of pulmonary artery band outcomes reported an overall hospital mortality of 8.1% for the palliative pulmonary artery band, deaths being largely among neonates, and almost 10% of survivors either died before, or were unsuitable for, definitive repair, a mean 9.5 months after palliation. Many failures are due to a loose band and/or band migration with pulmonary artery distortion and unprotected pulmonary vasculature. A pulmonary artery band that is adequate at placement can physiologically loosen with time as the pulmonary artery intima remodels. Post-stenotic dilatation, fibrosis, and pulmonary valve distortion over time can render the valve incompetent. These findings support the strategy that, when used, the use of a pulmonary artery band is safest when considered a short-term palliation, with a definitive repair performed as early as possible.

FURTHER READING

Bernstein HS, Brook MM, Silverman NH, Bristow J. Development of pulmonary arteriovenous fistulae in children after cavopulmonary shunt. *Circulation*. 1995; 92: 309–14.

Bradley SM, Simsic JM, Mulvihill DM. Hyperventilation impairs oxygenation after bidirectional superior cavopulmonary connection. *Circulation*. 1998; 98: 372–7.

Gladman G, McCrindle BW, Williams WG, et al. The modified Blalock–Taussig shunt: clinical impact and morbidity in Fallot's tetralogy in the current era. *J Thorac Cardiovasc Surg*. 1997; 114: 25–30.

Kawahira Y, Kishimoto H, Kawata H, et al. Optimal degree of pulmonary artery banding – adequate circumference ratio to calculated size from normal pulmonary valve dimensions. 1995; *Am J Cardiol*. 76: 979–82.

Mahle WT, Wernovsky G, Bridges ND, et al. Impact of early ventricular unloading on exercise performance in preadolescents with single ventricle Fontan physiology. *J Am Coll Cardiol*. 1999; 34: 1637–43.

Odim J, Portzky M, Zurakowski D, et al. Sternotomy approach for the modified Blalock–Taussig shunt. *Circulation*. 1995; 92: 256–61.

Shah MJ, Rychik J, Fogel MA, et al. Pulmonary AV malformations after superior cavopulmonary connection: resolution after inclusion of hepatic veins in the pulmonary circulation. *Ann Thorac Surg*. 1997; 63: 960–3.

41

Total anomalous pulmonary venous connection and cor triatriatum

JENNIFER C. ROMANO AND EDWARD L. BOVE

HISTORY

Total anomalous pulmonary venous connection (TAPVC) encompasses a group of anomalies in which the pulmonary veins drain into the systemic venous circulation via persistent splanchnic connections. The entity was first described in 1798 by Wilson. Muller performed the first partial correction at UCLA in 1951. The first complete correction was accomplished using inflow occlusion by Lewis and Varco in 1956.

TAPVC is a relatively uncommon congenital defect, representing approximately 2% of all congenital heart anomalies.

Cor triatriatum is a variant of TAPVC in which the common pulmonary vein fails to completely incorporate into the left atrium. Cor triatriatum is an uncommon entity, with only a few hundred cases reported since the initial description by Church in 1868.

EMBRYOLOGY AND ANATOMY

Total anomalous pulmonary venous connection refers to the circulation of pulmonary venous flow into the systemic venous system. This abnormality results from failed transfer, in the normal developmental sequence, of pulmonary venous drainage from the splanchnic plexus to the left atrium. The lungs arise as buds of the foregut with initial vascular supply based on the foregut splanchnic circulation. The venous branches of the lung buds ultimately coalesce to become the common pulmonary vein, which, in normal development, connects to the sinoatrial outpouching of the heart. This connection leads to pulmonary venous drainage entering the left atrium. After this connection is established, the primitive connections to the splanchnic circulation normally involute. In TAPVC, the connection with the left atrium fails to develop, and persistence of the splanchnic connections provides for venous drainage. Great variability

in pulmonary venous connections can result from the many combinations of persistent splanchnic communications. The most common classification system was originally described by Darling and consists of four types: supracardiac, cardiac, infracardiac, and mixed. Supracardiac TAPVC occurs in approximately 45% of patients. In this type, the common pulmonary vein drains superiorly into the left innominate vein or superior vena cava via an ascending vertical vein (**Figure 41.1a**). Cardiac TAPVC occurs in approximately 25% of patients. In the cardiac form, the common pulmonary vein drains into the coronary sinus, or, on rare occasions,

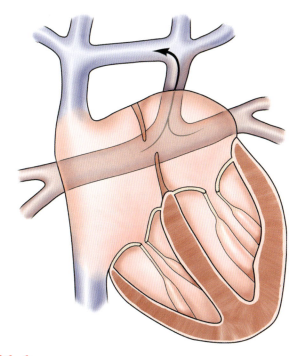

41.1a

individual pulmonary veins connect directly into the right atrium (**Figure 41.1b**).

In infracardiac TAPVC, which represents approximately 25% of patients, the common pulmonary vein drains through the diaphragm into the portal vein or ductus venosus (**Figure 41.1c**). Finally, a mixed type of TAPVC occurs in approximately 5% of patients and can involve any or all components of the previous three types.

In addition to the anatomical connections of the common pulmonary vein, TAPVC can be classified by the presence of obstruction. Impingement from surrounding structures or inadequate caliber of the draining pulmonary veins can result in obstruction of varying degrees. Obstruction in supracardiac TAPVC often occurs by compression of the

ascending vertical vein between the left main stem bronchus and left pulmonary artery. Obstruction is always present in the infracardiac type, because the pulmonary venous blood must pass through the sinusoids of the liver. Obstruction is uncommon in the cardiac type.

Partial anomalous pulmonary venous connection defines patients in whom some, but not all, venous drainage enters the left atrium, while the remaining veins drain via one or more persistent splanchnic connections.

Cor triatriatum results from failure of the common pulmonary vein to completely incorporate into the left atrium. The common pulmonary vein forms an accessory chamber, with a fibromuscular septum separating it from the left atrium. An orifice in this septum allows venous drainage to either enter the left atrium directly or enter the right atrium with flow into the left via an atrial septal defect (ASD) (**Figure 41.2a and b**). This entity can also be present with

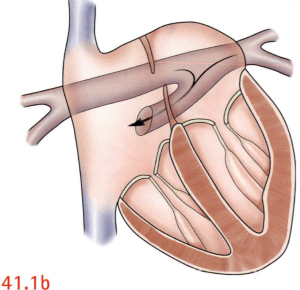

41.1b

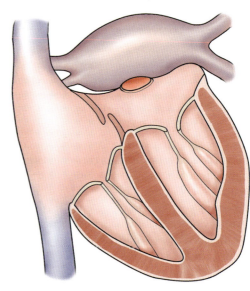

41.2a

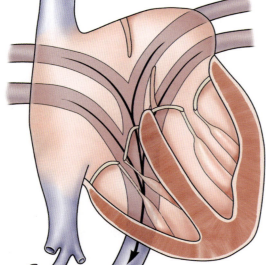
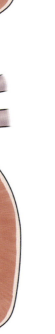

41.1c

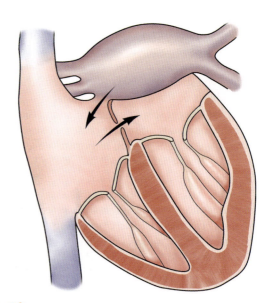

41.2b

various persistent splanchnic connections. The orifice for pulmonary venous drainage from the accessory chamber may be inadequate, with resultant obstruction leading to symptoms in the early newborn period.

PATHOPHYSIOLOGY

TAPVC produces a mixing lesion, because oxygenated blood from the pulmonary system drains back into the systemic venous circulation. The size of the ASD dictates the distribution of blood flow. Thus, a restrictive ASD results in decreased venous return to the left side of the heart, decreased cardiac output, and increased right-sided pressures. Rarely, these patients present early in life with cardiovascular collapse. With a non-restrictive ASD, which is most common, the distribution of blood flow at the atrial level depends on the relative ventricular compliance, as well as the relative resistance of the systemic and pulmonary vasculature. Most patients with unobstructed TAPVC have few to no symptoms in infancy and present with signs and symptoms similar to those of an ASD (i.e. large, atrial-level left-to-right shunt). In the neonatal period, the distribution of blood flow varies as pulmonary vascular resistance falls, resulting in increased pulmonary blood flow. Patients with excessive pulmonary blood flow present later in life with symptoms of congestive heart failure or pulmonary artery hypertension. This increase in flow can produce vascular changes, leading to pulmonary vascular occlusive disease over time. Elevated pulmonary vascular resistance in the presence of a non-restrictive ASD or patent ductus arteriosus can produce severe cyanosis from right-to-left shunting.

In the neonate with obstructed TAPVC, venous drainage from the pulmonary vasculature is impaired, leading to pulmonary venous hypertension and pulmonary edema. In severe cases, this increased pressure leads to reflexive vasoconstriction of the pulmonary vasculature with pulmonary hypertension and progressive cyanosis. Patients with obstruction present early in life with profound cyanosis.

PREOPERATIVE ASSESSMENT AND PREPARATION

Patients with TAPVC and significant obstruction present in the newborn period with pulmonary edema and, occasionally, right heart failure. Symptoms include poor feeding, tachypnea, and cyanosis that can be severe. Physical examination demonstrates a loud second heart sound due to pulmonary hypertension and hepatomegaly from congestive heart failure. Electrocardiographic abnormalities include right ventricular hypertrophy and, occasionally, an enlarged P wave (P pulmonale). A chest roentgenogram demonstrates

pulmonary edema with a normal heart size and represents a classic finding of obstructed TAPVC.

Patients with TAPVC in the absence of significant obstruction present later in life with symptoms of congestive heart failure, poor feeding, failure to thrive, and frequent respiratory infections. Physical examination demonstrates a hyperactive precordium with a widely split second heart sound and a systolic ejection murmur over the right ventricular outflow tract. Electrocardiogram findings of right ventricular enlargement are present. Chest roentgenogram shows increased pulmonary vascular markings along with cardiomegaly.

Diagnosis can be made with echocardiographic identification of the anomalous connection of the common pulmonary vein to the systemic venous system. The ASD can be delineated, as well as any other associated anomalies. Cardiac catheterization is rarely necessary, unless accurate measurement of pulmonary vascular resistance is needed in patients with late presentation.

The management of TAPVC is surgical repair. Medical management for stabilization and optimization of oxygenation and hemodynamics in patients with obstruction may be used, but they are often unsuccessful and should not delay surgical intervention. The use of prostaglandins to maintain ductal patency is generally not recommended in obstructed TAPVC in the newborn, because it results in a decrease in pulmonary blood flow as blood shunts from right to left across the duct.

OPERATION

The primary principles of operative repair are to establish a non-obstructed communication between the common pulmonary vein and the left atrium, to interrupt the connections with the systemic venous circulation, and to close the ASD. The specific repair is dependent on the type of anomalous connection.

The patient undergoes standard cardiac anesthesia. An umbilical or radial arterial line is placed for monitoring. Ventilatory measures to reduce pulmonary hypertension are used, including hyperventilation and 100% oxygen. The chest is opened via a median sternotomy. The presence of thymic tissue should be noted. Standard hypothermic cardiopulmonary bypass can be established with an arterial cannula in the ascending aorta and a single venous cannula in the right atrial appendage. The ductus arteriosus should be identified and ligated after establishing cardiopulmonary bypass. The patient is cooled to a core temperature of 18 °C. A dose of cold blood cardioplegia is administered at 30 mL/kg before circulatory arrest. Essential to successful repair is the proper identification of all four pulmonary veins and their anomalous connection before repair. Although preoperative studies are highly accurate, a mixed type of lesion may be missed.

For supracardiac connections, the optimal approach is to retract the superior vena cava and ascending aorta laterally to expose the common pulmonary vein. The vertical vein can then be ligated outside the pericardium at the level of the innominate vein. Care should be taken to avoid the phrenic nerve, which travels along the lateral aspect of the vertical vein and the entry of the left upper pulmonary vein. The dome of the left atrium and the pulmonary venous confluence are optimally exposed between the aorta and the superior vena cava. This approach provides excellent exposure without distortion of the heart or venous structures. A transverse incision is made in the common pulmonary vein confluence, and a parallel incision is placed on the dome of the left atrium beginning at the base of the left atrial appendage. The common pulmonary vein is then anastomosed to the left atrium, taking care not to narrow the orifice (**Figure 41.3a and b**). The anastomosis may be performed with either continuous monofilament absorbable suture or polypropylene. A right atriotomy is then made to identify and repair the ASD. Use of a prosthetic patch is often required. Attempts to enlarge the left atrium are rarely, if ever, needed.

An alternate approach uses a transverse right atriotomy that is extended across the atrial septum at the level of the ASD. The incision is then continued across the posterior aspect of the left atrium to the base of the left atrial appendage. A parallel incision is then made in the common pulmonary vein. The posterior wall of the left atrium can then be anastomosed to the common pulmonary vein, beginning at the most leftward extent of the atriotomy (**Figure 41.3c**). After the anastomosis is complete, the ASD is then closed with a prosthetic patch. Finally, the right atriotomy is closed with reinstitution of cardiopulmonary bypass and rewarming.

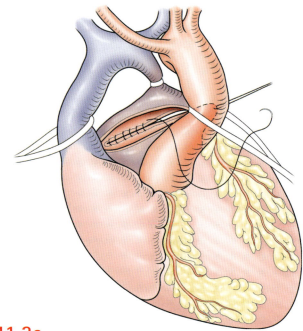

41.3a

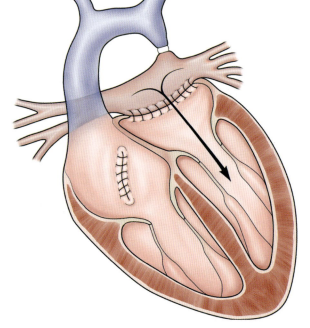

41.3b

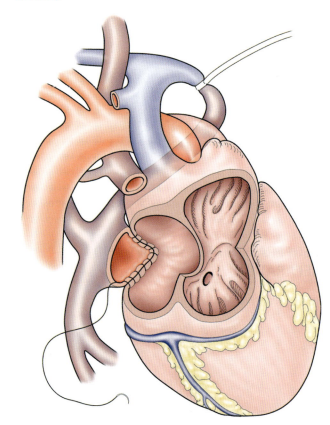

41.3c

For cardiac connections, bicaval cannulation with minimial hypothermia without circulatory arrest can be employed. After cardioplegic arrest of the heart, a right atriotomy is performed with identification of the ASD and the orifice of the coronary sinus (**Figure 41.4a**). The roof of the coronary sinus is excised into the left atrium (**Figure 41.4b**). A prosthetic or pericardial patch is then placed to close the enlarged ASD, effectively channeling the pulmonary venous return and the coronary sinus into the left atrium (**Figure 41.4c**). The conduction system travels in proximity to the coronary sinus; therefore, care must be taken while suturing the patch to avoid postoperative dysrhythmias.

For infracardiac connections, the heart is rotated superiorly. The connection to the descending vertical vein is ligated at the level of the diaphragm. An incision is made along the length of the common pulmonary vein with a parallel incision on the posterior wall of the left atrium (**Figure 41.5a**). The common pulmonary vein is then anastomosed to the left atrium, taking care not to narrow the orifice (**Figure 41.5b**). The heart can then be returned to its normal position. A right atriotomy can be performed, through which the ASD is closed.

The repair of mixed-type TAPVR involves a combination of the above approaches as dictated by the specific anatomy of the lesion.

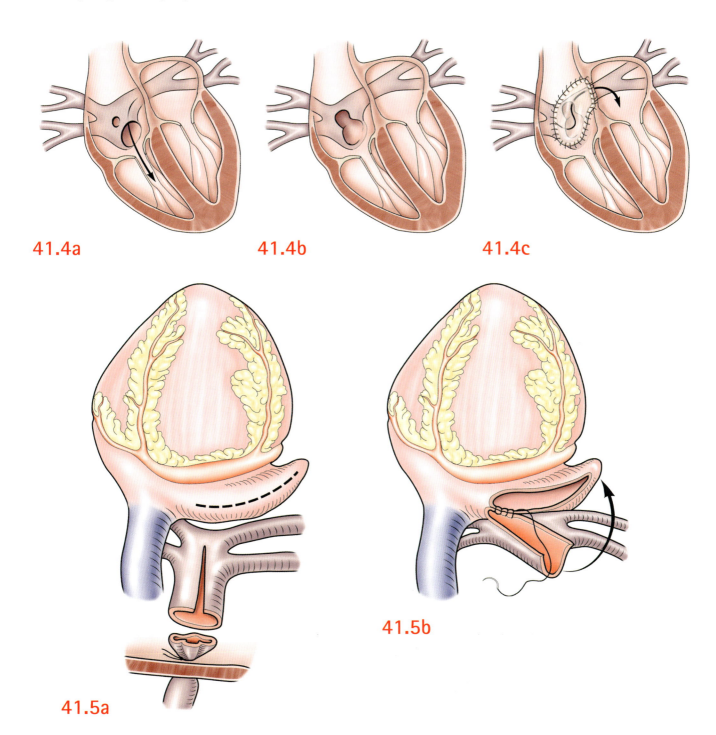

41.4a

41.4b

41.4c

41.5a

41.5b

Cor triatriatum with an accessory chamber in communication with the left atrium can be approached through a vertical incision in the accessory chamber (**Figure 41.6a**). The membrane separating the two chambers can be identified and excised to allow unobstructed communication (**Figure 41.6b**). The vertical incision in the accessory chamber is then closed.

Cor triatriatum with an accessory chamber in communication with the right atrium can be approached via a right atriotomy. The ASD can be enlarged into the orifice between the left atrium and the accessory chamber (**Figure 41.6c**). This step allows visualization and wide excision of the membrane. The interatrial septum can then be reconstructed using a prosthetic or pericardial patch (**Figure 41.6d**).

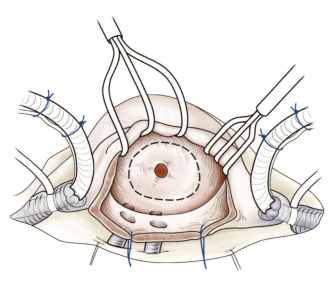

41.6a

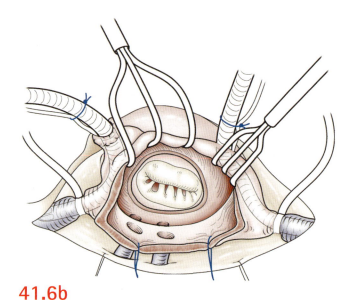

41.6b

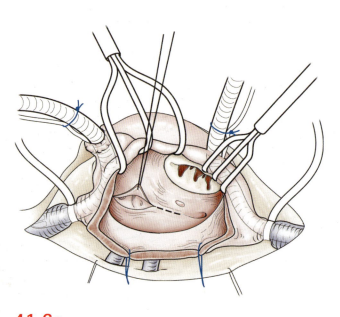

41.6c

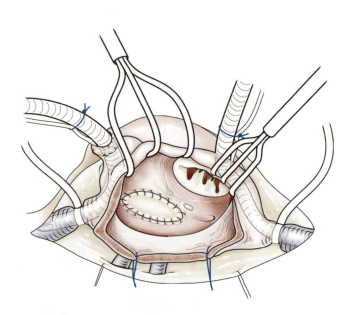

41.6d

POSTOPERATIVE CARE

Cardiac output and systemic vascular resistance are optimized through the use of inotropes and afterload reducing agents. A pulmonary artery catheter should be placed for postoperative monitoring. Pulmonary vascular resistance is kept as low as possible with hyperventilation and nitric oxide as needed. Fluids are minimized with judicious use of diuretics to optimize the respiratory status. Preoperative pulmonary edema may take several days to resolve, requiring prolonged postoperative mechanical ventilation. In severe cases of respiratory failure or persistent pulmonary hypertension, extracorporeal membrane oxygenation can be used while the pulmonary status improves.

Pulmonary hypertensive crises, manifested by sudden hypoxemia with rapid cardiovascular collapse and metabolic acidosis, can develop in patients with elevated preoperative pulmonary artery pressures. These crises can be precipitated by simple measures such as endotracheal suctioning. Measures to reduce the risk of such crises include fentanyl and/or paralysis for 24–48 hours. Interventions to circumvent a crisis include adequate sedation, hyperventilation, maintenance of oxygenation, and inhaled nitric oxide.

OUTCOME

Early mortality in patients undergoing repair of TAPVC is largely dependent on the initial degree of obstruction. The early mortality rate for initial repair in recent series range from 5% to 10% with higher mortality rates associated with patients presenting with obstruction. Early diagnosis and repair, as well as optimal methods of postoperative management including extracorporeal membrane oxygenation as required, have resulted in a dramatic reduction in operative risk. For patients surviving the perioperative period, the long-term survival and functional status are good. Recurrent pulmonary vein stenosis is the most common indication (10–20% of hospital survivors) for reoperation and tends to recur within the first 6–12 months following repair. It is most common in patients who initially present with obstruction or mixed type TAPVC.

Outcomes following the repair of cor triatriatum are excellent with postoperative mortality and morbidity primarily associated with associated cardiac defects requiring concomitant repair. The risk of recurrent obstruction or need for further intervention is low.

MANAGEMENT OF RECURRENT VENOUS OBSTRUCTION

An infrequent but challenging problem is the development of recurrent venous obstruction in 10–20% of patients. Obstruction can develop at the anastomosis or at the individual pulmonary vein ostia in the common pulmonary vein. The obstruction usually develops within the first several months after initial repair and is believed by many to be the result of an exuberant inflammatory response. Repair of this lesion is technically challenging, and recurrent early stenoses remain a problem. The mortality associated with reoperation can be in excess of 50% when bilateral stenoses are present.

The approach to recurrent venous obstruction is dependent on the level of obstruction. Isolated narrowing of the anastomosis between the common pulmonary vein and left atrium can be repaired with revision of the anastomosis. Many efforts have been used to prevent inadequate growth at the suture line, including the use of absorbable sutures or interrupted sutures, without significant differences in the rate of stenosis.

Obstruction of the individual pulmonary venous ostia can be a greater challenge. Although the obstruction often appears to be limited to the ostium initially, recurrence is common, with progressive narrowing along the length of the vein into the hilum of the lung. Results after balloon angioplasty and/or stent insertion have been disappointing, and recurrent stenoses are the rule. Individual patch angioplasty of the ostia has also been used with poor long-term results. Lung transplantation has been considered in severe cases of extensive, bilateral disease.

In the current era, the most commonly utilized surgical approach to recurrent pulmonary vein stenosis after repair of TAPVC involves a sutureless repair technique using *in situ* pericardium to create a neoatrium with marsupialization of the pulmonary veins. The theory behind this repair is based on the concept that pulmonary venous obstruction results from inflammation induced locally by suture placement. Repair involves wide unroofing of the narrowed portion of each involved pulmonary vein as well as the initial surgical connection extending from the left atrium to the hilum (**Figure 41.7a and b**). A wide flap of pericardium is then elevated, with care taken to avoid disruption of posterior adhesions and damage to the phrenic nerve. The flap of pericardium is rotated over the unroofed pulmonary veins and sutured to the left atrial wall away from the venous ostia (**Figure 41.7c**). A large neoatrium is created into which pulmonary venous return can drain.

A study from the University of Michigan evaluating outcomes associated with congenital or acquired pulmonary vein stenosis following TAPVC repair demonstrated marked superiority in restenosis free survival in both groups when the sutureless pericardial marsupialization technique was employed compared to conventional primary vein repair or anastomotic revision. Of the 22 patients with recurrent pulmonary vein stenosis following TAPVC repair, 91% of the sutureless repair patients were alive without restenosis compared to 45% in the primary repair group. Given the superior outcomes that have been demonstrated with the sutureless neoatrium technique, several centers have adopted this approach for primary repair of TAPVC when it is associated with a small pulmonary venous confluence or small individual pulmonary veins with excellent results for these higher risk patients.

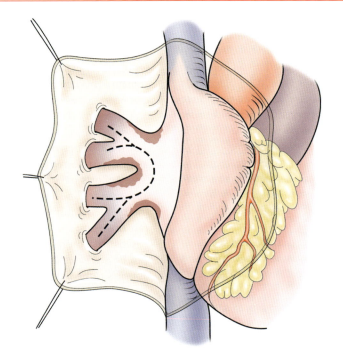

41.7a

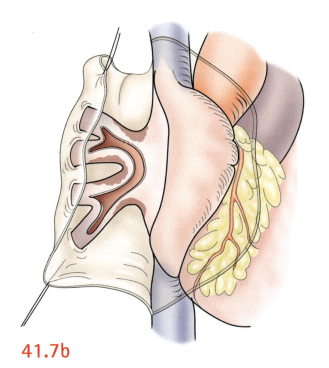

41.7b

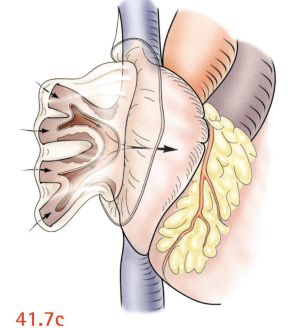

41.7c

FURTHER READING

Darling RC, Rothney WB, Craig JM. Total pulmonary venous drainage into the right side of the heart: report of 17 autopsied cases not associated with other major cardiovascvular anomalies. *Lab Invest.* 1957; 6: 44–64.

Devaney EJ, Chang AC, Ohye RG, Bove EL. Management of congenital and acquired pulmonary vein stenosis. *Ann Thorac Surg.* 2006; 81(3): 992–5.

Devaney EJ, Ohye RG, Bove EL. Pulmonary vein stenosis following repair of total anomalous pulmonary venous connection. *Semin Thorac Cardiovasc Surg Pediatr Card Surg Annu.* 2006; 9: 51–5.

Husain SA, Maldonado E, Rasch D, et al. Total anomalous pulmonary venous connection: factors associated with mortality and recurrent pulmonary venous obstruction. *Ann Thorac Surg.* 2012; 94(3): 825–31.

Kelle AM, Backer CL, Gossett JG, et al. Total anomalous pulmonary venous connection: results of surgical repair of 100 patients at a single institution. *J Thorac Cardiovasc Surg.* 2010; 139(6): 1387–94.

Saxena P, Burkhart HM, Schaff HV, et al. Surgical repair of cor triatriatum sinister: the Mayo Clinic 50-year experience. *Ann Thorac Surg.* 2014; 97(5): 1659–63.

Seale AN, Uemura H, Webber SA, et al. Total anomalous pulmonary venous connection: outcome of postoperative pulmonary venous obstruction. *J Thorac Cardiovasc Surg.* 2013; 145(5): 1255–62.

Yanagawa B, Alghamdi AA, Dragulescu A, et al. Primary sutureless repair for "simple" total anomalous pulmonary venous connection: midterm results in a single institution. *J Thorac Cardiovasc Surg.* 2011; 141(6): 1346–54.

42

Atrial septal defects

PETER B. MANNING

HISTORY

The management of atrial septal defects (ASDs) holds a special place in the history of congenital cardiac surgery and also serves as an example of current trends in treatment of congenital cardiac anomalies. Closure of a secundum ASD by Gibbon in 1952 was the first successful operation performed using cardiopulmonary bypass support. For many years ASD closure was the most frequently performed open-heart operation in children in most centers. Since 2001, the widespread availability of catheter-delivered devices for ASD closure has resulted in the management of the majority of secundum ASDs completely avoiding the need for surgical incision and cardiopulmonary bypass.

PRINCIPLES AND JUSTIFICATION

Occasionally an ASD results in a large enough shunt to cause symptoms of congestive heart failure in young children. Most isolated atrial level shunts, though, are asymptomatic during childhood. Closure is indicated to prevent long-term sequelae of pulmonary hypertensive vascular disease, atrial arrhythmias, congestive heart failure, and cerebrovascular accident from paradoxical embolization.

The preschool years are generally chosen for closure of most secundum ASDs. Spontaneous closure beyond 2 years of age is exceedingly rare. If diagnosed early, delaying until the child is 2–3 years (>12 kg) often allows the procedure to be done without need for any blood product transfusion. In older children the defect is repaired electively upon discovery. Primum ASDs, however, should be repaired earlier, generally around 1 year of age, as some studies have shown worse long-term AV valve function associated with older age at repair.

OPERATION

Surgical incisions

Median sternotomy is most commonly employed. Adequate exposure can be obtained using partial sternotomy or limited right thoracotomy, which may be chosen for cosmetic reasons.

Cannulation for bypass

Standard ascending aortic cannulation is used for arterial inflow. Bicaval cannulation for secundum ASD closure can be most easily obtained using two cannulae placed via the right atrial appendage, which is typically enlarged due to chronic volume overload (**Figure 42.1**). For sinus venosus defects, the superior cannulation is best placed directly into the superior vena cava (SVC), well above the entrance of any pulmonary veins (**Figure 42.2**). Preliminary dissection of the

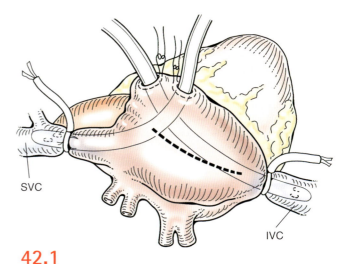

SVC

IVC

42.1

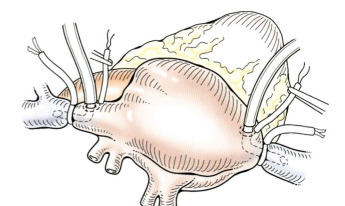

42.2

SVC should be performed before a cannulation site is chosen. When a persistent left SVC is present, it may be directly cannulated, or its return controlled using cardiotomy suction. Rarely, a communicating vein to the right SVC exists allowing tourniquet occlusion of the left SVC during repair.

Myocardial protection

Due to the short period of cardiac arrest needed for most repairs, systemic hypothermia may be avoided. Myocardial protection is most easily achieved using antegrade, cold blood cardioplegia with the addition of topical hypothermia.

Secundum ASD

A limited right atriotomy typically affords excellent exposure of the defect. An anterior retractor can hold the inferior vena cava (IVC) cannula out of the way if atrial appendage cannulation is employed. Defects in the fossa ovalis are the most commonly encountered. If the defect seems more superior or posterior in the septum than typical, a sinus venosus defect should be suspected and confirmation of the entry of the right pulmonary veins to the left of the septum should be made. Often thin, multifenestrated remnants of septum primum may partially cover the fossa ovalis (**Figure 42.3**). These can be resected to facilitate suture placement in stronger tissue. A left-sided vent is rarely needed and care should be taken to avoid suction into the left atrium to prevent air entrapment after closure of the defect.

In the past, the majority of defects could be closed by primary suture technique, partly due to the oval shape of most secundum defects. Since the advent of device closure of the majority of secundum ASDs, those referred for surgical closure are typically larger and more round in shape with deficient margins of atrial wall, requiring patch closure (see below). If primary closure is feasible, a double layer of polypropylene is begun at the inferior limit of the defect, as this margin is typically most difficult to define (**Figure 42.4a and b**). Prior to complete closure of the defect, entrapped air should be evacuated from the left atrium.

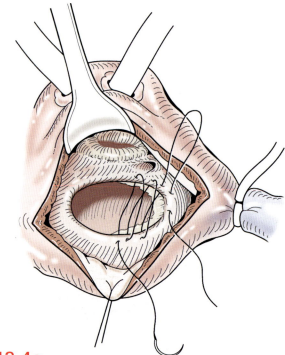

42.4a

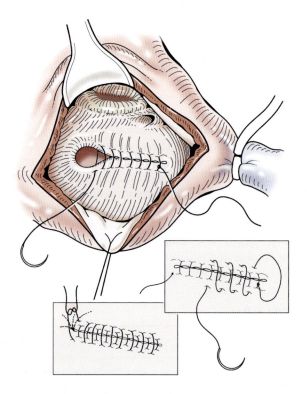

42.4b

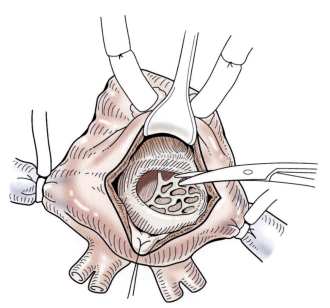

42.3

If the defect is large or more round in shape, patch closure should be performed to avoid closure under tension and distortion of atrial anatomy. A patch of autologous pericardium slightly smaller than the relaxed size of the defect may be used, again beginning the suture line inferiorly (**Figure 42.5**). Polytetrafluoroethylene (PTFE), Dacron, CorMatrix®, or bovine pericardium are also suitable patch materials.

With the septal defect securely closed, the aortic cross-clamp can be removed and the atriotomy closed using a double layer of polypropylene suture. Caval tourniquet snares are released after atriotomy closure, and cannulae that were placed via the right atrial appendage can be backed into the body of the atrium to improve venous drainage.

Maneuvers to evacuate any residual air from the left side of the heart using the left atrial vent (if employed) or the cardioplegic site should be performed during rewarming. Temporary pacing wires are generally not necessary unless the patient has exhibited evidence of arrhythmia or conduction delay during rewarming.

If the pulmonary veins drain to the cavoatrial junction area, baffle repair of the defect using a pericardial patch is performed. If there are pulmonary veins entering some distance up the SVC, or if the right SVC is unusually small (as seen in the presence of a persistent left SVC), the so-called Warden repair is performed, directing the lower SVC flow through the septal defect with translocation of the upper SVC to the right atrial appendage.

BAFFLE REPAIR

The right atrial incision is oriented longitudinally, and is angled superiorly toward the lateral aspect of the cavoatrial junction. If better exposure is needed, the incision may be extended onto the SVC to the upper limit of any anomalously connected pulmonary veins. The lateral placement of this incision is important to avoid injury to the sinus node, though its blood supply may still be compromised in some cases (**Figure 42.6a and b**).

The patch is sutured beginning superiorly at the junction of the highest pulmonary vein and the SVC, transitioning down and around the lower edge of the septal defect to direct the flow of pulmonary venous blood through the septal

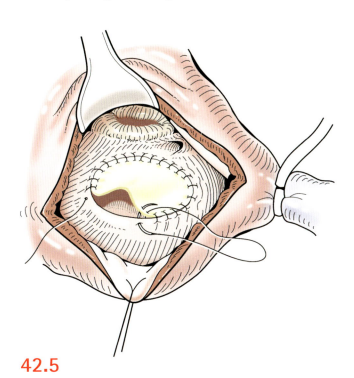

42.5

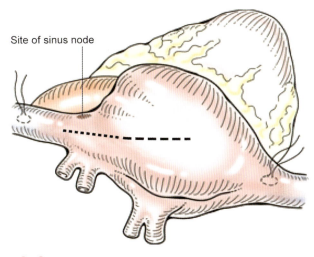

Site of sinus node

42.6a

Superior sinus venosus ASD

The ASD is more superior and posterior compared to the typical secundum ASD. The right upper pulmonary veins typically drain into the junction of the SVC and right atrium. Occasionally, multiple veins drain the right upper lobe and may enter the SVC some distance from its atrial junction. Careful, circumferential dissection of the SVC allows identification of these anomalous venous connections for cannulation site selection and planning of the repair. Injury to the right phrenic nerve must be avoided during dissection of the lateral aspect of the SVC.

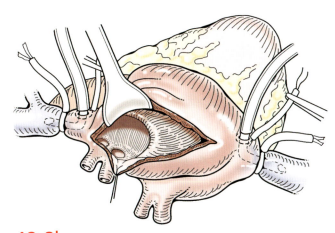

42.6b

defect to the left atrium (**Figure 42.7a**). The patch should be slightly redundant to avoid obstructing this pathway, especially when it is extended up the vena cava more than a few millimeters. A single small pulmonary vein branch draining high into the SVC may be ignored, as this amount of persistent left-to-right shunt will be of little consequence. If the incision has been carried onto the SVC, the atriotomy closure may be augmented with a patch superiorly to prevent stenosis of the SVC–right atrial junction (**Figure 42.7b**).

WARDEN REPAIR

A limited, longitudinal right atriotomy allows exposure of the septal defect and the cavoatrial junction (**Figure 42.8a**). The patch is sutured from the lower edge of the septal defect around the lateral aspect of the cavoatrial junction directing all SVC flow through the defect to the left atrium

(**Figure 42.8b**). The SVC is then transected just at the upper level of the highest pulmonary vein.

The cardiac end is oversewn avoiding stenosis of the highest pulmonary vein. The cephalic end of the SVC is mobilized further, if necessary, then anastomosed to a position on the right atrial appendage where it reaches without tension or angulation using fine, absorbable, monofilament suture (**Figure 42.8c**). Care must be taken to avoid pursestringing this anastomosis.

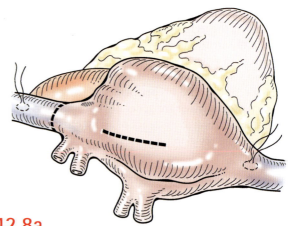

42.8a

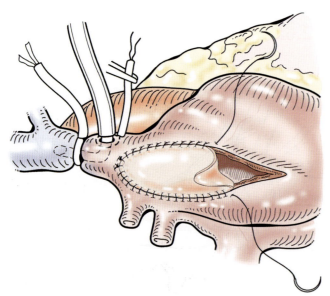

42.7a

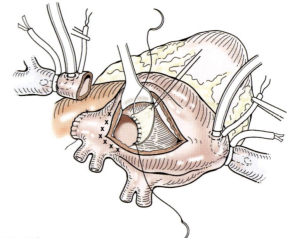

42.8b

42.7b

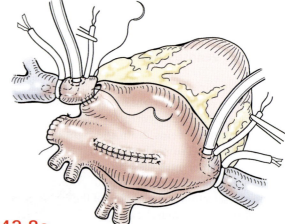

42.8c

Coronary sinus septal defect/unroofed coronary sinus

This defect is associated with persistence of a left SVC, typically without a communicating innominate vein to the right SVC (**Figure 42.9**). The coronary sinus is often completely unroofed with the left SVC draining to the roof of the left atrium just medial to the left atrial appendage.

In the rare case that the coronary sinus is partially unroofed, the defect may be closed either directly or with a patch. Care should be taken to avoid either narrowing the coronary sinus with direct closure or making the patch too redundant, obstructing left ventricular inflow.

When the coronary sinus is completely unroofed, the anomaly is best repaired using a pericardial baffle to direct the left SVC blood across the roof of the left atrium to the secundum ASD (**Figure 42.10**). This avoids the need to sew

near the pulmonary veins or the mitral valve annulus. The secundum ASD is enlarged superiorly to the roof of the atrium, if necessary to better expose the left SVC orifice. An oblong patch is attached to the far side of the left SVC orifice, typically between this opening and the opening into the left atrial appendage. The first suture line is run above the superior pulmonary vein orifices to the posterior aspect of the ASD. The other end of the suture is run more anteriorly across the roof of the left atrium to the anterior edge of the ASD. The suture lines converge at the inferior aspect of the ASD, thus directing the left SVC blood to the right atrium and closing the secundum ASD.

Primum atrial septal defect (partial AV canal)

Venous cannulation should allow unobstructed exposure of the intra-atrial anatomy, especially in the smaller child. This is accomplished using direct cannulation of the inferior cavoatrial junction with a thin-walled, right-angle cannula. Superior caval cannulation may be via the right atrial appendage or directly into the SVC. Venting of the left side of the heart via the right superior pulmonary vein facilitates exposure by capturing pulmonary venous return.

Initial careful inspection of the intracardiac anatomy must be carried out following right atriotomy (**Figure 42.11**). The limits of the primum ASD should be defined as well as the presence of any additional septal defect in the fossa ovalis region. The absence of interventricular communication should be confirmed by gentle inspection and probing of the subvalvar region using a fine right-angle clamp. Particular attention to the anatomy of the left-sided atrioventricular valve is crucial, as the most frequent need for reoperation in these patients is related to left AV valve dysfunction, usually regurgitation. The presence of the cleft in the anterior or septal leaflet is identified, the presence of two, well-separated

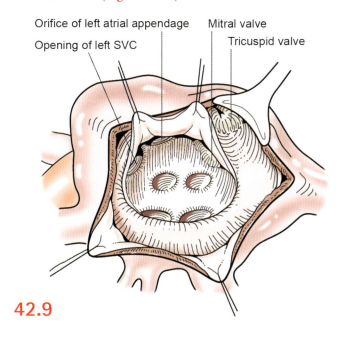

Orifice of left atrial appendage   Mitral valve

Opening of left SVC   Tricuspid valve

42.9

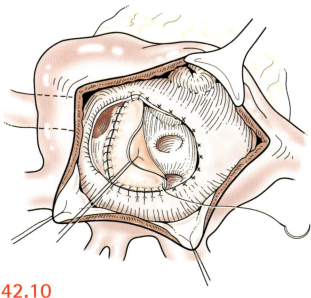

42.10

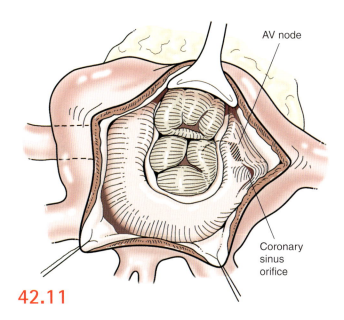

AV node

Coronary sinus orifice

42.11

papillary muscles within the left ventricle is confirmed, and anomalies such as a double orifice or parachute valve configuration are excluded.

The cleft in the anterior left AV valve leaflet is closed first, using fine sutures with an interrupted simple or mattress technique (**Figure 42.12**). Testing of the valve by instilling iced saline into the ventricle confirms competence of the repair and identifies the need for the addition of any annuloplasty stitches.

The septal defect is closed with a pericardial patch (**Figure 42.13**). The use of a non-smooth surfaced patch such as Dacron has been associated with postoperative hemolyisis in the presence of even a small regurgitant jet directed against the septal patch. A pledgeted mattress suture is placed at the midpoint of the base of the reconstructed anterior leaflet, passing the suture through some of the ventricular septal crest from the right ventricular side. One edge of the patch is cut without a curve and this edge is anchored to the heart using the mattress suture. A line of demarcation between the right- and left-sided components of the valve is usually easily appreciated, although this may be accentuated by traction on the mattress suture at the midpoint on the valve. Each end of

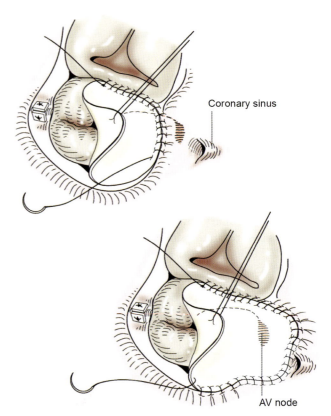

Coronary sinus

AV node

42.13

the suture is run to the atrioventricular annulus, securing the straight edge of the patch to the demarcation line between right- and left-sided valve tissue. The patch is now trimmed to the appropriate size to match the septal defect and the suture line continued at each end, attaching the patch to the inferior, free edge of the atrial septum. Inferiorly, care must be taken to avoid injury to the bundle of His. If the edge of the atrial septum is quite close to the site where the patch is attached to the valve leaflets, superficial bites may be used in this area. Alternatively, the patch may be cut with a projection to allow suturing directly toward the coronary sinus, then within the medial margin of the coronary sinus, and finally transitioning over to the free edge of atrial septum.

POSTOPERATIVE CARE

In most cases the patient can be extubated in the operating room. Close monitoring of the cardiac rhythm should be carried out particularly after repair of sinus venosus defects (sinus node dysfunction) and partial AV canal (heart block or accelerated junctional rhythms). In many centers blood product transfusion may be completely avoided for ASD repair even in children as small as 10 kg using small volume circuits and blood conservation techniques. Postoperative anemia to a hematocrit level in the low 20s is usually well tolerated, though monitoring for signs of poor perfusion or acidosis should be carried out to ensure adequate tissue oxygen delivery in the face of this anemia.

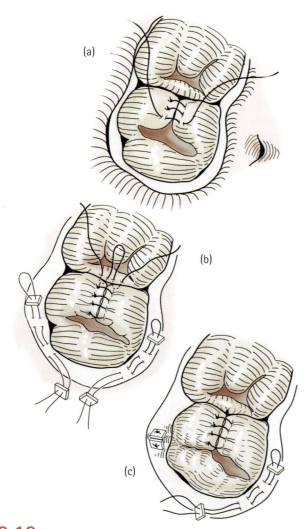

(a)

(b)

(c)

42.12a–c

OUTCOME

When repairs are made early in the patient's life, longevity and exercise capacity are no different from the general population. Although patients with isolated ASDs are not at an increased risk for bacterial endocarditis, SBE prophylaxis is recommended postoperatively for a period of 6 months following closure of a secundum defect. In older patients, when atrial arrhythmias have developed prior to repair, closure of the defect will often not reverse the atrial dilation that has developed, and ongoing dysrhythmia management may be necessary. Following repair of primum ASDs, up to 10% of patients will require later operation to repair or replace the left AV valve, usually related to regurgitation. Up to 5% of these patients will develop left ventricular outflow tract obstruction that will require reoperation.

FURTHER READING

Baskett RJ, Tancock E, Ross DB. The gold standard for atrial septal defect closure: current surgical results, with an emphasis on morbidity. *Pediatr Cardiol.* 2003; 4: 444–7.

Du ZD, Hijazi ZM, Kleinman CS, et al. with Amplatzer Investigators. Comparison between transcatheter and surgical closure of secundum atrial septal defect in children and adults: results of a multicenter nonrandomized trial. *J Am Coll Cardiol.* 2002; 39: 1836–44.

Gustafson RA, Warden HE, Murray GF, et al. Partial anomalous pulmonary venous connection to the right side of the heart. *J Thorac Cardiovasc Surg.* 1989; 98: 861–8.

Horvath KA, Burke RP, Collins JJ Jr, Cohn LH. Surgical treatment of adult atrial septal defect: early and long-term results. *J Am Coll Cardiol.* 1992; 20: 1156–9.

Meijboom F, Hess J, Szatmari A, et al. Long-term follow-up (9 to 20 years) after surgical closure of atrial septal defect at a young age. *Am J Cardiol.* 1993; 72: 1431–4.

Najm HK, Williams WG, Chuaratanaphong S, et al. Primum atrial septal defect in children: early results, risk factors, and freedom from reoperation. *Ann Thorac Surg.* 1993; 66: 829–35.

43

Atrioventricular septal defects

MICHAEL O. MURPHY AND THOMAS L. SPRAY

HISTORY AND ANATOMY

Atrioventricular septal defects (AVSDs) include deficiencies in the inferior portion of the atrial septum, the inflow portion of the ventricular septum, and the tissue forming the left and right atrioventricular (AV) valves.

Anatomically, AVSDs have been divided into partial, incomplete, and complete subtypes. Partial AVSDs have an ostium primum-type atrial septal defect (ASD) above the AV valve with a cleft or commissure between the superior and inferior cleft AV valve leaflets, associated with varying degrees of AV valve insufficiency. In incomplete AVSD, the atrial ostium primum defect is present, and the junction between the left and right AV valves is separated from the crest of the ventricular septum via a membrane of tissue (**Figure 43.1a**). In these patients, the left and right AV valves have separate orifices but with abnormal structure, and the ventricular septal defect (VSD) component beneath the AV valve leaflets may be restrictive and filled in by chordal tissue. In complete AVSD, the common AV valve bridges over the VSD. The AV valve apparatus and AVSD has what can be considered as five leaflets in the complete form and six leaflets in the partial form. In complete AVSD, a superior and inferior bridging leaflet is always present with two additional right-sided lateral and anterosuperior leaflets and a left lateral or "mural" leaflet.

The degree of bridging and chordal attachments of the common AV valve leaflets have been used to create the Rastelli classification of AVSDs.

In Rastelli type A defect (**Figure 43.1b**), the superior bridging leaflet is split at the ventricular septum, and the left superior leaflet is over the left ventricle and the right superior leaflet over the right ventricle, with chordal attachments to the ventricular septum.

In Rastelli type C (**Figure 43.1c**), the superior bridging leaflet floats freely over the ventricular septum without chordal attachments to the crest of the ventricular septum. The posterior bridging leaflet may be attached or free in either Rastelli type A or C classification. Rastelli type B is between the A and C extremes and is very rare.

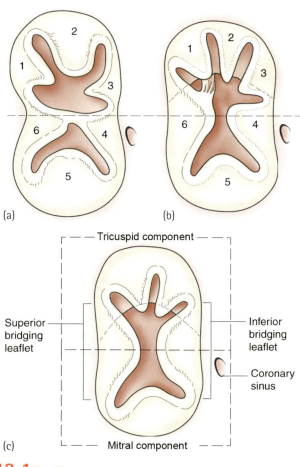

(a)   (b)

(c)

43.1a–c

An additional consideration in AVSD repairs is the location of the AV conduction tissue, which is displaced posteriorly in AVSD toward the coronary sinus. The conduction tissue generally lies between the coronary sinus and the VSD. The ostium primum ASD distorts the coronary sinus orifice more posteriorly and inferiorly toward the left atrium, distorting the triangle of Koch. The bundle of His generally travels from the location near the coronary sinus along the crest of the VSD, under the inferior bridging leaflet on the rim of the VSD (**Figure 43.2**).

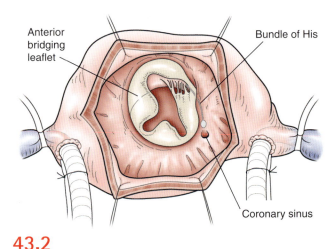

43.2

PRINCIPLES AND JUSTIFICATION

Patients with AVSDs have symptoms related to the magnitude of the associated left-to-right shunt and the magnitude of associated lesions such as AV valve insufficiency. Patients with partial AVSDs may have physiology similar to that of patients with secundum ASDs with no symptoms and a similar cardiac murmur, with right heart volume overload on echocardiography. When associated left AV valve insufficiency is present, cardiac failure and pulmonary congestion with dyspnea can occur. Because complete AVSD is associated with more significant left-to-right shunting, patients often have congestive heart failure, fatigue, and dyspnea with failure to thrive. Severe pulmonary hypertension eventually develops in the majority of patients, resulting in death in up to 65% of infants with the complete form before 1 year of age without surgery. The majority of patients with complete AVSDs have Down syndrome, which may exacerbate the development of pulmonary hypertension. Echocardiography is the diagnostic procedure of choice in patients with AVSDs; valve anatomy and function can be accurately assessed.

Patients with partial AVSD usually undergo elective repair before school age, unless symptoms of heart failure are present. If significant AV valve insufficiency is present, earlier operation is indicated. Patients with complete AVSDs generally require complete correction between 2 and 4 months of age. Operation at an early age may prevent the development of progressive pulmonary hypertension, which is a significant source of morbidity, and also may prevent early postoperative pulmonary hypertensive events that can increase postoperative morbidity and mortality. Patients who have significant congestive heart failure, failure to thrive, and poor weight gain can be operated on at any age, including the newborn period, although the requirement for operation in the neonatal period is rare and generally reserved for those patients with severe heart failure with associated significant AV valve insufficiency. Pulmonary artery banding is generally contraindicated, as complete anatomical repair can be performed at essentially any age in patients with AVSDs.

Contraindications to surgical intervention are based on the severity of pulmonary vascular resistance. Severely elevated pulmonary resistance above 10 Wood units may be a relative contraindication to repair, and significant unbalancing of the flow through the common AV valve to the left or right ventricle may be an indication for either delayed repair and preliminary pulmonary artery banding or consideration of a single-ventricle surgical strategy. Echocardiographic assessment of the adequacy of inflow, into the hypoplastic ventricle, is of critical importance in deciding the suitability for biventricular repair in unbalanced AVSDs.

PREOPERATIVE CARE

Patients with complete AVSDs often require aggressive medical management to control congestive heart failure. If weight gain is sluggish or non-existent, early operation is indicated. Prolonged attempts at feeding or placement of nasogastric tubes or gastrostomy tubes for continuous feeding in hopes of weight gain are generally ill-advised, as weight gain can continue to be poor, and progressive congestive heart failure may lead to more instability postoperatively.

If patients present late, after 4 months of age, and have signs of significant elevation of pulmonary vascular resistance, cardiac catheterization should be considered for assessment of the pulmonary vascular bed under conditions of oxygen, nitric oxide, and prostacycline to assess reversibility of the pulmonary vascular disease before initiation of complete repair.

ANESTHESIA

Anesthetic management for patients with AVSDs is similar to that for other neonates or infants undergoing complex cardiac procedures. Narcotic anesthesia is generally used and, because of the potential for pulmonary vascular resistance elevation, hyperventilation early postoperatively is generally preferred. Nitric oxide can be used if pulmonary resistance is significantly elevated in the early postoperative period. This strategy decreases the risk of pulmonary hypertensive crises that were a cause of significant morbidity and early mortality in early series of AV canal defect repairs when operation was undertaken at over 6 months of age.

OPERATION

A standard median sternotomy is performed, and thymic tissue is removed if necessary. A portion of the anterior pericardium is excised and set aside for use as a patch in the atrium. The pericardium can be fixed in glutaraldehyde solution if desired. The aorta and vena cavae are cannulated, and a cardioplegia needle is inserted into the aortic root. It is generally advisable to mobilize the ligamentum arteriosum and ensure complete ductal closure by ligation, as echocardiography may occasionally miss the presence of a small patent ductus arteriosus with the excess turbulent flow out the pulmonary outflow tract from the large left-to-right shunt. After cardioplegic arrest is accomplished, the caval tapes are tightened, and a right atriotomy incision is made parallel to the AV groove and extending downward near the inferior vena caval cannula to gain maximum exposure of the atrium. Stay sutures may then be placed to allow adequate exposure of the common AV valve. Resection of the atrial septal tissue between the primum defect and the secundum defect or patent foramen ovale can improve visualization of the left AV valve.

The AV valve is exposed, and saline is injected into the ventricle to float the AV valves to assess the areas of coaptation (**Figure 43.3a**). The area of coaptation between the left superior and left inferior bridging leaflet is then identified and secured with a suture (**Figure 43.3b**). Identification of this coapting area is important to prevent distortion of the AV valve during the repair and associated mitral regurgitation (**Figure 43.3c**). The size of the VSD is then examined, and a patch of Dacron material or Gore-Tex is cut in a semicircular fashion appropriate to the height of the defect from the right side of the ventricular septum to the bridging AV valves. The anterior posterior dimension is then measured. Inferiorly, a slightly larger length of the patch must be permitted to extend beyond the posterior aspect of the VSD underneath the inferior leaflet to protect the common bundle of His; superiorly, the patch is cut in a concave 'scooped-out' fashion to accommodate the common AV valve attachment.

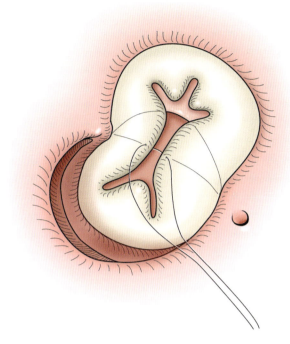

43.3b

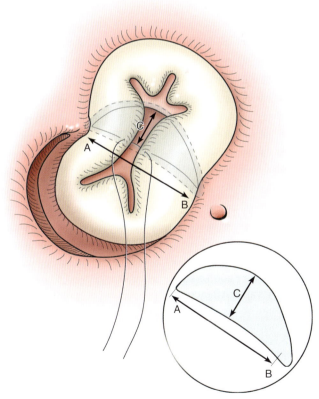

43.3c

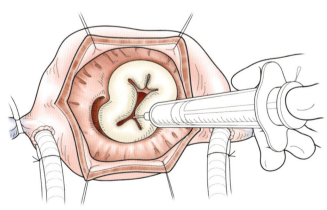

43.3a

The patch of Dacron material is then secured into the VSD starting at the midportion of the patch, inferiorly to the right of the crest of the ventricular septum (**Figure 43.4**). Using a running technique, the patch can then be anchored into place using traction on the suture to gain exposure superiorly and inferiorly near the hinge points of the bridging leaflets of the common AV valve. If chordal attachments of the inferior bridging leaflet obscure the margin of the septum, secondary chordae or the inferior bridging leaflet itself can be divided as the patch is inserted. Posteriorly, the suture is brought through the base of the bridging leaflet at the level of the annulus to avoid penetrating the bundle of His. Superiorly, the suture is brought through the annulus at the appropriate site of the superior bridging leaflet.

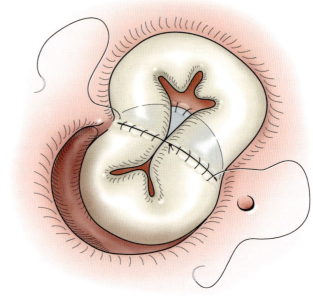

43.5

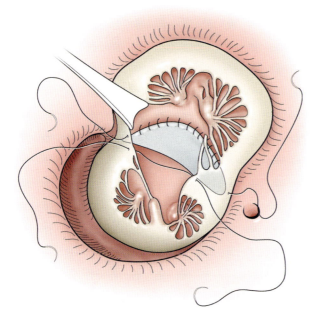

43.4

Next, the superior margin of the VSD patch is secured to the common AV valve leaflets using a running technique, incorporating the crest of the VSD patch below the AV valve tissue (**Figure 43.5**). A mattress technique may be necessary in some cases to avoid chordal attachments, and care must be taken to bring the coapting surfaces of the left superior and inferior bridging leaflets together at the initially marked point to ensure good coaptation of the left-sided component of the AV valve. After completion of the VSD patch implant, injection of saline into the left- and right-sided components of the common AV valve assesses the degree of insufficiency.

The commissure or cleft between the left superior and inferior bridging leaflet is then closed to the point of chordal attachments at the tip of the leaflet using a running suture, generally of 6-0 Gore-Tex material that does not cut through the delicate valve leaflet tissue (**Figure 43.6a**). AV valve competence is then assessed again with saline injection and, if additional regurgitation at the coaptation areas is present,

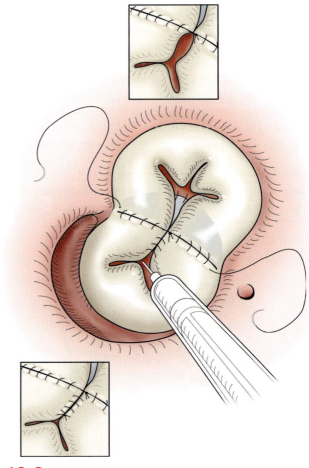

43.6a

small pledgeted annuloplasty sutures may be required at the commissures (**Figure 43.6b**).

After AV competence is assured, the ostium primum ASD component of the canal defect is closed with the homologous pericardial patch (**Figure 43.7**). The pericardium is cut to an appropriate size and shape, and then the suture line at the level of the common bridging AV valve leaflets is created using a running technique, reinforcing the VSD closure against the common AV valve with the suture to prevent valve dehiscence.

Posteriorly, the suture line is carried along the leaflet tissue at the annulus of the posterior bridging leaflet to allow the suture line to deviate away from the coronary sinus before connection to the atrial septum, to avoid the AV node and

leave the coronary sinus in the right atrial aspect of the repair (**Figure 43.8**). The ASD closure is completed, and then the right atrium is closed with a running suture.

Primary closure of ventricular septal defect component

An alternative to two-patch repair of AVSD has been popularized by Nunn. In this repair, the VSD patch is omitted, and pledgeted mattress sutures are taken from the right-sided aspect of the VSD and then brought directly through the bridging leaflets of the AV valves and through the lower portion of the atrial septal patch (**Figure 43.9**). When the sutures

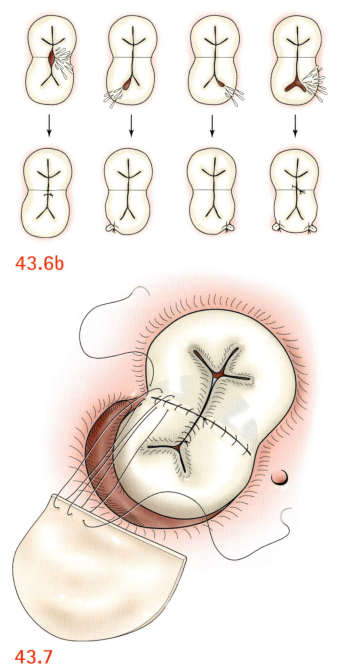

43.6b

43.7

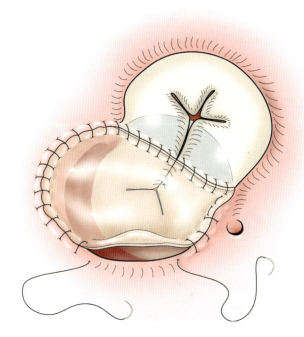

43.8

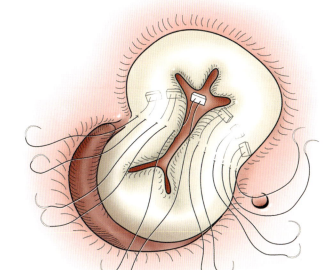

43.9

are tied, the common AV valve leaflets are brought down to the crest of the ventricular septum. Although this technique would seem to potentially distort the AV valve leaflets and possibly create subaortic stenosis, experience to date has shown that good results can be obtained with the technique, with achievement of AV valve competence and no higher incidence of subaortic obstruction. Care, however, must be taken to place the sutures accurately to avoid distortion of the AV valve. The technique appears to be most suitable in patients with Rastelli type C anatomy, but it has been used in all types of AVSDs with good success.

Repair of partial atrioventricular septal defect

The repair of partial AVSD involves the ASD patch as done in the complete form of AVSD. A pericardial patch is secured to the AV valve at the bridging tissue between the left and right valve orifices, and the cleft or commissure of the mitral valve between its left superior and inferior leaflets is closed with a running suture. After assessment of AV competence is performed, the ASD patch is completed, leaving the coronary sinus on the right atrial aspect of the repair (**Figure 43.10**).

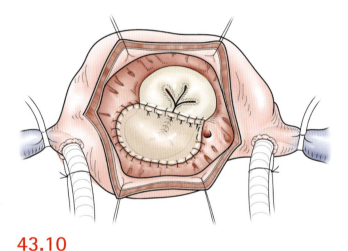

43.10

POSTOPERATIVE CARE

Postoperative complications include pulmonary hypertensive events, left AV valve insufficiency, and complete heart block. Intraoperative transesophageal echocardiography is used routinely to assess the competence of the AV valves after the repair. If significant regurgitation is present, immediate reoperation with additional attempts to create AV valve tissue coaptation is important to prevent postoperative pulmonary hypertension and increased operative mortality. Infant patients who are older at operation or have significant pulmonary hypertension preoperatively are generally kept sedated and paralyzed for 24 hours before emerging from anesthesia to decrease the risk of pulmonary hypertensive

events. Nitric oxide is used, if necessary, to control the pulmonary vascular bed. Younger patients and those without significant pulmonary hypertension generally are allowed to awaken from anesthesia and are extubated within 24 hours of surgery.

Postoperative AV valve insufficiency is a more prevalent problem than previously appreciated, with as many as 25% of patients having moderate or severe regurgitation postoperatively. Patients are often managed with inotropic support consisting of milrinone to decrease afterload and improve right ventricular function and are converted to oral afterload-reducing agents before discharge from the hospital.

OUTCOME

The surgical results with repair of AVSDs have progressively improved. Partial AVSD repairs have a mortality rate similar to that of isolated secundum ASDs, at 1% or less. Nevertheless, these patients may have an incidence of reoperation for left AV valve insufficiency or stenosis, and reoperation may be associated with significant mortality and morbidity if there is deficiency of left AV valve tissue resulting in either significant mitral stenosis or progressive mitral insufficiency. These patients may, on occasion, come to valve replacement after repair attempts have failed.

The surgical results with complete ASD repairs have also progressively improved. Most major centers now have an operative mortality of 3% or less for complete AV canal repair, with reoperation rates of 10–15%. When competence of the common AV valves has been achieved, long-term valve function has been excellent, with rare reoperation on late follow-up. Mild to moderate degrees of AV valve regurgitation are generally well-tolerated, although reoperation may be required if regurgitation progresses and the patient shows signs of congestive heart failure or pulmonary hypertension. Reoperation for secondary repair of the left AV valve has been associated with good results, with only a rare need for valve replacement in large series.

FURTHER READING

Canter CE, Spray TL, Huddleston CB, Mendeloff E. Interoperative evaluation of atrioventricular septal defect repair by color flow mapping echocardiography. *Ann Thorac Surg.* 1997; 63: 592.

Elliott MJ, Jacobs JP. Atrioventricular canal defects. In: Kaiser LR, Kron IL, Spray TL (eds). *Mastery of cardiothoracic surgery.* Philadelphia: Lippincott–Raven Publishers; 1997: pp. 742–58.

Kaza AK, Colan SD, Jaggers J, et al. Surgical interventions for atrioventricular septal defect subtypes: the pediatric heart network experience. *Ann Thorac Surg.* 2011; 92: 1468–75.

Miller OI, Tang SF, Keech A, et al. Inhaled nitric oxide and prevention of pulmonary hypertension after congenital heart surgery: a randomised double-blind study. *Lancet.* 2000; 356: 1464–9.

Rastelli GC, Kirklin JW, Titus JL. Anatomic observations on complete form of persistent common atrioventricular canal with special reference to atrioventricular valves. *Mayo Clin Proc.* 1966; 41: 296.

Rastelli GC, Ongley PA, Kirklin JW, McGoon DC. Surgical repair of the complete form of persistent common atrioventricular canal. *J Thorac Cardiovasc Surg.* 1968; 55: 299.

Szwast AL, Marino BS, Rychik J, et al. Usefulness of left ventricular inflow index to predict successful biventricular repair in right-dominant unbalanced atrioventricular canal. *Am J Cardiol.* 2011; 107: 103–9.

Thiene G, Wenink A, Anderson RH, et al. Surgical anatomy and pathology of the conduction tissues in atrioventricular septal defects. *J Thorac Cardiovasc Surg.* 1981; 82: 928.

44

Bidirectional Glenn and hemi-Fontan procedures

J. MARK REDMOND

The construction of an anastomosis between the superior vena cava (SVC) and the pulmonary artery (PA) is now well established in the management of the functional single ventricle either as a preliminary procedure in staged Fontan palliation or as an alternative procedure to the Fontan, occasionally as part of a one-and-a-half ventricle reconstruction.

HISTORY

Although Carlon in Italy first reported an experimental method for creating an anastomosis between the SVC and the right PA in 1951, the shunt bears the name of Glenn, whose pioneering research in right heart bypass in dogs paved the way for widespread clinical application of a direct end-to-end SVC to right atrium connection. In the Soviet Union, Meshalkin reported the first successful clinical use of the shunt in 24 children with 21 survivors in 1956. Glenn first performed the shunt on a 7-year-old boy with right ventricular hypoplasia and pulmonary stenosis in 1958.

As more complex intracardiac repairs became feasible and the safety of the shunt in infants was questioned, its popularity waned during the 1960s, only to be embraced once more in the 1970s as the logical first stage toward complete Fontan right heart bypass. In 1966, Haller and colleagues experimented with an end-to-side cavopulmonary shunt, without ligation of the right PA, in a canine model. Glenn had recognized that the normally occurring minute precapillary arteriovenous connections in the lung in patients with end-to-end SVC-to-PA shunts could enlarge, resulting in arterial desaturation. Because of Glenn's experience with the value of axillary arteriovenous fistulae, it was believed that the introduction of pulsatile flow into the pulmonary circuit could prevent the development of such fistulae. The end-to-side SVC-to-right PA modification was therefore adopted and became known as the bidirectional Glenn shunt (BDG).

To simplify the Fontan completion operation in patients with hypoplastic left heart syndrome (HLHS), further modification of the shunt was popularized by Norwood as the hemi-Fontan procedure.

PRINCIPLES AND JUSTIFICATION

The BDG is currently defined as an anastomosis that diverts systemic venous return from the SVC (or cavae) to both lungs. The value of the operation is as an intermediate stage to render the patient with single physiology as ideal a candidate as possible for later Fontan completion. The BDG removes the obligatory volume overload imposed on the ventricle by a systemic-to-PA shunt, allowing resolution of excessive ventricular hypertrophy and dilatation with concomitant increase in diastolic compliance before the Fontan completion procedure. Improvement in tricuspid regurgitation in some patients may also be achieved. Because augmentation of the PAs is occasionally required, particularly in patients with hypoplastic heart syndrome who have successfully undergone the first palliative stage, the hemi-Fontan operation, which also involves homograft patch enlargement of the PAs, is preferred by some surgeons. Although this latter procedure is more complex, involving placement of a dam between the right atrium and the PA, it facilitates the Fontan completion if the latter is performed using the intracardiac lateral tunnel technique. As intermediate procedures, the BDG or hemi-Fontan have been associated with improved ventricular function and decreased incidence of pleural effusions at the completion operation.

The BDG can be combined with intracardiac correction to incorporate a smaller tripartite pulmonary ventricle, and thereby create pulsatile pulmonary blood flow as the one-and-a-half ventricle repair. Direct visceral venous return containing the "hepatic factor" is preserved, which, together with preservation of pulsatile pulmonary blood flow, may prevent development of pulmonary arteriovenous fistulae.

Finally, the BDG may be used as definitive palliation in the management of complex cyanotic heart disease in patients not considered ideal candidates for Fontan physiology because of common atrioventricular valve insufficiency or congenital or iatrogenic abnormalities of PAs. Substantial improvement in systemic oxygen saturations can be achieved with reduction in cardiac workload.

PREOPERATIVE ASSESSMENT AND PREPARATION

Before performing the BDG or hemi-Fontan, it is critically important to identify physiological or anatomical problems that may have developed after the first-stage neonatal palliative procedure for single ventricle, whether it be a shunt, PA band, or more complex procedure such as a stage I Norwood operation for HLHS or a Damus–Kaye–Stansel procedure. Evaluation for congestive heart failure due to ventricular dysfunction and dilatation associated with progressive atrioventricular valve regurgitation in the presence of a systemic-to-PA shunt should be performed. Narrowing or distortion of the PAs should be ruled out, especially in patients who have undergone stage I palliation for HLHS, in whom progressive cyanosis may also be a manifestation of shunt narrowing or restriction of the atrial septal defect. Aortic arch obstruction in this latter group can cause pulmonary overcirculation and elevation of pulmonary vascular resistance. Early intervention for these problems may stabilize patients and lower the morbidity of the BDG or hemi-Fontan procedures. Although echocardiography and magnetic resonance angiography (MRA) are valuable tests for screening, cardiac cardiac catheterization is strongly recommended not only as a diagnostic test, but also for intervention when indicated. Residual arch obstruction can be dilated and stented, while aortopulmonary collateral vessels, if present, can be addressed. PA abnormalities can be delineated before surgery. Such an aggressive approach is of paramount importance to ensure that patients remain "ideal" Fontan candidates.

When performed as staged palliation for functional single ventricle, the BDG can be electively performed between 3 and 6 months of age. If the clinical condition of the infant mandates earlier intervention, such as ventricular dysfunction due to the volume overload of the systemic shunt or pressure overload due to recoarctation of the aorta not amenable to percutaneous intervention, then BDG as early as 2–3 months of age can be safely performed without significant additional morbidity or mortality.

ANESTHESIA

Patients are intubated using the nasotracheal or orotracheal route. They are ventilated using low mean airway pressures with long expiratory times and minimal positive end-expiratory pressure. A radial arterial line is preferable. Monitoring of cavopulmonary pressures can be achieved using a percutaneous internal jugular line, although we have found it convenient to place transthoracic 3 Fr lines in the common atrium and at the cavopulmonary connection through the appropriate suture lines intraoperatively.

OPERATION

Bidirectional Glenn shunt

The BDG anastomosis is performed using aortobicaval, normothermic cardiopulmonary bypass with a beating, decompressed heart. Cannulation of the SVC may be avoided by placing a pump sucker in the proximal orifice of the transected SVC. PA isolation and patch augmentation of the branch PAs can be performed if required at this stage. Moderate hypothermia (28°C), aortic cross-clamping, and cold blood cardioplegia are used if concomitant atrial septectomy or atrioventricular valve repair is necessary.

After median sternotomy, the aorta, PAs, and inferior vena cava (IVC) are dissected. The SVC is dissected and fully mobilized superiorly to the innominate and subclavian vein tributaries. The azygous vein is doubly ligated and divided. The medial and lateral aspects of the SVC are marked with 7-0 polypropylene monofilament suture (Prolene, Ethicon, Somerville, NJ) to ensure correct orientation for the BDG anastomosis. Similar marking sutures can be placed to delineate the location and extent of the incision on the superior aspect of the right PA. Control of a systemic-to-PA shunt, if present, is obtained. The aorta is cannulated using a single aortic pursestring. Cannulation of the IVC (DLP, Grand Rapids, MI, or RMI Research Medical, Midvale, UT) is followed by high SVC cannulation at the innominate vein junction using a right-angled cannula (DLP or RMI) (**Figure 44.1a**). Cardiopulmonary bypass is established, and

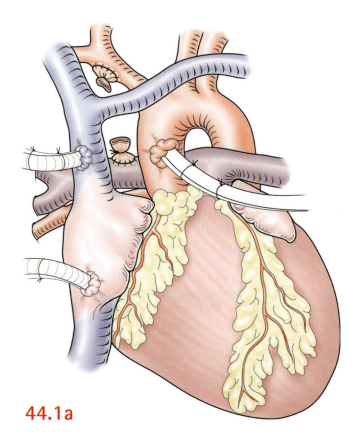

44.1a

the systemic-to-PA shunt is ligated and divided. The PA branches may be opened and patch augmentation performed at this point. Depending on the anatomy, the pulmonary trunk may need to be clamped during this maneuver to prevent air entry into the beating heart.

The tourniquet on the SVC is secured, and a clamp is positioned across the SVC–right atrial junction. The SVC is then transected (**Figure 44.1b**). If the SVC has not been cannulated, the SVC is transected and a pump sucker carefully positioned in the cephalic end of the SVC to maintain adequate exposure during cardiopulmonary bypass (**Figure 44.1c**). If an intracardiac procedure is required, the aorta is cross-clamped and cardioplegia administered. Then the IVC tourniquet can be secured and the right atrial incision made.

With the vascular clamp on the SVC–right atrial junction, the cardiac end of the transected SVC is closed in two layers, using a running horizontal mattress suture of 5-0 polypropylene, followed by a running suture line after removal of the clamp. The PA is incised and the back wall of the SVC-to-right PA anastomosis begun at the medial end using a running 6-0 absorbable monofilament suture (Polydioxanone, Ethicon, Somerville, NJ) (**Figure 44.1d**). The suture line is intermittently locked to prevent pursestringing of the anastomosis. The anterior aspect of the anastomosis is completed with a similar suture line or with

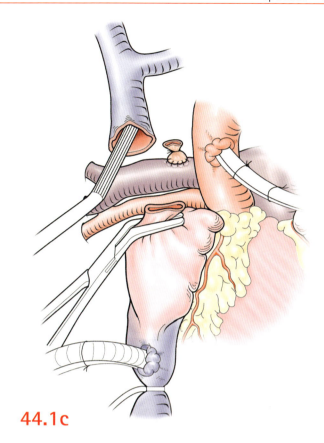

44.1c

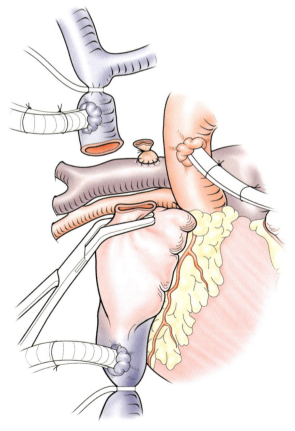

44.1b

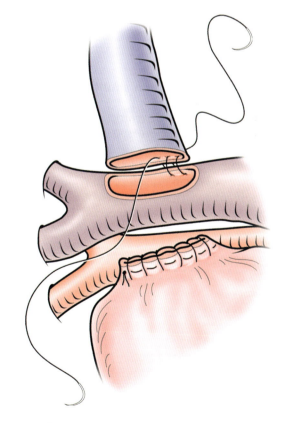

44.1d

interrupted sutures if desired (**Figure 44.1e**). Although rarely required, patch augmentation of the anterior aspect of the SVC-to-right PA anastomosis may be necessary to achieve a tension-free, large cavopulmonary connection. The tourniquet on the SVC is released, the heart allowed to fill and eject, and the patient separated from cardiopulmonary bypass. If an intracardiac procedure has been performed, de-airing of the heart before removal of the cross-clamp and during rewarming is required.

and the SVC is transected. The cardiac end of the transected SVC is closed in two layers, using a running horizontal mattress suture of 5-0 polypropylene, followed by a running suture line after removal of the clamp. The right PA is opened on its superior aspect, and an end-to-side cavopulmonary anastomosis is created using 6-0 polydioxanone suture as described previously (**Figure 44.2b**). All clamps and tourniquets are removed.

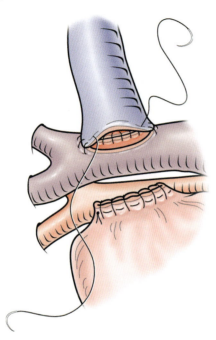

44.1e

Bilateral bidirectional Glenn shunt

Patients with a functional single ventricle, particularly those with heterotaxia, have anomalies of systemic and pulmonary venous return associated with splenic abnormalities. A high incidence of bilateral SVCs occurs in this group who, as suitable candidates for Fontan palliation, will require bilateral BDG shunts. If pulmonary atresia is present, a systemic-to-PA shunt is required in the neonatal period. If pulmonary stenosis is present, adequate pulmonary blood flow may be present initially, so that a bilateral BDG procedure may be the first intervention required, as in the example shown in **Figure 44.2a**. Such anatomy occasionally affords the surgeon an opportunity to perform the BDG shunts sequentially, obviating the need for cardiopulmonary bypass.

After median sternotomy and subtotal thymectomy, the pericardium is opened and suspended with stay sutures. The great vessels are dissected and mobilized fully.

Starting with the right SVC, marking sutures of 7-0 polypropylene are placed on the medial and lateral aspects. The right upper and lower PA branches in the hilum are encircled and tourniquets applied. The right PA is clamped medially, being careful to avoid distortion of the main and left PAs, and the tourniquets are secured laterally. Once oxygen saturations are stable, the SVC and cavoatrial junction are clamped,

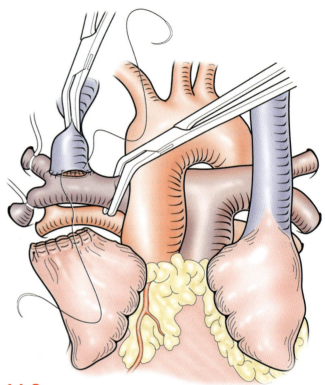

44.2a

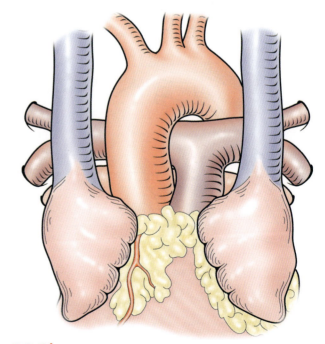

44.2b

After encircling the left upper and lower PAs in the left hilum, tourniquets are applied. The left SVC and the left-sided cavoatrial junction are clamped and the left SVC transected. Again, the cardiac end of the SVC is closed in two layers. The left PA is clamped medially, and the tourniquets are secured laterally. The left pulmonary is opened on its superior aspect, and once more, an end-to-side cavopulmonary anastomosis is created with 6-0 polydioxanone suture (**Figure 44.2c**). The clamps and tourniquets are removed.

A PA band is applied to reduce the blood flow through the stenotic main PA (**Figure 44.2d**). Transesophageal echocardiography and direct pressure measurements in the branch PAs can be used to guide tightening of the band.

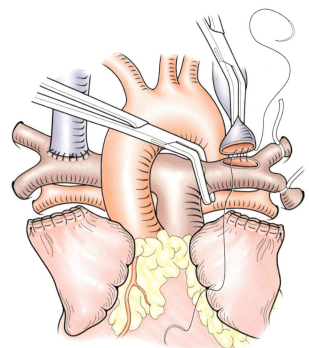

44.2c

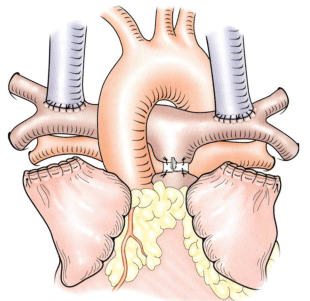

44.2d

Hemi–Fontan I

The great vessels and relevant cardiac structures are dissected. The neoaorta and right atrium are cannulated. The right modified Blalock–Taussig shunt is encircled with a braided polyester ligature. The pulmonary bifurcation is mobilized as completely as possible before initiation of cardiopulmonary bypass (**Figure 44.3a**). The shunt is ligated once bypass is established, and the PA dissection is completed, as the patient is cooled to a nasopharyngeal temperature of 18 °C. When cooling is complete, circulatory arrest is established, the neoaorta is cross-clamped, and cardioplegia is administered. The venous cannula is removed from the right atrium. The SVC is opened at the cavoatrial junction. The incision spirals cephalad around the medial border of the SVC and ends posteriorly, adjacent to the PA. Caudally, it extends across the cavoatrial junction toward the sinus nodal artery, transection of which can occasionally be avoided. The PA is opened on its anterior aspect from a point immediately posterior to the SVC to the branch point of the left PA.

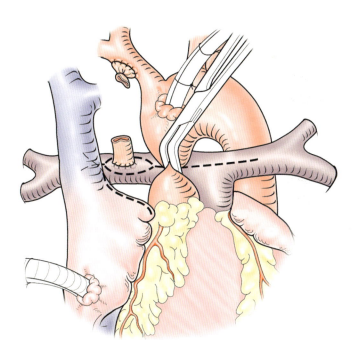

44.3a

A patch of Gore-Tex (Gore, Flagstaff, AZ, USA), appropriately tailored, is sewn into the right atrium immediately below the cavoatrial junction, through the incision, using 5-0 polypropylene suture (**Figure 44.3b**). This patch serves to separate the right atrium from the cavopulmonary anastomosis and is excised during the subsequent Fontan completion procedure.

The posterior border of the cavoatrial opening is then sutured to the inferior edge of the pulmonary arteriotomy using a running 6-0 polypropylene suture (**Figure 44.3c**).

A generous triangular-shaped patch of cryopreserved pulmonary homograft is cut to the appropriate size. Using 6-0 polypropylene suture, the patch is sewn to the remaining margins of the pulmonary arteriotomy, starting at its leftward extent (**Figure 44.3d**). The suture line is carried onto the cavoatrial junction, where it is completed (**Figure 44.3e**). The right atrial cannula is replaced and, after de-airing the heart, cardiopulmonary bypass is re-established and rewarming begun.

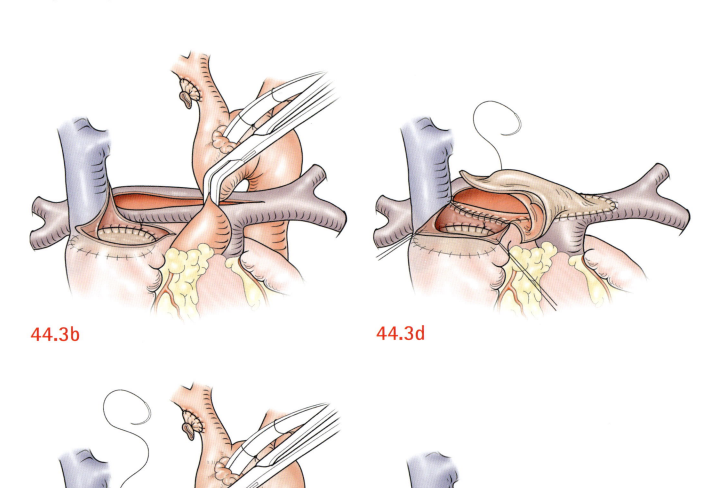

44.3b

44.3d

44.3c

44.3e

Hemi–Fontan II

After dissection of the great vessels and relevant cardiac structures, the neoaorta and right atrium are cannulated. Cardiopulmonary bypass is initiated, and ligation of the right modified Blalock–Taussig shunt is performed. The dissection of the pulmonary bifurcation is completed; and after neoaortic cross-clamping, cardioplegia is administered. Circulatory arrest is begun. An incision is made in the PA from hilum to hilum. An incision is also made on the medial aspect of the SVC extending from just below the innominate vein junction, across the cavoatrial junction, onto the right atrial appendage (**Figure 44.4a**).

The posterior margin of the SVC–right atrial incision is then sewn to the rightward end of the pulmonary arteriotomy using a running 6-0 polypropylene suture (**Figure 44.4b**). This maneuver ensures a wide opening between the SVC and PA.

A large triangular-shaped patch of cryopreserved pulmonary homograft is tailored for augmentation of the pulmonary bifurcation. Beginning at the left hilum, the patch is sewn to the margins of the pulmonary arteriotomy using a running 6-0 polypropylene suture. The suture line connecting the patch and the inferior margin of the pulmonary arteriotomy is carried onto the cavoatrial junction along the margin of the incision in the right atrial appendage (**Figure 44.4c**). The pulmonary homograft patch is then folded down, creating a dam at the level of the cavoatrial junction between the right atrium and the cavopulmonary anastomosis. This point is secured circumferentially with a 5-0 polypropylene suture (**Figure 44.4d**). Careful incorporation of the double flap of pulmonary homograft is important to prevent any baffle leaks entering the right atrium. The cannula is replaced in the right atrium, the heart is de-aired, and cardiopulmonary bypass is re-established.

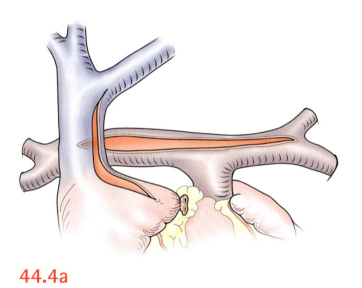

44.4a

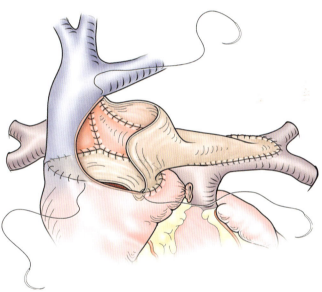

44.4c

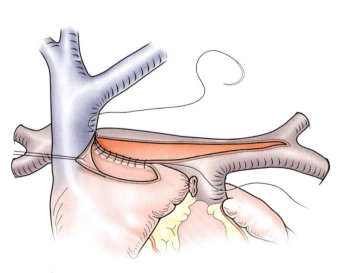

44.4b

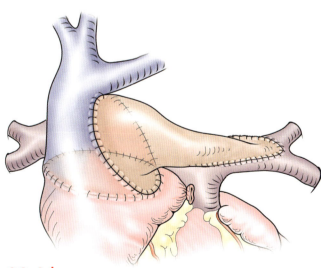

44.4d

Hybrid modification

Occasionally, prior to performing the BDG as a second procedure in the staged palliation for HLHS, significant central and proximal left pulmonary artery (LPA) hypoplasia is identified by preoperative echocardiographic or MRA assessment. The mechanism of this is often anterior compression of the PA by the substantial neoaorta. Patch augmentation of the central and proximal PA at the time of the bidirectional Glenn procedure or the hemi-Fontan procedure can address this. However, because the etiology is often arterial compression, recurrence is not unusual. It is possible to overcome this problem by a hybrid procedure involving intraoperative pulmonary balloon arterioplasty and stent placement during the Glenn procedure. Long-term, the stent prevents recompression of the central and LPA, simplifying the Fontan completion procedure.

Redo sternotomy, followed by arterial and venous cannulation, is performed as in a standard bidirectional Glenn procedure; the SVC is prepared for the Glenn anastomosis. The right PA is opened (**Figure 44.5a**).

The balloon/stent assembly is then prepared. The "indeflator" is connected to the inflation port of a suitable balloon catheter (e.g. 6 mm or 8 mm Powerflex, length 2 cm, Johnson & Johnson) and the balloon is inflated to de-air it (**Figure 44.5b**). Saline flush may also be used.

The operator hand-crimps the stent (e.g. PG 1910XD, Johnson & Johnson) and places it over the deflated balloon, and the balloon is then pressurized to 0.5–1.0 atm to create a "shoulder" to hold the stent securely (**Figure 44.5c**). A tongue wire is inserted into the guidewire lumen of the balloon/stent assembly, ensuring that the guide wire tip is projecting from the tip of the balloon by 3 cm or so.

The balloon/stent assembly with guidewire is then introduced through the right pulmonary arteriotomy into the retroaortic hypoplastic cental PA/LPA confluence (**Figure 44.4d**). Using a combination of predetermined landmarks from preoperative MRI/CT or cardiac catheterization, or theatre C-arm, along with direct visualization of the proximal end of the assembly, the stent is accurately positioned. In a hybrid operating room this is simplified by use of fluoroscopic control.

The stent is then deployed by inflating the balloon to 6–8 atm. The balloon is deflated and carefully removed from the stented area (**Figure 44.5e**) and, finally, the Glenn anastomosis is completed as described above (**Figure 44.5f**).

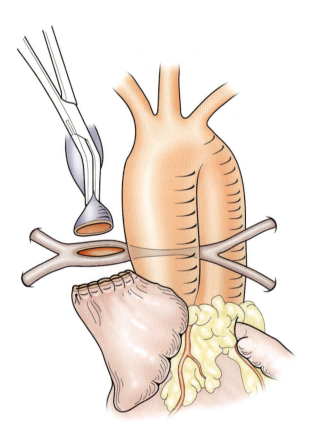

44.5a

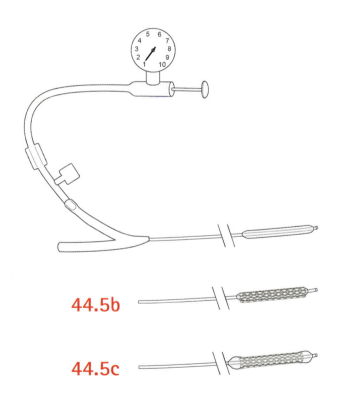

44.5b

44.5c

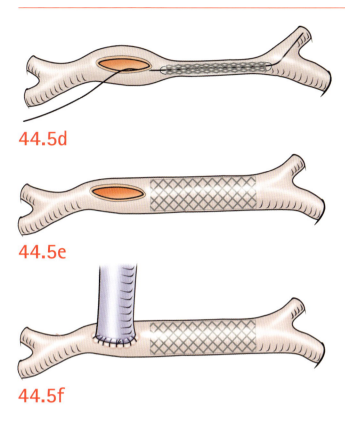

44.5d

44.5e

44.5f

POSTOPERATIVE CARE

After the procedure, patients are allowed to awaken and are extubated as early as possible. Expeditious removal from positive pressure ventilation improves hemodynamics across the pulmonary vascular bed. Head elevation and inhaled nitric oxide are used in the early postoperative phase if "Glenn" pressures are temporarily increased. Pressure monitoring lines are removed as soon as hemodynamics have stabilized. Oxygen saturations in the mid 80% range are typical after the procedure. Failure to wean rapidly from mechanical ventilation should initiate evaluation for phrenic nerve paralysis. Pleural effusions requiring intervention are unusual but should be ruled out. Although early sinus node dysfunction is not uncommon, normal sinus rhythm returns within 2 or 3 days of the procedure, and patients are generally ready for discharge by the fourth or fifth postoperative day.

OUTCOME

When used as an intermediate procedure in the staged palliation for HLHS, perioperative mortality for the BDG and hemi-Fontan procedures is 1–2%. With the use of modified ultrafiltration or aggressive postoperative diuresis, the incidence of pleural effusions requiring intervention is 5%. PA thrombosis and heart block occur in less than 5% of patients.

Our preference has been to perform the BDG rather than the hemi-Fontan. Some advantages of the BDG include the potentially lower incidence of dysrhythmias by avoiding incisions that interfere with sinus node function or blood supply. Hypothermic circulatory arrest and aortic cross-clamping can generally be avoided. If the surgeon's preference is ultimately to perform an extracardiac Fontan, then the BDG may be preferable. The improved energy conservation and hemodynamics obtained by offset of SVC and IVC flow are more readily accomplished when the BDG is used.

The hemi-Fontan, however, has several features that render it particularly suitable for patients with HLHS. PA distortion or hypoplasia is common in these patients, a problem readily addressed by use of a generous patch of pulmonary homograft across the pulmonary bifurcation or the insertion site of the modified Blalock–Taussig shunt in the hemi-Fontan procedure. In addition, when the surgeon's preference is to perform an intracardiac lateral tunnel completion, which facilitates more reliable fenestration, the hemi-Fontan may be more desirable. In the latter procedure, a dam is created at the SVC–right atrial junction either as part of the pulmonary bifurcation patch, as described by Jacobs and Norwood, or as a separate patch, as described by Bove. This patch can be easily resected at the time of the Fontan completion, rendering this procedure very straightforward.

A disadvantage of the hemi-Fontan is that the cavoatrial incision often transects the sinus nodal artery, with the potential for adverse consequences on sinus node function and for the development of late atrial dysrhythmias. The procedure requires hypothermic circulatory arrest with its attendant risk of neurological injury, although it does obviate the need for cannulation of the SVC.

When used as part of a one-and-a-half ventricle repair, the BDG has yielded favorable results, as long as the small or dysfunctional pulmonary ventricle is tripartite. Overall, survival of 90% at 5 years has been reported, with the majority of patients experiencing a good clinical outcome. When the pulmonary ventricle is non-tripartite, results have been unsatisfactory.

The commonest problem after the BDG procedure has been progressive cyanosis. This situation may be due to the development of systemic venous collaterals, which decompress the superior caval system into the inferior caval system. These collaterals usually can be treated by coil embolization. More difficult to deal with are the pulmonary arteriovenous collateral vessels arising from the brachiocephalic, bronchial, or intercostal arteries. Such left-to-right shunting can also place a hemodynamic burden on the systemic ventricle. Whereas discrete collaterals can be embolized, diffuse arteriovenous shunting is often not readily amenable to coil embolization. Presence of a BDG rather a completion Fontan procedure and older age are risk factors for these collaterals. Earlier Fontan completion may be indicated in such patients.

FURTHER READING

Bove EL, Lloyd TR. Staged reconstruction for hypoplastic left heart syndrome: Contemporary results. *Ann Surg.* 1996; 224(3): 387–95.

Douglas WI, Goldberg CS, Mosca RS, et al. Hemi-Fontan procedure for hypoplastic left heart syndrome: outcome and suitability for Fontan. *Ann Thorac Surg.* 1999; 68: 1361–8.

Jacobs ML, Norwood WI. Fontan operation: influence of modifications on morbidity and mortality. *Ann Thorac Surg.* 1994; 58: 945–52.

Koutlas TC, Gaynor JW, Nicolson SC, et al. Modified ultrafiltration reduces postoperative morbidity after cavopulmonary connection. *Ann Thorac Surg.* 1997; 64: 137–43.

Kreutzer C, de Mayorquim R, Kreutzer GOA, et al. Experience with one and a half ventricle repair. *J Thorac Cardiovasc Surg.* 1999; 117: 662–8.

Seliem MA, Baffa JM, Vetter JM, et al. Changes in right ventricular geometry and heart rate early after hemi-Fontan procedure. *Ann Thorac Surg.* 1993; 55: 1508–12.

45

Fontan procedure for functionally single ventricle and double-inlet ventricle

TARA KARAMLOU AND GORDON A. COHEN

HISTORY

In 1971, Fontan and Baudet published their landmark paper describing a surgical correction whereby the pulmonary and systemic circulations were placed in series in a patient with tricuspid atresia. Since that time, the indications for this procedure have been extended to include all defects with a functionally univentricular heart. Despite the early success of this procedure, longevity and efficiency of this circulatory arrangement have been of constant concern, leading to numerous modifications of the original operation. Some of the early modifications dispensed with the inlet and outlet valves and ultimately led to the direct connection of the functional right atrium to the pulmonary circulation.

The usefulness of the right atrium in this connection has been questioned, and this concern led to the concept of lateral tunnel or total cavopulmonary connection (TCPC). In this operation, the superior and the inferior caval veins are connected to the pulmonary arteries. However, the superior vena cava (SVC) undergoes a direct connection, whereas the inferior vena cava (IVC) is connected via a prosthetic conduit. The inferior connection takes the form of either an intra-atrial tunnel or an extracardiac conduit.

PRINCIPLES AND JUSTIFICATION

The basic principle of the original Fontan operation was to divert systemic venous return back to the pulmonary artery without the use of a functional ventricle. This arrangement then allowed the functional ventricle of the heart to be used for providing systemic blood flow. Since it was originally described in 1971, the operation has undergone numerous modifications. Despite the evolution of the procedure, that central principle remains the basis of the various techniques that are used to perform the operation today.

A number of factors influence the approach to the repair of the patient with a functionally single ventricle. The main considerations include:

- whether or not to perform a staged repair (bidirectional Glenn shunt or hemi-Fontan followed by completion Fontan procedure)
- the timing of the Fontan procedure
- the type of repair performed: lateral tunnel versus conduit, fenestrated versus non-fenestrated.

The product of these considerations is a short list of surgical options for a functional single ventricle that includes systemic–pulmonary artery shunting or pulmonary artery banding, bidirectional Glenn shunt (or hemi-Fontan), and fenestrated and completed Fontan procedures. Although the term "repair" is often used, it is important to remember that all of these procedures are really palliative, and have specific advantages and disadvantages that can be exploited in certain anatomic situations. Unfortunately, the indications and timing for some of the procedures remain poorly defined. As a result, utilization of these options remains highly variable, and they are often applied depending on surgeon or institutional-bias.

The initial Fontan procedure and early modifications attempted to use a contractile atrial chamber as a pump to assist blood flow into the pulmonary arteries. The atriopulmonary Fontan, however, was an inefficient system with important inherent energy losses, turbulence, and stasis. Furthermore, the original atriopulmonary Fontan operation exposed a large area of atrial wall to the elevated venous pressure of the Fontan circuit, which contributed to massive dilation and hypertrophy of the atrial chamber. Late sequelae of the atriopulmonary Fontan, not surprisingly, included arrhythmias, thrombosis, and accelerated failure. A contemporary modification, the TCPC does not depend on the contractile properties of the atrium, does not require *in situ* valves, and can be employed in patients with essentially all single ventricle morphologies. The TCPC directs, rather than pumps, systemic venous return into the pulmonary arteries.

The traditional approach to the patient with a functional single ventricle had been a neonatal palliative procedure (shunt, pulmonary artery band, or complex reconstruction) followed by a completed Fontan procedure later in life. However, Hopkins et al. from Duke published a landmark paper in 1985 chronicling the excellent outcomes of 21 patients who underwent an intermediate bidirectional Glenn shunt (superior cavopulmonary anastomosis). Based on these results, surgeons from the Children's Hospital in Boston advocated that the bidirectional Glenn shunt be employed as an intermediate step between a neonatal palliative procedure and a completion Fontan (TCPC) in high-risk cases. The staged repair was thought to reduce the morbidity and the mortality of the subsequent Fontan procedure. Consequently, the concept of performing a bidirectional Glenn shunt as an intermediate step has received relatively widespread acceptance.

The issue of timing for a Fontan procedure as definitive palliation is poorly defined. A review of the literature demonstrates published series with a broad spectrum of ages. Children younger than 1 year of age as well as adults in their mid-40s are among the patients who have undergone a successful Fontan procedure. However, the approximate average age of patients who undergo the operation in contemporary series is somewhere between 4 and 5 years. Despite the large number of patients who have undergone a Fontan procedure worldwide, no "ideal" age or "optimal" timing for the operation has yet been identified. Moreover, the timing of a Fontan procedure may differ depending on the underlying diagnosis (i.e. hypoplastic left heart syndrome vs tricuspid atresia, etc.) and the anticipated need for concomitant procedures.

The two most common modifications of the TCPC performed today are the lateral tunnel Fontan and the total extracardiac TCPC (extracardiac conduit). The most recent iteration of the extracardiac Fontan is the so-called intra/extracardiac Fontan, which may have potential benefit in particular anatomic situations. No prospective multi-institutional series has been published that demonstrates one modification to be superior to the other in terms of survival or postoperative morbidity, although recent studies have suggested improved in-hospital outcomes with the fenestrated lateral tunnel. Additionally, fluid computational studies from Bove et al. and de Leval et al. have shown reduced energy loss and more equivalent pulmonary artery distribution of IVC blood flow with the lateral tunnel Fontan. Despite excellent results with the lateral tunnel at selected centers, however, the standard extracardiac conduit is currently performed with greater frequency (63% vs 47% for the lateral tunnel) according to a review of the Society of Thoracic Surgeons Congenital Heart Surgery Database in 2012, with some centers performing exclusively the extracardiac conduit Fontan.

This enthusiasm for the extracardiac modification as compared to the lateral tunnel notwithstanding, theoretical concerns may favor one procedure over the other. The extracardiac conduit may be performed with normothermic cardiopulmonary bypass, without cardioplegic arrest. Most surgeons also feel that the extracardiac conduit is a conceptually and technically simpler operation to perform, and is more reproducible over time. The extracardiac conduit

also reduces the number of atrial suture lines, especially in the region of the sinoatrial node, and therefore has a reduced propensity for late atrial arrhythmias. Moreover, the extracardiac location removes all foreign material from within the systemic ventricle, potentially decreasing the risk of thrombosis. In contrast, the lateral tunnel Fontan procedure requires systemic cooling (most surgeons prefer to perform this procedure at 28–32 °C) and cardioplegic arrest. Foreign material, albeit a small amount, is required in the construction of the systemic venous baffle for the lateral tunnel. Perhaps the most important advantage of the lateral tunnel, however, is that it can be performed on children of all ages since part of the tunnel consists of the native atrial wall, allowing somatic growth. The extracardiac conduit, on the other hand, needs to be performed on larger children (usually at least 13 kg), who could accommodate at least an 18–20 mm conduit. Even in cases where there is adequate somatic size to place an extracardiac conduit, the issue of pulmonary artery distortion from vertical growth (i.e. the intercaval distance) must be considered carefully.

Anatomical issues can also be important in determining the ideal Fontan modification. The extracardiac conduit can be used to account for difficult pulmonary venous anatomy in cases in which obstruction of a pulmonary vein may occur with a lateral tunnel Fontan procedure. However, the lateral tunnel Fontan can account for difficult systemic venous anatomy when multiple systemic venous orifices drain into the right atrium. Finally, fenestration patency and construction are undoubtedly easier with the lateral tunnel than the extracardiac conduit, and the lateral tunnel allows catheter access to the atrium for future electrophysiologic or interventional procedures.

Another important technical issue in Fontan surgery is whether use of a fenestration is beneficial, and, if so, whether it be employed universally or selectively. Fenestration of the Fontan circuit was theorized to decrease specific morbidities following Fontan completion, including low postoperative cardiac output, pleural and pericardial effusions, ascites, ventricular dysfunction, and poor exercise performance. The placement of a fenestration between the systemic and pulmonary circulations at the atrial level as part of a TCPC results in decreased systemic venous pressures, decreased arterial oxygen saturations, and higher cardiac outputs. Despite the purported benefits, fenestration carries with it the risk of potential paradoxical embolization, cyanosis, and potential need for late catheter-based intervention for fenestration closure. There is also concern regarding the durability or patency of fenestration, especially with the extracardiac conduit modification.

A recent study from Texas Children's Hospital demonstrated equivalent outcomes among fenestrated and non-fenestrated Fontan procedures in 226 patients. Tweddell et al. reported, in their series of 256 consecutive Fontan patients, worse event-free outcomes among those receiving fenestrations. However, these data must be interpreted cautiously because of confounding by indication – in other words, many surgeons employ fenestration in less favorable anatomic or physiologic subtypes. Thus, the questions of whether fenestration is beneficial, and in which substrates, remain unclear.

PREOPERATIVE ASSESSMENT AND PREPARATION

Preoperative assessment of a patient for a Fontan procedure should include a thorough history, physical examination, chest X-ray, and electrocardiogram. However, more sophisticated tests are necessary to determine the precise anatomy and physiology of the congenital cardiac defect. Transthoracic echocardiography is useful for identifying the cardiac morphology. Color flow Doppler echocardiography is useful in providing information about the competence of the atrioventricular valve(s) and data regarding the presence and severity of left ventricular outflow tract obstruction, as well as other hemodynamic information. Cardiac catheterization is necessary to identify any unclear anatomy following the echocardiogram, provide a precise evaluation about the size and morphology of the pulmonary arteries, and provide precise hemodynamic and oximetric data. Specific measurements that are evaluated include the end-diastolic pressure in the systemic ventricle, the transpulmonary gradient, the pulmonary vascular resistance, and the mixed venous and systemic saturation.

Historically, the focus was on the *selection* criteria for a TCPC. In fact, in 1977, Choussat et al. published the so-called 10 commandments, which were the strict selection criteria for performing a Fontan procedure. With time, those criteria became more extended to include patients with more complex congenital cardiac defects and patients who fulfilled fewer of Choussat et al.'s original criteria. However, the emphasis has now evolved away from selection and into *preparation* for a Fontan procedure. Infants are currently palliated and staged, with early removal of the volume load from the systemic ventricle. Correctable hemodynamic lesions are dealt with before a TCPC is performed. This shift in attitude has most likely contributed in large part to the improvements in mortality and morbidity that have been seen with the Fontan procedure in contemporary times.

ANESTHESIA

Critical issues in the anesthetic management of a patient who is undergoing a Fontan procedure begin immediately upon entry into the operating room. Decisions regarding the type and location of venous access are critical to the long-term success of the operation. Because of the risk of venous thrombosis that is associated with indwelling central venous catheters, many centers have a policy of avoiding central lines in the SVC at any time. Intracardiac lines or femoral venous lines are considered more desirable for central venous access in a patient who is undergoing a TCPC.

After the surgical pathway has been constructed and the patient is weaned and separated from cardiopulmonary bypass, it is important to ensure that the patient has appropriate and adequate intravascular volume status. The goal is to optimize cardiac output at the lowest possible central venous pressure. To achieve this, it is necessary to minimize pulmonary vascular resistance. Measures to reduce the pulmonary vascular resistance include avoiding hypoxia and hypercarbia, correcting metabolic acidosis, and rewarming of the patient. Patients should also be ventilated with the lowest possible airway pressure to reduce intrathoracic pressure. Ideally, patients should be extubated in the operating room following a Fontan procedure.

Van Arsdell et al. have published their results on interventions that are associated with minimal Fontan mortality. They reported that the use of modified ultrafiltration after cardiopulmonary bypass was associated with a lower mortality and suggested that this was at least in part due to a reduction in pulmonary vascular resistance. In the same report, they also identified the institution of inotropic and vasodilator support at the time of separation from cardiopulmonary bypass to be associated with lower mortality. The authors suggested that this approach carried the potential benefit of avoiding a postoperative fall in cardiac output and the inherent delay in treatment that is associated with late recognition. They also noted that patients in their higher-mortality group arrived in the intensive care unit on lower doses of inotropic support but had reached equivalent doses to the lower-mortality group by 6 hours postoperatively.

Therapy in the perioperative period can be aided by the intraoperative placement of a left atrial line. Continuous evaluation of the atrial pressure and the transpulmonary gradient will facilitate informed pharmacological management of the patient. When the transpulmonary gradient is elevated, pulmonary vasodilators, such as inhaled nitric oxide, nitroglycerin, and phosphodiesterase inhibitors, can be used to reduce pulmonary vascular resistance. Alternatively, when the volume status is low, volume expanders can be safely used. Sound management of post-Fontan patients should always be guided by physiologic data and principles, whether in the operating room by the anesthesiologists, or in the intensive care unit.

OPERATION

As discussed earlier, the Fontan procedure has evolved and undergone a number of modifications. Numerous variations of the TCPC exist. For the purpose of this chapter, we describe the most common modifications.

Bidirectional cavopulmonary anastomosis

Staging of the Fontan procedure has become routine and is now an accepted standard in many institutions. Common to all modifications of the operation is a superior cavopulmonary anastomosis (bidirectional Glenn shunt). The superior cavopulmonary anastomosis is an end-to-side anastomosis of the SVC to the right pulmonary artery (or, in the case of a left SVC, to the left pulmonary artery).

The operation is performed via median sternotomy, with cardiopulmonary bypass and systemic cooling. Although the operation can be performed without the use of cardiopulmonary bypass, no studies have conclusively found the short period of normothermic bypass to be detrimental. The SVC and the right pulmonary artery are fully mobilized. Extreme care is taken to avoid injury to the phrenic nerve. Once the patient is heparinized, the aorta is cannulated in a routine fashion. Venous return to the bypass circuit is through a cannula placed into the right atrial appendage, and a second small cannula is placed high up on the SVC near the innominate vein. Cardiopulmonary bypass is initiated, and the patient is usually maintained at normothermia. Any systemic–pulmonary artery shunts that are present should be dissected and controlled. If a right systemic–pulmonary artery shunt is present at the time of surgery, it should be disconnected from the pulmonary artery immediately after the institution of cardiopulmonary bypass. The end of the shunt is then oversewn with a fine Prolene suture. When a shunt is present, the opening that is created in the right pulmonary artery by removing the shunt is extended centrally, and the anastomosis can later be performed to this area.

The operation itself is performed on a beating heart. A snare is passed around the SVC and snugged down onto the venous cannula. If azygos continuation of the IVC is not present, the azygos vein is ligated. Some surgeons choose to divide the azygos vein if further mobilization of the SVC is necessary to create a tension-free anastomosis.

A vascular clamp is then applied to the SVC, just above the cavoatrial junction, taking care not to injure the sinus node. The SVC is then divided above the clamp, and the atrial end of the SVC is oversewn with a running 6-0 Prolene suture. Once this step has been accomplished, the clamp is released. The right pulmonary artery is then fully mobilized all the way out to the first divisions. If the decision has been made to maintain forward flow in the patient, the main pulmonary artery is mobilized but not divided. However, if this is not to be the case, the main pulmonary artery is divided. The proximal pulmonary artery is then oversewn in two layers using a 4-0 Prolene suture, making sure to catch the valve leaflets with each stitch so that no dead space is left behind that could become a site of later emboli. Alternatively, the valve leaflets can be sharply excised. The distal end of the divided main pulmonary artery can then either be directly closed or be patched with a small piece of bovine pericardium or Gore-Tex®.

To perform the actual superior cavopulmonary anastomosis, a side-biting vascular clamp is applied along the superior surface of the right pulmonary artery starting at the point of its bifurcation from the main pulmonary artery. A long incision is then made on the superior aspect of the right pulmonary artery nearly the entire distance from its origin to its branching (**Figure 45.1**).

The cavopulmonary anastomosis is then carried out with a running 6-0 Prolene suture, which is interrupted in two areas to avoid a pursestring effect at the suture line and to maintain a widely patent anastomosis (**Figure 45.2**). Bypass is then discontinued.

In the case of bilateral SVCs, a bilateral, bidirectional, superior cavopulmonary anastomosis is necessary. In this instance, the cavae must be cannulated separately; three venous cannulae are therefore required to perform this operation. Alternatively, two venous cannulae can be used, and the superior cannula is repositioned during the operation to the side on which the anastomosis is being performed. In this situation, the hemiazygos vein is ligated and divided, unless there is hemiazygos continuation of the IVC.

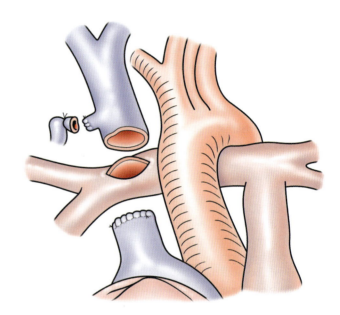

45.1

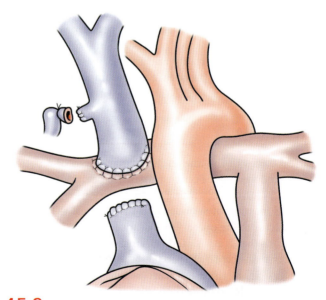

45.2

Lateral tunnel cavopulmonary anastomosis

Lateral tunnel cavopulmonary anastomosis is a modification of the Fontan operation that uses the placement of an intra-atrial Gore-Tex baffle to route blood from the IVC along the lateral wall of the right atrium through the previously oversewn orifice of the SVC up into the right pulmonary artery. This operation is performed following bidirectional cavopulmonary anastomosis and, as discussed earlier, usually occurs in a staged manner.

This operation is carried out by reopening the chest via the median sternotomy that was previously performed for the construction of the superior cavopulmonary anastomosis. Once the patient is fully heparinized, aortic cannulation is done in a routine fashion. Bicaval cannulation is performed by placing a venous cannula directly into the SVC, and an additional cannula is placed in the IVC just above the diaphragmatic surface. Cardiopulmonary bypass is initiated, and the patient is then cooled to 28–32 °C. Next, the aorta is cross-clamped, the cavae are snared, a right atriotomy parallel to the crista terminalis is performed, and cardioplegia is

administered. Care is taken to avoid the crista terminalis as they are important in maintaining sinus rythmn.

The intra-atrial baffle is then cut from a segment of Gore-Tex tube and is fashioned so that a smooth, tubular intra-atrial tunnel can be created. Before the creation of the intra-atrial tunnel, the portion of the atrial septum within the confines of the oval fossa is excised. Before the Gore-Tex baffle is sewn into place, a 4 mm fenestration is made using either a scalpel or an aortic punch. The superior cavoatrial junction, which had been previously oversewn at the time of the superior cavopulmonary shunt, is now opened (**Figure 45.3a–c**).

Once this step is complete, the baffle is sewn into position, starting at the orifice of the inferior cavoatrial junction, running the suture line posteriorly up to the superior cavoatrial junction. The suture line is then constructed around the entrance of the IVC into the atrium (**Figure 45.4a**). It is important to note that the coronary sinus should be left on the pulmonary venous atrial side of the baffle so as to avoid injury to the conduction system. When the suture line reaches the inferior cavoatrial junction at its lateral

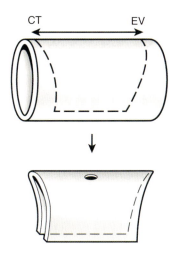

45.3a

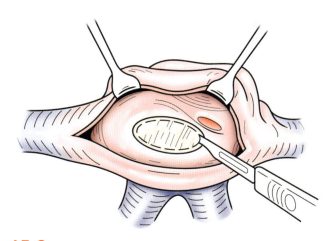

45.3c

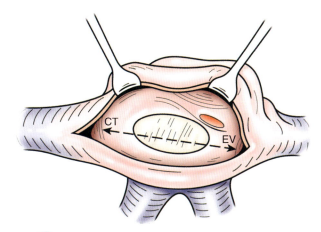

45.3b

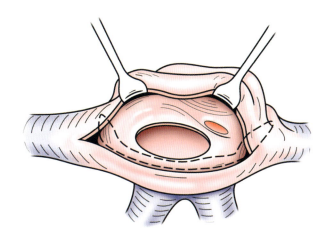

45.4a

aspect, the Gore-Tex baffle can be trimmed to optimize the fit (**Figure 45.4b**).

The suture line is then carried around so that the remainder of the baffle is sutured to the lateral wall of the atrium (**Figure 45.5**). The suture line to the lateral wall of the atrium can be incorporated into the closure of the right atriotomy. The right atriotomy is then closed in two layers. It is important to avoid placing sutures into the crista terminalis, as this is thought to contribute to the later development of atrial arrhythmias. Once this is complete, the previously transected and now open superior cavoatrial junction can be anastomosed to the undersurface of the right pulmonary

artery or to the site of the divided main pulmonary artery. This anastomosis is performed in a manner similar to that which was used to perform the superior cavopulmonary shunt. However, because the aorta is currently cross-clamped, it is not necessary to place an additional vascular clamp across the right pulmonary artery. The right pulmonary artery should be well mobilized before the creation of this anastomosis.

The completed lateral tunnel TCPC is demonstrated in **Figure 45.6**. Once this step is complete, the heart is de-aired, the aorta unclamped, and the patient fully rewarmed.

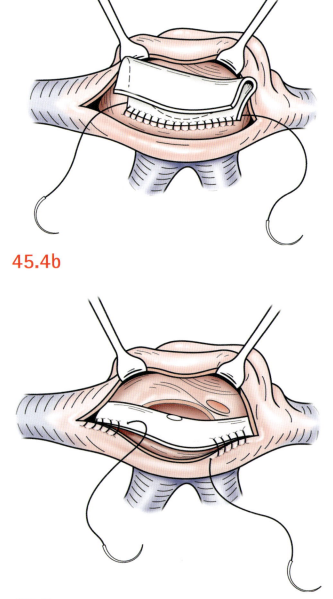

45.4b

45.5

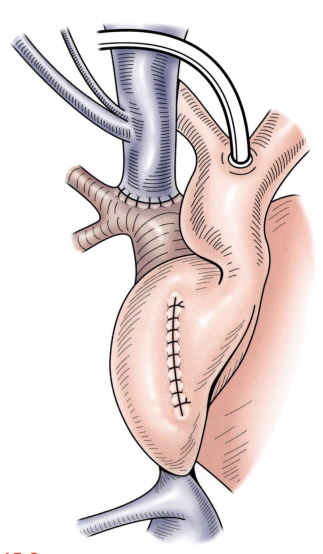

45.6

Extracardiac conduit

The extracardiac conduit is an anatomical option that allows the creation of an extra-atrial pathway from the IVC to the pulmonary artery. This operation is performed using a Gore-Tex tube as the conduit to divert the blood from the IVC to the right pulmonary artery. In general, this technique should be reserved for somewhat older patients so that growth and the long-term adequacy of the conduit size do not become an issue.

This technique is also performed using cardiopulmonary bypass. Although the procedure has been performed without cardiopulmonary bypass by some centers with encouraging results, we have continued to advocate the use of normothermic cardiopulmonary bypass for Fontan completion. As described earlier, the chest is re-entered through the previous median sternotomy. The right pulmonary artery is fully mobilized. The ascending aorta is cannulated in a routine fashion. Venous return to the pump is via bicaval cannulation, with a small cannula placed in the SVC and an additional cannula positioned in the IVC just above the diaphragmatic surface. Once cardiopulmonary bypass is initiated, the patient is kept at normothermia. One of the benefits of this technique is that it does not require cross-clamping of the aorta, unless fenestration is required and the atrium is not suitable for a partial-occluding clamp.

The IVC is snared down to the venous cannula. A vascular clamp is placed at the inferior cavoatrial junction, taking care not to injure the coronary sinus. The IVC is divided just below the vascular clamp. The atrial end of the IVC is then oversewn in two layers with a running 5-0 Prolene suture, and the clamp is released. Next, a Gore-Tex tube is sized to run from the cut end of the IVC up to the undersurface of the right pulmonary artery. The tube should be sized so that a gentle curve is formed just lateral to the heart. The IVC is then anastomosed to the Gore-Tex tube using a running 5-0 or 4-0 Prolene suture. Once this step is completed, a snare is placed around the SVC, which is snared down onto the venous cannula. Alternatively, a vascular clamp can be placed below the SVC cannula. If the main pulmonary artery is still intact, it is divided and oversewn as described previously. However, the opening on the pulmonary arterial side is left open, and this opening is used for the anastomosis. If the main pulmonary artery had previously been divided, an arteriotomy is then performed on the undersurface of the fully mobilized right pulmonary artery. A small sump-suction can be placed in the pulmonary arteriotomy to facilitate visualization of the anastomosis.

The end of the Gore-Tex tube is then spatulated, and an anastomosis is created between the tube and the undersurface of the right pulmonary artery using a running 6-0 Prolene suture (**Figure 45.7**). Once the connection is completed, the snare and ligatures are released, followed by removal of the vascular clamp. The patient can then be weaned from cardiopulmonary bypass.

If a fenestration is desired, this goal can be accomplished with a side-to-side anastomosis between the Gore-Tex conduit and the atrial wall. This anastomosis can be performed by using either a side-biting vascular clamp on the atrial wall or a very short period of aortic cross-clamping, if necessary.

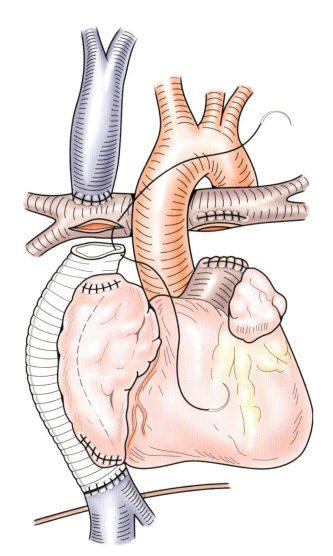

45.7

To create the anastomosis, a fenestration, using a 4 mm aortic punch, is made in the conduit adjacent to the atrium (**Figure 45.8a**). A small opening is then made in the right atrium, which is next anastomosed circumferentially around the fenestration in the conduit 3–4 mm outside the perimeter of the fenestration (**Figure 45.8b and c**). A 5-0 Prolene or Gore-Tex suture can be used, taking full-thickness bites through the edge of the atriotomy and partial-thickness bites in the wall of the Gore-Tex conduit.

Intra/extracardiac conduit

An intra/extracardiac conduit is an alternate technique that is particularly useful in patients with multiple hepatic venous orifices that drain into the right atrial chamber. As with the other techniques, this approach is undertaken via a median sternotomy. After full heparinization, the aorta is routinely cannulated. Venous drainage is via bicaval cannulation, with the inferior cannula placed low down in the IVC just above the diaphragmatic surface. The patient is placed on cardiopulmonary bypass and cooled to 22 °C to allow for reduction in flow. The cavae are snared, and the aorta is cross-clamped. Cold cardioplegia solution is administered to arrest the heart. A right atriotomy is performed toward the inferior cavoatrial junction. Flow is reduced, and the inferior caval cannula is clamped, removed, and replaced with a small sump sucker.

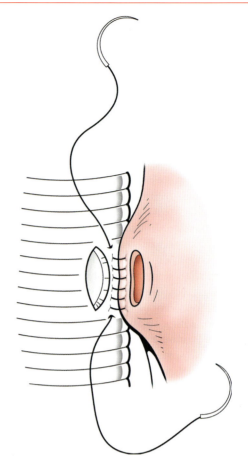

45.8b

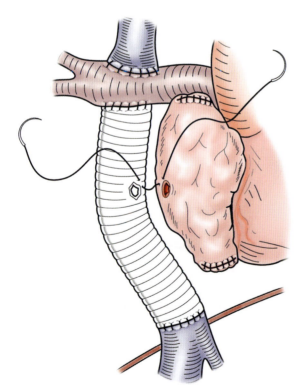

45.8a

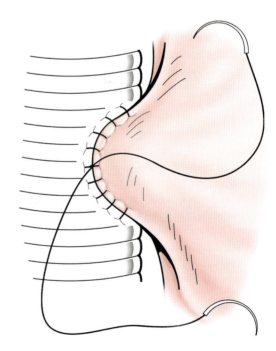

45.8c

The orifice to the IVC (or multiple orifices from hepatic veins and IVC) should be clearly visible. An appropriate-sized Gore-Tex tube is then spatulated to provide the inflow into the conduit and sewn into place around the IVC and/or hepatic vein orifices (**Figure 45.9a**). This step is most easily accomplished by starting at the most medial edge of the IVC orifice. Once the inferior caval end of the Gore-Tex is anastomosed, the conduit is brought outside the heart through the right atriotomy. An appropriate spot is picked for a fenestration inside the right atrium so that flow can occur easily into the atrial chamber. A 4 mm fenestration is created with either a scalpel blade or an aortic punch.

Once this opening is made, the edges of the atriotomy are sewn to the outer surface of the Gore-Tex tube using a running 5-0 or 6-0 Prolene suture (**Figure 45.9b**). The length of the conduit is then assessed so that it fits neatly to the undersurface of the right pulmonary artery. Once this distance has been estimated, the end of the conduit is cut in a spatulated fashion. The undersurface of the right pulmonary artery is then opened, and the incision is extended from just beyond the origin of the right pulmonary artery all the way out to the branching of the right pulmonary artery. (Depending on the anatomy, the divided main pulmonary artery can alternatively be used.)

An alternative as advocated by Jonas et al. is to use an inverted T-incision at the level of the bidirectional Glenn anastomosis, extending into both pulmonary arteries and the SVC. The superior end of the conduit can then be beveled appropriately and sutured to the opening using Prolene suture.

An anastomosis is then created using a running 6-0 Prolene suture (**Figure 45.9c**). Once this is complete, the sump sucker is removed from the pursestring in the IVC, and the venous cannula is replaced into this location. At this

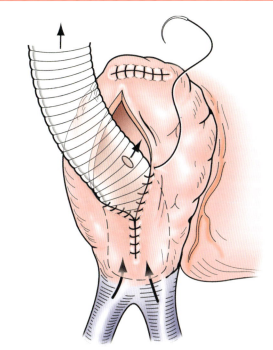

45.9b

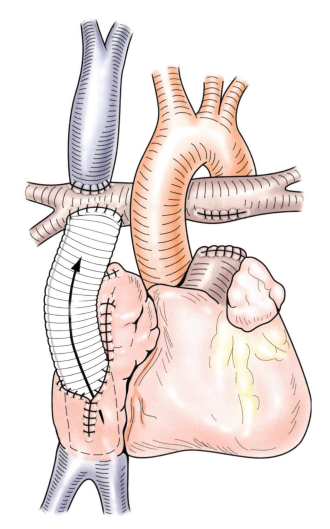

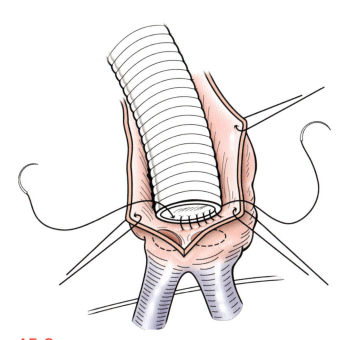

45.9a

45.9c

point the aorta is filled with blood and de-aired, the patient is fully rewarmed, and the aorta is unclamped.

POSTOPERATIVE CARE

The primary goal in the postoperative management of a patient having a Fontan procedure is to achieve the optimal cardiac output at the lowest possible central venous pressure. Although the preference is extubation in the operating room, if the patient remains intubated on arrival to the ICU, early weaning from the ventilator and extubation is expedited to achieve the optimal hemodynamics. Positive pressure ventilation increases mean airway pressures, and positive expiratory pressure can increase pulmonary vascular resistance and intrathoracic pressure, leading to decreased ventricular filling. Hence, a suboptimal cardiac output state may be improved simply by returning the patient to spontaneous ventilation. However, if a patient is in a relatively severe low cardiac output state, he or she should remain ventilated, as spontaneous breathing can make the situation worse.

The patient may have a relative degree of cyanosis due to right-to-left shunting through a fenestration secondary to increased pulmonary vascular resistance and high central venous pressures. Patients who cannot be weaned from ventilatory support should be evaluated early for diaphragmatic activity, as the phrenic nerve is at risk to injury, especially during performance of the extracardiac conduit. Injury to the phrenic nerve may have more dire consequences in patients with a Fontan circulation than in those with other types of cardiac repair. Other potential causes for failure to wean from ventilatory support should also be investigated, including pleural effusions, lung consolidation, pneumothorax, and an unsatisfactory repair. Arrhythmias following the Fontan procedure can be significantly problematic. As a result, it is imperative to place atrial and ventricular temporary pacing wires at the time of surgery. Loss of atrioventricular synchrony may result in a low cardiac output state due to increased dependence on the so-called "atrial kick" in patients with this anatomical arrangement. Tachycardias are also poorly tolerated and may result in severe hemodynamic deterioration. Ultimately, tachycardias result in a low cardiac output state due to an attenuated stroke volume secondary to reduced ventricular filling times.

As stated earlier, the primary objective in the early postoperative management of a Fontan procedure is achieving the optimal cardiac output at the lowest possible central venous pressure. Thus, a strategy of aggressive evaluation of low cardiac output states must be used. Factors such as mechanical ventilation and arrhythmias are obvious causes of a low cardiac output state. However, other factors, such as inadequate volume status (i.e. low preload due to hypovolemia), elevated pulmonary vascular resistance, ventricular failure, and an anatomical obstruction in the surgical pathway, are all additional causes of a low cardiac output state. To assist with postoperative management and the potential need to evaluate a low cardiac output state, intraoperative placement of a central venous catheter, and potentially a common atrial line, are imperative, as they are invaluable tools in the management of a postoperative Fontan patient. Postoperative echocardiography should also be used as an additional diagnostic tool in the management of these patients, to assess ventricular function and possible anatomical obstructions in the systemic venous pathway or pulmonary arteries. Echocardiography can also provide information about atrioventricular valve regurgitation, ventricular outflow obstruction, and tamponade, which can all be additional causes of low cardiac output states. In some cases, early cardiac catheterization may be necessary to evaluate the quality of the surgical repair. Aggressive therapy to correct any factors contributing to a low cardiac output state is mandatory in this group of patients, as the early postoperative period is a critical time in the longer-term durability of this operation.

Other postoperative issues in patients who have undergone a Fontan procedure can also complicate a patient's convalescence. Pleural and pericardial effusion are two of the more frequent causes of prolonged hospitalization. The use of modified ultrafiltration and fenestration may reduce the incidence and severity of pleural and pericardial effusions, but there are no clear data to support their efficacy. Most surgeons have adopted a policy of selective fenestration, although the criteria for selection remain contentious. Thus, chest drains should be placed in the mediastinum as well as both pleural spaces intraoperatively and should not be removed until the drainage has decreased to below 1 mL/kg. In patients in whom ongoing drainage to the chest tubes continues to occur, problems with protein losses, fluid losses, and electrolytes need to be addressed in an attentive manner. Often, ongoing pleural drainage that is chylous can be managed with the use of medium-chain triglyceride enteral feeds, total parenteral nutrition, or even ligation of the thoracic duct. In patients who experience prolonged drainage, upper extremity ultrasound should be performed to investigate upper extremity venous obstruction, and early cardiac catheterization may be necessary to look for surgically correctable causes of the persistent effusion.

Anticoagulation regimens to prevent thromboembolic complications in patients who have undergone a Fontan procedure are not uniform and often seem to be instituted as a matter of physician preference. After the Fontan procedure, patients can certainly be at increased risk of venous thrombosis. Low cardiac output, a foreign body in the circulation, and increased blood viscosity all contribute to the risk of thrombosis. Embolism, in the setting of fenestration, is also a related concern. Thus, anticoagulation therapy with warfarin or antiplatelet therapy with aspirin is often used in Fontan patients. However, no strict or uniform guidelines exist to date.

Finally, a late complication of the Fontan procedure is the development of protein-losing enteropathy. This problem can be severe and debilitating. The condition itself is poorly understood in this group of patients but can be so exaggerated that it is an indication for cardiac transplantation. Other late complications of the Fontan procedure include atrial arrhythmias, cyanosis due to the formation of arteriovenous fistulae, and late cardiac failure.

OUTCOME

Follow-up data from the Children's Hospital in Boston on 196 of 220 patients who underwent a lateral tunnel Fontan procedure over a 4-year period (1987–1991) provided some insight into 10-year outcomes of this particular modification of the operation. Kaplan–Meier estimated survival in their series was 93% at 5 years and 91% at 10 years. Freedom from failure was 90% at 5 years and 87% at 10 years. Freedom from new supraventricular tachyarrhythmia was 96% at 5 years and 91% at 10 years; freedom from bradyarrhythmia was 88% at 5 years and 79% at 10 years.

In 2012, Stewart et al. published a contemporary series of 2747 patients undergoing Fontan operation from 2008 to 2009, as reported by the Society of Thoracic Surgeons' Congenital Heart Surgery Database. The study included data from 68 participating centers. The authors demonstrated that, although the extracardiac conduit was the preferred operation, short-term early outcomes, including Fontan takedown or revision and postoperative length of stay, were improved in patients having a lateral tunnel procedure (**Table 45.1**).

These contemporary mortality data demonstrate a marked improvement as compared to data from the Pediatric Cardiac Care Consortium from 1984 to 1993 (30-day mortality 14.4%). However, as survival has improved, the focus has shifted to the long-term health-related quality of life and functional health status of Fontan patients. The Pediatric Heart Network sponsored Fontan Cross-sectional Study involved 546 children aged 6–18 years following Fontan operation. Anderson et al. reported that measures of cardiac function and functional health status were below average, but generally within two standard deviations of the mean compared to control subjects. Not surprisingly, patients with systemic right ventricles fared worse than those patients with systemic left ventricle morphology (**Table 45.2**).

Table 45.1 Summary data of patients undergoing a Fontan procedure in 2008–2009 (as reported by the Society of Thoracic Surgeons' Congenital Heart Surgery Database, 2012)

Total number of patients	2747
Age (years)	3 years (median 2.3 years, IQR 3.6)
Type of Fontan connection	
TCPC lateral tunnel	1017 (37%)
TCPC extracardiac conduit	1730 (63%)
Fenestration performed	1788 (65%)
In-hospital mortality	45 (1.6%)
Fontan takedown/revision	37 (1.4%)
Postoperative complication	1111 (40.4%)
Postoperative length of stay (days)	9 days (median 7 days; IQR 14)

Table 45.2 Summary data of patients 6–18 years of age who underwent a Fontan procedure (as reported by the Pediatric Heart Network Fontan Cross-sectional Study, 2003–2004)

Total number of patients	546
Previous Stage II operation	546 (75%)
Type of Fontan connection	
Atriopulmonary connection	13%
TCPC lateral tunnel	59%
TCPC Extracardiac conduit	13%
Other	15%
Measures of functional status	
Exercise performance (percent predicted peak VO$_2$)	65 ± 16
CHQ-PF Physical Summary Score	45.3 ± 11.9
CHQ-PF Psychosocial Summary Score	47.2 ± 10.8
Ejection fraction (%) by echocardiography	59 ± 10

FURTHER READING

Anderson PAW, Sleeper LA, Mahony L, et al. Contemporary outcomes after the Fontan procedure: a Pediatric Heart Network Multicenter Study. *J Am Coll Cardiol.* 2008; 52: 85–98.

Backer CL, Deal BJ, Kaushal S, et al. Extracardiac vesrus intra-atrial laterl tunnel Fontan: extracardiac is better. *Semin Thorac Cardiovasc Pediatr Card Surg Ann.* 2011; 14: 4–10.

Bove EL, de Laval MR, Migliavacca F, et al. Computational fluid dynamics in the evaluation of hemodynamic performance of cavopulmonary connections after the Norwood procedure for hypoplastic left heart syndrome. *J Thorac Cardiovasc Surg.* 2003; 126: 1040–7.

Brown JW, Ruzmetov M, Deschner BW, et al. Lateral tunnel Fontan in the current era: is it still a good option? *Ann Thorac Surg.* 2010; 89: 556–63.

Choussat A, Fontan F, Besse P, et al. Selection criteria for Fontan's procedure. In: Anderon RH, Shinebourne EA (eds). *Paediatric cardiology.* Edinburgh: Churchill Livingstone; 1977: pp. 559–66.

Cnota JF, Allen KR, Colan S, et al. Superior cavopulmonary anastomosis timing and outcomes in infants with single ventricle. *J Thorac Cardiovasc Surg.* 2013; 145(5): 1288–96.

de Leval MR, Kilner P, Gewillig M, Bull C. Total cavopulmonary connection: a logical alternative to atriopulmonary connection for complex Fontan operations. *J Thorac Cardiovasc Surg.* 1988; 96: 682–95.

Fontan F, Baudet E. Surgical repair of tricuspid atresia. *Thorax.* 1971; 26: 240–8.

Gentles TL, Mayer JE, Gauvreau K, et al. Fontan operation in five hundred consecutive patients: factors influencing early and late outcome. *J Thorac Cardiovasc Surg.* 1997; 114: 376–91.

Hagler DJ. Fontan. In: Moller JH (ed). *Perspectives in pediatric cardiology: Surgery of congenital heart disease: Pediatric Cardiac Care Consortium 1984–1995.* Vol. 6. Hoboken, NJ: Wiley-Blackwell; 1998: pp. 345–52.

Jonas R. Indications and timing for the bi-directional Glenn shunt versus the fenestrated Fontan circulation. *J Thorac Cardiovasc Surg.* 1994; 108: 522–4.

Jonas RA. The intra/extracardiac conduit fenestrated Fontan. *Semin Thorac Cardiovasc Surg Pediatr Card Surg Ann.* 2011; 14: 11–18.

Salazar JD, Zafar F, Siddiqui K, et al. Fenestration during Fontan palliation: now the exception instead of the rule. *J Thorac Cardiovasc Surg.* 2010; 140: 129–36.

Stamm C, Friehs I, Mayer JE, et al. Long-term results of the lateral tunnel Fontan operation. *J Thorac Cardiovasc Surg.* 2011; 121(1): 28–41.

Stewart RD, Pasquali SK, Jacobs JP, et al. Contemporary Fontan operation: association between early outcome and type of cavopulmonary connection. *Ann Thorac Surg.* 2012; 93: 1254–61.

Tweddell JS, Nersesian M, Mussatto KA, et al. Fontan palliation in the modern era: factors impacting mortality and morbidity. *Ann Thorac Surg.* 2009; 88(4): 1291–9.

Van Arsdell GS, McCrindle BW, Einarson KD, et al. Interventions associated with minimal Fontan mortality. *Ann Thorac Surg.* 2000; 70: 568–74.

46

Double-outlet ventricles

PASCAL R. VOUHÉ, OLIVIER RAISKY, AND YVES LECOMPTE

INTRODUCTION

Double-outlet ventricles encompass a wide spectrum of heart defects and include all anomalies of ventriculoarterial connection ranging from normal ventriculoarterial connection to complete transposition of the great arteries.

Some anomalies are not amenable to biventricular repair because of one or several of the following associated lesions: severe hypoplasia of one of the ventricles, multiple ventricular septal defects making ventricular septation impossible, severe anomalies of the atrioventricular valves. Such patients are usually candidates for a univentricular approach and they are excluded from further discussion.

PREOPERATIVE ASSESSMENT AND PLANNING

Choice of the type of repair

In order to classify double-outlet ventricles, it is usual to describe the ventriculoarterial alignment, the spatial relationship between the great arteries and the position of the ventricular septal defect (VSD). Identification of hearts with double-outlet right ventricle, double-outlet left ventricle, and transposition of the great arteries with VSD is then possible.

Although of value from a morphological point of view, this classification is of little help from a surgical standpoint.

In nearly all these malformations, there is a defect in the conotruncal septum (conoventricular VSD). Our surgical strategy is based on the individual analysis of the connection of each semilunar valve to the ventricles (i.e. existence and length of a muscular subvalvar conus). These anatomical features are extremely variable, since all combinations may occur, according to the relative development of the subaortic and subpulmonary conuses.

The choice of the surgical procedure which provides anatomical repair (i.e. connects the left ventricle with the aorta and the right ventricle with the pulmonary artery) depends upon the following two anatomical determinants:

- the distance between the tricuspid valve and the pulmonary valve (i.e. the length of the subpulmonary conus). When the distance is sufficient, an unrestricted left ventricle-to-aortic valve tunnel can be constructed and the pulmonary orifice can be left in its native position, as the natural outflow for the right ventricle
- the presence of pulmonary outflow tract obstruction (subvalvar and/or valvar).

Using these two anatomical determinants, the choice can be made between four types of anatomical repair (**Figure 46.1**).

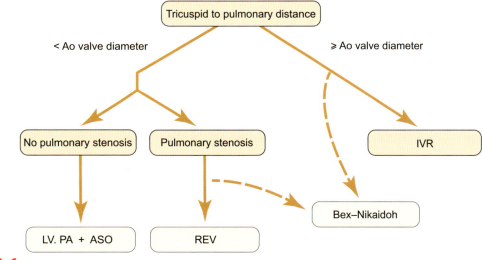

46.1

1. *Intraventricular repair (IVR)* (i.e. entirely within the ventricular cavity) when the tricuspid-to-pulmonary distance is long enough (i.e. at least equal to the aortic valve diameter). A baffle is constructed that creates an unobstructed pathway from the left ventricle to the aorta through the VSD, and the natural right ventricular outflow tract courses around the left ventricular baffle but remains within the right ventricle with the pulmonary orifice in its native position. In the presence of associated pulmonary outflow tract obstruction, the right ventricular outflow tract is enlarged using a prosthetic infundibular or transannular patch.

2. *Arterial switch operation* when the tricuspid-to-pulmonary distance is too short (i.e. inferior to the aortic valve diameter) and in the absence of pulmonary outflow tract obstruction. A tunnel is constructed to connect the left ventricle to the pulmonary orifice through the VSD, and an arterial switch procedure is performed.

3. *Réparation à l'étage ventriculaire (REV procedure)* when the tricuspid-to-pulmonary distance is too short and pulmonary outflow tract obstruction is present. A left ventricle-to-aorta tunnel is created including the pulmonary orifice; the main pulmonary artery is transected and translocated anteriorly onto the right ventricle.

   In potential candidates for a REV procedure, it has been suggested to preserve the native pulmonary valve (pulmonary translocation or en-bloc rotation of the truncus). It is our opinion that the indications for these procedures are very rare. When there is severe and diffuse pulmonary obstruction with a dysplastic and hypoplastic valve, the valve cannot be preserved usefully. On the contrary, in patients with a predominant subvalvar stenosis and a near-normal valve, a better approach may be relief of the subvalvar obstruction and arterial switch operation.

4. *Bex–Nikaidoh procedure* in some patients with pulmonary outflow tract obstruction, in whom IVR procedure or REV operation is technically difficult or impossible. Potential indications include:

   - very long subaortic conus on which most of the tricuspid subvalvar apparatus is attached
   - abnormal insertions of the mitral valve on the conal septum, making conal septal resection impossible
   - relative hypoplasia of the right ventricular cavity
   - remote position of the VSD (inlet or trabecular) without conoventricular extension.

The left ventricular outflow tract is enlarged while closing the VSD; the aortic root (with the coronary arteries) is translocated onto the enlarged left ventricular ostium; the pulmonary artery is translocated anteriorly onto the right ventricle. A major coronary artery crossing the right ventricular outflow tract close to the aortic root (right coronary artery from the left ostium or left anterior descending from the right ostium) is a potential contraindication to the Bex–Nikaidoh operation; both the harvesting of the aortic root and the reconstruction of the right ventricular outflow tract may be hazardous.

Principles of repair

Whatever the type of biventricular repair, the procedure always includes two main surgical steps.

1. An intracardiac tunnel is constructed to connect the left ventricle to one of the arterial orifices through the conoventricular VSD (aortic orifice in IVR and REV procedures, pulmonary orifice in arterial switch and Bex–Nikaidoh operations).

   To create an unobstructed left ventricular tunnel, enlargement of the VSD is often necessary. Enlarging the VSD is indicated in two circumstances:

   - When a portion of the interventricular septum (usually the conal septum) interposes between the VSD and the arterial orifice to which the left ventricle must be connected. To create a tunnel as straight, short, and large as possible, this portion of the interventricular septum must be resected extensively, even if the VSD is large.
   - When the VSD itself is small and represents a potential cause of postoperative subaortic stenosis. Depending upon the intracardiac anatomy, septal enlargement may involve either the conal septum or the muscular septum at the anterior margin of the VSD.

2. The right ventricle is connected to the pulmonary arteries. This can be performed either through an intracardiac channel (IVR procedure), or by reimplanting the main pulmonary artery on the native aortic root (arterial switch) or on the right ventricular ostium (Bex–Nikaidoh), or by using an extracardiac reconstruction (REV procedure).

   When extracardiac reconstruction is indicated, the option which is commonly used is to implant an extracardiac (valved or non-valved) conduit between the right ventricle and the pulmonary arteries (Rastelli procedure). In an effort to reduce the risk of reoperation, we favor extracardiac reconstruction of the right ventricular outflow tract by direct reimplantation of the pulmonary artery onto the right ventricle without prosthetic conduit, with, in most cases, anterior translocation of the pulmonary artery.

Preoperative evaluation

The type of symptoms and the age at which they appear are very variable, although, in most cases, the presence of congenital heart anomaly becomes evident very early in life. The information which is necessary to choose the type of repair and to plan the surgical procedure can almost always be provided by careful transthoracic echocardiographic evaluation alone. The echocardiographer should have extensive experience with the diagnosis and repair of conotruncal anomalies. Most importantly, the examination should be performed in the presence of the attending surgeon. The anatomy of the malformation should be fully delineated and the surgical repair carefully planned. Occasionally, other preoperative studies (transesophageal echocardiography, CT scan, MRI, cardiac catheterization) are necessary to define some features, such as anomalies of the atrioventricular valves, pulmonary arterial anatomy, pulmonary vascular resistances, or extracardiac anomalies. If a Bex–Nikaidoh operation is planned, the coronary anatomy must be determined precisely (by coronary angiography), because some coronary patterns may preclude such a procedure. In all cases, preoperative workup must be complete in order to avoid, as far as possible, unexpected intraoperative findings and the need for unplanned decisions.

The optimal age for anatomical correction depends on the type of repair and, particularly, on the anticipated difficulty of the intracardiac surgical step (length of the intracardiac tunnel, need for extensive resection of the conal septum, presence of abnormal insertions of the atrioventricular valves, multiple VSDs). Primary repair is possible during the neonatal period or during early infancy when the intracardiac repair is easy. On the contrary, if the anticipated construction of the intracardiac tunnel is more difficult, early palliative surgery (aortopulmonary shunt or pulmonary artery banding) is indicated if needed, and corrective surgery is performed a few months later. Bilateral systemicopulmonary shunts should, however, be avoided if extensive mobilization of the pulmonary arteries is anticipated during complete repair.

OPERATION

A median sternotomy is performed. The relative position of the great arteries is inspected. The decision to translocate anteriorly the pulmonary bifurcation is taken. As a rule, anterior translocation of the pulmonary artery (French maneuver) is necessary when the aorta is anterior to the pulmonary artery and should be avoided when the great arteries are strictly side by side. The great arteries are dissected and the pulmonary arteries are freed from their pericardial attachments, including division of the ligamentum arteriosum. Previous aortopulmonary shunts are controlled.

Cardiopulmonary bypass is instituted using two caval cannulae and an ascending aorta cannula. A left vent is placed directly into the left atrium. Cardiopulmonary bypass is carried out in normothermia and using conventional hemofiltration. Intraoperative myocardial preservation is achieved using multidose warm-blood cardioplegia.

Reconstruction of the left ventricular outflow tract

CARDIAC INCISIONS

In some patients (i.e. those with near-normal ventriculoarterial connection), intracardiac repair may be carried out through a right atrial approach. However, in most cases, a right ventricular approach is warranted as well.

The right atrium is opened. If an atrial septal defect (ASD) is present, it is partially closed; in most cases, a small calibrated ASD is left in order to allow temporary left or right ventricular unloading. Through the tricuspid orifice, the intraventricular anatomy is inspected. The right atrial approach may subsequently be used to secure to the inferior margin of the VSD the prosthetic patch used to construct the intracardiac tunnel.

The right ventricle is then opened (**Figure 46.2**) either below the aortic valve (incision 1) or below the pulmonary orifice (incision 2) when pulmonary outflow tract enlargement is anticipated. Care is taken to preserve as many coronary arteries as possible; a large conal coronary artery is often present and should be preserved. The incision is started at its caudal end and extended upwards, taking great care to preserve the aortic leaflets. The incision must be planned and performed to provide excellent exposure of the aortic orifice and perfect assessment of the intracardiac anatomy.

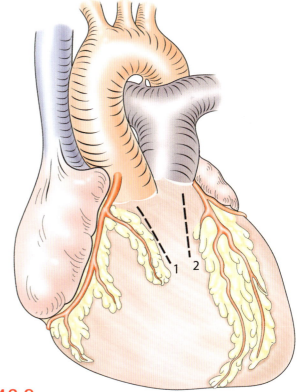

46.2

As previously stated, the intracardiac step of the surgical procedure is essentially the same, regardless of the arterial orifice to which the left ventricle is connected (aortic orifice in IVR and REV procedures, pulmonary orifice in arterial switch and Bex–Nikaidoh operations). The procedure is described in detail for the construction of a left ventricle-to-aorta tunnel. The principles are similar for a left ventricle-to-pulmonary orifice connection.

SEPTAL RESECTION: INDICATIONS

The next step is to decide whether septal resection is indicated.

When the distance between the tricuspid valve and the aortic valve is equal or greater than the tricuspid valve-to-pulmonary valve distance (i.e. when the subaortic conus is longer than the subpulmonary conus), the conal septum usually interposes between the VSD and the aortic orifice and, therefore, interferes with the intraventricular left ventricle-to-aorta tunnel (**Figure 46.3a**). The conal septum must be resected, even if the VSD itself is large.

On the contrary, when the subaortic conus is shorter than the subpulmonary conus, the conal septum lies anterior to the anticipated intracardiac tunnel (**Figure 46.3b**). The septum does not need to be resected and, actually, can be used to construct the anterior wall of the tunnel.

In some patients, the anterior margin of the VSD may bulge inside the anterior aspect of the left ventricle-to-aorta tunnel. It is then indicated to incise or resect the anterior margin of the VSD to avoid postoperative subaortic obstruction (**Figure 46.3c**). This type of septal resection is

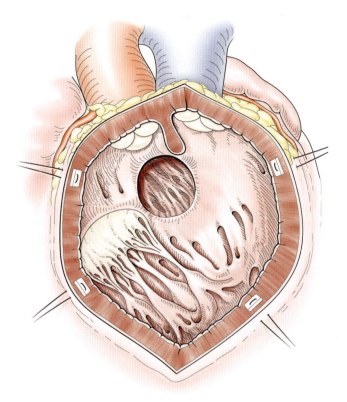

46.3b

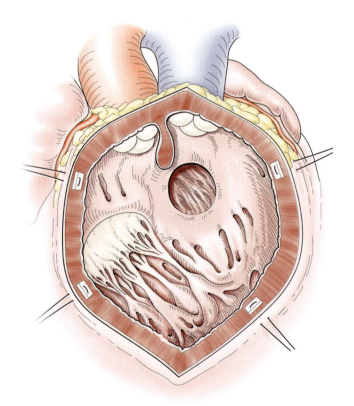

46.3a

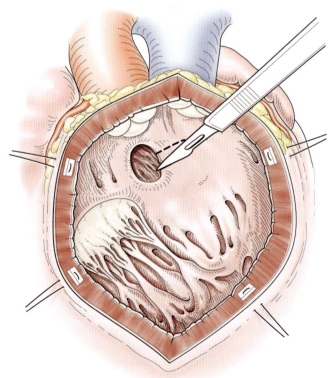

46.3c

hazardous, as this portion of the interventricular septum may include large septal coronary arteries participating in the vascularization of the conduction tissue.

SEPTAL RESECTION: TECHNIQUE

When resection of the conal septum is indicated, it must be complete; adequate alignment of the aortic orifice with the newly created left ventricular outflow tract depends upon the extensiveness of the septal resection. This step is facilitated by the introduction of a Hegar dilator through the pulmonary orifice into the left ventricular cavity. This maneuver improves the exposure of the conal septum and protects the mitral valve apparatus.

Three incisions are then made (**Figure 46.4a**): one anterior and one posterior from the upper margin of the VSD up to the aortic annulus (incisions 1 and 2), and one parallel to the aortic annulus (incision 3). The conal septum is resected "en bloc." It is crucial to carry out the upper incision in an oblique plane (and not in a horizontal plane) to avoid injury to the ventricular wall between both arterial orifices or to proximal coronary arteries.

When abnormal attachments of the tricuspid valve onto the conal septum are present, the conal septum cannot be resected. Only the incisions 1 and 3 are made (**Figure 46.4b**).

The conal septum is then mobilized as a flap and pulled back laterally. The left ventricle-to-aorta tunnel is constructed on the left ventricular side of the mobilized septum. After construction of the tunnel, the conal septum can be reattached on the prosthetic patch, if needed.

CONSTRUCTION OF THE INTRACARDIAC TUNNEL

The intracardiac tunnel is constructed using a prosthetic patch, made of either heterologous pericardium or glutaraldehyde-treated autologous pericardium. The important technical point is a perfect tailoring of the patch. It is sometimes recommended to oversize the patch, in order to prevent the development of subaortic stenosis. Actually, oversizing is ineffective, and potentially harmful. In most cases, there is an angulation between the lower part of the tunnel close to the tricuspid valve and the upper part close to the aortic valve. If the patch is oversized, the summit of the angulation may protrude to the left side and cause subaortic obstruction. Extensive resection of the conal septum and perfect tailoring of the prosthetic patch are the best ways to avoid subaortic obstruction, not oversizing of the patch.

The distance between the inferior margin of the VSD and the anterior margin of the aortic annulus is precisely

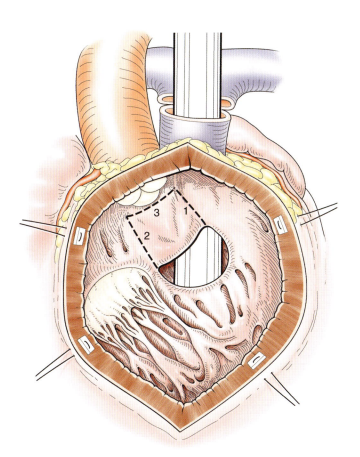

46.4a

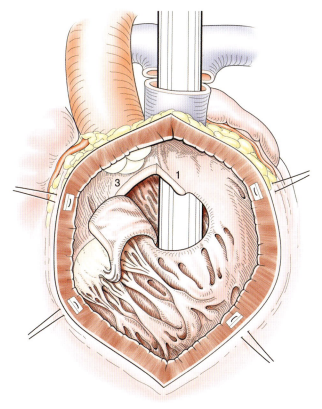

46.4b

measured (**Figure 46.5a**). A circle having this distance as its circumference is tailored in the prosthetic patch. The future right-sided margin of the patch is trimmed straight, whereas the left-sided margin is temporarily left intact and round (inset).

The patch is then secured to the inferior margin of the VSD using interrupted pledgeted mattress sutures (**Figure 46.5b**). The approach may differ according to the anatomy. When the margin is formed by the tricuspid annulus itself, the sutures are passed through the base of the septal leaflet of the tricuspid valve and we prefer to do it through the right atrium; great care is taken to avoid injury to the conduction tissue. Alternatively, if there is a muscular rim between the VSD and the tricuspid annulus, the sutures are placed in that rim through the right ventricular approach.

The suture line then goes up on the right side to reach to the right portion of the aortic annulus. For this portion of the suture, a continuous running suture is used, reinforced with a few interrupted pledgeted stitches.

At this point, the patch must be tailored definitively. This is done by trimming the left-sided margin of the patch such that it reaches the anterior limit of the tunnel without tension, but also without bulging. As previously stated, the anterior limit of the tunnel may vary according to the final procedure. However, in all instances, the rule to tailor the patch adequately remains valid.

When the tricuspid-to-pulmonary valve distance is long enough (at least equal to the diameter of the aortic valve), the anterior limit of the tunnel runs posterior to the pulmonary orifice (which, therefore, remains within the right ventricular cavity). The left-sided suture line is carried out up to the aortic annulus using a continuous running suture (**Figure 46.5c**).

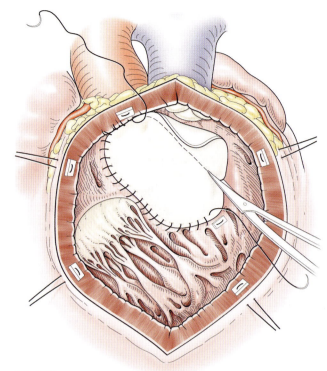

46.5b

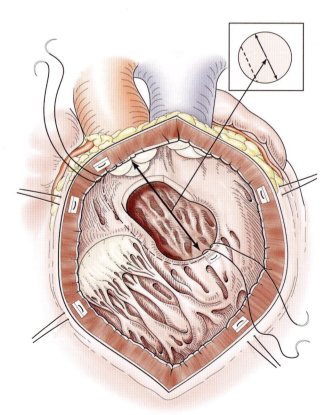

46.5a

46.5c

When the tricuspid-to-pulmonary valve distance is too short to allow IVR, the anterior limit of the tunnel runs anterior to the pulmonary orifice and the tunnel is constructed including the pulmonary valve (**Figure 46.5d**). The pulmonary artery must subsequently be translocated anteriorly (REV procedure).

The final step of the construction of the intracardiac tunnel is to secure the patch around the anterior margin of the aortic annulus. This is done using a series of interrupted mattress sutures (**Figure 46.5e**). To prevent the occurrence of "intramural" residual VSDs, the sutures must be placed very close to the aortic annulus, and not on trabeculations within the right ventricle. When the aortic annulus is not exposed adequately through the right ventricle, the sutures along the superior aspect of the VSD should be inserted through the aortic orifice, after opening of the ascending aorta. Mattress sutures are placed in the base of the aortic leaflets; pledgets are avoided to prevent any distortion of the valve.

INTRACARDIAC TUNNEL AND ARTERIAL SWITCH OPERATION

When an arterial switch operation is indicated (i.e. short tricuspid-to-pulmonary valve distance without pulmonary outflow tract obstruction), the intracardiac tunnel must be constructed between the left ventricle and the pulmonary orifice. Nevertheless, the principles regarding septal resection, as well as tailoring and anchoring of the patch, are very similar to those described for the construction of a left ventricle-to-aorta tunnel.

In most cases (i.e. when the subpulmonary conus is shorter that the subaortic conus), the conal septum is located anterior and to the right of the intracardiac tunnel. It does not need to be resected, and, actually, it can be used for the construction of the tunnel (**Figure 46.6a**).

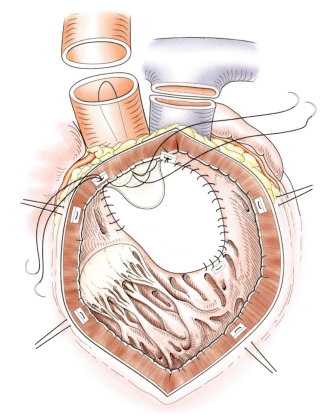

46.5e

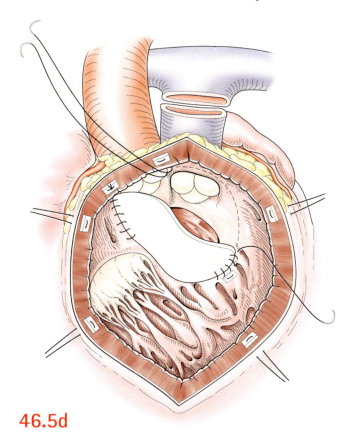

46.5d

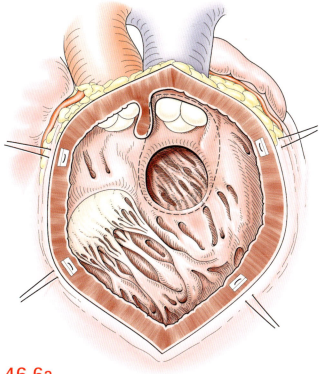

46.6a

Sometimes (i.e. in the rare cases in which the subpulmonary conus, although too short to allow IVR, is longer than the subaortic conus), the conal septum interposes between the VSD and the pulmonary orifice. It must then be resected extensively, using the same surgical principles as those previously described for the construction of a left ventricle-to-aorta tunnel (**Figure 46.6b**).

RECONSTRUCTION OF THE LEFT VENTRICULAR OUTFLOW TRACT IN A BEX–NIKAIDOH OPERATION

The ascending aorta is transected at its mid-portion. Although the aortic root may be harvested without detaching the coronary arteries, we prefer to excise the coronary ostia with a circular button of aortic wall, while preserving the sinotubular junction as a ring to prevent distortion of the aortic root (**Figure 46.7a**). The proximal coronary arteries are mobilized. The aortic root is harvested with a muscular rim of subaortic conus (exactly as during the harvesting of the pulmonary autograft for a Ross operation in normally related great arteries).

The pulmonary artery is transected above the level of the pulmonary valve. The pulmonary valve is excised. The pulmonary branches are extensively mobilized (**Figure 46.7b**).

If the Bex–Nikaidoh is indicated because of abnormal insertions of the tricuspid and/or mitral valve onto the conal septum with a conoventricular VSD, the conal septum is divided between the pulmonary orifice and the VSD, but not resected. Care is taken to preserve the abnormal valvular insertions (particularly in the case of abnormal mitral insertions).

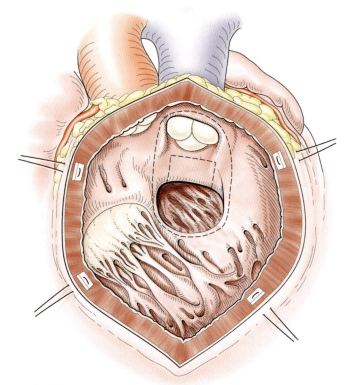

46.6b

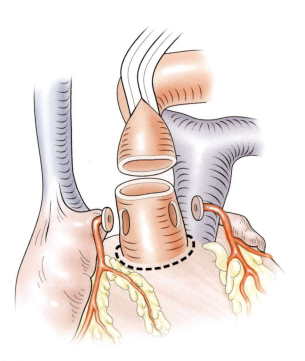

46.7a

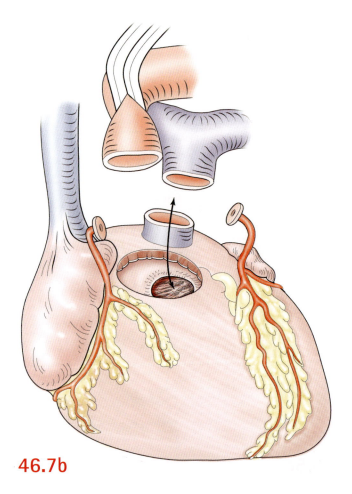

46.7b

When the VSD is muscular, it is closed separately (usually through a right atrial approach) and the conal septum is incised obliquely towards the base of the conal papillary muscle of the tricuspid valve (similar to a classical Konno operation) (**Figure 46.7c**).

A prosthetic patch (heterologous pericardium) is implanted to close the VSD and/or enlarge the conal septum (**Figure 46.7d**). The patch must be tailored precisely in order to obtain a left ventricular ostium which has the same size as the harvested aortic root.

The left ventricular outflow tract is reconstructed by reimplanting the aortic root onto the enlarged left ventricular ostium. The aortic root should be rotate 180 degrees, so that the defects from the coronary buttons face anteriorly towards the excised coronary ostia. Great care must be taken to reimplant the aortic root on the left ventricular ostium (pulmonary annulus posteriorly and prosthetic patch anteriorly) without any distortion of the aortic valve; interrupted sutures may be superior to a running suture.

The coronary buttons are then reinserted on the aortic root, either at the site of the coronary button defects or at the optimal reimplantation site in order to achieve adequate coronary perfusion (**Figure 46.7e**).

The distal orifice of the aortic root is anastomosed end-to-end to the distal ascending aorta, usually after the branch pulmonary arteries are mobilized extensively and translocated anteriorly (French maneuver). A generous piece of ascending aorta should be removed, in order to keep the reconstructed ascending aorta as short as possible and leave more space anteriorly for the translocated pulmonary artery.

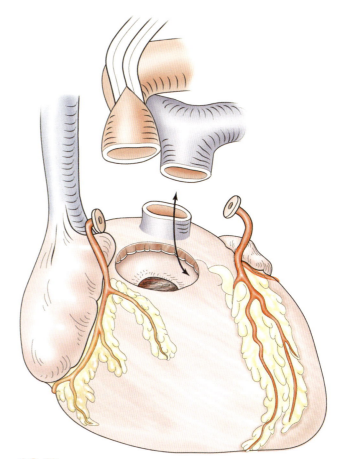

46.7c

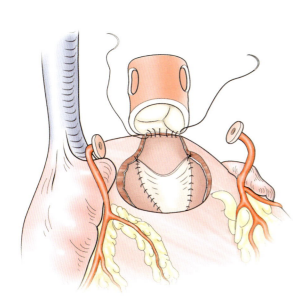

46.7d

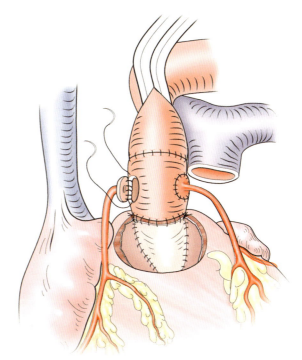

46.7e

Reconstruction of the right ventricular outflow tract

IN AN IVR PROCEDURE

In the absence of pulmonary outflow tract obstruction, the right ventriculotomy is closed primarily. If there is associated pulmonary stenosis, the right ventricular outflow tract is reconstructed using prosthetic patches (infundibular or transannular), exactly as for the repair of tetralogy of Fallot.

There is a situation in which the IVR procedure, although theoretically possible, should be avoided. In most patients, the subpulmonary conus is symmetrical; that means that the tricuspid-to-pulmonary distance is equal to the mitral-to-pulmonary distance. More uncommonly, the subpulmonary conus is asymmetrical; the mitral-to-pulmonary distance is then shorter than the tricuspid-to-pulmonary distance. The tricuspid-to-pulmonary distance may be long enough to allow IVR, but, because of the shorter mitral-to-pulmonary distance, the right ventricular outflow tract (with the pulmonary orifice in its anatomical position) may be long, angulated and potentially stenotic. In these circumstances, alternative options are preferable:

- left ventricle-to-pulmonary orifice connection with arterial switch in the absence of pulmonary stenosis, or
- left ventricle-to-aorta connection and REV procedure if pulmonary stenosis is present.

IN A REV OPERATION

The main pulmonary artery is divided as close as possible to the valvar commissures. The cardiac end is closed primarily using a series of interrupted sutures (**Figure 46.8a**). Care is taken not distort the proximal coronary arteries, which may course very close to the pulmonary annulus and be difficult to identify in case of previous operations.

In most patients, the spatial relationship between the great arteries is more or less anteroposterior. In this situation (approximately 75% of cases), the pulmonary bifurcation must be translocated anterior to the ascending aorta. The ascending aorta is divided. The pulmonary branches are mobilized extensively, well beyond the pericardial reflection, down to the second branches of division. The pulmonary bifurcation is translocated in front of the ascending aorta (French maneuver). The ascending aorta is reconstructed by end-to-end anastomosis. It is essential to remove a generous piece of ascending aorta in order to shorten the reconstructed ascending aorta and to push it in the back of the mediastinum, thus leaving more space anteriorly for the reimplanted pulmonary artery. The piece of ascending aorta may subsequently be interposed between the pulmonary artery and the right ventriculotomy to facilitate the direct reimplantation of the pulmonary artery.

Sometimes, the great arteries are strictly side by side. The French maneuver is then potentially harmful. After adequate mobilization of the pulmonary branches, the main pulmonary artery is left in its anatomical position (on the left or on the right of the undivided ascending aorta) and reimplanted directly onto the right ventricle.

The posterior half the circumference of the distal pulmonary trunk is directly anastomosed to the upper part of the right ventricular incision. The anterior wall of the pulmonary trunk is incised vertically up to the bifurcation. A prosthetic patch (heterologous or autologous pericardium), calibrated according to the patient's body surface area, is inserted to reconstruct the right ventricular outflow tract (**Figure 46.8b**).

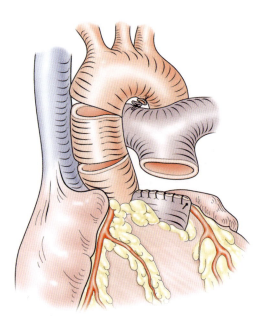

46.8a

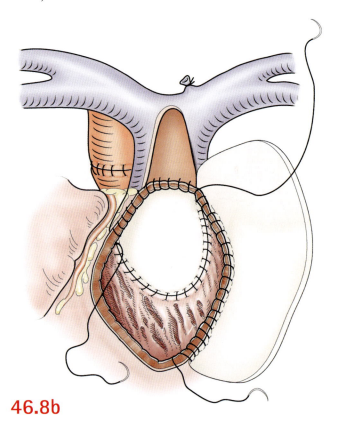

46.8b

It has been our practice to implant routinely a monocuspid pulmonary valve, made of heterologous pericardium, autologous pericardium, or polytetrafluoroethylene (PTFE) membrane. Most of these valves function for only a limited period of time and, subsequently, calcify and become stenotic, thus representing a major cause of reoperation. Most candidates have severe pulmonary stenosis and, therefore, low pulmonary arterial pressure and resistances; we currently recommend performing a valveless reconstruction. However, in patients with less severe pulmonary stenosis, implanting a well-functioning monocuspid valve is still indicated.

Unlike the intracardiac patch, the extracardiac patch, which reconstructs the right ventricular outflow tract, must be generous, particularly in its longitudinal axis. An obligatory angulation exists between the intracardiac portion of the right ventricular outflow tract and the extracardiac portion (**Figure 46.8c**). If the anterior patch is too flat (dotted line), this situation may create an obstruction at the level of the summit of this angulation.

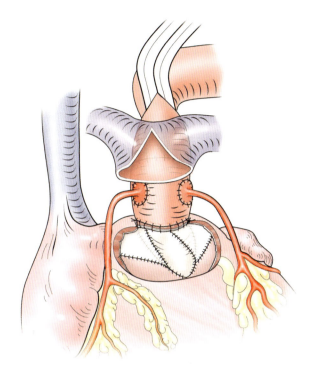

46.9a

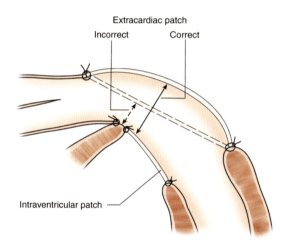

46.8c

IN A BEX–NIKAIDOH OPERATION

The reconstructed left ventricular outflow tract is protruding into the right ventricular outflow tract. The right ventricular ostium takes the shape of a bean (or kidney). To facilitate the reconstruction of the right ventricular outflow tract, we recommend implanting two triangular pericardial patches on each side of the septal patch. A circular right ventricular ostium is thus obtained, on which the pulmonary artery can be reimplanted (**Figure 46.9a**).

The posterior half of the pulmonary trunk is anastomosed directly. The anterior wall of the main pulmonary artery is incised vertically up to the pulmonary bifurcation. The right ventricle-to-pulmonary artery continuity is completed with an anterior prosthetic patch (**Figure 46.9b**).

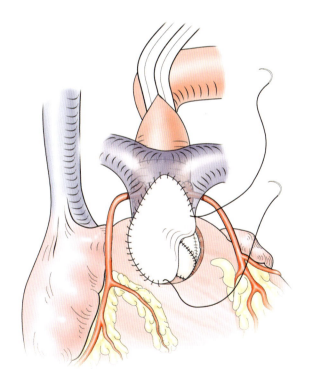

46.9b

POSTOPERATIVE CARE

Patients undergoing biventricular repair of double-outlet ventricle must be evaluated using intraoperative transesophageal echocardiography following separation from cardiopulmonary bypass. Potential residual defects are multiple: obstruction of the intraventricular tunnel (inadequate enlargement of a restrictive VSD or distortion of the prosthetic patch), residual VSD, obstruction of the right ventricular outflow tract (inadequate relief of native pulmonary stenosis or bulging of the intraventricular tunnel patch into the right ventricular outflow tract). Such residual anomalies must be recognized and corrected prior to leaving the operating room.

Biventricular repair of double-outlet ventricle usually requires a prolonged period of aortic cross-clamping, and temporary myocardial dysfunction may occur. Allowing residual shunting at the atrial level may be useful to maintain adequate systemic cardiac output, at the expense of some arterial desaturation. If the hemodynamic status is marginal, delayed sternal closure and extracorporeal membrane oxygenation (ECMO) assistance may be necessary.

In patients with preoperative excessive pulmonary blood flow, pulmonary hypertensive crises can occur. This may be particularly dangerous when valveless reconstruction of the right ventricular outflow tract is carried out. Careful monitoring of pulmonary arterial pressure and adequate management (using inhaled nitric oxide and/or sildenafil) are indicated.

OUTCOME

The early risk is currently low, whatever the type of anatomical repair; early mortality rate is less than 5%. Overall, the late functional results are satisfactory as well, although differences may occur according to both the malformation and the repair. As a rule, the best results are observed in patients who underwent repair early in life and are free from residual anomalies. On the other hand, in patients with residual lesions (such as subaortic stenosis and/or dilatation of the right ventricular outflow tract), severe arrhythmias are not rare and may cause late sudden deaths; they must be detected and managed aggressively.

In all types of repair, there is a risk of subaortic stenosis, particularly when the left ventricle-to-aorta tunnel is long and complex. Adequate resection of the conal septum when indicated and precise tailoring of the intracardiac patch are essential to decrease this risk. In our experience with the REV procedure (205 patients with a mean follow-up of 12.3 years), the actuarial risk of reoperation for left ventricular outflow tract obstruction was 5% at 25 years.

The long-term fate of the reconstructed right ventricular outflow tract remains a major issue. Recurrent obstruction of the right ventricular outflow tract is rare after IVR procedure or arterial switch operation. The experience accumulated with the REV operation shows that avoiding the use of a prosthetic conduit to reconstruct the right ventricular outflow tract decreases the need for reoperation but does not abolish it; the risk of reoperation on the right ventricular outflow tract was 33% at 25 years. Many reoperations were necessary because a prosthetic monocuspid valve had become stenotic; valveless reconstruction may decrease this problem. Interestingly, the need for pulmonary valve implantation has been, to date, very rare (2.7% of operative survivors). Similar results can be anticipated following the Bex–Nikaidoh operation.

Following arterial switch operation or Bex–Nikaidoh procedure in which the coronary arteries are transferred, a significant incidence of coronary obstructions can be anticipated and sought after by routine coronary evaluation. In both procedures, the long-term fate of the aortic valve (native pulmonary valve in ASO, translocated aortic valve in Bex–Nikaidoh) and the incidence of aortic regurgitation remain unknown.

FURTHER READING

Castaneda AR, Jonas RA, Mayer JE, Hanley FL. Double outlet right ventricle. In: *Cardiac surgery of the neonate and infant.* Philadelphia: Saunders; 1994: pp. 445–59.

Di Carlo D, Tomasco B, Cohen L, et al. Long-term results of the REV (réparation à l'étage ventriculaire) operation. *J Thorac Cardiovasc Surg.* 2011; 142: 336–43.

Lecompte Y, Vouhé P. Réparation à l'étage ventriculaire (REV procedure): not a Rastelli procedure without conduit. *Op Tech Thorac Cardiovasc Surg.* 2003; 8: 150–9.

Morell VO, Jacobs JP, Quintessenza JA. Surgical management of transposition with ventricular septal defect and obstruction to the left ventricular outflow tract. *Cardiol Young.* 2005; 15(Suppl 1): 102–5.

Sakata R, Lecompte Y, Batisse A, et al. Anatomic repair of anomalies of ventriculoarterial connection associated with ventricular septal defect. I. Criteria of surgical decision. *J Thorac Cardiovasc Surg.* 1988; 95: 90–5.

47

Ebstein's malformation of the tricuspid valve: surgical treatment and cone repair

JOSE PEDRO DA SILVA

INTRODUCTION

Ebstein's malformation (EM) was described by Wilhelm Ebstein in 1866. The patient was a 19-year-old cyanotic male with dyspnea, palpitations, jugular venous distension, and cardiomegaly. At autopsy, Ebstein described an abnormal tricuspid valve with enlarged and fenestrated anterior leaflet and hypoplasia of the other leaflets which thickened and adhered to the right ventricle (RV). A thin and dilated atrialized portion of the RV was present with a dilated right atrium and a patent foramen ovale (PFO).[1]

Clinical presentation depends on the severity of the disease and it may be apparent in infancy, childhood, or adulthood. If the atrial septum is intact the patient may present with symptoms of low cardiac output such as dizziness, especially during exercise. If an ASD is present, the patient may present with cyanosis, which generally gets worse as RV function deteriorates. Palpitations are common due to ventricular arrhythmias that are related to the RV cardiomyopathy and/or to supraventricular tachycardia, which is related to the presence of abnormal atrioventricular accessory conduction tissues, which are present in about 15% of Ebstein's anomaly patients.

ANATOMY

The normal TV anatomy may vary, but is usually formed by three leaflets, proximally attached to the tricuspid annulus located at the right atrioventricular junction and distally supported by a variable number of papillary muscles. The TV leaflets are: anterior leaflet (anterosuperior position); inferior leaflet (posterolateral position); and septal leaflet. The anterior papillary muscle is attached to the middle of the anterior leaflet distal edge; the posterior papillary muscle is located at the commissure between the anterior and inferior leaflets and, generally, presents a fan shape; the medial papillary muscle is usually related to the anteroseptal commissure and can be a single papillary muscle or a group of small papillary muscles that are attached to the medial edges of the septal and anterior papillary muscles. Distal attachments are to the septal portion of the moderator band.

EM is a congenital heart defect involving the TV and the RV. Its main features are downward displacement of the septal and inferior TV leaflets, redundant anterior leaflet with a sail-like appearance, dilation of the true right atrioventricular annulus, TV regurgitation, and right atrial and RV dilation. Tricuspid regurgitation is mainly due to severe restriction of tricuspid leaflet tissue, particularly involving the septal and inferior leaflets. There is also annular dilation; the available mobile anterior leaflet tissue is insufficient to cover the orifice during systole. Displacement of the septal and inferior leaflet divides the RV in two chambers: the atrialized RV, which is positioned between the normal atrioventricular junction and the displaced TV; and the functional RV located distal to the TV. The small capacitance of the functional RV also plays an important role in the pathophysiology of Ebstein's anomaly.

Other congenital heart defects are often associated with Ebstein's anomaly, the most common being atrial septal defect (ASD) (80–94%), allowing right-to-left flow, resulting in fall of systemic arterial saturation and cyanosis. Approximately 14% of patients have one or more accessory atrioventricular conduction pathways (Wolff-Parkinson-White syndrome). Congenitally corrected transposition of the great vessels, pulmonary atresia or stenosis, anomalies of the mitral valve, left ventricular septal defect, and left ventricular fibrosis are other less frequent associations.

DIAGNOSIS

The electrocardiogram is usually abnormal; however, it is not diagnostic. Complete or incomplete right bundle branch block and right-axis deviation are typically present. The P waves are large, and the R waves in leads V1 to V2 are small. The PR-interval is often prolonged and the QRS-complex is slurred. Arrhythmias are common. Ventricular pre-excitation (Wolff-Parkinson-White syndrome) is encountered in approximately 15% of patients and is almost always of the RV free wall or posterior septal type; a broad band or multiple pathways may be identified at intraoperative electrophysiologic mapping. In addition, atrioventricular nodal re-entry tachycardia is found in 1–2% of patients.

Chest X-ray

The cardiac silhouette may vary from almost normal to the typical configuration, which consists of a globular-shaped heart with a narrow waist similar to that seen in pericardial effusion. This appearance is produced by enlargement of the right atrium and displacement of the right ventricular outflow tract (RVOT) outward and upward. Vascularity of the lungs is either normal or decreased. Severe cardiomegaly is the usual finding in neonates.

Echocardiography

Echocardiography remains the standard for establishing the diagnosis, and 2D and 3D echocardiography allows an accurate evaluation of the tricuspid leaflets (displacement, tethering, dysplasia, and absence), the size of the right atrium, including the atrialized portion of the RV, and the size and function of the right and left ventricles. Doppler echocardiography and color-flow imaging allow detection of an ASD and the direction of shunt flow. The principal echocardiographic characteristic that differentiates EM from other forms of congenital tricuspid regurgitation is the degree of apical displacement of the septal leaflet at the crux of the heart ($> 0.8\,cm/m^2$). Importantly, the regurgitant jet is located at the functional tricuspid orifice (not necessarily at the true tricuspid annulus), which may be located up toward the RVOT and pulmonary valve. The most useful view for the surgeon is the 4-chamber view, which outlines the degree of delamination of the anterior, inferior (to a lesser degree), and septal leaflets and indicates mobility of the leading edges. Echocardiographic factors that are favorable for valve repair

include a large, mobile anterior leaflet with few free wall attachments and a free leading edge. Significant adherence of the edge of the leaflet to underlying endocardium (i.e. leaflet tethering) makes successful valve repair more difficult. Any delamination of inferior leaflet tissue is helpful, and the more septal leaflet tissue present, the more likely a successful valve repair (especially a cone type repair) can be obtained. In addition, color-flow imaging allows assessment of the site and degree of TV regurgitation and the presence of intracardiac septal defects.

In neonatal EM, the TV echocardiographic assessment using the Great Ormond Street Ebstein score (GOSE score) is helpful.[2] The GOSE score is calculated in the 4-chamber view to create a ratio of the combined areas of the right atrium and atrialized RV divided by sum of the functional RV, left atrial, and the left ventricular areas. Importantly, the RVOT must be evaluated to differentiate "anatomic" from "functional" pulmonary atresia. Anatomic RVOT obstruction (infundibulum, pulmonary valve, or branch pulmonary arteries) is a risk factor for both early and late mortality.

Magnetic resonance imaging (MRI)

MRI allows accurate assessment of size and function of both the right and left ventricles. Furthermore, it can distinguish and accurately determine size and function of the functional and atrialized RVs. It can also provide information about TV anatomy (**Figure 47.1**).

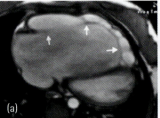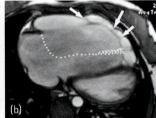

47.1a,b Preoperative magnetic resonance image of a 19-year-old girl with severe Ebstein's anomaly. The arrows point at abnormal papillary muscles and endocardial bands tethering the anterior leaflet of the tricuspid valve to the anterior wall of the right ventricle (a). The dotted line in (b) shows the aimed systolic position for the anterior leaflet after its extensive mobilization.

Cardiac catheterization

Catheterization is rarely necessary in the current era. In the setting of late presentation or when left ventricular dysfunction is present, it can be helpful to measure left- and right-sided pressures, especially if a bidirectional cavopulmonary shunt is being considered before a modified Fontan procedure.

Electrophysiologic studies

Atrial and ventricular arrhythmias are common in patients with EM. Holter monitoring is suggested for rhythm assessment in patients with palpitations or tachycardia. Invasive electrophysiological study is performed when pre-excitation is present on electrocardiogram or recurrent supraventricular tachycardia, undefined wide-complex tachycardia, or syncope is present.

SURGICAL TREATMENT

Early surgical procedures employed for the treatment of patients with Ebstein's anomaly have included the systemic-pulmonary anastomosis, the closure of ASD, and anastomosis of the superior vena cava to the right pulmonary artery (Glenn operation). Of these surgical procedures, only cavopulmonary connections resulted in the survival of some patients. This operation has the advantage of decreasing the cyanosis, reducing the tendency to polycythemia, and, consequently, the risk of paradoxical embolism and thrombosis.

The first survivor of TV regurgitation correction was an Ebstein's anomaly patient subjected to valve replacement, a case reported by Barnard and Schrire in 1962.[3] In this case, part of the valve prosthesis ring was sutured in the right atrium proximally to the coronary sinus; this maneuver intended to avoid the atrioventricular block. In 1964, Hardy et al.[4] published the first successful case with a TV repair technique and transverse plicature of the RV atrializade portion, using the technique that had already been proposed by Hunter and Lillehei in 1956.[5]

Despite the fact that TV replacement was the first successful surgical procedure for biventricular correction of Ebstein's anomaly, published results have been variable.[6,7]

Danielson et al. developed a TV repair technique, which was a modification of Hardy's technique, to which was added posterior tricuspid annuloplasty and the right atrium reduction plasty with transverse plication of the atrialized portion of the RV.[8] The displaced leaflets and the true tricuspid annulus were approximated, obliterating the atrialized RV (transverse plication). Next, the posterior part of the tricuspid annulus was also plicated in order to further reduce the tricuspid annulus circumference. This technique, which is based on the right atrioventricular valve functioning as monocusp valve, became one of the most common repair techniques in the treatment of Ebstein's anomaly. The Mayo Clinic group has accumulated great experience with this procedure. However, the necessity of having a large and mobile anterior leaflet to achieve the goal of correcting the tricuspid regurgitation limited the procedure to a restricted group of anatomical variations, requiring TV replacement in 36–65% of cases.

Many other surgical techniques have been developed, but the wide variety of anatomical and pathophysiological presentations of Ebstein's anomaly has made it difficult to achieve uniform results with surgical repair.

Carpentier et al. described a new technique in 1988.[9] In contrast to the transverse plication of the atrialized RV chamber, described by Danielson et al., they described vertical plications of the atrialized RV. The TV was brought to the anatomically correct level. The TV annulus was remodeled and reinforced with a prosthetic ring. Carpentier's group was able to apply this procedure to the vast majority of anatomical presentations of the disease, but the hospital mortality was high (14%) in their initial series, and long-term complications were also frequent. Quaegebeur performed a slight modification to this operation without the use of a prosthetic ring.[10] Despite good survival, there was still an observed high incidence of moderate and severe degree of tricuspid regurgitation. Hetzer and coworkers described a technique involving plication of the true tricuspid annulus, and exclusion of abnormally attached TV leaflets, creating one or two orifices.[11]

THE CONE PROCEDURE

Starting in 1989, our group has developed and subsequently gone on to routinely use a new surgical technique, which uses some principles of the Carpentier technique, but reconstructs the valve in a very different way.[12] The conical valve opening allows the central blood flow and complete coaptation of the valve. This technique, which was devised in order to obtain coaptation between valve tissue and the interventricular septum, was applied to the first 40 patients with mortality rate of 2.5%, and without any valve replacement, with significant reduction of the immediate degree of AV valve insufficiency. The follow-up, in the medium term, showed clinical improvement and a low incidence of reoperation.

The concept of the cone procedure is to cover 360 degrees of the right AV junction with leaflet tissue, allowing leaflet to leaflet coaptation, which mimics the normal TV anatomy and differs from previously applied procedures that result in a monocusp valve coapting with the ventricular septum.

Surgical technique

The operation is performed via median sternotomy. Cardiopulmonary bypass is instituted with aortic and bicaval cannulation. Moderate systemic hypothermia (25–28°C) and cold antegrade blood cardioplegia (30 mL/kg), followed by subsequent doses (10–15 mL/kg) at 20- to 30-minute intervals during the cross-clamp period, is used for myocardial protection. The main pulmonary artery can be closed by placement of a snare with the goal of maintaining a dry RV during the valve repair and to facilitate examination of the TV after repair when the RV is filled with saline solution via a bulb syringe or catheter placed inside the RV.

The main steps of the cone operation are as follows.

1. EXPOSURE AND ASSESSMENT OF THE TRICUSPID VALVE

This is done by transverse right atriotomy with placement of stay sutures just above the true valve annulus at the 10, 12, and 3 o'clock positions (10 and 12 go through the pericardium to avoid distortion of annular plane). The left heart is vented with a catheter inserted across the PFO or ASD.

2. MOBILIZATION OF THE TRICUSPID VALVE

The surgical methods to achieve TV mobilization in Ebstein's anomaly are based upon the degree of anterior leaflet tethering, septal leaflet size, degree of posterior and septal leaflets delamination failure, and the axis of the tricuspid opening in relationship to the RVOT and to the RV apex. Mobilization of the TV is done by complete sectioning of the abnormal tissues between the tricuspid leaflets and ventricular wall, leaving the leaflet tissues attached to the ventricle only at its distal margin (by normal papillary muscle, cords, or directly to muscle). In general, the majority of leaflet tissue is detached circumferentially except at the 10 to 12 o'clock

positions. This part should be attached to the true annulus with no tethering to the ventricular wall to allow free movement. The aggressive detachment of the leaflet down to its distal point is a critical part of the procedure, because it produces an adequate amount of tissue for construction of the cone and gives sufficient mobility of the leaflet body in the constructed cone, allowing it to move sufficiently during systole and close with a good coaptation surface.

The anterior and posterior leaflets of the TV are mobilized as single piece (**Figure 47.2**). This starts with an incision at its proximal attachment to the atrioventricular junction (12 o'clock position) and moves clockwise, toward the displaced posterior leaflet. The incision terminates when the posterior leaflet is completely released from its abnormal proximal attachment to the RV wall. This gives access to the space between these leaflets and the RV wall, allowing sectioning of all abnormal papillary muscle, myocardial bridges, and cordal tissues that tether these leaflets to the RV wall, restricting its movements. The posterior papillary muscle, usually positioned at the anteroposterior commissure, must be freed from its more proximal attachment to the RV wall, keeping only its supports near the RV apex. In some cases it is necessary to completely release the posterior leaflet from its abnormal attachments to the RV, taking only its membranous portion, in order to permit its medial rotation to join the septal leaflet for the composition of the septal aspect of the cone.

The TV anteroseptal commissure is approached with the goal of creating a future space between the ventricular septum and the septal aspect of the cone and to move the opening axis of the TV toward the RV apex. An incision is made at the proximal attachment line of anterior leaflet, approximately 1 cm anterior to the anteroseptal commissure, and continued counterclockwise down to the septal

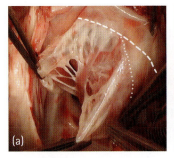 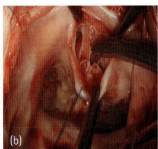 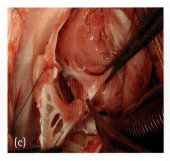 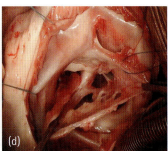

47.2a–d   Anterior and inferior leaflets of the tricuspid valve mobilized as a single piece. (a) Inferior and posterior leaflets anatomy: dotted line shows the displaced and the dashed line shows the true tricuspid annulus; (b) anterior leaflet mobilization; (c) section of inferior leaflet proximal connection to RV wall; (d) the completely mobilized anterior and inferior leaflets.

leaflet, which is mobilized to its lateral limit (**Figure 47.3**). Stay sutures are placed at the proximal edge of the leaflet, providing good exposure to the subvalvar apparatus of the septal aspect of the anterior leaflet, septal leaflet, and the anteroseptal commissure. The tissues that are holding the proximal portion of these leaflets to the septum are divided. In cases that present with the TV opening toward the RVOT, it is necessary to mobilize or cut the papillary muscle abnormally attached at the RVOT. In some cases, the medial papillary muscle, which is usually related to the anterior and septal leaflet at its commissure, is fused to the septum and can be mobilized deeply, giving improved mobility to that area of the future cone.

3. CONE CONSTRUCTION

The cone is constructed by using all the available tissue that has been mobilized. Basically, it is accomplished by two vertical suturing of leaflets: posterior to septal, and septal to anterior. A 5-0 polypropylene running suture technique is used for adults and a 6-0 polypropylene interrupted suture technique is applied in children. Typically, the cone tends to be narrower posteriorly where the leaflet tissue is more deficient; this area must be made wider by vertical plication of the leaflet tissue in the constructed cone. In some cases it is necessary to place some interrupted sutures at the anteroposterior commissure (proximal circumference) in order to widen that portion of the cone.

The septal leaflet is incorporated to the cone in such a way that the range length of the septal part of the cone is longer than the septal vertical distance between the final TV hinge line to its distal attachment to the ventricular septum. This is important in order to allow the septal component of the cone to move anteriorly in the coaptation process with the anterior component of the cone during systole. Also, this will prevent tension at the suture line at the septal aspect of the annular attachment of the cone.

The principal methods for the septal leaflet incorporation to the cone are as follows:

1. Placing a vertical suture joining the septal leaflet superior edge to the septal edge of the anterior leaflet, followed by a second suture line uniting the septal leaflet inferior edge to the lateral edge of the posterior leaflet (**Figure 47.4a–c**). This approach is used for septal leaflet that are large after been mobilized.
2. Combining the septal leaflet with the completely detached posterior leaflet. These leaflet plication and combining maneuvers will increase the depth of the cone and reduce its proximal circumference (**Figure 47.4d, e**).

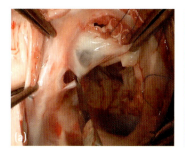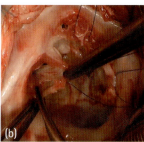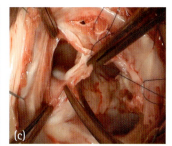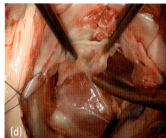

47.3a–d Anteroseptal commissure mobilization. (a) An incision made at the proximal attachment line of anterior leaflet continues anticlockwise (b), mobilizes the medial papillary muscle (c), and reaches the septal leaflet (d), which is mobilized as deep as possible.

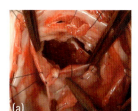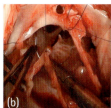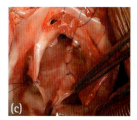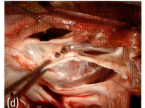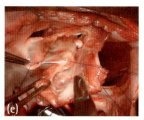

47.4a–e Septal leaflet incorporation. (a) A vertical suture joins the septal leaflet superior edge to the medial edge of the anterior leaflet (b), and a second suture line (c) unites the septal leaflet inferior edge to the lateral edge of the inferior leaflet. In cases with small septal leaflet it is combined with the completely detached inferior leaflet by a vertical suture (d), followed by a horizontal suture (e).

4. PLICATION OF THE RIGHT VENTRICLE AND THE TRUE TRICUSPID ANNULUS

This begins with the vertical plication of the thin and attenuated RV free wall. This usually aneurysmal portion of the atrialized component is defined by the area of attachment of the posterior leaflet as it enters the RV cavity and the septum. The RV plication starts by placement of a 4-0 polypropylene stitch at the distal part of this triangular shaped area, with the apex situated at the distal atrialized ventricle and the base at the true annulus (proximally). The vertical plication is performed using 4-0 polypropylene in two layers with gentle superficial bites to avoid coronary injury or distortion.

Additional RV plication

Since December 2013, we have plicated further the RV anteroposterior wall with the intention of preventing bulging of the area where the lateral portion of the anterior leaflet and the posterior leaflet were tethered.

The preparation of the true tricuspid annulus

If the tricuspid annulus requires additional reduction, this is performed at multiple sites: first at the anteroseptal and then at the anteroposterior position of the true tricuspid annulus. These multiple plications decrease the chance of right coronary artery distortion or kinking.

5. CONE ATTACHMENT TO TRUE TRICUSPID ANNULUS

The cone is attached proximally to the true annulus over 360 degrees and with no tension in either the horizontal or vertical plane (**Figures 47.5 and 47.6**).

Judgment is required so that the proximal cone circumference is correct for the true annular dimension. The true annulus can be further reduced by separate plication at 2–3 o'clock and 9 o'clock. The cone proximal circumference can be reduced by leaflet plication. The initial attachment and assessment is carried out with the placement of 5-0 polypropylene single sutures to obtain an even distribution of the valve in the tricuspid annulus. Then, the suture line is completed with a running suture. Special care should be taken when suturing the area of the annulus, just medial to the coronary sinus, due to the risk of heart block. The use of a prosthetic ring may be considered for reinforcement in patients with a fragile adult size annulus.

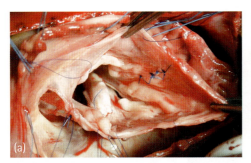 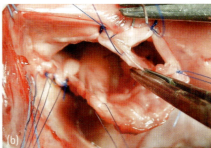 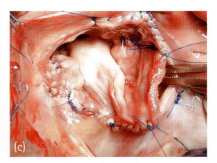

47.5a–c Cone attachment to true tricuspid annulus. The constructed cone (a) is reattached to the true tricuspid annulus starting at the anterior position (b) and completing the attachment (c), taking superficial bites when suturing near the atrioventricular node area (arrow).

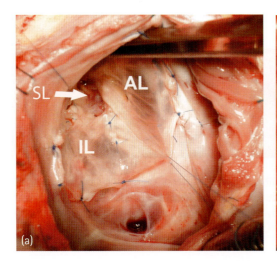 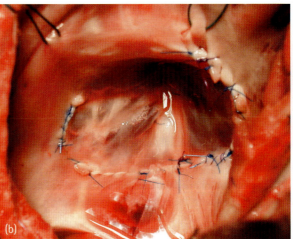

47.6a, b Cone construction done by rotation of the inferior leaflet, which was combined with the septal leaflet (a), before attachment to the true tricuspid annulus (b). AL, anterior leaflet; IL, inferior leaflet; SL, septal leaflet.

6. ATRIAL SEPTAL DEFECT TREATMENT

The ASD/PFO is closed in a valved fashion, in a way that allows blood shunting from right to left in the case of post-operative RV failure. The opening size of the resulting orifice should be proportional to the degree of RV dysfunction or enlargement. This can be accomplished with the single stitch technique in cases of PFO or using a polytetrafluoroethylene (PTFE) patch with an extension flap positioned inside the left atrium to allow unidirectional blood flow toward the left atrium. In cases of severe RV dysfunction, the single stitch technique can be performed with placement near the PFO anterior corner. This will result in a less restrictive PFO. The bidirectional Glenn procedure as an adjunct to Ebstein's anomaly repair is recommended in dysfunctional RV.

Special anatomic types of Ebstein's anomaly

In some anatomical situations, the three leaflets are connected at the commissures and the distal attachment of the TV to the RV is well formed. In these cases, after mobilization from their displaced hinge line and release of abnormal connections to the RV wall, some plications are made at the distal and proximal edges, reducing its proximal and distal circumferences and widening the septal and posterior leaflets to give a cone shape to the TV.

Patients presenting with Carpentier's type D anatomy of Ebstein's anomaly can also be treated with the cone technique. **Figure 47.9** depicts one of the four patients successfully repaired by taking down the leaflets as a single piece, keeping only the distal direct attachment of the leaflet to the RV. Vertical fenestrations were provided at the distal third of this large leaflet. Then, the lateral and medial edges of this leaflet were sutured together, resulting in a cone-like structure.

As in all other cases, the cone was revised, and any holes/fenestrations in the proximal two-thirds of the cone's membranous tissues are closed in order to have similar depth circumferentially and to prevent regurgitation leaks. Also,

fenestrations should be present, natural or surgically created, at the distal third of the cone to allow unrestricted forward blood flow from RA to RV in diastole.

From November 1993 to July 2018, 208 consecutive patients with Ebstein's malformation underwent surgical treatment in our department at the Beneficencia Portuguesa Hospital in Sao Paulo, Brazil and at UPMC Children's Hospital of Pittsburgh, all patients repaired with the Cone technique, except for one who required tricuspid valve replacement as the initial procedure (0.5%). The hospital mortality was 2.5%, excluding the eight patients submitted to biventricular treatment in the neonatal period, who presented a mortality rate of 25%. There were five late deaths (2.6%) and six patients required reoperation in the long term for re-repair (3%) and one for TV replacement (0.5%). Since January 2013, after we modernized our overall care, we have operated on 74 patients without mortality, excluding the neonatal patients.

Tricuspid regurgitation was markedly diminished after repair (**Figure 47.8**). TV stenosis was observed in only one patient during long-term follow-up, which was mild on echocardiogram and had no clinical consequences.

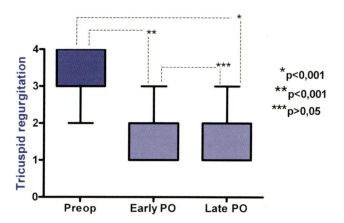

47.8 Tricuspid regurgitation degree: comparison of pre and postoperative echocardiographic data in patients subjected to the cone repair of Ebstein's anomaly.

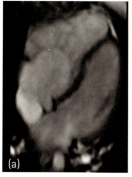
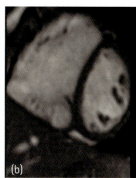
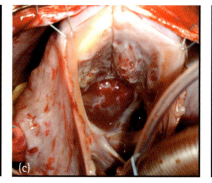
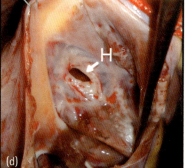

47.7a–d Preoperative magnetic resonance images and intraoperative photos depicts the heart's anatomy of a 4-year-old girl with type D Ebstein's anomaly (Carpentier's classification). Images (a), (b) and (c) show that the tricuspid valve leaflets are tethered to the right ventricle wall. Image (d) shows that there is only a small hole (H), communicating the atrialized to the functional right ventricle.

COMMENTS

Usually, the mechanism of tricuspid insufficiency in Ebstein's anomaly is related to restrictive leaflet movements. This is due to failure of leaflet delamination, which results in more distal attachment of their hinge line to the RV, and to the presence of muscular bridges and abnormal papillary muscles that tether the TV leaflets to the RV wall, restricting their movements. In order to create a competent TV using the cone technique, it is very important to perform extensive mobilization of the displaced or tethered leaflets; otherwise, repair will result in failure of leaflet coaptation or excessive tension in the leaflet suture line due to pulling of the leaflet that was kept improperly attached to the free RV wall, which will undergo strong tension when the RV is filled. We consider these concepts essential tools to minimize the incidence of tricuspid insufficiency after the cone procedure, and also to prevent postoperative dehiscence of the suture line due to diastolic tension. The incorporation of the septal leaflet construction of the septal aspect of the cone, which is frequently made by its combination with the inferior leaflet, is a very important component of the cone technique. It helps prevent both stenosis and insufficiency of the TV.

Because the cone technique gives a more anatomical design to the TV as compared to previous techniques, it has been adopted in most cardiac centers as the method of choice for the repair of Ebstein's anomaly.

Annuloplasty ring or suture reinforcement of the tricuspid valve annulus

It is a fallacy to think that it is unnecessary to reinforce the new tricuspid annulus after the cone repair because patients with Ebstein's anomaly tend to have low pulmonary pressure. We observed a few adult patients with postoperative systolic pulmonary pressures between 40 and 50 mm/Hg. Also, it is possible that the pulmonary pressure can increase temporarily in the presence of pulmonary complications. During our initial experience with the cone technique, some of our patients required reoperation related to postoperative tricuspid regurgitation due to suture dehiscence at the septal and posterior regions of the cone attachment to the new tricuspid annulus. These observations suggest that the new tricuspid annulus should be reinforced, either by extra interrupted sutures or by an annuloplasty ring for the adult tricuspid annulus.

Resection versus plication of the dilated atrialized RV

We adopted the vertical plication described by Carpentier et al., which consists of the thin atrialized RV exclusion by endocardial plicature. There are two concerns about this technique: 1) it can kink the right coronary artery trunk or damage its branches; and 2) because this technique does not electrically isolate the excluded area, it can maintain re-entrant circuits that may be the source of serious postoperative ventricular arrhythmias. This area would be difficult to reach with endocardial ablation catheter in the future. We have addressed these two issues by making a less extensive plication near the atrioventricular junction in order to cause less folding of the right coronary artery, therefore causing less coronary kinking. Regarding ventricular arrhythmias, we have isolated the area to be plicated by transmural cryoablation prior to plication in patients with preoperative ventricular arrhythmia. Some surgeons use surgical resection of the atrialized RV area, when the RV is massively dilated.

Bidirectional Glenn procedure to improve postoperative cardiac output

Early after the cone procedure, some RV dysfunction is expected. This occurs due to damage of the RV wall related to surgical maneuvers and to the myocardial injury caused by the extended ischemic time necessary to perform this somewhat complex operation, superimposed on a variable degree of RV impairment as part of the EM. Bearing in mind that many patients may present temporary postoperative RV dysfunction, we have routinely used a valved ASD that allows blood flow from the right to the left atrium aiming to reduce RV preload and increase LV preload, therefore helping to prevent low cardiac output in the early postoperative period due to severe RV dysfunction. The ASD stays functionally closed from the beginning of the postoperative course in the majority of patients, but in approximately 10% of cases there was important right to left blood shunting causing a moderate drop in oxygen saturation. Usually, oxygen saturation increases in a few days as RV function improves. Additionally, the resulting RV decompression may prevent (avoid) excessive tension at the TV, decreasing the risk of suture dehiscence and TV regurgitation.

Some authors have addressed the problems related to postoperative RV dysfunction by diverting the superior caval blood flow to the right pulmonary artery. This bidirectional cavopulmonary shunt (BCPS), also called the bidirectional Glenn (BDG) procedure, was reported by Chauvaud et al.,[13] who used it in 36% of patients with Ebstein's anomaly as an adjunctive procedure to Carpentier's operation in patients with severe RV dysfunction. According to their report, improved results were seen with this procedure. The BCPS was also reported by Quinonez et al.,[14] reporting on 14 patients from the Mayo Clinic who underwent surgical treatment of Ebstein's anomaly (TV replacement in 13 and TV repair in 1), having the creation of a BCPS as an adjunctive procedure. This approach was done mostly as a planned procedure in anticipation of RV failure, but was also done as a salvage procedure owing to postoperative hemodynamic instability. Considering the serious clinical situation of the patients, they had excellent results with only one death, outlining the relevance of this procedure for a subset of patient.

Liu et al. reported the performance of the BCPS procedure in addition to the cone operation.[15] The fact that they applied this method to a high proportion of patients (20 of 30) raised our attention. However, their series of young patients had good clinical outcome at mid-term follow-up.

We think that it is important to employ one of these two methods after the cone operation in order to prevent low postoperative cardiac output and also to protect the dysfunctional RV from distension. We prefer to use the valved closure of ASD routinely, despite initial cyanosis in some patients and the possibility of paradoxical thromboembolism, because the RV dysfunction is completely or partially reversible with time; consequently, oxygen saturation progressively improves. In case of low oxygen saturation ($< 75\%$) we would add a BCPS for older patients or a small (3.0 mm) modified Blalock-Tausig shunt for neonates. We tend to anticoagulate patients with a dilated RV and/or with right to left atrial shunting. Despite the BCPS advantage of providing better oxygenation, we do not use it routinely because it may be associated with pulsations of the head and neck veins and other complications.

Centers of excellence have recently shown excellent results by using the refinements of the cone technique that we developed over the years, applying updated concepts of perioperative care, and using high technology assist devices.[16–20] The indication for operation has been expanded, using a more rational indication criteria regarding the patient's age and clinical conditions. This was a consequence of the cone technique efficacy and the increased possibility of repairing instead of replacing the TV.

Some studies suggest that the cone technique has a valuable impact on RV remodeling, in the LV work and sustained benefits in long-term clinical results.[16–20]

REFERENCES

1. da Silva JP, Baumgratz JF, Fonseca L, et al. Anomalia de Ebstein: resultados com a reconstrução cônica da valva tricúspide. *Arq Bras Cardiol.* 2004; 82(3): 212–16.

2. Celermajer DS, Cullen S, Sullivan ID, et al. *J Am Coll Cardiol.* 1992; 19: 1041–6.

3. Barnard CN, Schrire V. Surgical correction of Ebstein's malformation with prosthetic tricuspid valve. *Surgery.* 1963; 54: 302–8.

4. Hardy KL, May IA, Kimball KG. Ebstein's anomaly: a functional concept and successful definitive repair. *J Thorac Cardiovasc Surg.* 1964; 48: 927–40.

5. Hunter SW, Lillehei CW. Ebstein malformation of the tricuspid valve: study of a case together with suggestions of a new form of surgical therapy. *Chest Dis.* 1958; 33: 297–304.

6. Danielson GK, Driscoll DJ, Mair DD, et al. Operative treatment of Ebstein anomaly. *J Thorac Cardiovasc Surg.* 1992; 104: 1195–202.

7. Kiziltan HT, Theodoro DA, Warnes CA, et al. Late results of bioprosthetic tricuspid valve replacement in Ebstein's anomaly. *Ann Thorac Surg.* 1998; 66: 1539–45.

8. Dearani JA, O'Leary PW, Danielson GK. Surgical treatment of Ebstein malformation: state of the art in 2006. *Cardiol Young.* 2006; (suppl 3): 1612–20.

9. Carpentier A, Chauvaud S, Mace L, et al. A new reconstructive operation for Ebstein's anomaly of the tricuspid valve. *J Thorac Cardiovasc Surg.* 1988; 96(1): 92–101.

10. Quaegebeur JM, Sreeram N, Fraser AG, et al. Surgery for Ebstein's anomaly: the clinical and echocardiographic evaluation of a new technique. *J Am Coll Cardiol.* 1991; 17: 722–28.

11. Hetzer R, Nagdyman N, Ewert P, et al. A modified repair technique for tricuspid incompetence in Ebstein's anomaly. *J Thorac Cardiovasc Surg.* 1998; 115: 857–68.

12. da Silva JP, Baumgratz JF, da Fonseca L, et al. The cone reconstruction of the tricuspid valve in Ebstein's anomaly. The operation: early and midterm results. *J Thorac Cardiovasc Surg.* 2007; 133(1): 215–23.

13. Chauvaud S, Fuzellier JF, Berrebi A, et al. Bi-directional cavopulmonary shunt associated with ventriculo and valvuloplasty in Ebstein's anomaly: benefits in high risk patients. *Eur J Cardiothorac Surg.* 1998; 13: 514–19.

14. Quinonez LG, Dearani JA, Puga FJ, et al. Results of the 1.5-ventricle repair for Ebstein anomaly and the failing right ventricle. *J Thorac Cardiovasc Surg.* 2007; 133: 1303–10.

15. Liu J, Qiu L, Zhu Z, et al. Cone reconstruction of the tricuspid valve in Ebstein anomaly with or without one and a half ventricle repair. *J Thorac Cardiovasc Surg.* 2011; 141(5): 1178–83.

16. Lange R, Burri M, Eschenbach LK, et al. Da Silva's cone repair for Ebstein's anomaly: effect on right ventricular size and function. *Eur J Cardiothorac Surg.* 2015; 48: 316–21.

17. da Silva JP, da Silva LFS. Ebstein's anomaly of the tricuspid valve: the cone repair. *Semin Thorac Cardiovasc Surg Pediatr Card Surg Annu.* 2012; 15: 38–45.

18. Li X, Wang SM, Schreiber C, et al. More than valve repair: effect of cone reconstruction on right ventricular geometry and function in patients with Ebstein anomaly. *Int J Cardiol.* 2016; 206: 131–7.

19. Holst KA, Dearani JA, Said S, et al. Improving results of surgery for Ebstein Anomaly: where are we after 235 cone repairs? *Ann Thorac Surg.* 2018; 105: 160–9.

20. Ibrahim M, Tsang V, Caruana M, et al. Cone reconstruction for Ebstein's anomaly: patient outcomes, biventricular function, and cardiopulmonary exercise capacity. *J Thorac Cardiovasc Surg.* 2015; 149: 1144–50.

48

Ventricular septal defect

CARL LEWIS BACKER

INTRODUCTION

If there is a single operation that "defines" congenital heart surgery, it is probably closure of a ventricular septal defect (VSD). This procedure in isolation is one of the most common congenital heart operations performed. In addition, it is also an important part of the repair of many complex congenital cardiac lesions including tetralogy of Fallot, common arterial trunk, and atrioventricular septal defect. Hence, understanding the anatomy and pathophysiology of VSDs along with the techniques of VSD closure is an integral and essential part of any congenital heart surgeon's repertoire.

HISTORY

The pathological finding of a VSD was first described by Roger in 1879. Eisenmenger in 1897 described the autopsy findings of a 32-year-old cyanotic patient with a large VSD and overriding aorta. The first surgical intervention for VSD was in 1952 when Muller and Dammann performed a pulmonary artery band to limit the pulmonary artery blood flow in a patient with a large VSD. The first intracardiac repair of a VSD was in 1954 by C. Walton Lillehei at the University of Minnesota. Lillehei used controlled cross-circulation with the child's parent acting as the pump oxygenator. John Kirklin and associates at the Mayo Clinic reported successful transventricular repair of a VSD using a mechanical pump oxygenator in 1956. In 1961 Kirklin reported successful repair of a VSD in infancy thereby eliminating the need for a pulmonary artery band.

ANATOMY AND NOMENCLATURE

A VSD is defined as an opening or hole in the interventricular septum. Isolated VSDs occur in approximately 2 out of every 1000 live births and constitute over 20% of all congenital heart defects. Because isolated VSD is one of the most commonly recognized forms of congenital heart disease, numerous nomenclature schemes have been utilized to describe and classify this lesion. This text attempts to unify the concept of VSD anatomy using the classification scheme advocated by Professor Robert Anderson. This classification divides VSDs into four main types (see **Table 48.1**):

- *perimembranous defects,* which are bordered directly by the fibrous continuity between the AV valves and an arterial valve
- *doubly committed juxta-arterial defects,* which are bordered directly by the fibrous continuity of the leaflets of the aortic and pulmonary valves
- *muscular defects,* which are completely embedded in the septal musculature
- *Gerbode defects,* which are rare defects in which there is a left ventricle to right atrium communication.

Table 48.1 Anatomy and nomenclature of VSD

1. Perimembranous (paramembranous, conoventricular)
   - Outlet extension
   - Trabecular extension
   - Inlet extension
2. Doubly committed juxta-arterial (subarterial, supracristal, conal)
3. Muscular
   - Outlet
   - Trabecular
   - Inlet
   - Apical
4. Gerbode (left ventricle to right atrium)

Perimembranous and muscular defects have been subdivided into three subgroups based on whether they extend into the inlet, trabecular, or outlet portion of the right ventricle (see **Figure 48.1**). Muscular defects are identified by their location in the septum (outlet, trabecular, inlet, apical). The anatomy of the VSD is quite important as the indications for VSD closure vary significantly depending on the anatomic location of the VSD. Perimembranous defects are the most common and account for 80% of all defects. Muscular and doubly committed juxta-arterial defects are equally split in most surgical series at 10% each. The Gerbode defect is quite rare and accounts for 1% of VSD procedures.

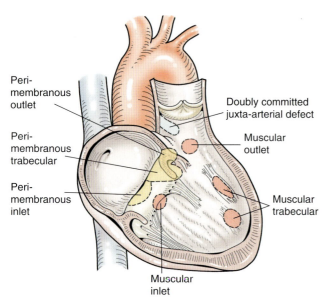

Peri-membranous outlet

Peri-membranous trabecular

Peri-membranous inlet

Doubly committed juxta-arterial defect

Muscular outlet

Muscular trabecular

Muscular inlet

48.1 Classification of VSDs.

INDICATIONS FOR VSD CLOSURE

With steadily improving results of VSD closure secondary to improvements in cardiopulmonary bypass techniques, myocardial protection, and postoperative intensive care unit management, the indications for VSD closure have been expanded and the age of the patients at the time of correction has steadily decreased. In general, the indications for VSD closure are based on a comparison between the natural history of VSD and the results of surgical intervention. For the individual patient, there are four main considerations: the anatomy of the defect, the child's age and symptoms, the pulmonary vascular resistance, and associated intracardiac anomalies. Our general indications for VSD closure are shown in **Table 48.2**.

Infants with a large VSD present with a loud systolic murmur and symptoms of congestive heart failure. These symptoms include sweating with feeds, failure to thrive, and frequent upper respiratory tract infections. Older children with a smaller VSD usually present with a harsh pansystolic murmur. They may be otherwise asymptomatic. The

Table 48.2 Indications for VSD closure

1. Non-restrictive VSD with congestive heart failure and pulmonary hypertension
2. Restrictive VSD with Qp:Qs > 1.5:1.0
3. Aortic valve prolapse or aortic valve insufficiency
4. All doubly committed juxta-arterial defects and Gerbode defects
5. Prior episode bacterial endocarditis

diagnostic evaluation of a child with a VSD includes chest X-ray, electrocardiogram, 2D color Doppler echocardiogram, and, in select cases, cardiac catheterization or cardiac MRI. Chest X-ray will help reveal the size of the cardiac silhouette. Patients with large VSDs have cardiomegaly and evidence of increased pulmonary blood flow. The electrocardiogram will show right and left ventricular hypertrophy if there is a large VSD. The 2D color Doppler echocardiogram is diagnostic in most cases. The echocardiogram will demonstrate the location of the VSD, the size of the VSD, the size of the left ventricle, and, by Doppler evaluation of tricuspid valve regurgitation, give an assessment of right ventricular pressure. Cardiac catheterization was historically performed for most patients with a VSD, but in the past 15 years this has become much less frequently employed with the increasing diagnostic accuracy of echocardiography. Cardiac catheterization will provide the precise degree of left-to-right shunt (Qp:Qs) and the exact pulmonary artery pressures in borderline cases. Cineangiography at the time of cardiac catheterization gives an anatomic "picture" of the defect. Also quite useful is cardiac MRI, which can give the accurate size of the ventricles and the Qp:Qs. MRI can calculate Qp:Qs by both stroke volume differential and net flows through the semilunar valves.

The size of the VSD and the pulmonary vascular resistance determine the magnitude of intracardiac left-to-right shunting. At birth the pulmonary vascular resistance is predictably high and blunts the potential left-to-right shunt. Within weeks to months after birth the pulmonary vascular resistance falls, resulting in increasing left-to-right shunt, which results in progressive manifestations of congestive heart failure as described above. If the patient has a large non-restrictive VSD, defined as a VSD the same size or larger than the aortic valve annulus, right ventricular and pulmonary artery pressures will be systemic. In these patients the VSD should be closed at 2–4 months of age to prevent the development of pulmonary vascular obstructive disease. Patients with this unrestricted pulmonary blood flow may develop irreversible pulmonary vascular obstructive disease by 1–2 years of age. This is referred to as Eisenmenger's syndrome. These patients have a progressive elevation of pulmonary vascular resistance that eventually leads to the shunt changing from a left-to-right shunt to a right-to-left shunt with resultant cyanosis and eventual right ventricular failure. Closure of a VSD when the pulmonary vascular resistance has progressed to a point where it is not reversible will result in right ventricular failure and death following VSD closure.

A restrictive VSD is one that is smaller than the aortic valve annulus. In these patients right ventricular and pulmonary artery pressures are less than systemic. These patients may be managed medically in infancy unless they meet other surgical criteria. Spontaneous closure is observed in nearly 80% of all small muscular and perimembranous VSDs. The mechanisms of spontaneous closure include fibrosis of the defect margins, muscle bundle hypertrophy, and tricuspid valve pouch adherence to the defect. The incidence of spontaneous closure is highest in the first year of life and continues to a lesser degree up to about 5 years of age, after which spontaneous closure is rare. For patients with a restrictive VSD not affecting the aortic valve I recommend closure after 3 years of age if the Qp:Qs by cardiac catheterization or MRI is greater than 1.5:1.

Patients with perimembranous and doubly committed juxta-arterial VSDs may develop aortic valve prolapse as the cusps of the aortic valve sag into the VSD. Left unrepaired, aortic valve prolapse may lead to progressive valve insufficiency. If the VSD is closed when the patient has only aortic valve prolapse or mild aortic insufficiency (AI), the aortic valve disease does not progress. If the AI is moderate or greater at the time of VSD closure, consideration should be given to resuspending the aortic valve at the time of VSD closure. All patients with aortic valve prolapse or aortic valve insufficiency associated with the VSD should undergo VSD closure. The morphology of the doubly committed juxta-arterial VSD is such that it cannot exist in the setting of the normal heart. In the normal heart, the free-standing muscular subpulmonary infundibulum lifts the pulmonary trunk away from the base of the heart. The leaflets of the aortic and pulmonary valves are separated, and are at different levels (**Figure 48.2a**). This infundibular sleeve is lacking in the presence of a doubly committed and juxta-arterial VSD; the aortic and pulmonary valves are at the same level, the phenotypic characteristic of the defect being fibrous continuity between the leaflets of the aortic and pulmonary valves (**Figure 48.2b**). Because of the lack of muscular support, the right coronary leaflet of the aortic valve tends to prolapse into the defect. That, combined with the Venturi effect pulling on the leaflet, results in AI. These patients have a very high incidence of aortic valve prolapse leading to aortic valve insufficiency. These VSDs should be closed even if they are small because of the high incidence of aortic valve prolapse leading to aortic valve regurgitation. We also recommend closing all Gerbode VSDs because they typically have a large shunt due to the low resistance of the right atrium. In our experience all patients with a Gerbode VSD have been symptomatic.

For children with a VSD, the incidence of bacterial endocarditis is 14.5 per 10 000 patient years. This is 35 times the normal population base rate for bacterial endocarditis. Surgical closure reduces the risk of subacute bacterial endocarditis (SBE) by over 50%. Prevention of SBE is a consideration for VSD closure in borderline cases. All patients with a VSD who have had a prior episode of SBE should have surgical closure of their VSD because of the risk of SBE recurrence.

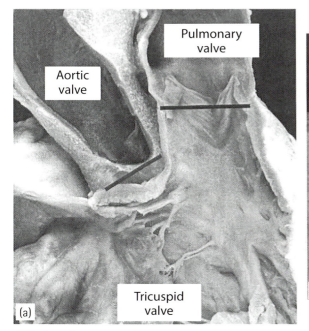

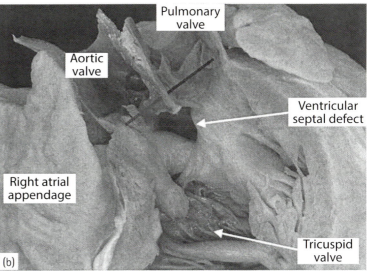

48.2a, b (a) Normal anatomic relationship of aortic and pulmonary valves, (b) Anatomy of doubly committed juxta-arterial VSD.

OPERATIVE TECHNIQUES

The operative approach to VSDs has evolved considerably over the past several decades. The current technique of VSD closure emphasizes an approach which is either transatrial or transpulmonary, hence avoiding a ventriculotomy in nearly all cases. There are several general principles of VSD closure which apply to nearly all VSDs. These will be covered first. Each individual anatomic subtype of VSD has technical points related specifically to that diagnosis. These will be covered as separate entities.

General principles

The general principles of surgical VSD closure are summarized in **Table 48.3**.

VSD closure is performed using cardiopulmonary bypass and hypothermia. Most VSDs can be successfully closed without the use of circulatory arrest, although this has been useful for some subgroups such as VSD with interrupted aortic arch and small premature babies less than 2 kg in weight. Bicaval venous cannulation allows cardiopulmonary bypass to continue during VSD closure and avoid the potential complications of circulatory arrest. Aortic cross-clamp with cold blood cardioplegia administration (we use del Nido solution) allows VSD closure to be performed in a quiet field. A vent in the right superior pulmonary vein makes for a bloodless field by suctioning blood from the left atrium and left ventricle. The operative approach varies according to the type of VSD. Perimembranous VSDs are usually repaired through a right atrial approach. Doubly committed juxta-arterial defects are approached through the main pulmonary artery. Muscular VSDs are usually approached through the right atrium, although they may also be approached through the main pulmonary artery or through a limited right or left ventriculotomy. The Gerbode defect is approached via the right atrium. Rarely, perimembranous and doubly committed juxta-arterial VSDs, particularly those with significant associated aortic valve insufficiency, may be best approached through the aorta and the aortic valve. These different approaches are summarized in **Table 48.4**.

Table 48.3 General principles of VSD closure

Aortic and bicaval venous cannulation
Cardiopulmonary bypass
Moderate hypothermia (28–32 °C)
Vent right superior pulmonary vein
Aortic cross-clamp
Cold blood cardioplegia

Table 48.4 Approaches for VSD closure

Type of defect	Approach
Perimembranous	Right atrium
Doubly committed juxta-arterial	Main pulmonary artery
Muscular	
• Outlet muscular	Right atrium or main pulmonary artery
• Trabecular muscular	Right atrium
• Inlet muscular	Right atrium
• Apical muscular	Right ventricle or left ventricle
Gerbode	Right atrium

Specific technique based on anatomy of VSD

PERIMEMBRANOUS VSD

Essentially all perimembranous VSDs are approached through the right atrium. A "medial" atriotomy provides the optimal exposure of the tricuspid valve orifice especially for closure of VSDs that extend into the outlet septum (**Figure 48.3a**). This atriotomy begins at the base of the right atrial appendage and extends parallel to the right coronary artery staying at least 1 cm away from the right coronary artery. The incision extends between the right coronary artery and the inferior caval vein cannula. Stay sutures placed on the edges of the atriotomy are used to hold open the right atrium and expose the tricuspid valve orifice.

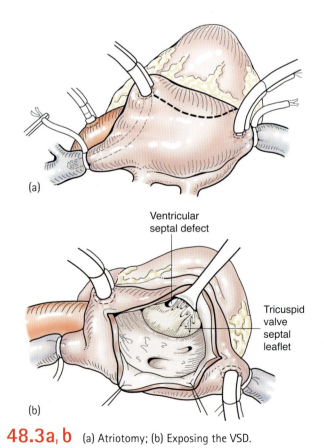

Ventricular septal defect

Tricuspid valve septal leaflet

(a)

(b)

48.3a, b (a) Atriotomy; (b) Exposing the VSD.

The perimembranous VSD is identified by retracting the septal and anterior leaflets of the tricuspid valve. One clue to the location of the VSD is a portion of the tricuspid valve that is pulled into the defect by the suction of the vent (**Figure 48.3b**). Another clue is fibrotic hemodynamic change in the right ventricular muscle adjacent to the VSD orifice.

In some instances the VSD perimeter cannot be completely identified because of the overlying tricuspid valve tissue. This is called a tricuspid valve pouch (**Figure 48.4**). It is advantageous in these situations to open the tricuspid valve in a radial fashion from the leading edge of the septal leaflet to the tricuspid valve annulus (**Figure 48.5**). This allows exposure of the entire perimeter of the VSD, although not necessarily all at one time – only a portion of the VSD

perimeter needs to be visualized at any one time. Fine stay sutures placed at the leading edge of the tricuspid valve prior to opening the leaflet will assist in precisely repairing the tricuspid valve following VSD closure. An alternative method of opening the tricuspid valve is to detach the valve along the annulus in a circumferential fashion. The next step is to inspect the VSD and in particular examine for the location of the aortic valve leaflets. The aortic valve leaflets may prolapse into the defect and need to be avoided during suture placement.

The technique of VSD closure that we have used at Ann & Robert H. Lurie Children's Hospital of Chicago for over 50 years is to encircle the perimeter of the VSD with multiple interrupted pledget based Dacron sutures. The sutures are then sequentially placed through an appropriately sized patch, the patch is lowered into the defect, and the sutures are tied and cut. The suture placement for a perimembranous VSD must avoid the area of the atrioventricular (AV) node and the conducting system. The location of the AV node is shown in **Figure 48.6**. To avoid injury to the conducting system the sutures should be placed superficially and carefully along the inferior and posterior margins of the defect and stay on the right ventricular side of the VSD. This begins from the area of the insertion of the muscle of Lancisi (medial papillary muscle of the conus) to the annulus of the tricuspid valve near the region of the apex of the triangle of Koch. The borders of the triangle of Koch are the tricuspid valve annulus, the orifice of the coronary sinus, and the tendon of Todaro. In some cases the sutures will be passed from the right atrial side of the tricuspid valve through the valve itself into the right ventricular side. Care must be taken when placing these sutures to avoid the aortic valve cusp, which is just on the other side of the tricuspid valve annulus.

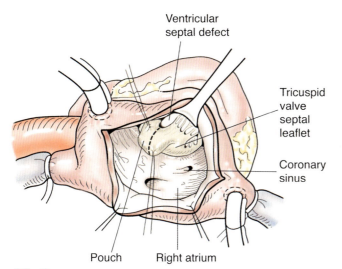

48.4 Incision in the tricuspid valve pouch.

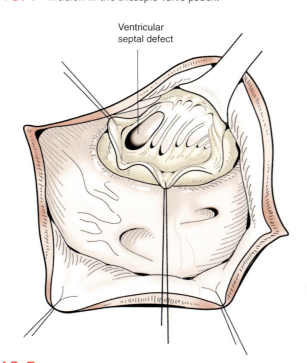

48.5 Exposure of ventricular septal defect.

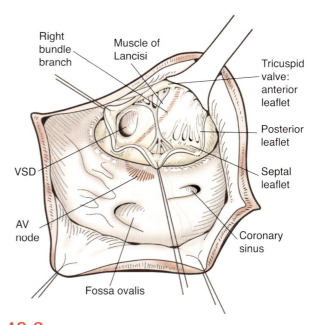

48.6 AV node.

Once all of the pledgeted sutures have been placed around the perimeter of the VSD, a polytetrafloroethylene (PTFE) patch is cut to the appropriate size. The size of the patch is usually approximately 1.5 times the size of the actual hole in the septum. This allows a space for the pledgeted sutures to be placed with a 2–3 mm rim of patch between the suture placement and the edge of the patch. **Figure 48.7** shows the sutures going through the patch. When all the sutures have been passed sequentially through the patch, the patch is lowered into the defect and care is taken to make sure that all the loops of the sutures are pulled up. The sutures are then tied and cut.

If the tricuspid valve has been incised in a radial fashion (or detached along the annulus), after the patch has been anchored the tricuspid valve is repaired. This is facilitated by the stay sutures placed at the leading edge of the tricuspid valve prior to dividing the tricuspid valve. The repair of the tricuspid valve is with multiple, interrupted, fine simple sutures (usually 6-0 Prolene) (**Figure 48.8**).

When the tricuspid valve repair is completed, the right ventricle can be irrigated with a bulb syringe filled with cold saline. This will give the surgeon an idea of whether significant tricuspid valve regurgitation has been caused by the tricuspid valve repair. This can then be addressed further as needed.

The completion of the VSD closure is to close the atrium. This is accomplished with two layers of running Prolene suture, the first layer placed as a mattress suture. The heart is de-aired by temporarily turning the vent off and allowing the bronchial collateral circulation to fill the left atrium with blood. Air is evacuated from the right side of the heart by temporarily occluding the IVC cannula, releasing the IVC tourniquet, and evacuating air through the right atrial suture line. The cardioplegia needle, which is at the high point of the left side, is then aspirated with a syringe, evacuating air from the left side of the heart. Once the heart is fully de-aired, then the aortic cross clamp is removed. As soon as the cross-clamp is removed, the vent is restarted in order to aspirate any residual air which might come up from the pulmonary veins during the rewarming and ventilating process. In addition, the cardioplegia needle in the ascending aorta can be converted to a vent to the bypass circuit to capture any other air bubbles that might go out of the aorta.

The patient is rewarmed and typically will resume a spontaneous normal sinus rhythm. If not, the heart is defibrillated (1 joule/kg). The patient is ventilated. When good cardiac action is restored, the vent is removed. This is done during lung inflation to increase the pressure in the left atrium and prevent aspiration of air through the vent site. The patient is then weaned from cardiopulmonary bypass with milrinone for inotropic support.

We have used intraoperative transesophageal echocardiography (TEE) for all VSD closures since 1992. TEE is used to confirm the preoperative diagnosis and to assure the integrity of the repair following the closure by evaluating for residual intracardiac left-to-right shunting. If there is residual shunting, the TEE can give the surgeon an idea of where the residual VSD is located, the size of the residual defect, and the magnitude of the residual shunting. TEE can also demonstrate significant postoperative tricuspid valve insufficiency if it is present. TEE is especially useful in those cases where aortic valve insufficiency is repaired, to assess the degree of AI pre- and postoperatively.

DOUBLY COMMITTED JUXTA-ARTERIAL VSD

Doubly committed juxta-arterial VSDs account for 5–10% of all VSDs closed surgically in Western countries. In reviews from Asian countries doubly committed juxta-arterial VSDs are more frequent, representing 25–30% of VSD closures. All patients with a doubly committed juxta-arterial VSD should

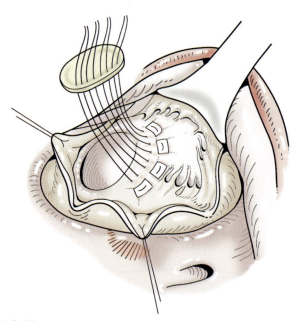

48.7 Pledgeted sutures and patch.

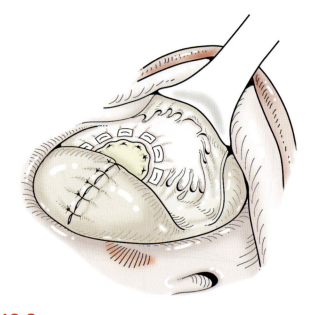

48.8 Repair of the tricuspid valve.

undergo closure because of the high risk of development of aortic valve prolapse followed by aortic valve insufficiency. The approach to these defects is through the main pulmonary artery and then the pulmonary valve. Cardiopulmonary bypass maneuvers are the same as for perimembranous VSD. However, after cardioplegia has been administered, the exposure of the defect is accomplished through a vertical incision in the main pulmonary artery. This incision typically extends from the distal main pulmonary artery into the sinus of the pulmonary valve anteriorly and to the patient's right. This is shown in **Figure 48.9**. Retraction of the pulmonary artery opening is accomplished with stay sutures. Small-vein retractors are used to gently retract the pulmonary valve and demonstrate the doubly committed juxta-arterial VSD.

Pledgeted sutures are placed circumferentially around the perimeter of the VSD. A critical part of the closure involves placing sutures directly in the base of the pulmonary valve cusps as an anchoring point where there is no muscular septum separating the aortic and pulmonary valves (**Figures 49.10 and 48.11**). **Figure 48.10** shows the location of the pledgeted sutures not only in the top of the muscular septum, but also in the base of the pulmonary valve cusp. **Figure 48.11** shows the lateral projection of the defect showing pledgeted sutures passing through the base of the pulmonary valve cusp and the relationship to the aortic valve cusp. These sutures must be very carefully placed to avoid injuring the aortic valve or the pulmonary valve.

Once sutures have been placed around the perimeter of the VSD they are passed through the patch, which is then lowered into the defect and all of the sutures are tied. Completed patch closure is shown in **Figure 48.12**. After the VSD has been closed, the opening in the pulmonary artery is closed with a running Prolene suture. The left and right sides of the heart are de-aired as for a perimembranous VSD prior to removing the aortic cross-clamp.

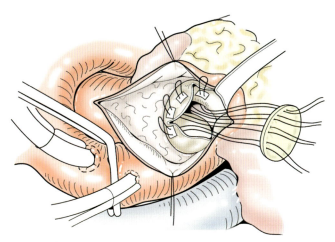

48.10 Pledgeted sutures – base of pulmonary artery cusp.

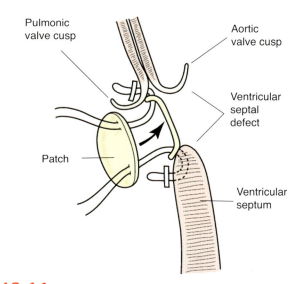

48.11 Lateral projection of pledgeted sutures in relation to the aortic and pulmonary valves.

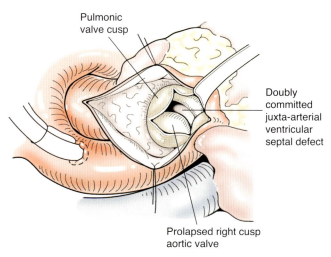

48.9 VSD exposure with pulmonary artery incision.

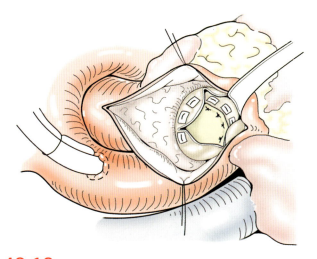

48.12 Completed VSD closure.

Right ventricular approach

An alternative approach for the patient with a doubly committed juxta-arterial VSD is through the infundibulum of the right ventricle. Of note is that some of these patients will have an associated right ventricular outflow tract stenosis which will require resection. Some surgeons have felt that the approach through the infundibulum facilitates the excision of infundibular stenosis and the exposure for the VSD closure. However, we have preferred to avoid a ventriculotomy and have not used it since the early 1980s. There are two types of right ventriculotomy incisions, transverse and vertical. The transverse incision may have the advantage of limiting injury to the circular muscular fibers. However, exposure through this approach may be restricted. This is also usually inadequate when enlargement of the infundibulum with a patch is required. If a vertical incision is used, it should be limited to the infundibular area (**Figure 48.13**). It is important to examine the coronary artery distribution before beginning any ventriculotomy. If there is a left anterior descending coronary artery (LAD) originating from the right coronary artery, ventriculotomy is dangerous and should be avoided because of the possible injury to the LAD itself, with resultant myocardial infarction. Infrequently, these arteries as they cross the infundibulum are intramyocardial and may not be seen on the myocardial surface. The preoperative aortic angiogram location of the coronary arteries should be evaluated. Alternatively, an echocardiogram can also show the location of the coronary arteries.

Transaortic approach

If the patient has associated aortic valve insufficiency, they may require a simultaneous aortic valve suspension. Vertical suspension in patients such as this was initially described in great detail by Dr George Trusler from Toronto. In our original series of doubly committed juxta-arterial VSD patients, four patients required aortic valve suspension. In three of these patients the VSD was closed through an aortotomy rather than through the pulmonary artery. This was because the primary indication for the procedure was the aortic valve insufficiency.

After cardioplegia, an obliquely curved incision is made starting on the anterior aspect of the ascending aorta curving down into the non-coronary sinus (**Figure 48.14**). This incision may be extended as needed transversely toward the left. The aortic valve leaflets are retracted carefully to expose the defect. Often there is an absence of a superior muscular or fibrous rim of the defect, making suture placement somewhat difficult. In this situation sutures may be passed through the aortic wall from the inside of the aortic valve sinus in a fashion analogous to the placement of suture through the base of the pulmonary valve cusp as described earlier. However, we do not usually use pledgets on the aortic side to prevent adhesions at the base of the aortic valve cusp with resultant AI. The transaortic approach to a VSD is illustrated in **Figure 48.14**.

MUSCULAR VSD

The operative approach to muscular VSDs is not as straightforward as for perimembranous and doubly committed juxta-arterial defects. Muscular defects are often multiple and are technically often difficult to reach. Historically, these lesions (especially when multiple) were managed by first placing a pulmonary artery band, and then 6–12 months later removing the band and closing the defects when the patient was older and larger. This often also required attention to reconstructing the pulmonary artery at the band site. More recently, there has been a distinct trend to repairing muscular defects in infancy, even if they are multiple. In one series reviewing 130 patients with multiple VSDs, 32% had a preliminary pulmonary artery band. The perimembranous septum was involved in 102 patients, the muscular septum in 121 patients, and the conal septum in 9 patients. Fifty patients had the "Swiss cheese" form of the lesion. In that

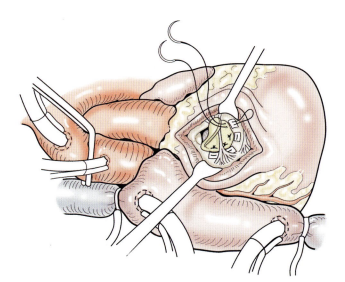

48.13 Right ventricle approach – vertical incision.

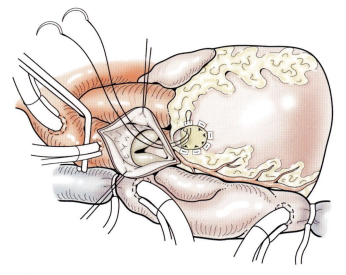

48.14 Transaortic approach.

same experience, right atriotomy was used in 82 patients (63%), right ventriculotomy in 32 patients (24%), and left ventriculotomy in 14 patients (10%). Left ventriculotomy was only used in low apical muscular VSDs. That series used the same technique for closure that we have used at Ann & Robert H. Lurie Children's Hospital of Chicago – interrupted pledget-based mattress sutures and a PTFE patch. The division of trabeculations within the body of the right ventricle facilitates the exposure and accurate closure of muscular VSDs. In particular, the moderator band can be divided in cases of mid-trabecular muscular VSDs. However, this may cause right bundle branch block. These trabeculations become hypertrophied with a pulmonary artery band and hence an increasing number of surgeons are electing to repair these lesions in infancy rather than placing a pulmonary artery band first. An alternative approach to these defects is the use of catheterization-delivered devices.

Left ventricular approach

Use of this operative exposure is limited to certain muscular VSDs, particularly those with multiple apical openings (Swiss cheese). These defects may be easier to patch on the left ventricular side because of the relatively smooth septum, lack of heavy trabeculations, and single orifice compared to multiple orifices on the right ventricular side. The ventricular incision is usually a vertical one starting in a relatively avascular left ventricular apical area with limited extension (**Figure 48.15**). The coronary artery distribution must be carefully analyzed in order to minimize injury to the coronary arteries. Left ventricular incisions, however, may be associated with significant long-term ventricular dysfunction and should be avoided whenever possible except for small apical incisions that are probably well tolerated.

GERBODE VSD

The so-called Gerbode ventriculoatrial defect is a rare defect that permits shunting of blood from the left ventricle to the right atrium. It occurs when there is a deficiency of the AV membranous septum (**Figure 48.16a and b**). From 1990 to

2008, we identified six patients who had undergone surgical closure of a congenital defect of the AV component of the membranous septum. Median age at repair was 1.6 years. All patients were symptomatic, with three having congestive cardiac failure, two failing to thrive, and two having intolerance to exercise. All had a dilated right atrium. All were closed by insertion of a patch. No patient had a residual defect or heart block.

Alternative techniques

Although our experience at Ann & Robert H. Lurie Children's Hospital of Chicago has been using pledgeted interrupted sutures for the majority of VSDs, there are certain exceptions to this. For very tiny infants (i.e. <3 kg) the VSD is often surrounded by relatively friable neonatal

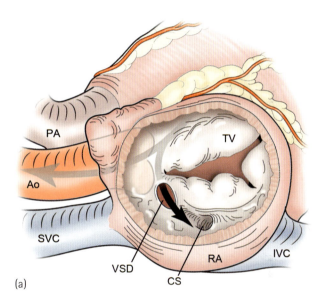

(a)

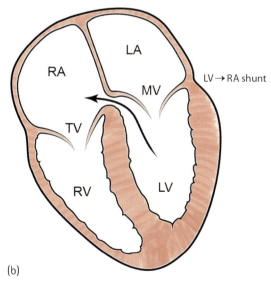

(b)

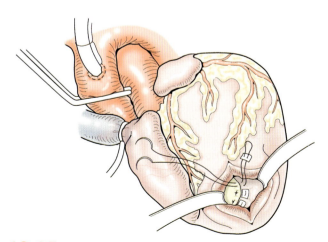

48.15 Left ventricle apical approach.

48.16a, b Gerbode VSD.

muscle. Placement of sutures with pledgets and then tying all of the sutures separately may actually increase the chances of the sutures pulling through the delicate neonatal myocardium. In this circumstance we have employed a running suture technique using 6-0 Prolene suture. The suture is anchored with a pericardial pledget and we then use a pericardial patch fixed in glutaraldehyde for the VSD closure. The technique is illustrated in **Figure 48.17a and b**. The pericardial pledget is passed through the portion of the VSD which is furthest away from the surgeon. The suture is passed through the tanned pericardium and then tied. The two remaining ends of the sutures are then used in a running fashion, one superiorly and one inferiorly, and the pericardial patch is sutured to the edge of the VSD. The suture is completed on the tricuspid valve annulus and the knot tied outside the tricuspid valve. Again, we have found this most useful for neonates.

Our reasoning for using the interrupted pledgeted technique has been to minimize the incidence of residual VSD. However, some centers use a running suture technique for essentially all VSDs. Some surgeons have recommended using a strip of pericardium as a pledget to reinforce a portion of the VSD repair.

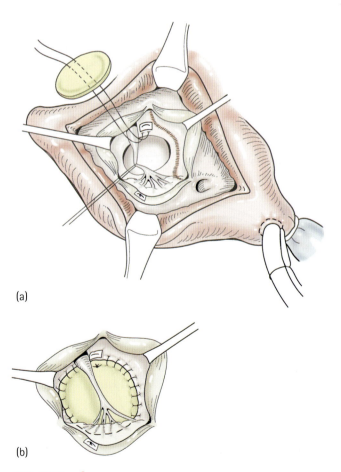

(a)

(b)

48.17a, b Running suture technique with pericardial pledget: (a) initial suture placement; (b) knot on the RA side of the TV annulus.

POSTOPERATIVE CARE

The postoperative care of the patient with a VSD is dictated by the age of the patient and the size and morphology of the VSD. Infants with large VSDs have the potential to develop pulmonary hypertensive crisis and are treated differently from older children with small VSDs where the patients are often extubated in the operating room. There is a wide spectrum of potential postoperative strategies between these two extremes. For the small infant with a large non-restrictive VSD, we keep the patient paralyzed and ventilated for the first 12–24 hours postoperatively. These patients are also treated expectantly with pulmonary vasodilators, afterload reduction, and inotropic support. This would typically include low-dose epinephrine (0.02–0.05 mcg/kg/min) and intravenous milrinone (0.5 mcg/kg/min). These patients would also be kept on Versed (midazolam) and fentanyl drips along with a vecuronium drip for the first 12–24 hours. In severe cases we would use inhaled nitric oxide (20 ppm). We then stop the vecuronium infusion and, if the child does not have pulmonary hypertensive crisis, we wean the sedation and the ventilation and extubate the child at 48–72 hours following the procedure. If the child shows evidence of pulmonary hypertensive crisis (arterial desaturation, hypotension), we reinstate their paralysis. In the current era where most babies with large VSDs undergo a prompt operative repair within the first several months of life pulmonary hypertensive crisis are really quite rare. This was more common when children were allowed to go to an age of 1–2 years (or older) prior to closure of large VSDs. Most patients with a non-restrictive VSD will have been on Digoxin, Lasix, and Catopril prior to the surgery. We discontinue their Digoxin and Catopril, but do keep them on Lasix for several weeks following the procedure. Usually after 4–6 weeks following the operation they are off all medications. An older child with a restrictive VSD who is being repaired for indications of aortic valve prolapse or aortic valve insufficiency is often weaned off cardiopulmonary bypass with only milrinone. These patients are frequently extubated in the operating room.

RESULTS

At Ann & Robert H. Lurie Children's Hospital of Chicago between 1990 and 2013, 709 patients had closure of a VSD: perimembranous (591), doubly committed juxta-arterial (59), muscular (53), and Gerbode (6). There was no operative mortality. Thirteen patients had heart block and required a pacemaker (2%); 11 of these 13 patients had a chromosomal abnormality. The incidence of heart block in patients with normal chromosomes was 0.3%. Fourteen patients required reoperation while in the intensive care unit (2%), and one patient had a significant residual VSD requiring reoperation. Between 1980 and 2012, 106 children with a doubly committed juxta-arterial VSD underwent intracardiac repair at Lurie Children's. Median age at repair was 1.1 years. There was no mortality and no patient had heart block. In patients undergoing "elective" VSD closure (i.e. patients over 1 year of age, with a pulmonary to systemic flow ratio <2) there were almost no complications. Between 1980 and 1991, 141 patients at Lurie Children's had closure of a restrictive VSD at an age over 1 year. The mean pulmonary artery pressure was 26 mmHg and the mean pulmonary to systemic flow ratio was 1.6 : 1. Aortic valve prolapse was present in 45% of patients, aortic valve insufficiency in 18% of the patients, and 3.5% of the patients had prior bacterial endocarditis. There were no early or late deaths and no major morbidity. No patient required a ventriculotomy to accomplish VSD closure. The mean hospital stay was 5 days. There were no instances of permanent complete AV dissociation. There were no reoperations for bleeding and no postoperative wound infections. There were no reoperations for residual or recurrent VSDs.

This review led us to call for a re-evaluation of historical indications for VSD closure. The surgical risk of VSD closure (as defined by this experience) when compared with the known natural history studies is less than the lifetime risks of developing bacterial endocarditis or progressive aortic valve prolapse leading to aortic valve insufficiency. VSD closure also removes the socioeconomic stigma associated with living with an uncorrected cardiac defect (which is not insignificant).

Special consideration: heart block

If in the operating room following full rewarming the patient is not in sinus rhythm, temporary pacing wires should be placed on the surface of the right atrium and ventricle. These temporary wires can be used to pace the ventricle safely in order to wean the child from cardiopulmonary bypass. Many times as the child recovers from the cardioplegia or is started on inotropic support the heart block will resolve. However, if the heart block does not resolve, we recommend using the temporary wires to pace the child and then recommend observing the child for a period of 7–10 days. We have not urgently reoperated to revise the patch in this situation. During the period of observation frequently many children will resume sinus rhythm. Should this occur, we then perform a 24-hour Holter monitor to establish the resolution of heart block and resumption of sinus rhythm before discharging the patient. However, after 7 days the chances of the child resuming normal sinus rhythm become remote and at this point, somewhere between 7 and 10 days, we would recommend placement of a dual-chamber pacing system. Currently, we would recommend placement of steroid eluting epicardial leads and dual-chamber pacing. This would be performed in an epicardial fashion for the majority of patients who have VSD closure as these patients are usually less than 1–2 years of age.

Residual VSD

If a residual VSD is suspected in the operating room either because of a thrill palpable on the anterior surface of the right ventricle or a color jet seen on the TEE, there are several considerations. The TEE can estimate the size of the color Doppler jet, i.e. tiny, mild residual, moderate residual, or severe residual. Residual defects that are 2 mm or less in diameter will close over time. The surgeon should consider a re-exploration for moderate or severe residual defects. If TEE is not available, or in cases that are not easily classified, one can measure the intracardiac shunt in the operating room and use this information to decide whether to re-explore. Two separate syringes with fine needles are used to aspirate blood from the right atrium and the pulmonary artery. The oxygen saturation of the blood in the right atrium versus the pulmonary artery along with the known aortic saturation (usually 100%) can then be used to calculate the shunt (Qp : Qs), using the following formula.

$$\frac{AoSat - PASat}{AoSat - RASat} = \frac{Qp}{Qs}$$

Unless the residual shunt is more than 1.5 : 1, the residual defect will probably close over time.

SUMMARY

Anatomically, the four main types of VSD are perimembranous (80%), doubly committed juxta-arterial (10%), muscular (10%), and the Gerbode (left ventricle to right atrium) defect (1%). Indications for VSD closure include congestive heart failure, Qp : Qs > 1.5 : 1, aortic valve prolapse, aortic valve insufficiency, all doubly committed juxta-arterial and Gerbode defects, and prior episode of SBE.

The results of operative closure of VSDs in the current era are extremely good. The risk of death for all patients including those with pulmonary hypertension approaches zero. The risk of major morbidity such as heart block, emergent reoperation, or significant residual VSD is extremely low. Nearly all patients who have VSD closure will have an excellent outcome, and the long-term prognosis for these patients is very close to that of a normal child.

FURTHER READING

Backer CL, Idriss FS, Zales VR, et al. Surgical management of the conal (supracristal) ventricular septal defect. *J Thorac Cardiovasc Surg.* 1991; 102: 288–96.

Backer CL, Winters RC, Zales VR, et al. Restrictive ventricular septal defect: how small is too small to close? *Ann Thorac Surg.* 1993; 56: 1014–19.

Beerbaum P, Körperich H, Barth P, et al. Noninvasive quantification of left-to-right shunt in pediatric patients: phase-contrast cine magnetic resonance imaging compared with invasive oximetry. *Circulation.* 2001; 103: 2476–82.

Devlin PJ, Russell HM, Mongé MC, et al. Doubly committed and juxta-arterial ventricular septal defect: outcomes of the aortic and pulmonary valves. *Ann Thorac Surg.* 2014; 97: 2134–40.

Dodge-Khatami A, Knirsch W, Tomaske M, et al. Spontaneous closure of small residual ventricular septal defects after surgical repair. *Ann Thorac Surg.* 2007; 83: 902–5.

Fraser CD, Zhou X, Palepu S, et al. Tricuspid valve detachment in ventricular septal defect closure does not impact valve function. *Ann Thorac Surg.* 2018; 106: 145–50.

Gaynor JW, O'Brien JE Jr, Rychik J, et al. Outcome following tricuspid valve detachment for ventricular septal defects closure. *Eur J Cardiothorac Surg.* 2001; 19: 279–82.

Gersony WM, Hayes CJ, Driscoll DJ, et al. Bacterial endocarditis in patients with aortic stenosis, pulmonary stenosis, or ventricular septal defect. *Circulation.* 1993; 87(Suppl I): I121–I126.

Jacobs JP, Burke RP, Quintessenza JA, Mavroudis C. Congenital heart surgery nomenclature and database project: ventricular septal defect. *Ann Thorac Surg.* 2000; 69: S25–S35.

Kelle AM, Young L, Kaushal S, et al. The Gerbode defect: the significance of a left ventricular to right atrial shunt. *Cardiol Young.* 2009; 19(Suppl 2): 1–4.

Russell HM, Forsberg K, Backer CL, et al. Outcomes of radial incision of the tricuspid valve for ventricular septal defect closure. *Ann Thorac Surg.* 2011; 92: 685–90.

Serraf A, Lacour-Gayet F, Bruniaux J, et al. Surgical management of isolated multiple ventricular septal defects. *J Thorac Cardiovasc Surg.* 1992; 103: 437–43.

Trusler GA, Moes CAF, Kidd BS. Repair of ventricular septal defect with aortic insufficiency. *J Thorac Cardiovasc Surg.* 1973; 66: 394–403.

Trusler GA, Williams WG, Smallhorn JF, Freedom RM. Late results with repair of aortic insufficiency associated with ventricular septal defect. *J Thorac Cardiovasc Surg.* 1992: 103; 276–81.

49

Tetralogy of Fallot

TOM R. KARL AND NELSON ALPHONSO

HISTORY

Tetralogy of Fallot (TOF) is one of the most frequently encountered congenital cardiac surgical lesions, occurring in 3 of every 10 000 live births. It is the commonest cause of cyanotic cardiac disease in patients beyond the neonatal age, and accounts for up to one-tenth of all congenital cardiac lesions. TOF is, therefore, an important entity for all paediatric cardiac surgeons. In fact, TOF was the first cyanotic lesion to be formally described, and some of the initial palliative and definitive operations for congenital heart disease were performed for TOF. Probably more is known about TOF than about any other complex cardiac malformation and, consequently, the lesion has served as a model for the natural history of cyanotic congenital heart disease and our ability to alter that history with surgery. Our understanding of cardiac physiology, myocardial protection, cardiopulmonary bypass (CPB), developmental anatomy, molecular biology, genomics, and other areas has been enhanced by the study of TOF. Finally, TOF is a potentially lethal lesion without treatment, but one that now has a quite favorable natural history when an appropriate surgical strategy is employed.

The first operations for TOF were performed by Blalock and associates at Johns Hopkins Hospital in 1948. The Blalock strategy was to divert blood from the systemic circulation to the pulmonary circulation to reduce the physiologic effect of right-to-left shunting within the heart. A more direct approach to TOF was first used by Lillehei and associates at the University of Minnesota in 1954. Open correction of TOF was performed by Lillehei's group using cross-circulation between the child and a support patient, and later using CPB with a bubble oxygenator. Although numerous strategic and technical modifications have been introduced since these initial efforts, Lillehei's work set the standard for our modern surgical approach to TOF.

The anatomical features of TOF are described in detail by Anderson (see Chapter 39, "The anatomy of congenital cardiac malformations"), whose general approach to congenital heart disease and its nomenclature has improved our surgical understanding significantly. The basic anatomical features relevant to the surgical repair of tetralogy are shown in **Figure 49.1**. Anterior and cephalad displacement of the infundibular (muscular outlet) septum results in a malalignment ventricular septal defect (VSD), right ventricular outflow tract obstruction (RVOTO), and RV hypertrophy. The pulmonary valve (PV) and pulmonary arterial (PA) tree may show any degree of hypoplasia.

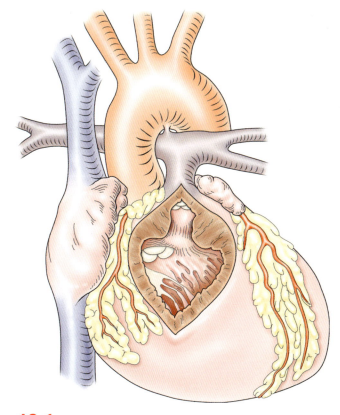

49.1

PRINCIPLES AND JUSTIFICATION

For most patients with TOF, the diagnosis can be established with echocardiography in the neonatal period, or prenatally. Depending on the anatomy of the RVOT and PAs, as well as the degree of collateral circulation and other factors, a plan for timing and strategy can be developed. The images in **Figure 49.2a–d** show the features of TOF.

PREOPERATIVE ASSESSMENT AND PLANNING

Preoperative investigation is based primarily on 2D echocardiography, which provides information about the RVOT, VSD, central PA tree, and proximal coronaries. In some cases, angiography may be required to delineate unusual features. The decision to perform a definitive intracardiac repair is predicated on the presence of an adequate PA tree (i.e. one which can accept the full cardiac output after septation, with a subsystemic RV pressure, in the face of increasing cardiac output). Many formulae have been proposed to assess this feature, but none is infallible. Surgical judgment and experience remain critically important.

Treatment strategy is determined by assessment of a number of factors (**Figure 49.3**). In the current era, most cardiac surgical teams elect definitive intracardiac repair whenever possible for unacceptably cyanotic patients. Although the strategy of routine intracardiac repair (as opposed to a palliative operation) in stable neonates with acceptable oxygenation has little to recommend it, the perceived best age for elective repair varies from birth to 1 year of age. The trend worldwide over the past decade has been toward earlier elective repair (at 3–6 months of age), but there are many outliers. Other factors that may influence timing of repair in a given cardiac center include the general condition of the baby, prematurity, very low birth weight, genetic syndromes, possible need for

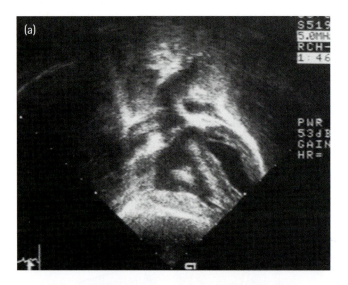
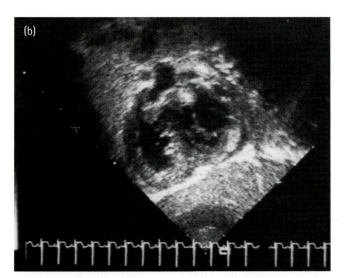
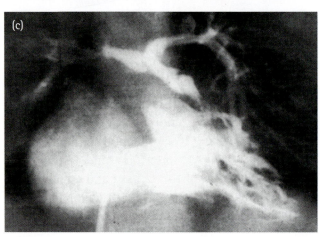
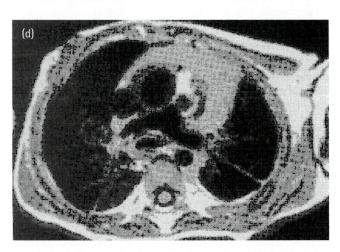

49.2 Imaging in tetralogy of Fallot. (a) and (b) 2D echocardiograms demonstrating aortic override of the large VSD, RV hypertrophy, and malalignment of ventricular septal segments that generates the VSD, with approximately 50% of the aorta arising from the RV; Figure (c) Right ventriculogram demonstrating hypoplasia of the PA tree with severe RVOTO. (d) Cardiac gated T-1 weighted spin echo (magnetic resonance imaging) showing confluent branch PAs with a severe stenosis just proximal to the LPA bifurcation. Pulmonary stenosis and aortic enlargement are also demonstrated.

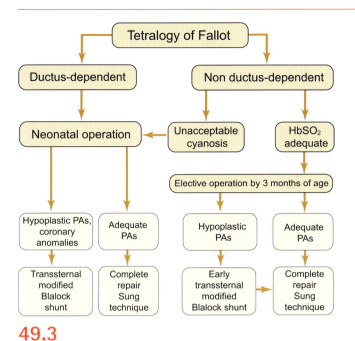

49.3

an extracardiac conduit, the presence of additional intracardiac problems, and discontinuous PAs. However, good early results have been achieved in most centers with diverse timing strategies, involving both single- and two-staged approaches (i.e. primary definitive repair, or modified Blalock–Taussig shunt followed by repair at an interval).

OPERATION

Modified Blalock–Taussig shunt

The indication for a modified Blalock–Taussig shunt procedure is cyanosis of an unacceptable degree in a patient believed to be unsuitable for intracardiac repair for one of a variety of reasons (see above). The best approach is via median sternotomy, which can be limited to the upper half of the sternum if desired. Use of the transsternal approach allows continuous ventilation during the operation and a generally more stable hemodynamic situation, as well as good access for CPB should it become necessary. The thymus is resected, and the upper pericardium is opened longitudinally. The preferred side for the shunt is the right in all cases, irrespective of arch anatomy (i.e. arch to right or left of trachea). Performing the shunt at this site facilitates closure at subsequent definitive repair and protects the phrenic nerves. The polytetrafluoroethylene (PTFE) shunt can be easily dissected medially to the superior caval vein, clipped, and divided immediately after the commencement of CPB (see below).

The transsternal approach is used for a modified Blalock shunt. The brachiocephalic artery and PA are dissected with electrocautery and isolated within Silastic loops (**Figure 49.4a**). Heparin is administered systemically (1 mg/kg), and the brachiocephalic artery is controlled with a vascular clamp. A PTFE graft (3.5 mm or 4.0 mm, for infants

under and over 3.5 kg respectively) is cut on a bevel and anastomosed to the brachiocephalic artery with running 7-0 polypropylene suture. The clamp is left in place while the distal end of the shunt is sutured to the right PA using either a second clamp or traction on the vessel loops (**Figure 49.4b**). Excessive length of the shunt may result in a kink, which can

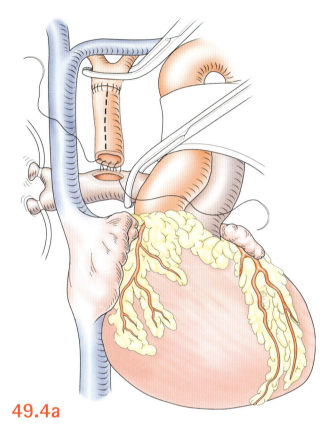

49.4a

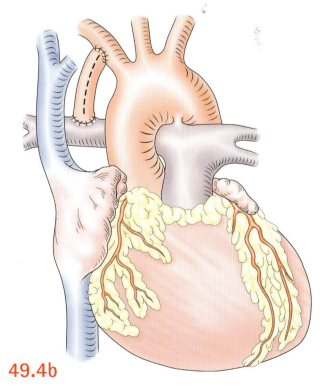

49.4b

lead to occlusion. Clamps are removed, and the pericardium and sternum are closed over a Silastic drain.

Common early postoperative problems include low diastolic systemic arterial pressure, and mild metabolic acidosis and unilateral hyperemia on chest X-ray, both usually transient. Chylous or serous effusions may also occur, but the incidence of either may be decreased by limiting the extent of mediastinal dissection and avoiding direct instrumentation of the shunt respectively. Postoperatively, patients receive heparin (1 unit/kg/hour) until oral aspirin (5 mg/kg/day) can be started.

Definitive intracardiac repair of tetralogy of Fallot

In the early era of TOF repair, a large right ventriculotomy and transannular patch were usually employed both for relief of RVOTO and repair of the VSD. Over ensuing decades, the resultant PV insufficiency and volume loading sometimes led to RV failure, dilation, fibrosis, and arrhythmias. PV replacement may not be curative in such situations. Conversely, residual severe RVOTO may limit PV insufficiency but is a risk factor for late RV hypertrophy and death.

The goals of repair, therefore, are to provide adequate relief of RVOTO, to septate the heart completely, and to preserve contractile, electrical, and valvular function as much as possible. A different approach to TOF repair using transatrial VSD closure and limited or no ventriculotomy was promoted by Hudspeth, Edmunds, and others. The best strategy available today for most patients is the transatrial–transpulmonary repair, described in **Figure 49.5a–g**, with preservation or reconstruction of the PV.

The operative approach is via full median sternotomy, using a relatively short skin incision. The thymus is resected, and the pericardium is opened to the right of the midline. A suitable pericardial patch adequate for RVOT reconstruction is excised, immersed for 2 minutes in 0.1% glutaraldehyde solution, and rinsed several times in saline. The patient is heparinized (3 mg/kg) and cannulated for CPB via the superior and inferior caval veins and the ascending aorta (at the base of the brachiocephalic artery). The modified Blalock–Taussig shunt, if present, is dissected, clipped, and divided as CPB is commenced. The patient is cooled systemically to 34 °C. The arterial ligament (or duct) is dissected and ligated. The aorta is clamped, and sanguinous cardioplegia is delivered into the aortic root. The caval vein snares are tightened around the venous cannulae, and the right atrium (RA) and pulmonary trunk are opened longitudinally. A vent sucker is placed through the ASD, which may require opening with a scalpel. The pulmonary valve is inspected, and fused commissures are opened right back to the sinotubular junction (**Figure 49.5a**). A 3 mm 45-degree Hegar dilator is passed retrogradely into the RV to facilitate identification and inspection of the RVOT, which is done through the transtricuspid valve approach. With the anterior leaflet of the tricuspid valve (TV) retracted, the RVOT is exposed. The

septoparietal trabeculations of the muscular outlet septum (parietal extension of the infundibular septum) are excised as completely as possible (**Figure 49.5b(i) and (ii)**), taking care to avoid the rim of the VSD and aortic valve leaflets.

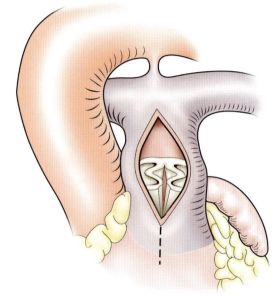

49.5a

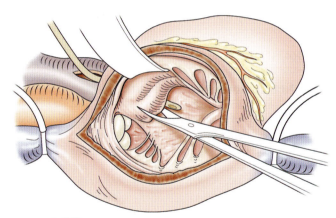

49.5b(i)

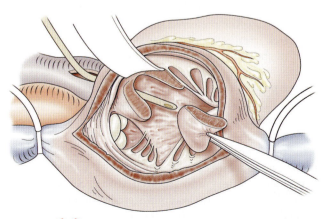

49.5b(ii)

Additional obstructing muscle bands in the RVOT are mobilized and excised as well, and this exercise may be repeated working through the pulmonary valve. The goal of RVOT resection is to allow free passage of a dilator that is 2 mm larger than predicted for the normalized pulmonary valve diameter. In approximately 75% of cases, a small, transannular extension of the PA incision (10–20 mm) will be required, and this extension should be made through the middle of the anterior cusp of the pulmonary valve, extending onto the free wall of the RV (**Figure 49.5c**). Care should be taken to avoid injuring coronary artery branches.

The VSD is then closed, working through the TV (**Figure 49.5d(i) and (ii)**). Polypropylene mattress sutures (5-0 or 6-0 with pledgets) are placed through the base of the septal tricuspid leaflet and around the rim of the VSD. The aortic leaflets should again be identified through the VSD and protected, as should the area of the atrioventricular (AV) conduction tissue along the posterior rim. In the conduction area, a distance of 5 mm from the VSD rim is maintained (as in other perimembranous defects). The sutures are passed through a PTFE or pericardial patch, which is tucked beneath the TV septal leaflet, and then tied and cut. The patch size approximates that of the aortic diameter at the junction with the left ventricle (LV). Proper apposition of the TV leaflets is checked and adjusted with a septal–anterior commissural suture as required. The atrial septal defect is closed with a polypropylene suture, and the heart is de-aired via the aorta. The aortic clamp is removed, and the patient is warmed to 37 °C. The remainder of the operation can be performed with the heart beating at normothermia.

The RA incision is closed with running polypropylene, and the caval vein tapes are removed. If a transannular incision has not been used, the PA is either closed directly (if the caliber has been judged to be adequate) or repaired with a second small oval pericardial patch (**Figure 49.5e**).

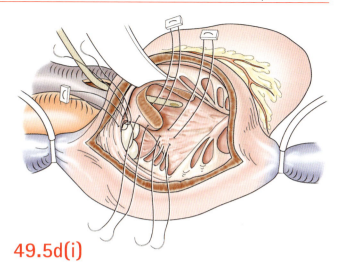

49.5d(i)

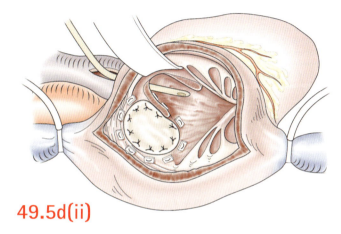

49.5d(ii)

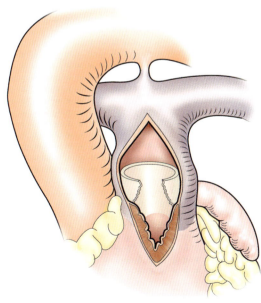

49.5c

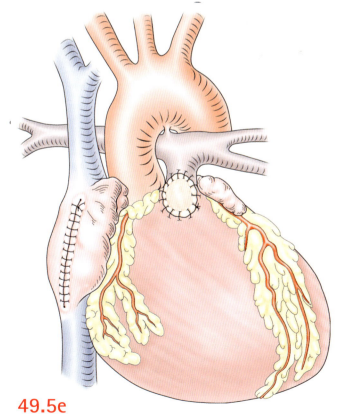

49.5e

When a transannular extension has been required, we employ a standard technique for RVOT reconstruction based on the technique of Sung et al. (**Figure 49.5f**). A triangular patch of pericardium is sutured to the cut edges of the anterior PV cusp, and the suture line is extended onto the endocardium of the RV incision. The size of the cusp is calibrated to enlarge the anterior leaflet and annulus to an acceptable normalized diameter, with creation of a sinus of Valsalva. A second larger pericardial patch is then used to augment the PA and RVOT, with the inferior suture line running along the epicardial edge (**Figure 49.5g**). We sometimes prefer a CardioCel (Admedus, Western Australia) bovine pericardial patch for this purpose. This reconstruction technique usually eliminates the RVOT gradient, with a high degree of preservation of the PV function. CPB is discontinued after application of atrial and ventricular pacing wires.

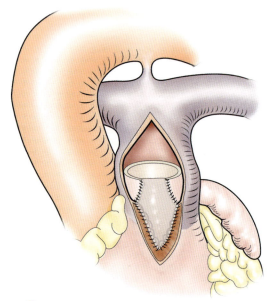

49.5f

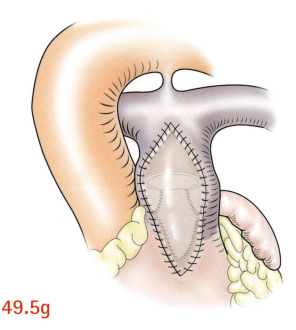

49.5g

Special considerations for tetralogy of Fallot repair

CORONARY ARTERY ANOMALIES

Coronary artery anatomy in TOF deviates from the expected pattern for normal hearts in 5–30% of cases. Of concern to the surgeon are cases in which an abnormal coronary branch crosses the RVOT, imposing limitations on the safe extent of the ventriculotomy (should it be required).

Figure 49.6 illustrates patterns of anomalous coronary arteries in 36 cases encountered in the Royal Children's Hospital (RCH) series (Melbourne). The most frequently appearing anomaly was an anterior descending branch from the right coronary artery. All patterns shown theoretically could preclude a classical transventricular approach to repair.

Coronary abnormalities can usually be imaged preoperatively with 2D echocardiography, although both CT angiograms and contrast aortography with steep caudocranial angulation may be more sensitive. Ultimately, responsibility for identification lies with the surgical team at the time of operation. A number of strategies have been proposed for dealing with anomalous coronaries during TOF repair, including the use of extracardiac RV–PA conduits. Mobilization of the coronary to accommodate a patch beneath it is not recommended. In our experience, most cases can be handled with the general transatrial–transpulmonary repair strategy described above without compromising the adequacy of RV–PA reconstruction (see Outcome).

Figure 49.7 shows transatrial–transpulmonary repair in the presence of an anomalous coronary (anterior descending from right coronary). The small transannular patch stops short of the coronary branch and can be deviated leftward. In patients with the anterior descending coronary artery arising from the right coronary artery, extension of a transannular patch laterally may be possible. In those with the right coronary artery arising from the left anterior descending, the patch must stop short of the transverse pathway of the coronary, and a more extensive muscle resection may be required. There may be a role for intraoperative balloon dilation of the annulus. In a minority of patients, alternative strategies such as extracardiac conduits can be used with acceptable outcome.

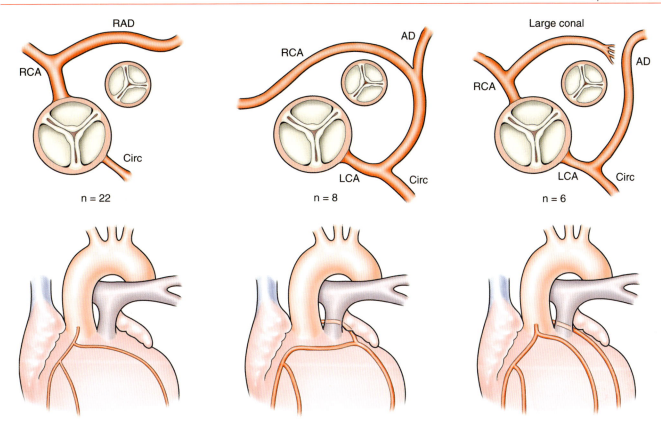

49.6

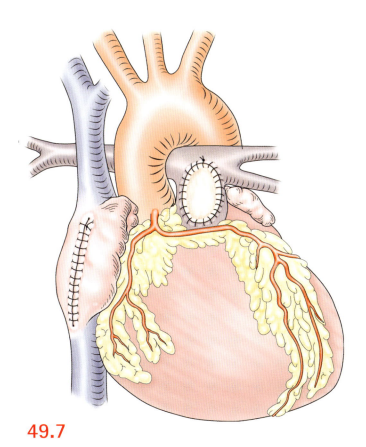

49.7

TETRALOGY OF FALLOT WITH ATRIOVENTRICULAR SEPTAL DEFECT

Atrioventricular septal defect (AVSD) complicates TOF in 1.0–6.5% of cases. Conversely, TOF occurs in 2.7–10.0% of cases of AVSD. The combination of two lesions is therefore relatively rare, and has a strong (greater than 75%) association with Down syndrome. Basic anatomical features of both AVSD and TOF are present, but there is a wide spectrum of AV valve and RVOT and PA anatomy. The VSD typically (but not invariably) extends under the inferior bridging AV valve leaflet, which makes the anatomy distinctly different from that of TOF. The superior bridging leaflet is freely floating (Rastelli type C).

The surgical procedure for TOF and AVSD is an extensive one. Definitive intracardiac repair is possible at any age but, in general, the results are not as good as those for either lesion in isolation. If possible, the operation should be performed after 3–4 months of age, when the AV valve repair is more reliable and more surgical options are available. In practice, an earlier operation is often required due to severity of the RVOTO and/or AV valve insufficiency. The main operative considerations are maintenance of AV and pulmonary valve competence.

The operative strategy for repair of TOF with AVSD is a combination of techniques used for isolated AVSD and TOF. It is helpful for the surgeon to understand the spatial relationships (**Figure 49.8a**). Initial steps of the operation are similar to those for isolated TOF, up to the point of VSD closure. For this part of the operation, a comma-shaped patch is used. Pledgeted sutures are placed around the aortic valve and the inlet portion of the VSD and then through the patch, which is seated beneath the tricuspid chords. Sutures are placed through the crest of PTFE or pericardial VSD patch, through the AV valve leaflets, and through one edge of a second autologous pericardial patch, to partition the single large AV valve into two non-stenotic orifices (**Figure 49.8b**). This septation can also be done using the Nunn technique, in which the bridging leaflet tissue is attached directly to the crest of the VSD with interrupted pledgeted sutures (**Figure 49.8c(i) and (ii)**).

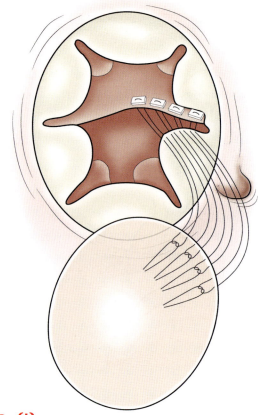

49.8c(i)

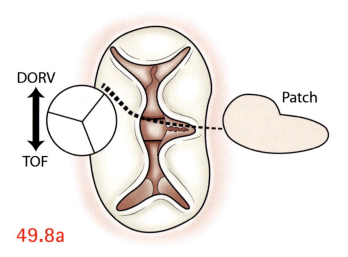

49.8a

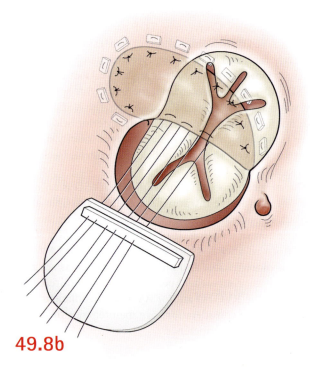

49.8b

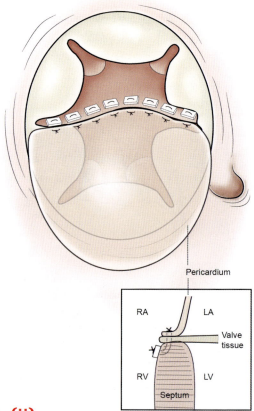

49.8c(ii)

The LV is then filled with cold saline to assess AV valve competence. Sutures are placed in the accessory septal commissure (or AV valve cleft) as required. Other valve repair techniques, such as commissuroplasty or semicircular annuloplasty, may be required.

A similar exercise is used to assess the RV and tricuspid portion of the partitioned AV valve, with the PA temporarily occluded. The ostium primum is then closed with a patch (autologous pericardium or CardioCel), leaving the coronary sinus in the RA. The heart is de-aired, and the aortic clamp is removed. RVOT reconstruction is then performed as for isolated TOF according to the Sung technique. We have also used homograft or bovine xenograft RV-to-PA conduits as pulmonary valve replacements in patients who would otherwise have important pulmonary incompetence due to lack of leaflet tissue or extent of right ventriculotomy, as the hemodynamic burden of residual AV valve and pulmonary valve incompetence may result in an unstable postoperative course.

ABSENT PULMONARY VALVE SYNDROME

Absent pulmonary valve syndrome (APVS) is considered by many to be a Fallot variant, although there are important differences. APVS is characterized by moderate pulmonary stenosis and severe incompetence, with variable (sometimes extreme) dilation of the main and branch PAs. The dilation usually extends to the main lobar branches in the lung hilum. The pulmonary valve is rudimentary, and the annulus is moderately hypoplastic. Intrinsic abnormalities of the PA wall and ventriculoarterial junction are also encountered. Some infants with APVS have tracheobronchomalacia and airway compression of the major lobar branches. Intrinsic airway and vascular abnormalities may extend to the level of the small bronchi. Repair may be required within the first few months of life if airway abnormalities are severe. In stable patients, the timing of surgery can be similar to that for elective repair of balanced TOF.

For APVS with massively dilated main and branch PAs (**Figure 49.9a**) the basic operative strategy consists of transatrial–transpulmonary repair, as outlined for TOF. An approach which we have favored in more recent years involves division of either the RPA or the aorta, full mobilization of the branch pulmonary arteries, and a modified Lecompte maneuver (anterior or preaortic translocation of the pulmonary arteries) (**Figure 49.9b and c**). Reduction-plasty of the branches may not be necessary in all cases if the Lecompte maneuver is employed. The RPA (or aorta) is then reconstructed, and central tracheobronchial compression is thereby reduced. A bovine xenograft valved conduit is then used to reconstruct the RVOT, as continued pulmonary insufficiency may contribute to further dilation of the abnormal PAs. The Sung repair may not be effective in APVS due to lack of native leaflet tissue.

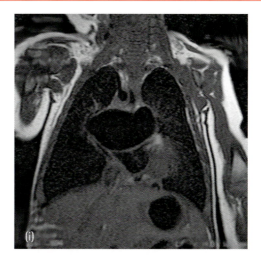

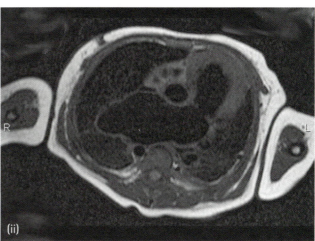

49.9a

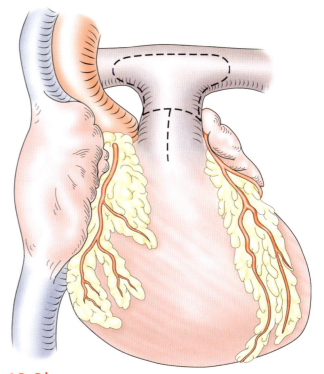

49.9b

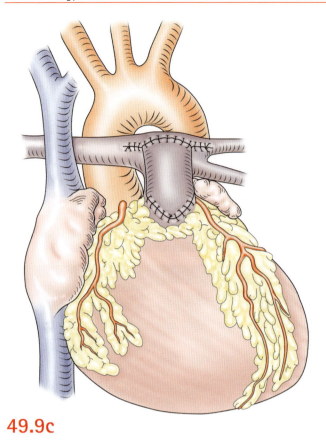

49.9c

The postoperative course may be difficult in infants with APVS, with a requirement for prolonged ventilator support due to established tracheobronchomalacia.

OLDER PATIENTS WITH TETRALOGY OF FALLOT

In some less-developed parts of the world, cardiac surgical teams may be faced with very late diagnosis or referral of patients with TOF. Teams receiving and treating patients from such areas face similar problems. Typically, older patients may present with four different clinical scenarios:

- *Patients who have been previously well palliated with an additional blood supply (e.g. a Blalock–Taussig or Waterston shunt).* The LV has been adequately volume loaded, and the RV is hypertrophied but well developed, so that can be undertaken at minimal risk. An aortogram may be indicated to exclude the presence of aortopulmonary collaterals. Attention to the possibility of left PA (previous Waterston shunt) or right PA (previous Blalock–Taussig shunt) distortion is advised.
- *Patients who have had no palliation but are minimally cyanotic.* The anatomy is usually that of predominantly valvular stenosis with well-developed PA branches. The repair as described is well tolerated, and the postoperative course is fairly simple. These patients can be quite old by TOF standards, even up into the fifth decade of life.
- *Patients who have had no palliation and are deeply cyanotic.* SaO_2 is less than 70%, and hematocrit may be greater than 65%. The anatomy is usually favorable for a repair, with

well-developed PA branches and predominantly severe infundibular stenosis. However, complete repair may be contraindicated in some cases, as the risk is significantly higher than that of patients with other clinical presentations. The threshold for temporary palliation depends on the culture of the unit, past experience with such patients, and the availability of reliable extracorporeal life support. In this group, the LV can be small relative to the RV and, at times, very echogenic, with depressed function. A very small heart on the chest X-ray is suggestive of very low Qp:Qs, with total systemic flow supported by two ventricles.

The RV may not adapt to receive a full cardiac output postoperatively. The pathophysiology of right or global ventricular failure after total repair in such cases is multifactorial. High LV preload may be required, which may not be tolerated by the failing RV, especially in the presence of a PI and/or TI. The failure of the RV can be systolic, diastolic, or both. Underdevelopment of the pulmonary lymphatic system may contribute to pulmonary edema with moderately elevated left atrial pressure. LV failure can be due to intrinsic myocardial properties or to the shift of the septum to the left. The systemic resistances are low preoperatively (as an adaptation to the high blood viscosity), and they may remain pathologically low postoperatively. The role of an atrial septal defect placed initially or after the onset of the failure is not clear, and may not prevent or solve all of the above problems. Finally, CPB for patients with extremely high hematocrit is challenging in terms of blood viscosity, hemostasis, and systemic resistance.

All these risk factors can be neutralized to a large extent by a systemic–PA shunt or a percutaneous pulmonary valvotomy for a period of a few weeks to a few months, associated with a cautious hemodilution.

- *Patients deeply cyanotic after a very recent history of deterioration.* Bronchopulmonary infection, viral or bacterial pneumonitis, and endocarditis must be ruled out with certainty before total repair can be undertaken. In the presence of infection and persistent life-threatening cyanosis, palliation is indicated, and total repair is usually delayed. The risk–benefit ratio of a shunt over a total repair, even in a compromised patient, is a subject of ongoing debate, and individual patient factors must be taken into account.

POSTOPERATIVE CARE

Basic principles of postoperative management for infants apply. Low-dose inotropic support (dopamine 5 μg/kg/minute) and a period of mechanical ventilation may be required, but early extubation is usually preferable. We extubate our patients in the operating theatre in about two-thirds of cases. The main problems encountered are moderately low cardiac output due to right heart failure and atrial arrhythmias. Both may be due to a combination of factors, including systemic inflammatory response, RV damage during resection and ventriculotomy, induced tricuspid insufficiency, and intrinsic myocardial abnormalities specific to TOF. RV pressure may be greater than 50% of LV pressure transiently after transatrial–transpulmonary repair, due to high endogenous catecholamine levels. These problems are usually self-limited, and most infants can be supported with fluid restriction, diuretics, low-dose inotropes, and avoidance of excessive beta agonist stimulation. In all cases with persistent hemodynamic problems, an assiduous search should be made for a residual VSD and/or anatomical components of RVOTO, which may require early revision.

CONTEMPORARY RESULTS OF TETRALOGY REPAIR

TOF repair

In the Congenital Databases of both the Society of Thoracic Surgeons (STS) (n = 2535) and European Congenital Heart Surgeons Association (ECHSA) (n = 6654), the transventricular approach to TOF repair remains prevalent (53% and 57.5% respectively). Thirty-day and hospital mortality for TOF repair in the ECHSA Congenital Database is summarized in **Table 49.1**, stratified by anatomic variant and repair type (current to February 2018).

Table 49.1 Thirty-day and hospital mortality for TOF repair in the ECHSA Congenital Database

Operation	n	30–day mortality (%)	Hospital mortality (%)
TOF repair, right ventriculotomy, transannular patch	8354	2.4	2.62
TOF repair, right ventriculotomy, non-transannular patch	2875	1.32	1.43
TOF + atrioventricular septal defect repair	390	10.03	11.05
Absent pulmonary valve syndrome repair	387	9.3	12.66

TOF with AVSD

In general, while the early results in the current era are excellent, the mid- to long-term results in this group of patients are less favorable. A 2012 report from the Royal Children's Hospital (RCH), Melbourne, summarized a 30-year experience (1980 to 2010). Forty-eight consecutive patients with AVSD and TOF (n = 26) or double-outlet right ventricle (DORV) (n = 22) were operated at a median age of 1.8 years (0.2-14.8 years). Previous palliative procedures were performed in 40% of patients and 60% had trisomy 21. The preferred technique was the transatrial–transpulmonary approach using two patches (for the AVSD), and 43% of patients required a transannular incision. There were four hospital deaths (8.4%), two of which were related to repair of the left AV valve. The

actuarial survival was 82% at 2 years, 76% at 5 years and 71% at 20 years. The overall freedom from reoperation was 65% at 2 years, and 55% at both 5 years and 20 years. The main reoperative indication was left AV valve insufficiency.

TOF with abnormal coronary artery

Using the transatrial–transpulmonary repair, results for patients with an abnormal coronary artery crossing the RVOT have been favorable. Operative risk for 36 such patients (operated at the RCH, Melbourne) was 0% (95% confidence interval 0–11%), with a late RV-to-PA gradient of ±19 mm. The presence of an anomalous coronary was not a risk factor for poor outcome, either early or late after repair.

Absent pulmonary valve syndrome

Results for APVS have improved considerably in recent years but early outcome continues to be influenced adversely by the presence of tracheomalacia and the need for preoperative ventilation. Late results are also less favorable.

In 2007, results from Toronto were reported for 62 consecutive patients following repair of APVS (1982–2006) at a median age of 1.4 years. A third of patients required preoperative ventilation. Nearly all patients had a valve implanted in the RVOT and half underwent pulmonary artery plication or reduction. There were three (5%) early deaths, all before 1995. Seven infants with persistent postoperative airway obstruction required additional airway interventions in the early postoperative period. Prolonged ventilation was more frequently required in neonates and in those who required preoperative ventilation. The mean ICU stay for neonates was more than 1 month. Five- and 10-year survival probability was 93% and 87%.

The RCH, Melbourne, experience in 36 consecutive patients was reported in 2006. The proportion of patients requiring preoperative ventilation was 28%, and median age at repair was 0.8 years. Forty-seven per cent of patients had a valve inserted in the RVOT and 86% underwent pulmonary artery reduction-plasty. There were five hospital deaths (14%), and actuarial survival was 82% at 1 year and 79% at 5, 10, and 15 years. Postoperative survival was adversely affected by preoperative ventilator dependency (50% mortality). At a median follow-up of 9.2 years, 11% of patients were in NYHA 3. None of the 17 patients without a valve in the pulmonary position required reoperation at a median follow-up of 13.7 years.

LONG–TERM OUTCOME

Lillehei himself published results for 106 hospital survivors, six of whom were operated with cross-circulation. The 30-year survival probability was 77%, with a 91% freedom from reoperation.

Nollert et al. reported follow-up for 490 survivors of hospitalization, operated between 1958 and 1977. The 10-, 20-, 30-, and 36-year survival probabilities were 97%, 94%, 89%, and 85%. The annualized risk of death increased from 0.0024 to 0.0094 during the follow-up period, primarily due to congestive heart failure or (presumed) arrhythmia. Mortality risk factors were operation before 1970, polycythaemia, and the use of an RVOT patch ($P < 0.01$). For patients without these risk factors ($n = 164$), the 36-year actuarial survival probability was 96%.

In 1998, Knott-Craig et al. reported a 20-year postoperative survival probability of 98% for 294 tetralogy patients. Primary complete repair was done in 199 patients (68%), and a staged repair in 62 patients (21%). The freedom from reintervention at latest follow-up was 85% in patients who received a primary repair and 91% in those who had a staged repair. Additionally, there was no increased risk of reintervention in the group of patients who were repaired during infancy.

In 2001, Bacha et al. from Boston reported a series of 57 consecutive patients undergoing repair of TOF (1972–1977) at a median age of 8 months. The repair was performed through an infundibulotomy and 65% had a transannular patch. There were eight (14%) early deaths and one death 24 years after repair. Median follow-up was 23.5 years. Freedom from reintervention was 93% at 5 years and 79% at 20 years. Patients with a transannular patch required significantly fewer interventions. Only one patient required pulmonary valve implantation. Despite pulmonary regurgitation, 41 (84%) of 49 long-term survivors were in NYHA class 1. Actuarial survival was 86% at 20 years.

A recent comprehensive long-term study from Rotterdam included 144 patients with a minimum postoperative follow-up time of 30 years (median 36 years). The survival probability at 40 years was 72% (25% event-free survival).

Contemporary results for the Sung repair of TOF have been favorable in terms of preservation of PV and RV function at mid-term, as documented in several series from Korea, India, and the USA. This technique is straightforward and reproducible, and is currently preferred by the authors and most of their trainees for the majority of TOF cases.

CONCLUSION

In conclusion, although some problems remain unsolved, surgical treatment has effectively altered the natural history for all Fallot variants. The most problematic patients are those with AVSD and APVS. The long-term outlook for less complex cases, even those with a coronary artery crossing the RVOT, is excellent.

FURTHER READING

Alsoufi B, Williams WG, Hua Z, et al. Surgical outcomes in the treatment of patients with tetralogy of Fallot and absent pulmonary valve. *Eur J Cardiothorac Surg.* 2007; 31(3): 354–9.

Anagnostopoulos P, Nolke L, Alphonso N, et al. Pulmonary valve cusp augmentation may improve results for repair of tetralogy of Fallot. *Ann Thorac Surg.* 2007; 83: 1458–62.

Bacha EA, Scheule AM, Zurakow D, et al. Long-term results after early primary repair of tetralogy of Fallot. *J Thorac Cardiovasc Surg.* 2001; 122: 154–61.

Brizard CPR, Sohn YS, Mas C, et al. Trans-atrial trans-pulmonary repair of tetralogy of Fallot with anomalous coronary arteries. *J Thorac Cardiovasc Surg.* 1998; 116: 770–9.

Cuypers JA, Menting ME, Konings EE, et al. Unnatural history of tetralogy of Fallot: prospective follow-up of 40 years after surgical correction. *Circulation.* 2014; 130: 1944–53.

Dharmapuram A, Ramadoss N, Verma S, et al. Preliminary experience with the use of an extracellular matrix to augment the native pulmonary valve during repair of tetralogy of Fallot. *World J Pediatr Congenit Heart Surg.* 2017; 8: 174–81.

European Congenital Heart Surgeons Association (ECHSA) Congenital Database: www.echsacongenitaldb.org

Geva T. Tetralogy of Fallot repair: ready for a new paradigm. *J Thorac Cardiovasc Surg.* 2012; 143: 1305–6.

Karl TR. Tetralogy of Fallot. In: Laks H (ed.). *Glenn's thoracic & cardiovascular surgery, Vol 2.* 6th edn. New York: Appleton-Century-Crofts; 1995: pp. 1345–67.

Karl TR. Atrioventricular septal defect with tetralogy of Fallot or double outlet right ventricle: surgical considerations. *Semin Thorac Cardiovasc Surg.* 1997; 9: 26–34.

Karl TR. Tetralogy of Fallot: current surgical perspective. *J Pediatrics.* 2008; 1: 93–100.

Karl TR, Provenzano SC, Nunn GR, Anderson RH. The current surgical perspective to repair of atrioventricular septal defect with common atrioventricular junction. *Cardiol Young.* 2010; 20(Suppl 3): 120–7.

Karl TR, Sano S, Pornvilawan S, Mee RBB. Transatrial transpulmonary repair of tetralogy of Fallot: favourable outcome of non-neonatal repair. *Ann Thorac Surg.* 1992; 54: 903–7.

Kim H, Sung SC, Choi KH, et al. Long-term results of pulmonary valve annular enlargement with valve repair in tetralogy of Fallot. *Eur J Cardiothorac Surg.* 2018; 53(6): 1223–9.

Knott-Craig CJ, Elkins RC, Lane MM, et al. A 26-year experience with surgical management of tetralogy of Fallot: risk analysis for mortality or late reintervention. *Ann Thorac Surg.* 1998; 66: 506–11.

Kopic S, Stephensen SS, Heiberg E, et al. Isolated pulmonary regurgitation causes decreased right ventricular longitudinal function and compensatory increased septal pumping in a porcine model. *Acta Physiol.* 2017; 221: 163–73.

Lillehei CW, Varco RL, Cohen M, et al. The first open heart corrections of tetralogy of Fallot: a 26–31 year follow-up of 106 patients. *Ann Surg.* 1986; 204: 490–502.

Mertens LL. Right ventricular remodelling after tetralogy of Fallot repair: new insights from longitudinal follow-up data. *Eur Heart J Cardiovasc Imaging.* 2017; 18: 371–2.

Nölke L, Azakie A, Anagnostopoulos PV, et al. The Lecompte maneuver for relief of airway compression in absent pulmonary valve syndrome. *Ann Thorac Surg.* 2006; 81: 1802–7.

Nollert G, Fischlein T, Bouterwek S, et al. Long-term survival in patients with repair of tetralogy of Fallot: 36-year follow-up of 490 survivors of the first year after surgical repair. *J Am Coll Cardiol.* 1997; 30: 1374–83.

Norgaard MA, Alphonso N, Newcombe AE, et al. Absent pulmonary valve syndrome: surgical and clinical outcome with long-term follow-up. *Eur J Cardiothorac Surg.* 2006; 29: 682–7.

Ong J, Brizard CP, d'Ukedem, et al. Repair of atrioventricular septal defect associated with tetralogy of Fallot or double-outlet right ventricle: 30 years of experience. *Ann Thorac Surg.* 2012; 94: 172–8.

Sarris GE, Comas JV, Tobota Z, Maruszewski B. Results of reparative surgery for tetralogy of Fallot: data from the European Association for Cardio-Thoracic Surgery Congenital Database. *Eur J Cardiothorac Surg.* 2012; 42: 766–74.

50

Pulmonary atresia with ventricular septal defect

MICHAEL MA AND FRANK L. HANLEY

HISTORY

Definition

Pulmonary atresia with ventricular septal defect (PA-VSD) is an uncommon complex congenital cardiac lesion in which no luminal continuity exists between the right ventricle (RV) and the pulmonary arteries. PA-VSD represents the most severe end of the spectrum of Tetralogy of Fallot and is often referred to as "Tetralogy of Fallot with pulmonary atresia." The intracardiac anatomy is consistent and similar to that of Tetralogy of Fallot with an anteriorly malaligned VSD, a well-developed left ventricle (LV), and a variable degree of RV infundibular hypoplasia. The extracardiac pulmonary blood supply, however, has great morphological variability as a hallmark characteristic.

Collaterals

Blood flow to the lungs is supplied from the systemic arterial circulation via a patent ductus arteriosus (PDA) or aortopulmonary collaterals. This feature represents the greatest challenge to surgical reconstruction. If a PDA is present, normally sized and arborizing confluent pulmonary arteries are typically found. Surgical repair is relatively straightforward, with closure of the VSD, ligation of the PDA, and creation of unobstructed continuity between the RV and central pulmonary arterial system. When the ductus arteriosus is absent, major aortopulmonary collateral arteries (MAPCAs) provide systemic blood flow to the lungs. Great variation in the number, origin, size, course, and destination of these MAPCAs exists. MAPCAs frequently have intrinsic stenoses. Additionally, MAPCAs may be the exclusive source of blood flow to both lungs, one or more lobes of each lung, or particular lung segments, or they may be part of a dual supply along with the true pulmonary arteries. The morphology of the true pulmonary arteries themselves varies widely, ranging from complete absence to normal caliber, although typically they are markedly hypoplastic and centrally confluent, exhibiting distinct arborization abnormalities. The

morphological and physiological details of the true pulmonary arteries and MAPCAs are of critical importance in designing the reconstructive operation.

Because of the morphological and physiological complexity of the pulmonary blood supply in PA-VSD/MAPCAs, attempts at surgical repair have been undertaken only relatively recently. Before the 1980s, this entity was considered inoperable. In the 1980s, several groups began to approach the lesion using multiple-staged palliative procedures. In 1995, a systematic approach for one-stage complete repair, including reconstruction of the pulmonary blood supply and intracardiac repair, was described.

PRINCIPLES AND JUSTIFICATION

The natural history of PA-VSD hinges on the adequacy of pulmonary blood flow. Based on this principle, patients can be loosely categorized into three anatomical subgroups. Patients with well-developed confluent pulmonary arteries and a large PDA represent 50% of those with PA-VSD. With the ductus arteriosus as the sole or dominant source of pulmonary blood flow, these infants typically present soon after birth with profound cyanosis as the ductus closes. Due to the ductal-dependent source of the pulmonary blood flow, 90% die within the first year of life if untreated. The second category, representing 25% of patients, have moderately developed pulmonary arteries with a moderate number of MAPCAs. Clinical presentation may be later in life compared to that of the first group, but the majority become symptomatic within the first year. Untreated, mortality approaches 90% by the tenth year of life. The third category, representing 25%, are those patients with extremely hypoplastic or absent central pulmonary arteries and extensive systemic collaterals to the lungs. Presentation may be delayed beyond early infancy. Patients in this anatomical subgroup also typically present within the first year of life with cyanosis. However, these patients generally have a longer life expectancy if untreated, with mortality near 90% by the third decade of life. Conversely, in a small number of cases with large aortopulmonary collaterals and few stenoses, the clinical presentation may be with heart failure rather than cyanosis, which develops at 4–6 weeks of life as pulmonary vascular resistance falls. However, many patients with MAPCAs do not fall easily within specific categories, but rather the morphological variability of the pulmonary arteries and MAPCAs describes a spectrum.

The size of the central pulmonary arteries may vary from complete absence to normal size. This situation depends on the degree of communication between the MAPCAs and the pulmonary arteries. Non-confluent right and left pulmonary arteries are found in approximately 30% of cases. A particular segment of the lung may receive blood flow solely by either the true pulmonary arteries or the aortopulmonary collaterals, or dually by both. Connections between the two systems may be located at central or peripheral points and at single or multiple sites. Although collaterals originate most commonly from the anterior aspect of the descending thoracic aorta, they may also arise from the ascending aorta, transverse aortic arch major neck branches of the aorta, the intercostal or coronary arteries or rarely from the abdominal aorta or its branches.

MAPCA stenoses commonly follow a course of progression to severe stenosis or occlusion. Stenoses may play an early protective role in preventing overcirculation and development of hypertensive pulmonary vascular disease, but, untreated, they often result in distal arterial hypoplasia and underdevelopment of its supplied lung segment. When stenoses are absent or mild, unrestricted systemic pulmonary blood flow at systemic pressures can promote pulmonary vascular disease in those patients surviving beyond infancy.

Surgical goals

The ultimate surgical goal in repair of PA-VSD is to establish completely separated, in-series pulmonary and systemic circulations, with the lowest possible pressure in the RV. Achieving these goals is based on four objectives. First, the true pulmonary arteries and MAPCAs must be "unifocalized," with a goal of achieving the maximal possible cross-sectional "neopulmonary" artery area to supply the total pulmonary capillary bed. Second, reconstruction of the central pulmonary arteries may be required, depending on the extent of central pulmonary hypoplasia. Third, RV-to-pulmonary artery continuity must be established via right ventriculotomy and placement of a valved conduit. Fourth, the VSD is closed to separate the systemic and pulmonary circulations.

The actual repair performed is tailored to the individual patient based on the morphological severity of the defect. The most important physiological factor signifying a favorable outcome after complete repair is the postrepair peak RV pressure, which should be as low as possible. This factor is dependent on the number of lung segments unifocalized, the status of the pulmonary microvasculature in those segments, and the absence of obstruction in the pathway from the RV to the lung microvasculature.

Staged approach

The traditional surgical approach to the management of PA-VSD has generally been based on the concept of staged unifocalization of the pulmonary blood supply, followed by central pulmonary artery reconstruction and VSD closure, thus requiring multiple operations before complete repair is achieved. Although associated with excellent long-term results in selected patients, this approach has a number of theoretical and practical disadvantages.

- Multiple procedures are required to achieve complete repair, including thoracotomy to access the lung hilum for peripheral pulmonary arterial reconstruction.
- Staged repair results in delay in achieving normal circulatory physiology.
- Iatrogenic loss of lung segments often occurs by occlusion using a staged approach.
- Some lung segments may be exposed for long periods to high-pressure MAPCAs.
- Peripheral conduits have no growth potential and tend to calcify, leading to difficulty in centralizing these grafts when reconstructing the RV outflow tract from a midline approach at a subsequent operation.

Rationale for one-stage repair

The longer a given lung segment is exposed to MAPCA physiology, the higher the likelihood that it will develop either hypertensive pulmonary vascular obstructive disease or will atrophy. Because stenoses with MAPCAs progress over time, even a vessel with the perfect degree of stenosis at birth will not remain that way. The pulmonary vascular bed is healthiest at birth and declines thereafter. Thus, the earlier the repair can be made, the greater the chance of incorporating the largest number of healthy lung segments into the unifocalized pulmonary circuit. The number of lung segments recruited into the pulmonary arterial system correlates strongly with low postrepair pulmonary arterial pressures and calculated pulmonary vascular resistance.

Based on this argument, we have adopted a strategy of early complete unifocalization of the pulmonary blood flow with intracardiac repair and an RV-to-pulmonary artery conduit in a single stage as the procedure of choice for repair of PA-VSD. Prosthetic material in the lung periphery is eliminated with a single-stage approach. Native tissue-to-tissue apposition provides better theoretical growth potential and is given priority in planning reconstruction. The ideal age of repair of this lesion is unknown. If the patient is well balanced physiologically, we prefer to perform this procedure at 3–4 months of age. However, if the patient is severely cyanotic or is overshunted and in heart failure, repair is feasible as early as the first week of life.

The morphological variability of the lesion, the timing of referral, and prior interventions sometimes preclude adoption of a single-stage approach. In patients whose collaterals are not adequate to allow one cardiac output because of distal stenosis, either naturally occurring or secondary to shunt procedures, we prefer to completely unifocalize the collaterals but not close the VSD. In the small subgroup of patients with small true pulmonary arteries and a paucity of MAPCAs, we have performed an aortopulmonary window as a palliative step to promote growth of the pulmonary arteries and facilitate later repair. Very rarely unifocalization is performed electively in stages via thoracotomy.

PREOPERATIVE ASSESSMENT AND PREPARATION

Investigation and decision-making

Echocardiography provides the initial diagnosis and identifies any additional associated cardiac malformations. The echocardiographic appearance of PA-VSD is similar to that of Tetralogy of Fallot but differs in lack of continuity between the RV and pulmonary artery. Difficulty may exist in delineating the presence and extent of the true pulmonary arteries or the sources of systemic arterial supply with echocardiography. Because of this deficiency, detailed angiography is essential in all cases to clearly assess the anatomical and hemodynamic characteristics of the true pulmonary arteries and MAPCAs and to plan the optimal surgical management of patients. Angiography provides critical information regarding MAPCA numbers, size, location, presence and location of stenoses, and sites of communication with the true pulmonary arteries (see Figure 50.1). Each MAPCA is selectively injected to demonstrate whether it connects with a true pulmonary artery or enters the lung parenchyma as a sole supply to a particular lung segment. Identification of stenoses and pressure measurements is important. Pulmonary vein wedge angiography may be useful to visualize the central pulmonary arteries. In selected cases with well-developed confluent central pulmonary arteries and a large PDA, angiography may not be required. However, one should be certain that no evidence of significant collateral vessels is seen by echocardiography.

Angiography or CT scan is performed at diagnosis in the neonatal period to define the anatomy of the pulmonary arteries and MAPCAs and to identify ductal tissue. If ductal tissue is present with MAPCAs, the ductus typically provides flow to either the left or right pulmonary artery. In these cases, neonatal repair is undertaken, as the entire ductal-dependent lung is in jeopardy of being lost if surgery is delayed. If surgery is electively scheduled at 3–4 months of age, then repeat angiography is mandatory, because new stenoses may develop.

Preparation

Thorough preoperative planning of MAPCA reconstruction is a necessity. One must have a "mental image" of MAPCA numbers, origins, and courses before surgery, as well as an idea of how they may be best unifocalized. Selected angiographic images or cineangiograms may be helpful to have available for review during the reconstruction. The total cross-sectional area of the neopulmonary arterial unifocalization is the most important determinant of the postrepair RV/LV pressure ratio (pRV/pLV); however, flawless technical execution of the unifocalization procedure is also necessary, as poorly constructed anastomoses and/or kinking of unifocalized MAPCAs can add critical amounts of resistance to the pulmonary vascular circuit.

If the patient is ductal-dependent, infusion of prostaglandin E_1 maintains stability before surgery. Ductal closure results in hypoxemia and cyanosis and necessitates emergent repair if adequate systemic collateral vessels are absent. In contrast, in the few cases with a large PDA or collateral shunt, patients may manifest clinical features of congestive heart failure. To optimize the preoperative pulmonary status, diuresis, inotropic support, and mechanical ventilation may be needed.

EXAMPLE CASE

Figure 50.1 shows a case that illustrates the importance of careful angiography in a characteristically complex and heterogeneous anomaly. This patient has multiple unusual collaterals to the right lung and a single collateral to the left lung. No true central pulmonary arteries are

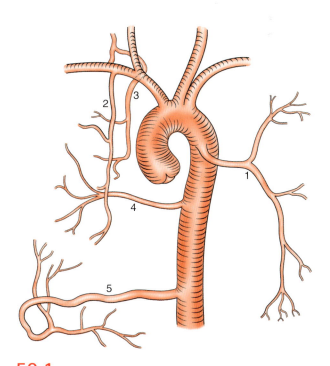

50.1

present. The left lung is supplied by a single collateral (1) originating from the lower aspect of the aortic arch. This collateral arborizes into a near-normal pulmonary arterial pattern to supply all segments of the left lung. This supply was originally thought to be of ductal origin, but intraoperative findings failed to demonstrate the presence of the recurrent laryngeal nerve below its origin, thus confirming that this vessel is an embryological collateral rather than ductal tissue. The right lung is supplied by four collaterals without any segmental stenoses. A collateral of pericardiophrenic artery origin (2) arising from the internal mammary artery pedicle supplies three medial segments of the right lower lobe. A collateral originating from the thyrocervical trunk (3) supplies most middle and upper lobe segments. A small collateral from the descending aorta (4) supplies several medial lung segments. A dominant and large intercostal artery (5) originates from the descending aorta and travels to its lateral-most extent before penetrating the lung and branching to supply the majority of the right lower lobe. The collateral supply to the right lung in this case is similar to that seen in pulmonary sequestration. This patient underwent one-stage complete repair as a neonate.

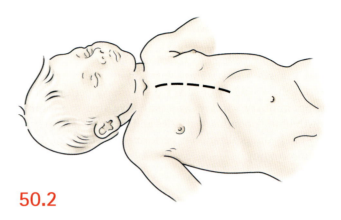

50.2

OPERATION

Incision and exposure

EXTENDED MIDLINE INCISION AND STERNOTOMY, SUBTOTAL THYMECTOMY

Wide exposure is obtained by extended midline incision and median sternotomy (**Figure 50.2**). Combined with generous sternal retraction, this approach improves exposure of both lungs. A subtotal thymectomy is performed, and both pleural spaces are opened widely. Care is taken to avoid the phrenic nerves, particularly where they are located more anteriorly in the upper mediastinum.

WIDE HARVEST OF PERICARDIAL PATCH, PERICARDIAL EDGES SUSPENDED

A large anterior patch of pericardium is harvested, and the pericardial edges are suspended with stay sutures (**Figure 50.3**). These sutures can then be moved and pinned appropriately to greatly improve exposure and facilitate hilar dissection in both lungs.

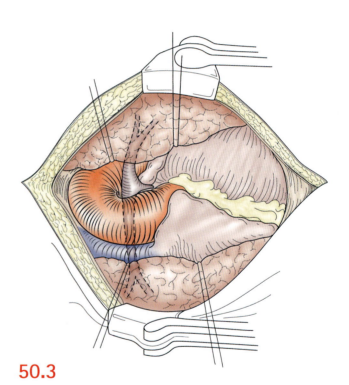

50.3

Mediastinal dissection

MEDIASTINAL DISSECTION OF TRUE PULMONARY ARTERIES AND MAJOR AORTOPULMONARY COLLATERAL ARTERY ORIGINS

The aorta and central pulmonary arteries (if present) are widely dissected (**Figure 50.4**). Extensive dissection is performed in the posterior mediastinal space superior to the left atrium (asterisk in **Figure 50.4**). This critical maneuver provides space for mobility during relocation of collateral vessels. This area is best approached through the space between the aorta and superior vena cava. The transverse sinus is widely opened, and the posterior mediastinal soft tissues are dissected. The central collaterals are identified and dissected over their entire course, extending toward their aortic origins. The descending aorta itself is dissected as needed in the posterior mediastinal space to expose MAPCA origins. Any further collaterals in the subcarinal space from the proximal descending aorta, transverse aortic arch, and ascending aorta are identified and dissected.

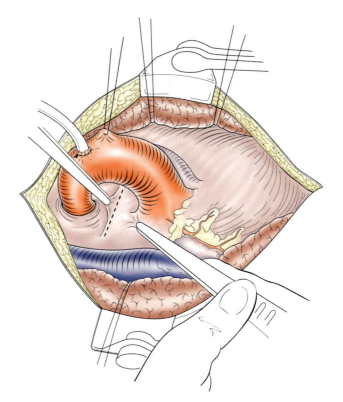

50.5a

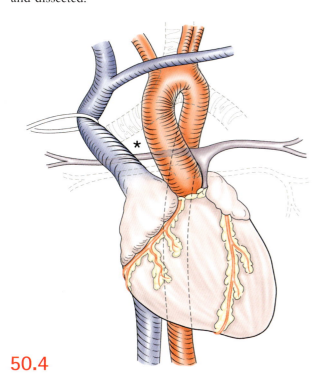

50.4

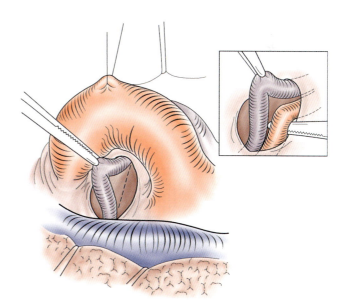

50.5b

RIGHT HILAR DISSECTION

The right lung is left *in situ*, and the right pulmonary artery is dissected as peripherally into the hilum as possible (**Figure 50.5a**). This dissection usually extends into the lung parenchyma to the first- or second-level bifurcation of the true pulmonary artery. The right collaterals are identified and mobilized into the hilum (**Figure 50.5b**). This step is often achieved as a natural progression of the central mediastinal dissection. At times, however, the right lung is retracted anteriorly out of the right chest cavity, and the collateral is dissected along its posterior route into the right hilum.

LEFT HILAR DISSECTION

The left lung is left *in situ,* and the left pulmonary artery is dissected as peripherally into the hilum as possible, similar to right lung dissection (**Figure 50.6a**). The left collaterals are identified and mobilized into the hilum (**Figure 50.6b**).

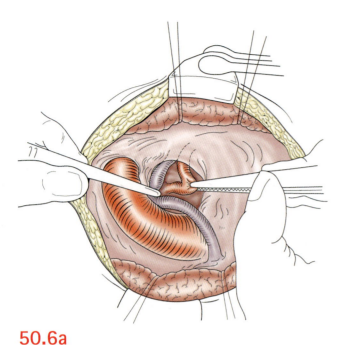

50.6a

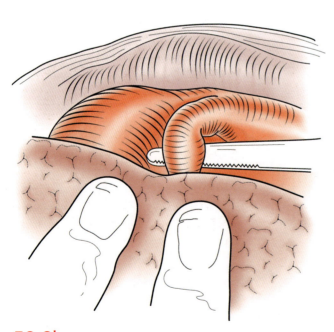

50.6b

Institution of cardiopulmonary bypass and control of collaterals

All collaterals are identified, dissected completely, and controlled with vessel loops before initiation of cardiopulmonary bypass (CPB) (**Figure 50.7**). This approach prevents damaging pump flow run-off into the lungs and maximizes systemic perfusion. The patient is systemically heparinized and prepared for aortic and bicaval cannulation. Before initiating CPB, as many collaterals as possible are permanently ligated at their origin, mobilized, and unifocalized to minimize pump time. When oxygen saturations approach a compromising level, the remaining MAPCAs are snared or occluded, the patient is cannulated, and CPB is initiated. The remainder of the collaterals are then unifocalized at mild to moderate hypothermia with the heart beating.

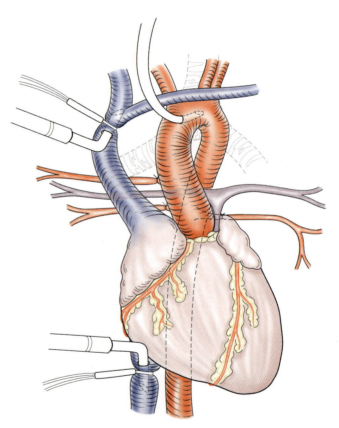

50.7

Peripheral unifocalization

ANASTOMOTIC TECHNIQUES TO MAXIMIZE NEOPULMONARY ARTERY CROSS-SECTIONAL AREA

Achieving the best reconstruction depends on advanced planning, flexibility in reconstruction, aggressive mobilization, and creative rerouting of MAPCAs. Reconstruction of the pulmonary arteries is performed with the highest priority given to maximally using the length of the MAPCAs in the anastomoses, preservation of autologous tissue apposition, and avoidance or minimizing use of synthetic conduits or allograft tissue in the periphery. Non-absorbable fine (7-0 or 8-0) monofilament suture is used for anastomoses. Mobilized collaterals are typically routed through the transverse sinus and delivered to the true pulmonary arteries for subsequent unifocalization; however, occasionally they are best routed above the hilum. Even collaterals that are part of a dual supply to a lung segment also supplied by a native pulmonary artery are often unifocalized to maximize the cross-sectional area of the reconstructed neopulmonary arteries. Techniques that generally maximize the neopulmonary artery area include the following (illustrated in **Figure 50.8**):

1. Side-to-side anastomosis of collaterals to central pulmonary artery (augments the hypoplastic central pulmonary artery)
2. Side-to-side anastomosis of collateral to collateral
3. End-to-side collateral to peripheral native pulmonary artery
4. End-to-side collateral to collateral
5. End-to-end or end-to-side of collateral to central allograft conduit
6. Allograft patch augmentation of collateral stenosis
7. Button of aorta giving rise to multiple unobstructed collaterals to native pulmonary arteries
8. Reconstruction of neocentral pulmonary arteries with allograft tissue patch.

The use of allograft tissue patch material is common; however, a patch is used non-circumferentially to augment the

central pulmonary arteries out to the level of the hilum on both sides so that the growth potential of the native tissue is maintained. Rarely, the central pulmonary arteries are of adequate size, and patch augmentation is unnecessary.

EXAMPLE CASE

Figure 50.9 illustrates the completed unifocalization of the case illustrated earlier in **Figure 50.1**. Collateral 2 was taken from its origin and transposed across the central mediastinum to create central continuity with the left lung collateral. The remaining right-sided collaterals were carefully anastomosed to collateral 2 to create an unifocalized right-lung vascular supply. A central pulmonary arterial augmentation was created with homograft patch material.

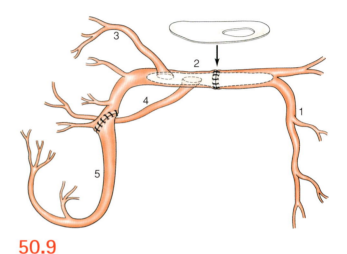

50.9

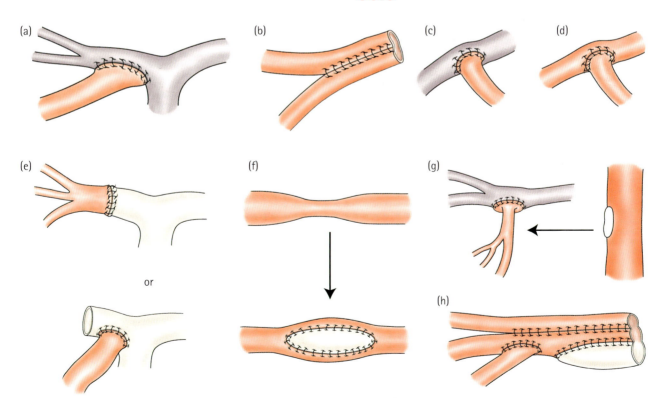

50.8a–h

INTRAOPERATIVE FLOW STUDY

At this point, a decision must be made regarding VSD closure and conduit placement. In patients who are completely unifocalized, the total resistance of the neopulmonary artery vascular bed is estimated by an intraoperative flow study. After complete unifocalization, while the patient is still supported by bypass, a pulmonary artery (PA) pressure catheter and a perfusion cannula are placed through the allograft conduit into the central neopulmonary bed. The left atrium is vigorously vented (**Figure 50.10**). Incremental volumes of gradually increasing blood flow up to at least one cardiac index ($3.0\,L/min/m^2$) are pumped through the unifocalized pulmonary arteries with the use of a standard roller pump. Mean pulmonary artery pressures are recorded at each steady state. If the pulmonary arterial pressure is less than or equal to $25\,mmHg$ at a flow equivalent to one cardiac output, a decision is made to close the VSD and establish antegrade

RV to PA connection. If the flow study demonstrates elevated neopulmonary vascular resistance, an appropriately sized central shunt from ascending aorta to neopulmonary bed is created and the patient weaned from cardiopulmonary bypass.

RIGHT VENTRICULOTOMY AND CLOSURE OF THE VSD

The aorta is cross-clamped, and cardioplegia is administered. A longitudinal ventriulotomy is made in the RV infundibulum. The anatomy of the infundibulum is inspected, and any obstructive tissue and/or hypertrophic muscle bundles are resected. The VSD is closed through the ventriculotomy with a bovine or glutaraldehyde-treated autologous pericardial patch using pledgeted, braided, polyester interrupted mattress sutures or running non-absorbable monofilament sutures, as preferred (**Figure 50.11**). The right atrium is opened to inspect the atrial septum. If an atrial septal defect

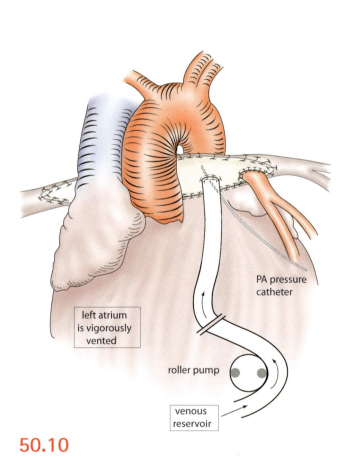

PA pressure catheter

left atrium is vigorously vented

roller pump

venous reservoir

50.10

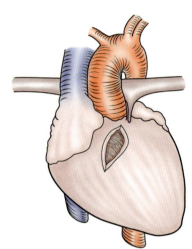

50.11a

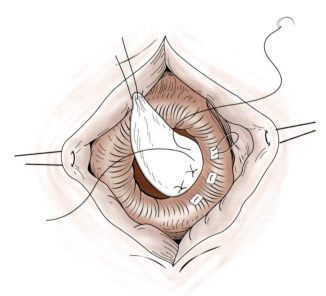

50.11b

or patent foramen ovale is present, it is closed. After right atrial closure, the cross-clamp is removed, and rewarming is started.

COMPLETION OF THE RV-TO-PULMONARY ARTERY CONDUIT AND CLOSURE

An appropriate-sized allograft valved conduit is then selected to connect the RV to the unifocalized neopulmonary arterial system. Because of the possibility of somewhat elevated right-sided pressures, an aortic allograft is preferred. The distal end is typically anastomosed end-to-side to the centrally augmented, reconstructed neopulmonary arteries (see **Figure 50.12a–f**). Rarely, a second non-valved conduit is needed to reconstruct the central left and right pulmonary arteries, usually in older patients with completely absent true pulmonary arteries and inadequate collateral tissue.

Circumferential allograft conduits are always limited to the pericardial cavity due to concerns over growth potential.

The proximal RV-to-pulmonary artery conduit anastomosis is completed with running non-absorbable monofilament suture. A pericardial or allograft tissue hood is fashioned to complete the infundibulotomy closure. A

pressure-monitoring line is placed through the right atrial free wall, across the tricuspid valve, to monitor the RV pressure.

After separation from CPB, the aortic, RV, and left and right atrial pressures are monitored continuously. Intraoperative transesophageal echocardiography is routinely performed. Bilateral pleural and mediastinal drains are placed, and the sternum is closed. If bleeding or ventilation is an issue, the sternum is electively covered with a silicone rubber patch (Silastic). Secondary closure is then performed on the second or third postoperative day.

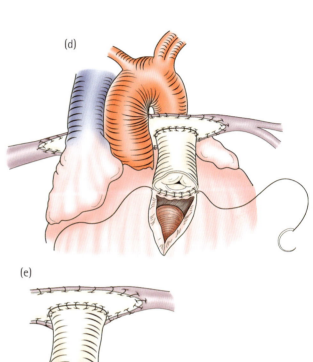

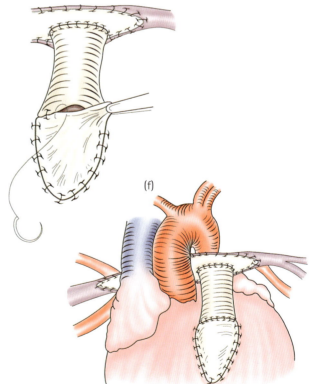

(a)
(b)
(c)
(d)
(e)
(f)

50.12a–c

50.12d–f

POSTOPERATIVE CARE AND FOLLOW-UP

RV pressure monitoring, as well as right and left atrial pressure monitoring, is routinely performed. Maneuvers to minimize the RV afterload and optimize pulmonary function include maintenance of a mild respiratory alkalosis and relatively high arterial oxygen concentrations, as pulmonary hypertension or high peak RV pressures are often an issue in the early postoperative period. Sedation and paralysis are maintained during the critical phase of the patient's recovery. Inotropic support is used routinely in the early postoperative period. Our typical regimen includes low-dose epinephrine, moderate-dose dopamine, and moderate-dose amrinone or milrinone.

Postoperative bleeding is managed similarly to that in other instances in which prolonged and extensive operations have been performed, with aggressive correction of coagulation abnormalities. Fresh frozen plasma, platelet, packed red blood cell transfusions, and anti-inhibitor coagulant complex may be required. Antifibrinolytic medications are not used because of concerns over thrombosis in the neopulmonary arterial circuit, which has many fresh suture lines.

Minor lung hemorrhage is common and is managed expectantly. Catastrophic bleeding is rare. Fiber-optic bronchoscopy is sometimes performed if evidence of tracheobronchial obstruction exists before the operation. Postoperative bronchoscopy is sometimes performed for pulmonary toilet or to rule out tracheobronchomalacia. Lung reperfusion injury is seen commonly and is almost always self-limiting. Injury has been limited to segments that are severely underperfused before unifocalization. Recovery is evident within the first few postoperative days.

Phrenic nerve injury often is not apparent until attempting to wean the patient from the ventilator. Phrenic nerve praxia is typically temporary, and the incidence has markedly diminished as we have gained experience with the operation. In an occasional patient, pulmonary vasoreactivity is of concern, and inhaled nitric oxide may be used. This problem is more prevalent older patients with an unprotected pulmonary vascular bed or large shunts. Monitoring of serum electrolytes, glucose, and hepatic enzymes in the perioperative period is strongly recommended, especially in the younger age groups. Splanchnic end-organ injury, manifested by acute hepatic insufficiency and, rarely, bowel necrosis, has been encountered on occasion in our experience.

Predischarge echocardiography and perfusion lung scanning are routinely performed in all patients and repeated at 6-month intervals thereafter. If the tricuspid regurgitation jet suggests elevated RV pressure and/or the lung scan shows maldistribution of flow, cardiac catheterization is performed promptly. Completely repaired patients are followed clinically and scheduled for cardiac catheterization approximately 1 year after surgery, or earlier if symptoms develop. Patients who do not undergo closure of the VSD and conduit placement at the time of the unifocalization are catheterized electively at 3 months postoperatively to assess the feasibility of complete repair. Growth of the unifocalized bed is visually assessed by angiography, and pulmonary artery pressures throughout the neopulmonary bed are measured. Further reconstruction can be performed as needed, until an adequate pulmonary vascular bed is achieved for complete repair.

OUTCOME

Early postoperative reactive airway problems resolve over several weeks. Lung function is otherwise normal in all patients. Due to the early postoperative lung issues, we have avoided repair in the neonatal period except in those who are severely overcirculated. In a recent report from our institution we reported 27 infants under 60 days of age who underwent complete repair and had excellent results with no early mortality. This is often due to MAPCAs, which are large and unobstructed.

The most commonly observed postoperative events in our series have included phrenic nerve palsy, pulmonary parenchymal reperfusion injury, pulmonary hemorrhage, and bronchospastic hyperreactivity. Bleeding requiring re-exploration has been minimized due to the use of delayed sternal closure and mediastinal packing in selected cases (rate less than 5%). Phrenic nerve praxia has been seen in approximately 5% of cases; however, the incidence has declined as experience has been gained. Diaphragmatic plication has been required in a few patients. The rate of reintervention for pulmonary arterial stenoses, either percutaneous or surgical, is approximately 20–30%. In our review of patients who underwent cardiac catheterization postoperatively at Stanford since 2002 we also found that the unifocalized collaterals grow and the RV pressure continues to be low.

RV-PA conduit obstruction occurs at the same rate as that for other procedures requiring RV outflow tract conduit reconstruction. The smaller conduits get replaced at an average of about 15 months after initial surgery and longevity is inversely proportional to the pulmonary artery pressure.

Our most recent single-center experience exceeds 450 patients, of which roughly 65% were primarily managed at our center, and 35% referred for secondary intervention after prior outside surgical intervention. At a median follow-up of 3.0 years (0.6–7.9 years), estimated Kaplan-Meier 5-year survival was 85% ± 2%. Eighty-three per cent of this cohort achieved complete repair (unifocalization with intracardiac septation) at one year, and 93% by five years. The median RV:LV pressure 0.35 (0.30–0.42), with only four patients persisting with an RV:LV > 0.6. Mortality subsequent to complete repair was influenced by chromosomal abnormalities, increasing age at repair, elevated RV pressure, RV:LV pressure > 0.35, and an increasing number of unifocalized MAPCAs. Prior outside interventions and presence/absence of native intrapericardial PAs did not influence survival.

FURTHER READING

Bauser-Heaton H, Borquez A, Han B, et al. Programmatic approach to management of Tetralogy of Fallot with major aortopulmonary collateral arteries: a 15-year experience with 458 patients. *Circ Cardiovasc Interv.* 2017; 10:e004952.

Carrillo SA, Mainwaring RD, Patrick WL, et al. Surgical repair of pulmonary atresia/ventricular septal defect/major aortopulmonary collaterals with absent intra-pericardial pulmonary arteries. *Ann Thorac Surg.* 2015; 100: 606-14.

Ma M, Mainwaring RD, Hanley FL. Comprehensive management of major aortopulmonary collaterals in the repair of Tetralogy of Fallot. *Semin Thorac Cardiovasc Surg Ann.* 2017; 21: 75-82.

Mainwaring RD, Patrick WL, Punn R, et al. Fate of right ventricular to pulmonary artery conduits after complete repair of pulmonary atresia and major aortopulmonary collaterals. *Ann Thorac Surg.* 2015; 99: 1685-91.

Mainwaring RD, Reddy VM, Peng L, et al. Hemodynamics assessment after complete repair of pulmonary atresia with major aortopulmonary collaterals. *Ann Thorac Surg.* 2013; 95: 1397-402.

Reddy VM, Liddicoat JR, Hanley FL. Midline one-stage complete unifocalization and repair of pulmonary atresia with ventricular septal defect and major aortopulmonary collaterals. *J Thorac Cardiovasc Surg.* 1995; 109: 832-45.

Reddy VM, Petrossian E, McElhinney DB, et al. One-stage complete unifocalization in infants: when should the ventricular septal defect be closed? *J Thorac Cardiovasc Surg.* 1997; 113: 858-68.

Watanabe N, Mainwaring RD, Reddy VM, et al. Early complete repair of pulmonary atresia with ventricular septal defect and major aortopulmonary collaterals. *Ann Thorac Surg.* 2014; 97: 909-15.

51

Right ventricular outflow tract obstruction with intact ventricular septum

STEPHANIE FULLER

INTRODUCTION TO PULMONARY STENOSIS AND PULMONARY ATRESIA

Although obstructive lesions of the right ventricular outflow tract (RVOT) are found in 25–30% of children with congenital heart disease such as atrial and ventricular septal defects, isolated pulmonary stenosis at the valvular level with an intact ventricular septum accounts for approximately 8–10% of all congenital heart defects. The clinical presentation is variable, ranging from asymptomatic mild stenosis to complete atresia of the pulmonary valve, occurring in approximately 4.5 per 100 000 live births. Common genetic syndromes associated with pulmonary stenosis include Noonan's, Williams, and Leopard syndromes.

The initial pathological description of pulmonary stenosis is credited to Morgagni in 1761 yet the first attempt at surgical treatment of this lesion was by Doyen in 1913. The report describes a transventricular valvotomy using a tenotomy knife with an unsuccessful outcome. Subsequent reports followed in 1948 by Sellors and Brock describing successful blunt valve dilatation using a transventricular approach. Several successful reports of open pulmonary valvotomy using systemic hypothermia and ventricular fibrillation followed. In 1953, with the advent of cardiopulmonary bypass (CPB), open pulmonary valvotomy was introduced as a successful approach to this lesion. Open valvotomy remained the primary therapy for patients with pulmonary stenosis until the technique of balloon valvotomy was introduced by Semb and associates in 1979. Currently, balloon valvotomy is used as the initial therapy in most patients with pulmonary stenosis and is highly successful. Pulmonary atresia, however, is initially treated by a combination of interventional and surgical methods depending on the nature of the lesion.

PULMONARY STENOSIS

Pulmonary stenosis can be valvular, subvalvular or infundibular, or supravalvular. Valvular pulmonary stenosis is the most common form and can present in isolation or with either the sub- or supravalvular features. In the cases of isolated pulmonary valve stenosis, subvalvular obstruction forms secondary to infundibular hypertrophy and can often be dynamic. Supravalvular pulmonary stenosis occurs commonly in the setting of pulmonary atresia, in which the most severe cases also have an atretic main pulmonary artery segment with a variable degree of branch pulmonary artery hypoplasia.

In patients with valvular pulmonary stenosis, the pulmonary valve is typically dome-shaped with fusion of the leaflets at the commissures and a small central orifice. The pulmonary annulus may be normal in size or smaller than predicted. The timing of presentation and intervention is usually determined by the severity obstruction to pulmonary blood flow and subsequent clinical findings. The clinical findings are directly related to the severity of the stenosis as well as the degree of shunting across the atrial septum and the patent ductus arteriosus. While most patients with mild to moderate pulmonary stenosis are asymptomatic, neonates with critical pulmonary stenosis or pulmonary atresia develop severe tricuspid regurgitation, cyanosis due to right-to-left shunting across the patent foramen ovale, and congestive heart failure. Neonates with critical pulmonary stenosis benefit from the treatment with prostaglandin E1 (PGE1) therapy to maintain ductal patency. Older patients typically present when a murmur is auscultated or when they exhibit symptoms of exertional dyspnea and fatigue.

PREOPERATIVE ASSESSMENT

On physical examination, most children with pulmonary stenosis present with a harsh holosystolic ejection murmur or ejection click, and a palpable thrill over the pulmonic valve region. A murmur associated with the ductus arteriosus may be heard in the upper sternal region, left axilla or back as well. An electrocardiogram reveals right axis deviation, prominent P waves, and right ventricular strain indicative of right ventricular hypertrophy. A chest radiograph often reveals prominent pulmonary artery shadows secondary to poststenotic dilatation, diminished pulmonary vascular markings, and cardiomegaly.

An echocardiogram establishes the severity of the stenosis and identifies any associated anomalies. The anatomy and function of the pulmonary valve, tricuspid valve, and right ventricle (RV) and patency of the foramen ovale and ductus arteriosus can be determined. Often an estimate of the RVOT gradient or right ventricular pressure can be made as well. Cardiac catheterization is performed for additional diagnostic information and potential intervention using balloon valvotomy or valve ablation in cases of critical pulmonary stenosis and pulmonary atresia.

ANESTHESIA

The anesthetic management of these patients is similar to that for any neonate or child with a right ventricular outflow tract obstruction (RVOTO). In the neonate with severe obstruction, the ductus must be kept patent by administration of PGE1 therapy and pulmonary vascular resistance reduced to ensure adequate pulmonary blood flow. Systemic hypotension is avoided, as it may result in reduced ductal flow and subsequent hypoxemia. These patients may also have dynamic obstruction in the infundibular region secondary to right ventricular myocardial hypertrophy. Inotropes must be used with caution as increased contractility may cause increased functional obstruction across the pulmonary outflow tract and further compromise pulmonary blood flow.

OPERATIONS

The goal of therapy is to relieve RVOTO and provide ample pulmonary blood flow while relieving the pressure-loaded RV. Both balloon valvuloplasty and surgical valvuloplasty or valvotomy are associated with low morbidity and mortality rates and excellent long-term survival. Each procedure has a significant incidence of recurrent stenosis requiring interventions for either recurrent stenosis or regurgitation. For those patients with significant infundibular or supravalvular pulmonary stenosis, often surgical intervention is necessary.

Valvuloplasty is performed by catheterization via the femoral veins. The valve is often dilated multiple times to achieve a gradient of <30 mmHg. Complications, albeit rare, include transient bradycardia and hypotension, tricuspid valve injury, and tears in the pulmonary artery. Restenosis requiring repeat intervention is common with more severe forms of obstruction. The main indication for surgical treatment is unsuccessful balloon valvuloplasty. Currently, an open valvulotomy or commissurotomy is performed through the pulmonary trunk via a vertical incision. Valvular tissue is excised when other methods fail to achieve relief of obstruction.

Open pulmonary valvotomy using cardiopulmonary bypass

Open pulmonary valvotomy is performed through a median sternotomy using CPB and bicaval cannulation. The patent ductus arteriosus is ligated or snared at the initiation of CPB. An aortic cross-clamp is applied, and antegrade cardioplegia is administered through the aortic root to achieve myocardial arrest. A vertical or transverse arteriotomy is then performed on the anterior wall of the main pulmonary artery (**Figure 51.1**).

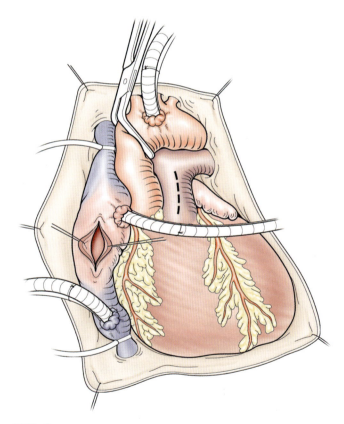

51.1

The stenotic valve is inspected, and the fused commissures are carefully incised with an 11 scalpel blade or fine vascular scissors (**Figure 51.2a**). The incisions in the valve should extend to the annulus (**Figure 51.2c**). Any valvular adhesions to the pulmonary arterial wall are sharply incised. A partial valvectomy may be necessary to remove thickened valve tissue or dense fibrous scarring on dysplastic leaflets. The infundibulum is then inspected through the valve for any subvalvular stenosis (**Figure 51.2c**). Sharp infundibular resection may be performed if necessary. The arteriotomy is closed using a running polypropylene suture.

In cases of subvalvular stenosis, a vertical incision is made and a vein retractor is used to suspend the annulus, allowing for exposure of the right infundibulum. Muscle is sharply resected underneath the valve. In cases of supravalvular stenosis, a patch of homograft, native, or bovine pericardium or another tissue substitute is used to augment the pulmonary artery. Often this patch is carried onto the left pulmonary artery beyond the ductal insertion site.

Off-pump transventricular pulmonary valvotomy

If no atrial septal defect is present, a pulmonary valvotomy may be performed through a median sternotomy using an off-pump transventricular technique. A pursestring suture is placed in the anterior wall of the RV. An angiocatheter connected to a pressure transducer is first introduced through the pursestring in the RV and into the pulmonary artery. Using the same technique, progressively larger metal dilators are then introduced across the valve membrane (**Figure 51.3**). If the valve tissue does not dilate easily, a long vascular clamp may be sued to initially disrupt the valve tissue. After adequate dilation, the pursestring is tied and reinforced.

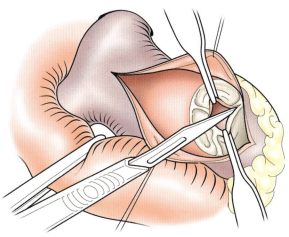

51.2a

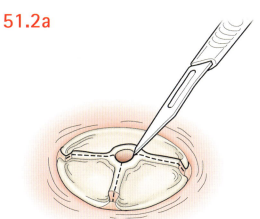

51.2b

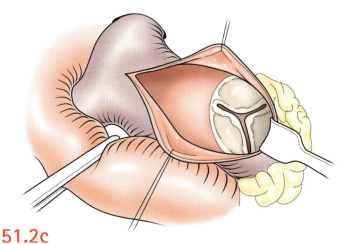

51.2c

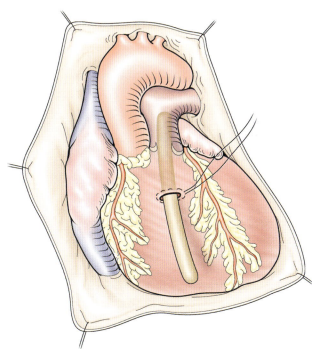

51.3

POSTOPERATIVE CARE

Most patients with pulmonary stenosis are operated on electively and require routine preoperative and postoperative care. In neonates, the management of acidosis, electrolyte derangements, and congestive heart failure should begin preoperatively and continue postoperatively. A residual gradient often exists across the RVOT. Inotropic support should be used judiciously to avoid exacerbation of any residual infundibular obstruction. Transesophageal echocardiography may be performed to assess any residual gradient. In cases of cyanosis, infusion of PGE1 may be maintained until antegrade flow is improved. Mild and moderate residual gradients often resolve with increasing age and growth of the patient. However, for children who remain cyanotic or with a significant gradient, catheterization should be repeated for assessment of hemodynamics.

OUTCOME

Long-term outcome and survival after both balloon valvuloplasty and surgery are excellent, with survival rates exceeding 90%. Reintervention is more likely after balloon valvuloplasty with approximately 85% 10-year freedom from reintervention. The only prospective multicenter trial assessing outcome among infants with critical pulmonary stenosis was conducted by the Congenital Heart Surgeons Society (CHSS) and the results were reported in 1993. Neonates from 27 institutions were evaluated and overall survival was 89% at 1 month and 81% at 4 years for all modes of intervention in neonates with critical pulmonary stenosis. Unfortunately, 26% of these patients required reintervention within 2 years for residual stenosis (defined as a gradient greater than or equal to 30 mmHg) regardless of whether undergoing surgical valvotomy or balloon valvuloplasty. Risk factors for requiring a systemic-to-pulmonary artery shunt were small right ventricular cavity and the use of closed surgical valvotomy. After successful pulmonary valvotomy (after either initial intervention or reintervention), right ventricular size approaches normal in more than 90% of these neonates. Surgical intervention in older children is associated with minimal morbidity and mortality and excellent short-and long-term outcomes. Postoperative pulmonary valve regurgitation is common, however. Life-long surveillance of these patients is recommended.

PULMONARY ATRESIA WITH INTACT VENTRICULAR SEPTUM

In contrast to other forms of RVOTO, pulmonary atresia with intact ventricular septum (PA-IVS) is an uncommon congenital cardiac malformation representing between 1% and 3% of all congenital heart defects. It is characterized by atresia of the pulmonary valve with no forward flow from the RV to the pulmonary arteries. This is associated with varying degrees of RV and tricuspid valve hypoplasia as well as hypoplasia or absence of the main pulmonary artery. Historically, surgical treatment of this defect was associated with a very high morbidity and mortality depending on the severity of right-sided hypoplasia. The low incidence of the defect, combined with its extreme morphologic variability, delayed the development of a standardized approach to surgical therapy. Instead, both interventional and surgical approaches to PA-IVS have been based primarily on a quantitative Z-score assessment of the tricuspid valve diameter as well as the size of the RV. These vary between biventricular repairs for those with adequate tripartite right ventricular size and normal tricuspid valve size and morphology to a single ventricle pathway for patients with diminutive right-sided structures. Cardiac transplantation is reserved for those patients who fail traditional therapies.

Without early surgical intervention, children with PA-IVS have an extremely high mortality rate. The natural history is a 50% mortality rate at 2 weeks and approximately 85% mortality at 6 months. Death occurs secondary to severe hypoxemia and progressive metabolic acidosis secondary to closure of the ductus arteriosus. In general, most children with PA-IVS require multiple interventions.

Neonates with PA-IVS are initially separated into three groups of *mild*, *moderate*, and *severe right ventricular hypoplasia*. In patients with *mild right ventricular hypoplasia*, the tricuspid valve and right ventricular cavity are approximately two-thirds or greater of calculated normal size, and the RVOT is well developed. In patients with *moderate right ventricular hypoplasia*, the tricuspid valve and the right ventricular cavity are approximately one-half of calculated normal size (with a range of one-third to two-thirds of normal), and the pulmonary outflow tract is usually developed enough to perform an effective pulmonary valvotomy. In patients with *severe right ventricular hypoplasia*, the tricuspid valve and right ventricular cavity are one-third or less of calculated normal size, and the pulmonary outflow tract is not amenable to an effective pulmonary valvotomy.

During the initial evaluation of patients with PA-IVS, special attention must be directed towards the anatomy of the coronary circulation. Right ventricle-to-coronary artery fistulae are present in 45% of cases and are more common in those patients with a severely hypoplastic RV and a small competent tricuspid valve. These connections are frequently accompanied by the development of fibrous intimal hyperplasia, resulting in stenosis or complete obstruction of the native coronary circulation. The presence of obstructive lesions in the proximal coronaries may produce a "right ventricle-dependent coronary circulation" (RVDCC). Such patients are at high risk for myocardial ischemia, as desaturated blood from the RV perfuses a significant portion of the myocardium. A greater risk of myocardial ischemia is incurred by reduced diastolic aortic pressure resulting from the creation of a systemic-to-pulmonary artery shunt. In such patients, decompression of the RV by an outflow tract patch, pulmonary valvotomy, or tricuspid valvotomy is poorly tolerated and may lead to acute myocardial infarction.

In addition, an Ebstein's malformation of the tricuspid valve is present in 10% of patients with PA-IVS. This group of neonates should be considered separately. Most of these patients have severe tricuspid valve insufficiency and a normal-sized or enlarged RV. Massive dilation of the right atrium also exists. The left ventricle is often compromised in these infants because of the dilated dysfunctional RV. Although an aorta-to-pulmonary artery shunt may establish adequate pulmonary blood flow, left ventricular output remains compromised by the dilated RV.

PREOPERATIVE ASSESSMENT

Echocardiography remains the initial diagnostic study to identify the anatomic abnormalities and to assess the right ventricular morphology. Because of the complexity and variability of PA-IVS, the anatomy and morphology must be defined by echocardiography and right and left heart cardiac catheterization. Selective coronary injections and an injection into the RV to determine the presence of fistulae are also required for a complete evaluation. Classification is determined from these studies, and an appropriate operative procedure is selected based on the right ventricular morphology, the tricuspid valve size, the RVOT, and the coronary circulation.

SELECTION OF OPERATION

Initial surgical management of most neonates with PA-IVS involves the establishment of a reliable and adequate source of pulmonary blood flow and optimizing the potential growth and development of the RV and tricuspid valve. The selection of appropriate operations in these neonates is based primarily on the degree of right ventricular hypoplasia as well as the presence of a main pulmonary artery segment. While there is no consensus on which therapeutic approach is most appropriate for all cases, the increasing role of interventional therapies such as valve plate perforation and radiofrequency ablation as well as ductal stenting has customized the initial therapy for this lesion and offered a variety of palliative strategies.

In neonates with PA-IVS and mild right ventricular hypoplasia, the goal is to achieve a biventricular repair. These patients may be treated either by interventional or open surgical therapies or a combination thereof. RV decompression with radiofrequency perforation and balloon pulmonary valvuloplasty may be successful. Alternatively, these patients are treated with a pulmonary valvotomy and placement of a RVOT patch. In some patients a pulmonary valvotomy alone restores adequate pulmonary blood flow. Experience

has shown that initial valvotomy alone often fails to produce effective palliation despite favorable anatomy due to a small RV with diastolic dysfunction. In most instances, addition of a systemic-to-pulmonary artery shunt with ligation of the ductus arteriosus or ductal stenting is necessary to ensure adequate pulmonary blood flow and promote subsequent growth of the branch pulmonary arteries.

Neonates with PA-IVS and moderate right ventricular hypoplasia are best treated with a pulmonary valvotomy, augmentation of the pulmonary outflow tract, insertion of a systemic-to-pulmonary artery shunt, and ligation of the ductus arteriosus versus ductal stenting if augmented pulmonary blood flow is still required. Pulmonary valvotomy and augmentation of the pulmonary outflow tract relieve right ventricular hypertension, reduce tricuspid regurgitation, and potentiate the growth of the tricuspid annulus and the right ventricular cavity. This approach may allow for a subsequent biventricular repair as the definitive procedure. This procedure can be performed off-pump without using CPB or with the use of CPB at the discretion of the surgeon.

Those neonates with severe right ventricular hypoplasia are likely to proceed down a single ventricle pathway. Pulmonary valvotomy is usually not effective in relieving right ventricular hypertension. These neonates are best treated with a systemic-to-pulmonary artery shunt versus ductal stenting and atrial septostomy either by balloon or surgically. In cases with RVDCC, decompression of the RV may result in myocardial ischemia thus systemic right ventricular pressure must be maintained to ensure adequate coronary perfusion to the myocardium. In patients with RVDCC and severe right ventricular dysfunction, early shunt placement may be followed by orthotopic heart transplantation.

Infants with PA-IVS are followed closely after their initial palliative procedures. With improving results, an increasing number of patients are presenting for later interventions. A cardiac catheterization is performed at 3–6 months of age depending on the infant's initial morphology and the subsequent echocardiographic findings. In patients with severe right ventricular hypoplasia, the selection of operative procedures is once again based primarily on right ventricular morphology and an assessment of the tricuspid valve and RV growth since the previous intervention. Whereas in neonates the size of the tricuspid valve and the RV usually correlate, in older children a significant discrepancy may exist between these two structures.

In patients with moderate right ventricular hypoplasia, later intervention is dictated by the previous growth of the RV and the tricuspid valve. If the RV is one-half to two-thirds normal size, then repair includes closure of the atrial septal defect, enlargement of the right ventricular cavity by myocardial resection, and a valved connection between the RV and pulmonary artery versus a transannular patch. If the right ventricular volume and the tricuspid valve diameter are marginal (one-third to one-half normal) for a two-ventricle repair, a bidirectional cavopulmonary shunt (Glenn shunt) is performed. This shunt allows the channeling of one-third of the systemic venous return from the superior vena cava directly to the pulmonary arteries while the inferior vena cava (two-thirds of the systemic venous return) continues to pass through the tricuspid valve and RV. This approach has been termed the one and one-half ventricle or partial biventricular repair. This plan limits the volume load on the RV and provides obligatory pulmonary blood flow directly to the pulmonary arteries. A two-ventricle repair (with takedown of the Glenn shunt) or a completion Fontan reconstruction may follow based on the subsequent growth of the RV and the tricuspid valve.

In patients with PA-IVS and severe right ventricular hypoplasia, a biventricular repair is usually not feasible. Most of these patients have a systemic-to-pulmonary artery shunt in the neonatal period with or without tricuspid valvotomy. The bidirectional cavopulmonary shunt is performed in the first 3–6 months of life with a plan for a Fontan procedure within the first 2–3 years. The principles and techniques of the Glenn and Fontan procedures are discussed in Chapter 44, "Bidirectional Glenn and hemi-Fontan procedures," and Chapter 45, "Fontan procedure for functionally single ventricle and double-inlet ventricle."

ANESTHESIA

The management of neonates with PA-IVS is similar to that described for neonates with severe pulmonary stenosis. Because no blood flow is pumped from the RV to the pulmonary arteries, these patients are completely ductal-dependent. Careful modulation of the pulmonary vascular resistance is essential to ensure adequate oxygenation. Patients with RVDCC must be carefully monitored for evidence of myocardial ischemia. Older children undergoing biventricular repairs should be managed to optimize antegrade pulmonary blood flow. Patients undergoing one and one-half and staged single ventricle repairs often require higher inotropic support. They also need reduction of their pulmonary artery pressures to maintain adequate flow in the Glenn and Fontan shunts. In multiple series, RVDCC was associated with high (up to 60%) early interstage mortality and consideration of transplant is thus advocated.

OPERATIONS IN NEONATES

Shunts

The principles and techniques of systemic-to-pulmonary artery shunts are discussed in Chapter 40, "Palliative procedures: shunts and pulmonary artery banding."

OFF-PUMP INSERTION OF A PULMONARY TRANSANNULAR PATCH

A median sternotomy is performed, and a primed CPB pump is made available. A pediatric cross-clamp is placed immediately beneath the bifurcation of the main pulmonary artery. The ductus is kept patent to provide pulmonary blood flow.

A vertical incision is made in the anterior aspect of the main pulmonary artery and extended down to the junction of the RV (**Figure 51.4a**). A partial thickness incision is continued down to the area over the right ventricular cavity. Epicardial muscle is resected to a depth of 2–3 mm to thin out of superficial wall of the RV.

A pericardial patch or alternate tissue such as homograft or synthetic pericardium is now sutured to the edges of the pulmonary artery and to the edges of the right ventricular

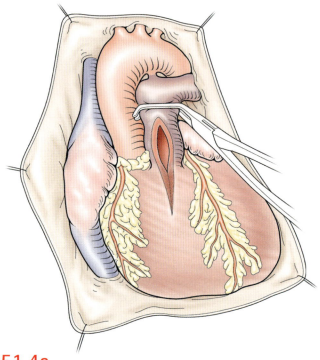

51.4a

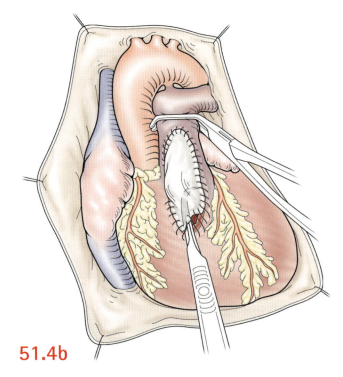

51.4b

incision. The sutures are left loose inferiorly, and a scalpel is used to incise the valve membrane and the remaining myocardium over the right ventricular cavity (**Figure 51.4b**).

The sutures are pulled up to control the bleeding, and the cross-clamp is removed (**Figure 51.4c**). Flow is re-established through the RVOT. As long as saturation is maintained, the ductus arteriosus is ligated.

OFF-PUMP TRANSARTERIAL PULMONARY VALVOTOMY

An open pulmonary valvotomy can be performed with or without the use of CPB. The main pulmonary artery is cross-clamped immediately below the bifurcation. Pulmonary perfusion is maintained through the ductus arteriosus. A pursestring suture is placed in the anterior wall of the main pulmonary artery. The main pulmonary artery is incised vertically within the pursestring and retracted to expose the valve (**Figure 51.5a**). The fused commissures are identified and incised sharply with an 11 scalpel to the level of the annulus (**Figure 51.5b**).

The pursestring is tightened, and a thin-bladed vascular C-clamp is quickly applied to the incision (**Figure 51.5c**). The cross-clamp on the pulmonary artery is removed.

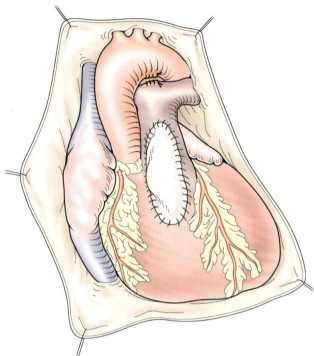

51.4c

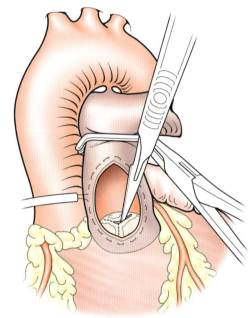

51.5b

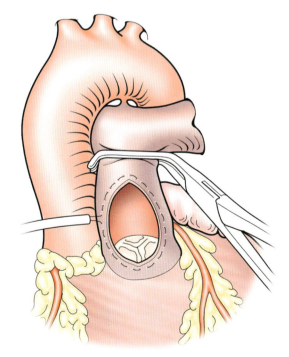

51.5a

51.5c

Enlargement of the right ventricular cavity and outflow tract

Enlargement of the right ventricular cavity is performed through a median sternotomy using CPB with bicaval cannulation. The heart is arrested with antegrade and retrograde delivery of cardioplegic solution. The right atrium is incised and opened. A second incision is made vertically from the main pulmonary artery, through the pulmonary annulus, and across the infundibulum to the main right ventricular cavity. The cavity is enlarged by extensive sharp resection of trabecular right ventricular myocardium through both incisions. A right-angle clamp is used to avoid injury to underlying myocardium and the papillary muscles of the tricuspid valve. A transannular patch of pericardium, homograft, or an alternative tissue is then sutured to the RV and pulmonary artery. The atriotomy is closed using a running polypropylene suture in a two-layered technique. Please refer to **Figures 51.4b and 51.4b** as performed for pulmonary stenosis.

Transannular patch with valve insertion

Insertion of a bioprosthetic valve and transannular patch is performed through a median sternotomy using CPB with bicaval cannulation. Myocardial arrest with cardioplegia is often used but may not be necessary. A transannular incision is made vertically across the pulmonary outflow tract and extended distally on to the left pulmonary artery and proximally down into the RV (**Figure 51.6a**). Any residual membrane in the region of the pulmonary annulus is resected. An oversized (relative to the normal valve size of the child) porcine bioprosthetic valve is placed under a pericardial or Gore-Tex patch within the RVOT (**Figure 51.6b**). If pericardium is used, it is treated with glutaraldehyde for 5 minutes and rinsed with saline. The sewing ring of the porcine bioprosthetic valve is seated below the level of the true pulmonary annulus. This approach allows a larger valve to be implanted and reduces the amount of compression that may result from sternal closure. A running polypropylene suture is used to anchor the porcine valve sewing ring to the RVOT posteriorly. The transannular patch is sewn to the edges of the pulmonary artery, and the porcine valve is anchored to the patch anteriorly. Implantation of the patch is completed by suturing the proximal edges to the remaining myocardial defect in the RVOT (**Figure 51.6c**).

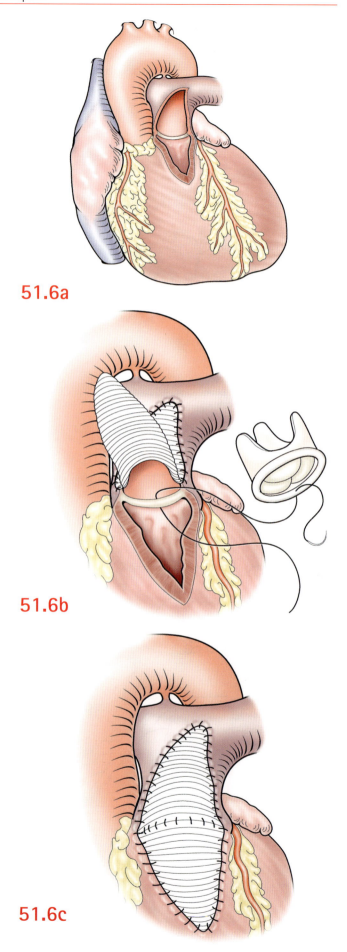

51.6a

51.6b

51.6c

Transannular patch with monocusp valve insertion

Insertion of a transannular patch with a monocusp valve is performed through median sternotomy using CPB and bicaval cannulation. After harvesting, the pericardium is treated with glutaraldehyde for 5 minutes and then rinsed in saline. The transannular patch and the monocusp valve leaflet are marked on the harvested pericardium using a sterile marking pen (**Figure 51.7a**). Sizing of the monocusp valve is made using a metal dilator that approximates the expected "normal" diameter of the pulmonary annulus. The width of the monocusp leaflet at its base should be approximately one-half of the circumference of the dilator. This width should also correspond with the width and shape of the proximal end of the transannular patch. The superior edge of the monocusp valve leaflet should be attached to the edges of the incised pulmonary artery several millimeters distal to the area of the true valve annulus (**Figure 51.7b**). The monocusp valve is attached to the edges of the pulmonary artery and the RV using the same suture that attaches the edges of the transannular patch (**Figure 51.7c**).

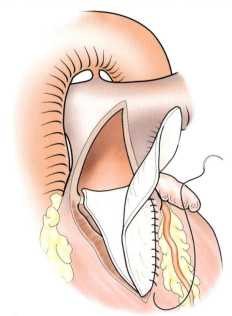

51.7b

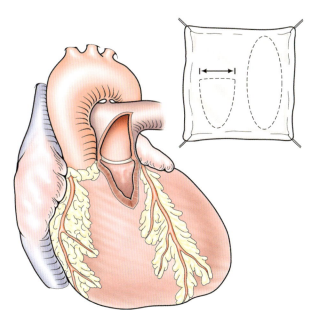

51.7a

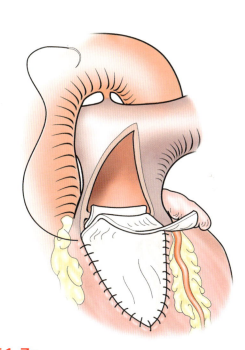

51.7c

Homograft valve insertion

The insertion of an aortic or pulmonary homograft is performed through a median sternotomy using CPB and bicaval cannulation. Cardioplegic arrest of the heart may or may not be necessary. An appropriately sized aortic or pulmonary homograft is selected, thawed, and trimmed to the correct length. The pulmonary artery is opened, and a running polypropylene suture is used for the distal anastomosis of the homograft to the pulmonary artery bifurcation (**Figure 51.8a**).

Proximally, the posterior edge of the homograft is sutured to the RVOT just below the pulmonary valve annulus using a running polypropylene suture (**Figure 51.8b**).

The remaining anastomosis of the anterior edge of the homograft to the right ventriculotomy can be performed using the anterior leaflet of the mitral valve of an aortic homograft (**Figure 51.8c**). Alternatively, this anastomosis may require a rectangular hood of Gore-Tex or pericardium (**Figure 51.8d**). This hood enlarges the RVOT and avoids residual obstruction at the junction of the homograft.

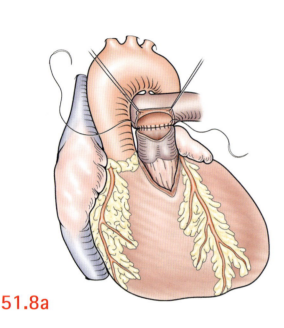

51.8a

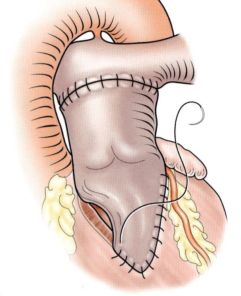

51.8c

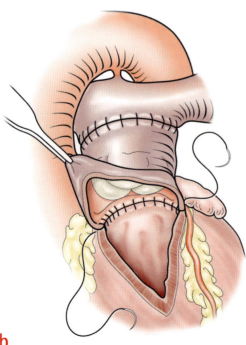

51.8b

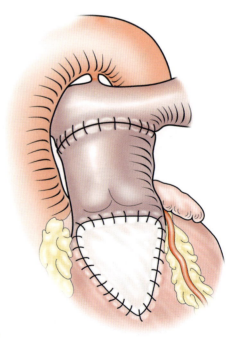

51.8d

POSTOPERATIVE CARE

Neonates may be critically ill in the early postoperative period after operative intervention for PA-IVS. The presence of low cardiac output may require substantial inotropic support. In the presence of an aorta-to-pulmonary artery shunt, balanced pulmonary and systemic blood flow must be achieved. The management of pulmonary and systemic vascular resistance is critical to maintaining adequate oxygenation and cardiac output. Episodes of pulmonary hypertension must be managed quickly and may require the use of inhaled nitric oxide. An excessively large shunt may lead to pulmonary overcirculation and require adjustment or replacement of the shunt. Postoperative ischemia can develop due to unrecognized RVDCC and may be associated with electrocardiogram changes, ventricular dysrhythmias, and segmental wall dyskinesis on echocardiography. In patients with persistent hypoxemia despite adequate medical management, residual RVOTO or severe tricuspid hypoplasia should be excluded.

OUTCOME

The only study of sufficient size to compare initial management strategy is the prospective multicenter study conducted by the CHSS consisting of 171 neonates treated from 1987 to 1991. There was considerable management variability with little use of what are now common hybrid strategies. The overall survival was 81% at 1 month and 64% at 4 years. Size of the tricuspid valve expressed as a Z value correlated to right ventricular cavity volume and was a marked predictor of outcome when the initial procedure included right ventricular decompression in the presence of RVDCC. Additional studies question the long-term outcomes with respect to borderline biventricular repairs as opposed to one and a half ventricle or single ventricle outcomes.

PA-IVS remains a formidable congenital heart defect that requires surgical intervention early in life. In the neonate with PA-IVS, we have found that surgical classification of right ventricular hypoplasia into mild (greater than two-thirds of normal), moderate (one-third to two-thirds of normal), and severe (less than one-third of normal) is useful in selecting a surgical approach. In older children, a similar classification is used, and patients are stratified into those who will benefit from an attempt to achieve a biventricular repair and those who are best suited to a Fontan procedure. By using this approach, the surgical mortality and morbidity have been markedly reduced, and long-term survival has been excellent.

For both pulmonary stenosis and pulmonary atresia, catheter-based intervention has evolved as an increasingly prominent choice for neonatal therapy. While it is difficult to standardize pathways, the significance of individual approach to unique patients is key. Transplant remains an option for those neonates with the most severe form of pulmonary atresia.

FURTHER READING

Ashburn DA, Blackstone EH, Wells WJ, et al. Determinants of mortality and type of repair in neonates with pulmonary atresia and intact ventricular septum. *J Thorac Cardiovasc Surg.* 2004; 127: 1000-7.

Cheung EW, Richmond ME, Turner ME, et al. Pulmonary atresia/intact ventricular septum: influence of coronary anatomy on single-ventricle outcome. *Ann Thorac Surg.* 2014; 98: 1371-7.

Chubb H, Pesonen E, Sivasubramanian S, et al. Long-term outcome following catheter valvotomy for pulmonary atresia with intact ventricular septum. *J Am Coll Cardiol.* 2012; 59: 1468-76.

Cuypers JA, Witsenburg M, van der Linde D, Roos-Hesselink JW. Pulmonary stenosis: update on diagnosis and therapeutic options. *Heart.* 2013; 99(5): 339-47.

Daubeney PE, Wang D, Delany DJ, et al. Pulmonary atresia with intact ventricular septum: predictors of early and medium-term outcome in a population based study. *J Thorac Cardiovasc Surg.* 2005; 130: 1071.

Hanley FL, Sade RM, Blackstone EH, et al. Outcomes in neonatal pulmonary atresia with intact ventricular septum: a multi-institutional study. *J Thorac Cardiovasc Surg.* 1993; 105: 406-27.

Hu R, Zhang H, Dong W, et al. Transventricular valvotomy for pulmonary atresia with intact ventricular septum in neonates: a single-centre experience in mid-term follow-up. *Eur J CardioThorac Surg.* 2015; 47: 168-72.

John AS, Warnes CA. Clinical outcomes of adult survivors of pulmonary atresia with intact ventricular septum. *Internat J of Cardiol.* 2012; 161: 13-17.

Kan JS, White RO, Mitchell SE, Gardner TJ. Percutaneous balloon valvuloplasty: a new method for treating congenital pulmonary stenosis. *N Engl J Med.* 1982; 307: 540.

Karamlou T, Poynter JA, Walters III HL, et al. Long-term functional health status and exercise test variables for patients with pulmonary atresia and intake ventricular septum: a Congenital Heart Surgeons Society study. *J Thorac Cardiovasc Surg.* 2013; 145: 1018-27.

Laks H, Plunkett MD. Pulmonary stenosis and pulmonary atresia with intact septum. In: Kaiser LR, Kron IL, Spray TL (eds). *Mastery of cardiothoracic surgery.* Philadelphia: Lippincott-Raven Publishers; 1998: pp. 805-18.

Mallula K, Vaughn G, El-Said H, et al. Comparison of ductal stenting versus surgical shunt for palliation of patients with pulmonary atresia and intact ventricular septum. *Catheter Cardiovasc Interv.* 2015; 85: 1196-202.

Merino-Ingelmo R, Santos-de Soto J, Coserria Sanchez F, et al. Long-term results of percutaneous balloon valvuloplasty in pulmonary valve stenosis in the pediatric population. *Rev Esp Cardiol.* 2014; 67(5): 374-9.

Moore JW, Vincent RN, Beekman RH, et al. Procedural results and safety of common interventional procedures in congenital heart disease: initial report from the National Cardiovascular Data Registry. *J Am Coll Cardiol.* 2014; 64(23): 2439-51.

Polansky DB, Clark EB, Doty DB. Pulmonary stenosis in infants and young children. *Ann Thorac Surg.* 1985; 39: 159.

Rychik J, Levy H, Gaynor JW, et al. Outcome after operation for pulmonary atresia with intact ventricular septum. *J Thorac Cardiovasc Surg.* 1998: 116(6): 924–31.

Sehar T, Qureshi AU, Kazmi U, et al. Balloon valvuloplasty in dysplastic pulmonary valve stenosis: immediate and intermediate outcomes. *J Coll Physicians Surg Pak.* 2015; 25: 16–21.

Schneider AW, Blom NA, Bruggemans EF, Hazekamp MG. More than 25 years of experience in managing pulmonary atresia with intact ventricular septum. *Ann Thorac Surg.* 2014; 98: 1680–6.

Schwartz MC, Glatz AC, Dori Y, et al. Outcomes and predictors of reintervention in patients with pulmonary atresia and intact ventricular septum treated with radiofrequency perforation and balloon pulmonary valvuloplasty. *Pediatr Cardiol.* 2014; 35: 22–9.

Shinebroune EA, Rigby ML, Carvalho JS. Pulmonary atresia with intact ventricular septum: from fetus to adult. *Heart.* 2008; 94: 1350–7.

Zampi JD, Hirsch-Romano JC, Goldstein BH, et al. Hybrid approach for pulmonary atresia with intact ventricular septum: early single center results and comparison to the standard surgical approach. *Catheter Cardiovasc Interv.* 2014; 83(5): 753–61.

52

Left ventricular outflow tract obstruction

ROSS M. UNGERLEIDER AND IRVING SHEN

INTRODUCTION

Left ventricular outflow tract obstruction (LVOTO) can be caused by a spectrum of lesions that obstruct the flow of blood from the left ventricle into the aorta. The site of obstruction is often classified anatomically as valvular, subvalvular, or supravalvular. Although these lesions usually occur separately, patients can present with combinations of the anatomic varieties. In this chapter, common presentations of LVOTO are considered, and the surgical management is discussed.

CRITICAL AORTIC STENOSIS OF THE NEONATE

Aortic stenosis in the newborn is a very serious defect. In contrast to aortic stenosis in adults, which can be followed for years as it progresses toward the need for intervention, aortic stenosis in neonates can present as an acute, life-threatening problem. The anatomy of the aortic valve leaflets can be very abnormal, ranging from bicuspid, with fusion of the commissures, to unicuspid, with an eccentrically located orifice and no obvious discernible commissural fusion. The valve annulus is usually small and produces a significant component of the stenosis. Because left ventricular outflow is restricted, systemic perfusion is impaired. In severe cases, perfusion to the body requires right-to-left shunting across a patent ductus arteriosus; thus, critical aortic stenosis of the newborn can be considered a "ductal-dependent" lesion (**Figure 52.1**).

Ductal-dependent systemic perfusion explains why some infants may present *in extremis* shortly after birth when the ductus arteriosus closes. Left heart failure and poor cardiac output result in decreased systemic perfusion, delayed capillary refill, and severe metabolic acidosis. When they present in this manner, these infants are usually tachypneic to compensate for their metabolic acidosis. All peripheral pulses may be indiscernible, in contrast to infants with aortic coarctation where the pulses are usually strong in the right arm. These critically ill infants appear ashen "gray" and need immediate intensive resuscitation and simultaneous diagnostic workup. Infants with less severe LVOTO may present in the first few weeks of life with less acute left heart failure, irritability, and failure to thrive.

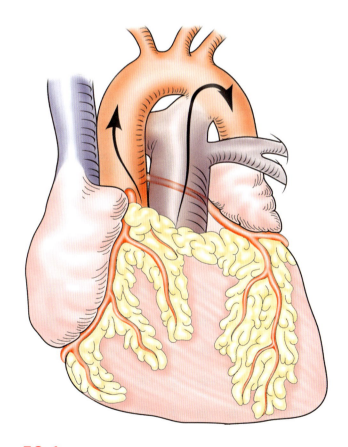

52.1

DIAGNOSIS OF AORTIC STENOSIS

Echocardiography is the single most useful diagnostic modality to establish the diagnosis. A parasternal long-axis view demonstrates a small aortic valve annulus (usually 4–6 mm) with abnormal or thickened valve leaflets. A minor axis view may help define the anatomy of the valve leaflets as being bicuspid or unicuspid, although this distinction may not be necessary to guide management. The left ventricle may be dilated and demonstrate decreased contractile function, or shortening fraction, consistent with poor ejection and low cardiac output. Echocardiography is also useful in estimating left ventricular size and whether other commonly associated cardiac anomalies are present. Hypoplasia of the left ventricle can exist in combination with critical neonatal aortic stenosis and may be severe enough to warrant staging to a univentricular palliation. The most commonly used calculator to help guide the decision for one- vs two-ventricle repair is based on research from the Congenital Heart Surgeons Society (CHSS) and can be located on the internet at http://www.chssdc.org/content/chss-score-neonatal-critical-aortic-stenosis. This calculator can help predict the survival advantage for employing a single- vs two-ventricle pathway in the management strategy of neonatal critical aortic stenosis. Also commonly used to predict whether patients with critical aortic stenosis are best treated with a one- vs two-ventricle strategy are the Rhodes criteria, first reported in 1991, and later revised by Colan and colleagues in 2006. Essentially, these criteria use the following equation:

10.98 (body surface area) + 0.56 (aortic annulus z-score) + 5.89 (left ventricular to heart long-axis ratio) – 0.79 (grade 2 or 3 endocardial fibroelastosis) – 6.78

With a cutoff of –0.65, outcome was predicted accurately in 90% of patients reviewed from a single center. Significant associated anomalies that may coexist with critical neonatal aortic stenosis include *mitral stenosis* (mitral valve annulus diameter less than 9 mm in a normal size infant), *endocardial fibroelastosis* (EFE) of the left ventricle (signifying severe subendocardial ischemia with fibrosis of the left ventricular endocardium), *aortic coarctation*, and *atrial septal defect* (ASD) or *ventricular septal defect* (VSD). The combination of many of these left-sided outflow obstructions can increase the risk of survival when a two-ventricle pathway is selected and may favor selection of a univentricular staging procedure. A ductus arteriosus may be present; and if the patient has been started on prostaglandin E1, knowing whether the ductus is patent as well as the direction of the ductal shunt is helpful. In 1963, Shone described a complex of left-sided outflow tract obstructions that included *sub*aortic stenosis, parachute mitral valve, supravalvar mitral ring, and aortic coarctation. In the current era, many infants with multiple areas of LVOTO, including mitral stenosis, aortic stenosis (valvar or subvalvar), and aortic coarctation are often considered to have Shone's complex. Many of these infants also have ASDs and VSDs and datasets of critical aortic stenosis will therefore often include a subset of these complex patients.

Cardiac catheterization to gain additional anatomic information is seldom necessary. Measurement of the gradient across the valve is not useful because, in severely ill patients, the greatly reduced cardiac output may not generate a gradient commensurate with the severity of the LVOTO. However, when a balloon aortic valvotomy is chosen as the best treatment option for a specific infant with critical aortic stenosis, a cardiac catheterization may be performed as a part of that procedure and can enable measurement of pulmonary artery pressures, degree of intracardiac shunting (when an ASD or VSD is present), and determination of end diastolic pressures in the ventricular chambers. It is important to carefully consider the role of valvotomy when an infant appears to be a better candidate for staging to a single-ventricle pathway, since any systemic semilunar valve insufficiency in these patients may complicate long-term management.

PREOPERATIVE MANAGEMENT OF AORTIC STENOSIS

Management requires simultaneous resuscitative measures to stabilize these very ill patients and diagnostic efforts to define the anatomic abnormalities and to plan intervention strategy. Resuscitation requires management in the intensive care unit with central venous and arterial access, endotracheal intubation, and mechanical ventilation. These infants should be started on an infusion of prostaglandin E1 to open or maintain ductal patency. Inotropic support may often be necessary. The patient should be sedated to minimize overall body oxygen consumption. Arterial blood gases should be monitored, and acidosis or hypoxia should be corrected to ensure adequate tissue oxygen delivery. In critical neonatal aortic stenosis, ductal patency can be assured by seeing a right-to-left ductal shunt by echocardiography, with restoration of femoral pulses, diminishment of acidosis, and recovery of some ventricular function.

Once the infant is stabilized, the team can proceed with the treatment plan, which can range from balloon or surgical valvotomy to Norwood-type palliation (see Chapter 62, "Hypoplastic left heart syndrome") with creation of a Damus–Kaye–Stansel, a source of pulmonary blood flow (from an aortopulmonary shunt or an RV–PA conduit), and an atrial septectomy (which is sometimes limited in patients where growth of the LV is hoped to occur that can lead to late conversion to a two-ventricle path).

INDICATIONS FOR SURGERY FOR AORTIC STENOSIS

Neonates with critical aortic stenosis should be treated with urgency. Once they are stabilized and anatomic diagnosis has been established, therapeutic options are considered to formulate a treatment plan. Neonates with critical aortic stenosis and adequate left ventricular volume (see calculator above) should proceed with balloon or surgical valvotomy. If the left ventricular volume is inadequate or if the aortic stenosis is part of the hypoplastic left heart syndrome, these patients eventually may need to be staged to a Fontan procedure. Patients with less severe aortic stenosis, who present weeks to months after birth, can be treated more electively depending on the degree of LVOTO and whether they have important associated defects.

VALVULAR AORTIC STENOSIS

OPERATION – AORTIC VALVOTOMY

If the infant has "isolated" valvular aortic stenosis without significant associated defects, the preferred treatment is to enlarge the aortic valve opening. This can be achieved either by catheter-based balloon valvotomy or by surgical open valvotomy. Results with balloon valvotomy have improved in recent years, and non-operative dilation is becoming the preferred technique at most institutions. Currently, surgical open valvotomy is rarely performed on infants with critical aortic stenosis, except at a few centers which believe that a surgical approach can provide a more anatomically directed valvotomy; however, the data supporting surgical over balloon valvotomy in critically ill neonates are not conclusive and the advantages of a catheter-based approach (avoidance of a sternotomy and exposure to cardiopulmonary bypass (CPB)) have led to catheter-based treatment emerging as the most commonly employed option.

A few approaches are available for open aortic valvotomy. Some centers have employed inflow occlusion with open valvotomy without the use of CPB. This is performed by occluding the superior and inferior cavae with snares for a few cardiac cycles to allow the heart to empty. The aorta is then cross-clamped, a transverse aortotomy is made, and the appropriate valvotomy is performed. The aortotomy is then rapidly closed in one layer, and the aortic cross-clamp and caval snares are removed. Because this procedure requires speed and subjects a compromised heart to added stress, we believe this approach should only be utilized in extraordinary circumstances (e.g. a critically ill infant where catheter-based intervention or open valvotomy using CPB are either unavailable or contraindicated).

When used (rarely in the past 25 years) our technique of open valvotomy employs CPB. The heart is approached through a median sternotomy. After systemic heparinization, the patient is cannulated for CPB with an arterial cannula in the distal ascending aorta and a single venous cannula in the right atrium (**Figure 52.2**). Shortly after inception of CPB, the patent ductus arteriosus, if one is present, should be temporarily occluded with a snare. Mild hypothermia (34 °C) is employed. The aorta is cross-clamped, and the heart is arrested with antegrade cardioplegia. A

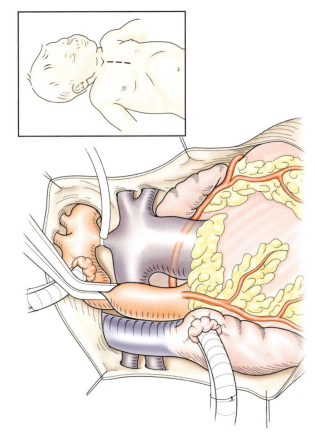

52.2

transverse aortotomy is made to gain access to the aortic valve. Rewarming on bypass can begin immediately after the aorta is cross-clamped.

The stenotic aortic valve is inspected carefully, and the areas of commissural fusion are identified. In some patients, inserting a small cardiotomy sucker through the valve orifice can facilitate inspection of the stenotic aortic valve. In many neonates, simply placing a cardiotomy sucker through the valve and using it to open the commissural fusion is sufficient to open the valve and sharp valvotomy is not required. The fused commissures can also be gently opened with an 11 scalpel blade. The incision should extend toward, but not into, the annulus to minimize postvalvotomy aortic insufficiency

(**Figures 52.3, 52.4a, b, and 52.5**). Moderate to severe aortic insufficiency is poorly tolerated and leads to early valve replacement more often than mild residual stenosis.

After performing the valvotomy, the aortotomy is repaired with a single line of continuous suture (**Figure 52.6**), the aorta is de-aired, the aortic cross-clamp is removed, and the patient is weaned from CPB. The ductus arteriosus should be ligated if the patient is stable. However, if the left ventricular output is inadequate even on aggressive inotropic support, the ductus can be left open and maintained patent on a prostaglandin E1 infusion during the early postoperative period. This maneuver allows additional systemic perfusion from the right ventricle through the ductus arteriosus. If necessary, mechanical support of the left ventricle can be employed (either as isolated left ventricular assist or, more commonly in neonates, as extracorporeal membrane oxygenation (ECMO)). Failure to wean from mechanical support after several days may invite consideration for conversion to a single-ventricle palliation (such as atrial septectomy, Damus–Kaye–Stansel, and source of pulmonary flow – a Norwood-type procedure).

POSTOPERATIVE MANAGEMENT AFTER AORTIC VALVOTOMY

After surgical aortic valvotomy, infants may remain critically ill and require inotropic support for several days. The left ventricle may have significant diastolic dysfunction that leads to decreased ventricular filling and low cardiac output. This syndrome is manifested by tachycardia with marginal distal perfusion. Pulmonary hypertension can be managed by maintaining adequate oxygenation and ventilation to lower PCO_2 and achieve respiratory alkalosis. In some extreme

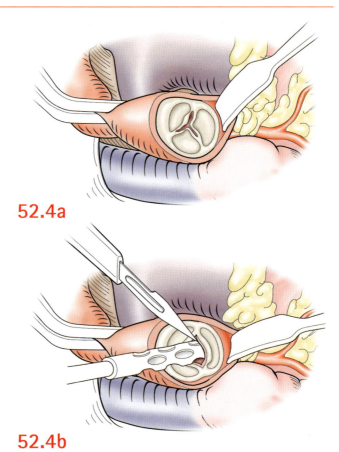

52.4a

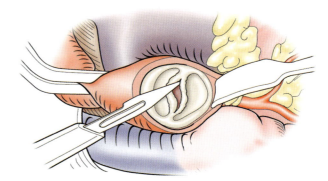

52.4b

52.5

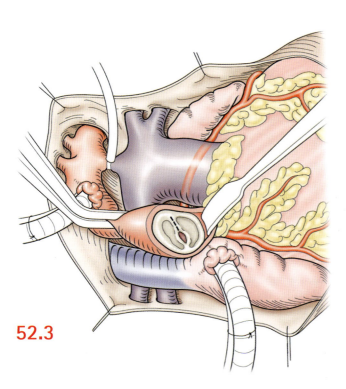

52.3

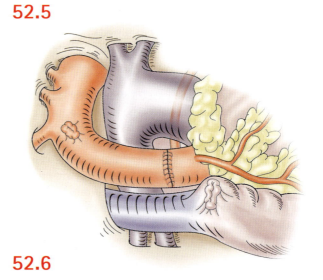

52.6

cases, the patient may require prostaglandin E1 infusion to assist with distal perfusion. Nitric oxide can be tried but, if the pulmonary hypertension is from LV diastolic or systolic dysfunction, the pulmonary hypertension is unlikely to resolve until the left ventricle recovers.

Most infants with a properly performed aortic valvotomy and an adequate size left ventricle should improve over several days. The heart rate decreases as left ventricular compliance improves and allows an increase in stroke volume to maintain cardiac output. Prostaglandin can be stopped, and inotropes can be weaned. Ventilation can be normalized, and the patient can be removed from mechanical ventilatory support and allowed to begin oral feeding. Echocardiography demonstrates improved flow across the aortic valve, and there may actually be an increase in left ventricular outflow gradient compared to preoperatively as cardiac output across the aortic valve increases. A mild amount of aortic insufficiency is not uncommon if the valvotomy was adequate. The patient's clinical course is more important than these echocardiographic findings as long as the clinical course is one of continued improvement and progress.

If the patient is not progressing through an expected course of convalescence, further diagnostic tests must be performed to evaluate the importance of other associated defects. A large VSD may require closure or pulmonary artery banding. Severe aortic coarctation may exist, although it may not have been apparent when the ductus was maintained patent with prostaglandin E1. If the valvotomy is inadequate, the patient may require repeat valvotomy or aortic valve replacement.

OUTCOME AFTER AORTIC VALVOTOMY

Complications of aortic valvotomy are few. Mild aortic insufficiency is common, but usually well tolerated. If the aortic annulus is small or if the valve is extremely dysplastic, the infant may have persistent severe LVOTO after the valvotomy. The infant can be treated by repeat valvotomy or by aortic valve replacement. Dissection of the aorta during advancement of balloon catheters has been encountered and may require surgical treatment. Local vascular complications at the insertion site of the balloon catheters can lead to pulse loss in the leg, but this problem can be treated with thrombolytic agents, or heparin, often with good resolution. Injury to the iliac artery by percutaneous attempt to gain arterial access in neonates with low cardiac output has been reported and can lead to massive retro- or intraperitoneal bleeding, shock and fatality; so this potential complication should be monitored following catheter-based aortic valvotomy with serial hematocrits and attentiveness to increasing abdominal girth. If iliac artery injury is suspected, urgent surgical exploration may be necessary.

The majority of infants with critical aortic stenosis benefit from open or balloon valvotomy and can be discharged from the hospital. However, aortic valvotomy is only palliative because the aortic valve remains anatomically abnormal in these patients. Eventually, all patients probably will require aortic valve replacement. For infants and children, our preferred choice for aortic valve replacement is the pulmonary autograft (Ross procedure, see below) unless the patient has a contraindication for using their pulmonary valve.

OPERATION – AORTIC VALVE REPLACEMENT IN INFANTS

Using the pulmonary autograft for pediatric aortic valve replacement (Ross procedure) is attractive because the valve has the potential to grow with the patient. The procedure is conducted through a median sternotomy and moderate hypothermic (32 °C) CPB. A single venous cannula can be used, although we prefer bicaval cannulation for venous drainage. Bicaval venous drainage also enables placement of a retrograde coronary sinus catheter under direct vision, which is a benefit when a repeat dose of cardioplegia is required in smaller patients. In infants and young children, we prefer to place a loose pursestring around the coronary sinus catheter to help prevent it from dislodging during the operation, and to help keep it in place with minimal inflation of the balloon. A left ventricular vent is extremely helpful and administration of cardioplegia through the retrograde fashion protects the myocardium during the procedure.

After cross-clamping the aorta, the aorta is transected at the level of the sinotubular junction (**Figure 52.7a and b**). The aortic valve is inspected and, once a decision has been made that the valve is not repairable, the pulmonary valve is

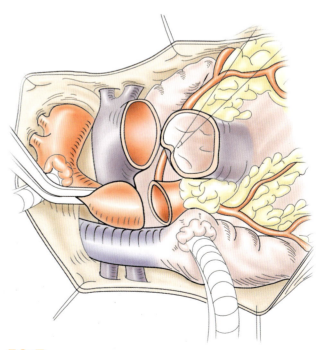

52.7a

harvested to use for replacement. The main pulmonary artery is transected just proximal to the bifurcation of the right and left pulmonary artery. The pulmonary valve is inspected to ensure no abnormality exists that would exclude its use as an aortic valve replacement. We have encountered a bicuspid pulmonary valve in occasional patients (approximately 1% of those referred for pulmonary autograft) and believe that, in selected patients, a bicuspid pulmonary valve may be preferable to other current aortic valve replacement options for young patients. In normal trileaflet pulmonary valves, there is always a commissure anteriorly lined up with the RV outflow tract. We generally float the valve leaflets with saline in order to facilitate inspection (**Figure 52.7b**).

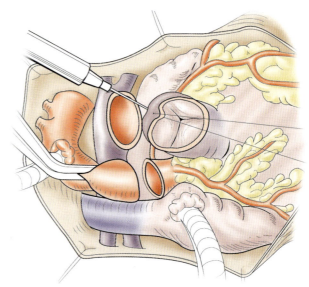

52.8

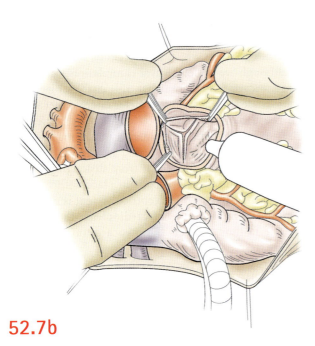

52.7b

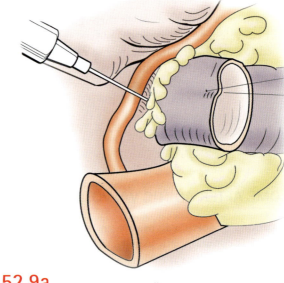

52.9a

By pulling the main pulmonary artery anteriorly, the posterior investment of the valve is dissected free from the right ventricular muscle (**Figure 52.8**). A right-angle clamp is then placed across the pulmonary valve, directly below the anterior commissure and used to identify the spot on the anterior right ventricular wall just inferior to the nadir of the adjacent sinuses. This opening is carefully extended in both directions around the base of the pulmonary valve in order not to damage the valve leaflets (**Figure 52.9a and b**). A dissection plane usually develops along the posterior aspect of the valve where the region of previous posterior dissection is encountered; staying in this plane prevents deep incision into the interventricular septum and injury to the first septal perforating branch of the left descending coronary artery. We find it helpful to "score" the epicardium with electrocautery near the pulmonary outflow near the left anterior descending coronary artery to create a clear guide for the dissection in this region.

After the anterior incision is made, we are able to visualize the pulmonary valve from the inside of the RV and we essentially follow the annulus staying about 3 mm below

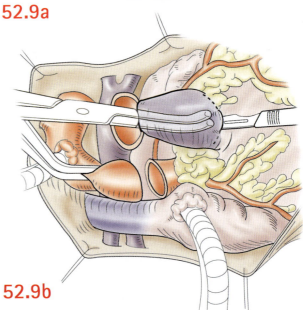

52.9b

the valve and valve sinuses. Once we have incised the valve medially and laterally (the posterior dissection separating the posterior pulmonary valve from the back of the heart makes this fairly simple), we often use a 15 blade to score the endocardium below the posterior pulmonary valve leaflet, which then creates a well-defined plane for the posterior incision to free the pulmonary valve from the back of the heart.

When the pulmonary valve has been harvested, it is checked to be certain that the leaflets are intact, and the valve is trimmed so that there is a small proximal cuff of muscle around the annulus for sewing. Once it is ascertained that the autograft is in good shape, we thaw a pulmonary homograft for reconstruction of the RV outflow tract. More recently, as an alternative, we have been reconstructing the RV outflow tract with polytetrafluoroethylene (PTFE) valved conduits which we make on a back table prior to the operation.

Attention is returned to the aortic root and the coronary arteries are removed as buttons with a large amount of adjacent sinus wall (**Figure 52.10**). The aortic valve leaflets and the excess aortic wall tissue are removed. The pulmonary autograft is then sutured to the left ventricular outflow tract opening using continuous or interrupted sutures. Over our experience with more than 250 Ross procedures, we have developed a highly reproducible technique for this proximal suture line that we have come to prefer. First, we place a double-armed suture that connects each sinus of the autograft to the appropriate sinus region of the aortic root (**Figures 52.11 and 52.12**). By orienting the autograft in this manner, the right and left sinus will line up with the coronary arteries and the non-coronary sinus will be properly located without distortion. Orientation of the autograft in such a way that the coronary buttons can be situated in the sinuses of the autograft without excessive tension or kinking is important.

We then place a suture at each commissure. We begin by tying the suture in the left coronary sinus. We sew this in a continuous fashion towards the suture, orienting the right coronary sinus. Putting mild tension on the right coronary sinus suture and the commissural suture between the left and right sinus creates a "straight line" which facilitates the suturing and sizing. Next we do the same, running the suture from the left coronary sinus towards the suture in the non-coronary sinus. This leaves the final suture line running from

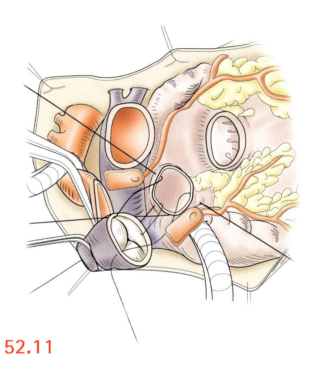

52.11

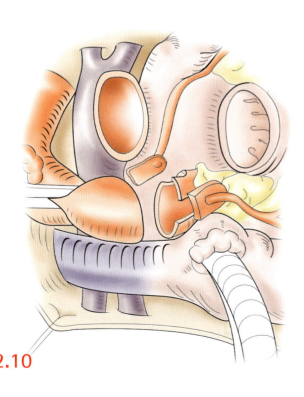

52.10

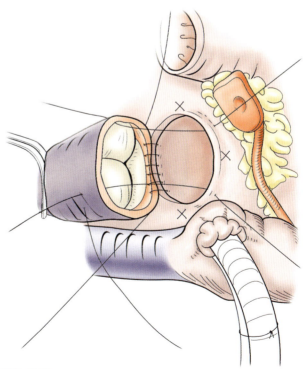

52.12

the non-coronary to the right coronary sinus. We try to finish this suture line at the commissure between the non- and the right coronary since "blind" sutures placed in this location are at a commissure and less likely to injure a valve.

After the proximal suture line is completed, the coronary arteries (left first and then right) are anastomosed to appropriate locations on the posterior and anterior walls of the autograft (**Figure 52.13a and b**). We used to wait until the autograft was reconnected to the ascending aorta and distend it before placing the right coronary artery, but over the last several years we have found it simpler to place both coronary buttons before completing the distal aortic repair.

Next we place the conduit selected for replacement of the RV outflow tract. Typically this has been an appropriate

size allograft that has been thawed once the autograft has been safely harvested. However, more recently, we have been attracted to PTFE conduits that we handsew at the time of surgery. We believe that these PTFE valved grafts – we fashion them as trileaflet valves, although some groups have reported bileaflet construction – will have good durability and will provide an excellent "landing zone" for a percutaneous pulmonary valve replacement in the future should that become necessary (**Figure 52.14**). The autograft is then anastomosed to the distal aorta using a continuous suture (**Figure 52.15**).

After completing the distal anastomosis, the neoaortic root can be distended with a dose of cardioplegia solution to demonstrate autograft valve function is adequate. The proximal suture line for the RV–PA conduit is then performed

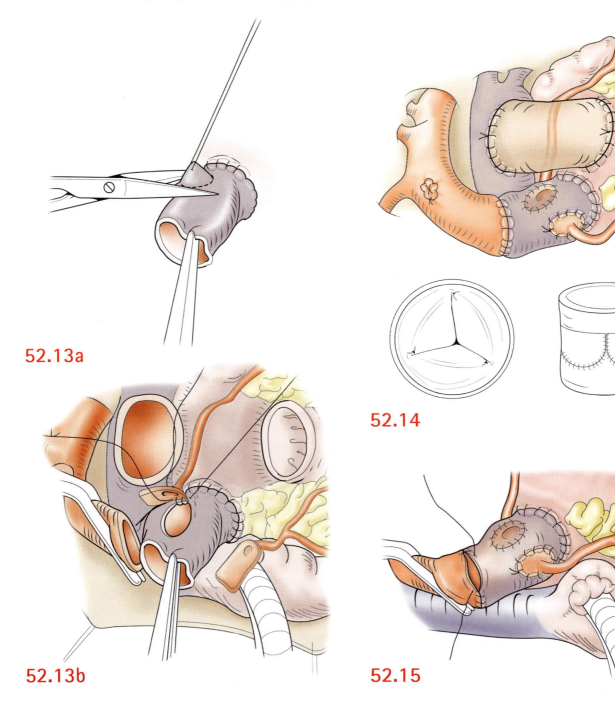

52.13a

52.14

52.13b

52.15

with the aortic cross-clamp still in place (**Figure 52.16**). The right and left sides of the heart are then carefully de-aired prior to removing the aortic cross-clamp.

Occasions exist, especially in neonates, in which significant LVOTO is caused by annular or subannular narrowing. In these circumstances, an aortoventriculoplasty can be performed to enlarge the left ventricular outflow tract in addition to valve replacement using a pulmonary autograft. In many cases, the LVOT can be enlarged simply by resection through the open aortic root after the diseased valve leaflets have been excised. However, when more extensive subaortic enlargement is required, our preference is to incorporate the aortoventriculoplasty with the Ross procedure (Ross–Konno procedure). This procedure is performed using moderate hypothermic CPB through a median sternotomy. Protection of the myocardium using additional retrograde coronary sinus cardioplegia

perfusion is extremely useful, particularly in neonates and infants. After cross-clamping the aorta and arresting the heart, the ascending aorta is transected at the level of the sinotubular junction. After examining the aortic and pulmonary valves, the pulmonary autograft is harvested. For the Ross–Konno procedure, extra tissue is harvested from the anterior right ventricular free wall with the pulmonary autograft. This extra tissue is used to repair the VSD resulting from performing the aortoventriculoplasty (**Figure 52.17**).

The coronary arteries are then harvested from the aortic root with large amounts of sinus tissue. After the coronary arteries are removed from the aortic root, even tiny aortic roots seem to open up and allow easy visualization for a perpendicular incision to be made across the commissure between the right and left coronary artery. This incision is carried into the interventricular septum creating a VSD (**Figure 52.18**).

The pulmonary autograft is then sutured to the base of the aortic annulus using a continuous suture. The pulmonary autograft is oriented in such a way so that the extra right ventricular free wall tissue is placed anteriorly to close over the VSD (**Figure 52.19**). The apex of this additional infundibular tissue is aligned with the commissure between the right and left coronary arteries and this means that the right coronary

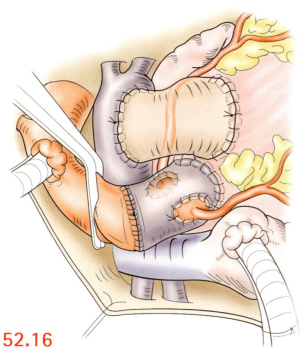

52.16

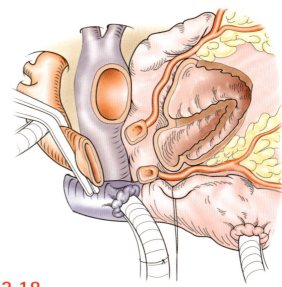

52.18

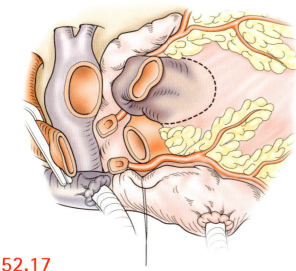

52.17

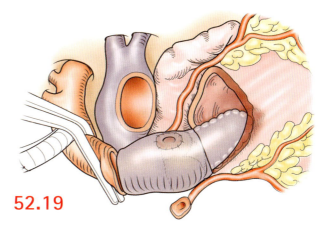

52.19

artery will be attached to the autograft just to the right of this commissure on the autograft wall. After reattaching the coronary artery buttons to the pulmonary autograft, the distal end of the selected RV–PA conduit is anastomosed to the pulmonary artery bifurcation.

Next the distal autograft is attached to the transected aorta using a continuous suture. Finally, the proximal conduit is attached to the right ventricle. A gusset using extra pulmonary artery tissue from the homograft or a piece of PTFE patch may be needed for the proximal anastomosis of the pulmonary homograft to the right ventricle, although this maneuver is frequently not necessary in neonates and infants (**Figure 52.20**).

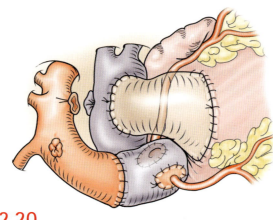

52.20

Success with the pulmonary autograft procedure has led many authorities to recommend aortic valve replacement for any child with critical aortic stenosis, and some use this procedure in lieu of aortic valvotomy. However, many infants with critical aortic stenosis not only survive a simple balloon valvotomy, but thrive and live for years before aortic valve replacement is necessary. Therefore, despite the attractiveness and success of the pulmonary autograft procedure, we recommend reserving aortic valve replacement for those patients in whom it is the only or distinctly the best option for survival. The pulmonary autograft procedure has generally been contraindicated for patients with collagen vascular disease, rheumatic heart disease, or abnormality of the pulmonary valve, although use of a bicuspid pulmonary valve is reasonable. Use of a rare quadricuspid pulmonary valve is not advisable. We have also encountered a patient with an anomalous origin of the left descending coronary artery from the right coronary artery crossing the right ventricular outflow tract near the pulmonary valve annulus, for whom harvesting the pulmonary valve was not possible. Patients with conal septal VSD and aortic insufficiency may not have adequate muscle under the pulmonary valve to allow for safe harvest of the pulmonary valve. In these cases, it may be more prudent to replace the aortic valve with a homograft, biologic valve (stentless), or mechanical valve rather than to attempt using an autograft.

Many patients who receive balloon valvotomy in infancy do not present for aortic valve replacement until they are older, often teenagers or young adults. There is concern that over time the pulmonary autograft may dilate, especially in patients with bicuspid aortic valve (BAV) disease, who may have an associated aortopathy, which is commonly the scenario with these patients. This has led some authorities to criticize the Ross operation as being contraindicated for these patients. In 2005, we described a technique for older patients, whose autograft no longer needed growth, in which the autograft could be placed inside a non-expandable conduit (e.g. Dacron) (**Figures 52.21a–e and 52.22a–c**). In this

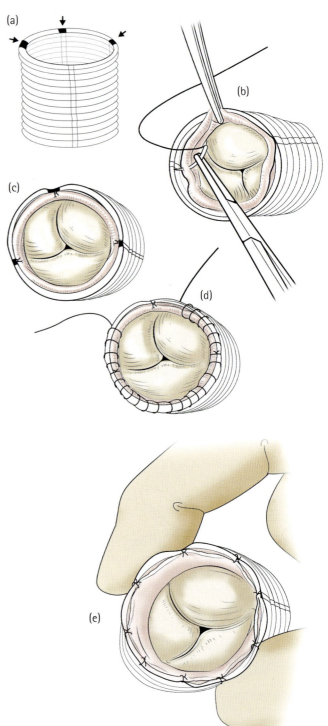

52.21a–e

technique, the coronary buttons are placed into slits that are cut into the appropriate sinuses (**Figure 52.23a–c**). The ascending aorta is generally replaced with Dacron, but if it is not, we recommend prevention of splaying at the coronary

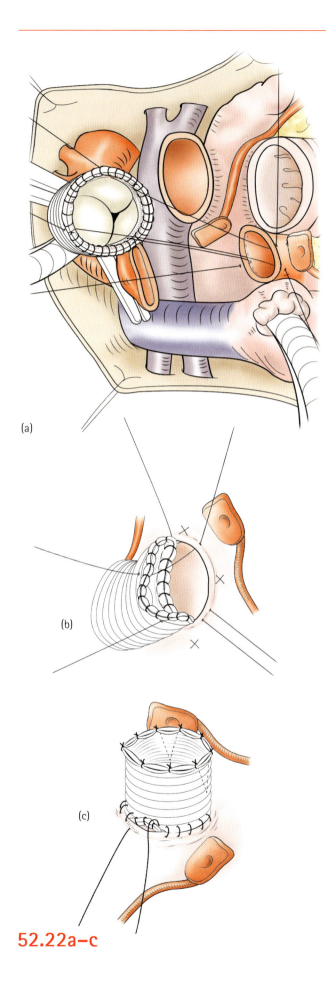

52.22a–c

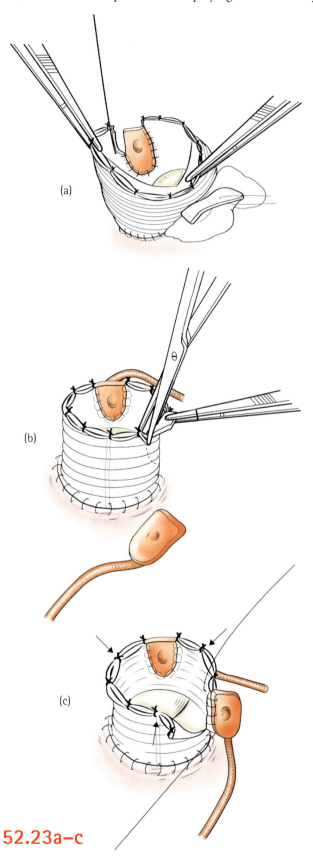

52.23a–c

slits with an overlay of Dacron strips (**Figure 52.24a–c**). With over 12 years follow-up, this technique has shown great promise with good autograft function, especially with modifications to the original technique reported more recently in 2008, and no dilation of the autograft, even in a patient with Marfan syndrome now 12 years on from his autograft procedure. This modified Ross operation may be useful for older patients (including adults with aortic insufficiency) who might otherwise be considered poor candidates for a traditional Ross operation because of their risk of autograft dilation and also may allow patients with collagen vascular disease to be candidates for a Ross procedure.

As new "tissue-engineered" valves become clinically available, some advantage may exist in using biologic valves (stented or stentless) for aortic valve replacement with the plan to replace these with adult-size tissue engineered valves at a subsequent setting. This strategy preserves the pulmonary valve. The use of mechanical valves in children and young adults has limited application owing to the long-term complications from anticoagulation and limitations in lifestyle.

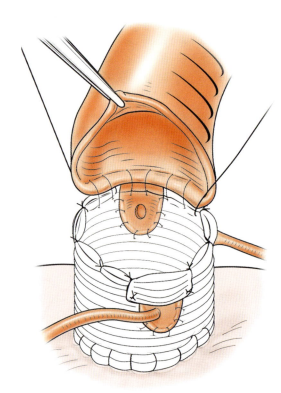

52.24b

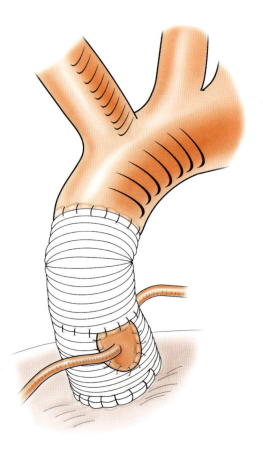

52.24a

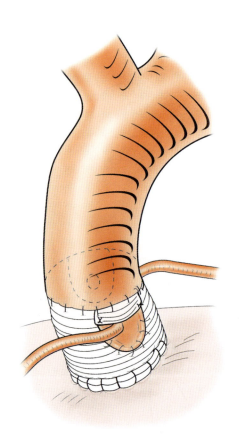

52.24c

OUTCOME AFTER AORTIC VALVE REPLACEMENT

Outcome after aortic valve replacement using a pulmonary autograft is excellent. Mortality is less than 2% with good long-term functional results. Greater than 90% of patients should still have a functioning autograft 15 years after implantation. The need to replace the pulmonary homograft depends on the size inserted as much as the duration of follow-up, but the need for replacement should also be approximately 10% at 15 years. We have recently reported intermediate-term outcomes for PTFE valved conduits in the RV–PA position with 0% valve failure and these results are similar to those reported in series from Japan, with excellent valve function past 18 years.

OPERATION – AORTIC VALVE REPAIR

Some authorities with experience in LV outflow tract reconstruction have been attracted to newer techniques of aortic valve repair for children with LVOTO. The most attractive techniques involve *tricuspidization* of the aortic valve using leaflet extension. Although the long-term outcome of these techniques remains to be shown, they may help children grow to larger sizes and older age as options for LV outflow tract reconstruction continue to evolve, including more data on the modified Ross procedure using a Dacron graft to prevent autograft dilation, the emergence of a tissue-engineered valve, or even placement of suitable valves using percutaneous techniques. Even if none of the above options turns out to be available or suitable with more follow-up, delay of aortic valve replacement for a prolonged period of time may be beneficial if only to allow placement of a larger valve.

Tricuspidization requires careful myocardial protection, since these procedures can be time-consuming. We prefer to approach these cases with similar cannulation used for a pulmonary autograft aortic valve replacement (which is generally our contingency plan if valve repair does not work). In particular, we recommend delivery of additional doses of cardioplegia via a retrograde catheter in the coronary sinus, and placement of a vent into the left ventricle (through the right superior pulmonary vein).

The procedure begins with careful inspection of the valve. We try to identify the three commissures and, depending on the previous valvotomy, there may be a fused raphe separating two leaflets which can be divided, resulting in two leaflets that are slightly smaller than the one larger leaflet on the other side of the valve opening (**Figure 52.25**). In a normal aortic valve, each leaflet length is equal to the diameter of the aortic annulus. The height of the valve is 40% of the total valve (horizontal plus vertical portion) or more simply, two-thirds of the annular radius. For example, if an aortic annulus is 20 mm, the horizontal portion of the valve is 10 mm (radius of the annulus) and the vertical portion of the valve is 6.6 mm (two-thirds of the annular radius, or horizontal portion of the valve). When performing a leaflet extension, the commissures (including the fused raphe) are incised to the annulus to create three leaflets (see **Figure 52.25**). The thickened and dysplastic

vertical portions of the valve leaflets are excised (**Figure 52.26**) and replaced with strips of material cut to the appropriate length (valve annular diameter, *D*) and height (2/3 valve annular radius, *R*) (**Figure 52.27**). We generally add a couple of millimeters to the height in order to accommodate the loss of material taken up by the sutures. We then begin suturing in the middle of the leaflet and continue out towards each commissure, with the height being slightly reduced towards the end.

The biggest challenge confronting the option to repair a valve is the uncertainty of what material to use. Pericardium (untanned), collagen matrix, and even membrane thin (0.1 mm) PTFE have all been described with inconsistent outcomes. Nevertheless, all of these materials can provide reasonable aortic valve function for a period of time that can enable patient growth and perhaps the emergence of other options for aortic valve replacement. Future options may include leaflet "scaffolding" that can recelluarize with recipient cells.

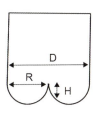
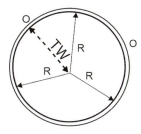

Leaflet length = 2 R

Total Leaflet Width (TW) = R+H
TW = R x 1.5

52.25

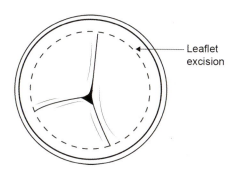

Leaflet excision

52.26

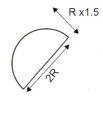
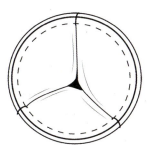

R x1.5

2R

52.27

SUBVALVULAR AORTIC STENOSIS

The left ventricular outflow tract can also be obstructed by tissue inferior to the aortic valve. The most common form of this obstruction is by a discrete ridge of fibromuscular tissue or membrane located within a few millimeters below the aortic valve annulus. This shelf of tissue extends in a counterclockwise direction from the membranous septum around the muscular septum to the region of the mitral valve below the commissure that separates the left and the non-coronary leaflet. In some cases, the subvalvar tissue can present as diffuse thickening or scarring of the muscle of the LVOT that extends proximally into the ventricle creating a tunnel outflow for the LVOT. This is different from asymmetric septal hypertrophy that is seen in hypertrophic obstructive cardiomyopathy (HOCM) and is often associated with previous resection of discrete (membranous) subvalvar obstruction or with the presence of a previous subvalvar resection with a small residual VSD. Usually, the aortic valve itself is normal, although the turbulence created by the subvalvular stenosis may result in some degree of valve thickening and insufficiency. A less common cause of subvalvar LVOTO is duplication of the anterior leaflet of the mitral valve.

DIAGNOSIS OF SUBVALVULAR AORTIC STENOSIS

These patients usually present outside of infancy and commonly after 2 years of age. They have decreased exercise capacity and a classic systolic murmur on physical examination. Echocardiography usually demonstrates the subvalvular ridge with turbulent flow beginning at the level inferior to the aortic valve. Doppler measurements of the LVOTO can quantify the gradient. Some of these patients also have mild to moderate degrees of aortic insufficiency. A cardiac catheterization is usually not necessary because echocardiography is diagnostic and displays the anatomy of the defect quite well.

INDICATIONS FOR SURGERY FOR SUBVALVULAR STENOSIS

Indications for surgery are controversial. The presence of subvalvular stenosis eventually leads to compromised aortic valve function, but this fact cannot be proven aside from individual patient experiences. Nevertheless, a discreet subvalvular stenosis should be resected if the gradient is greater than 30–40 mmHg or if the patient develops new aortic insufficiency compared to previous echocardiograms.

OPERATION – SUBVALVULAR AORTIC STENOSIS

Discrete subaortic stenosis is best treated by resection of the fibromuscular ridge through a median sternotomy on CPB and moderate hypothermia. A left ventricular vent placed through the right superior pulmonary vein is helpful during the procedure. The heart is arrested and protected with a dose of antegrade cardioplegic solution given after cross-clamping the distal ascending aorta. The aortic valve is exposed through a transverse or oblique aortotomy, and the aortic leaflets are retracted to expose the fibromuscular ridge (**Figure 52.28**). Extreme caution must be exercised so that the aortic valve leaflets are not damaged during the resection. This maneuver is particularly challenging in patients with bicuspid aortic valves. The fibromuscular ridge is excised sharply starting from the area near the membranous septum and working in a counterclockwise fashion toward the region of the commissure that separates the left and the non-coronary leaflet (**Figure 52.28**). The location of the conduction tissue near the membranous septum should be identified, and deep incision in this region must be avoided (**Figure 52.29**). We have found that a helpful technique is to first separate the membrane from below the annulus of the aortic valve with a longitudinal incision at the separation point. Then the knife blade (we prefer a 11 blade) can be turned away from the annulus and the incision can extend out to the edge of the membrane. This will detach the

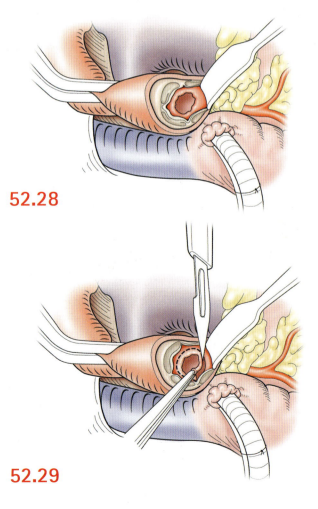

52.28

52.29

membrane near the conduction area. The membrane can then be sharply and bluntly dissected all the way around to the mitral valve area.

After excising the ridge, performing a septal myectomy by sharply excising a wedge of muscle from the interventricular septum below the right and left coronary leaflet is beneficial (**Figure 52.30**). Many surgeons believe that adding this septal myectomy improves outcome and reduces the likelihood for recurrence.

In diffuse (tunnel) subvalvar obstruction, the surgical techniques need to be more extensive. If the aortic valve is also small or abnormal, then a Konno aortoventriculoplasty can be employed using the techniques described above for the Ross–Konno (with pulmonary autograft) if the pulmonary valve is available. In some cases of diffuse subvalvar LVOTO, the aortic annulus and valve are normal and a "modified Konno" can be performed, with resection of the subvalvar muscle and preservation of the aortic valve. In this procedure, after a transverse aortic incision has been performed at the sinotubular level of the aorta, the right ventricle is opened in the infundibulum and a right-angle clamp is placed through the aortic valve and pushed into the septum below the sinuses of the right and left coronary leaflets (**Figure 52.31**). This corresponds to the thickened and obstructive area of the septum.

The muscle of the septum overlying the right angle is then carefully resected from the right ventricular side, creating a VSD which is carefully enlarged. Usually we enlarge first away from the aortic and pulmonary valve, towards the base of the heart (**Figure 52.32**). We remove as much muscle as we can and this removes the muscular subvalvar obstruction. We constantly work through both the aortic valve annulus

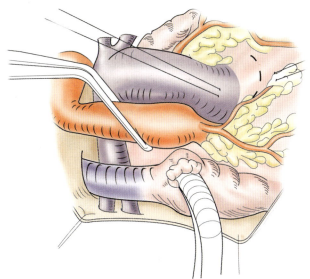

52.31

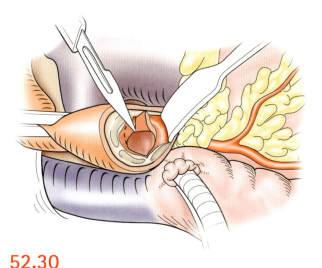

52.30

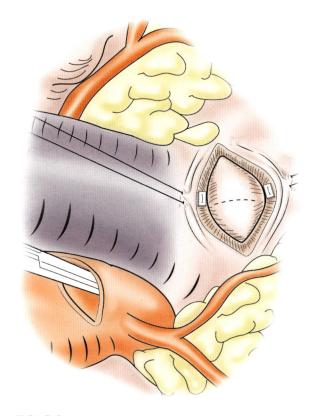

52.32

and the newly created VSD to ensure that we remove the muscle from the LVOT that is creating the obstruction (with the leaflets of the aortic valve carefully protected). We then place our clamp at the level of the aortic valve sinuses and identify this superior margin of resection through the right ventricular septal incision, allowing removal of muscle from the septum up to but not into the aortic valve (**Figure 52.33a and b**).

After sufficient muscle has been removed from the LVOT, the resulting VSD is repaired with a patch from the RV side (**Figure 52.34a and b**). Inspection through the aortic valve should confirm that the subaortic area is now greatly

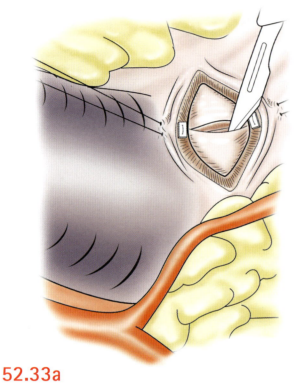

52.33a

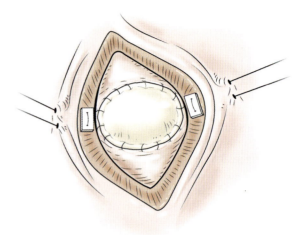

52.34a

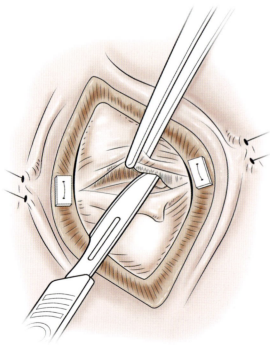

52.33b

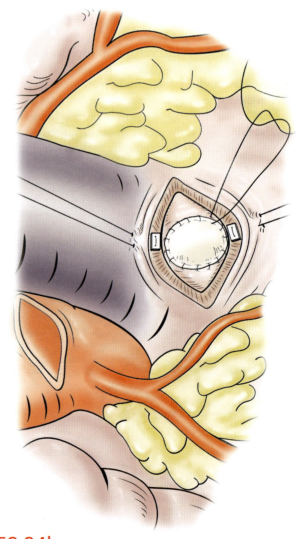

52.34b

enlarged. The aortotomy and the RV incisions are closed (**Figure 52.35**) and the heart is de-aired. We do not hesitate to use a patch to close the right ventriculotomy in order to prevent RV outflow obstruction.

When the LVOTO is caused by duplication of the anterior leaflet of the mitral valve, the redundant tissue can be resected through the aortic valve and is usually easily identified as a

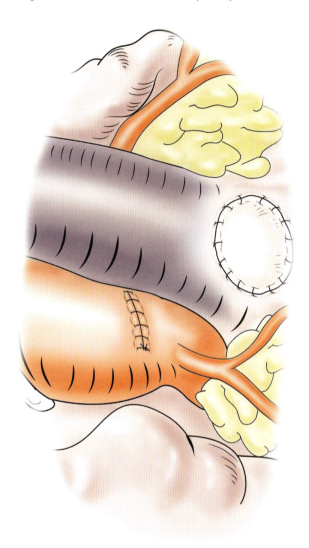

52.35

windsock of tissue that can be delivered through the aortic annulus.

Occasionally, LVOTO is created by posterior malalignment of the infundibular septum in association with a VSD and frequently is accompanied by aortic coarctation, aortic arch hypoplasia or even interruption of the aortic arch. The severity of the LVOTO becomes an important factor in determining the treatment strategy for these patients and is covered in Chapter 60, "Coarctation of the aorta: repair of coarctation and arch interruption."

Complications of these procedures include creation of heart block, VSD, and aortic insufficiency owing to injury to the aortic valve leaflet. Recurrence is reported in as many as 15–20% of patients with discrete subvalvar obstruction and may be reduced by adding a septal myectomy to the resection of the membrane. When a VSD is created as a complication of the procedure, the VSD can be easily recognized on the postrepair intraoperative echocardiogram. Creation (and repair) of such a VSD has a high risk of concomitant complete heart block. In patients with significant aortic insufficiency and subvalvular stenosis, resection of the subaortic ridge can be performed as a part of the pulmonary autograft replacement of the aortic valve. If the major component of outflow obstruction is caused by subvalvular pathology, performing an aortoventriculoplasty and replacing the aortic valve with an autograft can enlarge the left ventricular outflow tract substantially.

OUTCOME FOR SUBVALVULAR AORTIC STENOSIS

Although operative mortality for resection of a subaortic membrane approaches 0%, the risk of recurrent subaortic stenosis can approach 20%, especially when the resection is performed in patients under 3 years of age. Complete heart block requiring implantation of a permanent pacing system is a real risk of the procedure. Aortic valve pathology is also common with the presence of a BAV or thickening of the leaflets, presumably from the turbulent subvalvular flow. For these reasons, many of these patients may eventually need aortic valve replacement later in life.

SUPRAVALVULAR AORTIC STENOSIS

LVOTO can be a result of a discreet or diffuse narrowing of the supravalvular aorta. This form of obstruction is uncommon and can be part of Williams syndrome, which includes elfin features, mental retardation, and failure to thrive. Congenital discrete supravalvular narrowing usually occurs at the level of the sinotubular junction, and variable amounts of intimal thickening can create an internal shelf similar to aortic coarctation. The aortic valve leaflets are

usually normal in this lesion, although mild thickening can occasionally occur. Discrete narrowing in other parts of the ascending aorta can be due to complication from previous cardiac surgery (at prior aortic cannulation site) or from intimal disruption after interventional catheterization. An isolated diffuse form of supravalvular aortic stenosis is less common, and can extend throughout the length of the ascending aorta and even into the aortic arch. Supravalvular aortic stenosis, whether in the discrete or the diffuse form, imposes an increased afterload to the left ventricle. This lesion most often presents later in childhood and is rarely seen in neonates and young infants.

DIAGNOSIS OF SUPRAVALVULAR AORTIC STENOSIS

Diagnosis might be suggested by echocardiography, but cardiac catheterization, CT angiography, or MRI is usually necessary to fully delineate the features of the lesion. In the diffuse form, the entire ascending aorta, transverse arch, and descending aorta can be narrowed. In these patients, there is often narrowing of the branch pulmonary arteries. The discrete form usually presents with an intimal shelf at the sinotubular junction, although stenosis can be found in the distal ascending aorta if it is related to previous aortic cannulation or in the mid ascending aorta if it is related to intimal injury from catheterization. Whereas an angiogram can delineate the nature of the obstruction, pressure measurements can quantify its physiological significance.

INDICATIONS FOR SURGERY FOR SUPRAVALVULAR AORTIC STENOSIS

The presence of discrete supravalvular stenosis with a pressure gradient greater than 30 mmHg is probably an indication for surgery. Patients with lesser gradients, but who exhibit echocardiographic signs of left ventricular hypertrophy, can also be referred for surgical correction. In the diffuse form of the defect, surgical repair is more extensive, and good results are less likely. The indications for repair of the diffuse form therefore need to be individualized for each patient.

OPERATION – SUPRAVALVULAR AORTIC STENOSIS

Surgical approach to the discrete form of supravalvular aortic stenosis requires CPB with aortic cannulation in the distal ascending aorta beyond the area of stenosis. If the area of stenosis is high in the ascending aorta, then it may be necessary to cannulate the femoral, axillary, or even carotid artery for CPB.

The heart is protected with hypothermic cardioplegic arrest after cross-clamping the distal ascending aorta. A longitudinal aortotomy is made across the area of stenosis and extends into the non-coronary sinus of Valsalva. Typically, another incision is made branching off from the initial aortotomy incision at the area of the tightest stenosis and extending into the right coronary sinus on the opposite

side of the right coronary artery (**Figures 52.36 and 52.37**). We do not recommend routine excision of the intimal shelf because this procedure may weaken the integrity of the aortic wall and can lead to aneurysmal formation in the future.

Most surgeons recommend placing a generous piece of either prosthetic or homograft patch on the ascending aorta to enlarge the narrowed area. In the typical situation in which the obstruction is at the sinotubular junction, the patch should be "pantaloon"-shaped and extends into the right and non-coronary sinuses (**Figure 52.38**). In neonates and infants, we have preferred the use of three separate patches to enlarge all three sinuses, as described by Brom (**Figure 52.39a–i**).

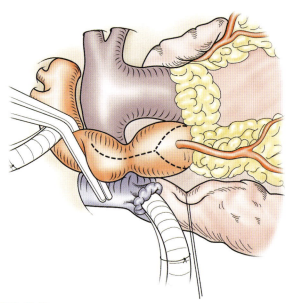

52.36

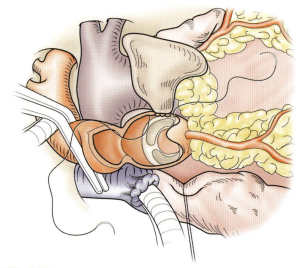

52.37

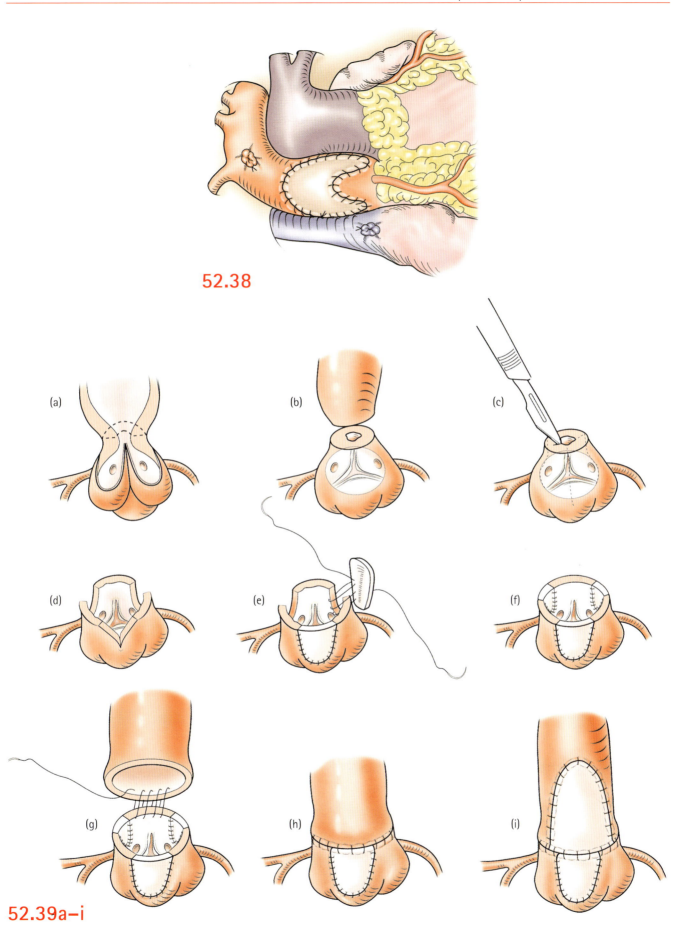

52.38

52.39a–i

An alternative to the Brom, three-sinus repair, described by Myers (**Figure 52.40a and b**) uses contralateral incisions in the ascending aorta to fit into and enlarge the sinus incisions in the proximal aorta, as a method to repair supravalvar aortic stenosis using autologous tissue. We have been concerned that this technique, particularly in neonates, can foreshorten the aorta and put pressure posteriorly on the right pulmonary artery (which can also be involved in this disease and might need concomitant enlargement). We have developed a technique (**Figure 52.41a–d**) that combines the Brom three sinus repair with the Myers technique, by allowing the sinus patches to extend above the sinus so that they

can be used to fit into contralateral incisions in the ascending aorta, and we have found that this nicely enlarges the area of stenosis in neonates and prevents the ascending aorta from compressing on posterior structures. The diffuse form of supravalvular aortic stenosis is most commonly repaired by suturing a generous piece of homograft or polytetraflouroethylene (Gore-Tex) patch from the sinotubular junction all the way around the aortic arch using a period of deep hypothermic circulatory arrest. If the descending aorta needs to be enlarged, this procedure is more easily accomplished through a left thoracotomy with placement of an additional patch.

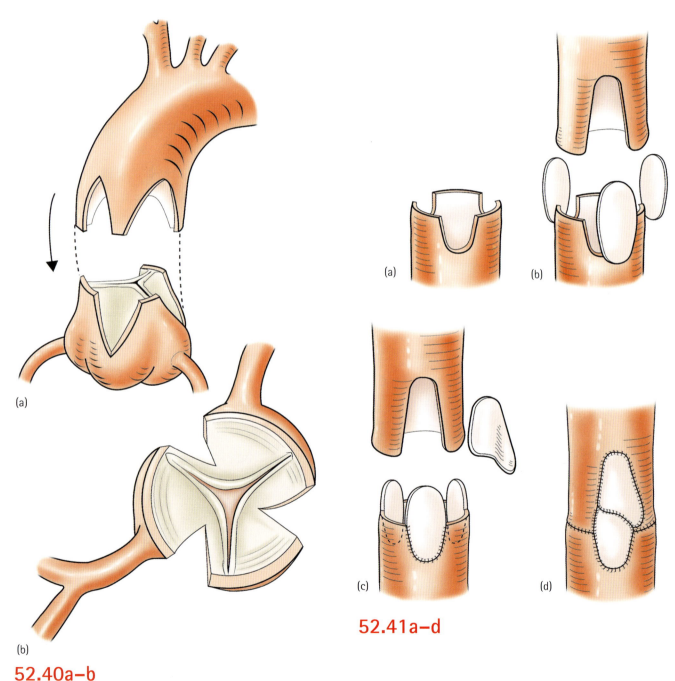

(a)

(b)

52.40a–b

(a)

(b)

(c)

(d)

52.41a–d

OUTCOME FOR SUPRAVALVULAR AORTIC STENOSIS

Few complications occur after repair of the discrete form of supravalvular LVOTO. However, bleeding from the suture line in the aortic sinuses is a risk of which the surgeon should be aware. As with any procedure on the ascending aorta, a risk of air or particulate embolism exists resulting in a stroke. The risks of repair for the diffuse form are similar, although probably at greater risk of bleeding due to the more extensive suture line and the longer period of hypothermic circulatory arrest.

FURTHER READING

Congenital Heart Surgeons Society (CHSS) Calculator for neonatal critical aortic stenosis: http://www.chssdc.org/content/chss-score-neonatal-critical-aortic-stenosis.

Gaynor JW, Bull C, Sullivan ID, et al. Late outcome of survivors of intervention for neonatal aortic valve stenosis. *Ann Thorac Surg.* 1995; 60: 122–6.

Ootaki Y, Welch AS, Walsh MJ, et al. Medium-term outcomes after implantation of expanded polytetrafluoroethylene valved conduit. *Ann Thorac Surg.* 2018; 105(3): 843–50.

Slater M, Shen I, Welke K, et al. Modification to the Ross procedure to prevent autograft dilatation. *Semin Thorac Cardiovasc Surg Pediatr Card Surg Annu.* 2005; 181–4.

Ungerleider RM, Ootaki Y, Shen I, Welke KF: Modified Ross procedure to prevent autograft dilation. *Ann Thorac Surg.* 2010; 90: 1035–7.

53

Transposition of the great arteries with left ventricular outflow tract obstruction

CHRISTO I. TCHERVENKOV AND PIERRE-LUC BERNIER

HISTORY

The arterial switch has become the procedure of choice for d-transposition of the great arteries (TGA) with intact ventricular septum (IVS) or with ventricular septal defect (VSD). It was initially successfully performed by Jatene in 1975 and applied to the treatment of early repair in neonates by Castaneda. The atrial switch (Mustard or Senning operations) is rarely performed nowadays for d-transposition and has become an historical procedure with very limited indications.

The presence of left ventricular outflow tract obstruction (LVOTO) can significantly complicate the surgical treatment of TGA and alternative treatment options have to be entertained in such cases. Indeed, in the context of significant fixed LVOTO, the arterial switch operation (ASO) is contraindicated as the obstructed subpulmonic area becoming the neosubaortic area would create severe outflow obstruction to the systemic left ventricle (LV).

This chapter summarizes the various lesions that can lead to LVOTO in patients with TGA and details the various surgical techniques that can be used to achieve anatomical repair in these complex variants of TGA with LVOTO.

LEFT VENTRICULAR OUTFLOW TRACT OBSTRUCTION

Multiple anatomical abnormalities can cause LVOTO in patients with TGA. LVOTO can be dynamic or fixed and can be valvular or subvalvular, or a combination of both.

Dynamic LVOTO is predominantly encountered in patients with TGA-IVS. It results from bowing of the interventricular septum into the outflow tract of the low-pressure LV due to the systemic pressure in the right ventricle (RV). Depending on how narrow the effective left ventricular outflow tract (LVOT) becomes, the obstruction may also be exacerbated by abnormal systolic anterior motion of the mitral valve. In the absence of fixed LVOTO it is still amenable to anatomic correction by the ASO, as the dynamic

obstruction resolves when the LV is connected to the systemic circulation. Indeed, after performing the ASO, the systemic LV pressure associated with falling RV pressure results in the interventricular septum moving towards the RV opening of the LVOT.

Fixed forms of LVOTO are much more complex to manage. The presence of a VSD is frequent in patients with TGA and fixed LVOTO. The obstruction may be valvular, subvalvular, or result from a combination of multiple processes. Subvalvular LVOTO may be due to one or a combination of the following: posterior malalignment of the infundibular septum, fibromuscular bands or shelves, abnormal chordal insertions of the atrioventricular (AV) valves into the LVOT, or prolapsing of the AV valve tissue through the VSD. In cases in which LVOTO is caused by accessory tissue, or abnormal insertions of the mitral valve, resection of that tissue or mitral valve repair may be performed with an ASO.

Patients with TGA, IVS with LVOTO present a unique and formidable surgical challenge in the absence of a VSD to channel the blood flow to the systemic circulation and allow for anatomical correction of the lesion. One option is to create a VSD surgically in the subaortic area and then proceed with the Rastelli operation. Another option is to proceed with an aortic root translocation (Nikaidoh operation).

PREOPERATIVE ASSESSMENT AND PLANNING

Preoperative preparation requires a complete understanding of the intracardiac and great vessel anatomy to plan the optimal surgical repair. Although echocardiography is sufficient in the majority of cases, cardiac catheterization may be indicated in some situations. Magnetic resonance imaging (MRI) is increasingly showing promise in the investigation of this lesion. Echocardiography can accurately define the morphology of the LVOTO, the size of the VSD and its location with respect to the great vessels, and the anatomy and size of the pulmonary arteries (PAs). The echocardiogram is also useful to identify any factors that may alter the surgical approach, such as abnormal insertions of the AV valves into the LVOT or right ventricular outflow tract (RVOT) or around the edges of the VSD. Cardiac catheterization may be useful to rule out branch PA stenoses or distortions caused by prior palliative procedures.

Very importantly, a discussion must take place with the family explaining the surgical options and the associated risks and expected outcomes. For the Rastelli operation, early mortality in experienced centers is low, but late morbidity and mortality may be significant. Parents must understand that the majority of patients undergoing the Rastelli operation will require reintervention in the future as a result of conduit obstruction. Patients undergoing the Nikaidoh procedure probably have a higher upfront risk for mortality and significant morbidities than those undergoing the Rastelli operation. However, their likelihood of requiring a reintervention may be lower.

GENERAL PRINCIPLES

Patients with VSD and LVOTO have traditionally been palliated with a systemic-to-pulmonary artery (PA) shunt. This strategy allows babies with such lesions to grow to a size allowing placement of a larger conduit at the time of the Rastelli operation or to a point where the weight is more favorable for a successful translocation procedure. While this approach is still valuable in specific cases, it also presents some clear disadvantages. Indeed, it leads to persistent cyanosis and ventricular volume overload. Ventricular function may suffer as a result of this. Moreover, the shunt may cause some PA distortion, scarring, and stenoses that will subsequently complicate the Rastelli operation and most certainly the Nikaidoh operation. Because of this possibility, we prefer to perform the Rastelli operation in early life as a primary procedure, even in the newborn period if required, consistent with the philosophy of early primary repair adopted by multiple institutions including ours.

In the operating room, standard principles of neonatal cardiac anesthesia are followed. Some specific points still deserve to be mentioned. Systemic steroids (methylprednisolone 30 mg/kg) are administered just after induction of anesthesia. Blood conservation techniques such as hemofiltration and limitation of cardiopulmonary bypass circuit volume are employed. This permits us to reach a high hematocrit (35–40%) at the time of separation from cardiopulmonary bypass (CPB). Importantly, these measures, and others, have limited the degree of extracellular fluid accumulation associated with CPB.

OPERATION

The Rastelli operation (including the REV modification)

After median sternotomy, the patient is prepared for cannulation for CPB. Patients are heparinized to achieve an activated clotting time greater than 400 seconds. In first-time operations, the pericardial sac is opened, and a piece of autologous pericardium is harvested for later use as a hood to augment the connection between the conduit and the RVOT if one is planning to use a homograft. This will not be necessary if one is planning to use an internal jugular venous conduit. In the case of a redo sternotomy, the administration of heparin is delayed to allow the dissection of most of the adhesions in the pericardial cavity and the identification of the key structures prior to the initiation of anticoagulation. The distal ascending aorta is cannulated through a purse-string suture, snared in place, and connected to the arterial line. Both venae cavae are cannulated with right-angle cannulae and connected to the venous line with a Y-connector. CPB is instituted followed by immediate ligation or control of the patent ductus arteriosus, if present. Likewise systemic-to-pulmonary shunts are dissected, controlled, clamped, and divided. The aorta is cross-clamped, cardioplegia is delivered antegrade in the ascending aorta, and the venae cavae are snared. The right atrium is opened to avoid distension of the heart. A cardiotomy suction is placed into the left atrium through an atrial septal defect or patent foramen ovale to decompress the left heart. After administering a full dose of cardioplegia, a transverse incision is made in the proximal PA. The pulmonary valve and the LVOTO are then inspected and the decision to perform a Rastelli operation is finalized. A vertical right ventriculotomy also assists us in making that decision (**Figure 53.1**).

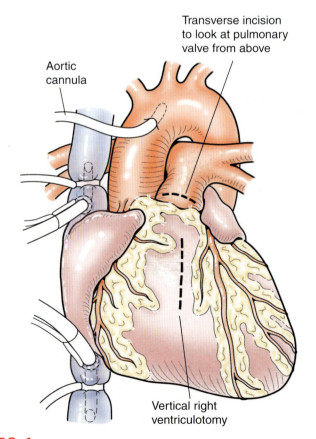

Aortic cannula

Transverse incision to look at pulmonary valve from above

Vertical right ventriculotomy

53.1

After examining the LVOTO and confirming that a Rastelli repair will be performed, an appropriately sized valved pulmonary homograft is thawed, rinsed, and prepared for later use. Alternatively, an internal jugular venous conduit may be used. Pledgeted stay sutures are placed on the edges of the ventriculotomy to provide traction and aid in exposure (**Figure 53.2**). The intracardiac anatomy is carefully examined. Particular attention is given to the size and location of the VSD relative to the size and location of the aortic valve annulus. Importantly, if the VSD is smaller than the diameter of the aortic valve annulus, it is enlarged at its leftward and anterior margin by resecting a wedge of interventricular septum. The VSD can be further enlarged by resection of part of the infundibular septum.

Patients with IVS and fixed LVOTO may still be candidates for the Rastelli operation by surgically creating a VSD in the subaortic area. Using this new VSD, an intracardiac tunnel can then be used to baffle the LV blood to the aorta. Similarly, in patients with a VSD remote to the aorta, baffling of the LV to the aorta is difficult. In these circumstances, a new VSD can be created in a suitable location after having closed the native VSD using a standard technique.

To create the intracardiac baffle, interrupted sutures of pledgeted 4-0 braided polyester are placed circumferentially to encompass the VSD and the aortic valve annulus (**Figure 53.3a**). Superiorly, great care is used to keep the suture close to the aortic valve annulus and thus avoid leaving trabeculations or myocardial crevices which would result in a significant residual VSD. Inferiorly, the suture line may need to be placed directly through the annulus

of the tricuspid valve in the absence of a muscle band. The sutures may be placed through the right atrial aspect into the tricuspid valve annulus. Along the rightward and inferior border of the VSD, the sutures are placed several millimeters away from the edge to avoid affecting the conduction system. In order to decrease the myocardial ischemia time, this suture line can also be performed with a continuous running technique using 4-0, 5-0, or 6-0 polypropylene. To close the VSD and create the intracardiac baffle, our preference is to use a 0.6 mm thick Gore-Tex patch (W.L. Gore and Associates, Flagstaff, Arizona, USA) (**Figure 53.3b**). To avoid

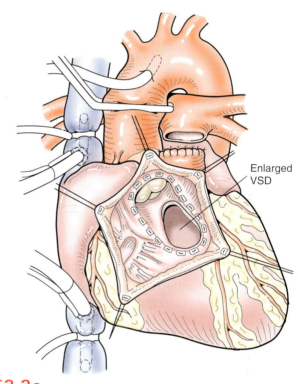

Enlarged VSD

53.3a

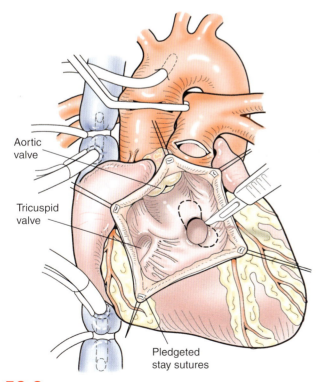

Aortic valve

Tricuspid valve

Pledgeted stay sutures

53.2

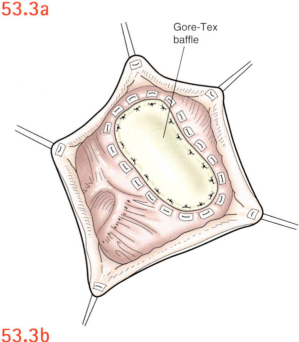

Gore-Tex baffle

53.3b

obstruction of the baffle, the patch is cut with greater width therefore allowing bowing into the RV. With a pressurized LV, the baffle therefore assumes a semicircular shape, bowing into the RV.

Following, the construction of the intraventricular tunnel and VSD closure, the proximal PA is transected and the pulmonary valve and PA stump are then oversewn. In the classic Rastelli operation, RV to PA continuity is then re-established with a size-appropriate pulmonary homograft, which has been trimmed to an adequate length. A small rim of muscle at the proximal end is intentionally preserved to facilitate implantation. The distal anastomosis is constructed using a 6-0 polypropylene suture in the neonate or young infant, using 5-0 in the older child. We prefer to perform these anastomoses with the heart arrested, believing that the slight increase in myocardial ischemia time is worth the increased accuracy of the anastomosis. Proximally, the pulmonary homograft is sutured to the distal end of the ventriculotomy incision with a running 5-0 polypropylene suture in the neonate or young infant, using 4-0 in the older child. We routinely use a patch of autologous pericardium to augment the proximal anastomosis, creating a smoother unobstructed transition between the homograft and the right ventricular surface (**Figure 53.4**).

In the last several years we have preferred to use an internal jugular valved venous conduit (Contegra: Medtronic, Minneapolis, Minnesota, USA) due to the ability to cut it in a way as to move the conduit valve more distal, closer to the PA bifurcation and thus away from the undersurface of the sternum, minimizing the chance of sternal conduit compression. Furthermore, the proximal end can be placed in an oblique fashion, obviating the need for a proximal augmentation with autologous pericardium.

The patient is rewarmed during the insertion of the pulmonary conduit. The cardiotomy suction is removed from across the atrial septum and any residual septal defect is closed after filling the left side with saline, inflating the lungs, and making sure a hole is venting the ascending aorta. The patient is then placed in the Trendelenburg position, and the aortic cross-clamp is removed, making sure that the ascending aorta is vented. We continue to vent the aorta until CPB is weaned off and most of the intracardiac air has been expelled by the ejecting heart. Intracardiac lines are placed as needed and the patient is separated from CPB when the core temperature reaches 36°C. A transesophageal echocardiogram is performed by the cardiologists. If the repair is deemed satisfactory and the hemodynamic parameters acceptable, protamine is administered and the heart is decannulated in the usual fashion.

The Lecompte modification (also known as réparation à l'étage ventriculaire, REV) was proposed to avoid the use of a conduit by directly anastomosing the PA to the right ventriculotomy. To do so, a Lecompte maneuver has to be performed. The PAs are extensively mobilized to avoid excessive stretching. The aorta is transected, and the mobilized PA confluence is transferred anterior to the ascending aorta. The intracardiac repair remains identical to the Rastelli operation. The main differentiating feature is that the PA confluence is anastomosed directly to the right ventriculotomy incision. As with the classic Rastelli, a patch of autologous pericardium is utilized to augment that connection (**Figure 53.5**). Obviously, the transected aorta is re-anastomosed using a

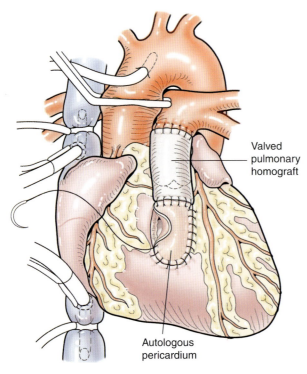

Valved pulmonary homograft

Autologous pericardium

53.4

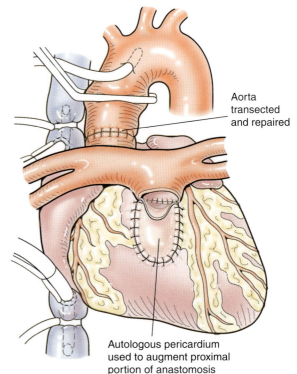

Aorta transected and repaired

Autologous pericardium used to augment proximal portion of anastomosis

53.5

running 6-0 polypropylene suture. Other similar modifications have been proposed such as the Metras procedure. A downside of the REV operation proposed by Lecompte is the absence of a pulmonary valve after the surgical repair. However, the need for reoperation for conduit obstruction may be decreased. Late reoperations may be necessary for severe pulmonary regurgitation and right ventricular dilatation and dysfunction.

Aortic translocation procedure

Despite the application of the Rastelli operation, surgical management of d-TGA, VSD, or TGA, IVS with LVOTO remains a challenge. In order to avoid long-term complications associated with the Rastelli operation, such as conduit stenosis or intracardiac baffle obstruction, the aortic translocation procedure was proposed by Nikaidoh in 1984. The Nikaidoh procedure is undoubtedly a more technically challenging and riskier procedure, but lessons learnt over the years have allowed for a reduction in the early mortality risk. The operation may yield superior long-term outcomes compared to the Rastelli operation, but proper patient selection is absolutely imperative.

The surgical procedure consists of complete dissection and mobilization of the aortic root from the outflow tract of the anatomical RV and translocation to the widely opened outflow tract of the LV. In the original description proposed by Nikaidoh, the right ventricular outflow is normally reconstructed without a conduit using a pericardial hemipatch in order to diminish the risk of requiring a reoperation. However, multiple options exist to re-establish RV–PA continuity. These options include a RV–PA valved conduit, a REV-type RV–PA connection, and a modified REV anastomosis using a valveless tube graft. The surgeon's preference and case-specific anatomical variations will dictate which option is preferable.

The Nikaidoh operation is well suited for patients with d-TGA, associated with a VSD and a stenotic pulmonary valve annulus. In our opinion, at the present time we believe that the Nikaidoh operation is most appropriate and superior to the Rastelli operation in patients with TGA with a remote VSD, LVOTO, or for TGA, IVS, with LVOTO.

After median sternotomy, a thymectomy is performed, the pericardial sac is opened, and systemic heparinization is achieved. The ascending aorta and both venae cavae are cannulated. Cardiopulmonary bypass is instituted. The ductus arteriosus or ligamentum is isolated, ligated, and divided. Systemic pulmonary shunts, if present, are dissected, clamped, and divided. The aorta is cross-clamped and the heart is arrested by delivering cold-blood cardioplegia in the aortic root. The aortic root is then carefully dissected and mobilized with great care to protect the coronary arteries and the aortic valve. The right and left coronary arteries are carefully mobilized to gain enough length and allow transfer

of the aortic root (**Figure 53.6a**). In cases of side-by-side great vessels, the right coronary may need to be detached and re-anastomosed to allow aortic root translocation without compromising coronary perfusion (as demonstrated in **Figures 53.8a** and **53.8b**).

The PA is transected above the level of the valve. The severely stenotic or atretic pulmonary annulus is divided at the point of continuity with the aortic annulus. This incision is carried down through the conal septum (if present) (**Figure 53.6b**).

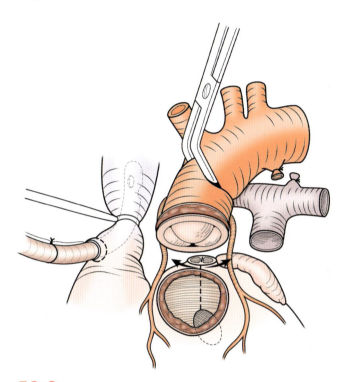

53.6a

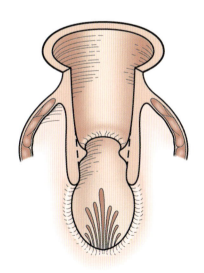

53.6b

Interrupted sutures of pledgeted 4-0 braided polyester are placed circumferentially on the rim of the VSD and passed to a previously tailored patch of Gore-Tex. The anterior portion of the translocated aortic root is similarly anastomosed to the superior edge of the VSD patch (**Figure 53.7a and b**).

As mentioned previously, multiple approaches exist to re-establish RV to PA continuity. The classic Nikaidoh operation does not entail the use of a conduit. The right lateral wall of the distal main PA is sutured to the external wall of the aortic root. A patch of autologous pericardium (preferably) is utilized to baffle the right ventriculotomy externally to the PA confluence using the anterior portion of the aortic root as the "back wall". Alternatively, a valved conduit (homograft of Contegra) can be employed. Placement of this conduit should be carefully guided by the geometry of the great vessels and coronary arteries in order to avoid hemodynamically significant compression (**Figure 53.8a and b**).

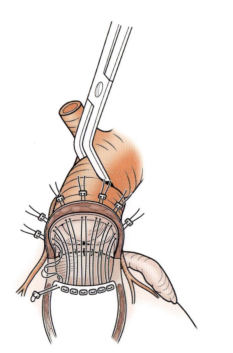

53.7a

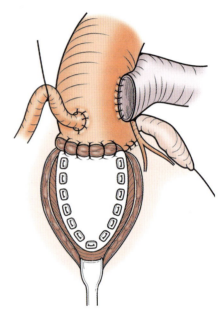

53.8a

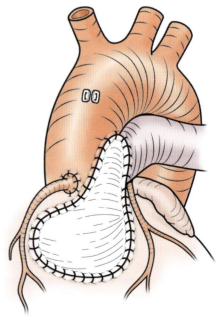

53.7b

53.8b

CONCLUSION

Transposition of the great arteries with left ventricular outflow tract obstruction is a complex lesion for which multiple treatment options have been proposed over the years. The anatomic variations of this lesion dictate the most appropriate surgical option. Both the Rastelli and the Nikaidoh procedures offer good short- and mid-term results. Recent data may demonstrate superior long-term results with the aortic translocation procedure, mostly in terms of increased long-term survival and reduced rate of re-intervention. Optimal patient selection is most important. More definitive prospective studies are needed to demonstrate convincingly which procedure offers the better overall long-term treatment for this patient population. It may be that each procedure has a specific place in the surgical treatment within the spectrum of TGA, VSD, or TGA, IVS with LVOTO.

FURTHER READING

Bautista-Hernandez V, Marx GR, Bacha EA, del Nido PJ. Aortic root translocation plus arterial switch for transposition of the great arteries with left ventricular outflow tract obstruction intermediate-term results. *J Am Coll Cardiol.* 2007; 49: 485–90.

Hazekamp MG, Gomez AA, Koolbergen DR, et al. Surgery for transposition of the great arteries, ventricular septal defect and left ventricular outflow tract obstruction: European Congenital Heart Surgeons Association multicentre study. *Eur J Cardiothorac Surg.* 2010; 38: 699–706.

Jatene AD, Fontes VF, Paulista PP, et al. Successful anatomic correction of transposition of the great vessels: a preliminary report. *Arq Bras Cardiol.* 1965; 28: 461–4.

Kreutzer C, De Vive J, Oppido G, et al. Twenty-five year experience with Rastelli repair for transposition of the great arteries. *J Thorac Cardiovasc Surg.* 2000; 120: 211–23.

Lecompte Y, Neveux JY, Leca F, et al. Reconstruction of the pulmonary outflow tract without prosthetic conduit. *J Thorac Cardiovasc Surg.* 1982; 84: 727–33.

Nikaidoh H. Aortic translocation and biventricular outflow tract reconstruction: a new surgical repair for transposition of the great arteries associated with ventricular septal defect and pulmonary stenosis. *J Thorac Cardiovasc Surg.* 1984; 88: 365–72.

Rastelli GC, Wallace RB, Ongley PA. Complete repair of transposition of the great arteries with pulmonary stenosis: a review of a case corrected by using a new surgical technique. *Circulation.* 1969; 39: 83–95.

Yeh T Jr, Ramaciotti C, Leonard SR, et al. Strategy for biventricular outflow tract reconstruction: Rastelli, REV, or Nikaidoh procedure? *J Thorac Cardiovasc Surg.* 2008; 135: 331–8.

54

Transposition of the great arteries with right ventricular outflow tract obstruction

ERGIN KOCYILDIRIM, MAHESH S. SHARMA, AND VICTOR O. MORELL

BACKGROUND

In 1797, Scottish pathologist Matthew Baillie first described the morphologic details of transposition of the great arteries (TGA)[1] in which the aorta arises entirely or largely from the right ventricle and the pulmonary trunk arises entirely or largely from the left ventricle (ventriculoarterial discordant connection). Surgical correction for this lesion was attempted during the 1950s either at the atrial or great artery levels.[1] The first successful anatomic correction was performed in 1975,[2] when Jatene and colleagues applied the arterial switch operation to infants with TGA and ventricular septal defect (VSD).

TGA is the most common cyanotic congenital heart defect that presents in neonates[3, 4] and accounts for 9.9% of all cases of congenital heart disease.[5] In contrast to left ventricular outflow tract obstruction (LVOTO), right ventricular outflow tract obstruction (RVOTO) is encountered much less frequently in patients with TGA. It is rare in patients with TGA-intact ventricular septum (IVS), but may occur in 20–30% of patients with TGA-VSD.[6] RVOTO is due to an anterior-cephalad malalignment of the conal septum and varying degrees of aortic annular hypoplasia. The resultant increased right ventricular pressure promotes hypertrophy of the ventricular muscle and progressive RVOTO. Hypertrophied septoparietal trabeculations, prominence of the ventriculoinfundibular fold, and abnormal insertions of the atrioventricular (AV) valves into the right ventricular outflow tract (RVOT) may contribute as well. Occasionally, tricuspid insufficiency and hemodynamic deterioration may be observed as a consequence of the elevated right ventricular pressure.[8] RVOTO results in subaortic stenosis (SAO), which may lead to preferential streaming of blood flow through the pulmonary artery (PA) and patent ductus arteriosus (PDA) during fetal life. This, in turn, leads to underdevelopment of the aortic arch resulting in tubular hypoplasia, coarctation of the aorta (CoA), or interrupted aortic arch in 10% of the cases.[7] The presence of RVOTO may complicate attempts at arterial switch operation (ASO) or even preclude its use. This chapter details surgical techniques that have been devised to achieve an unobstructed RVOT in TGA.

OPERATION

Right ventricular outflow tract obstruction in TGA

The technical details of the arterial switch operation and aortic arch reconstruction have been described in Chapter 55. Cardiopulmonary bypass (CPB) is carried out using an appropriate cannulation scheme and the patient is cooled to 28 °C, or 20 °C if aortic reconstruction is necessary. At the Children's Hospital of Pittsburgh we use a proprietary cold-blood cardioplegia solution which is reinfused every 30 minutes. The VSD is most commonly approached through an infundibulotomy in the presence of SAO recognizing that combined approaches through the tricuspid valve, native aorta, or pulmonary valve might be necessary. However, approach through the pulmonary valve is associated with late aortic regurgitation. The RVOT must be carefully inspected. Frequently, at the time of ASO, all that is required is direct resection of the obstructing muscle bundles (**Figure 54.1**), followed by a patch augmentation of the RVOT incision after the VSD closure (**Figure 54.2**). Usual precautions are taken in the setting of a right coronary artery (RCA) or left anterior descending (LAD) from the RCA crossing the infundibulum including strategic positioning of the ventriculotomy or use of an RV–PA conduit. Moderate RV hypoplasia may exist, but it is usually not significant enough to preclude biventricular repair. In such cases, we elect to leave a limited atrial level communication.

In certain circumstances, infundibular resection is not suitable or coronary anatomy is unfavorable for ASO, necessitating an alternate approach such as the Damus-Kaye-Stansel procedure (DKS).[9–13] This operation has the advantage of restoring ventriculoarterial concordance without the need for coronary artery relocation, but it has the disadvantage of requiring the use of an extra-anatomic conduit between the RV and the PA. Such patients will require periodic conduit changes due to somatic growth and conduit stenosis or regurgitation. Of note, as the aortic pressure remains higher than the right ventricular pressure throughout the cardiac cycle in this arrangement, the aortic valve remains closed. The aortic valve, which is in a statically closed position, is subject to clot formation and insufficiency.

We perform a classic end-to-side DKS connection, although others have advocated a "double-barrel" technique for the prevention of postoperative pulmonary (neoaortic)

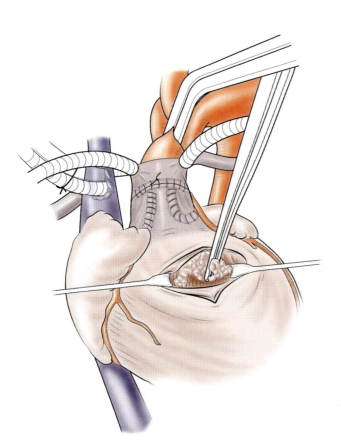

54.1   Muscle resection of the right ventricular outflow tract.

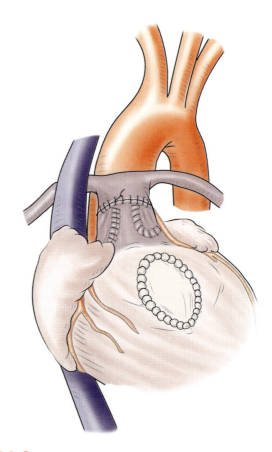

54.2   Right ventricular outflow tract reconstruction completed.

(a)

(b)

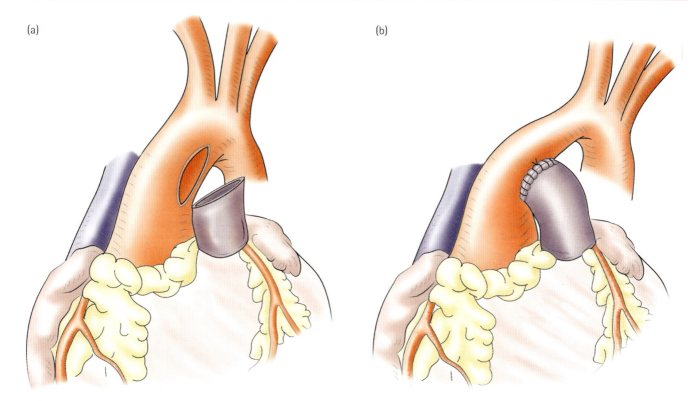

54.3a,b Damus–Kaye–Stansel operation. (a) Main pulmonary artery is transected; (b) end-to-side anastomosis between the main pulmonary artery and aorta.

regurgitation.[14] After CPB has been established, a vertical right ventriculotomy is created, and the VSD is closed with a prosthetic patch. The main pulmonary trunk is then transected just proximal to the bifurcation, and a matching aortotomy is made in the adjacent ascending aorta (**Figure 54.3a**). The proximal end of the transected PA is anastomosed end-to-side to the aorta (**Figure 54.3b**). A pericardial or prosthetic hood is usually interposed in this anastomosis to prevent distortion of the great arteries or semilunar valves. We prefer the application of a valved conduit to re-establish RV–PA continuity, although non-valved connections may be used (**Figure 54.4**).

After repair, RV pressure should be less than half systemic with tricuspid valve competency especially in the face of non-valved RV–PA connection.

Postoperative care is routine with an emphasis on managing obligatory right ventricular dysfunction. Surveillance should be vigilant for coronary patency, recurrent aortic arch obstruction, and late neoaortic (pulmonary) insufficiency in DKS connections.

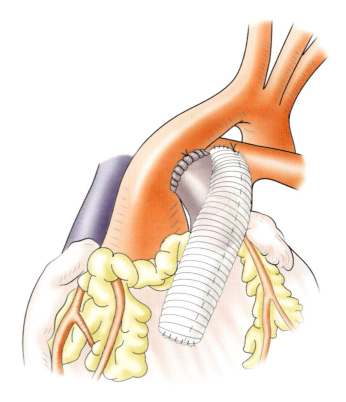

54.4 Damus–Kaye–Stansel operation. Aortopulmonary anastomosis and conduit interposition between the right ventricle and the distal main pulmonary artery.

REFERENCES

1. Baillie M, Wardrop J. The morbid anatomy of some of the most important parts of the human body: to which are prefixed preliminary observations on diseased structures. London: Longman, Rees, Orme, Brown, Green, & Longman; 1833.
2. Jatene AD, Fontes VF, Paulista PP, et al. Successful anatomic correction of transposition of the great vessels: a preliminary report. *Arq Bras Cardiol.* 1975; 28(4): 461–4.
3. Šamánek M, Voříšková M. Congenital heart disease among 815,569 children born between 1980 and 1990 and their 15-year survival: a prospective Bohemia survival study. *Pediatr Cardiol.* 1999; 20(6): 411–17.
4. Ferencz C, Rubin JD, McCarter RJ, et al. Congenital heart disease: prevalence at livebirth. The Baltimore-Washington Infant Study. *Am J Epidemiol.* 1985; 121(1): 31–6.
5. Talner NS. Report of the New England Regional Infant Cardiac Program, by Donald C. Fyler, MD, Pediatrics, 1980; 65(suppl): 375–461. *Pediatrics.* 1998; 102(1 Pt 2): 258–9.
6. Moene RJ, Oppenheimer-Dekker A. Congenital mitral valve anomalies in transposition of the great arteries. *Am J Cardiol.* 1982; 49(8): 1972–8.
7. Vogel M, Freedom RM, Smallhorn JF, et al. Complete transposition of the great arteries and coarctation of the aorta. *Am J Cardiol.* 1984; 53(11): 1627–32.
8. Huhta JC, Edwards WD, Danielson GK, Feldt RH. Abnormalities of the tricuspid valve in complete transposition of the great arteries with ventricular septal defect. *J Thorac Cardiovasc Surg.* 1982; 83(4): 569–76.
9. Damus PS. Letter to the editor. *Ann Thorac Surg.* 1975; 20: 724–5.
10. Kaye MP. Anatomic correction of transposition of great arteries. *Mayo Clinic Proc.* 1975; 50(11): 638–40.
11. Stansel HC Jr. A new operation for d-loop transposition of the great vessels. *Ann Thorac Surg.* 1975; 19(5): 565–7.
12. Alvarez Díaz, F, Hurtado E, Perez de León J, et al. Técnica de corrección anatómica de la transposición completa de grandes arterias. *Rev Esp Cardiol.* 1975; 28: 255–7.
13. Damus PS, Thomson NB Jr, McLoughlin TG. Arterial repair without coronary relocation for complete transposition of the great vessels with ventricular septal defect. Report of a case. *J Thorac Cardiovasc Surg.* 1982; 83(2): 316–18.
14. Fujii Y, Kasahara S, Kotani Y, et al. Double-barrel Damus-Kaye-Stansel operation is better than end-to-side Damus-Kaye_Stansel operation for preserving the pulmonary valve function: the importance of preserving the shape of the pulmonary sinus. *J Thorac Cardiovasc Surg.* 2011; 141: 193–9.

55

Anatomical repair of transposition of the great arteries

FRANCOIS LACOUR-GAYET

Anatomical repair, by restoring ventriculoarterial concordance, offers the optimal long-term survival to patients born with transposition of the great arteries. The arterial switch operation (ASO) has become, with time, a simplified and safe operation, with an operative mortality approaching 0%.[1] Almost all technical problems raised by an abnormal coronary artery anatomy and by associated cardiac lesions have found adapted solutions. The aim of this chapter is to describe the current surgical technique and some useful "tricks" adopted during a 25-year experience with this operation. This chapter focuses on management of transposition of the great arteries with intact ventricular septum (TGA-IVS) and describes the anatomical classification of coronary arteries and the technique of coronary transfer in complex anatomy.

HISTORY

The first successful arterial switch was achieved in patients with TGA-VSD by Abib Jatene in Sao Paolo in 1975. Arterial switch in TGA-IVS was first reported by Donald Ross in 1976 in a 20-month-old child with persistent ductus arteriosus. A two-stage arterial switch in TGA-IVS was reported by Yacoub et al. in 1976, whereas the first successful neonatal arterial switch attempted in a patient with TGA-IVS was reported by Aldo Castaneda in 1984. The description of the French maneuver by Yves Lecompte in 1981, avoiding the use of foreign material to reconstruct the pulmonary artery (PA), and our suggestion in 1985 to use a single posterior autologous pericardial patch, contributed to the wide success of the ASO.

CLASSIFICATION OF CORONARY ARTERIES

The classification[2] described in 1978 by Magdi Yacoub, remains valid today. We are following a classification[3] that is based on the course of the coronary arteries vessels and not

on the origin. The main interest of this classification is that the coronary relocation techniques depend on these different courses. The coronaries are defined in situs solitus with a left and a right ostium. Four groups are recognized according to the following coronary courses:

1. Normal course
2. Looping courses
3. Intramural course
4. Miscellaneous course.

Normal course (60%)

The normal course of the coronary arteries is the most frequent and represents 60% of cases. The left ostium gives the left anterior descending and the circumflex artery (CX), and the right ostium gives the right coronary artery (RCA). No vessel is crossing either in front of or behind the great vessels (**Figure 55.1**).

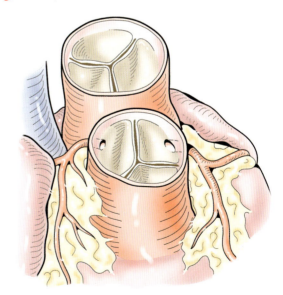

55.1

Looping courses (35%)

The looping courses are those in which a coronary runs in front of and/or behind the great vessels, and represent 35% of cases. Three subgroups exist: the posterior looping course, the anterior looping course, and the double looping course.

POSTERIOR LOOPING COURSE (20%)

The posterior looping course is one in which a coronary runs posterior to the PA, and two subtypes exist. One is frequent, with the posterior looping coronary being the CX arising from the RCA (Yacoub type D), and the other is a single coronary ostium (1%) (**Figure 55.2**).

ANTERIOR LOOPING COURSE (1%)

The anterior looping course is one in which a coronary runs anterior to the aorta, and three subtypes exist, including two single ostium forms (**Figure 55.3**). A strictly anterior looping is very rare.

DOUBLE-LOOPING COURSE (14%)

Two forms are frequent: one with a posterior loop, done by the common left trunk (8%) (called inverted coronary artery by A. Castaneda) and one with a posterior loop done by the CX (5%). One rare form is a single coronary ostium (1%). Notice some malalignment of the commissures present on the three forms (**Figure 55.4**).

Intramural course (5%)

The intramural course is one in which one or both coronary arteries have an abnormal intramural course in the posterior aortic wall, crossing behind or above the posterior commissure (**Figure 55.5**).

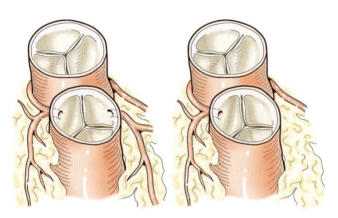

55.2

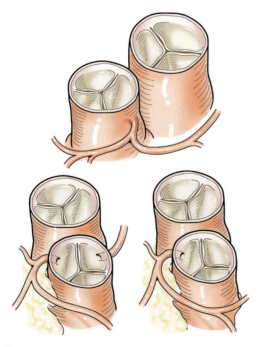

55.3

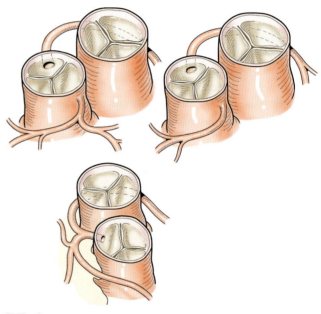

55.4

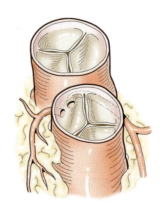

55.5

Miscellaneous course (0.1%)

The miscellaneous course is one which associates an intramural course with a looping course and/or a single coronary ostium (**Figure 55.6**). One deserves to be identified as being the most challenging anatomic pattern to manage; it is the one where a single coronary ostium is associated with an intramural course (Yacoub type B).

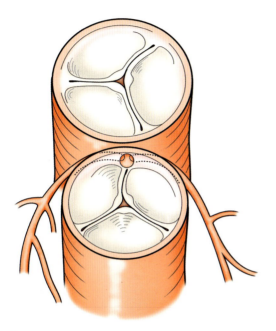

55.6

PREOPERATIVE MANAGEMENT OF TRANSPOSITION OF THE GREAT ARTERIES WITH INTACT VENTRICULAR SEPTUM

Antenatal diagnosis is obtained in 50–80% of the patients and allows optimal management, with a delivery organized close to a pediatric cardiology unit. The protocol for patients with TGA-IVS routinely includes a Rashkind septostomy and prostaglandin E1 infusion at a minimal dose to maintain patency at the ductus arteriosus. Preoperative angiography is not necessary to define the coronary anatomy. Echocardiography is superior, particularly for the diagnosis of intramural coronary. The left ventricular myocardial mass is evaluated when the patient presents beyond 2 weeks of age. A myocardial mass over $35 \pm 5 \, g/m^3$ is required for safe anatomical repair. The arterial switch is electively undertaken at the end of the first week of life.

CARDIOPULMONARY BYPASS AND MYOCARDIAL PROTECTION

Anesthesia follows the principles of neonatal cardiac surgery. The optimal cardiopulmonary bypass (CPB) in neonates remains controversial. The principle uniformly followed is to avoid circulatory arrest. CPB is achieved using full flow at 100–150 mL/kg/minute with bicaval cannulation. The priming volume is currently less than 200 mL, using short tubing and miniaturized membrane oxygenators. The priming solution uses exclusively reconstituted blood, including fresh frozen plasma and red blood cells, to obtain a hematocrit around 30%. The CPB is run at a temperature between 25 °C and 32 °C according to the complexity of the procedure. Myocardial protection uses routinely Custodiol crystalloid cardioplegia injected at a dose of 30 mL/kg for the first injection, and repeated every 40 minutes at a dose of 10 mL/kg by direct injection in the coronary ostia, using a DLP® cannula (Medtronic, Minneapolis, MN). Others are using blood cardioplegia. Modified ultrafiltration and steroids are exceptionally used.

OPERATION

Uniform arterial switch technique

With time, the technique has been simplified and standardized. The technique described here is applicable to all coronary anatomy.

After median sternotomy, the thymus gland is partially resected, keeping a residual superior segment (**Figure 55.7**).

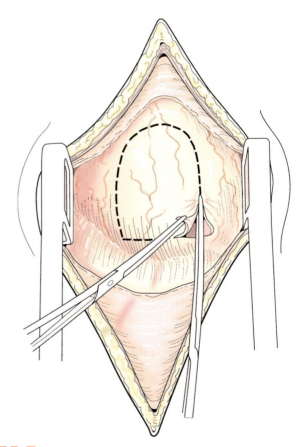

55.7

A large rectangular patch of anterior pericardium is harvested (**Figure 55.8**) and kept in iced saline solution. The pericardium is used fresh.

INSPECTION

The patient pericardium is suspended, avoiding undue traction. Gentle retraction on the right atrial appendage helps to expose the great vessels. The anatomy is carefully analyzed, evaluating the following:

- Origin and courses of the coronary arteries, recognizing abnormal loopings and single ostium. (Full evaluation of the coronary anatomy requires intra-aortic inspection.)
- The relationship of the great vessels, either anteroposterior or side-by-side. (The relationship is most frequently a d-transposition [aorta anterior and to the right].)

The technique is first described in the most frequent and simple condition, with normal coronary artery course, anteroposterior great vessels relationship, and no significant diameter size mismatch.

DISSECTION OF PULMONARY ARTERY BRANCHES AND DUCTUS ARTERIOSUS

All dissection is performed using electrocoagulation. The aorta and the right and left PAs are dissected and controlled by vessel loops (**Figure 55.9**). The ductus arteriosus wall is extremely fragile under prostaglandin and its dissection is started below the right side of the aorta, on its right border. Traction on the left PA vessel loop helps to dissect the left border. The ductus is carefully controlled by a 3-0 suture, which will be tied when going on bypass. In case of torrential pulmonary flow by a large ductus arteriosus, occlusion of the right pulmonary branch with a tourniquet is helpful to increase the aortic diastolic pressure and improve the coronary blood flow.

CANNULATION

Continuous bypass requires an accurate cannulation technique (**Figure 55.10**). The aorta is cannulated very close to the brachiocephalic artery, using a small (size 8 or 10), straight cannula. The superior vena cava venous cannula (straight, reinforced venous cannula, size 12 or 14) is introduced into the atrial appendage and placed in the right atrium. CPB is instituted with one venous cannula. After establishing bypass, the inferior vena cava venous cannula is introduced close to the inferior vena cava and snared. A left atrial (LA) venting cannula (Medtronic) is further introduced through the Sondergard sulcus, distant from the right pulmonary vein ostia. The superior venous cannula is then introduced into the superior vena cava and snared.

DUCTUS ARTERIOSUS DIVISION AND PROXIMAL AORTA DISSECTION

During cooling, the ductus arteriosus, which has been ligated at the onset of CPB, is divided. Following

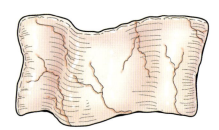

55.8

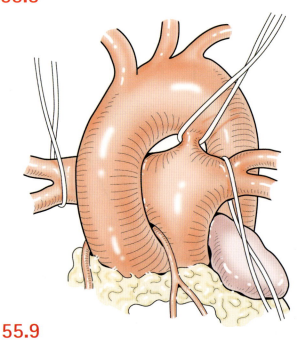

55.9

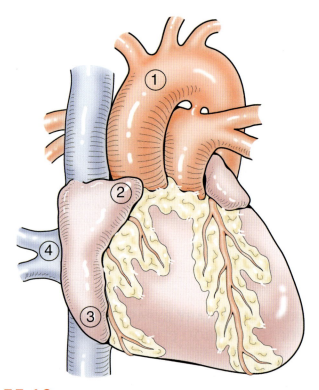

55.10

prostaglandin infusion, the ductus wall is very fragile and should be managed carefully. The ductus is doubly ligated (**Figure 55.11**) and then divided, with suturing of both ends (**Figure 55.12a and b**). The aortic end can also be occluded by a vascular clip. Any tear or needle puncture of

the ductal wall proximal to the ligation should be avoided, as a tear of the origin of the ductus arteriosus is difficult to control. Additional direct stitching usually worsens the hemorrhage, or it may create an isthmus stenosis. Serious hemorrhage at this stage is better controlled under circulatory arrest.

The space between the aortic and pulmonary roots is carefully dissected. This dissection is performed more easily when the aorta is filled. This dissection runs close to the origin of the coronary trunks that are dissected, carefully using very low coagulation intensity. When the coronary trunks are not well seen, this dissection should not be done.

CROSS-CLAMPING, CARDIOPLEGIA, AND CLOSURE OF ATRIAL SEPTAL DEFECT

The aortic cross-clamp is placed very close to the aortic cannula. The cardioplegia is given through a needle placed at the level of the aortotomy. A short, longitudinal, right atriotomy allows good access to the atrial septal defect, which is closed using running suture. In case of a large atrial septal defect, patch closure is preferred to prevent potential arrhythmias.

GREAT VESSELS TRANSECTION

This step is an important step, defining all landmarks of the arterial switch. The aorta is transected exactly at a middle point between the clamp and the aortic annulus. *This incision should be high*, to reduce the length of the reconstructed aorta that will lie behind the PA (**Figure 55.13**).

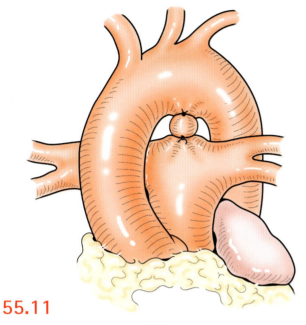

55.11

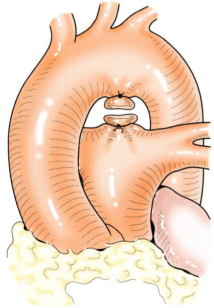

55.12a

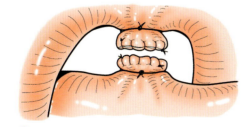

55.12b

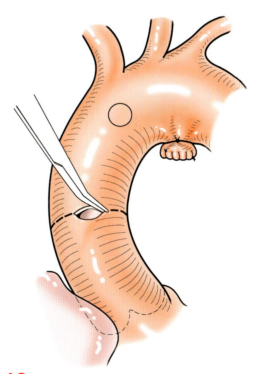

55.13

For the same purpose, *the PA is transected in a low position*, a few millimeters above the pulmonary commissures (**Figure 55.14**). This inferior incision reduces the length of the future neoaortic root, allowing the Lecompte maneuver without compression on the pulmonary branches.

DISSECTION OF PULMONARY ARTERY BRANCHES AND LECOMPTE MANEUVER

Helped by gentle traction on the vessel loops, the PA branches are fully dissected until the lobar branches are clearly seen. The pulmonary bifurcation is then pulled up

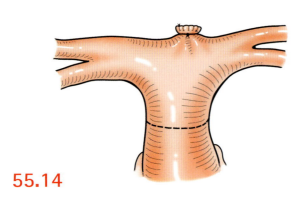

55.14

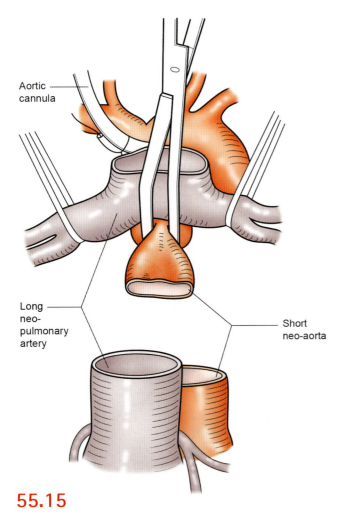

55.15

in front of the ascending aorta. Using a second clamp or forceps, the aortic cross-clamp is mobilized and placed below the pulmonary bifurcation, closely in contact with the aortic cannula, to expose the maximum length of distal ascending aorta. Notice in **Figure 55.15** that, after optimal transection of the great vessels, the future neoaorta is short, and the future neopulmonary artery long. The aortic clamp is blocked on the surgical field at 12 o'clock to stabilize the distal aorta.

HARVESTING OF CORONARY BUTTONS

The harvesting of coronary buttons is crucial (**Figure 55.16**). The general principle is to *take the largest possible button*, removing almost all the sinus of Valsalva, to perform safe anastomoses sufficiently distant from the coronary ostia. *These coronary buttons are in fact aortic buttons containing the coronary ostium*. Two traction sutures, one anterior and one posterior, help exposure. The locations of the ostia are carefully evaluated, particularly their proximity with the commissures and with the aortic annulus. The left button is taken first. An anterior and vertical incision is made in the direction of the left lateral commissure, and the incision stays in close contact with the commissure until the bottom of the sinus. The second incision, which is posterior and vertical, similarly follows the posterior commissure. The last incision is horizontal and follows the aortic annulus. Depending on the location of the ostium, this incision is more or less in contact with the aortic annulus. In rare instances, when the ostium is very low, the aortic annulus itself should be resected. The origin of the left coronary trunk is dissected for 2–3 mm from the myocardium using coagulation until the button can be mobilized posteriorly without affecting the course of the left anterior descending and CX arteries. The right button is then harvested. Similarly, the incisions follow the commissures and the aortic annulus. The button is mobilized for a few millimeters using electrocoagulation to allow a posterior translation without distortion of the right coronary. Three particular coronary anatomical conditions require appropriate management, as discussed below.

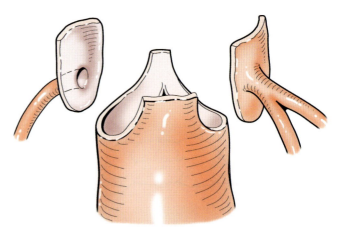

55.16

OSTIUM NEXT TO A COMMISSURE

In some instances, one ostium is eccentric and located very close to or in contact with a commissure (**Figure 55.17**). This usually involves the posterior commissure and rarely the anterior commissures. In these cases deliberate detachment of the posterior commissure and harvesting a large button that could include part of the annulus are crucial (**Figure 55.18**). It will be further reimplanted on the neopulmonary artery.

EARLY INFUNDIBULAR BRANCH

In other instances, an early branching of the infundibular artery arises from the left main trunk. This early branch may limit the posterior translation and can create a stenosis through kinking of the left main trunk (**Figure 55.19**). The branch should be dissected and mobilized if it is large (**Figure 55.20**). Otherwise, and in most instances, however, it must be sacrificed and divided. More rarely, this early infundibular branching comes from the RCA but it should be managed the same way and sacrificed if necessary.

STABILIZATION AND EXPOSURE OF THE NEOAORTA

Starting the operation with three or four posterior stitches on the aortic anastomosis between the distal ascending aorta and the neoaorta is very useful (**Figure 55.21**). This maneuver places the aorta in its final position and greatly helps the exposure. At the same time, a traction stitch is placed on the anterior edge of the PA at the site of the anterior commissure. The aortic clamp is blocked at 12 o'clock.

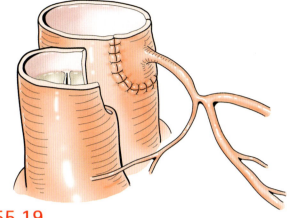

55.19

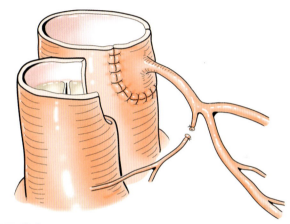

55.20

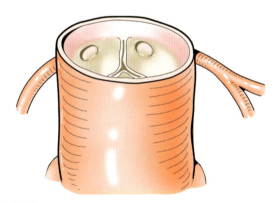

55.17

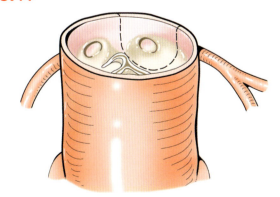

55.18

55.21

CORONARY TRANSFER PRINCIPLES

There are two techniques of coronary transfer.

- *The closed aorta technique* is to complete the aortic anastomosis first, then open the aortic cross-clamp and figure out the best place to relocate the coronary buttons on the neoaorta. This technique does not increase the diameter of the neoaortic root. The risk is injury to the neoaortic valve, as the exposure is quite limited.
- *The open aorta technique* is to implant the coronary buttons prior to completing the aortic anastomosis. It is our preferred technique. It offers an excellent exposure on the neoaortic valve.

Trapdoor or no trapdoor? Long-term results of the ASO[4] show that the neoaortic root dilates significantly with time with a risk of aortic valve regurgitation. The trapdoor technique enlarges the neoaortic root and could possibly impact on the stability of the commissures. We have abandoned the trapdoor technique for many years.[1, 3] The technique of rectangular resection does not increase or may decrease the diameter of the neoaortic root and stay away from the commissures.

OPEN AORTA TECHNIQUE WITHOUT TRAPDOOR

Three points to consider are:

1. Place the buttons laterally to avoid compression by the PA, which lies anteriorly.
2. Use rectangular resections of a size equal or superior to the buttons to be reimplanted.
3. Place the left button in a low position and the right button in a higher position, across the aortic anastomosis, using the long length of the button to limit the mismatch between the distal ascending aorta and the neoaortic root.

LEFT CORONARY BUTTON

A rectangular resection is made on the left sinus of Valsalva. It should be equal in size or larger than the left coronary button. The base of the resection stays 2–3 mm above the neoaortic annulus. The left button is anastomosed in a low left lateral position. The anastomosis is performed using a 7-0 or 8-0 suture and starts at the base of the button (**Figure 55.22**).

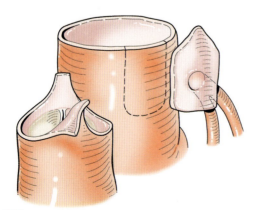

55.22

RIGHT CORONARY BUTTON

A similar rectangular resection is made on the right sinus of Valsalva. It is not as deep: from 2 mm to 8 mm according to the free movement of right coronary. The right coronary button is transferred in high lateral right position (**Figure 55.23**). It will always be placed high in posterior and double loops.

AORTIC ANASTOMOSIS AND INCLUSION OF THE RIGHT BUTTON

The distal aortic anastomosis is then performed. When reaching the anterolateral aorta, suturing in such a way that the left button remains located laterally on the left is important. When reaching the middle anterior line, the stay suture should be exactly at 12 o'clock. Crossing the line in the right anterior part, the suture comes next to the right button. The right button is included in the distal aorta by an incision directed vertically, close to the aortic clamp (**Figure 55.24**). This maneuver allows limiting the diameter

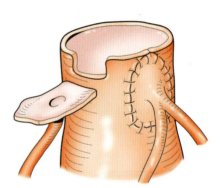

55.23

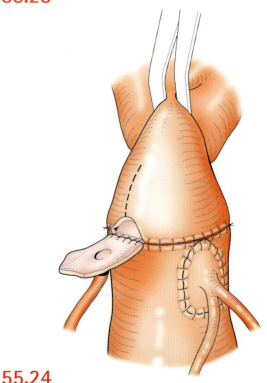

55.24

mismatch between the neoaortic root, which is always large, and the distal aorta (**Figure 55.25**). After de-aeration, the anastomosis is checked. Any bleeding requires additional stitches. A shallow layer of biological glue is placed on the suture lines.

This technique is uniformly used in all coronary anatomy.

RECONSTRUCTION OF THE NEOPULMONARY ROOT

Reconstruction of the neopulmonary root is easier to perform with the aorta maintained cross-clamped. A large, rectangular, fresh patch of autologous pericardium is used. The patch is sutured on the remnant of the previous aortic annulus (**Figure 55.26a**). This suture line requires particular attention, as any posterior bleeding on the beating heart is difficult to manage. When detached, the posterior commissure is reattached on the pericardial patch posteriorly (**Figure 55.26b**).

REMOVAL OF THE AORTIC CLAMP AND CHECKING OF THE CORONARIES REPERFUSION

In favorable coronary anatomy, the cross-clamp can be removed before the completion of the proximal pulmonary reconstruction.

The quality of the reperfusion is carefully evaluated, based on the coloration of the myocardium and on normal filling of the coronary arteries. The courses of the proximal coronary trunks are carefully checked. The presence of poor filling of a coronary, poor coloration, ventricular arrhythmia, and major ECG changes indicate a coronary issue. This requires to be immediately corrected including reclamping the aorta and redoing a coronary button. When this evaluation is completed, the patient is rewarmed.

DISTAL PULMONARY ARTERY ANASTOMOSIS

The distal anastomosis is performed during rewarming (**Figure 55.27a**). The final anatomical repair is shown in **Figure 55.27b**.

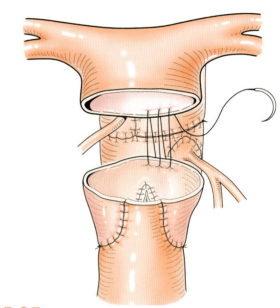

55.27a

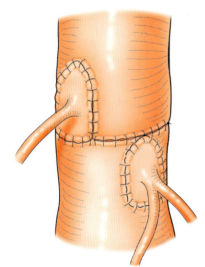

55.25

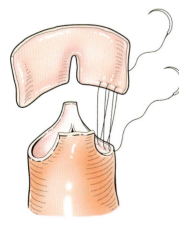 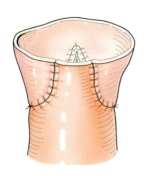

55.26a   **55.26b**

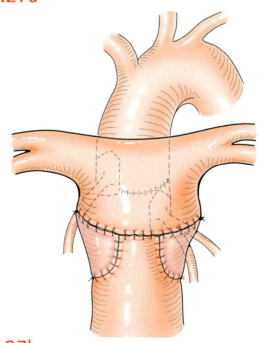

55.27b

COMING OFF BYPASS AND HEMOSTASIS

Before coming off bypass, the ECG, the coloration, and the contractions of all myocardial segments should be normal. Bleeding should be minimal. A left atrial (LA) line is routinely placed. Atrial pacing is used to obtain a sinus rhythm of around 140 beats/minute. The need for inotropic support depends on the quality of LV function, varying from small doses of dopamine and milrinone to epinephrine. Pulmonary hypertension can occur, requiring nitric oxide. Any suspicion of myocardial ischemia related to a kinking of a coronary trunk requires going back on bypass and redoing the anastomosis. The sternum can be closed when the hemodynamics are satisfactory and when the heart is not distended. Otherwise, the sternum should be left open and the skin closed with a patch of polytetrafluoroethylene (Gore-Tex).

Hemostasis is a major complication of the ASO. With experience, major hemostatic problems are rare. When the bleeding cannot be easily controlled, going back on bypass and eventually taking down the distal pulmonary anastomosis to gain access to all bleeding is preferable.

POSTOPERATIVE MANAGEMENT

In the simple forms, the postoperative course is frequently straightforward.[1] When the hemodynamics remain instable, it is preferable to go on extracorporeal membrane oxygenation (ECMO) rather than to increase the inotropes. Extubation should be undertaken only when the LV function is back to normal on transthoracic echocardiogram.

Management of complex anatomy

Basically, the same coronary transfer technique is applied to all coronary anatomy. In complex forms of TGA, the surgical technique is more demanding and requires a sort of "second" learning curve. Complex anatomies include the following:

- looping courses
- intramural course
- single coronary ostium
- the case of single ostium with intramural course
- malaligned commissures
- major diameter mismatch between PA and aorta.

LOOPING COURSES

It is important to understand the risk inherent to coronary transfer in complex coronary patterns. The risk of transfer follows the type of looping courses. *The posterior loop is associated with a risk of kinking (Figure 55.28) and the anterior loop with a risk of stretching (Figure 55.29). Extensive dissection of the coronary trunks is necessary* to avoid kinking or stretching of the coronary trunks.

In posterior loop, with the circumflex coming off the right coronary and looping posteriorly, the circumflex is at risk

of kinking when placed in a low position. The circumflex is dissected far away, behind the PA, to allow a safe mobilization. The button is placed in a high position to increase the distance and prevent kinking (**Figure 55.30**).

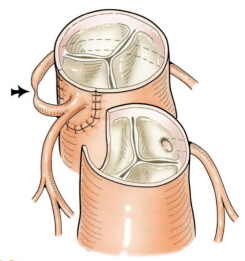

55.28

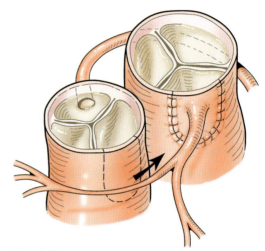

55.29

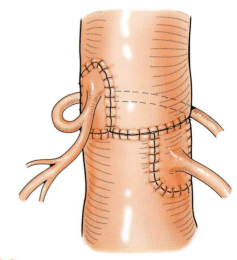

55.30

In double loop, the posterior loop is either the circumflex or the left main trunk. The risk of kinking is controlled in placing the button in a supra-anastomotic position. The main issue is the anterior loop made by the RCA, which crosses in front of the aorta and is many times adherent to the wall. The RCA should be dissected on a long distance from the aorta and the RV to prevent stretching (**Figure 55.31a**). Others are using trapdoor to control the stretching of the RCA.

Figure 55.31b shows a double loop, with posterior circumflex (right) and posterior left main trunk (left). In both cases, the right button is placed in a supra-anastomotic position. The RCA that crosses in front of the aorta should be extensively dissected free.

Side-by-side vessels are almost constant in double loop and in Taussig–Bing hearts. After the Lecompte maneuver, the reconstruction of the pulmonary bifurcation can compress the right coronary that is looping anteriorly. Mobilization of the pulmonary bifurcation to the right is necessary to prevent a compression of the RCA. The right PA is incised for 20 mm, and the PA trunk is directly anastomosed to the right PA to free the RCA course. The left part of the PA trunk is then patched. The other option is not to do the Lecompte maneuver.

The patch reconstruction of the PA bifurcation can compress the left button, particularly the RCA that crosses in front of the previous aorta. The PA bifurcation is realigned on the right by an incision of the right PA (**Figure 55.32**).

The distal pulmonary anastomosis uses a large patch. The PA trunk reconstruction is done before the left coronary button relocation in double-loop coronary with side-by-side vessels (**Figure 55.33**).

INTRAMURAL COURSE OF CORONARY ARTERIES

Coronary transfer with intramural course represents a major surgical difficulty. Preoperative echocardiogram is superior

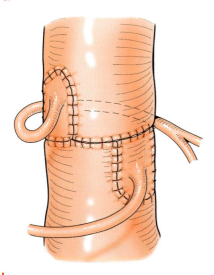

55.31a

55.31b

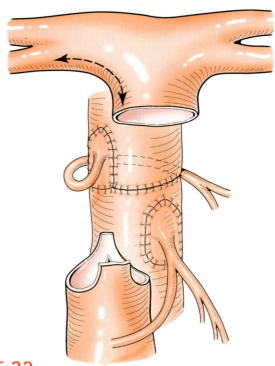

55.32

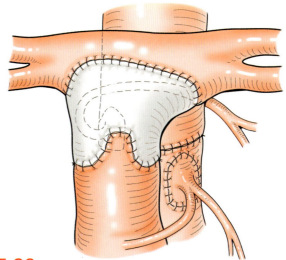

55.33

to angiocardiography for recognizing this rare pattern. In many instances, this anomaly is discovered intraoperatively. The technique described by T. Asou and R. Mee is the preferred one.[5] The anomaly is due to an abnormal course of the coronary arteries inside the posterior aortic wall. The ostia are found very close to each other, either in the right sinus or above the posterior commissure. It is most often an abnormal location of the left ostium, with intramural course of the left coronary artery. The intramural course can be very long and is at great risk when harvesting the button. The technique is to create two buttons. First, the posterior commissure is totally detached. The intramural course is evaluated using a coronary probe. It can be extremely long, measuring more than 20 mm. The left ostium, which is frequently stenotic, is incised and "unroofed" for a distance of 5 mm (**Figure 55.34**). After this opening, the two ostia are sufficiently distant to allow the creation of two buttons. The harvesting of the left button should be very cautious, considering the very long intramural course. It is the entirety of the sinus that is harvested. Then, two buttons are created in dividing the common button in its middle. The incision should stay as distant as possible from the ostia to allow safe suturing. Using 8-0 Prolene, the two buttons are relocated on each sinus according to the basic technique. The posterior commissure will be reattached on the pericardial pulmonary patch.

Note that the worst form of intramural coronary is when there is a single ostium with intramural course of both coronary arteries (see **Figure 55.6**), which is addressed below (see **Figure 55.39**).

SINGLE CORONARY OSTIUM

All cases of single coronary ostium have an abnormal looping course: anterior, posterior, or double loop. Their relocation follows the same principles. Extensive dissection of the looping coronary trunks is essential, either the posterior or the anterior one. The risks are the same: stretching of the anterior vessel and kinking of the posterior one. The right buttons are transferred in a high position and the left button in a low position.

There are three forms of single right coronary and one form of single left coronary:

- single right coronary ostium:
  - posterior looping from the right button (**Figure 55.35**)
  - double looping from the right button (**Figure 55.36**)
  - anterior looping from the right button (**Figure 55.37**)
- single left coronary ostium:
  - anterior looping from the left button (**Figure 55.38**).

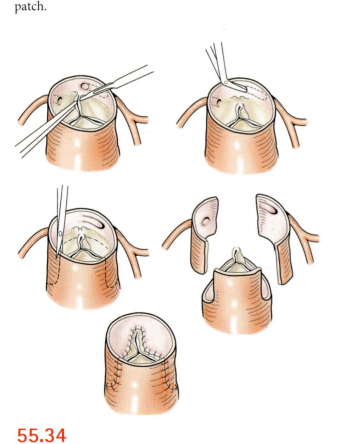

55.34

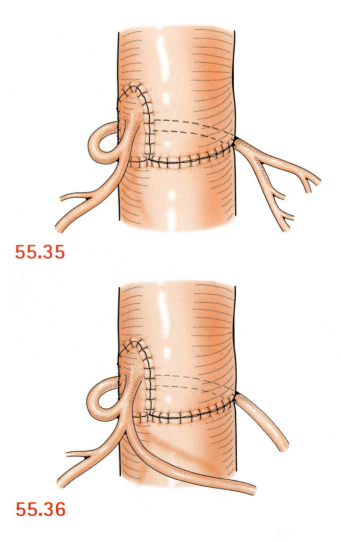

55.35

55.36

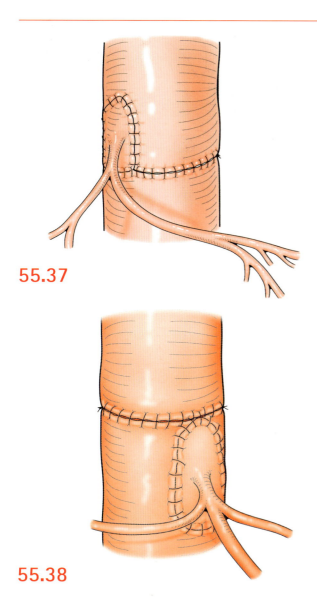

55.37

55.38

THE CASE OF SINGLE OSTIUM WITH INTRAMURAL COURSE

This is the worst form to deal with. This Yacoub type B (see **Figure 55.6**) includes both a single ostium and an intramural course. Several solutions are proposed. The technique proposed by Magdi Yacoub[2] is to rotate the button 180 degrees and to place a hood anteriorly. This technique is at risk for having the button compressed by the PA lying anteriorly, following the Lecompte maneuver. The other technique was described by Moat and Pawade,[6] following proposals by Aubert and Takeuchi. It is to create a fistula between the posterior wall of the aortic root and the anterior wall of the pulmonary root, in order to reroute the coronary flow without doing a coronary relocation. This technique leaves the coronary in place and avoids any dissection and rotation (**Figure 55.39**). The risk is that the coronary arteries remain between the aorta and PA and could ultimately been compressed and cause sudden death. Creating two buttons would be the ideal solution in favorable forms. Finally, this anatomy could be the only contraindication of arterial switch and to proceed to an atrial switch.

MALALIGNED COMMISSURES

This is a major abnormality when severe. It was the only cause of late death in our recent series of ASOs.[1] It can be seen in all coronary patterns, but it is more frequent in complex anatomy. The malalignment impacts on the coronary relocation, not really on the right button, which could be placed above the commissure, but very much on the left button, which could have to be reimplanted exactly on the abnormally located commissure. We have used a technique of commissures realignment. Prior to transferring the coronary, the distal ascending aorta and the PA trunk are rotated in opposite directions in order to realign the anterior and posterior commissures. (In **Figure 55.40** the distal aorta is rotated counterclockwise and the pulmonary trunk clockwise to realign the commissures.) As the rotations are distributed evenly on the two vessels, the torsion is well tolerated. Then the aortic clamp is repositioned at 12H (12 o'clock position) to stabilize the new setting.

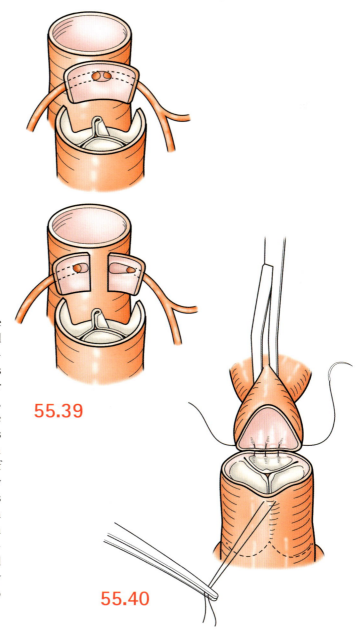

55.39

55.40

MAJOR DIAMETER MISMATCH AND AORTIC ARCH RECONSTRUCTION

Major diameter discrepancy between the aorta and PA is seen in TGA-VSD and particularly in TGA-VSD-coarctation. This has an important impact on the coronary transfer. The solution is to enlarge the distal aorta to correct the mismatch, which is done during the arch repair, now performed under antegrade brain perfusion and no circulatory arrest.

Figure 55.41 shows major PA-to-aorta diameter mismatch associated with side-by-side vessels and double-loop coronary course. This feature is seen in TGA-VSD coarctation or Taussig–Bing with coarctation. The coarctation is resected, and the ascending aorta and the transverse arch entirely incised (**Figure 55.42**). The distal ascending aorta and transverse arch are enlarged using a homograft or Cormetrix patch. This step corrects the diameter mismatch. Placing the extremity of the right and left button above the aortic anastomosis also allows correction of the mismatch (**Figure 55.43**).

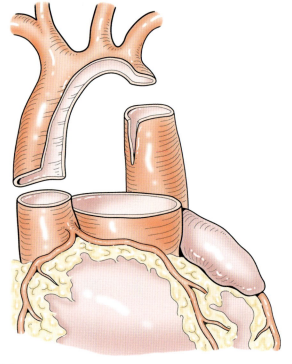

55.42

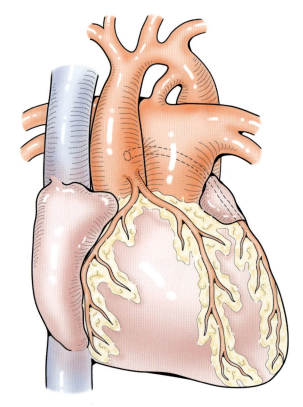

55.41

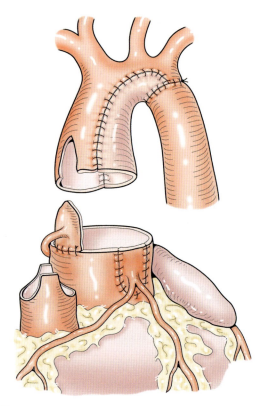

55.43

OUTCOME

The arterial switch technique is now standardized, the coronary transfer being nearly always the same. The arterial switch is currently achieved with minimal operative mortality: from 0%[1] to 5% in simple forms. Arterial switch performed in complex forms, including looping courses or intramural courses, is associated with an increased risk. The long-term results can be complicated by reoperation on the pulmonary branches that could be stretched, by coronary artery stenosis in complex coronary patterns and by aortic regurgitation. The main long-term issue remains the late dilation of the neoaortic root that requires close follow-up.

REFERENCES

1. Stoica S, Campbell D, Lacour-Gayet F, et al. Morbidity of the arterial switch operation. *Ann Thorac Surg.* 2012; 93: 1977–83.

2. Yacoub M, Radley-Smith R. Anatomy of the coronary arteries in transposition of the great arteries and methods for their transfer in anatomical correction. *Thorax.* 1978; 33: 418–24.

3. Lacour-Gayet F, Anderson R. A uniform surgical technique for transfer of both simple and complex patterns of the coronary arteries during the arterial switch procedure. *Cardiol Young.* 2005; 15: 93–101.

4. Co-Vu JG, Ginde S, Bartz PJ, et al. Long-term outcomes of the neoaorta after arterial switch operation for transposition of the great arteries. *Ann Thorac Surg.* 2013; 95(5): 1654–9.

5. Asou T, Karl TR, Pawade A, Mee RB. Arterial switch: translocation of the intramural coronary artery. *Ann Thorac Surg.* 1994; 57: 461–5.

6. Moat N, Pawade A, Lamb R. Complex coronary arterial anatomy in transposition of the great arteries: arterial switch procedure without coronary relocation. *J Thorac Cardiovasc Surg.* 1992; 103: 872–6.

56

Congenitally corrected transposition

DAVID J. BARRON

HISTORY

This rare condition (0.5% of all congenital heart disease) is characterized by both atrioventricular (AV) and ventriculoarterial (VA) discordance. Thus, physiologically the circulation is "corrected" in the sense that the systemic venous blood is directed to the lungs (via a morphological left ventricle) and the pulmonary venous return is directed to the aorta. However, the systemic ventricle is a morphological right ventricle (mRV), guarded by a tricuspid valve. The condition was first described by Rokitansky in 1875 and is typified by *laevo-* or *L*-transposition in which the transposed aorta sits anterior and to the left of the pulmonary artery.

Congenitally corrected transposition of the great arteries (ccTGA) is characterized by its variety of associated lesions, and by unusual cardiac position, which makes classification complex and accounts for its great heterogeneity in terms of clinical presentation and symptoms – which is further complicated by the unpredictable nature of the performance of the mRV and the tricuspid valve within the systemic circulation. However, the most important classification is in the presence or absence of left ventricular outflow tract obstruction (LVOTO) either as pulmonary stenosis or atresia, which is almost always associated with a ventricular septal defect (VSD). Approximately half of cases will fall into this group and will therefore be cyanosed. There is considerable geographical variability in this feature, being much commoner in the Far East, whereas unobstructed LVOTO is commoner in the Western hemisphere.

Over 85% of cases will have associated cardiac abnormalities, the most common being VSD, and the management will be dependent on their nature and severity, so that a neonate with a large VSD might need immediate intervention yet some cases of isolated ccTGA (i.e. no associated lesions) may live into old age without ever requiring any treatment. Surgical intervention was traditionally focused on correcting the associated lesions, achieving so-called "*physiologic repair*" which left the mRV in the systemic circulation, but overall results were disappointing with a high incidence of systemic ventricular failure and tricuspid regurgitation (TR) during follow-up. These concerns over the systemic mRV, coupled with the recognition that even isolated ccTGA could exhibit unpredictable mRV dysfunction at any age, led to the concept of "*anatomic repair*" in the early 1990s, which would restore the (mLV) to the systemic circulation. This required both atrial inversion (the Mustard and Senning procedures) and arterial switch or Rastelli, together with correction of any associated lesions – these are known as the double-switch procedures. These anatomic repair procedures have the advantage of restoring the mLV to the systemic circulation but are a complex undertaking and require careful case selection and preparation. Although the outcomes are substantially better than the natural history of uncorrected ccTGA, the long-term performance of the mLV in the double switch remains under scrutiny.

PRINCIPLES AND JUSTIFICATION

The principles of management are based on the associated lesions, the underlying ventricular function (of both mRV and mLV), and the age of the patient.

Anatomy and associated lesions

There is AV- and VA-discordance with the transposed aorta being to the left with the majority of cases being situs solitus (Van Praagh classification of S,L,L), although situs inversus is relatively common compared to other cardiac lesions, occurring in 5–8% of cases.

The aorta is anterior and to the left, although the great vessels tend to be more side-by-side in comparison to the more AP relationship seen in d-TGA. The coronaries arise from the facing sinuses and are usually suitable for translocation as part of the arterial switch.

Abnormal positioning of the heart is common with dextrocardia or mesocardia seen in 20–25%. The ventricular mass tends to be more anterior in these cases, making access to the atria and the AV valves more difficult. The venous connections are usually normal. The landmarks of the right atrium are normal, but it leads into the mLV through a mitral valve. The left atrium leads through a tricuspid valve into the mRV.

Ventricular septal defect occurs in up to 85% of cases and is most commonly perimembranous outlet and variable in size. When there is associated LVOTO, the VSD is large but occasionally can be committed more to the inlet, making it remote from the aorta. Anatomic repair can be possible only if the mLV can be committed through to the aorta with a Rastelli procedure, with or without VSD enlargement. Coarctation, arch hypoplasia, and, rarely, interruption can occur (10%) in the presence of a VSD and require neonatal intervention, typically with arch repair and pulmonary artery (PA) band. Associated pulmonary stenosis or atresia requires provision of additional pulmonary blood flow according to the severity of cyanosis – usually with a modified Blalock–Taussig shunt, allowing for definitive repair when the child is older.

The conduction system is very abnormal in ccTGA. The AV node is displaced anteriorly and superiorly so that it does not lie in the triangle of Koch. The bundle takes a long course around the free wall of the left ventricle, anterior to the pulmonary valve, before sweeping down onto the ventricular septum in the mLV. This long course predisposes to heart block and 40% of patients will develop conduction abnormalities as part of the natural history, some requiring early pacemaker for congenital heart block. Note that in situs inversus the topology of the heart reverts to normal and, with it, so does the conduction pathway, with the AV node reverting to its usual position in the triangle of Koch.

Abnormalities of the tricuspid valve are common, the commonest being an exaggeration of the offsetting of the AV valves resulting in an "Ebsteinod" displacement of the valve (although not associated with the failed delamination or extreme leaflet anomalies seen in true Ebstein anomaly) and regurgitation is common. The aetiology of TR in ccTGA is complex, being related to ventricular dysfunction, annular dilatation, and morphological abnormalities of the valve.

Ventricular function

Deteriorating mRV function is common and is frequently part of the indication for surgery, often associated with variable degrees of TR. Good function of the mLV is essential for anatomic repair to be successful. Patients with ccTGA and a large VSD have always had an mLV exposed to systemic pressures and its ability to support the systemic circulation is not usually in question. Patients who have required pulmonary artery banding prior to double switch usually have equal pressure between the two ventricles.

Age

Neonates with large VSDs may require PA banding and any arch obstruction repaired. These measures palliate the circulation and prepare for potential anatomic repair later in childhood. Similarly, pulmonary stenosis or atresia can be palliated with BT shunt. Anatomic repair is typically performed at 2–6 years of age. The decision-making in older children can be more difficult as they may not be symptomatic, yet have evidence of mRV dysfunction and TR. Some will require pre-emptive PA banding to retrain the mLV, as discussed below.

The justification for intervention in symptomless patients is a cause for considerable debate. These patients typically have no associated lesions or a small VSD. In this situation, if there is well preserved mRV function then they should be left well alone and managed expectantly. However, any evidence of mRV dysfunction and ≥mod TR will almost certainly lead to congestive heart failure over the next 5 years and warrants early intervention in the form of pre-emptive PA banding to retrain the mLV and splint the interventricular septum to preserve tricuspid valve function. If the mLV responds well to the band, then double-switch may be performed within the next 6-18 months. However, older children or adolescents may have lost the fundamental plasticity in ventricular remodelling to be able to respond to banding and may never be suitable for anatomic repair, being better diverted to management on a heart failure programme and consideration for transplantation if required. A small subset of adolescents with well preserved mRV function and ≥mod TR may benefit from isolated tricuspid valve replacement but need careful surveillance of mRV function. Tricuspid valve repair in this setting has been universally disappointing and direct replacement is recommended.

PREOPERTIVE ASSESSMENT AND PLANNING

The heterogeneity of the condition is reflected in the very variable age and condition of the patients when they come forward for surgery. These factors will dictate what initial procedure is undertaken, as discussed above. Neonates with duct-dependent lesions require standard supportive care and treatment with prostaglandin to stabilize their condition and may require preoperative ventilation. However, most patients coming forward for anatomic repair are older children and are clinically stable, being able to plan the surgery as an elective procedure.

Most information can be obtained from transthoracic echocardiography and cardiac catheterization. Most cases will need hemodynamic data from catheterization, particularly if a pulmonary artery band has been placed previously. A CT scan or cardiac MRI is not strictly necessary unless there is concern regarding the location of the VSD or to delineate the branch pulmonary arteries if there has been a previous Blalock–Taussig shunt. Each component of the anatomy and physiology should be carefully assessed on echo, paying particular attention to the position of the cardiac chambers and to the function and morphology of the AV valves. The position of the VSD should be carefully delineated, together with the positioning of a PA band and the presence of any associated pulmonary root dilatation and/or pulmonary incompetence. A preoperative ECG is essential to document any pre-existing conduction abnormalities.

ANESTHESIA

The anesthetist must be fully aware of the morphology (particularly situs) in terms of placement of lines and the monitoring should be set up to accommodate a left atrial pressure line at the end of the procedure. Standard cardiac anesthetic protocols should be used, taking into account that this is likely to be a relatively long procedure. Ideally, venous pressure monitoring in both the superior vena cava (SVC) and inferior vena cava (IVC) territories is helpful in assessing the Senning pathways at completion of the procedure.

OPERATION: PULMONARY ARTERY BANDING

Banding can be indicated for a variety of reasons. If the VSD is large, then a band is necessary to balance the circulation and protect the lungs from overcirculation; in the case of smaller VSDs or intact septum the band is used to retrain the mLV to become suitable for a subsequent double switch. Banding also has a therapeutic role in splinting the ventricular septum and reducing the degree of TR.

The band can be applied via right thoracotomy or sternotomy, but we prefer the sternotomy approach. A pressure line is floated into the mLV via a sheath in the right internal jugular vein. A limited opening is made in the pericardium and the main PA is carefully dissected so that the position of the branch PAs are clearly seen, placing the band immediately above the sinotubular junction. The circumference of the main PA is measured and the band is initially fixed at half of the initial circumference. We use a 3 mm Silastic impregnated nylon tape, but Gore-Tex® can also be used.

If there is a large VSD, we alter the band to achieve a pressure of one-third systemic in the PAs distal to the band and confirm good position on epicardial echo to ensure there is no distortion of the pulmonary valve and ensure that the mLV function remains unchanged. In smaller (restrictive) VSD or intact septum we alter the band to achieve 60–70% systemic pressure in the mLV. Epicardial echo is helpful to assess mLV function and the septal positioning. The band should create some straightening of the ventricular septum and help reduce the degree of TR. If pressures do not reach this level, the band can be incrementally tightened maintaining careful assessment of mLV function on echo. The band should not be so tight that it causes right-to-left shunting at the VSD with desaturation. Finally, the band diameter is secured with an additional suture and fixed to the adventitia with 6-0 Prolene to prevent it migrating distally over time.

Patients are monitored carefully on the intensive care unit for the next 24 hours with the mLV line *in situ*. It may be necessary to loosen the band if there is any subtle deterioration in mLV function, which can occur particularly in older children. Equally, it may be necessary to tighten the band if the pressure drops to below half systemic.

OPERATION – THE DOUBLE-SWITCH PROCEDURES

Anatomic correction can be divided according to the management of the LVOT. Those with normal LVOT dimensions and normal pulmonary valve annulus are suitable for double-switch whereas those with pulmonary stenosis or atresia require atrial switch with Rastelli procedure to commit the mLV to the aorta. The atrial switch is common to both procedures and either the Mustard or Senning techniques can be used according to preference. The Senning is the more commonly used option and is the technique described here; the Senning does not require any artificial material to create the intracardiac baffles and has generally had a better freedom from late arrhythmias and baffle obstructions in comparison to the Mustard. In contrast, the Mustard procedure involves complete excision of the atrial septum and the use a dumbbell-shaped prosthetic patch to create the intra-atrial baffle.

The preparation and initial steps of the operation are common to both the double-switch and the Rastelli–Senning.

Preparation

The variability and complexity of anatomy in ccTGA necessitates extensive and careful preoperative assessment, and each component of the repair needs to be carefully considered as outlined above. Most cases will have undergone previous palliative or preparatory procedures and great attention must be placed on extensive and thorough dissection of all components of the heart free from any adhesions as complete mobility of the heart is essential to enable successful creation of both the venous and the arterial pathways. The pulmonary artery and its branches must be fully mobilized and separated from the aorta, dissecting out the pulmonary artery band, if present. The cavae should be extensively mobilized, identifying the azygos vein superiorly and freeing up the IVC as inferiorly as possible onto the diaphragmatic surface.

Initial incisions

Cardiopulmonary bypass is established using high aortic cannulation and bicaval cannulation. The SVC should be cannulated high (above the azygos vein if possible, snaring the azygos separately) and the IVC at the diaphragm as low as possible. In the presence of mesocardia or dextrocardia it may be easier to cannulate the right atrial appendage initially (the same pursestring can be used to site a left atrial pressure line at completion) to allow the heart to decompress and then cannulate the IVC with the heart collapsed. Moderate hypothermia to 25°C is used to ensure thorough cooling and allow for short periods of low flow or arrest in assessing the pathways. Waterston's groove is then developed as much as possible to facilitate the layers of the Senning (**Figure 56.1**).

The aorta is then cross-clamped and the heart arrested: we use St Thomas's crystalloid cardioplegia given at 20–25-minute intervals during the case. The initial incision in the right atrium is then made, staying well anterior to the crista terminalis and parallel to the AV groove. It is important not to make this incision too long initially and a good guide is to leave a length superiorly approximately equivalent to the width of the SVC (marked as "*x*" in **Figure 56.1**) and a similar length inferiorly short of the IVC junction equivalent to the width of the IVC (marked as "*y*" in **Figure 56.1**). This allows for sufficient atrial wall to allow the free wall to fold inwards to create the systemic venous baffle at the next stage. This incision can be completed later after the intra-atrial anatomy has been fully assessed.

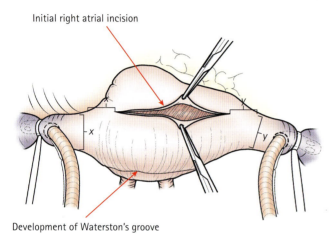

Initial right atrial incision

Development of Waterston's groove

56.1

The intracardiac anatomy should now be carefully assessed to confirm the VSD position and define the outflow tracts such that the surgeon is confident that anatomic repair will be achievable. It is much easier to revise the surgical strategy at this point if things are not as expected. The mitral valve should be examined as simple anomalies such as cleft anterior leaflet have been reported and can be readily repaired at this point.

Creation of the septal flap

The atrial septal flap is now created, starting with a stab incision at the medial border of the fossa ovalis (i.e. closest to the mitral valve). This is then continued inferiorly across the floor of the heart and superiorly under the limbus. This is beginning to create a trapdoor-shaped flap based on the lateral wall of the heart. The incision now has to be extended superiorly along the dotted line shown in **Figure 56.2a**; this is a bold incision taken across the full thickness of the limbus, immediately beneath the root of the SVC. It is not a comfortable incision to make as it is carrying the scissors outside the heart. A right-angled instrument can now be passed

under the flap and the tip should appear in fresh air, sitting in Waterston's groove (**Figure 56.2b**). Having developed Waterston's groove extensively at the outset of the procedure greatly facilitates this maneuver.

This opening created by the passage of the instrument can now be extended inferiorly, staying immediately above the right pulmonary veins. This creates a wide opening into the pulmonary venous atrium and leaves the flap hinged on the lateral wall of the heart. This final incision can be facilitated by working back and forward from inside and outside the atrium, using the surgical assistant to hold the free edge of the flap taught. This prevents inadvertently disconnecting the flap from the heart laterally. The flap is little bigger than a postage stamp and will be used to create the first layer of the Senning. We have not found it necessary to augment this flap with additional tissue, which has been suggested by some authors.

We leave the Senning at this stage and return to it towards the end of the procedure.

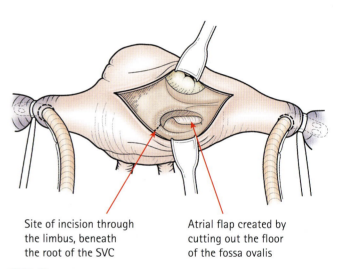

Site of incision through the limbus, beneath the root of the SVC

Atrial flap created by cutting out the floor of the fossa ovalis

56.2a

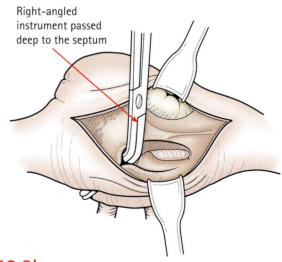

Right-angled instrument passed deep to the septum

56.2b

VSD closure

Attention is now turned to the VSD. **Figure 56.3** shows the typical position of a perimembranous outlet VSD in ccTGA. The defect is usually closed transatrially, working through the mitral valve as shown here, but it can be closed working through the aorta after the coronary arteries have been excised. Interrupted or continuous suture techniques can be used according to personal preference but we prefer interrupted pledgeted sutures. The abnormal path of the conduction tissue in ccTGA means that placement of the sutures is critical to avoid damage to the bundle. The sutures around the superior and lateral margins of the defect should be placed from within the VSD (i.e. from the morphologic right ventricular side) to avoid the bundle that runs along the edge of the defect on the leftward surface of the septum.

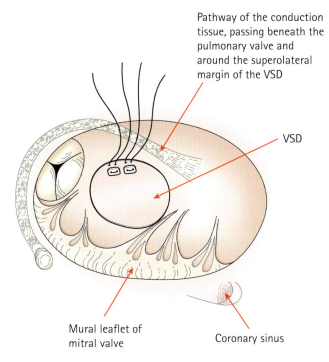

Pathway of the conduction tissue, passing beneath the pulmonary valve and around the superolateral margin of the VSD

VSD

Mural leaflet of mitral valve

Coronary sinus

56.3

Rastelli procedure

A longitudinal ventriculotomy is made into the body of the right ventricle, choosing a suitable site free from coronaries and starting well below the aortic valve. At this point the anatomy should be carefully assessed to confirm the position of the AV valves and VSD. Usually, the VSD is large but occasionally there may be some trabeculations to the leftward side beneath the aorta that can be resected to enlarge the pathway. The remnant of the outflow septum between the aorta and small pulmonary annulus should never be resected as the conduction tissue passes through here in ccTGA. We use a curved patch taken from a Gore-Tex vascular graft and fixed in place around the tricuspid valve with four or five pledgeted sutures before completing the suture line with a double layer

of running suture. There is no risk to the conduction tissue inferiorly and the sutures can pass close to the edge of the defect as the patch comes past the mitral valve.

In cases of pulmonary stenosis (rather than atresia) the main pulmonary artery must be ligated to exclude it from the mLV. If possible, we also oversew the pulmonary valve leaflets from within the ventricle. This seals off what would otherwise be a small cul-de-sac of the PA stump, which can occasionally fill with thrombus postoperatively.

A conduit is then placed between the ventriculotomy and the pulmonary arteries. We prefer a strong material such as Dacron (the Hancock® conduit) which is less likely to be deformed when the chest is closed and has adequate length for what can be a longer distance than standard pulmonary atresia morphology. The conduit can be placed either to the left or right of the aorta but we prefer to place it to the left (which may require considerable mobilization of the left PA) as this prevents the conduit from lying directly behind the sternum (**Figure 56.4**).

If the VSD is predominantly inlet and remote from the aorta, a Nikaidoh procedure has occasionally been used in place of the Rastelli. However, division of the conaI septum will carry a very high risk of creating heart block.

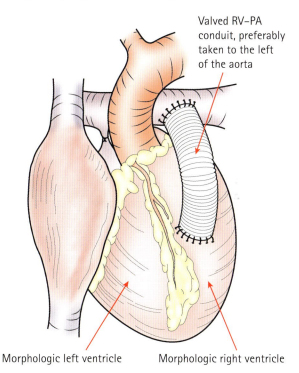

Valved RV–PA conduit, preferably taken to the left of the aorta

Morphologic left ventricle

Morphologic right ventricle

56.4

The arterial switch

The principles of arterial switch and coronary transfer are similar to those in a neonatal switch in d-TGA but the surgery is rotated through 90 degrees compared to the "usual" orientation that the surgeon might be used to in a neonatal switch. However, the slightly more side-by-side nature of the great vessels requires attention. Both the aorta and pulmonary artery are transected, dividing the PA through the site of the band (if present) to retain as much height as possible. The aorta is transected well above the sinotubular junction and the coronary positions confirmed. The coronaries arise from the facing sinuses with the posterior coronary (equivalent of the right coronary artery) tending to run directly posteriorly and the anterior coronary (equivalent of the left coronary) dividing into two main branches, which can arise from dual orifices. The coronaries are excised on generous buttons of aortic tissue and mobilized until they are free-floating; this is particularly important with the anterior coronary, which needs a little more distance to rotate than the posterior vessel. The defects in the aorta are repaired with a patch of autologous pericardium or pulmonary homograft leaving plenty of patch tissue sitting above the height of the transected root (**Figure 56.5**). The coronary buttons are then implanted into the neoaorta-facing sinuses, keeping the incisions as high as possible. We tend to cut out a small V incision for the posterior coronary and create a medially hinged trapdoor incision for the anterior coronary (**Figure 56.6**).

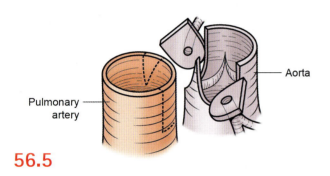

56.5

Note that, although the pulmonary artery is narrowed at the site of the band, making these incisions for the coronary buttons allows the pulmonary root to open out like the petals of a flower and it is not usually necessary to augment the banded region.

PA reconstruction

A decision now has to be taken whether or not to perform the Lecompte maneuver. Although this would be the preferred method, the side-by-side nature of the great vessels and the older age of the patients (compared to a neonatal switch) can mean that it is not possible to gain adequate mobility of the branch pulmonary arteries to safely bring the PAs anteriorly. If there is sufficient length to the PAs, they can be brought forward and the aortic anastomosis completed behind them (**Figure 56.7**). It may be necessary to move the opening in the branch PAs leftwards to accommodate for the side-by-side nature of the vessels and avoid undue tension on the RPA. Leaving plenty of tissue in the patch used to repair the coronary defects may help to give a little more laxity to this anastamosis (as shown in **Figure 56.7**). If the PAs do not have sufficient laxity, it may be necessary to leave them behind the aorta. In this situation it may be easier to reconstruct the pulmonary anastomosis first, before reconstructing the aorta; this affords an opportunity to assess the tension on the main PA, which can potentially distort the anterior coronary, and it may help to place an additional patch into the PA anastomosis anteriorly to reduce any tension. Leaving a relatively long neo-PA (by transecting the aorta well above the sinotubular junction) also helps give added flexibility to this anastomosis.

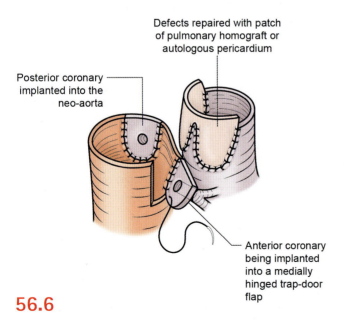

Defects repaired with patch of pulmonary homograft or autologous pericardium

Posterior coronary implanted into the neo-aorta

Anterior coronary being implanted into a medially hinged trap-door flap

56.6

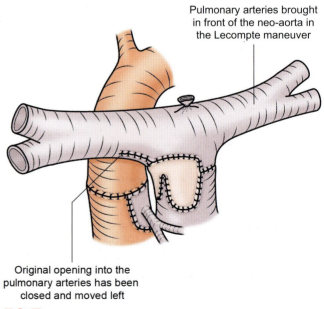

Pulmonary arteries brought in front of the neo-aorta in the Lecompte maneuver

Original opening into the pulmonary arteries has been closed and moved left

56.7

First layer of the Senning

Attention is returned to the atrium and the Senning is now created. The procedure is performed in three layers, creating a Y-shaped systemic venous pathway that is encircled by a C-shaped pulmonary venous pathway. It is a three-dimensional procedure, with each layer impacting on the shape and volume of the next layer. The first layer utilizes the septal flap created in **Figure 56.2**. The assistant's retractor is placed across the remnant of the interatrial septum to provide a clear view of the pulmonary venous atrium. A useful starting landmark is the base of the left atrial appendage and the free long edge of the septal flap is attached here with a running Prolene suture (**Figure 56.8**). It is important to use more of the flap for the superior limb of this suture line than for the inferior component. This ensures that the suture line can take a dog-legged pathway along the roof of the atrium, keeping as deep as possible to create plenty of volume above it for the SVC pathway. Thus, starting from the base of the left appendage, approximately two-thirds of the flap circumference should be used for the superior direction and one-third for the inferior direction, gathering up the floor of the left atrium towards the IVC.

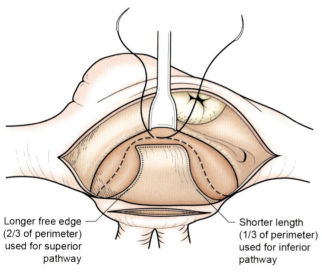

Longer free edge (2/3 of perimeter) used for superior pathway

Shorter length (1/3 of perimeter) used for inferior pathway

56.8

Second layer of the Senning: the systemic venous baffle

The retractor is now replaced in the mitral valve and the free edge of the right atrial wall is folded in to meet the cut edge of the interatrial septum to create the Y-shaped systemic venous baffle (**Figure 56.9**). Inferiorly, the flap can be folded down onto the Eustachian valve, leaving the IVC behind it (this is the advantage of having cannulated the IVC very inferiorly,

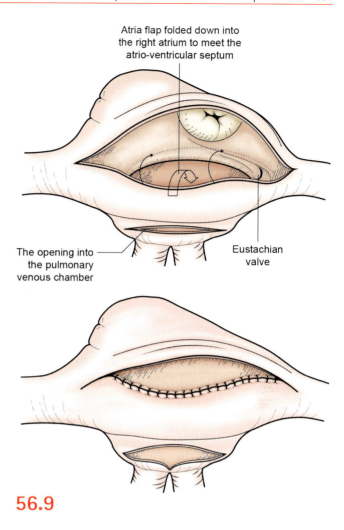

Atria flap folded down into the right atrium to meet the atrio-ventricular septum

The opening into the pulmonary venous chamber

Eustachian valve

56.9

below the level of the Eustachian valve), and then run superiorly to meet the cut edge of the interatrial septum. Superiorly, the flap is rolled in around the SVC inflow, trying to create as much volume as possible with the tissue available. As the AV node is not found in the triangle of Koch in ccTGA, the suture line can pass anterior to the coronary sinus (in contrast to the Senning in d-TGA where the suture line comes posteriorly, leaving the coronary sinus in the pulmonary venous atrium) and so incorporates the coronary sinus into the systemic venous channel. If necessary, the coronary sinus can be laid open into the floor of the left atrium to further enlarge the IVC pathway.

Third layer of the Senning: the completion of the pulmonary venous pathway

The Senning is completed by bringing the anterior free wall of the right atrium down onto the opening into the pulmonary venous chamber, like closing the lid on a suitcase. The suture lines can easily "strangle" the limbs of the systemic venous pathway so it is essential that enough tissue is available to give adequate length to these running sutures. This is achieved as shown in **Figure 56.10a and b**, bringing point A to B and point X to Y. The suture lines just pick up the adventitia as they cross the SVC and IVC limbs and then the central portion of the flap is secured to the cut edge of the left atrium. If necessary, an additional incision can be made down between the right pulmonary veins to give further volume to this opening.

If this layer is too tight, the pulmonary venous pathway can become obstructed laterally. This is a particular risk in cases of mesocardia or dextrocardia when the cardiac malposition creates a relatively small surface area to the free wall of the right atrium. If there is concern that there is insufficient tissue for this layer, it can be augmented with a patch of autologous pericardium or pulmonary homograft as shown in **Figure 56.11**. We usually fold X to Y to seal off the inferior part of the layer and then use the patch to augment the mid and superior part of the repair. A further incision can be made (point p in **Figure 56.11**) to open out the cavity if it feels tight.

An alternative way to augment this layer is to create a pericardial well to accommodate the pulmonary venous pathway, sewing the opened edges of the atria to the parietal pericardium (the Shumacher technique).

The one-and-a half repair

An alternative technique to the complete atrial switch is to perform a bidirectional Glenn first, as a means of simplifying the atrial switch. The atrial septum is excised and then a single patch is used to direct the IVC flow back to the tricuspid valve. This is sometimes referred to as a "hemi-Mustard" procedure (**Figure 56.12**).

A large, circular patch of Gore-Tex is used to baffle the IVC orifice across the remnant of the interatrial septum and then around the margins of the tricuspid valve. It is recommended to lay open the coronary sinus to provide additional volume to the pathway and reduce the ridge of the remnant of the atrial septum. This simplifies the atrial repair and can be particularly useful if there is concern over the size of the right ventricle; another advantage is that it may also give greater longevity to the RV–PA conduit used in the Rastelli as it has to carry only the IVC flow. The bidirectional Glenn could be performed as a palliative initial procedure in cases with pulmonary stenosis/atresia, and so delay the need to progress to Rastelli. However, the PA pressures must be low to tolerate the Glenn and the anatomy will deny access to the atrium should subsequent pacing or ablation procedures be required in the future. There is also some evidence that the functional capacity

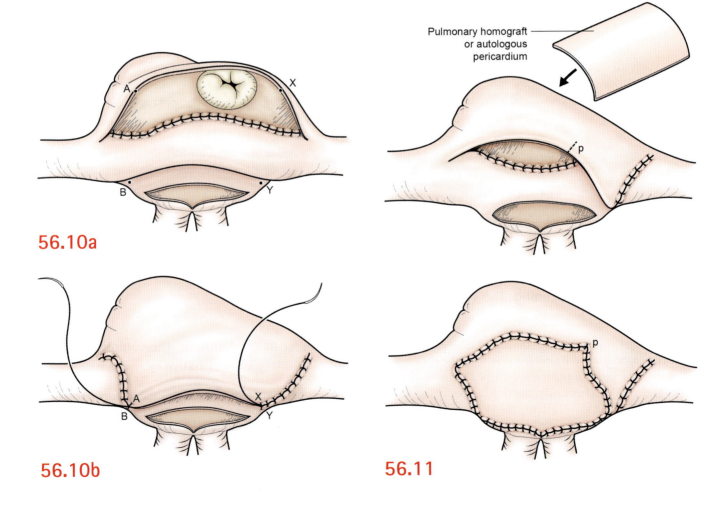

56.10a

56.10b

Pulmonary homograft
or autologous
pericardium

56.11

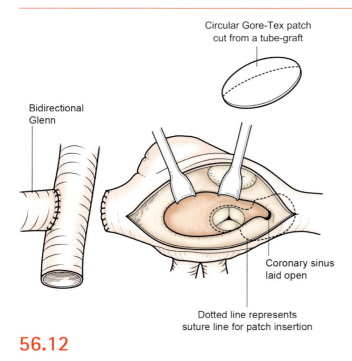

Circular Gore-Tex patch
cut from a tube-graft

Bidirectional
Glenn

Coronary sinus
laid open

Dotted line represents
suture line for patch insertion

56.12

of the one-and-a-half circulation is not as good as that of true biventricular circulation and, if the patient has two good-sized ventricles, then our preference is to aim for biventricular repair.

POSTOPERATIVE MANAGEMENT

A degree of low cardiac output is not unusual and we commonly leave the chest open for the first 24 hours. Monitoring of SVC and left atrial pressure is important and we routinely use milrinone 0.5–0.7 µg/kg/minute and adrenaline 0.05–0.1 µg/kg/minute support. Careful assessment of the venous baffles, outlet tracts, and ventricular function using transesophageal echocardiography (TEE) is essential. High SVC pressures with facial suffusion and pleural effusions can be seen, related to high SVC pressures in the Senning pathway, but these tend to settle over 48–72 hours, partly helped by natural decompression through the azygos vein. TEE is helpful in postoperative assessment of the pathways, but unless severe obstruction is seen these do not usually need surgical revision. Ventilation and inotropes are continued until cardiac output has stabilized. Atrial tachycardias can occur in relation to the Senning but are rare in the early postoperative phase. Mechanical support by extracorporeal membrane oxygenation (ECMO) has been used successfully for refractory low cardiac output state in a handful of reported cases.

OUTCOME

Surgical outcomes for the double-switch procedures in ccTGA-VSD are excellent with early mortality in the modern era of typically 2–5%. The outcomes can be stratified according to the nature and complexity of presentation: the highest risk procedures tend to be in neonates and infants who are clinically unstable and in heart failure preoperatively, often requiring arch repair in addition to double switch (mortality 8–15%) but in elective repairs in older children with well-preserved ventricular function the mortality approaches 0–2%. Most series report lower mortality among the Rastelli–Senning group compared to double switch as the former tend to include more elective procedures with no concerns over mLV function and no need for coronary transfer.

The commonest early complications are heart block (new pacemaker required in 5–10%), and low cardiac output, which is partly related to long bypass and cross-clamp times. Pleural effusions may occur in association with high SVC pressures.

Longer-term follow-up is now becoming available and survival is dramatically better than the natural history of symptomatic ccTGA managed conventionally (i.e. leaving the mRV as the systemic ventricle) with actuarial survival of 90–95% at 10 years. Freedom from reintervention is lower at 80–85% at 10 years. Although some of this is conduit replacement in the Rastelli group, there is still significant incidence of reoperation for a mixture of other lesions including Senning baffle obstruction, PA stenoses post-switch, and aortic valve repair and replacement. (Most baffle stenoses can be successfully managed with balloon dilatation or stenting.) However, reoperations on the tricuspid valve are very rare and simply removing the tricuspid valve from the systemic circulation universally improved function. A recent study from Boston emphasizes the importance of assessing the tricuspid valve at the time of surgery and even simple repairs of anatomically abnormal valves further improve the late tricuspid valve performance. Baffle obstruction and late atrial tachycardias are commoner with the Mustard procedure than the Senning, which has contributed to the popularity of the Senning technique. In summary, the freedom from reintervention is strikingly similar in both the double-switch and Rastelli–Senning groups.

As longer follow-up results are reported there is an emerging concern over the incidence of late mLV dysfunction, which occurs in 15–20% of patients at 20 years post surgery. This has been reported by several groups with similar findings and occurs in spite of what appears to be good mLV function early postoperatively. The etiology appears to be multifactorial but it certainly appears to be commoner in the double-switch group than the Rastelli–Senning group. Aortic regurgitation may be a factor, and is commoner in the double-switch group, in which the old pulmonary valve becomes the new aortic valve, but the relationship with mLV dysfunction is far from consistent. There is increasing interest in the fate of the mLV retrained by application of the pulmonary artery band, and the interaction with late LV dysfunction. However, this relationship is also inconsistent: the Boston group has shown a greater risk of late mLV dysfunction in patients who were initially banded when over 2 years of age whereas there was no incidence of late dysfunction in patients banded before they were 2 years old. This group of retrained mLVs will certainly require careful follow-up and these findings have fuelled interest in the controversial concept of early "prophylactic" PA banding in symptomless infants, which might protect the mLV in these patients from late failure.

It has also been noted that LV dysfunction is associated with a high incidence of patients requiring pacing and of patients who have a prolonged QRS interval. There are several reported successes with resynchronization using biventricular LV and right ventricular pacing improving mLV function in these patients, with some individual cases of dramatic improvement. This may be of value in patients requiring pacemaker insertion after a double-switch procedure.

Despite these concerns, the outcomes of the double-switch operations in ccTGA remain substantially better than both the natural history and for traditional physiological repair, with more than 75% of patients sustaining good mLV function at 20 years. It is also important to note that the group of "high-risk" patients who present with severe cardiac failure has done particularly well, with no incidence of late mLV failure.

FURTHER READING

Anderson RH, Becker AE, Arnold R, Wilkinson JL. The conducting tissues in congenitally corrected transposition. *Circulation.* 1974; 50: 911–24.

Bove EL, Ohye RG, Devaney EJ, et al. Anatomic correction of congenitally corrected transposition and its close cousins. *Cardiol Young.* 2006; 16: 85–90.

Connelly M, Liu PP, Williams WG, et al. Congenitally corrected transposition of the great arteries in the adult: functional status and complications. *J Am Coll Cardiol.* 1996; 27: 1238–43.

De Leva IMR, Basto P, Stark J, et al. Surgical technique to reduce the risks of heart block following closure of ventricular septal defect in atrioventricular discordance. *J Thorac Cardiovasc Surg.*1979; 78: 515–26.

Duncan BW, Mee RB, Mesia CI, et al. Results of the double switch operation for congenitally corrected transposition of the great arteries. *Eur J Cardiothorac Surg.* 2003; 24(1): 11–19.

Graham TP Jr, Bernard YO, Mellen BG, et al. Long-term outcome in congenitally corrected transposition of the great arteries: a multi-institutional study. *J Am Coll Cardiol.* 2000; 36: 255–61.

Langley SM, Winlaw OS, Stumper O, et al. Midterm results after restoration of the morphologically left ventricle to the systemic circulation in patients with congenitally corrected transposition of the great arteries. *J Thorac Cardiovasc Surg.* 2003; 125: 1229–41.

Malhotra SP, Reddy VM, Qiu M, et al. The hemi Mustard/ bidirectional Glenn atrial switch procedure in the double-switch operation for congenitally corrected transposition of the great arteries: rationale and midterm results. *J Thorac Cardiovasc Surg.* 2011; 141(1): 162–70.

Metton O, Gaudin R, Ou P, et al. Early prophylactic pulmonary artery banding in isolated congenitally corrected transposition of the great arteries. *Eur J Cardiothorac Surg.* 2010; 38(6): 728–34.

Murtuza B, Barron OJ, Stumper O, et al. Anatomic repair for congenitally corrected transposition of the great arteries: a single-institution 19-year experience. *J Thorac Cardiovasc Surg.* 2011; 142(6): 1348–57.

Myers PO, Bautista-Hernandez V, Baird CW, et al. Tricuspid regurgitation or Ebsteinoid dysplasia of the tricuspid valve in congenitally corrected transposition: is valvuloplasty necessary at anatomic repair? *J Thorac Cardiovasc Surg.* 2014; 147(2): 576–80.

Myers PO, del Nido PJ, Geva T, et al. Impact of age and duration of banding on left ventricular preparation before anatomic repair for congenitally corrected transposition of the great arteries. *Ann Thorac Surg.* 2013; 96(2): 603–10.

Quinn DW, McGuirk SP, Metha C, et al. The morphologic left ventricle that requires training by means of pulmonary artery banding before the double-switch procedure for congenitally corrected transposition of the great arteries is at risk of late dysfunction. *J Thorac Cardiovasc Surg.* 2008; 135(5): 1137–44.

Sano T, Riesenfeld T, Karl TR, Wilkinson JL. Intermediate-term outcome after intracardiac repair of associated cardiac defects in patients with atrioventricular and ventriculoarterial discordance. *Circulation.* 1995; 92: II272–8.

Shin'oka T, Kurosawa H, Imai Y, et al. Outcomes of definitive surgical repair for congenitally corrected transposition of the great arteries or double outlet right ventricle with discordant atrioventricular connection: risk analyses in 189 patients. *J Thorac Cardiovasc Surg.* 2007; 133: 1318–28.

57

Persistent truncus arteriosus

MARTIN J. ELLIOTT AND VICTOR T. TSANG

HISTORY

Truncus arteriosus is an uncommon congenital anomaly accounting for 1–4% of patients born with congenital heart disease. First described by Wilson in 1798, anatomic classifications were introduced by Collett and Edwards based on the presence of a main pulmonary trunk or the separation of the pulmonary arteries from the arterial trunk in 1949. A widely used classification has been the scheme developed by Van Praagh in 1965, which describes four subtypes with and without the presence of a ventricular septal defect (VSD). The detailed morphology is reviewed by Professor Robert H. Anderson in Chapter 39, "The anatomy of congenital cardiac malformations."

Classification

The Van Praagh classification is illustrated in **Figure 57.1**.

Type A: VSD present
Type B: VSD not present

1. Partially formed aortopulmonary septum (main pulmonary artery [PA] segment present)
2. Absent aortopulmonary septum (both pulmonary arteries originate directly from the aorta)
3. Absence of one PA branch from the trunk (ductal origin of one PA)
4. Interrupted aortic arch associated with truncus arteriosus.

In the past, patients were palliated by single or bilateral PA banding followed by definitive repair at a later age. This approach resulted in a high early mortality and morbidity. McGoon reported the first single-stage repair in 1968 using a valved homograft. Paul Ebert from San Francisco demonstrated, in a classic series published in 1984, that primary repair in infancy could be performed with a low mortality (11%) and advocated this as the preferred approach. Primary one-stage repair is now the treatment of choice, but even now few centers have achieved the results that Ebert produced so long ago.

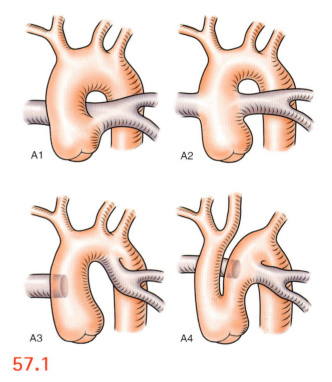

A1　A2　A3　A4

57.1

PRINCIPLES AND JUSTIFICATION

The majority of infants born with truncus arteriosus present with severe congestive heart failure within the first week of life. Without surgical treatment, a 75–85% mortality occurs during the first year of life. Excessive pulmonary blood flow results in severe pulmonary vascular disease very early in life. Further "run-off" from the truncal artery into the low resistance pulmonary circuit can result in a low diastolic blood pressure and therefore decreased coronary perfusion, affecting ventricular performance. Corrective surgery should be undertaken once the diagnosis is established, certainly within the first month of life. Operative risk increases after 100 days of life, and some experts suggest that waiting until after 7 days of age is best. In the presence of severe truncal valvar regurgitation or aortic arch interruption, emergency surgery may be needed.

PREOPERATIVE ASSESSMENT AND PREPARATION

Echocardiography usually establishes the diagnosis without difficulty. Assessment of truncal valve function, coronary arterial origins, aortic arch anatomy, and pulmonary arteries is crucial. On the rare occurrence of late referral, when irreversible pulmonary vascular disease needs to be ruled out or when echocardiography is inconclusive, cardiac catheterization may be warranted. If pulmonary vascular disease is identified, detailed physiological studies on pulmonary vascular resistance and its manipulation may be helpful for postoperative management.

If a child needs preoperative resuscitation and ventilatory support, careful clinical assessment is needed. Avoiding an acute decrease in pulmonary vascular resistance, which could alter ventricular performance, is important. Indeed, to maintain adequate diastolic pressure, management is directed at maintaining a degree of pulmonary vascular resistance by reducing ventilatory rates, using smaller tidal volumes, and increasing pulmonary vasoconstriction with lower inspiratory oxygen (FIO_2). Thus, the situation is very like a preoperative "Norwood" for duct-dependent hypoplastic left heart syndrome.

ANESTHESIA

Anesthetic management does not differ from operations for most congenital heart defects. Manipulations that increase the already excessive pulmonary blood flow should be avoided. A significant number of patients with persistent truncus arteriosus have DiGeorge syndrome; therefore, irradiated blood products must be used to avoid graft-versus-host reactions after blood transfusions. Blood calcium concentrations need particular attention intra- and postoperatively.

OPERATION

Surgical approach

The heart is exposed via a median sternotomy. The thymus (if present) is excised, taking care to avoid damage to the phrenic nerve. The pericardium is opened longitudinally, and a patch is harvested if needed. The aorta is dissected beyond the innominate artery. The pulmonary arteries are mobilized, and vessel loops are placed around both branch pulmonary arteries but are not tightened at this stage. A ligature is placed around the duct (if present) for later ligation. The external anatomy (in particular the coronary arteries) must be assessed.

Conduct of cardiopulmonary bypass

The aorta is cannulated at the level of the transverse arch, and bicaval venous return is established, so that circulatory arrest can be avoided during the intracardiac repair. Venus cannulation is best done via the right atrium in small children. Some surgeons prefer to use venous return via a single angled cannula in smaller children (less than 2.0 kg), and the patient is cooled slowly down to 18°C over 20 minutes. Vacuum-assisted venous drainage permits the use of smaller venous cannulae for adequate venous return and may permit bicaval cannulation even in very small infants.

As soon as bypass is initiated, the pulmonary arteries must be snared closed (we use looped vascular slings [vessel loops], **Figure 57.2**) to prevent run-off into the pulmonary circulation. Such run-off, associated with a drop in diastolic blood pressure, could cause significant cardiac or cerebral hypoperfusion.

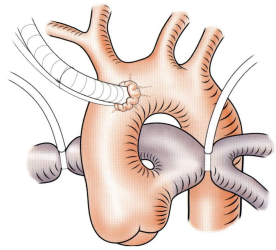

57.2

Pulmonary artery detachment from truncus arteriosus

The aorta is cross-clamped as high as possible, and cardioplegic solution is infused before transection of the common arterial trunk. Continued occlusion of branch pulmonary arteries ensures that cardioplegia perfuses the coronary arteries. If significant truncal valve incompetence exists, the trunk should be opened and cardioplegic solution infused directly into the coronary arteries with a small cannula. Retrograde cardioplegia delivery via the coronary sinus may also be used. The line of incision should be chosen carefully so as not to damage the coronary ostia, which may originate higher than usual, even from the branch pulmonary arteries. Sudden ST-segment changes on snaring the pulmonary arteries or failure to deliver adequately antegrade cardioplegia should alert the surgeon to this possibility.

For detachment of the pulmonary arteries from the aorta, a number of important steps should be performed. The first step is to observe the coronaries, their origin, and course, because abnormal origin of the coronary arteries is not infrequent. The second step is the inspection of the pulmonary arteries, their origin, and course. This inspection allows the surgeon to make a decision as to how to make the detachment of the pulmonary arteries from the trunk. Our preferred approach is simple transverse transection of the aorta, starting slightly above the origin of the pulmonary arteries from the common trunk, making an incision approximately halfway around the aorta (**Figure 57.3a**). This maneuver provides excellent exposure of the PA origins, coronary artery anatomy, and the truncal valve. The incision is continued around the pulmonary arteries, leaving a generous cuff around their origins.

After placing stay sutures of 6-0 Prolene above each commissure, the truncal valve is assessed, and a repair or replacement is undertaken if required (**Figure 57.3b–d**). Aortic reconstruction after a transection approach may be complicated because of the mismatch between the proximal aorta and the much smaller distal aorta.

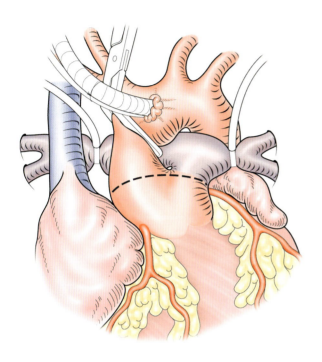

57.3a

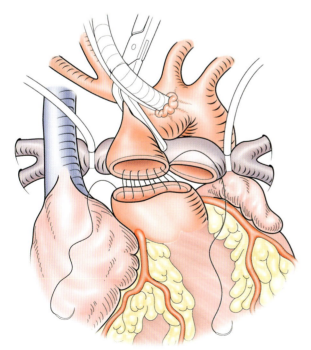

57.3b

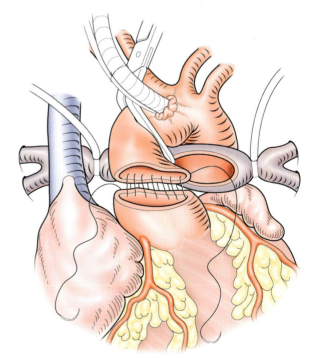

57.3c

57.3d

However, in most circumstances the reanastomosis can be performed easily by making minor alterations to the continuous suture line, for example using a horizontal mattress suture proximally and a vertical mattress suture distally (**Figure 57.4**).

The alternative method of separation is to dissect and detach the PA from the aorta. This approach is most suitable for a true type I truncus arteriosus, in which the pulmonary arteries have a common origin. However, this method runs the risk of damaging important structures such as the left coronary ostium, the aortic sinuses, and the truncal valve itself. Dissection has to be taken slowly and carefully. Detachment by this technique leaves a hole in a difficult posterior and leftward position.

The pulmonary arteries are excised from the common trunk with a generous cuff, and the defect in the aorta is closed either primarily or with a patch (**Figure 57.5a and b**). A patch is usually required to avoid distortion, particularly of the truncal valve and coronary arteries.

Truncal valve repair/replacement

Mild-to-moderate truncal valve regurgitation can be well tolerated and may improve postoperatively after corrective surgery. Significant truncal valve stenosis (gradient greater than 30 mmHg) and severe truncal valve regurgitation often necessitate surgery to the valve. As with all other heart valves, repair is better than replacement if it can be done successfully.

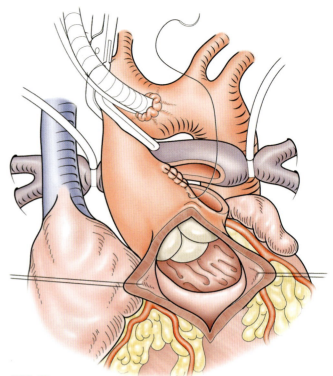

57.5a

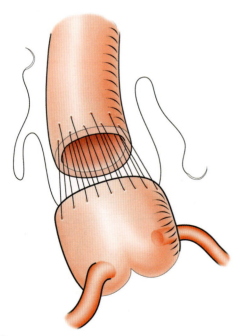

57.4

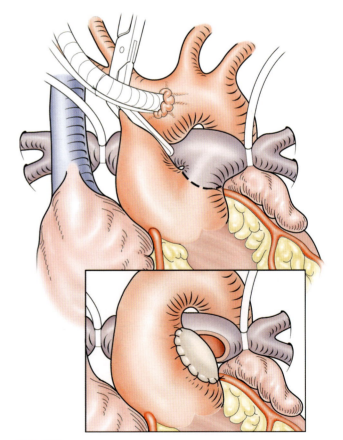

57.5b

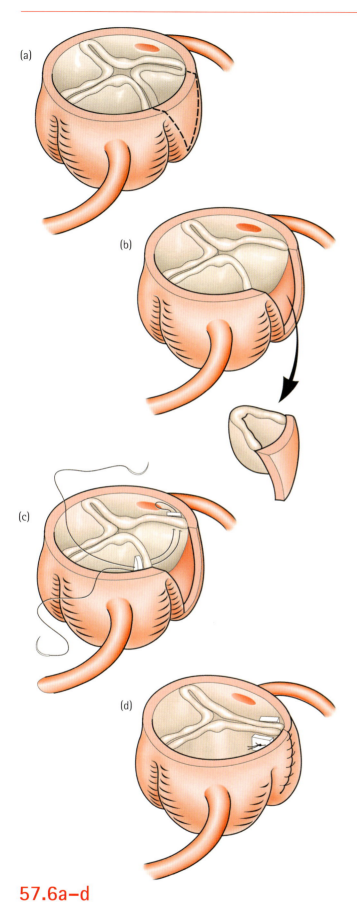

57.6a–d

Truncal valve stenosis

The stenotic truncal valve is often thickened and dysplastic. Thus, principles learnt from the surgical management of congenital aortic stenosis (e.g. commissurotomy and shaving [thinning] techniques) can be applied.

Truncal valve regurgitation

Several publications from the Cleveland Group have provided very helpful new techniques for truncal valve repair. In quadricuspid valves, repair may be possible by reducing the number of leaflets. Quadricusp valves can also be remodeled by excising the smallest cusp. The created defect is closed with pledgeted subcommissural sutures (**Figure 57.6a–d**).

If repair of the truncal valve fails, valve replacement may need to be undertaken. In this setting, a primary aortic root replacement using a cryopreserved homograft is probably the only viable procedure (**Figure 57.7a–d**). The homograft should be sized to the age of the child; therefore, preoperative echo diagnosis is mandatory, because the homograft has to be ordered in advance. We have used homografts as small as 6 mm in 1.5 kg children and sizes from 10–15 mm in children weighing up to 5 kg. If an aortic homograft is inserted, the mitral leaflet can sometimes be used to close the VSD (**Figure 57.7c**). The coronary arteries are excised from the

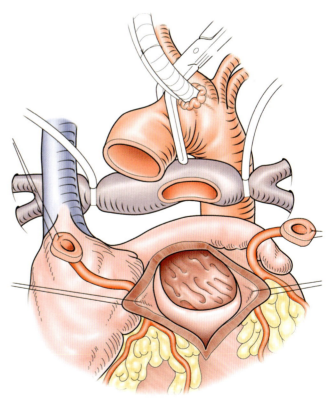

57.7a

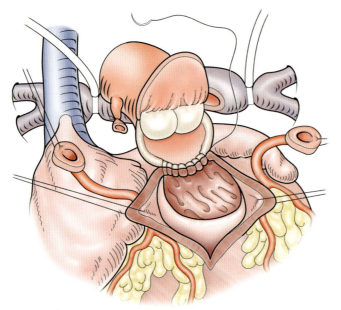

57.7b

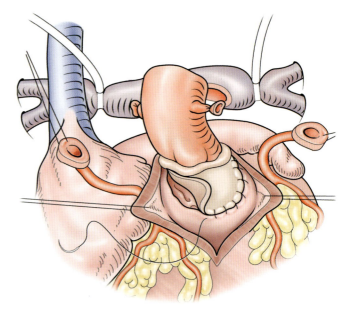

57.7c

truncal wall and reimplanted onto the homograft using fine suture material (**Figure 57.7a–d**). The right coronary artery is best sited after filling the aortic root with cardioplegia to identify the sinuses better.

Closure of ventricular septal defect

The VSD is approached through a vertical right ventricular infundibular incision between stay sutures (5-0 Prolene) approximately 0.5 cm apart and 1 cm below the truncal valve (which is closer than one expects). Care must be taken not to damage any crossing major coronary artery branches. The incision in the right ventricle (RV) should be large enough to create a good outlet for the conduit, but not so large as to damage the function of the RV. Gentle retraction of the incision using eyelid, nerve root retractors, or special VSD retractors gives good exposure of the VSD. The truncal valve can be inspected through the ventriculotomy to ensure that no damage has been done. Any obstructing right ventricular muscle bundles are divided, leaving the supporting apparatus for the tricuspid valve intact.

The VSD may be muscular (approximately 70%) or perimembranous (approximately 30%). In the more common muscular defects, suturing in this area can be performed without risk to the conduction tissue. A patch of Gore-Tex®, Dacron™, bovine pericardium, or glutaraldehyde-treated autologous pericardium can be used to close the defect to direct left ventricular blood to the aorta (**Figure 57.8**). The size of the patch should be big enough not to obstruct the pathway towards the aorta and to avoid truncal valve distortion. Our preference is to close these defects with interrupted 5-0 Surgilene sutures, reinforced with Teflon™ pledgets (**Figure 57.8** inset). The muscle in these small neonates is often very friable. At the upper part of the VSD the sutures

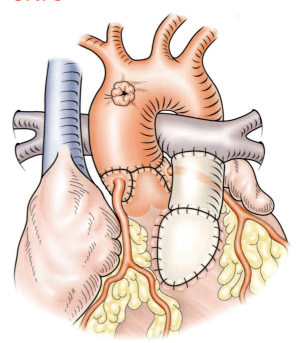

57.7d

are passed from the inside to the outside, leaving the pledgets on the outside of the heart. Usually, three or four stitches need to be placed like this.

If the VSD is perimembranous, the placement of the sutures in the depth of the RV is similar to a transventricular approach for a perimembranous VSD in tetralogy of Fallot. The interrupted Teflon-pledgeted sutures can be placed by passing the needle through the open tricuspid valve, inserting the suture through the atrial aspect of the anteroseptal leaflet close to the annulus of the tricuspid valve. The tricuspid valve annulus itself is avoided, bringing the sutures into the ventricular cavity.

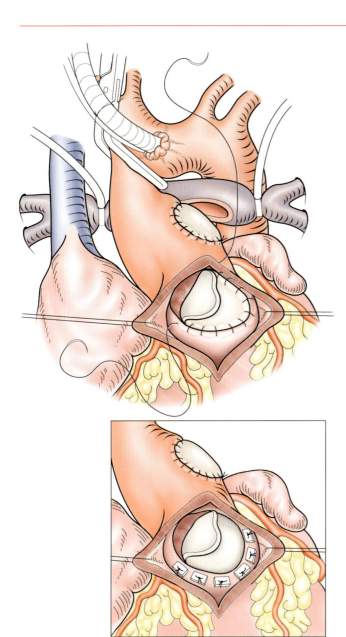

57.8

Three sutures are placed in this fashion, leaving the Teflon pledgets on the atrial side. The remainder of the VSD closure can proceed as usual. The conduction tissue sits at the inferior border, where the muscular rim meets the tricuspid valve. At this point a further suture should be placed *away* from the margin of the VSD, behind the chordae, to avoid damage of the bundle.

Atrial septal defect/Patent foramen ovale

A simple patent foramen ovale (PFO) is left open, and a larger concomitant atrial septal defect can be closed partially so as to leave the equivalent of a small PFO. This opening can be very useful in the postoperative period during pulmonary hypertensive episodes to maintain cardiac output by diverting some desaturated blood to the left atrium. If forward failure of the RV occurs and blood flow to the lungs is reduced, right ventricular and central venous pressures increase. Cardiac output can be maintained up to a certain level by right-to-left shunting through the PFO ("blue output is better than no output").

If the decision is not to leave a PFO, de-airing of the left side of the heart could then be undertaken, leaving a vent in the right superior pulmonary vein. The cross-clamp is taken off, and the rest of the procedure is done on the beating heart to reduce aortic cross-clamp time. If the PFO is going to be left open, the right atrium needs to be closed before removal of the cross-clamp.

Insertion of right ventricle–to–pulmonary artery conduit

After completion of the intracardiac repair, the left ventricle is de-aired, and RV-to-PA continuity is restored with a cryo-preserved homograft or other suitable conduit (Contegra, Medtronic, Minneapolis, MN; Hancock, Medtronic). Placing an intracardiac sucker in the right atrium is useful to obtain a bloodless field for suturing.

Most centers use valved conduits, because several studies suggest that the use of a non-valved conduit is another risk factor for adverse outcome. Some individual surgeons report good results from direct connection (described below). Pulmonary homografts seem to do better in the mid-term than aortic homografts. The choice of conduit size is very important and should match the size of the child. Excessively large conduits can produce an adverse hemodynamic outcome and are of no advantage in duration of valve survival. Closure of the chest may be made impossible as the conduit may be compressed after delayed chest closure.

If a homograft of an appropriate size is not available, a slightly larger one could be downsized by converting it from a tricuspid valve to a bicuspid valve, removing one of the cusps with the associated circumference of conduit and resuturing the homograft longitudinally. Smaller homograft sizes (8–12 mm, adjusted to the patient's body weight) are not disadvantageous and should be preferred because of better postoperative hemodynamic tolerance and no increased risk of early failure. The valve is often best placed distally, close to the bifurcation to avoid sternal compression, although opening of the left pleura may help in positioning. The distal anastomosis to the pulmonary arteries is constructed during rewarming using fine suture material (7-0 Prolene). If the pulmonary arteries are tiny, a bifurcated pulmonary homograft as a spatulated onlay allows extension into each branch to widen narrow segments. The conduit should lie leftwards without excess length to avoid kinking at the distal end. Next, the posterior proximal conduit wall is sutured directly to the ventriculotomy. A strip of Teflon, pericardium, or Dacron can be used to buttress the suture line. The anterior aspect is augmented with a patch of autologous or bovine pericardium. Gore-Tex, Dacron, and other materials can be used to create a large enough hood for the RV-to-conduit connection (**Figure 57.9**).

In a number of patients, a direct anastomosis of PA–right ventricular outflow tract (RVOT) incision may be used, as proposed by Barbero-Marcial et al. in 1990. The pulmonary arteries must be thoroughly mobilized to allow the partition wall of the distal transected main PA to be anastomosed to the upper end of the incision in the RVOT. A Lecompte (French) maneuver may be needed to achieve this goal. Once the posterior wall has been anastomosed, the anterior part of the RVOT–PA connection can be roofed with autologous or heterologous pericardium, creating a valveless connection.

Truncus arteriosus with discontinuous pulmonary arteries

Occasionally, the left PA originates from the ductus arteriosus, and the right PA arises from the truncus arteriosus. Both arteries are detached from their aortic connections. The larger artery is connected to the homograft with an end-to-end anastomosis, and the other is sewn end-to-side to the newly constructed PA (**Figure 57.10a–d**).

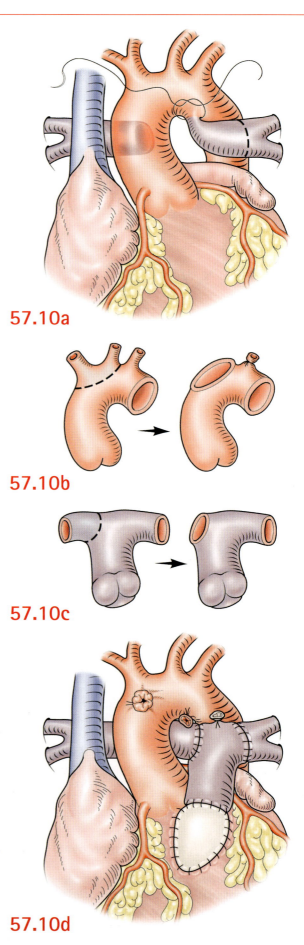

57.10a

57.10b

57.10c

57.10d

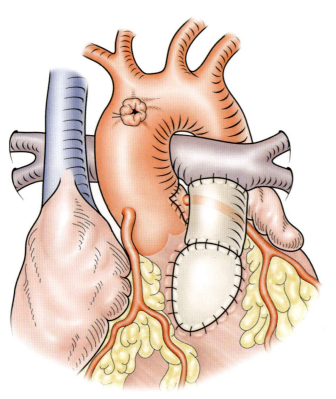

57.9

Alternatively, a bifurcated pulmonary homograft can be used. Continuity is restored with an end-to-end anastomosis (**Figure 57.11**).

Suturing the back wall of the two pulmonary arteries together provides the patient with a bifurcation of native tissue. The anterior aspect is enlarged using the bifurcated homograft as an onlay-patch (**Figure 57.12a–c**).

Truncus arteriosus with interrupted aortic arch

Approximately 10% of patients present with aortic arch interruption. All three types of interruption have been described, but interruption between the common left carotid and subclavian artery (interruption of aortic arch type B) is found most commonly (**Figure 57.13**). After extensive mobilization

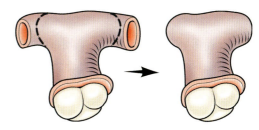

57.12b

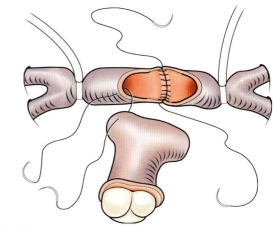

57.12c

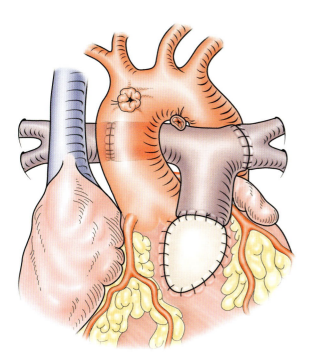

57.11

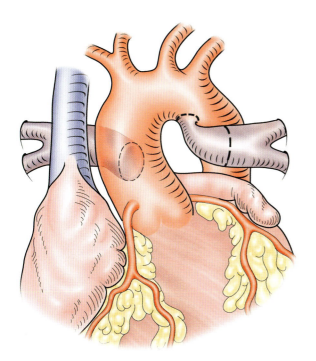

57.12a

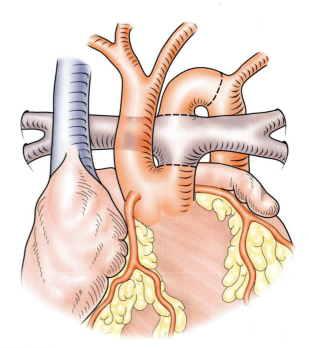

57.13

of the ascending and descending aorta, the pulmonary arteries, the ductus, and the head and neck vessels, the repair is undertaken under deep hypothermic circulatory arrest. The patient's temperature is lowered to 18 °C, the circulation arrested, and the head vessels snared. If one wishes to avoid deep hypothermic circulatory arrest, antegrade perfusion of the right carotid artery can be achieved by repositioning the aortic cannula at reduced flow to approximately 10 mL/kg/minute. The truncal root is transected as described above. Ductal tissue is resected from the descending aorta. Continuity between the small ascending aorta and normal sized descending aorta can be achieved in several ways.

End-to-end anastomosis is feasible if the gap between the two vessels is not too large (**Figure 57.14a and b**). Extensive mobilization of the head and neck vessels and the descending aorta can be improved by disconnecting the left subclavian artery in some rare patients.

The hypoplastic ascending aorta and aortic arch can be enlarged with a homograft patch after end-to-end connection of the posterior vessel wall (**Figures 57.15a and b and 57.16**).

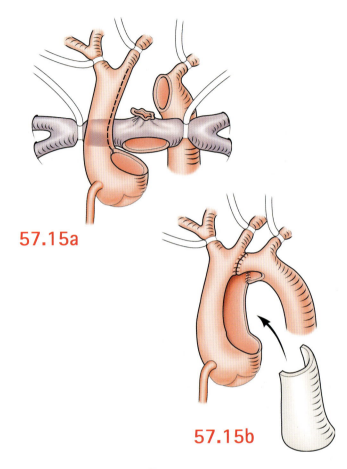

57.15a

57.15b

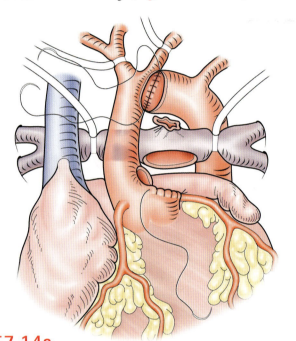

57.14a

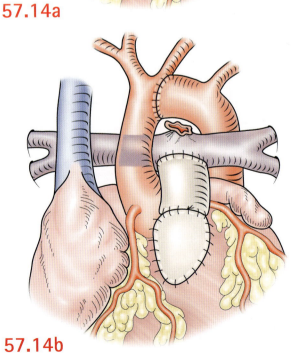

57.14b

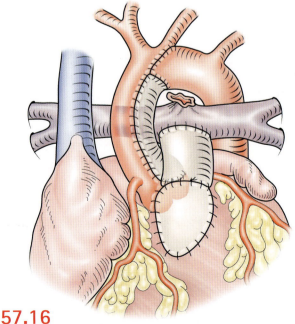

57.16

POSTOPERATIVE CARE

Intraoperatively placed monitoring lines (PA, left atrium) are used to assess postoperative hemodynamic variables of the patients. Most infants require some form of inotropic support with low doses of milrinone and dopamine or dobutamine for approximately 48 hours. High doses of inotropes (particularly adrenaline) and pulmonary vasoconstrictors should be avoided. Patients are kept paralyzed or heavily sedated for 24–72 hours to avoid a pulmonary hypertensive crisis. Typical triggers such as hypercarbia, hypoxia, acidosis, and unnecessary manipulations must be avoided. The core temperature is maintained below 37°C by active cooling if necessary to avoid arrhythmias. Junctional ectopic tachycardia is treated with further cooling and sequential pacing or amiodarone if required.

Vasodilators, such as nitroglycerine, nitroprusside, prostaglandin, and, most effectively, nitric oxide, can be used when PA pressures are elevated. Since early repair has become established, pulmonary hypertensive crises have become rare in the postoperative period, which has reduced the procedure-related mortality and morbidity significantly.

OUTCOME

The operative risk is somewhere between 10% and 20%, even in experienced centers. Important risk factors are severe truncal valve incompetence, interrupted aortic arch, coronary artery anomalies, and older age at repair (more than 100 days old) in most large series. Early repair dramatically reduces the incidence of pulmonary hypertensive crises in the postoperative period; and, thus, the overall results have improved. Despite the trend towards operations in smaller and more complex patients, the Society of Thoracic Surgeons (STS) congenital heart disease database, including almost 600 patients, showed an overall mortality of 11%.

Follow-up data spanning more than 20 years after surgical repair of truncus arteriosus are now available. Large studies confirm that hemodynamic results and long-term survival are excellent. The major potential of morbidity and mortality after the initial repair is related to reoperations such as conduit replacements or procedures on the truncal valve.

Replacement of obstructed, calcified RV-to-PA conduits is common several years (mean, 5.5 years) after the initial operation. Surprisingly, the incidence of conduit replacement is not related to the size of the first placed conduit, whereas aortic allografts fail earlier than pulmonary allografts. Obstructive lesions in the pulmonary arteries can be ballooned and stented.

Worsening regurgitation or stenosis of the dysplastic truncal valve may make repair or replacement necessary during follow-up of these children. A significant number of children develop aneurysmatic enlargement of the newly constructed aortic root, requiring root replacement with a Bentall-type procedure.

FURTHER READING

Barbero-Marcial M, Riso A, Atik E, Jatene A. A technique for correction of truncus arteriosus types I and II without extracardiac conduits. *J Thorac Cardiovasc Surg.* 1990; 99; 364–9.

de Leval MR. Persistent truncus arteriosus. In: *Surgery for congenital heart defects.* 2nd edn. Philadelphia, PA: Saunders; 1994: pp. 539–48.

Hanley FL, Heinemann MK, Jonas RA, et al. Repair of truncus arteriosus in the neonate. *J Thorac Cardiovasc Surg.* 1993; 105: 1047–56.

Heinemann MK, Hanley FL, Fenton KN, et al. Fate of small homograft conduits after early repair of truncus arteriosus. *Ann Thorac Surg.* 1993; 55: 1409–12.

Imamura M, Drummond-Webb JJ, Sarris GE, Mee RBB. Improving early and intermediate results of truncus arteriosus repair: a new technique of truncal valve repair. *Ann Thorac Surg.* 1999; 67: 1142–6.

Kirklin JW, Barratt-Boyes BG. Truncus arteriosus. In: *Cardiac surgery.* 2nd edn. New York: Churchill Livingstone; 1993: pp. 1131–51.

Russell HM, Pasquali SK, Jacobs JP, et al. Outcomes of repair of common arterial trunk with truncal valve surgery: a review of the STS congenital heart disease database. *Ann Thorac Surg.* 2012; 93: 164–9.

Spray T. Truncus arteriosus. In: Kaiser LR, Kron IL, Spray TL (eds). *Mastery of cardiothoracic surgery.* Philadelphia, PA: Lippincott-Raven; 1998: pp. 759–70.

58

Persistent ductus arteriosus

WILLIAM M. DECAMPLI

HISTORY

Dr John Munro, in 1907, presented a paper before the Philadelphia Academy of Surgery proposing ligation of the patent (persistent) ductus arteriosus (PDA), but the first successful ligation was performed by Robert Edward Gross on August 26, 1938, on a 7-year-old girl. Indications were expanded to include ligation in premature infants with the separate reports of Powell and Decancq in 1963. Video-assisted thoracoscopic (VATS) PDA clip ligation was first reported by Laborde and colleagues in 1993. DeCampli, in 1998, described VATS suture ligation of PDA with routine discharge of the patient on the day of operation.[1]

PRINCIPLES AND JUSTIFICATION

The ductus arteriosus, arising from the distal portion of the embryonic sixth aortic arch, is a vascular communication between the systemic and pulmonary vasculature, usually between the isthmus of the aortic arch and the origin of the left pulmonary artery, which forms a vital part of fetal anatomy. The ductus normally closes spontaneously within 72 hours after birth in full-term infants. The resulting non-patent ductus is called the *ligamentum arteriosum*. The *persistent ductus arteriosus* (PDA) is defined as persistent patency of the fetal ductus beyond its normal time of spontaneous closure. The most common risk factor for persistence of ductal patency is prematurity. The probability of PDA is inversely proportional to birth weight and gestational age (EGA), reaching 77% at 28 weeks EGA. The risk is further increased by the presence of infant respiratory distress syndrome (RDS), reaching 90% for EGA of less than 32 weeks. In these subsets, spontaneous closure can occur beyond 1 week but the risk of late patency is substantial.

When pulmonary vascular resistance normalizes, PDA results in a left-to-right shunt which, if substantial, results in congestive heart failure (CHF). In premature infants findings can include pulmonary congestion, tachypnea, ventilator dependence, peripheral edema, and compromised organ perfusion. In older infants and children, failure to thrive, recurrent respiratory infections, and fatigue with exertion are common. A large shunt may produce pulmonary vascular disease within 6–12 months. With progressive vascular injury, pulmonary hypertension becomes irreversible, resulting in Eisenmenger's syndrome. Occasionally, adults may present with endocarditis, ductal aneurysm, or aortic dissection.

The treatment of PDA is PDA closure. In general, the indication for PDA closure is the presence of symptoms attributable to the left-to-right shunt, as described above. PDA closure is indicated in any patient with an audible "machinery murmur" with or without echocardiographic evidence of cardiac chamber enlargement. Closure of the "silent ductus" – one which is inaudible but detected incidentally by echocardiography – is controversial but sometimes performed to eliminate the small risk of endocarditis. Infants and children undergoing other cardiothoracic procedures should have simultaneous PDA ligation. Premature neonates should have PDA closure if they have refractory or worsening ventilator dependence and/or poor tissue perfusion in the absence of another dominating cause and have failed a trial of cyclooxygenase inhibitors. Indications for PDA closure in premature infants, however, continue to evolve due to persistent lack of high-quality studies in this population, and therefore remain largely institution-dependent. Indications for PDA closure in adults are described in the American College of Cardiology/American Heart Association 2008 Guidelines for Adults with Congenital Heart Disease.[2]

In patients other than premature infants, if PDA flow is bidirectional or right-to-left, cardiac catheterization should be performed. PDA closure is contraindicated if pulmonary vascular resistance index exceeds 8 Woods units/m^2 and does not decrease with oxygen, nitric oxide, or other vasodilators. PDA ligation is, of course, contraindicated as an isolated procedure in the presence of "ductal-dependent" congenital cardiac disease. Catheter-based closure is the preferred approach in an adult with calcified PDA and/or with significant other medical problems.

Complications of PDA closure in all age groups include pneumothorax, chylothorax, bleeding, residual flow, wound infection, and vocal cord paresis (VCP). Age-related risks and complications include the following:

- *Premature neonates:* VCP is a potentially serious complication of PDA ligation in this subset. In a series published since 2008 the incidence has ranged from 5% to 67% and may increase the risk for comorbidities such as bronchopulmonary dysplasia, tube feeding, ventilator support, and length of stay. In one study VCP persisted in 65% of patients with median 16-month follow-up. Some studies have demonstrated an increased risk of scoliosis, retinopathy of prematurity, and neurosensory impairment in this subset.
- *Infants and children:* Ranges of incidences for residual flow are 0–8%, chylothorax 0.2–4%, and VCP 0–12%. Obstruction of the aorta or pulmonary artery has been reported.
- *Adults:* In one recent report of 34 adult patients undergoing PDA ligation, complications included VCP (14.7%), hemorrhage (8.8%), residual flow (5.9%), and pneumothorax (5.9%).

PREOPERATIVE ASSESSMENT AND PREPARATION

Echocardiography is sufficient to establish the diagnosis of PDA. Additionally, the echocardiogram should establish the arch anatomy, presence of coarctation, direction of ductal flow, and any associated cardiac anomalies. Premature newborns with PDA should be free of active infection at the time of ligation. Many premature newborns will have abnormal coagulation times; an attempt to correct them with fresh frozen plasma subjects them to a volume load and is not necessary prior to operation. Operation can be performed in the neonatal intensive care unit in the baby's warming bed, avoiding the risk of transport and problems with temperature control.

In full-term infants, children, and adults, echocardiography suffices for diagnosis. If a videoscopic (VATS) approach is entertained, the size and position of the ductus should be ascertained to minimize videoscopic dissection. Additionally, very large and short PDAs should probably be closed with an open technique. Presence of bidirectional or right-to-left ductal flow should prompt cardiac catheterization to assess pulmonary resistance, as described above. Aortic angiography or magnetic resonance imaging is indicated in cases of ductal or periductal aneurysm or calcified ductus. Patients with a short, calcified ductus should undergo PDA closure via a transpulmonary approach, as described below. Patients with acute endocarditis and PDA should undergo a trial of antibiotic therapy. If the infection is controlled, the ductus can be ligated a few months thereafter. If infection cannot be controlled with antibiotics, prompt ligation is carried out.

ANESTHESIA

For low birth-weight babies, one unit of blood should be available for operation. An arterial monitoring catheter is not necessary, but a pulse oximeter and blood pressure cuff should be placed on the lower extremity. An end tidal CO_2 monitor is useful to determine whether lung retraction is affecting pulmonary blood flow, although this technique is unreliable in small babies. Babies on an oscillator ventilator can undergo operation without preoperative conversion to conventional ventilation.

Older children and adults undergoing PDA ligation with thoracotomy can undergo standard intravenous anesthetic, but a regional technique, as described by Peterson et al., is also well suited for this operation.[3] Single-lung ventilation is preferable, but not necessary. This can be achieved by selective right mainstem bronchus intubation in small children and by use of a double lumen tube (or single lumen tube with bronchial blocker) in children greater than 25 kg in weight. Sufficient time should be allowed before incision to allow the lung to collapse. When the VATS technique is employed, intravenous anesthetic is used and single-lung ventilation is preferred in older patients. Adults undergoing transpulmonary approach for a large calcified ductus should be prepared in the standard manner for patients undergoing sternotomy and cardiopulmonary bypass.

OPERATIONS

PDA in the very low birth–weight (<1000 g) newborn

POSITIONING OF PATIENT AND INCISION

The baby is positioned in the right lateral decubitus position and biased toward the side of the surgeon (**Figure 58.1**). A pulse oximeter is placed on a toe. A temperature-regulated radiant heater is used. A custom-made electrocautery ground pad is applied. Adherent drapes should be avoided. An approximately 2 cm transverse incision is made just caudal to the palpable tip of the scapula.

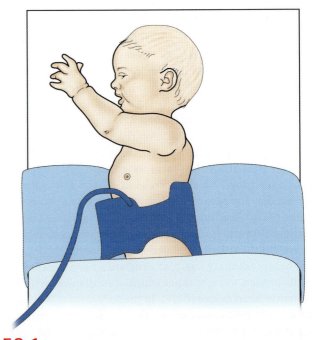

58.1

EXPOSURE OF THE DUCTUS

The chest wall muscles can be mobilized and preserved, or the latissimus muscle can be partially divided. The pleura is entered in the fourth interspace. Care should be taken to avoid violation of the visceral pleura, as this will cause an air leak and the necessity of a chest tube. A rib retractor is placed.

The lung lobes are swept anteriorly by the first assistant using two rubber-coated malleable retractors (**Figure 58.2a**). The position of these retractors is determined by the surgeon, as the assistant cannot see into the wound, and is based on exposure and the hemodynamic and respiratory status of the patient, which can change rapidly. The ductus arteriosus is readily identified as the structure around which the recurrent nerve loops (**Figure 58.2b**).

Using low-power needlepoint cautery, small incisions are made in the pleural reflection just caudal and cephalad to the ductus toward its aortic end. A Jacobson clamp is then used to gently bluntly dissect to the deep (medial) margin of the ductus. The ductus itself should not be dissected out, nor should it be grasped or otherwise put on traction. Small

cotton swabs can be used for blunt dissection and to keep the field dry. The course of the recurrent laryngeal nerve is determined.

LIGATION

An appropriate-sized metal clip on a manual applier is tested on the drapes to assure no scissoring. It is then carefully positioned around the ductus at its aortic end and then applied without traction on the ductus (**Figure 58.3a and b**). Spring-loaded or "autoclip" applicators should never be used. A rise in blood pressure sometimes, but not always, occurs. The lower extremity pulse oximeter should continue to show a strong signal. A second clip should be applied only if there is sufficient ductal length and the recurrent nerve can be avoided.

Because the risk of VCP may be hypothetically increased with clip ligation, suture ligation may be preferred. After ductal exposure as described above, a small right-angle clamp is used to gently undermine the ductus in a cephalad-to-caudal direction. Under the caudal side, one can readily see the clamp tip deep to the ductus and superficial to the

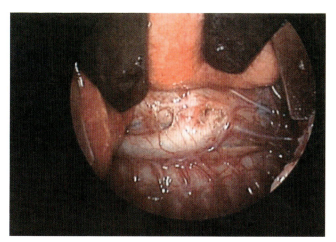

58.2a

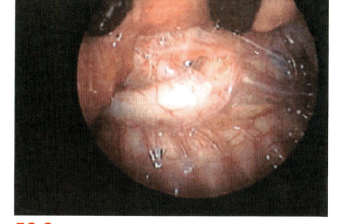

58.3a

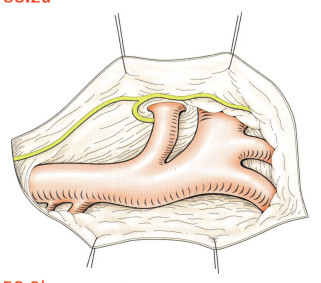

58.2b

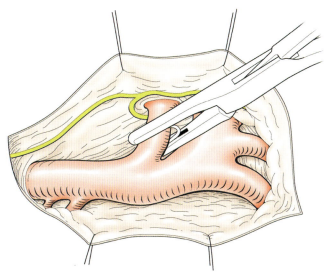

58.3b

recurrent nerve. The clamp is used to draw through a 3-0 non-absorbable suture which is used to ligate the ductus. This technique may be more hazardous in infants weighing less than 500 g and the choice is left to the individual surgeon's judgment.

CLOSURE

Hemostasis is confirmed, then the lung retractors removed. A 5 French pigtail catheter or 8 French pleural tube is placed and set to 10–15 cm water suction only if the lung was injured during the procedure. The pleural reflection over the aorta does not need to be reclosed. The ribs are approximated with three 2-0 absorbable stitches during manual inflation of the lungs, then the soft tissue layers closed with running absorbable suture.

PNEUMOTHORAX

If, shortly after chest closure, oxygen saturation decreases and inspiratory pressure requirements increase, the most likely diagnosis is pneumothorax. The diagnosis is confirmed by auscultation and transillumination and the air is evacuated with a needle or by placement of a pigtail catheter. A chest film is then obtained.

TORN DUCTUS

If the ductus tears during mobilization or ligation, a "peanut" gauze or Q-tip should be used to directly compress the tissue, assuring continued aortic and pulmonary artery blood flow. Blood should be made ready to infuse by the anesthesiologist. The thoracotomy incision is enlarged as needed, and the chest suctioned of blood. After sufficient duration of compression, release of the Q-tip usually does not result in immediate bleeding. During this time the proximal and distal ends of the ductus can be suture ligated with a 6-0 polypropylene suture. Alternatively, the aorta proximal and distal to the ductus can be quickly mobilized, and curved occluding clamps applied at both locations. The ductal orifice at the aorta is obliterated with a pursestring or running 6-0 polypropylene suture, then the aortic clamps released. The pulmonary artery end of the defect can be repaired with a 6-0 polypropylene stitch with or without a small Potts clamp in place, or by slowly rolling the Q-tip off the defect.

PDA ligation in patients >1000 g

"Double" or "triple ligation" is performed in all but the smallest infants. The positioning, incision, and exposure of the ductus are performed as described above. Somewhat more dissection is carried out cephalad and caudal to the ductus, and the pedicle containing the vagus and recurrent nerves is mobilized more medially. Traction sutures may be placed on this pedicle. The recurrent nerve is identified. A right-angle clamp is passed medial to ("underneath") the ductus as described above (**Figure 58.4a and b**). This many require some patience, as the pleural reflection is relatively firm in older infants.

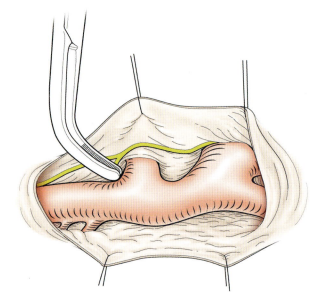

58.4a

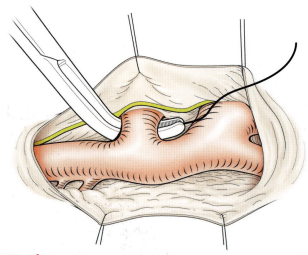

58.4b

A 5-0 monofilament polypropylene pursestring stitch is taken around the aortic base of the ductus, taking only bites of adventitia. Each end is pulled through under the ductus and an additional bite is taken on the ductal adventitia (**Figure 58.5a**). The suture is then tied (**Figure 58.5b**).

If the ductus is somewhat large, some surgeons prefer to temporarily apply a clamp across the aortic isthmus to lower the pressure in the ductus while tying down the first suture. Gentle lateral traction is then applied to the aorta, and a 2-0 non-absorbable polyester free tie or second pursestring suture is secured toward the pulmonary artery end (**Figure 58.5c**).

If the visceral pleura is injured or if drainage is anticipated, a 5 Fr or 8 Fr pigtail catheter can be placed. An intercostal block at the third, fourth, and fifth interspaces can be achieved using 0.4% Marcaine. Interrupted absorbable sutures are used to approximate the ribs, then running absorbable suture used to close the soft-tissue layers.

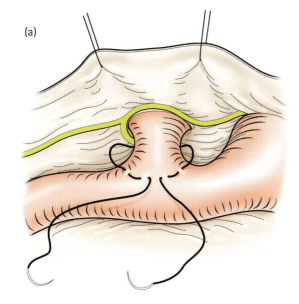

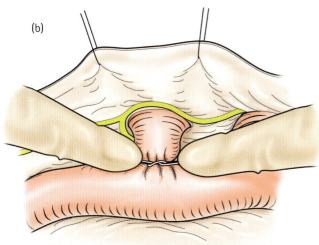

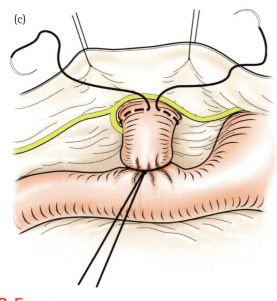

58.5a–c

Ligation and division for short ductus

Division of the ductus should be performed whenever the ductus is so short as to make it difficult to place two ligatures separated by at least a few millimeters. In this case, the vagus nerve pedicle flap should be mobilized thoroughly and traction sutures placed on its edges. The ductus, isthmus, and proximal descending aorta are mobilized. In particular, the aorta should be retracted anteriorly and dissection under the ductus performed under direct vision and with visualization of the recurrent nerve, which should be swept deep to the ductus.

APPLICATION OF CLAMPS

A multi-toothed, atraumatic partial occlusion clamp is then placed across the aortoductal junction, with the handles caudal. A similar straight clamp is then placed across the ductus keeping the recurrent nerve medial. Traction should not be placed on these clamps. On the contrary, they should be "pushed into" the pulmonary artery and aorta to avoid slippage (**Figure 58.6a**). Alternatively, occlusion clamps are placed on the aorta proximal and distal to the ductus when the latter is very short (**Figure 58.6b**).

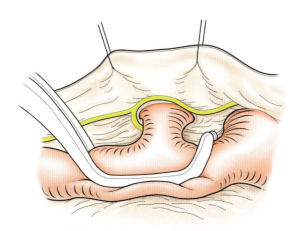

58.6a

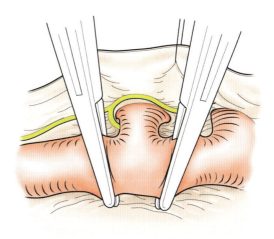

58.6b

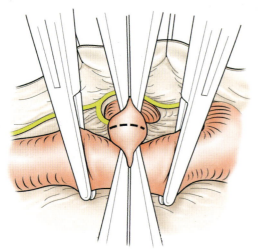

58.6c

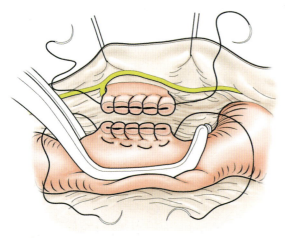

58.6d

The ductus is then divided and each end oversewn with a 5-0 polypropylene suture using a mattress technique followed by an over-and-over stitch (**Figure 58.6c and d**).

PDA ligation using VATS technique

The technique of video-assisted thoracoscopic ligation of PDA can be applied, in principle, to any ductus that does not need to be divided, regardless of age or weight. A very short or large ductus, evidence of pulmonary adhesions, ductal calcification, or recent endocarditis are contraindications to using the technique. Proper training in the general techniques of video-assisted surgery is, of course, essential.

Specialized instruments allow for safe, efficient exposure and ligation of the ductus and include those shown in **Figure 58.7**: (A) "fan" lung retractor, (B) ring forceps, (C) tissue grasper, (D) clip applier, (E) "diamond-dusted" suture grasper, (F) right angle, (G) suture scissors, (H) large right angle, (I) tissue scissors, (J) small grasper, and (K) small clip applier. Additionally, a cautery device and a 2.5–5.0 mm zero angle thoracoscope with attached camera are employed.

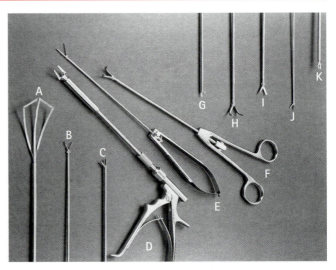

58.7

The technique described here is taken from DeCampli (1998)[1] and can be applied to patients weighing 2 kg or greater.

POSITION OF PATIENT AND INCISIONS

The patient is placed in the standard position for a left thoracotomy, with the area of the fourth, fifth, and sixth interspaces prepped. Standard thoracotomy instruments are available on the operating table, in case conversion to open thoracotomy is necessary. Two units of blood should be available. Four small (5 mm) incisions are made as shown in **Figure 58.8**. The most anterior incision (site 1) is at the posterior axillary line, third interspace. The second (site 2) is just anterior to the scapular tip, fourth interspace. The most posterior incision (site 4) lies between the medial edge of the scapula and the vertebral column. The last incision (site 3) lies between the latter two.

Each incision is deepened by muscle-splitting blunt dissection, and the pleura is entered. A 5 mm port is placed at

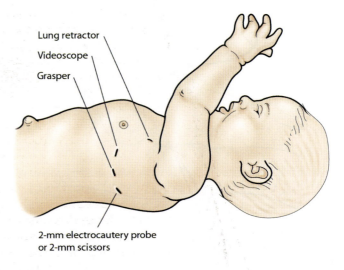

Lung retractor
Videoscope
Grasper

2-mm electrocautery probe
or 2-mm scissors

58.8

site 2 and a thoracoscope advanced. The lung retractor is placed through site 1. The retractor sweeps the upper lobe in an inferomedial direction. If the lower lobe obscures the juxtaductal area, a second fan retractor can be placed through site 1. A grasper is placed through site 3, and the cautery through site 4. Either the camera or the retractor, or both, can be held by an adjustable support bar to avoid the necessity of two assistants.

DISSECTION OF DUCTUS

With the juxtaductal area exposed, the pleural reflection on the aorta is grasped and opened along the aorta with cautery. The anterior flap is developed with blunt and sharp dissection, and the ductus is exposed (**Figure 58.9a**).

An appropriate balance of blunt and sharp dissection further mobilizes the cephalad and caudal borders of the ductus. A standard cotton tip applicator ("Q-tip") placed through sites 3 or 4 is useful for blotting blood and for blunt dissection.

A right-angle instrument is used, coming from the cephalad border, to undermine the ductus (**Figure 58.9b**). This step requires patience, as the medial connective tissue ("behind" the ductus) is firm. The thoracoscope should focus on the caudal border of the ductus to ensure that the right angle is passing through the proper plane.

SUTURE LIGATION

The right angle is used to pass a 1 polyfilament silk tie around the pulmonary end of the ductus (**Figure 58.9c**). Smaller gauge suture material tends to fray with the instrument tie technique. The ductus is ligated using an intracorporeal instrument tie technique. The preferred instruments for this are a pair of non-ratcheted suture graspers with diamond-dusted jaws, as shown in **Figure 58.7**. The first two throws form a sliding knot. The third throw forms a square knot with the second, and the fourth throw forms a square knot with the third. Although this tie may not always completely occlude the ductus, it serves to gather up ductal tissue for precise clip ligation without entrapment of the recurrent nerve.

APPLICATION OF CLIP

The thoracoscope is now replaced via a port into site 3. A nasal speculum is used to spread parallel to the rib through site 2 so that the clip applier can be advanced into the chest (**Figure 58.9d**).

The aorta is retracted laterally with the grasper through site 4, then the clip advanced onto the aortic end of the ductus and fired. Care should be taken to have a good thoracoscopic view of the ductus during this phase, and not to exert traction on the ductus by the applier.

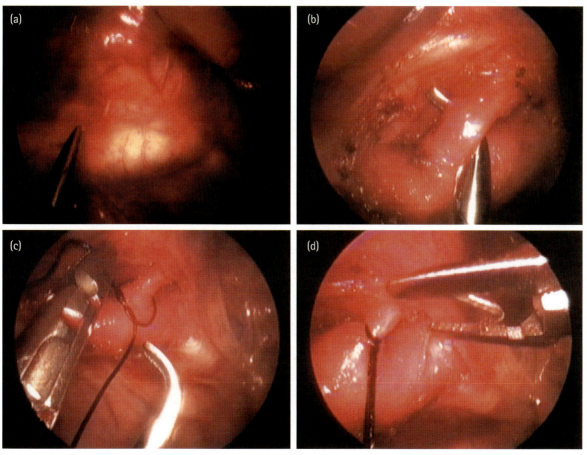

58.9a–d

Hemostasis is checked. A transesophageal echocardiogram is obtained to confirm ductal closure. An additional clip can be applied if residual ductal flow is detected. All instruments are removed except the thoracoscope. An 8 Fr pigtail catheter is placed using the Seldinger technique. The lung is then inflated and the thoracoscope is removed. The wounds are closed in two layers using absorbable sutures, and band-aids are applied. The patient is turned to the supine position and, if there is no active air leak or excessive drainage, the pleural catheter is removed. The patient is awakened, extubated, and taken to the recovery area. In a few hours, when the patient is able to get out of bed, void, and take liquids, he/she is discharged from the hospital.

If bleeding occurs during the VATS procedure, the procedure can be converted to open by joining the three lateral most port access incisions. Prior to making this incision a sponge stick can be inserted into the anterior port to control bleeding.

Robotic-assisted VATS ligation

Use of robotic assistance to perform VATS PDA ligation is widely reported. DeCampli, while at the Children's Hospital of Philadelphia, used a voice-controlled robotic arm to control the videoscope position, as shown in **Figure 58.10**. In this procedure, the incisions and instruments are the same as used for VATS PDA ligation. Alternatively, the camera position can be fixed and the dissecting instruments controlled from a remote location by robotic arms.

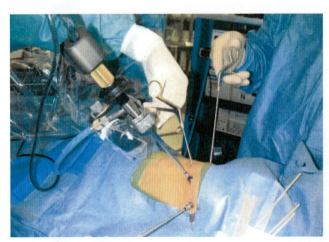

58.10

Calcified ductus

In the older adult patient, or the patient with a history of endocarditis, the ductus and/or periductal area may be calcified and thinned, typically near the aortic end. Simple ligation may be difficult or hazardous. Division may also be unwise if clamps cannot be applied to calcified or friable pulmonary arterial or aortic tissue. In this case, a transpulmonary

approach is used and is preferable to a transaortic approach. A full or partial upper median sternotomy is performed, and the patient placed on cardiopulmonary bypass using a single two-stage venous cannula. Ductal flow, if prolific, should be controlled with tourniquets around the branch pulmonary arteries, or occasionally by direct pressure on the ductus.

In the absence of active endocarditis, aneurysm or dissection, mild hypothermia is induced, and the main pulmonary artery is opened distally, extending slightly onto the left branch (**Figure 58.11a**). Bleeding is controlled using a short period of low-flow CPB or using balloon occlusion of the orifice.

The ductal orifice is closed within the pulmonary artery primarily (**Figure 58.11b**), or using a polytetrafluoroethylene patch. The pulmonary artery is closed and the patient weaned from cardiopulmonary bypass.

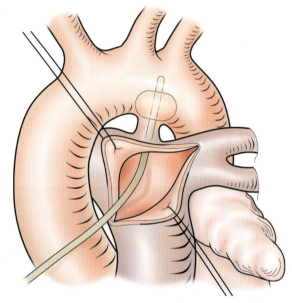

58.11a

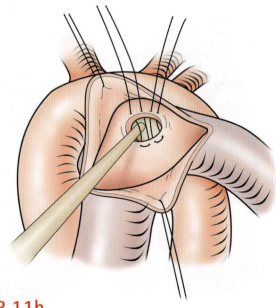

58.11b

If the ductal orifice is large, or if extensive debridement or repair is necessary to treat endocarditis, aneurysm or dissection, circulatory arrest with selective cerebral perfusion is utilized. Minimal dissection is carried out in the ductal area. The patient is cooled to 18 °C. An arterial cannula is placed in the innominate artery. The circulation is arrested and selective cerebral perfusion is begun. The proximal innominate and left carotid arteries are controlled with tourniquets or clamps, the aorta is clamped, and cardioplegic arrest is achieved. The pulmonary artery is opened and the necessary repair of the aorta and pulmonary artery is carried out, with obliteration of the ductal communication. In the Trendelenberg position aortic flow is reinstituted and the ascending aorta is de-aired. The carotid tourniquets and aortic cross-clamp are removed. The repair is checked and the patient warmed and weaned off cardiopulmonary bypass.

POSTOPERATIVE CARE

Low birth-weight neonates undergoing PDA ligation are returned to their preoperative ventilator settings. Pain is controlled by small doses of intravenous morphine. A drain tube, if placed, is removed in 12–24 hours. The most common early complication is pneumothorax, manifested by hypoxemia and increased inspiratory pressure requirements. This is treated with catheter drainage. Pleural effusion is infrequent and is also treated with catheter drainage. Wound infection is treated with drainage, and antibiotic treatment is begun according to wound culture results. Residual or recurrent ductal flow is usually restrictive and can be observed, then coil occluded by trans-catheter technique later in infancy. Recurrent nerve palsy can cause aspiration in small infants and is treated with nasogastric or gastrostomy feeding until the infant is stronger.

The older patient undergoing ligation of isolated PDA should be mobilized within hours of the procedure. Pain is controlled with small doses of intravenous morphine sulfate, oral acetometophen, or (when a thoracotomy has been performed) agents administered through an epidural catheter. The chest tube can be removed within 24 hours and the patient discharged in 1–2 days. When VATS is used, the patient can be discharged on the day of surgery, and oral acetometophin provides good pain control.

OUTCOME

The outcome following simple PDA ligation is good. Patients beyond infant age are routinely discharged the same day as the procedure if a VATS technique is used. Early mortality, even in premature infants, is nearly zero. Late mortality in premature infants is related to associated pulmonary disease, but is now less than 10%. Most normal-weight infants and children undergoing PDA ligation go on to have a normal life expectancy. Older adults with calcified ductus or ductal aneurysm have higher risk of death and complications, often related to associated cardiovascular disease.

REFERENCES

1. DeCampli WM. Video-assisted thoracic surgical procedures in children. In: Spray TL (ed.). *Pediatric cardiac surgery annual 1998 of the seminars in thoracic and cardiovascular surgery.* Philadelphia: W.B. Saunders; 1998: pp. 61–73.
2. Warnes CA, Williams RG, Bashore TM, et al. ACC/AHA 2008 guidelines for the management of adults with congenital heart disease: a report of the American College of Cardiology/American Heart Association Task Force on Practice Guidelines (Writing Committee to Develop Guidelines on the Management of Adults With Congenital Heart Disease). Developed in Collaboration With the American Society of Echocardiography, Heart Rhythm Society, International Society for Adult Congenital Heart Disease, Society for Cardiovascular Angiography and Interventions, and Society of Thoracic Surgeons. *J Am Coll Cardiol.* 2008; 52(23): e1–121.
3. McNamara PJ, Sehgal A. Towards rational management of the patent ductus arteriosus: the need for disease staging. *Arch Dis Child Fetal Neonatal Ed.* 2007; 92(6): F424–7.

FURTHER READING

Bixler GM, Powers GC, Clark RH, et al. Changes in the diagnosis and management of patent ductus arteriousus from 2006 to 2015 in United States neonatal intensive care units. *J Paediatr* 2017; 189: 105-112.

Dutta S, Mihailovic A, Benson L, et al. Thoracoscopic ligation versus coil occlusion for patent ductus arteriosus: a matched cohort study of outcomes and cost. *Surg Endosc.* 2008; 22(7): 1643–8.

Nezafati MH, Soltani G, Vedadian A. Video-assisted ductal closure with new modifications: minimally invasive, maximally effective, 1,300 cases. *Ann Thorac Surg.* 2007; 84(4): 1343–8.

Suematsu Y, Mora BN, Mihaljevic T, et al. Totally endoscopic robotic-assisted repair of patent ductus arteriosus and vascular ring in children. *Ann Thorac Surg.* 2005; 80(6): 2309–13.

59

Aortopulmonary window

WILLIAM M. DECAMPLI

HISTORY

Aortopulmonary window (AP window) was described by Elliotson in 1830. Gross, while operating for a presumed patent ductus arteriosus, encountered an AP window and successfully ligated it in 1948. Cooley and associates reported division of an AP window using cardiopulmonary bypass in 1957. Johansson and coworkers, in 1978, first described anterior incision into the AP window itself for exposure.

PRINCIPLES AND JUSTIFICATION

AP window is a rare anomaly, found in 0.1–0.2% of patients with congenital heart disease. The disorder consists of a direct connection between the aortic root or ascending aorta and main pulmonary artery. In the developing embryo, the aortopulmonary foramen is the space between the distal end of the cushions that divide the lumen of the primitive outflow tract and the dorsal wall of the aortic sac. According to Anderson, failure to close the embryonic aortopulmonary foramen is the best explanation for the morphogenesis of AP window (see Chapter 42, Atrial septal defects). AP window is usually classified according to its proximal and distal extent along the ascending aorta (**Figure 59.1a–d**).

Although it is frequently an isolated defect, AP window occurs with other lesions in one half of cases, most commonly type A interrupted aortic arch (IAA). The lesion is not associated with DiGeorge syndrome. Other associated anomalies include ventricular septal defect (VSD), transposition of the great arteries, and tetralogy of Fallot. In some patients, anomalous origin of either coronary artery from the pulmonary artery can occur. Lastly, aortic origin of the right pulmonary artery (AORPA) can occur and is an important association (Berry syndrome) to assess pre- or intraoperatively, as it influences the operative plan.

The physiology of AP window is similar to that of persistent patent ductus arteriosus (PDA), namely a left-to-right shunt in both systole and diastole. Occasionally, the defect is restrictive, and patients may present with an asymptomatic murmur. More often, the defect is moderate or large, giving rise to symptoms of congestive heart failure (CHF) in early infancy. As in the case of PDA, late complications of unrepaired AP window include heart failure, pulmonary hypertension with pulmonary vascular obstructive disease leading to Eisenmenger's syndrome, and endocarditis.

The treatment of AP window is repair that eliminates the left-to-right shunt and corrects associated anomalies. Repair should occur shortly after diagnosis is made. Repair is performed with cardiopulmonary bypass (CPB) and may require

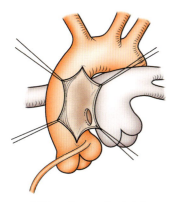 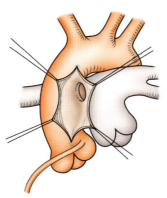 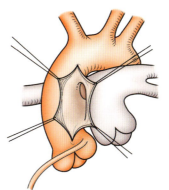 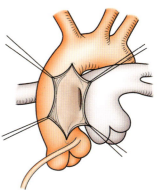

(a) Type I – proximal defect   (b) Type II – distal defect   (c) Type III – total defect   (d) Type IV – Intermediate defect

59.1a–d

deep hypothermia with circulatory arrest or selective perfusion, especially when there are associated arch anomalies. Potential complications include early or late coronary stenosis, arch obstruction, and branch pulmonary artery (branch PA) stenosis, in addition to central nervous system injury, recurrent nerve injury, airway compression, and residual VSD. Isolated cases of closure of AP window using transcatheter devices have been reported, but the indications for safety and intermediate and long-term complications remain unclear.

PREOPERATIVE ASSESSMENT AND PREPARATION

The anomaly is suspected in any infant with signs of CHF. A murmur may be heard, but large AP windows may lack a murmur. Babies with associated IAA will require prostaglandin to assure ductal patency. Echocardiography is sufficient for diagnosis and operative planning, but computed tomographic angiography may be a useful adjunct in complex anatomy. The echocardiogram should carefully delineate the location of the window, the anatomy of the aortic arch, branch PAs, and any other anomalies. Patients older than young infants or with oxygen desaturation with large AP window should undergo cardiac catheterization to clarify the magnitude and reactivity of pulmonary vascular resistance.

ANESTHESIA

In patients undergoing repair of AP window, the anesthetic considerations for CPB apply. With IAA, upper and lower extremity arterial monitoring is recommended. The upper extremity arterial catheter should be on the side of the more proximal arch branch. If deep hypothermia with circulatory arrest or selective cerebral perfusion is to be used, cerebral oximetry using infrared spectroscopy should be employed. For the patient with pulmonary hypertension, inhaled nitric oxide occasionally may be necessary post-CPB.

OPERATIONS

The operative approach depends on the details of the preoperative echocardiogram and intraoperative inspection. This section describes repair for (i) "simple" or isolated AP window, and (ii) AP window with IAA, with or without AORPA or coronary artery anomaly.

Isolated AP Window

EXPOSURE AND CANNULATION

The position is supine for all patients. A median sternotomy is performed and the thymus gland subtotally excised. The

ascending aorta, proximal arch, main and branch PAs are dissected out. The defect varies in distal extent, but an arterial cannula usually can be placed in the distal ascending aorta. If the defect is large and extends distally, the cannula may be placed through a 6-0 polypropylene pursestring suture on the mid-innominate artery. Single venous cannulation is sufficient, but bicaval cannulation is used if there is a VSD to close. CPB is initiated, then the branch PAs are controlled with tourniquets or small neuroaneurysm clips to avoid run-off through the window. The latter are small metal clips placed with an applier and are less traumatic than tourniquets, especially in small neonates. The patient is cooled to 28 °C. A small multi-holed vent is placed through the right superior pulmonary vein into the left ventricle and a cardioplegia catheter into the proximal aorta. The aorta is cross-clamped and cardioplegic solution is given (**Figure 59.2a**).

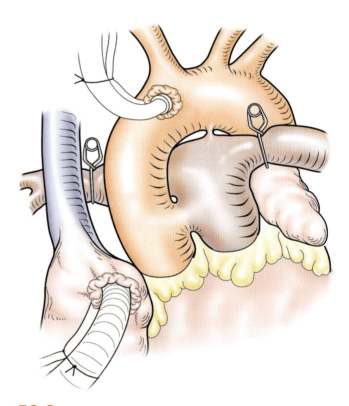

59.2a

ONE-PATCH CLOSURE TECHNIQUE

The anterior border of the AP window is opened along its length, representing one-third to one-half of the circumference (**Figure 59.2b**). Within the lumen, the branch pulmonary ostia, coronary artery ostia, and aortic valve leaflets and commissures should be located. A prosthetic patch is used to close the communication within the vessels. Its anterior edge is sandwiched between the walls of the aorta and pulmonary artery (**Figure 59.2c**).

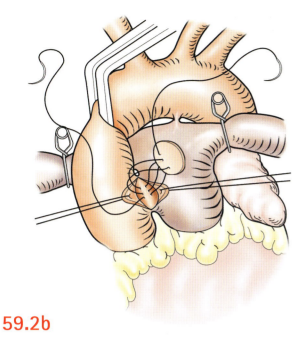

59.2b

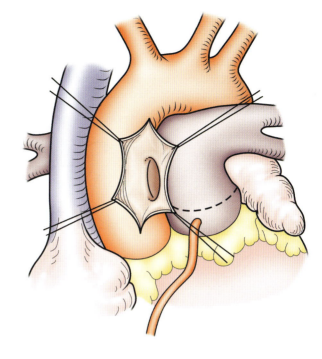

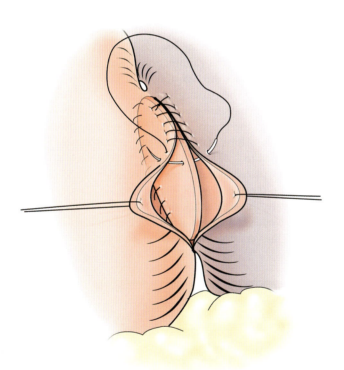

59.2c

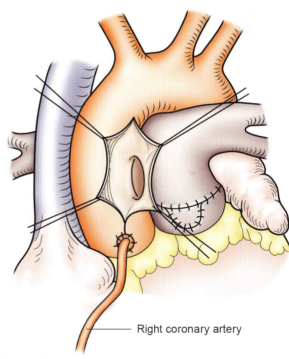

Right coronary artery

59.2d

If a coronary is located close to or within the pulmonary artery lumen, then the patch that closes the window can be positioned to baffle the aortic flow to that ostium. Rarely, a coronary ostium must be excised and transferred to the appropriate position (**Figure 59.2d**), as in repair of anomalous origin of the coronary artery from the pulmonary artery

(see Chapter 63, Coronary anomalies). If a VSD is present, it may be closed at this time in the manner described in Chapter 48, Ventricular septal defect. The aortic root is vented through the cardioplegia catheter and the cross-clamp removed. Clips or tourniquets are removed from the branch PAs. The patient is warmed. CPB is weaned at 37 °C.

TWO-PATCH CLOSURE TECHNIQUE

Alternatively, the window may be divided, and the defects in the aorta and pulmonary artery repaired with separate pericardial or homograft patches (**Figure 59.3**). As with the single-patch technique, the window should be partially divided first and the pulmonary and coronary ostial anatomy carefully inspected.

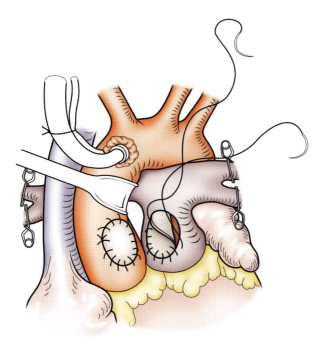

59.3

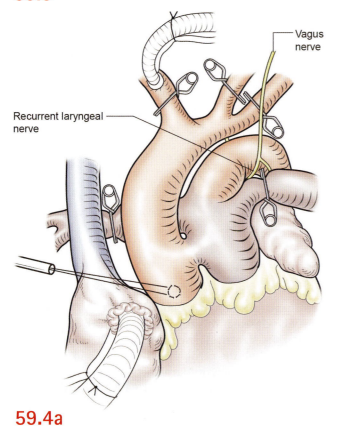

Vagus nerve

Recurrent laryngeal nerve

59.4a

AP Window with IAA

EXPOSURE, CANNULATION, AND CARDIOPULMONARY BYPASS

In AP window with IAA, the arch interruption is usually type A, and the window may be large and have distal extent. The anatomy is exposed as described above. Particular attention should be paid to the right pulmonary artery to see if it arises anomalously from the rightward aspect of the ascending aorta (AORPA).

The proximal arch and its branches are exposed. The ductus is carefully mobilized down to the descending aorta. During this step the recurrent nerve should be visualized and protected from cautery or excessive traction (**Figure 59.4a**). A 6-0 polypropylene pursestring suture is placed on the mid-innominate artery. An ink mark or silk tie is placed 3 mm distal to the tip of an 8 Fr wire-wound cannula. After giving heparin, a partially occluding clamp is placed on the mid-innominate artery and this cannula is placed through the pursestring stitch with the tip pointing toward the arch. The cannula and tourniquet are secured with a tie. Advancement to only 2–3 mm allows the cannula to be rotated readily for selective cerebral perfusion. Either a single venous cannula is placed into the right atrium, or bicaval cannulation is completed (in the case of a VSD) and CPB is initiated. Small neuroaneurysm clips are used to occlude the branch PAs. In contrast to isolated IAA, dual arterial cannulation is not required because aortic flow can pass through the AP window into the PDA (**Figure 59.4b**). The patient is cooled to 18 °C over at least 20 minutes. Ice bags are placed around the head to facilitate brain cooling. Intravenous phentolamine may be used for vasodilation. "Alpha stat" blood gas is used down to 28 °C then switched to "pH stat". Hematocrit is kept at 25–30 mg/dL. A vent is placed through the right superior pulmonary vein through a 6-0 polypropylene suture into the left ventricle or, alternatively, through either the left atrial appendage or the foramen ovale via the right atrium. A cardioplegia catheter is placed in the very proximal ascending aorta.

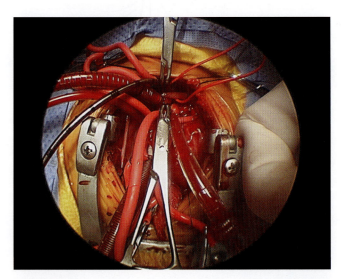

59.4b

After cooling to about 22 °C, the PDA is doubly ligated and divided, permitting exposure and mobilization of the isthmus and proximal descending aorta (**Figure 59.4c**). Depending on the distance between this and the arch, substantial mobilization may be required, including cautery division of several pairs of intercostal vessels. During this maneuver constant attention must be paid to the recurrent nerve. An angled vascular clamp is placed across the descending aorta. Ductal tissue is then excised from the aorta.

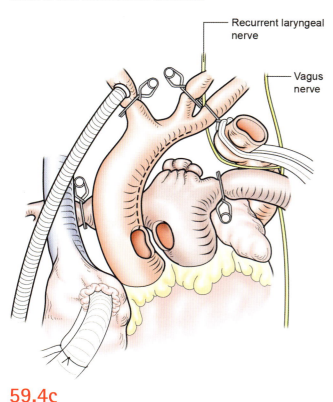

Recurrent laryngeal nerve

Vagus nerve

59.4c

SELECTIVE CEREBRAL PERFUSION

The arterial cannula is now carefully reoriented so the tip is pointed toward the distal artery. This should be achievable by a simple 180-degree "flip" of the arterial line. Small neuroaneurysm clips (or tourniquets) are placed to occlude the arch branches as the CPB flow rate is reduced to selective cerebral perfusion rate. The protocol for this flow depends on surgeon or institution preference. Typically, the flow is maintained in the range 30–60 mL/kg/minute to keep radial artery mean blood pressure 25–30 mmHg and relative cerebral oxygen saturation 90–95%. Some centers may also prefer to use transcranial Doppler measurements of the middle cerebral artery to adjust flow. Alternatively, some surgeons prefer use of circulatory arrest.

The aorta is cross-clamped and cardioplegic solution is administered. The cross-clamp is then removed.

METHODS OF REPAIR

At this point there are several possible choices of repair, depending on the surgeon's assessment of the anatomy.

Method 1

If there is not AORPA and the descending aorta can be easily advanced to the arch, then the AP window is divided, carefully checking for the coronary and pulmonary ostia. If a coronary ostium is located near or within a branch PA, division of the window must leave the ostium on the aortic side. The aortic defect is extended distally to and somewhat onto the leftward aspect of the left subclavian artery (or the left carotid artery in the infrequent case of type B IAA). The descending aorta is pulled up and the lateral third of its circumference sutured to the distal arch (**Figure 59.5a**).

The arch and aorta are then augmented with a patch of cryopreserved pulmonary homograft material. The defect in the pulmonary artery is repaired with a separate patch (**Figure 59.5b**).

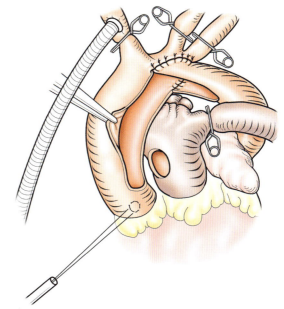

59.5a

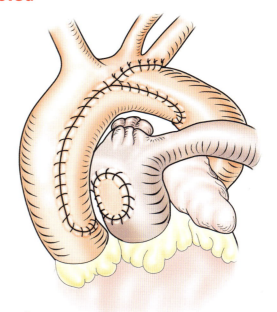

59.5b

Alternatively, when the AP window does not have too much distal extent, the descending aorta can be sutured primarily to the arch, then the AP window repaired as described in the section "Isolated AP window."

Method 2

If there is AORPA and the descending aorta can be advanced to the arch, then the anterior aspect of the AP window is opened and the incision extended distally to the distal arch vessel. A traction suture is placed on the side walls of the window for exposure (**Figure 59.6a**). The ostial anatomy

is inspected. About a third of the circumference of the descending aorta is sewn to the posterior edge of the arch incision.

A pulmonary homograft patch is then fashioned and sutured around the remaining circumference of the descending aortic edge (**Figure 59.6b**), and the suture is continued within the aortic lumen around the ostium of the right PA and brought to the caudal extent of the window (**Figure 59.6c**).

The anterior edge of this patch is then sewn to the edge of the ascending aorta. Lastly, the anterior edge of the PA is sutured directly to the outside of the patch (**Figure 59.6d**).

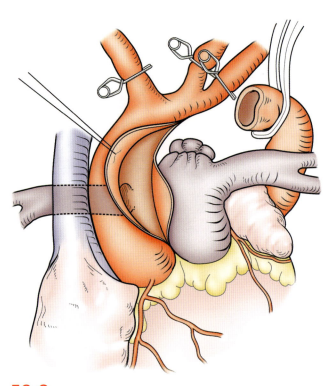

59.6a

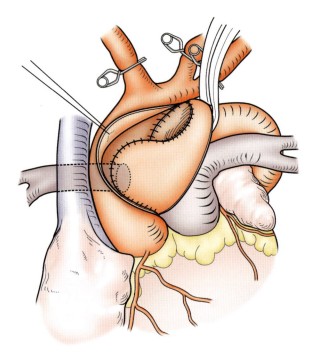

59.6c

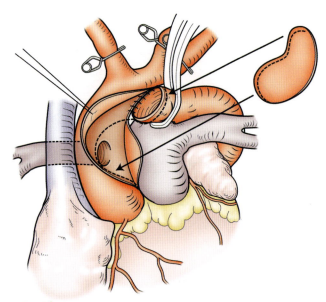

59.6b

59.6d

Alternatively, when the AP window does not have too much distal extent, the descending aorta can be directly sutured to the arch (**Figure 59.6e**). The aorta is divided proximal and distal to the window and the pulmonary artery is repaired with the anterior aortic flap (**Figure 59.6f**).

The proximal arch is pulled down and sewn directly to the proximal ascending aorta, with or without an anterior pericardial or homograft patch (**Figure 59.6g**).

Method 3

In rare instances the descending aorta cannot reach the arch without undue tension. This may occur with type A IAA with aorta descending to the right of midline. When this is the case and there is AORPA, a long gap between the arch and descending aorta can be bridged by using the left sub-clavian artery as a pedicle flap. Repair can then proceed as in Method 2 (**Figure 59.7a**).

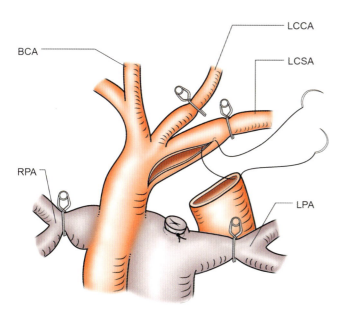

59.6e

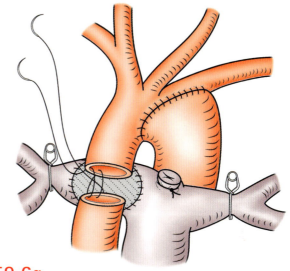

59.6g

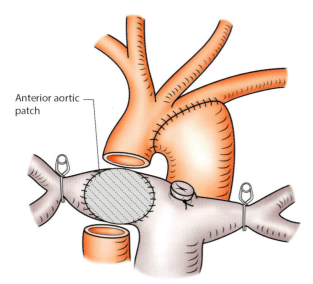

59.6f

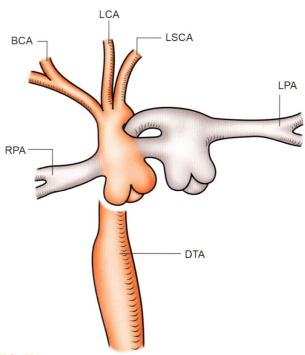

59.7a

Alternatively, the ascending aorta can be divided first distal then proximal to the AP window and PA ostium. PA repair can be completed with native aortic tissue or a homograft patch (**Figure 59.7b**). The PAs are then brought anterior to the aorta (as in a LeCompte maneuver).

The descending aorta is pulled up and part of its circumference sutured to the posterior lip of the aortic root. The distal ascending aorta is then pulled down and sutured around the composite circumference, with or without an anterior pericardial or homograft patch (**Figure 59.7c and d**).

Just prior to completion of the suture line, the descending

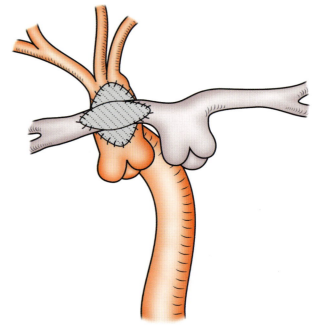

59.7d

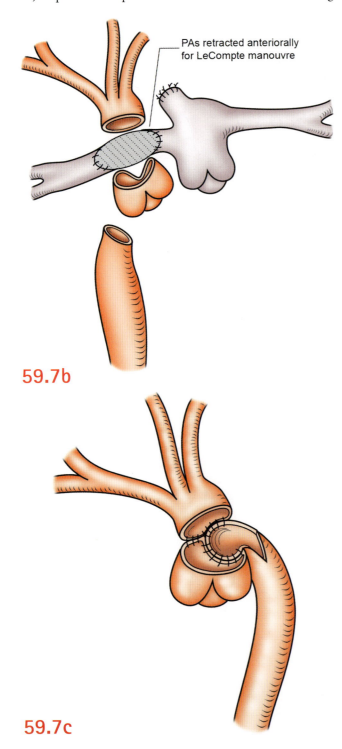

PAs retracted anteriorly for LeCompte manouvre

59.7b

59.7c

aortic clamp is released and the arch distended with saline through the suture line to assess the lie of the repair and to de-air. The suture line is then completed.

REPERFUSION

The cardioplegia catheter is set to low suction and the patient placed in the Trendelenberg position. The innominate artery clip is removed, and the arterial cannula is reoriented so the tip is pointing into the arch. The flow is increased as the clips or tourniquets are removed from the remaining arch vessels.

If there is a VSD, the ascending aorta can be clamped, cardioplegic solution given, the VSD closed through a right atriotomy, and then the clamp removed after de-airing through the cardioplegia catheter.

Warming is started. Clips are removed from the branch PAs. CPB is weaned at 37 °C. An umbilical artery catheter, together with a right radial arterial catheter or direct measurement through the aortic cannula provides a measure of the transaortic gradient. A right atrial catheter can be advanced into the right ventricle to assess pulmonary artery resistance. Unless there is a repaired VSD, transesophageal echocardiography is of limited use in assessing the repair.

POSTOPERATIVE CARE

Postoperative care of the infant following AP window repair (and associated anomalies) follows the general guidelines of infant care following CPB. If circulatory arrest or selective cerebral perfusion was used, temperature should be assiduously kept below 37.5 °C for the first 24 hours. Large AP windows in older infants and children subject the patient to the risk of pulmonary hypertension. This can be treated with adequate sedation, mechanical ventilation, and paralysis if necessary during the initial 24 hours. Nitric oxide should be available to treat recurrent or refractory episodes and should be weaned over several days. Delay in recovery should prompt cardiac catheterization to assess residual or recurrent lesions.

OUTCOME

Outcome following repair of isolated AP window is good and mortality approaches zero. All series of AP window with IAA are small but recent reports show mortality less than 10%. Late morbidity is rare with isolated AP window. With AP window and IAA, late complications include arch obstruction and branch pulmonary stenosis. The incidence of arch obstruction requiring catheter or surgical intervention after IAA repair alone is 10–36%. The incidence with AP window and IAA is not well known but is probably comparable to or slightly higher than that of IAA alone.

FURTHER READING

Barnes M, Mitchell M, Tweddell J. Aortopulmonary window. *Semin Thorac Cardiovasc Surg Pediatr Card Surg Ann.* 2011; 14: 67–74.

Konstantinov I, Oka N, d'Udekem Y, Brizard C. Surgical repair of aortopulmonary window associated with interrupted aortic arch: long-term outcomes. *J Thorac Cardiovasc Surg.* 2010; 140(2): 483–4.

Leobon B, Bret E, Roussin R, et al. Technical options for the treatment of anomalous origins of right or left coronary arteries associated with aortopulmonary windows. *J Thorac Cardiovasc Surg.* 2009; 138(3): 777–8.

Nayak HK, Islam N, Bansal BK. Transcatheter closure of aortopulmonary window with Amplatzer duct occluder II. *Ann Pediatr Cardiol.* 2017; 10(1): 93-94.

Talwar S, Agarwal P, Choudhary SK, et al. Aortopulmonary window: morphology, diagnosis, and long-term results. *J Card Surg.* 2017; 32(2): 138-44.

Yoshida M, Yamaguchi M, Oshima Y, et al. Single-stage repair of aortopulmonary window with interrupted aortic arch by transection of the aorta and direct reconstruction. *J Thorac Cardiovasc Surg.* 2009; 138: 781–3.

60

Coarctation of the aorta: repair of coarctation and arch interruption

CHRISTOPHER E. MASCIO AND ERLE H. AUSTIN III

HISTORY

Crafoord was the first to successfully repair coarctation of the aorta in 1944. The techniques of resection and end-to-end anastomosis had been thoroughly studied in laboratory animals by Gross, who soon followed with his own clinical success in 1945. The procedure had been limited to older children until 1955, when Mustard succeeded in repairing the lesion in a newborn infant. Resection and end-to-end anastomosis in small infants, however, often resulted in inadequate vessel growth at the circumferential suture line, leading to a high incidence of recurrent coarctation. In response to this problem, Waldhausen introduced the subclavian flap technique in 1966. Other surgeons, emphasizing the need to resect all ductal tissue, continued to obtain satisfactory results with the end-to-end technique. Neither technique specifically addressed the problem of arch hypoplasia, which was being seen at an increased frequency as more neonates with critical coarctation came to surgery. The maintenance of ductal patency with prostaglandin E1, introduced by Elliott in 1975, permitted stabilization of many newborns who otherwise would not have survived to surgical intervention. Zannini and colleagues in 1985 introduced the concept of an extended end-to-end anastomosis to deal with the hypoplastic aortic arch.

The first successful repair of an interrupted aortic arch was performed by Samson in 1955 in a 3-year-old child with type A interruption. The child's ventricular septal defects (VSDs) were closed 4 years later when cardiopulmonary bypass (CPB) became available. Simultaneous repair of the interrupted arch and VSD was performed by Barratt-Boyes in 1970 using a period of deep hypothermic circulatory arrest and a Dacron™ conduit to bridge the interruption. Complete single-stage repair with direct primary anastomosis of the interrupted segments and closure of the VSD was first performed successfully by Trusler in 1975.

PRINCIPLES AND JUSTIFICATION

Congenital obstruction of the aortic arch encompasses a broad spectrum from discrete coarctation distal to the left subclavian artery through tubular hypoplasia of the aortic arch to complete arch interruption. The presence of coarctation or arch interruption is sufficient indication for operative repair. The clinical presentation and natural history of coarctation segregates into two groups: infants presenting in the first weeks of life and children diagnosed after 3 months of age.

Neonates and very young infants typically present with severe congestive heart failure that can rapidly progress to acidosis and death. More than one-third of these infants have an associated cardiac anomaly such as VSD, transposition of the great arteries, or some form of univentricular heart. The outcome without repair in neonates with coarctation or interrupted arch is almost uniformly fatal.

In contrast, older infants and children rarely have associated defects, are often asymptomatic, and may go undiagnosed until a routine physical examination uncovers upper extremity hypertension and diminished lower extremity pulses. Repair of coarctation is indicated in these older children and young adults to avoid the long-term complications of upper body hypertension, which include aortic dissection, hypertensive heart failure, atherosclerosis, myocardial infarction, and cerebral vascular disease.

Careful preoperative assessment of aortic anatomy by echocardiography and/or angiography is required to determine the exact site of obstruction and the degree and sites of associated arch hypoplasia. Associated cardiac defects must also be identified with these studies. In older children and young adults, satisfactory imaging of the aorta may be obtained using computed tomography or magnetic resonance imaging. The image obtained must provide a reliable measurement of the ascending aorta, the proximal arch (between the innominate artery and the left carotid artery), the distal arch (between the left carotid and the left subclavian artery), and the isthmus (between the left subclavian artery and the ductus or ligament).

The overriding principle of surgical repair is to maximally reduce afterload on the systemic ventricle by eliminating any obstruction to flow between the ascending and descending aorta. Ideally, therefore, at the completion of the repair, no pressure gradient should exist between the left ventricle and the descending aorta. The operative technique chosen should result in a pathway that is at no point less than 50% of the diameter of the ascending aorta just before the innominate artery. As a rule of thumb in neonatal repairs, the final minimum pathway diameter in millimeters should be no less than the infant's weight in kilograms plus 1 (i.e. a diameter of at least 4.6 mm in a 3.6 kg infant). If this rule of thumb cannot be attained, the approach should be via median sternotomy utilizing CPB and deep hypothermia (with or without cerebral perfusion) as is done for interrupted aortic arch.

PREOPERATIVE ASSESSMENT

Newborns with coarctation or interrupted aortic arch require non-elective operation after a period of stabilization with prostaglandin E1. Other resuscitative techniques including mechanical ventilation, pharmacological paralysis, sodium bicarbonate, inotropic agents, and diuretics are also used to stabilize the child. If ductal patency cannot be achieved and acidosis worsens despite these measures, operative repair is performed emergently.

Asymptomatic infants undergo elective repair after 6 months of age after ductal remodeling has stabilized. Older infants and children with discrete coarctation are repaired electively at the time of diagnosis. Waiting until 3–5 years of age is unnecessary.

ANESTHESIA

All procedures are performed with general orotracheal anesthesia. Intraoperative monitoring should include a right radial arterial line. Placement of the arterial line in the left radial or in either femoral artery results in loss of the waveform during the period of aortic cross-clamping. If an umbilical artery line is present in a neonate, it is left in place to permit direct measurement of the post-repair flow gradient. A right radial artery catheter is still required for monitoring during the repair.

A left thoracotomy without CPB is the approach of choice for the majority of coarctation repairs. Rectal and/or nasopharyngeal temperature is monitored, and the patient is allowed to cool to as low as 34 °C for spinal cord protection during the period of aortic clamping.

A median sternotomy with CPB and a brief period of deep hypothermic circulatory arrest is used for most cases of interrupted aortic arch, coarctations requiring concomitant intracardiac repairs, and coarctations with hypoplasia of the proximal arch that cannot be safely approached from a left thoracotomy. With this approach, the patient is cooled actively on CPB to 18 °C for the period of hypothermic circulatory arrest required to repair the arch.

OPERATIONS FOR DISCRETE COARCTATION

Resection with end–to–end anastomosis

This technique is most commonly applied to infants and young children with discrete coarctation and a normal aortic arch.

After performing a left posterolateral muscle-sparing thoracotomy via the fourth intercostal space, the lung is retracted anteriorly and inferiorly. The parietal pleura overlying the aorta is incised from the descending aorta up along the subclavian artery dividing the superior intercostal vein between ligatures. The pleura is tacked up to further retract the lung and to create an operative "well" (**Figure 60.1a**). The vagus and recurrent laryngeal nerves are identified and carefully preserved. The aorta is dissected and mobilized from the left carotid artery to the second set of intercostal arteries. Although not always necessary, one or two levels of intercostals may be ligated (clipped) and divided to facilitate mobilization, clamping, and anastomosis. Because the ligamentum occasionally is patent, it is ligated. A vascular clamp is placed proximally across the aorta and base of the subclavian artery, and distally across the descending aorta (**Figure 60.1b**). The coarctation segment is excised leaving

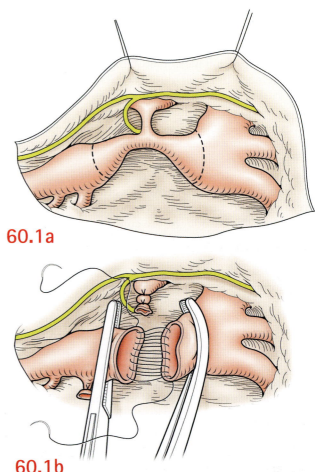

60.1a

60.1b

wide orifices proximally and distally. A double-armed polypropylene suture is used to perform the posterior portion of the anastomosis, sewing from the inside and beginning with the ends apart. The clamps are used to approximate the vessels, and the anterior portion of the anastomosis is completed with the other arm of the suture. The caliber of the suture is adjusted to the size of the patient. A 7-0 suture is used in neonates and a 4-0 suture in young adults, with intermediate choices for patients between these ages. The anterior segment of the anastomosis may be performed with interrupted sutures to prevent pursestringing and to minimize narrowing. Interrupting a portion of the suture line may also permit diameter growth, although fine-caliber polypropylene (6-0 and 7-0) tends to fracture over time after adequate healing has occurred and, as evidenced by the arterial switch experience, is unlikely to limit growth.

At completion of the anastomosis, the distal clamp is released first, and the suture line is carefully inspected (**Figure 60.1c**). Any significant bleeding is controlled with additional simple sutures. The proximal clamp is slowly released. An excellent pulse should be visible and palpable in the distal aorta. When concern exists, distal aortic pressure can be directly measured using a needle through a fine pursestring. When adequate hemostasis is achieved, the pleura is closed over the repair with a continuous suture of fine polypropylene or Dexon. After placing a single chest tube, the lung is re-expanded, and the thoracotomy incision is closed in the standard manner.

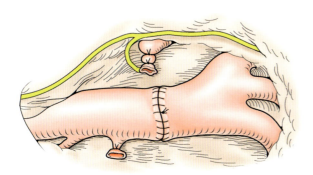

60.1c

Resection with insertion of tubular Dacron graft

In young adults and older patients, the area of coarctation may be long and/or the mobility of the aorta too restricted to allow a tension-free primary anastomosis. In these cases, a tubular graft of Dacron is inserted to bridge the gap (**Figure 60.2**). The size graft chosen should match the diameter of the descending aorta. Polypropylene (4-0 or 5-0) is used for the two suture lines.

Patch aortoplasty

Another technique used is the placement of a diamond-shaped patch across the segment of narrowing. Because

aortoplasty can be performed quickly, it may be the procedure of choice when coarctation repair must be performed emergently in a desperately ill infant whose ductus cannot be reopened with prostaglandin E1. This technique is also used in older children and young adults.

After dissecting the area of the coarctation as well as the distal arch, subclavian artery, and proximal descending aorta, the ligamentum is tied, and clamps are placed. The aorta is incised longitudinally across the area of coarctation (**Figure 60.3a and b**). A coarctation membrane is typically encountered at the narrowest point. This fibrous thickening should be left intact, because resecting it tends to significantly

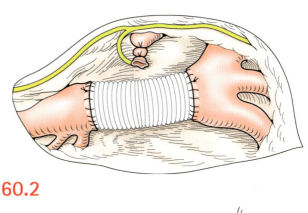

60.2

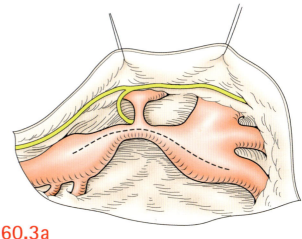

60.3a

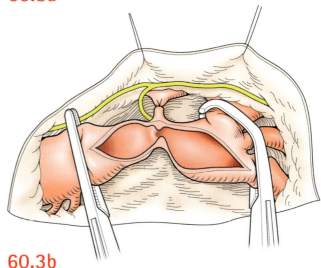

60.3b

weaken the aortic wall at this point. A large diamond-shaped patch is then fashioned from autologous or heterologous pericardium (neonates) or from a Dacron tube graft (older children or adults). The patch is sewn in place with a continuous polypropylene suture (**Figure 60.3c**). The posterolateral aspect of the anastomosis is sewn first within the vessel. The anastomosis is completed, bringing the two suture ends together on the anteromedial aspect of the patch.

Patch aortoplasty offers a reproducible and easily performed correction of coarctation with excellent short-term results. Unfortunately, the technique has been associated with a high incidence of late aneurysm formation. For that reason, this author prefers to use resection and tubular graft insertion for older patients requiring coarctation repair.

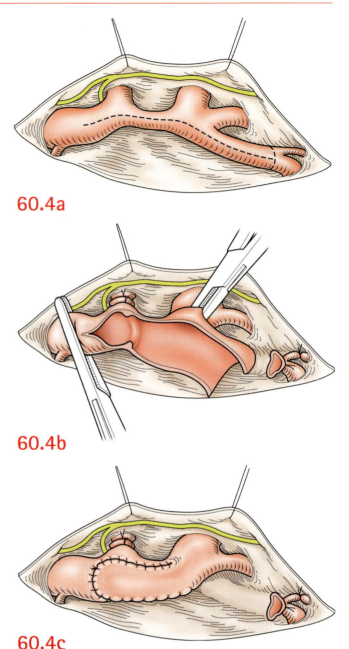

60.4a

60.4b

60.4c

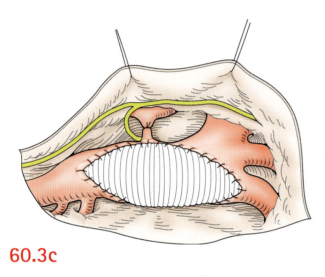

60.3c

Subclavian flap aortoplasty

The subclavian flap aortoplasty technique was introduced to eliminate the circumferential scar thought to be responsible for recurrence noted after resection and end-to-end anastomosis in small infants. Flap aortoplasty is primarily used in infants younger than 3 months of age who do not have arch hypoplasia. This procedure requires less overall dissection than the end-to-end technique and avoids tension on the suture line. On the other hand, the primary blood supply to the left arm is interrupted, potentially affecting its growth, and abnormal ductal tissue is retained, presenting the potential for recurrent coarctation or late aneurysm formation.

With this technique, in addition to the usual exposure, the subclavian artery is dissected to the point of its first branch, usually the vertebral artery, which is ligated (**Figure 60.4a**). The subclavian artery is ligated at this point. After ligating the ductus arteriosus, a proximal clamp is applied across the arch between the left carotid and left subclavian artery. A distal clamp is placed at least 1 cm distal to the coarctation. A longitudinal incision is made, beginning in the descending aorta, and is carried across the coarctation and the isthmus and along the lateral border of the subclavian artery, which is divided just proximal to the ligature (**Figure 60.4b**). If a

discrete intimal shelf exists, it may be carefully excised, but care must be taken to preserve the aortic media. The subclavian flap is then folded down into the aortic incision with a loose stay suture and sewn into place with a running of 7-0 polypropylene suture (**Figure 60.4c**).

OPERATIONS FOR COARCTATION WITH ARCH HYPOPLASIA

Reverse subclavian flap aortoplasty

When the site of arch hypoplasia is confined to the segment between the left carotid artery and the left subclavian artery, reverse subclavian flap aortoplasty may be used in combination with the standard resection and anastomosis procedure.

For all procedures dealing with arch hypoplasia, the dissection proximally and distally must provide extensive mobilization of the head vessels and the descending aorta. The arch is clearly exposed to the base of the innominate artery, and the distal aorta is dissected down to the fourth set of intercostals (**Figure 60.5a**). The left subclavian artery is ligated just before it branches, as previously described. A curved clamp is placed between the innominate artery and the left carotid in such a way as to occlude the left carotid distally. A second clamp is placed across the aortic isthmus, allowing distal perfusion through the ductus arteriosus if it is open (**Figure 60.5b**). The subclavian artery is divided proximal to the ligature and is incised along its medial border onto the superior aspect of the distal arch to the base of the left carotid artery. The flap of subclavian artery is turned in a reverse direction into the proximal aortic incision and sewn into place with 7-0 polypropylene suture (**Figure 60.5c**). The distal clamp is removed from the isthmus, and the proximal clamp is repositioned just distal to the left carotid. The ductus is now ligated, a second clamp is placed across the descending aorta, and a standard coarctation resection and end-to-end anastomosis is performed (**Figure 60.5d**).

Resection with extended end-to-end anastomosis

When arch hypoplasia extends proximal to the left carotid artery, a reverse subclavian technique does not eliminate the arch obstruction, and a more extensive approach is required. The extended end-to-end approach is now preferred by many surgeons because it results in complete removal of all ductal tissue and preserves normal blood flow to the left arm. This technique does, however, present a greater degree of technical difficulty and requires more extensive dissection to achieve a tension-free anastomosis.

After thorough dissection and mobilization of the head vessels, isthmus, ductus arteriosus, and descending aorta, the ductus arteriosus is ligated and divided. This step often improves exposure of the most proximal arch, including the distal ascending aorta and innominate artery. A large curved clamp is then positioned in such a way as to include the left subclavian artery, the left carotid artery, and part of the innominate artery. The tip of the clamp is positioned well down the left wall of the ascending aorta, but it must not obstruct flow to the innominate artery. If a significant change in the radial artery tracing occurs with application of the clamp, it must be repositioned. Other methods to assure

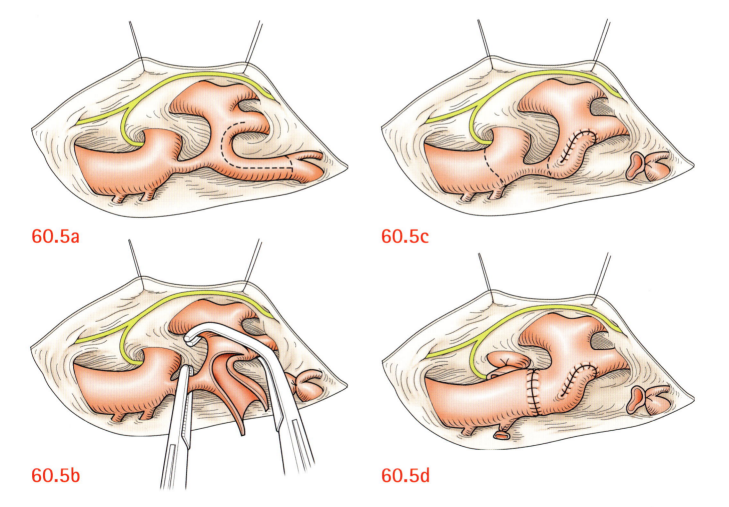

60.5a

60.5b

60.5c

60.5d

unobstructed cerebral blood flow include palpation by the anesthesiologist of the right carotid or right temporal artery and/or assessment of a pulse oximeter placed on the right ear. Although not commonly available, continuous transcranial Doppler monitoring of the right middle cerebral artery provides the most reliable feedback regarding cerebral blood flow during this critical period. A second clamp is placed across the mobilized descending aorta, often including several intercostal vessels. The coarctation is completely excised, and an incision is made along the undersurface of the aortic arch to within a few millimeters of the tip of the clamp (**Figure 60.6a**). Failure to bring this incision proximal to the origin of the left carotid artery is likely to result in a residual flow gradient. The orifice of the descending aorta is enlarged with a posterior longitudinal incision to match the extent of the opened aortic arch and to receive the tongue of the arch containing the left subclavian artery. An anastomosis is performed with 7-0 polypropylene suture, beginning medially and posteriorly with the vessels separated, then approximating the two clamps to reduce tension as the anastomosis is completed (**Figure 60.6b**). A continuous suture technique is usually satisfactory, although interrupted simple sutures can be used for the anterior aspect of the anastomosis.

End-to-side anastomosis to the aortic arch

An end-to-side anastomosis of the divided descending aorta to the underside of the proximal aortic arch has recently evolved as a modification of the extended end-to-end technique. This procedure is designed to assure apposition of normal aortic tissue at the site of anastomosis as well as to bypass all hypoplastic structures proximal to the discrete coarctation.

Initial exposure, dissection, and extensive mobilization are carried out as in the extended end-to-end technique (**Figure 60.7a**); however, after ligation and division of the ductus arteriosus, the aortic isthmus is ligated. After a distal descending aorta clamp is placed, the aorta is divided distal to the coarctation, leaving no ductal tissue at the edge of the divided descending aorta (**Figure 60.7b**). Lateral traction on the isthmus provides excellent exposure for placement of the arch clamp, which is placed as proximally as possible, preserving innominate artery flow. A longitudinal incision is made on the underside of the aortic arch beginning only millimeters from the tip of the clamp and is brought distally to a length slightly larger than the cross-sectional diameter of the descending aorta. An end-to-side anastomosis is performed

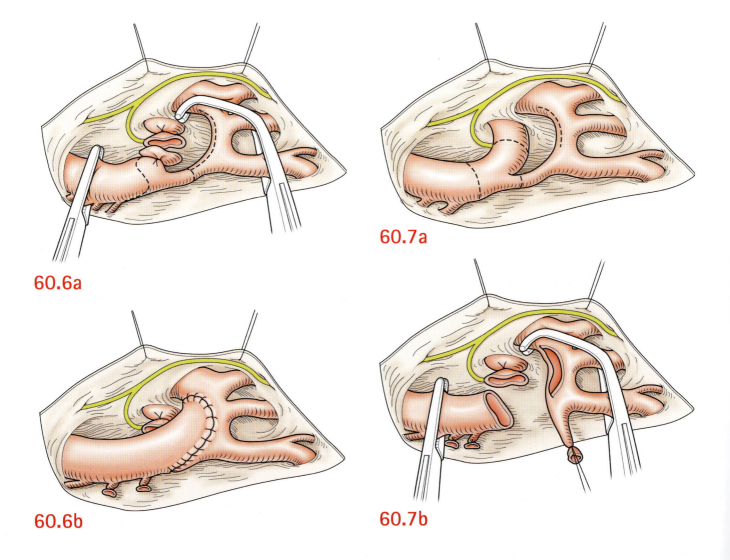

60.6a

60.6b

60.7a

60.7b

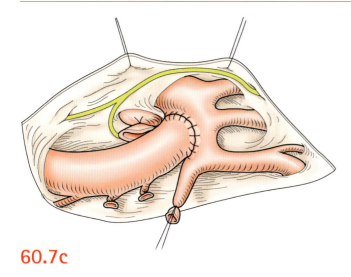

60.7c

with 7-0 polypropylene suture, bringing the descending aorta up to the underside of the arch (**Figure 60.7c**).

Aortic arch advancement

Approaching a coarctation via left thoracotomy will not adequately correct significant aortic arch hypoplasia (where the aortic arch measures less than the infant's weight in kilograms + 1) (**Figure 60.8a**). In these cases, the aortic arch advancement technique, performed via median sternotomy and utilizing CPB and deep hypothermia, will address both the coarctation and the arch hypoplasia.

Median sternotomy is performed. Dissection of the ascending aorta and the aortic arch and its branches is completed. Arterial cannulation is performed on the greater curvature of the aorta at the base of the innominate artery and can be single or dual (if preferred can use polytetrafluoroethylene graft sutured to innominate artery) (**Figure 60.8b**). CPB is commenced and the patient is cooled to 18 °C prior to deep hypothermic circulatory arrest. After cardioplegic arrest, ductal tissue is removed from the descending aorta, which is mobilized after commencing bypass and cooling. An incision is made on the undersurface of the arch opposite the innominate artery and is carried distally. The descending aorta is anastomosed to this incision in an end-to-side fashion using polypropylene (**Figure 60.8c**).

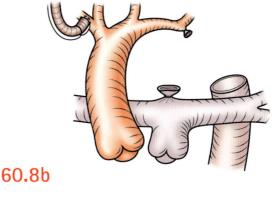

60.8b

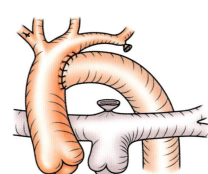

60.8c

Ascending sliding arch aortoplasty

In children beyond infancy the descending aorta is less mobile. In these cases, an ascending sliding arch aortoplasty, done via median sternotomy utilizing CPB and deep hypothermia can be employed to correct both the arch hypoplasia and coarctation.

Median sternotomy is performed. Dissection of the ascending aorta, the aortic arch and its branches, and the proximal descending aorta is completed. Arterial cannulation can be single or dual and can be in the ascending aorta or through a polytetrafluoroethylene graft sutured to the innominate artery. The patient is cooled to 18 °C for deep hypothermic circulatory arrest. After cardioplegic arrest, a coarctectomy is done if necessary and a partial anastomosis is done between the distal aortic arch and the proximal descending thoracic aorta (**Figure 60.9a**). The ascending

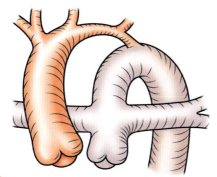

60.8a

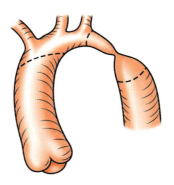

60.9a

aorta is transected just proximal to the innominate artery and is incised on the anterolateral aspect of the greater curvature (**Figure 60.9b**). The lesser curvature of the arch and descending aorta is then incised and the ascending aorta is advanced and anastomosed to the aortic arch and proximal descending aorta with continuous polypropylene (**Figure 60.9c**).

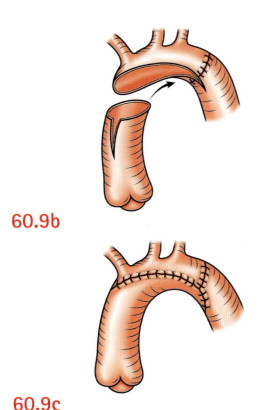

60.9b

60.9c

OPERATIONS FOR INTERRUPTED AORTIC ARCH

Repair of simple interrupted arch with ventricular septal defect

Although an interrupted aortic arch can be repaired in stages, currently the preferred approach is a single-stage complete repair with primary anastomosis of the descending aorta to the side of the ascending aorta and VSD closure. The procedure is performed through a median sternotomy and requires CPB and a brief period of deep hypothermic circulatory arrest. If the head vessels that come off the ascending aorta are large enough, a small (6 Fr or 8 Fr) cannula is placed in one of the carotid arteries to provide antegrade cerebral blood flow while the aortic anastomosis is performed. This technique eliminates the requirement for circulatory arrest but may give rise to overperfusion of the brain and may result in stenosis at the cannulation site. Because the aortic anastomosis is easy to perform in an expeditious fashion, the use of circulatory arrest in this circumstance introduces minimal risk and greatly facilitates this portion of the procedure.

After routine median sternotomy, the thymus, if present,

is excised and the pericardium opened. The brachiocephalic vessels, branch pulmonary arteries, ductus arteriosus, and the proximal portion of the descending aorta are thoroughly dissected. The recurrent laryngeal nerve should be clearly identified and protected. To achieve relatively uniform and complete cooling, two 8 Fr arterial cannulae are used, one in the ascending aorta and one in the main pulmonary artery (MPA) or ductus. The ascending aortic cannula is positioned in the right lateral aspect directly opposite the anticipated site of the aortic anastomosis. Tourniquets are placed around the right and left pulmonary arteries or around the duct to be tightened at commencement of CPB to direct flow from the second cannula through the ductus to the descending aorta. Venous cannulation can be single or double, depending on the surgeon's preference. If closure of the VSD requires exposure through the right atrium, double venous cannulation will permit this visualization while on CPB (**Figure 60.10a**).

Once CPB has been instituted, further mobilization of the aortic branches is performed while the patient is cooled to 18 °C. Although the left subclavian artery can be preserved in type B interruption, ligation and division of this vessel improves mobility of the descending aorta and minimizes tension on the final anastomosis. If an aberrant right subclavian artery exists, this vessel should also be ligated and divided. When rectal and tympanic temperatures reach 18 °C, bypass is discontinued. Tourniquets around the innominate and carotid arteries are tightened, whereas those around the pulmonary artery branches are removed. Cardioplegic solution is infused into the aortic root, and the arterial cannulas are removed. The ductus is ligated and divided where it joins the descending aorta. All ductal tissue is excised. Placing a small C-clamp on the descending aorta

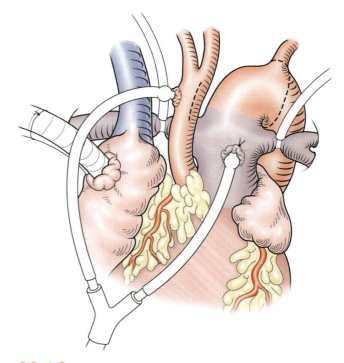

60.10a

at this point helps pull the divided end up to the level of the ascending aorta. After a longitudinal incision is made on the left posterior aspect of the ascending aorta, an end-to-side anastomosis is performed with 7-0 polypropylene suture (Figure 60.10b). If very little circulatory arrest time has elapsed at this point, the VSD is closed before reinstituting bypass. Alternatively, cerebral and systemic blood flow can be resumed at this point by reinserting one of the arterial cannulae into the aortic site and recommencing bypass. An additional dose of cardioplegic solution is infused into the aortic root for the VSD closure. Systemic rewarming can begin at this point.

In most cases, the VSD is best approached through a transverse incision in the proximal MPA, just distal to the pulmonary valve (**Figure 60.10c**). Using interrupted pledget-reinforced mattress sutures of 5-0 Tevdek, a Dacron or pericardial patch is positioned such that its superior margin is placed on the left ventricular side of the conal septum to promote deflection of the conal septum away from the left ventricular outflow tract (**Figure 60.10d**). Once the VSD is closed, the interatrial septum should be inspected, and any large communication closed down to the size of a 4 mm patent foramen ovale. After appropriate de-airing, the clamp on the aortic root is removed, and the pulmonary and atrial incisions closed in a routine fashion. A left atrial line is typically placed for postoperative monitoring. When the patient is adequately rewarmed (36 °C), separation from CPB is usually accomplished with minimal inotropic support.

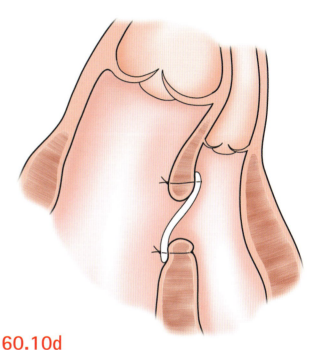

60.10d

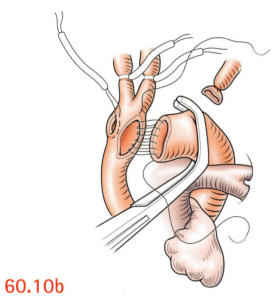

60.10b

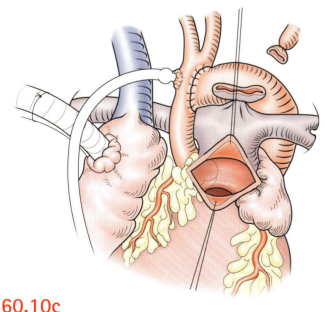

60.10c

Repair of interrupted aortic arch with severe left ventricular outflow tract obstruction

After instituting CPB, cooling to 18 °C is commenced, and the ductus is ligated and divided. Once hypothermic, cardioplegia is delivered and circulatory arrest is commenced. Tourniquets are carefully tightened around the arch branches. The pulmonary artery is transected just proximal to the bifurcation. A right ventriculotomy is created just inferior to the pulmonary valve and to the right of and parallel to the left anterior descending coronary artery. The VSD will be visible and can be enlarged in an anterosuperior direction if necessary. A Dacron graft is opened longitudinally and fashioned to an appropriate size and shape. This graft is sutured over the VSD and the pulmonary annulus with running polypropylene so that left ventricular blood has an unobstructed path through the VSD to the pulmonary valve (**Figure 60.11a–d**).

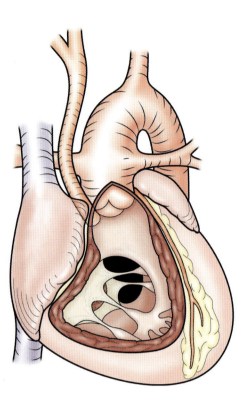

60.11a

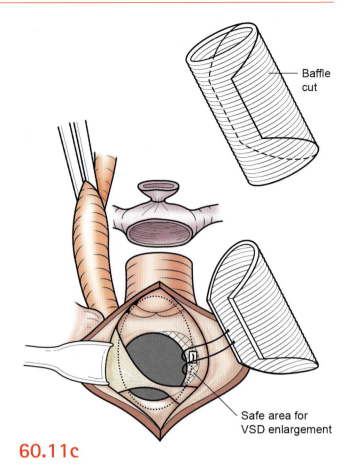

Baffle cut

Safe area for VSD enlargement

60.11c

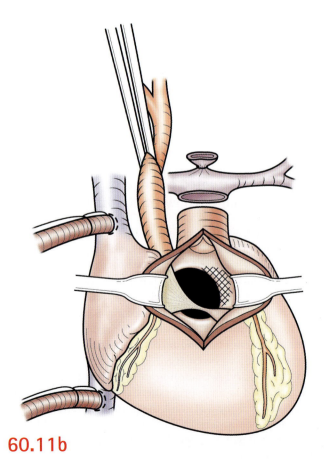

60.11b

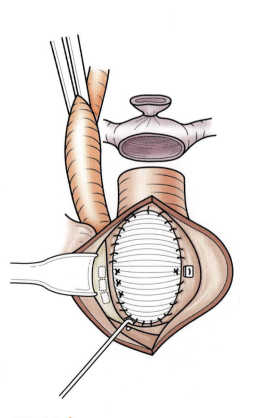

60.11d

Attention is then turned to amalgamating the ascending aorta and the MPA. A cutback incision is made on the pulmonary trunk, and the ascending aorta and MPA are anastomosed side-to-side using interrupted 7-0 polypropylene. A clamp is then placed on the distal descending aorta. All ductal tissue is excised. The descending aorta is incised 1 cm beyond the ductal insertion. The left subclavian artery is incised on its medial aspect and the proximal aorta is anastomosed to the distal aorta with running 7-0 polypropylene. A piece of homograft is cut to an appropriate size and shape and is used to complete the neoaortic reconstruction. A valved homograft is then used to re-establish right ventricle-to-pulmonary artery continuity (**Figure 60.12a–e**).

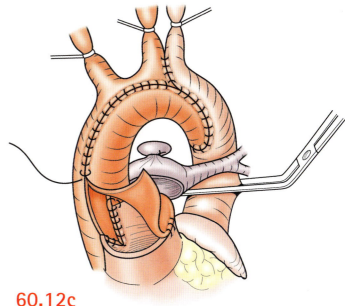

60.12c

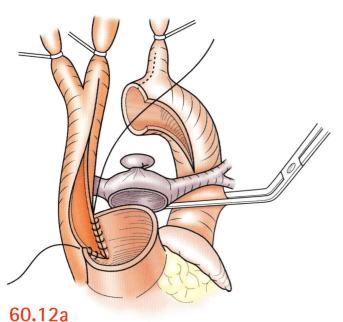

60.12a

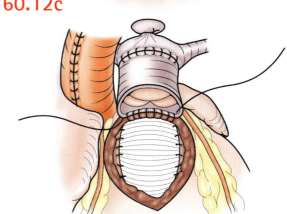

60.12d

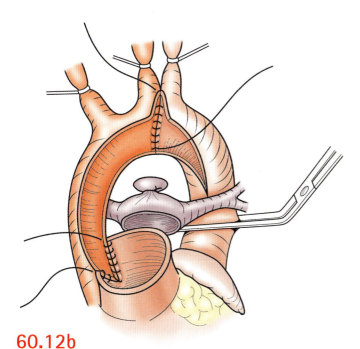

60.12b

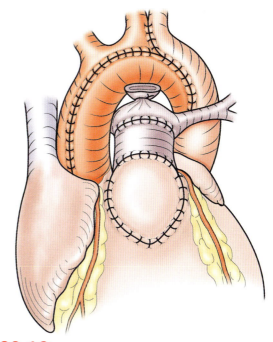

60.12e

Repair of interrupted aortic arch with truncus arteriosus

Other than VSD, truncus arteriosus is the most common coexistent cardiac anomaly associated with interrupted aortic arch. When these two lesions coexist, operative repair can successfully address both lesions. Arterial cannulation is simplified with the use of a single cannula placed in the distal ascending aorta or main pulmonary artery component of the trunk. The branch pulmonary arteries are occluded with tourniquets at the initiation of CPB. Once a temperature of 18 °C is reached, the head vessels are occluded, and circulatory arrest is achieved. The ductus is ligated and divided, and the pulmonary artery component of the truncus is separated from the truncal root. The ascending aorta is incised to include the first 5 mm of the left carotid artery. All ductal tissue is removed from the descending aorta, but the left subclavian artery is left in place. An incision in the base of the left subclavian artery of approximately 5 mm is made (**Figure 60.13a and b**).

With adequate mobilization of the left carotid and left subclavian arteries and the proximal descending aorta, the incisions in the left subclavian and left carotid arteries are brought together with 7-0 polypropylene suture. A gusset of allograft pulmonary artery or aorta, similar to that used in first stage reconstruction for hypoplastic left heart syndrome, is then implanted to create the lesser curvature of this aortic reconstruction from truncal valve to descending aorta (**Figure 60.13c**).

At this point, the arterial cannula is replaced, CPB is resumed, and the patient is rewarmed. Closure of the VSD is then performed through a longitudinal incision in the right ventricle, just below the truncal valve. Continuity between the right ventricle and the pulmonary artery bifurcation is achieved with a valved pulmonary or aortic allograft (**Figure 60.13d**).

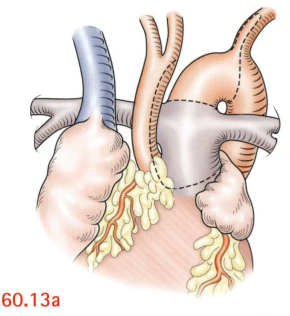

60.13a

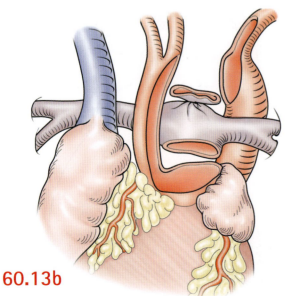

60.13b

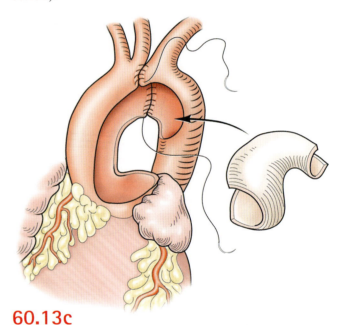

60.13c

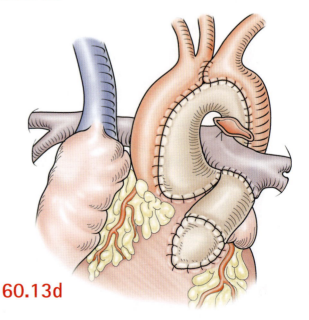

60.13d

Repair of interrupted aortic arch with transposition of the great arteries

When interrupted aortic arch is associated with transposition of the great arteries or Taussig–Bing anomaly (double-outlet right ventricle with subpulmonic VSD), arch reconstruction is combined with an arterial switch procedure. To address the marked disparity in the size of the great vessels in these patients, the arch repair is performed by dividing the ascending aorta just above the sinuses of Valsalva and swinging it to the left and posteriorly to be anastomosed end-to-end to the descending aorta. A longitudinal incision is made in the underside of this neoaortic arch (**Figure 60.14a and b**). The

large proximal neoaorta with its implanted coronary buttons is then anastomosed to this incision in an end-to-side fashion. After resumption of bypass, the VSD is closed through a right ventriculotomy, the atrial septal defect is closed through a small right atriotomy, and the proximal neopulmonary artery is anastomosed to the pulmonary bifurcation or right pulmonary artery with (anterior-posterior great arteries) or without (side-by-side great arteries) a Lecompte maneuver (**Figure 60.14c**).

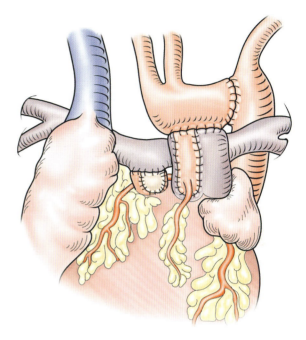

60.14c

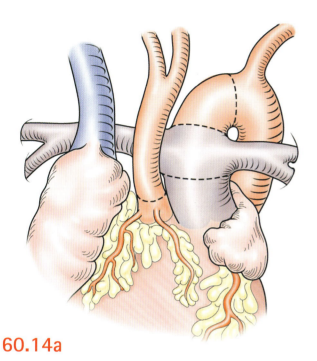

60.14a

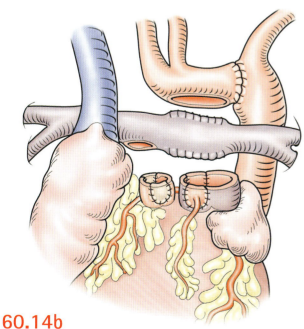

60.14b

OPERATIONS FOR COMPLEX COARCTATION OF THE AORTA

Ascending aorta–to–descending aorta bypass

Alternative strategies are sometimes necessary for patients, especially adults, with complex coarctation of the aorta. Exposure of the descending aorta through a median sternotomy for ascending-to-descending aorta extra-anatomic bypass can be done with low mortality. After median sternotomy, the ascending aorta is mobilized. Arterial cannulation is performed in the distal ascending aorta/proximal aortic arch. After cardioplegia administration, the posterior pericardium is exposed by retracting the apex of the heart. The pericardium is opened longitudinally from the left inferior pulmonary vein to the diaphragm to expose the descending aorta. A transesophageal echocardiography probe will aid in identifying the esophagus. An appropriate graft size is chosen and a partial occlusion clamp is applied to the descending aorta. Continuous polypropylene is used to perform the distal anastomosis. The graft is routed posterior to the inferior vena cava and around the right atrium to the greater curvature of the ascending aorta. The length of the graft is best estimated with a full heart and full aorta. The proximal anastomosis is also done under cardioplegic arrest. An aortotomy is created along the greater curvature of the ascending aorta and the end-to-side anastomosis is completed with running polypropylene (**Figure 60.15**).

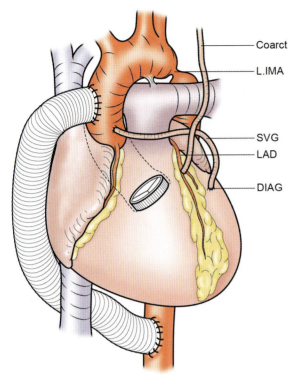

Coarct
L.IMA
SVG
LAD
DIAG

60.15

POSTOPERATIVE CARE

Care of patients after repair of coarctation differs little from that for any patient after a thoracotomy. The chest tube is generally removed on the first postoperative day. Systemic arterial hypertension is common and is generally treated with intravenous nitroprusside for the first 24 hours if the systolic blood pressure exceeds 120 mmHg in neonates or 150 mmHg in older patients. The patient is then rapidly weaned off the nitroprusside as an oral beta-blocker (e.g. propranolol) or angiotensin-converting enzyme inhibitor (e.g. captopril) is begun. Some patients are discharged on these agents, which are to be discontinued some time over the first 3 postoperative months. Neonates with residual cardiomegaly, especially those with cardiovascular lesions, such as a VSD, may also require digoxin and a diuretic at discharge.

Neonates and young infants are allowed to feed within the first 24 hours after coarctation repair. Older patients may have abdominal discomfort within the first few postoperative days secondary to some degree of splanchnic vasospasm. In these patients, oral intake should be instituted slowly.

Occasionally, abdominal distension may require nasogastric decompression and intravenous fluids. A chest radiograph is obtained before discharge to rule out the occasional chylothorax which, if present, is treated conservatively with chest tube drainage and a diet restricted in fat.

As with coarctation, the postoperative management of neonates after repair of interrupted aortic arch and VSD is relatively routine. To minimize hemodynamic lability, the infant is paralyzed and anesthetized with a continuous infusion of fentanyl (10–15 μg/kg/hour) for the first 24 hours. Beginning on the first postoperative day, these agents are weaned and progress toward extubation occurs over the next 48–72 hours. Infants with DiGeorge syndrome (common in infants with type B interruption) are likely to exhibit significant hypocalcemia in the postoperative period. Ionized calcium levels, therefore, must be frequently monitored and treated accordingly with infusions of calcium chloride or gluconate. After successful extubation, oral nutrition is begun, and caloric intake is increased as tolerated until the infant is feeding well and gaining weight appropriately. Most infants require digoxin and a diuretic at discharge and for the first few months postoperatively.

OUTCOME

Hospital mortality after coarctation repair in newborns with simple coarctation with or without a VSD is less than 5%. The mortality is significantly increased, however, if other major cardiac defects, especially other obstructive lesions of the left heart–aorta complex, are also present. Hospital mortality for repair of simple coarctation in older infants, children, and young adults is less than 1%. Recurrent coarctation requiring reoperation or balloon angioplasty occurs in 3–9% of neonates and in less than 1% of older children or adults. In a recent multicenter study of neonatal coarctation repair, no significant difference in recoarctation rate was noted between the techniques of resection and end-to-end anastomosis and the subclavian flap operation. In this study, the recoarctation rate after patch aortoplasty, however, was significantly higher at 21%.

Most reports describing outcomes after repair of interrupted arch and VSD are from single institutions with relatively small patient numbers and significant variation in hospital mortality. The Congenital Heart Surgeons Society did conduct a multi-institutional study, enrolling 183 neonates with this lesion between 1987 and 1992. In this study, the hospital mortality for repair was 27%. More recent experience reported from single institutions indicates that hospital mortality for repair of this lesion currently ranges between 5% and 15%. Residual or recurrent obstruction of the repaired aortic arch requiring reintervention occurs in 15–20% of patients, with a peak time of occurrence 4 months after the initial repair. In most cases, percutaneous balloon dilation provides satisfactory relief.

FURTHER READING

Connolly HM, Schaff HV, Izhar U, et al. Posterior pericardial ascending to descending Aortic bypass: an alternative surgical approach for complex coarctation of aorta. *Circulation.* 2001; 104(Suppl 1): I133–7.

Elgamal MA, McKenzie ED, Fraser CD Jr. Aortic arch advancement: the optimal one-stage approach for surgical management of neonatal coarctation with arch hypoplasia. *Ann Thorac Surg.* 2002; 73(4): 1267–72.

Kanter KR. The Yasui operation. *Oper Tech Thorac Cardiovasc Surg.* 2010; 15(3): 206–22.

Kanter KR, Kirshbom PM, Kogon BE. Biventricular repair with the Yasui operation (Norwood/Rastelli) for systemic outflow tract obstruction with two adequate ventricles. *Ann Thorac Surg.* 2012; 93(6): 1999–2005.

Kaushal S, Backer CL, Patel JN, et al. Coarctation of the aorta: midterm outcomes of resection with extended end-to-end anastomosis. *Ann Thorac Surg.* 2009; 88(6): 1932–8.

McKenzie ED, Klysik M, Morales DL, et al. Ascending sliding arch aortoplasty: a novel technique for repair of arch hypoplasia. *Ann Thorac Surg.* 2011; 91(3): 805–10.

Ungerleider RM, Pasquali SK, Welke KF, et al. Contemporary patterns of surgery and outcomes for aortic coarctation: an analysis of the Society of Thoracic Surgeons. *J Thorac Cardiovasc Surg.* 2013; 145: 150–8.

61

Congenital anomalies of the aortic arch

NHUE DO, LUCA VRICELLA, AND DUKE E. CAMERON

HISTORY

Abnormalities of the aortic arch are rare congenital anomalies commonly known as *vascular rings*, a term coined by Gross in 1945. The first report of a vascular ring was by Hommel in 1737, who described a double aortic arch. The first successful treatment of a vascular ring was by Gross in 1945 for a right aortic arch with left ligamentum. He also performed the first innominate artery "pexy" to the sternum for innominate artery compression syndrome in 1948. Recent advances for the most part have been in non-invasive diagnostic imaging.

An understanding of embryological origins is probably more important in the treatment of aortic arch anomalies than in any other group of congenital cardiovascular diseases. The Edwards classification system, based on the progression of a double arch to a single one, is the most widely used. Early in development, six pairs of aortic arches connect the ventral and dorsal aortae, although at no time do all six coexist. These arches variously recede, fuse, and remodel to form the typical left-sided aortic arch and its major branches. Inappropriate persistence or resorption of these arches may result in a vascular ring. Most of the first, second, and fifth arches regress, whereas the third pair evolves into the carotid arteries. The sixth arches become the pulmonary arteries, and the seventh intersegmental arteries become the subclavian arteries. The ventral portion of the left sixth arch becomes the ductus arteriosus, usually on the left side because of involution of the right sixth arch. The "sidedness" of the aortic arch is determined by which fourth arch persists, usually the left. A double arch is the result of bilateral persistence of the fourth arches (**Figure 61.1a and b**).

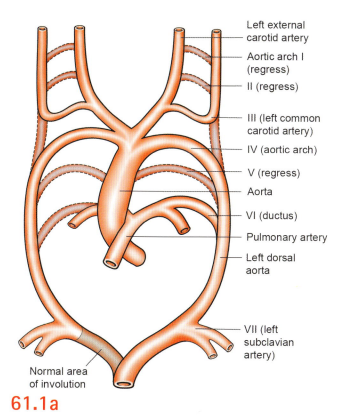

Left external carotid artery
Aortic arch I (regress)
II (regress)
III (left common carotid artery)
IV (aortic arch)
V (regress)
Aorta
VI (ductus)
Pulmonary artery
Left dorsal aorta
VII (left subclavian artery)
Normal area of involution

61.1a

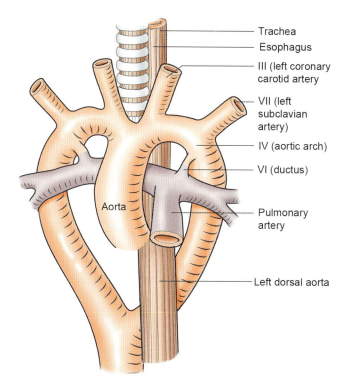

Trachea
Esophagus
III (left coronary carotid artery)
VII (left subclavian artery)
IV (aortic arch)
VI (ductus)
Aorta
Pulmonary artery
Left dorsal aorta

61.1b

Another classification scheme has recently been endorsed by the Congenital Heart Surgery International Nomenclature and Database Project for the Society of Thoracic Surgeons. The most commonly seen vascular anomalies include:

1. aberrant right subclavian artery with left aortic arch
2. aberrant left subclavian artery with right aortic arch
3. double aortic arch
4. right aortic arch with left ligamentum
5. tracheal compression by the innominate artery
6. pulmonary artery sling.

PRINCIPLES AND JUSTIFICATION

Vascular rings typically present because of compression of the trachea or esophagus with symptoms correlating with the degree of compression. Tracheal compression will manifest as stridor, tachypnea, or frequent respiratory infections, whereas esophageal compression leads to dysphagia or aspiration. The presence of symptoms attributable to the vascular ring is an indication for surgery; the asymptomatic patient is sometimes identified incidentally on CT scan for other pathology and probably best left untreated if completely asymptomatic. Most patients present within the first 2 years of life, with neonates mostly presenting with signs of tracheal compression, whereas infants will most often manifest esophageal compression symptoms. The prevalence of vascular rings is not known, but it is estimated to represent 1–3% of congenital anomalies requiring surgical intervention, with 15–20% of patients presenting with concomitant congenital heart disease.

PREOPERATIVE ASSESSMENT AND PREPARATION

The goals of evaluation and treatment are the following:

1. Confirm the diagnosis of a vascular ring and determine if other cardiac abnormalities are present.
2. Characterize the anatomy of the ring to plan the operative approach.
3. Divide the ring and mobilize the compressed structures.

Clinical history and examination

The initial clinical presentation is usually intolerance of feeds or respiratory distress, sometimes triggered by trivial pulmonary infections. Physical findings are frequently absent, but examination may reveal noisy breathing, wheezing, tachypnea, stridor, cough, or retractions.

Imaging

CHEST RADIOGRAPH

The plain chest film should show the side of the aortic arch; ambiguity suggests a double arch. Infiltrates and hyperinflation raise the possibility of tracheobronchial compromise. The lateral chest film should be reviewed for narrowing of the tracheal air column.

BARIUM ESOPHAGRAM

Historically, a barium esophagram was the most powerful tool used to confirm the diagnosis and even to delineate the anatomy of the vascular ring, but it is rarely used today with the existence and wide use of advanced imaging technologies (of chest tomography and magnetic resonance imaging). However, it is still utilized by some institutions. Vascular rings will often produce a posterior indentation of the esophagus, whereas a pulmonary artery sling will be associated with an anterior indentation.

CHEST TOMOGRAPHY/MAGNETIC RESONANCE IMAGING

Chest tomography and magnetic resonance imaging produce accurate images with 3D reconstructions incorporating surrounding mediastinal structures, but they might miss small atretic arch segments. Small infants may require sedation and endotracheal intubation for these studies, which carry significant risk in a patient with airway compromise.

ECHOCARDIOGRAPHY

Approximately 15–20% of vascular ring patients have congenital heart disease, an incidence that justifies routine echocardiographic screening. Imaging of the ring itself is often possible, and precision is improving with experience.

ENDOSCOPY

Although not usually necessary, bronchoscopy may confirm the site of airway compression and evaluate the severity of malacia. Mainly, it is useful in the setting of innominate artery compression of the trachea. Esophagoscopy is rarely necessary, but it may be useful to exclude other potential diagnoses.

ANGIOGRAPHY

Catheterization is rarely necessary for diagnosis, but, as with echocardiography, it may be part of the evaluation of concomitant congenital heart disease.

ANESTHESIA

General anesthesia and endotracheal intubation are routinely used. In older children and adults, a double-lumen endotracheal tube or "bronchial blocker" with single-lung ventilation can improve operative exposure. Bilateral radial artery pressure monitoring and intraoperative palpation of the carotid arteries may help to determine which limb of the double aortic arch should be divided in cases in which neither limb is strongly dominant. Spinal catheters for perioperative narcotic infusion minimize post-thoracotomy pain and ease ventilation.

OPERATION

General principles

Left thoracotomy is the preferred incision for the majority of vascular rings. Other approaches are possible depending on anatomy:

- right thoracotomy for innominate artery compression
- right thoracotomy or sternotomy for reimplantation of an anomalous origin of the right subclavian artery from a left-sided aortic arch
- right thoracotomy for a double aortic arch with a diminutive right-sided aortic arch descending thoracic aorta and right-sided ligamentum arteriosum.

Median sternotomy is chosen for repair of concomitant congenital heart disease as well as repair of pulmonary artery sling (**Figure 61.2a**). Posterolateral thoracotomy should be serratus-sparing through the fourth intercostal space (**Figure 61.2b**). The mediastinal pleura is incised posterior to the vagus nerve, and the major aortic branches are dissected out. No vascular structures should be divided until all are identified with certainty and the hemodynamic consequences of division known from pressure monitoring catheters or carotid palpation. The ligamentum is divided even if not part of the ring. Fibrous bands are lysed, and the trachea and esophagus are freed from surrounding tissues. Kommerell's diverticulum should be dissected out and, if necessary, resected or "pexed" to the prevertebral fascia. Lymphatic leaks should be controlled by suture or biological sealant.

Aberrant right subclavian artery

The aberrant right subclavian artery arising from a leftward descending thoracic aorta is the most common aortic arch anomaly (**Figure 61.3a and b**). Similar to innominate artery

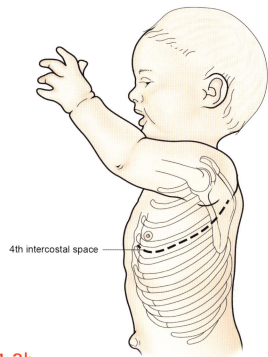

4th intercostal space

61.2b

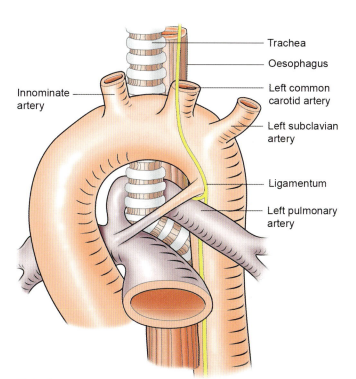

Innominate artery

Trachea

Oesophagus

Left common carotid artery

Left subclavian artery

Ligamentum

Left pulmonary artery

61.2a

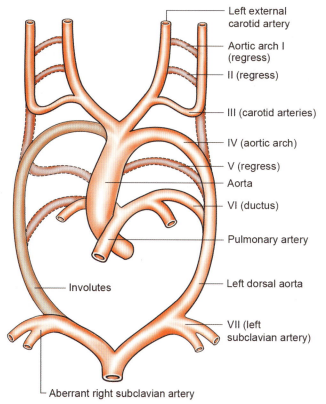

Left external carotid artery

Aortic arch I (regress)

II (regress)

III (carotid arteries)

IV (aortic arch)

V (regress)

Aorta

VI (ductus)

Pulmonary artery

Involutes

Left dorsal aorta

VII (left subclavian artery)

Aberrant right subclavian artery

61.3a

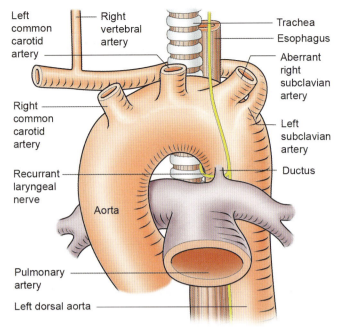

61.3b

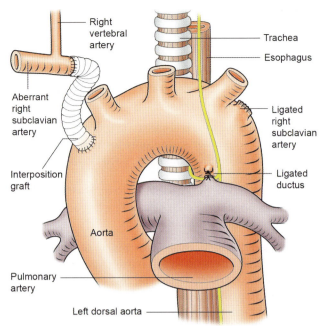

61.3c

compression, this entity is not a true vascular ring, but may cause compression nonetheless. Most patients with this entity are asymptomatic. Through a right thoracotomy, the subclavian artery may be ligated, divided, and mobilized in infants and small children. In older patients, or when a large vertebral artery arises from the anomalous subclavian artery, reimplantation of the subclavian artery to the ascending aorta is recommended. A prosthetic interposition graft is sometimes necessary (**Figure 61.3c**). Division of the ductus is not necessary and may be difficult to achieve through a right thoracotomy approach.

Aberrant left subclavian artery

When the left subclavian artery arises anomalously from a right-sided arch, it may compress the esophagus as it passes posteriorly and to the left, being drawn anteriorly by the left-sided ligamentum (**Figure 61.4a and b**). Division of the ligamentum is usually sufficient; but, as it is the mirror image situation to the above (anomalous right subclavian artery from the contralateral descending thoracic aorta), division and reimplantation may be required.

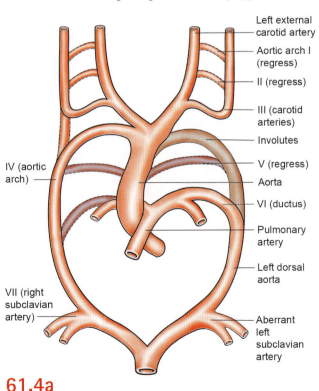

61.4a

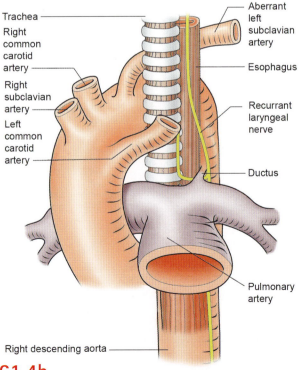

61.4b

Double aortic arch

Persistent left and right fourth arches result in an encircling ring formed by an anterior and leftward arch and a posterior and rightward arch that join to form the descending aorta posteriorly. In 75% of cases, the right aortic arch is the dominant one. The left subclavian and carotid arteries usually arise from the smaller left arch. Atretic or hypoplastic segments occur in the lesser arch approximately a third of the time and can be anywhere along the arch's curve, but they are usually distal at the junction with descending aorta (**Figure 61.5a and b**). In 15% of cases, the left arch is dominant, and in the remaining 10%, the arches are of equal size. The right recurrent laryngeal nerve must pass around the right aortic arch, rather than around the right subclavian artery.

After mobilization of the arches, ligamentum, esophagus, and trachea, the lesser arch should be test occluded, typically at the apparently atretic portion located at the insertion to the descending aorta (**Figure 61.6a**). Preservation of brachiocephalic flow is confirmed. Clamps are applied to the narrowest part of the lesser arch, the segment divided, and each end oversewn with continuous polypropylene suture in two layers. The arches are then reflected away from the

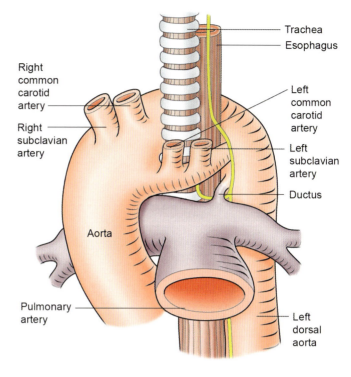

61.5b

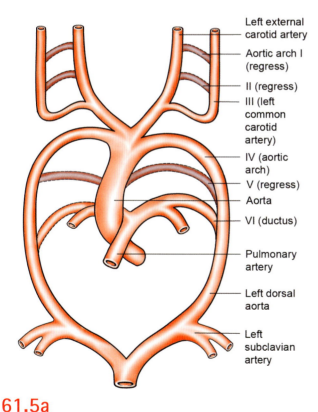

61.5a

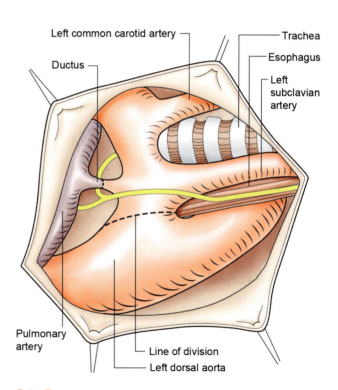

61.6a

trachea and esophagus, which are mobilized completely. The ligamentum is divided between ligatures (**Figure 61.6b**). The left recurrent laryngeal nerve must be identified and preserved.

Right aortic arch/left ligamentum

In this situation, the aorta passes to the right of the trachea and esophagus, coursing posteriorly and leftward behind them, and then usually descends on the left. The ring is formed by a left-sided ligamentum between the left subclavian artery or descending thoracic aorta, depending on the pattern of branching of the ascending aorta (**Figure 61.7a–d**). Treatment is simple division of the ligamentum and mobilization of the aorta and branches. If there is mirror image branching (which is the common pattern), the ligamentum inserts under the innominate artery, and no ring is formed. Similarly, in the rare instances in which the aorta descends on the right and the ligamentum connects the arch undersurface to the right pulmonary artery, no ring exists.

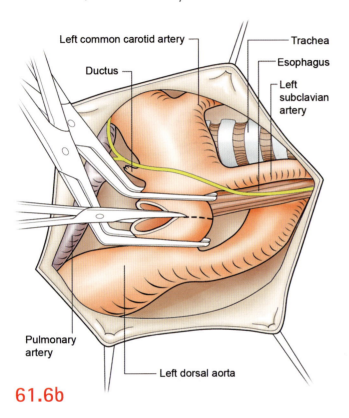

61.6b

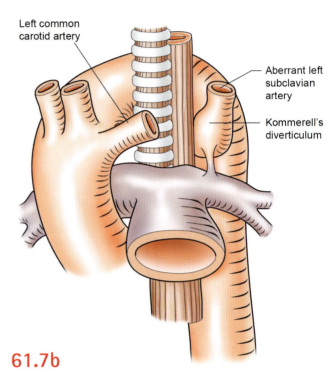

61.7b

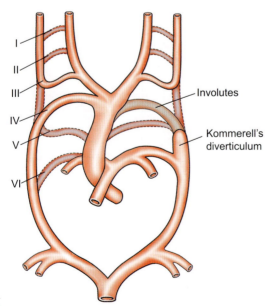

61.7a

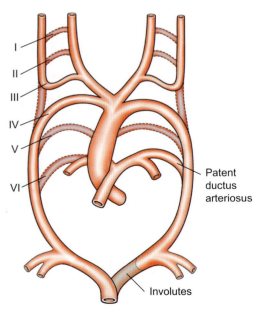

61.7c

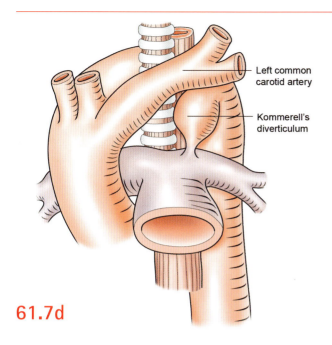

61.7d

Left common
carotid artery

Kommerell's
diverticulum

Innominate artery compression

In innominate artery compression (which, strictly speaking, is not a vascular ring), the innominate artery arises from the aortic arch far to the left. The body of the innominate artery is thus stretched across the anterior tracheal wall and compresses the airway as it passes rightward. Via right thoracotomy, the right lobe of the thymus is excised, and the adventitia of the anterior wall of the innominate artery is fixed to the periosteum of the sternum, elevating the artery off the trachea, which is dissected from the posterior wall of the artery (**Figure 61.8a–c**). Reimplantation may be necessary if the thoracic inlet is compressed so that insufficient room exists to "pexy" the artery to the sternum. Bronchoscopy is performed after the suspension to confirm airway compression has been relieved.

POSTOPERATIVE CARE

Early extubation is possible in most cases, but it should be followed by careful attention to pulmonary toilet, airway humidification, treatment of bronchospasm, and pain control. Potential concerns about recurrent laryngeal or phrenic nerve injury should be communicated to the intensive care unit team. Management of chest drains and the thoracotomy wound are the same as for other thoracotomy patients.

OUTCOME

Operative mortality is low (less than 5%) but not zero. One of the largest series on vascular rings by Backer et al. over a 57-year period had no deaths for 44 years with 12.4% of the patients with associated cardiac lesions. Deaths are usually related to coexistent cardiac disease or severe tracheomalacia.

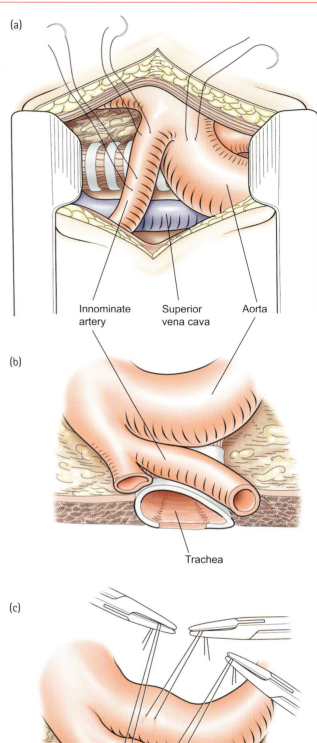

(a)

(b)

Innominate
artery

Superior
vena cava

Aorta

Trachea

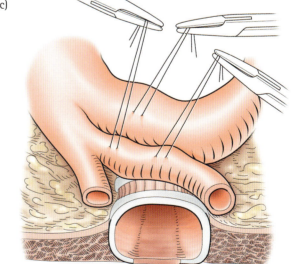

(c)

61.8a–c

Complications include hemorrhage, infection, esophageal and tracheal leaks, and chylothorax. Relief of symptoms occurs in 70–80% of patients, slightly greater in those with esophageal compression, and slightly less in those with tracheal compression. Benefit of surgical division of the ring may not be immediate, as some patients require several months to achieve their ultimate result. Persistent or recurrent symptoms beyond several months should prompt re-evaluation for incomplete mobilization of compressed structures from surrounding fibrous bands, Kommerell's diverticulum, esophageal stricture, or irreversible airway damage.

FURTHER READING

Arciniegas E, Hakimi M, Hertzler JH, et al. Surgical management of congenital vascular rings. *J Thorac Cardiovasc Surg.* 1979; 77: 721–7.

Backer CL, Mavroudis C. Congenital heart surgery nomenclature and database project: vascular rings, tracheal stenosis, pectus excavatum. *Ann Thorac Surg.* 2000; 69(4 Suppl): S308–18.

Backer CL, Mavroudis C, Rigsby CK, et al. Trends in vascular ring surgery. *J Thorac Cardiovasc Surg.* 2005; 129: 1339–47.

Edwards JE. Anomalies of the derivatives of the aortic arch system. *Med Clin North Am.* 1948; 32: 925–49.

Gross RE. Surgical relief for tracheal obstruction from a vascular ring. *New Engl J Med.* 1945; 233: 586–90.

62

Hypoplastic left heart syndrome

AARON ECKHAUSER AND THOMAS L. SPRAY

INTRODUCTION AND HISTORY

The term *hypoplastic left heart syndrome* (HLHS) has been used to describe a group of cardiac malformations that consists of hypoplasia or absence of the left ventricle and hypoplasia of the ascending aorta. In the most extreme form, HLHS refers to aortic valvar atresia, with a very diminutive ascending aorta and diminutive left ventricle. Like other single ventricle malformations of the heart, HLHS has a circulation dependent on patency of the ductus arteriosus and obligatory mixing of pulmonary and systemic venous blood. The single ventricle (in this case, an anatomic right ventricle (RV)) supplies the pulmonary circulation by the branch pulmonary arteries (PAs) and the systemic circulation via the patent ductus arteriosus. Flow in the ascending aorta is usually primarily retrograde, and in aortic atresia, the ascending aorta acts as a common coronary artery supplying coronary perfusion.

HLHS is the most common severe congenital heart defect, representing 7–9% of all congenital heart anomalies diagnosed within the first year of life. Untreated, HLHS is fatal, accounting for 25% of all cardiac deaths in the first week of life. Early attempts to provide palliative therapy for infants with HLHS were described by Cayler and Freedom. Continuity was created between the RV and descending aorta by placement of a graft, and pulmonary arterial banding was used to limit pulmonary blood flow. Initial attempts were unsuccessful, due primarily to distortion of the pulmonary vascular bed. Evolution of these initial therapies continued, and much of the development of successful first stage reconstruction is credited to Dr William I. Norwood, who gradually refined and developed the surgical principles we use today. Neonatal heart transplantation, pioneered by Leonard Bailey and his colleagues, has been used as an alternate form of therapy. However, the limitation of donor heart availability and the increased success with staged reconstruction have made primary transplantation less desirable. The first successful palliation with staged reconstruction as described by Norwood has changed little over the past 20 years; however, several new technical modifications have been proposed to limit the use of prosthetic material in the reconstruction and to decrease the use or duration of deep hypothermic circulatory arrest.

PRINCIPLES AND JUSTIFICATION

The principle of the staged reconstruction operations for HLHS is similar to that for other single ventricle malformations of the heart. The goals of the first stage reconstructive procedure (known commonly as the Norwood procedure) are:

1. creation of an unobstructed connection between the systemic ventricle (the right ventricle) and the aorta in a fashion that permits growth
2. regulation of pulmonary blood flow to permit growth of the pulmonary vascular bed and to limit the development of pulmonary vascular obstructive disease while minimizing the volume load on the single ventricle
3. creation of an unobstructed interatrial communication to avoid restriction of the pulmonary venous return to the heart.

These principles must be performed technically in such a fashion as to prevent distal arch obstruction and limit or interfere with coronary perfusion. Because successful first-stage reconstruction creates a situation where pulmonary blood flow is dependent on an aortopulmonary or RV–PA shunt, the single RV is subjected to an increased volume load as the entire systemic and pulmonary cardiac output passes through the right atrium, RV, and PA to the aorta. Tricuspid valve regurgitation can be a consequence of ischemic damage due to the diminutive aorta supplying coronary blood flow, true coronary anomalies, or a secondary effect of the increased volume load. Significant tricuspid regurgitation may require intervention at the first- or second-stage operation and, if associated with severe ventricular dysfunction, may be an indication for conversion to transplantation as a second-stage operation.

Completion of the first-stage operation creates a somewhat unstable physiological situation, with shunt-dependent pulmonary blood flow and a significant volume load on an anatomical RV. For this reason, a second-stage reconstruction operation (performed at 3–6 months of age) consisting of either a bidirectional Glenn shunt or hemi-Fontan procedure (see Chapter 44, "Bidirectional Glenn and hemi-Fontan procedures") is undertaken to decrease the volume load of the single ventricle and improve effective pulmonary blood flow. The third stage in the reconstruction, as in other single ventricle malformations, is a modification of the Fontan–Kreutzer procedure. The systemic and pulmonary circulations are separated, often with the use of a single fenestration to permit right-to-left shunting at the atrial level to maintain ventricular preload in the postoperative period and during times of stress or elevated pulmonary vascular resistance.

PREOPERATIVE ASSESSMENT AND PREPARATION

As in other single ventricle malformations with duct-dependent physiology, signs of HLHS may be minimal. Typically, tachypnea and mild cyanosis are the primary early signs but the diagnosis becomes more apparent when ductal constriction begins and systemic perfusion is severely compromised, resulting in metabolic acidosis, organ dysfunction, and shock. If ductal patency is maintained and the atrial septal defect is unrestrictive, significant pulmonary overcirculation can occur, resulting in a severely volume-overloaded ventricle and congestive heart failure, which also leads to systemic organ dysfunction, and metabolic acidosis with compromised peripheral perfusion. In rare cases, a severely restrictive atrial communication is present (2–5%), resulting in severe hypoxemia with a congestive pattern on chest X-ray. These patients often require emergent intervention to create an unrestrictive atrial communication in the catheterization laboratory or in the operating room.

The diagnosis of HLHS is confirmed by two-dimensional (2D) echocardiography with color-flow Doppler mapping. Cardiac catheterization is rarely necessary unless intervention is required to create less restriction at the atrial septal level or to document unusual pulmonary venous return. In patients without severe restriction of venous return at the atrial level, dilation of the atrial septal defect should not be undertaken, as the procedure increases the pulmonary blood flow and can potentially cause hemodynamic deterioration in an otherwise stable balance of pulmonary and systemic blood flow. Echocardiography is also used to evaluate the degree of hypoplasia of the aortic arch, retrograde flow in the ascending aorta, the presence or absence of coarctation, the presence or absence of significant tricuspid valve regurgitation, and restriction at the atrial septal defect.

Initial medical support for infants with HLHS involves maintaining patency of the ductus arteriosus and balancing the pulmonary and systemic blood flows to prevent significant abnormalities of systemic perfusion or pulmonary overcirculation. Prostaglandin E1 (PGE) is infused at a low dose (0.025–0.05 µg/kg/minute) to maintain patency of the ductus arteriosus. A balance of systemic and pulmonary circulation is best maintained with spontaneous ventilation on room air. However, if intubation is necessary due to PGE-induced apnea, then ventilation with 21–30% oxygen is used to prevent pulmonary consolidation and pulmonary vasodilation. Blending carbon dioxide or nitrogen into the gas mixture on the ventilator is rarely necessary but may be useful to increase pulmonary vasoconstriction and improve systemic cardiac output. If ventricular dysfunction is present, low doses of inotropic agents may be added. However, the lowest possible levels of inotropic support should be sought to limit the effects of unbalancing the systemic and pulmonary vascular resistance. Ventricular function generally recovers after initial acidosis and hemodynamic compromise has been corrected. The addition of diuretics and digoxin is often useful perioperatively to help deal with the volume effects on the single ventricle as pulmonary resistance decreases. Judicious use of these agents may permit a significant period of stabilization and recovery of renal and hepatic function and assessment of neurological status. In addition, both genetic anomalies and non-cardiac malformations can be assessed. Despite significant volume loads, the resuscitated single ventricle can provide quite stable physiology for several days to weeks before surgical intervention. Surgery is generally performed non-emergently after both the hepatic and renal function has normalized.

ANESTHESIA

Anesthesia for infants with HLHS can require delicate manipulations of systemic and pulmonary vascular resistances during induction and maintenance. Anesthesia is achieved with administration of narcotics (typically fentanyl) and muscle relaxants (typically non-depolarizing agents). Endotracheal intubation is typically performed. If the patient has unrestricted pulmonary blood flow, care is taken to avoid high oxygen gas mixtures to maintain the stable balance of pulmonary and systemic resistance. Anesthesia-induced vasodilation very rarely requires the addition of nitrogen or carbon dioxide to the gas mixture to maintain systemic perfusion in this critical stage. Monitoring with an umbilical arterial and venous line is used, and blood gases are monitored frequently to correct imbalances in perfusion and acidosis.

OPERATION

Exposure is performed through a midline sternotomy incision, and the majority of thymic tissue is excised to gain access to the superior mediastinum and the aortic arch vessels. The pericardium is opened in the midline. Because of the significant volume loading of the ventricle and hypothermia (body temperature is generally 34 °C due to low room temperature in the operating room), the myocardium can be extremely irritable and even minor retraction or irritation of the ventricle can result in instability and ventricular fibrillation. Therefore, care is taken to avoid manipulation of the ventricle as much as possible during the dissection, which is done with low-power electrocautery (**Figure 62.1a**). The very diminutive ascending aorta is separated from the PA to which it is adherent down proximal to the takeoff of the right PA. The entire aortic arch is mobilized, and the head vessels are encircled with snares for control. The ductus arteriosus is mobilized, as is the descending thoracic aorta beyond the ductus, with care being taken to avoid direct retraction on the ductal tissue, which is friable and can easily tear. The pulmonary bifurcation is also mobilized freely, and the right and left pulmonary arteries are encircled with snares for control when bypass is initiated. Pursestring sutures are placed in the proximal main PA below the pulmonary bifurcation and in the right atrial appendage for cannulation for cardiopulmonary bypass (CPB) (**Figure 62.1b**).

After heparinization, the PA and right atrium are cannulated, and CPB is initiated. After the initiation of bypass, the tourniquets on the right and left pulmonary arteries are tightened to prevent pulmonary blood flow during the cooling phase of the operation. The patient is typically cooled for 15 minutes to a temperature of 18°C. Given the undistorted anatomical relationships of both the innominate artery and the right PA, a polytetrafluoroethylene (PTFE) tube graft of an appropriate size (3.5–4.0 mm in diameter) is cut to size. A diagonal cut is made for the proximal anastamosis and a partial occluding vascular clamp is placed on the proximal innominate artery. The proximal anastomosis of the graft is created using a running 7-0 monofilament suture. The

vascular clamp can be released to ensure unrestricted inflow into the shunt (**Figure 62.1c**). A small Hegar dilator can be passed retrograde through the shunt to ensure that there is no distal narrowing in the innominate artery.

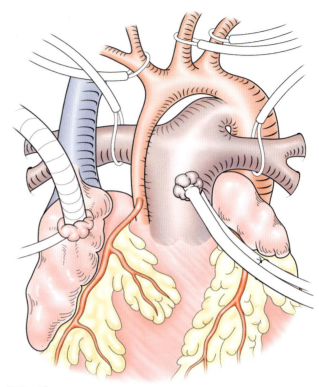

62.1b

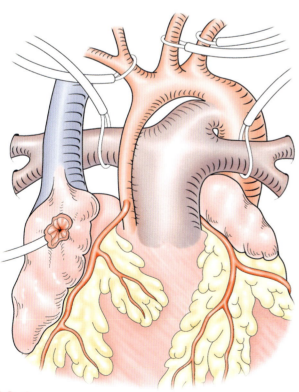

62.1a

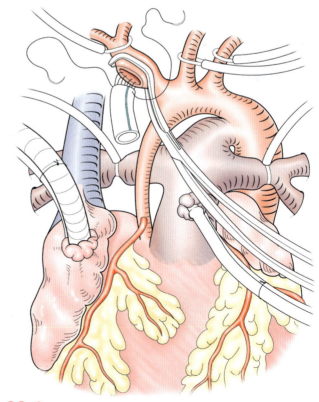

62.1c

The shunt is controlled with a hemoclip during the remainder of the procedure or, in alternative techniques, the shunt can be cannulated and bypass continued to maintain perfusion of the arch during the remainder of the operation (**Figure 62.2a**). Cardioplegia is connected to a side arm in the arterial cannula and, after cooling to 18 °C has been achieved over a 15–20-minute period, the circulation is arrested and the tourniquets on the arch vessels are tightened (**Figure 62.2b**).

A clamp is placed on the descending thoracic aorta below the ductal insertion site. Cardioplegia can then be injected retrograde through the aortic cannula and ductus into the ascending aorta to provide diastolic arrest of the heart (**Figure 62.3a**). After all the venous blood has been returned to the reservoir, both the aortic and venous cannula are removed. The tourniquets on the pulmonary arteries are removed, and the ductus arteriosus is ligated and divided distally on the aortic end (**Figure 62.3b**). Working through

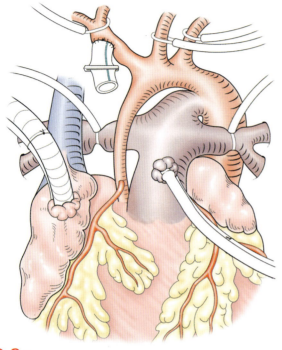

62.2a

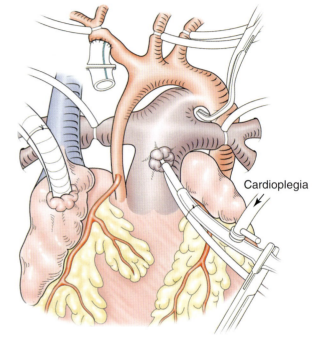

Cardioplegia

62.3a

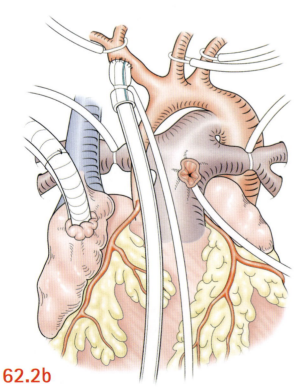

62.2b

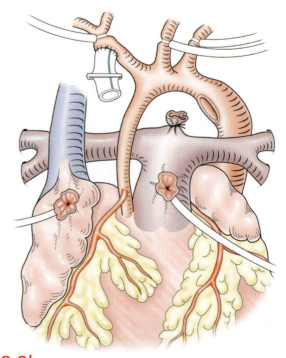

62.3b

the atrial pursestring suture, the atrial septum can be widely excised. If exposure is limited, a small right atriotomy is made and the septum primum, which is commonly displaced to the left, can be excised to create a widely unobstructed atrial opening (**Figure 62.3c**). The atrium is then closed with monofilament suture.

Next, the PA is divided transversely at the origin of the right pulmonary artery (**Figure 62.3d**). This incision leaves slightly more PA on the left side, unless the cut is made in an oblique fashion up to the origin of the left PA. Making the PA transection at the origin of the right PA ensures that the connection between the proximal PA and aorta is high enough to avoid sewing near the coronary artery origin from the diminutive ascending aorta. The bifurcation of the PAs is then closed primarily if the PAs are large or, more commonly, the bifurcation is closed with an oval-shaped patch of pulmonary homograft material using a running monofilament technique (**Figure 62.3e**).

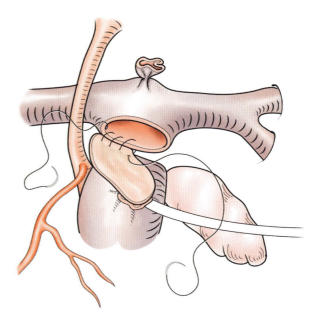

62.3d

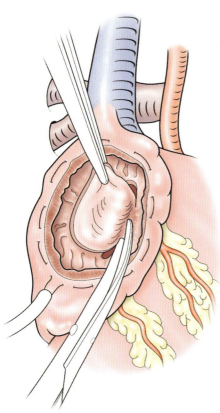

62.3c

62.3e

The distal anastomosis of the shunt is constructed at the origin of the right PA near the takeoff from the main PA bifurcation (**Figure 62.4**). This technique permits the shunt to connect more medially behind the reconstructed aorta and avoids having to create this anastomosis with the large neoaorta distended, making exposure difficult. Meticulous technique during creation of the shunt is essential to avoid cyanosis or early shunt thrombosis.

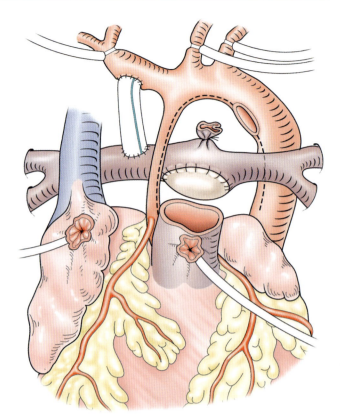

62.5a

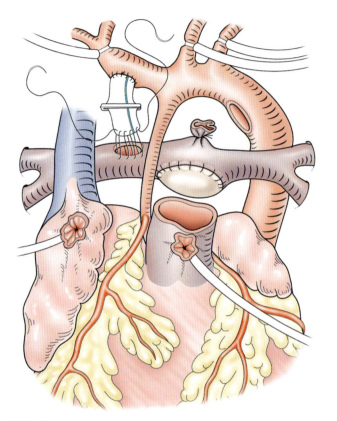

62.4

Next, an incision is made in the medial aspect of the diminutive ascending aorta and carried across the under-surface of the arch or the aorta beyond the last of the ductal insertion site (**Figure 62.5a**). Redundant ductal tissue is debrided, and the ridge of coarctation opposite the ductus is excised if present (**Figure 62.5b**). Proximally, the aortic incision is carried down to the level of the transection of the pulmonary bifurcation. In some cases a small incision into the proximal PA to allow adequate connection between the PA and ascending aorta may be necessary to prevent compression of the aorta (**Figure 62.5c**). The proximal PA is then sutured delicately to the diminutive ascending aorta with interrupted 7-0 monofilament sutures to prevent a pursestring effect and to create meticulous hemostasis at this critical junction (**Figure 62.5d**). At this time, it must be assured that no restriction to inflow into the coronary arteries is present. Mobilization of the tissue between the aorta and PA is performed so that epicardial adhesions

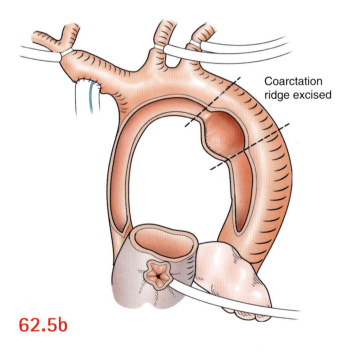

Coarctation ridge excised

62.5b

do not potentially kink the origin of the coronary arteries when the neoaorta expands.

The final stage of reconstruction is performed by augmenting the aortic arch with a patch of pulmonary homograft material using a running 7-0 monofilament suture. Care

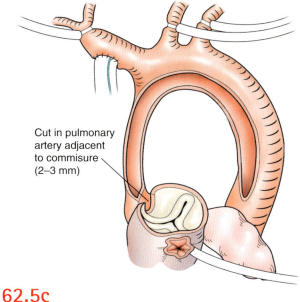

Cut in pulmonary artery adjacent to commisure (2–3 mm)

62.5c

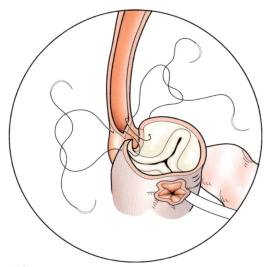

62.5d

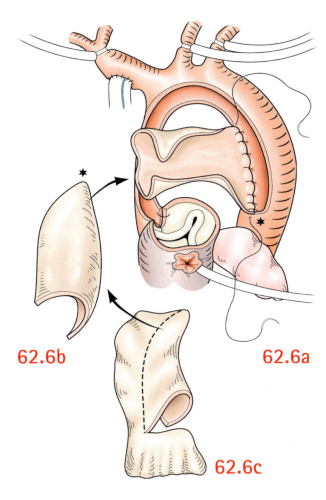

62.6b

62.6a

62.6c

must be taken to avoid creating an overly redundant patch (**Figure 62.6a–c**). When the neoaorta fills and systolic pressure increases, torsion of the reconstruction can occur, causing impingement on the origin of the innominate artery, limiting inflow into the shunt, coronary torsion causing ischemia or twisting in the descending aorta causing distal arch obstruction.

In general, making the patch too narrow rather than too wide is preferable. The posterior part of the pathway is generally shorter in length than the anterior portion. The patch is generally scooped out on the inferior incision to prevent excessive length, which can cause kinking of the pulmonary root at the connection to the patch and restriction to ejection from the heart with creation of neoaortic insufficiency through the pulmonary valve. The patch shape will often need to be tailored for different variations of HLHS in which the size of the ascending aorta is variable (**Figure 62.6d**).

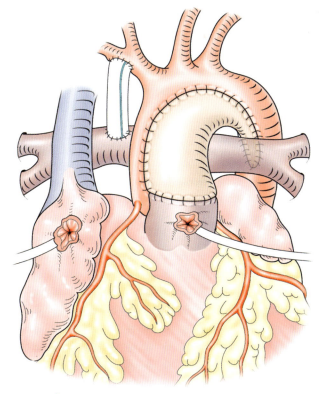

62.6d

After completion of the reconstruction, de-airing is performed by injection of saline into both the right atrial and the aortic cannulation site. The venous and arterial cannulae are reinserted and the infant is then placed back on CPB and rewarmed to 37 °C. The tourniquets on the arch vessels are released. At this time, prompt return of myocardial perfusion should be assessed to ensure that no restriction to coronary inflow exists. Significant dilation of the heart at this stage generally represents distortion of the pulmonary valve and neoaortic insufficiency, and needs to be addressed. After rewarming has been completed, atrial lines are brought through the chest wall and positioned in the pursestring suture in the right atrial appendage for pressure measurement and volume infusion. The patient is typically started on low-dose inotropic support using dopamine or epinephrine. Milrinone is commonly loaded into the bypass circuit to create vasodilation and improve right ventricular performance. For maintenance of systemic perfusion, it is critical to decrease elevated systemic vascular resistance. Other centers have alternatively used powerful alpha-blocking agents, such as phenoxybenzamine, to accomplish the same goal. Ventilation is initiated at high tidal volumes to ensure full lung recruitment and to minimize pulmonary resistance. The hemoclip is then removed from the shunt, and the patient is weaned off CPB. Modified ultrafiltration is routinely used in our center to decrease myocardial edema, improve systolic ventricular performance, and minimize the volume load on the circulation in the early postoperative period.

After cannulae have been removed from the heart and hemostasis is achieved, the chest is drained and the sternum is typically closed before transport to the intensive care unit. If concerns exist about myocardial function or if hemorrhage is a concern, the chest is left open, and a silicone patch is used to approximate the skin edges.

Variations in operative technique can be used depending on the particular cardiac anatomy. If the aorta and PA are transposed, or when the aorta is large in relation to the PA, reconstruction of the aortic arch may be simplified by division of the aorta and PA proximally with a side-to-side "double-barrel" connection over a short distance, followed by augmentation of the aortic arch with a triangular-shaped patch of cryopreserved pulmonary homograft material. The aorta is reconstructed to the double-barrel using continuous monofilament suture (**Figure 62.7a and b**). This approach avoids potential distortion and twisting of the reconstructed arch and can avoid too large a patch with compression of the posteriorly located pulmonary bifurcation.

An additional modification avoids the use of prosthetic material in the arch reconstruction. In this approach, rather than reconstruction of the aortic arch with cryopreserved homograft material, a direct connection is performed between the proximal PA and the undersurface of the aortic arch (**Figure 62.8a and b**). In this procedure, the arch vessels must be extensively mobilized to allow them to come down to the PA, and the division of the PA is created high towards the origin of the right PA. This avoids kinking of the diminutive ascending aorta, which acts as a common

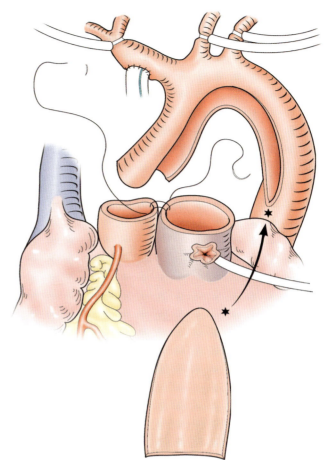

62.7a

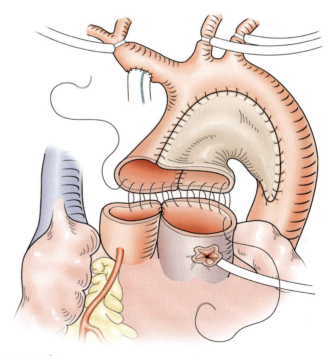

62.7b

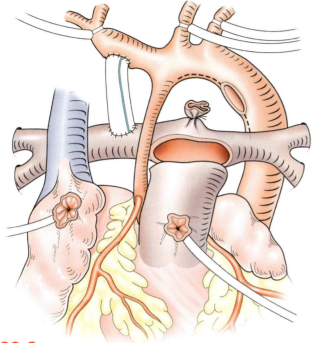

62.8a

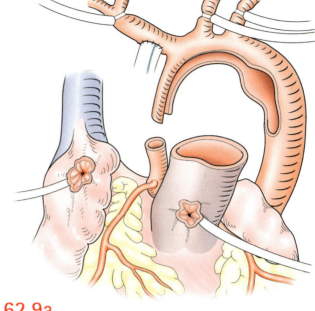

62.9a

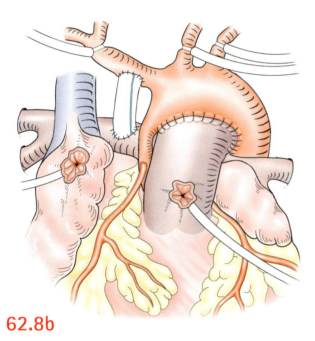

62.8b

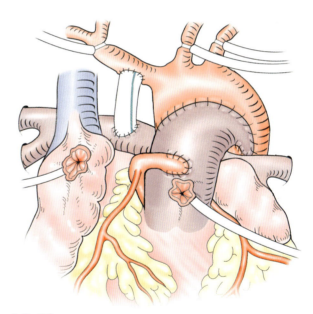

62.9b

coronary vessel. Problems with coronary inflow have led many centers to divide the diminutive ascending aorta and reimplant it directly onto the anterolateral aspect of the PA with interrupted or running monofilament sutures to avoid this complication.

If significant coarctation is present, division of the distal aorta beyond the subclavian artery and excision of all ductal tissue with direct connection posteriorly before arch reconstruction is also advisable to avoid leaving ductal tissue, which can cause recurrent arch obstruction (**Figure 62.9a and b**).

A recent modification of the stage one operation for HLHS

developed by Sano uses a RV–PA shunt instead of an aortopulmonary shunt to provide pulmonary blood flow. The Sano modification has the advantage of providing systolic antegrade flow into the PAs and avoiding diastolic run-off into the pulmonary vascular bed, which may decrease the diastolic pressure and potentially decrease coronary perfusion pressure. The Sano modification has gained rapid acceptance in many centers due to an improvement in early postoperative stability in patients in whom the RV–PA connection has been established. The early postoperative elevation of systemic vascular resistance which causes low cardiac output after the standard stage one Norwood operation has less physiologic impact with an RV–PA shunt, where the elevated systemic resistance results actually in improvement in forward flow into the pulmonary vascular bed as the right ventricular pressure increases. The theoretical disadvantages of the use of an RV–PA shunt are the need for an incision in the right ventricular infundibulum (which may have impact on long-term right ventricular function) and the potential for narrowing of the shunt at the origin from the RV due to the thick ventricular muscle.

Sano modification

The arch reconstruction is performed in the standard fashion (**Figure 62.10a**). An incision is then made in the infundibulum of the right ventricular outflow tract at least a half centimeter below the pulmonary valve which is bluntly dilated (**Figure 62.10b**). A piece of 5 mm externally reinforced PTFE is measured to length and cut approximately 4 cm from the start of the Silastic ribs. The depth of the ventricular free wall is measured and the ribbed portion of the graft is passed through the ventriculotomy so that 1–2 mm of graft protrudes into the ventricle. The graft is secured in each quadrant with an interrupted Prolene suture. A Hegar dilator is passed through the graft to ensure that it is not kinked where it enters the ventricle. A Prolene pursestring suture is placed circumferentially around the graft for hemostasis. The pulmonary bifurcation is closed partially, and then the distal anastomosis of the shunt is sewn superiorly into the pulmonary bifurcation to avoid interference with the reconstructed neoaorta and to allow for good growth of the pulmonary bifurcation. Alternatively, the distal end of the shunt can be

sutured to a tailored piece of homograft, which can then be sewn to the divided pulmonary bifurcation, assuring that the anastomosis is widely patent.

When using the Sano modification, no obstruction to the inflow of the RV–PA shunt should be present and the length of the shunt should be tailored appropriately so that it does not push posteriorly and cause kinking and potential occlusion of the pulmonary bifurcation. Postoperative diastolic pressures are higher and systolic pressures are often slightly lower compared to the standard Norwood operation. Oxygen saturations may be higher with the RV–PA connection; however, the higher oxygen saturations are well-tolerated and "steal" of coronary flow does not occur in diastole as has been seen in the standard Norwood aortopulmonary shunt connection.

A further modification of the technique involves the limited use or the lack of use of circulatory arrest. This approach can be done by initial cannulation of the PA through the ductus arteriosus with snaring of the ductus to maintain systemic perfusion or creation of the proximal modified Blalock–Taussig shunt before initiation of CPB with cannulation of the shunt for arterial inflow. In general, creation of the proximal shunt anastomosis is difficult without distortion of a very diminutive ascending aorta and temporary myocardial dysfunction; therefore, bypass support is generally preferable. The proximal anastomosis of the modified Blalock–Taussig shunt is created to the origin of the innominate artery. Then, with a brief period of circulatory arrest, cannulation is moved to the distal end of the shunt to provide retrograde flow into the innominate artery to perfuse the brain and, through collaterals, the distal vascular bed. Snares are tightened on the carotid and subclavian vessels, and the descending aorta is clamped while flow is maintained at approximately 30% of

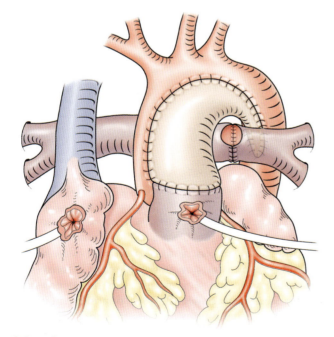

62.10a

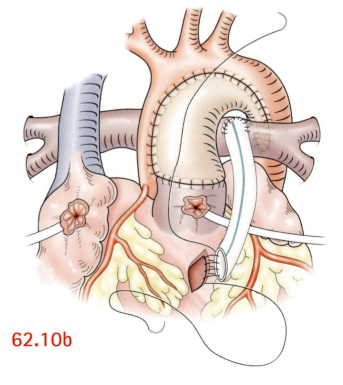

62.10b

normal. Monitoring of radial perfusion pressures is advisable when this technique is used. Venous return is evacuated either through a patent venous cannula or sump suction placed in the right atrium. After reconstruction of the aortic arch is complete, arch cannulation can be performed, and the distal anastomosis of the shunt is created to the PAs during rewarming.

The hybrid approach

The hybrid approach for management of HLHS is an alternative, less invasive technique that involves both the surgeon and the interventional cardiologist. Patients undergo standard anesthetic induction and the heart is approached through a median sternotomy. The right branch PA is circumferentially dissected between the SVC and the aorta and the left PA is dissected free immediately after its takeoff. Bilateral branch PA bands are placed using 1–2 mm rings of a 3.5 mm Gore-Tex® tube graft. The bands are sutured to surrounding adventitia with 6-0 Prolene suture. Accurate tightening of the bands is difficult and is guided by angiographic imaging and a step up in systemic blood pressure and a decrease in oxygen saturations.

Next, a pursestring suture is placed in the main PA immediately distal to the valve and a sheath is introduced into the PA (**Figure 62.11**). An appropriate-sized stent is deployed

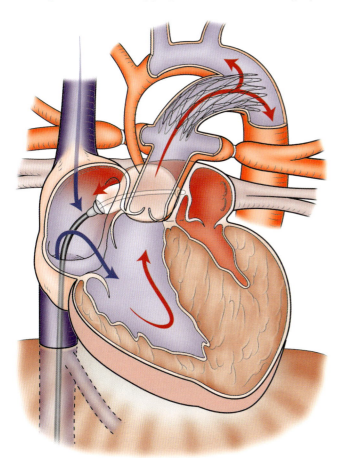

62.11

covering the entire length of the patent ductus arteriosus (PDA). Once the stent is confirmed to be in good position, a balloon atrial septostomy or stent is performed at this time. Depending on the degree of restriction at the atrial level, the septostomy can be performed as a separate procedure prior to discharge. Delaying the septostomy for several days allows for a more aggressive septostomy in a more stable patient. In 4–6 months patients undergo a comprehensive stage two procedure in which the atrial septum is fully excised, the PDA stent is removed, and a Damus–Kaye–Stansel (DKS) anastomosis with arch augmentation is created and a Glenn anastomosis for pulmonary blood flow. (For further details, see Galantowicz et al. 2008 in Further reading.)

POSTOPERATIVE CARE

The major advancement in the management of patients with HLHS has been the refinement of postoperative care, which has decreased the occurrence of early myocardial dysfunction and cardiovascular collapse.

Maintenance of systemic vascular perfusion by vasodilation of the systemic vascular bed is the primary goal in the early postoperative period. Early approaches to balancing systemic and pulmonary circulations after the first-stage reconstruction operation focused on preventing pulmonary overcirculation by limiting pulmonary blood flow with manipulation of vascular resistance. Oxygen was rapidly decreased; and occasionally, carbon dioxide was blended into the gas mixture to raise pulmonary vascular resistance. However, studies performed by Tweddell and associates have suggested that pulmonary blood flow is restricted by the shunt sufficiently so that significant manipulation of pulmonary vascular resistance is rarely necessary. Oxygen is weaned as appropriate to non-toxic levels of less than 40% as the patient recovers from the operative procedure and, with a satisfactory size shunt, weaning to 30–40% oxygen can generally be done fairly rapidly. However, strict attention to base deficit is important, and significant development or progression of base deficits suggests significant systemic perfusion abnormalities that require intervention with increasing inotropic support or more significant vasodilation, or both. The use of inodilators such as milrinone has significantly improved the maintenance of systemic output while improving right heart function. Postoperatively, we currently use 3 μg/kg/minute of dopamine for baseline inotropic and renal support and add 0.5–1.0 μg/kg/minute of milrinone to improve vasodilation and systemic output. Ventilation is maintained with slight hypocarbia in the 35–38 mmHg range to prevent alveolar hypoxemia and hypercarbia, and high tidal volumes are generally used to prevent atelectasis. The infant is kept sedated and paralyzed overnight, although patients who are in good condition preoperatively and have a stable balance of systemic and pulmonary flow can be allowed to awaken and extubate within 24–48 hours after surgery. Nutritional support is begun as early as possible after surgery, initially intravenously with early transition to enteral feeds as tolerated.

OUTCOME

Clinical outcomes have improved dramatically over the last decade, much of which is attributed to significant improvements in postoperative care. According to the Society of Thoracic Surgeons Congenital Heart Surgery Database, hospital survival for patients with HLHS improved from 68.6% in 2002 to 81.4% in 2009. Pooled data from multiple high-volume centers report current survival rates between 74% and 93%.

The SVR (single ventricle reconstruction) trial was a multi-center, NIH–sponsored, randomized trial comparing the BT shunt and RV–PA conduit in patients undergoing the Norwood operation. Patients were randomized to either a BT shunt or RV–PA conduit (Sano) and the primary endpoint was death or transplantation at 1 year. The RV–PA conduit was found to be superior to the BT shunt (26% vs 36%, $p = 0.01$) for the primary endpoint of death or transplant at 12 months. The increased risk of mortality in the BT shunt was no longer significant after 12 months. Additionally, the need for CPR during the postoperative course was greater in the BT shunt group (20% vs 13%, $p = 0.04$), whereas unintended cardiovascular interventions on the shunt or neoaorta were more common in the RV–PA group (92 vs 70 per 100 infants, $p = 0.003$).

Despite improvements in overall mortality, patients are at risk for significant morbidity postoperatively. These children are at risk for neurodevelopmental delay for multiple reasons such as cyanosis, congestive heart failure, and pre-existing central nervous system abnormalities, in addition to the effects of CPB and hypothermic circulatory arrest on an immature brain. Children with HLHS score statistically lower than non-HLHS children with single ventricles on scales of infant development and intelligence quotient testing; however, the majority remain in the normal range. Verbal tests tend to have higher scores than motor skill tests, as has been noted in other patients with congenital heart disease who undergo surgical intervention. The primary determinant of poor neurodevelopmental outcome is the presence of genetic syndromes or the presence of a seizure disorder in the perioperative or preoperative period. Clinical seizures are the most common neurological abnormality postoperatively (4–17%). Stroke or intracerebral hemorrhage occurs in approximately 5% of patients. Phrenic and recurrent laryngeal nerve injuries are not uncommon, and occur in 5% and 10% of patients respectively. Renal failure, depending on clinical definition, occurs in 10–15% of patients.

Clinical results from the hybrid approach are preliminarily encouraging. Galantowicz et al., with the largest North American experience ($N = 40$), report a hospital mortality rate of 2%, an interstage mortality of 5%, and a reintervention rate of 36%. A significant concern with the hybrid approach is development of a reverse coarctation, or retrograde stenosis of the tranverse aortic arch. This complication occurred in 10% of their patients, and all were successfully treated by placing a retrograde aortic stent. The hybrid approach clearly requires an experienced multidisciplinary team to navigate a very steep learning curve. However, the hybrid procedure has definitely carved a niche in our armamentarium for the treatment of patients with HLHS.

FURTHER READING

Bove EL, Lloyd TR. Staged reconstruction for hypoplastic left heart syndrome: contemporary results. *Ann Thorac Surg.* 1996; 224: 387–94.

Feinstein JA, Benson W, Martin GR, et al. Hypoplastic left heart syndrome: current considerations and expectations. *J Am Coll Cardiol.* 2012; 59(Suppl): S1–42.

Galantowicz M, Cheatham JP, Phillips A, et al. Hybrid approach for hypoplastic left heart syndrome: intermediate results after the learning curve. *Ann Thorac Surg.* 2008; 85: 2063–71.

Hoffman GM, Ghanayem NS, Kampine JM, et al. Venous saturation and the anaerobic threshold in neonates after the Norwood procedure for hypoplastic left heart syndrome. *Ann Thorac Surg.* 2000; 70: 1515–21.

Mahle WT, Spray TL, Wernovsky G, et al. Survival after reconstructive surgery for hypoplastic left heart syndrome: a 15-year experience from a single institution. *Circulation.* 2000; 102(Suppl III): III136–41.

Ohye RG, Sleeper LA, Gaynor JW, et al. Comparison of shunt types in the Norwood procedure for single-ventricle lesion. *New Engl J Med.* 2010; 362: 1980–92.

Tweddell JS, Hoffman GM, Fedderly RT, et al. Patients at risk for low systemic oxygen delivery after the Norwood procedure. *Ann Thorac Surg.* 2000; 69: 1893–9.

Weinstein S, Gaynor JW, Bridges ND, et al. Early survival of infants weighing 2.5 kilograms or less undergoing first-stage reconstruction for hypoplastic left heart syndrome. *Circulation.* 1999; 100(19 Suppl): II167–70.

Weinstein S, Gaynor JW, Wernovsky G, et al. Survival of low birth weight infants undergoing stage I Norwood reconstruction for hypoplastic left heart syndrome or single ventricle physiology. *Circulation.* 1998; 98(17 Suppl): I62.

63

Coronary anomalies

JULIE BROTHERS AND J. WILLIAM GAYNOR

INTRODUCTION

Most common variations in the number, origin, and distribution of the coronary arteries are of intellectual interest only. Although clinically significant congenital coronary artery anomalies are rare, they may result in myocardial ischemia, left ventricular dysfunction, and sudden death.

Important anomalies include:

- anomalous origin of a coronary artery from the pulmonary artery
- anomalous course of a coronary artery between the aorta and the pulmonary artery
- coronary artery fistulae
- congenital ostial atresia of the left main coronary artery.

ANOMALOUS ORIGIN OF A CORONARY ARTERY FROM THE PULMONARY ARTERY

The most important coronary anomaly is anomalous origin of the left main coronary artery (LMCA) from the pulmonary artery. Anomalous origin of the LMCA from the pulmonary artery (ALCAPA) occurs more frequently than anomalous origin of the right coronary artery (RCA). Anomalous origin of both the LMCA and RCA from the pulmonary artery is very rare and almost uniformly fatal. Infrequently, either the left anterior descending coronary artery (LAD) or the circumflex coronary artery may arise separately from the pulmonary artery. Associated anomalies are uncommon. Without surgical correction, anomalous origin of the LMCA is usually lethal during infancy with a mortality of 90% by 1 year of age.

Children with ALCAPA usually develop symptoms after closure of the ductus arteriosus and the postnatal fall in pulmonary vascular resistance. Before ductal closure, pulmonary artery pressure is elevated, and perfusion of the anomalous coronary artery is maintained. The clinical course after ductal closure is determined largely by the presence or absence of collaterals from the RCA to the left coronary system. If the collaterals are inadequate, myocardial ischemia and ventricular dysfunction result from inadequate perfusion. If the collaterals are adequate, perfusion of the left coronary system is maintained; however, as the pulmonary vascular resistance falls, a significant left-to-right shunt develops from the RCA to the pulmonary artery with progressive dilatation of the RCA and left coronary systems. Children with significant collaterals may survive past infancy, but they usually develop progressive left ventricular dysfunction. Severe mitral regurgitation is often present secondary to papillary muscle dysfunction and ventricular dilation.

The origin of the anomalous LMCA may be located almost anywhere on the main pulmonary artery or branch pulmonary arteries (**Figure 63.1a-c**). Most commonly, the anomalous

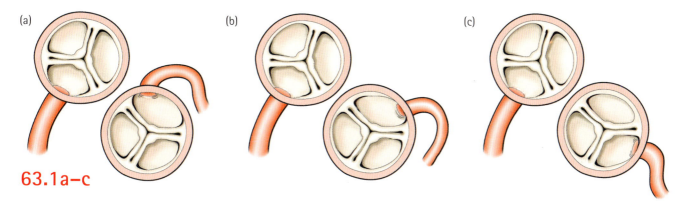

(a)　　　　　(b)　　　　　(c)

63.1a–c

LMCA originates from the rightward posterior sinus (facing) of the pulmonary artery; however, the anomalous coronary may originate from the left or posterior (non-facing) or, rarely, from the anterior (facing) sinus of the main pulmonary artery. An anomalous RCA most commonly originates from the anterior portion of the pulmonary artery.

The first successful surgical therapy for ALCAPA was simple ligation of the anomalous artery. Ligation prevents the left-to-right shunt and allows perfusion of the left ventricle through collaterals from the RCA. However, because of concern over early mortality and an increased risk of late sudden death, a variety of techniques were developed to create a dual coronary artery system, including bypass grafting with the left subclavian artery, the internal mammary artery, and saphenous vein. Takeuchi and associates described creation of an aortopulmonary window and intrapulmonary artery baffle using a flap of pulmonary artery to direct blood from the aorta to the anomalous coronary. In recent years, direct reimplantation of the anomalous coronary into the aorta has become the procedure of choice at most centers.

Because of the high mortality associated with medical therapy in these children, surgical intervention is indicated at the time of initial diagnosis. The goal of surgery is restoration of a two-coronary system. Severe left ventricular dysfunction and mitral insufficiency are not contraindications to revascularization in infants because significant recovery usually occurs. Mitral valve repair is rarely indicated at the time of the initial procedure. Even if severe mitral regurgitation is present preoperatively, the severity of mitral regurgitation almost always improves following reimplantation. In rare occurrences, transplantation may be necessary if ventricular function does not improve after reimplantation.

OPERATION

Aortic reimplantation

After induction of anesthesia and placement of monitoring lines, the chest is prepped and draped. A median sternotomy is performed, and the thymus is resected. The pericardium is opened and suspended with stay sutures. Because the left ventricle is usually dilated with significant dysfunction secondary to myocardial ischemia and mitral regurgitation, contact with the myocardium should be minimized until the patient is placed on cardiopulmonary bypass (CPB) to avoid ventricular fibrillation.

The aortic pursestring suture is placed distally, near the innominate artery, and a pursestring suture is placed in the right atrial appendage (**Figure 63.2**). Heparin is administered, the aorta is cannulated, a single right atrial cannula is inserted, and CPB is initiated. The operation may be performed using either continuous low-flow CPB with moderate hypothermia (25–30 °C) or deep hypothermic circulatory arrest (18 °C) in very small infants. A left ventricular vent should be placed via the right superior pulmonary vein to decompress the dilated left ventricle.

The pulmonary artery is mobilized, and the epicardial course of the left coronary artery is carefully inspected. If the anomalous coronary originates far to the left or anteriorly on the pulmonary artery, direct reimplantation may not be possible. The aorta is fully mobilized, as are the right and left pulmonary arteries. The ligamentum arteriosum is ligated and divided to improve mobility of the pulmonary artery. Tourniquets are placed around the right and left branch pulmonary arteries.

A cannula is placed in the ascending aorta for administration of cardioplegia solution (**Figure 63.3**). The aorta is

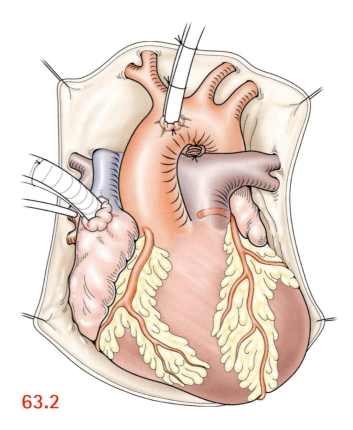

63.2

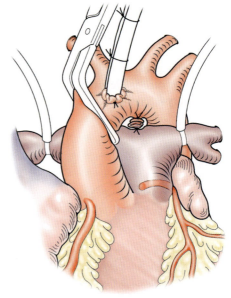

63.3

cross-clamped, and cold cardioplegia solution is administered via the aortic root. Occlusion of the branch pulmonary arteries with tourniquets prevents run-off of cardioplegic solution into the lungs. Alternatively, the ostium of the coronary artery may be compressed and occluded.

The pulmonary artery is opened transversely immediately above the sinotubular junction. The orifice of the anomalous coronary is identified, and the pulmonary artery is divided. The coronary ostium is excised from the pulmonary artery, as in the arterial switch operation, with a generous button of arterial wall. If the coronary ostium is located near a commissure, takedown of the commissure may be necessary to excise the coronary button. The excised pulmonary artery wall allows extension of the proximal end of the coronary, so that the anastomosis can be constructed without tension. The proximal portion of the coronary artery is mobilized using cautery, with care being taken to avoid small branches (**Figure 63.4**).

If the anomalous coronary arises anteriorly from the pulmonary artery, a portion of the pulmonary artery wall may be excised and used to create a tubular extension of the coronary artery (**Figure 63.5**).

The aorta is opened transversely just above the sinotubular junction (**Figure 63.6a**). The incision is carried posteriorly above the left posterior sinus. The sinus is incised vertically to accept the coronary button. The coronary button is carefully aligned with the incision in the aorta to avoid twisting or kinking. Alternatively, a medially based trapdoor incision may be performed as in the arterial switch operation to reduce tension on the anastomosis.

The anastomosis begins at the most inferior aspect of the coronary button, which is attached to the most inferior portion of the incision in the sinus with a continuous suture of

7-0 Prolene. The suture line is carried to the top of the incision anteriorly and posteriorly (**Figure 63.6b**). The aorta is closed with a continuous suture of 7-0 Prolene, which is tied to the coronary button suture as the anastomosis is

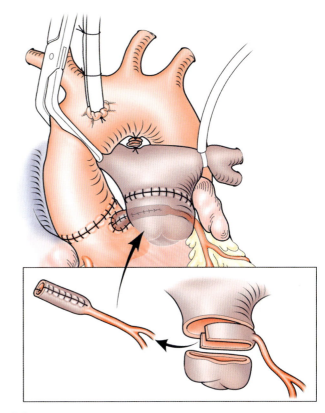

63.5

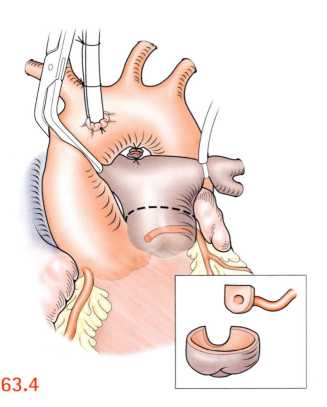

63.4

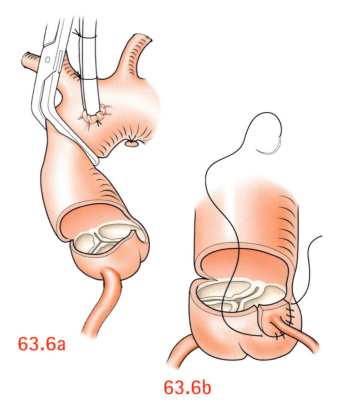

63.6a

63.6b

completed. After completion of aortic closure, cardioplegic solution is administered via the aorta root. The anastomosis is inspected to insure adequate filling of the coronary artery.

The defect in the pulmonary artery is usually repaired with a patch of autologous pericardium (**Figure 63.7**). The reconstructed proximal pulmonary artery is then anastomosed to the distal pulmonary artery confluence with a continuous suture of 7-0 Prolene. Occasionally, the pulmonary artery may be repaired with a direct anastomosis of the proximal pulmonary artery to the distal pulmonary artery confluence. If a commissure was taken down during excision of the coronary button, the pulmonary artery should be reconstructed with pericardium and the commissure resuspended. The aortic cross-clamp is removed, and the patient is rewarmed. If preferred, the cross-clamp may be removed before pulmonary artery reconstruction to decrease the ischemic time.

At the end of the procedure, the left ventricle is inspected to assess perfusion and function. The suture lines are inspected for hemostasis. Right and left atrial lines are inserted for pressure monitoring and drug administration. Atrial and ventricular pacing wires are also placed. After full rewarming, the patient is separated from CPB, and modified ultrafiltration is performed. The electrocardiogram should be monitored during reperfusion and after separation from bypass for evidence of ischemia. Temporary inotropic support is often necessary in infants or children with severe preoperative left ventricular dysfunction. Support with a left ventricular assist device or extracorporeal membrane oxygenation may occasionally be necessary in the postoperative period.

Modified Takeuchi repair

An alternative method for repair of ALCAPA is the intrapulmonary artery tunnel or Takeuchi repair. In the original repair, an aortopulmonary window was created, and a portion of the anterior pulmonary wall was used to create a baffle directing blood from the aorta to the ostium of the anomalous coronary. In the modified repair, the baffle is constructed with a polytetrafluoroethylene (Gore-Tex®) patch. This technique may be particularly useful if the origin of the coronary artery is located leftward on the pulmonary artery. Creation of a baffle may not be possible if the ostium is located near a commissure or arises from a branch pulmonary artery. Complications of the Takeuchi repair include baffle obstruction, baffle leaks, and supravalvar right ventricular outflow tract obstruction.

The modified Takeuchi repair may be performed with either continuous low-flow CPB (25–30 °C) or deep hypothermic circulatory arrest (18 °C). Cannulation is performed as for direct reimplantation, with a left ventricular vent to decompress the ventricle. Cardioplegia is administered via the aortic root with occlusion of the branch pulmonary arteries. After cardioplegic arrest of the heart, an anterior longitudinal pulmonary arteriotomy is performed. The ostium of the aberrant coronary artery is identified (**Figure 63.8**).

Using a punch, a 5 mm diameter opening is made in the aorta above the sinotubular junction, on the leftward aspect of the aorta. If any question exists concerning placement of the aortic opening, an anterior aortotomy should be performed, and the punch hole should be performed under direct vision

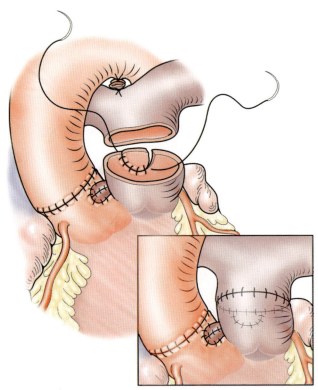

63.7

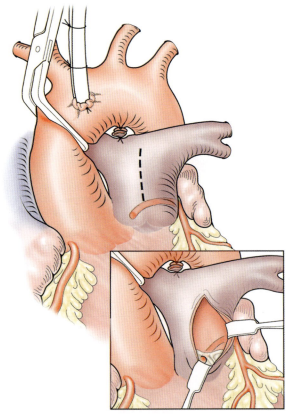

63.8

to avoid damage to the aortic valve. Placement of the aortopulmonary window above the sinotubular junction allows the baffle to angle downward into the sinus if the coronary ostium is located deep within the sinus (**Figure 63.9**).

A similar punch hole is made in the pulmonary artery directly opposite the punch hole in the aorta, and an aortopulmonary window is created with a continuous suture of 7-0 Prolene (**Figure 63.10**).

A 4 mm polytetrafluoroethylene (PTFE) graft is split longitudinally and tailored to an appropriate length. This graft is used to create an intrapulmonary tunnel, baffling

blood from the aortopulmonary window to the coronary ostium. The suture line begins at the coronary ostium and is continued inferiorly along the pulmonary artery wall to the aortopulmonary window. The suture line is completed by starting again at the coronary artery ostium and completing the superior portion of the baffle (**Figure 63.11**).

After creation of the baffle, the pulmonary artery should be repaired with a patched autologous pericardium to avoid supravalvar right ventricular outflow tract obstruction (**Figure 63.12**). The cross-clamp is removed, and the patient

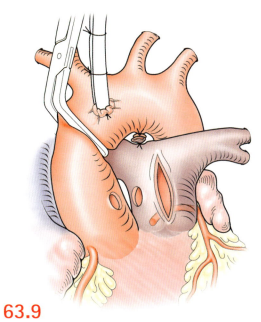

63.9

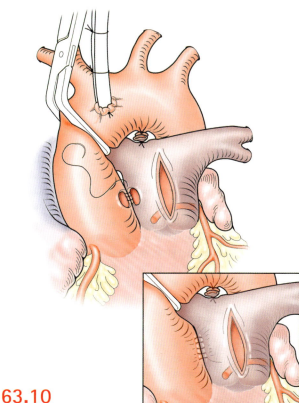

63.10

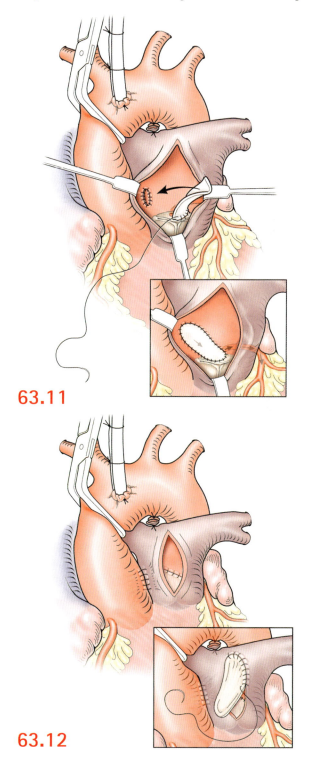

63.11

63.12

is rewarmed. Monitoring lines are inserted, and the patient is separated from CPB as after direct reimplantation.

Additional procedures for anomalous origin of a coronary artery from the PA

Coronary bypass grafting with the left subclavian artery, saphenous vein, or left internal mammary artery has been used for treatment of ALCAPA. The most common indication for use of a left internal mammary artery graft is creation of a dual coronary system after a previous ligation or because of stenosis or occlusion after a previous attempt at repair. Because of the risk of occlusion and poor long-term results, saphenous vein should be used only if no other conduit is available.

If anomalous origin of the LAD is present, excision of the ostium of the coronary artery with a portion of the pulmonary artery may be possible to create a tube graft to elongate the coronary artery for implantation. However, as the origin of the LAD is frequently anterior on the pulmonary artery, this maneuver may be difficult. The reimplanted artery may drape over the pulmonary artery and is at increased risk of occlusion. An alternative procedure is ligation with left internal mammary artery grafting. Isolated origin of the left circumflex coronary artery from the pulmonary artery is rare, and the optimal therapy (ligation or reimplantation) is not known. In patients with anomalous origin of the RCA from the pulmonary artery, the coronary artery usually arises anteriorly from the pulmonary artery and direct reimplantation is the treatment of choice.

ANOMALOUS COURSE OF A CORONARY ARTERY BETWEEN THE AORTA AND PULMONARY ARTERY

Anomalous course of a coronary artery between the aorta and the pulmonary artery occurs when the RCA or LMCA arises from a separate ostium in or above the opposite sinus and courses between the great vessels. An anomalous course also occurs when a single coronary arises from or above the right aortic sinus and the LMCA or LAD passes between the great vessels or when a single coronary arises from or above the left aortic sinus and the RCA courses between the great vessels. The anomalous LMCA or LAD course between the two great vessels should be distinguished from those that course within the ventricular septum caudad to the pulmonary valve. This is important because the latter is generally benign and is managed quite differently from those with an interarterial course. This section will focus solely on the course between the aorta and pulmonary artery.

When two ostia are present in the same sinus, the ostium of the anomalous coronary artery is frequently elliptical and slit-like. Anomalous course of a coronary artery between the aorta and pulmonary artery is associated with a high incidence of sudden death, particularly with exercise. This risk is significantly higher in those with anomalous aortic origin of the LMCA from the right sinus compared to the anomalous RCA from the left. These patients are often asymptomatic until an episode of syncope or sudden cardiac death. The incidence and natural history of anomalous course of a coronary artery between the great vessels are unknown. Surgical intervention is indicated in any patient with angina, syncope, or sudden death who is found to have an anomalous course of the coronary between the great vessels. The indications for surgery in asymptomatic patients have not been defined.

When two ostia are present, repair of this defect consists of enlargement and remodeling of the anomalous ostium to prevent compression between the great vessels

and to relieve the ostial obstruction. Bypass grafting may not be successful as normal flow usually is present in the coronary artery; therefore an increased risk of poor flow and occlusion in the graft exists secondary to competitive flow. However, when a single coronary artery exists and the LMCA or RCA courses between the great vessels, relief of obstruction by reimplantation or remodeling of the ostium may not be possible, and bypass grafting may be the only therapeutic option.

OPERATION

Remodeling of abnormal ostium

A median sternotomy is performed, the pericardium is opened, and the anatomy is inspected. The aorta is cannulated near the innominate artery, and a two-stage venous cannula is inserted via the right atrial appendage. CPB with moderate hypothermia is instituted, and a left ventricular vent is placed in the right superior pulmonary vein. A cannula for administration of cardioplegia solution is placed in the ascending aorta. The aorta is cross-clamped, and cold cardioplegia solution is administered.

After an adequate arrest is obtained, a transverse aortotomy is performed, and the coronary ostia are identified. The origin of the anomalous coronary is usually small and slit-like. Because the anomalous coronary usually arises from the opposite sinus, detachment of the aortic valve commissure may be necessary to remodel and enlarge the ostium (**Figure 63.13 a and b**).

After detachment of the commissure, the slit-like ostium is opened along the longitudinal axis of the coronary artery, and a portion of the common wall between the aorta and coronary is excised (**Figure 63.13c**). The intimal surfaces are

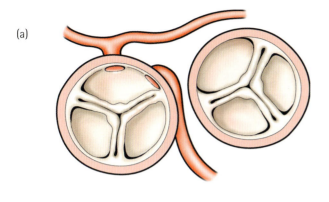

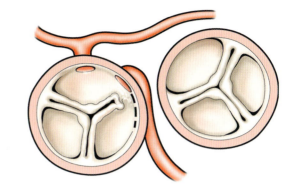

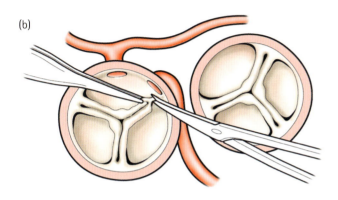

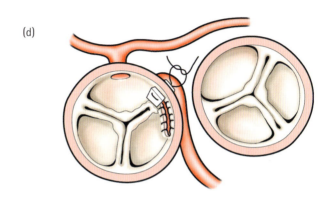

63.13a–d

approximated with sutures of 7-0 or 8-0 Prolene. The aortic valve commissure is resuspended with a pledgeted suture (**Figure 63.13d**). The aortotomy is repaired. The cross-clamp is removed after de-airing, and the patient is rewarmed.

The electrocardiogram is monitored for signs of ischemia. Monitoring lines are inserted. The patient is separated from CPB in the usual fashion.

CORONARY ARTERY FISTULAE

A coronary artery fistula is a communication between a coronary artery and a cardiac chamber, the coronary sinus, the venae cavae, a pulmonary artery, or a pulmonary vein. Coronary artery fistulae may arise from the right or left coronary artery. The most common sites of termination are the right ventricle and the right atrium. Most fistulae arise from a coronary artery with an otherwise normal distribution; they may arise in the midportion of the vessel with a normal vessel continuing past the origin or they may arise at the most distal portion of the vessel as an end artery.

Most patients with coronary fistulae are asymptomatic, and the fistula is discovered during an evaluation for a murmur. Rarely, the fistula may "steal" flow from the coronary circulation. The natural history of coronary fistulae has not been fully delineated but fistulae are most likely present early in life and gradually increase in size. All patients with symptomatic fistulae should undergo closure. While patients with very small fistulae may not require surgical closure,

they should be followed because progressive enlargement may occur.

OPERATION

The coronary artery anatomy must be clearly defined before surgical closure and before the operation is individualized. Many fistulae can be closed without the use of CPB and frequently can be ligated or oversewn at their origin or termination. Transcatheter coil embolization has been used for closure in some coronary artery fistulae.

After a median sternotomy, the thymus is resected, and the pericardium is opened. The coronary artery is carefully inspected, and the distribution of the coronary arteries at the site of the enlarged vessel is noted. If the fistula is located at the distal end of a coronary artery and no viable myocardium exists distal to the fistula, the fistula may be closed by ligation without the use of CPB. The ligature is placed around the coronary artery immediately proximal to the fistula, and the fistula is occluded temporarily. The heart is observed for signs of ischemia. If no signs of ischemia are present and myocardial perfusion remains adequate, the ligature is tied (**Figure 63.14a**).

If the fistula arises from the midportion of a coronary artery and the course cannot be fully defined, CPB should be used. The cannula is placed in the ascending aorta, both venae cavae are cannulated, and CPB is initiated. If opening a coronary artery or cardiac chamber is necessary, cardioplegic arrest should be used. The fistula should be compressed during administration of cardioplegia to prevent run-off into the heart. If inadequate arrest is not obtained because of run-off into the fistula, retrograde administration of the cardioplegia solution may be helpful.

A variety of techniques may be used to close the fistula. If the fistula arises from the midportion of the dilated aneurysm of coronary artery, the fistula's communication may be obliterated by placing multiple pledgeted sutures beneath the coronary artery with care being taken to avoid compromising the distal perfusion (**Figure 63.14b**).

Alternatively, the enlarged coronary artery may be opened, and the fistula identified and oversewn from within the coronary artery. The coronary artery is closed primarily (**Figure 63.15**). If distal perfusion of the coronary bed is compromised and the fistula is closed, CABG may be necessary.

If the fistula terminates in the right atrium, right ventricle, or other cardiac chamber, the fistula may be closed directly from within the chamber (**Figure 63.16**).

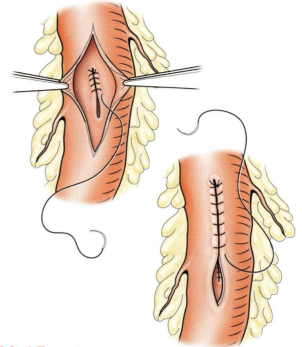

63.15

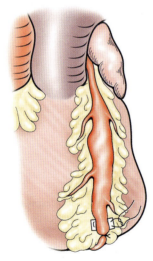

63.14a

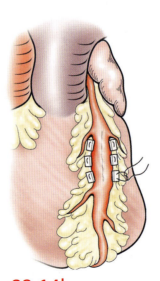

63.14b

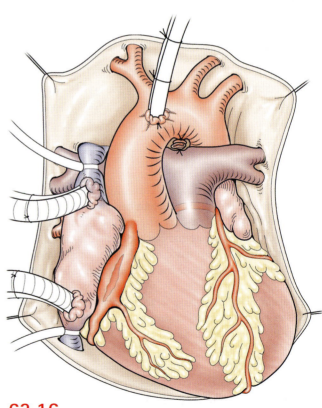

63.16

A right atriotomy is performed, and the termination site of the fistula is identified. Administration of cardioplegia solution may be helpful for localization. The termination site of the fistula may be closed primarily or with a pericardial patch (**Figure 63.17a and b**).

After complete closure of the fistula, the cross-clamp is removed. The patient is rewarmed. The electrocardiogram is monitored for signs of ischemia. Intraoperative echocardiography may be helpful to assess myocardial function and to document closure of the fistula.

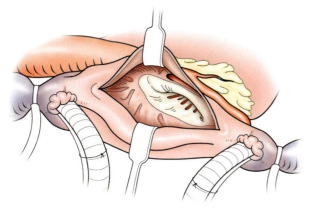

63.17a

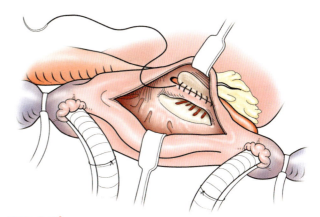

63.17b

CONGENITAL OSTIAL ATRESIA OF THE LEFT MAIN CORONARY ARTERY

Congenital atresia of the LMCA ostium is a rare congenital coronary anomaly with less than 50 cases reported in the literature. In this disease, there is no LMCA ostium; the LAD and circumflex coronary arteries, which are located in the correct position, end blindly and receive blood flow solely retrograde through the RCA, usually through at least one collateral vessel. However, these collateral vessels are generally inadequate to perfuse the left side of the heart and these patients are almost always symptomatic. Left main ostial atresia usually occurs alone; however, there have been associations noted with supravalvar aortic stenosis, VSD with pulmonic stenosis, right coronary ostial stenosis, and PDA and aortic regurgitation.

Clinically, there appear to be early-, middle-, and late-onset presentations with this congenital coronary anomaly. Nearly every patient reported in the literature was symptomatic, irrespective of age at presentation. The infants and toddlers generally present with clinical signs and symptoms similar to ALCAPA or dilated cardiomyopathy, including feeding difficulty, failure to thrive, emesis, and dyspnea. The older children and adolescents tend to present with syncope, dyspnea, angina, and ventricular tachyarrhythmias. The adults are likely to have dyspnea and angina. Sudden death may be the first presentation at any age.

SURGICAL MANAGEMENT

Because of the high risk of sudden death with ostial atresia of the LMCA, surgery should occur once the diagnosis is made. Coronary artery bypass grafting (CABG) is generally what has been described in the literature for both children and adults. Recently, however, there have been reports of surgical revascularization to create a dual coronary artery system, with the belief that, like patients with ALCAPA, long-term outcomes should be improved. This is especially important in children and young adults where the longevity of the bypass graft is of concern.

A few slightly different surgical techniques have been described for the creation of a dual coronary artery system. First, an autologous pericardial patch repair can been used to attain surgical revascularization. Under CPB, the aorta is transected, locating a dimple where the normal left coronary ostium should be. The aorta is incised vertically to the location of the ostium and the incision extended down the LMCA ending before the bifurcation into the LAD and circumflex coronary arteries. If there is an atretic membrane, it is removed. An autologous pericardial or homograft patch is then used to reconstruct the atretic LMCA ostium.

A second method is the enlargement of the LMCA and creation of a "funnel-shaped" neo-ostium. In this technique, after standard CPB, hot-induction blood cardioplegia, followed by cold-blood cardioplegia, and warm reperfusion are used to help attain myocardial preservation. To visualize the aortic root and left coronary artery system, the main PA is transected. The aortic incision begins on the anterior portion of the aortic root, extending toward the coronary orifice and beyond the atretic portion. Then, the two incisions (aortic and coronary) are connected using an onlay patch, consisting of saphenous vein, autologous pericardium, or PTFE. This patch not only enlarges the LMCA but also extends onto the portion of the aorta that was incised, creating a "funnel-shaped" neo-ostium.

Third, homograft patch ostioplasty may be used in the treatment of LMCA ostial atresia (**Figure 63.18a and b**). Bicaval cannulation is used and CPB established. After identifying the blind-ending LMCA on the surface of the heart, an incision is made in the aortic wall, directed inferiorly to the aortic sinus; an incision is then made in the LMCA until its division into LAD and circumflex coronary arteries. The ostium is then enlarged using a pulmonary homograft patch that also joins the aortic sinus to the proximal LMCA. Alternatively, the blind-ending LMCA can be sewn onto the posterior aortic wall with anterior augmentation. Confirmation of coronary patency should be achieved using coronary probes and with evidence of back bleeding. The aortotomy is closed and the patient is removed from bypass.

OUTCOMES FOLLOWING REPAIR OF CORONARY ANOMALIES

Outcomes following surgical repair of anomalous coronary artery arising from the pulmonary arteries have improved significantly, even in patients with significant left ventricular dysfunction and mitral regurgitation. Overall survival is greater than 90%. Mitral valve repair is rarely necessary, even in patients with significant preoperative mitral regurgitation. There are few data available on the long-term outcome in these patients, particularly in terms of left ventricular function and late mortality. The existing data, however, suggest that establishment of a two-coronary system is associated with improved survival and improved left ventricular function compared to simple ligation of the anomalous artery.

Operative mortality for repair of a coronary with an anomalous course between the aorta and the pulmonary artery is low. However, there are few data on the long-term prognosis for these patients. It is unclear if these reconstructive techniques reduce the incidence of syncope and sudden cardiac death. Mortality following surgery after closure of coronary artery fistulae is low with a low incidence of recurrence and excellent long-term outcome. No long-term data are available for operative mortality of LMCA coronary atresia. However, if the anomaly is recognized early and the patient has enough collateral vessels, short-term results are encouraging after surgical revascularization, notably with those procedures that establish a dual coronary system.

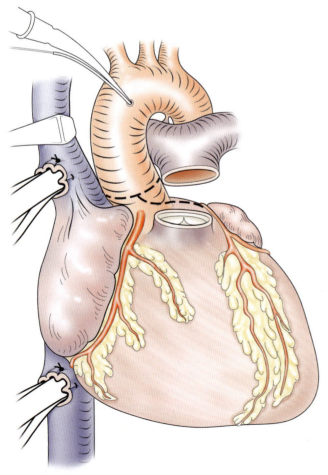

63.18a

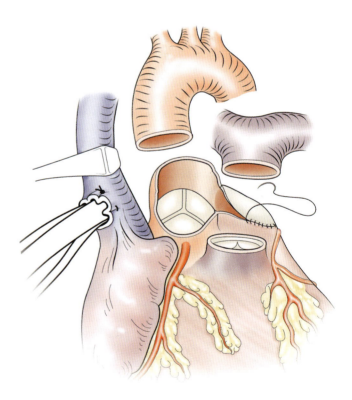

63.18b

FURTHER READING

Backer CL, Stout MJ, Zales VR, et al. Anomalous origin of the left coronary artery: a twenty-year review of surgical management. *J Thorac Cardiovasc Surg.* 1992; 103: 1049.

Davis JT, Allen HD, Wheeler JJ, et al. Coronary artery fistula in the pediatric age group: a 19-year institutional experience. *Ann Thorac Surg.* 1994; 58: 760.

Gaynor JW. Coronary artery anomalies in children. In: Kaiser LR, Kron IL, Spray TL (eds). *Mastery of cardiothoracic surgery.* Boston: Little, Brown and Company; 1998.

Kaczorowski DJ, Sathanandam S, Ravishankar C, et al. Coronary ostioplasty for congenital atresia of the left main coronary artery ostium. *Ann Thorac Surg.* 2012; 94: 1307.

Rinaldi RG, Carballido J, Giles R, et al. Right coronary artery with anomalous origin and slit ostium. *Ann Thorac Surg.* 1994; 58: 828.

Turley K, Szarnick RJ, Flachsbart KD, et al. Aortic implantation is possible in all cases of anomalous origin of the left coronary artery from the pulmonary artery. *Ann Thorac Surg.* 1995; 60: 84.

Vouhé PR, Tamisier D, Sidi D, et al. Anomalous left coronary artery from the pulmonary artery: results of isolated aortic reimplantation. *Ann Thorac Surg.* 1992; 54: 621.

64

Cardiac transplantation for congenital heart disease

JAMES A. QUINTESSENZA

BACKGROUND

Excellent results can be expected after cardiac transplantation for children and adults with congenital heart disease.[1] In order to achieve these excellent results in recipients with complex cardiac anatomy, the surgical team must have a variety of specific technical strategies available in their armamentarium.[2-9] This chapter will review the technical strategies that may be necessary for successful cardiac transplantation in those recipients.

Recipients with complex cardiac anatomy can be categorized into the following groups:

1. Abnormalities of systemic or pulmonary venous return
2. Abnormalities of the sidedness of the atrial chambers, or, in other words, the atrial "situs"
3. Abnormalities of the relationship of the great arteries (including transposition of the great arteries, malposition of the great arteries, and previous Lecompte maneuver)
4. Abnormalities of the main or branch pulmonary arteries (including hypoplasia, discontinuity, and anatomy altered by previous surgical and transcatheter interventions)
5. Abnormalities of the ascending aorta and aortic arch (including hypoplasia and interruption)
6. Abnormalities of the orientation of the ventricular mass (including dextrocardia, dextroversion, mesocardia, mesoversion)
7. Abnormalities secondary to previous operations that have altered the pathways of systemic venous return, pulmonary venous return, and/or pulmonary arterial anatomy (including previous superior cavopulmonary anastomosis(es), previous Fontan operations, previous atrial switch operations, previous arterial switch operations, and previous double-switch operations).

A variety of technical strategies designed to facilitate cardiac transplantation in these groups of patients are reviewed below.

TECHNICAL STRATEGIES

Organ procurement for the recipient with complex cardiac anatomy

Planning and communication between procuring surgeon, implanting surgeon, anesthesia, and the other organ-procuring teams is crucial. The location of the arterial line and central line in the organ donor is important. Femoral lines may be the best choice.

For recipients with a left superior vena cava (SVC), procurement includes the entire innominate vein, with parts of the left and right internal jugular veins, as necessary. The pulmonary arteries may be procured from hilum to hilum. This strategy will impact potential lung procurement.

The entire aortic arch may be procured. This dissection is enhanced by division of the donor innominate vein (if it is not needed for subsequent reconstruction), ligamentum arteriosum, as well as the brachiocephalic vessels, all prior to cross-clamping (**Figure 64.1**).

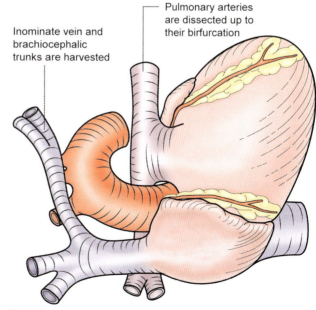

Inominate vein and brachiocephalic trunks are harvested

Pulmonary arteries are dissected up to their birfurcation

64.1

Surgical procedure – recipient

As always, careful induction of anesthesia is carried out with specifics related to the individual patient characteristics. Commonly these are reoperative patients with dilated hearts making re-entry sternotomy quite challenging. Preoperative imaging with MRI or CT scan is useful and a specific plan for re-entry is established. Prior to the initial skin incision, it is essential to ascertain what sites for arterial and venous cannulation are available and what specific method of peripheral institution of bypass is to be used, should the need arise. Thoughtful planning will optimize institution of emergent or semi-elective cardiopulmonary bypass (CPB) during re-entry. At times, this is a critical and life-saving process. The dissection of the recipient heart and necessary structures to be reconstructed should be carried out in a well-planned and meticulous manner.

Frequent communication between the harvesting and implanting team is needed to keep the process coordinated. Unexpected issues with the donor or recipient need to be discussed. The timing of organ arrival should be coordinated so that donor heart cold ischemic time as well as recipient operative and CPB times are minimized.

Abnormalities of systemic or pulmonary venous return

For recipients with an isolated left SVC, the donor innominate vein is anastomosed to the left SVC (**Figure 64.2**). Similarly, for patients with bilateral SVC anastomosis, the donor internal jugular and innominate vein is used (**Figure 64.3**). The neoaorta connection is kept short to minimize tension within the venous structures. For isolated left inferior vena cava (IVC), a generous portion of recipient right atrium is left attached to the recipient IVC. These recipient structures are mobilized toward the midline, and the extra

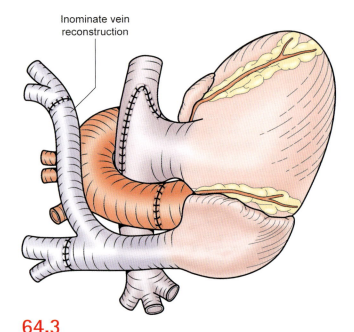

Inominate vein reconstruction

64.3

right atrial tissue can be used to create a tension-free connection to the donor heart. Abnormal hepatic venous drainage can be reconstructed by utilizing a common patch of atrium containing the IVC and the isolated hepatic veins using this extra tissue to create a tension-free connection, similar to isolated left IVC.

For extracardiac anomalous pulmonary venous connections,[10] the recipient pulmonary venous confluence is filleted open. The donor left atriotomy is modified to match the recipient pulmonary venous opening. Utilizing the original pulmonary venous openings or creating new ones as needed, the recipient pulmonary venous confluence is anastomosed to the created donor left atriotomy.

Abnormalities of the sided-ness of the atrial chambers or atrial "situs" including "situs inversus totalis"[11]

As stated by Montalvo and Bailey,[9] the "key in situs inversus is to position all anastomoses toward the midline." Generally, a malpositioned aorta can be mobilized and anastomosed to the normally related donor aorta. The donor pulmonary artery can be anastomosed to the undersurface of the recipient left or right pulmonary artery as needed. If this technique is used, the main pulmonary artery of the recipient is oversewn and the undersurface of the branch pulmonary arteries of the recipient is opened longitudinally to receive the donor main pulmonary artery. The left SVC and left IVC are reconstructed as they are when found in isolated cases (**Figure 64.4**). Generous opening of the pericardium, avoiding the phrenic nerve, is often helpful to accommodate the normal donor levocardic orientation.

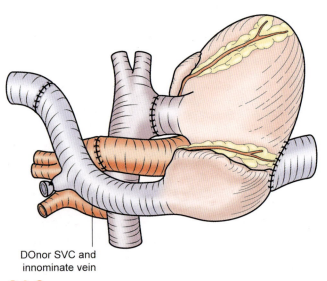

DOnor SVC and innominate vein

64.2

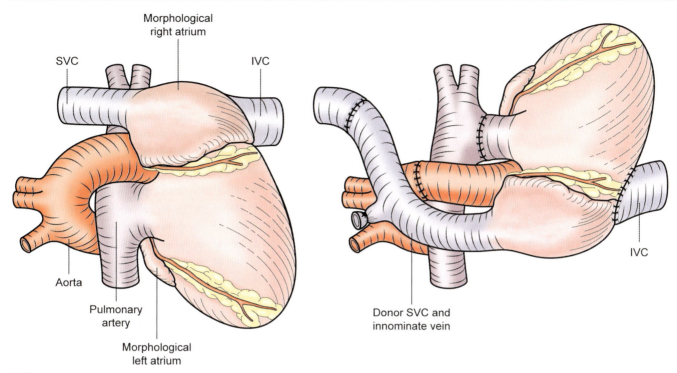

SVC

Morphological
right atrium

IVC

Aorta

Pulmonary
artery

Morphological
left atrium

Donor SVC and
innominate vein

IVC

64.4

Abnormalities of the relationship of the great arteries (including transposition of the great arteries, malposition of the great arteries, and previous Lecompte maneuver)

With abnormal relationships of the great arteries, reconstruction is similar to situs inversus. Generally, a malpositioned aorta can be mobilized and anastomosed to the normally related donor aorta. The donor pulmonary artery can be anastomosed to the undersurface of the recipient left or right pulmonary artery as needed.

Taking down a Lecompte maneuver can be accomplished by dividing the pulmonary and aortic trunks and relocating the pulmonary artery back to its normal position. Donor pulmonary artery can be used to facilitate the reconstruction.

Abnormalities of the main or branch pulmonary arteries (including hypoplasia, discontinuity, and anatomy altered by previous surgical and transcatheter interventions)

The technique of recipient pulmonary arterial reconstruction can vary from using the donor pulmonary artery to perform patch arterioplasty on a segment of the intrapericardial portion of the pulmonary artery to replacing the entire recipient intrapericardial pulmonary artery with donor branch pulmonary arteries. When the entire intrapericardial pulmonary arterial branches need replacement

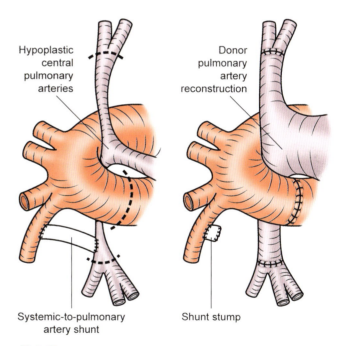

Hypoplastic
central
pulmonary
arteries

Donor
pulmonary
artery
reconstruction

Systemic-to-pulmonary
artery shunt

Shunt stump

64.5a

or reconstruction, it is usually best accomplished by procuring the donor pulmonary branches from hilum to hilum (**Figure 64.5a**). This requires careful planning and discussions with all involved so that competition for the intrapericardial pulmonary artery by a lung procurement team will not be an issue. When simultaneous lung procurement results in the non-availability of branch pulmonary arteries for the cardiac transplant team, an alternative method such as onlay patching of the branch pulmonary arteries can be utilized (**Figure 64.5b**).

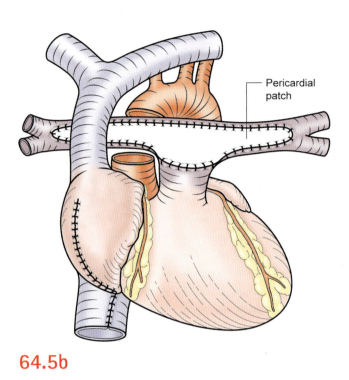

Pericardial patch

64.5b

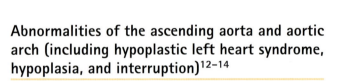

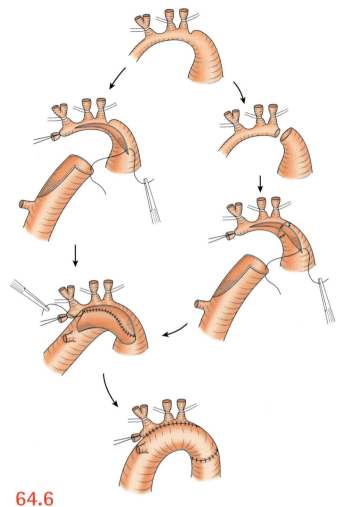

64.6

Abnormalities of the ascending aorta and aortic arch (including hypoplastic left heart syndrome, hypoplasia, and interruption)[12–14]

In neonates with hypoplastic left heart syndrome (HLHS), a diminutive ascending aorta requires establishing CPB with pulmonary arterial cannulation and systemic perfusion through duct. Pulmonary arterial run-off is controlled with a tourniquet around the duct or the branch pulmonary arteries.

Arch reconstruction can be performed with a short period of circulatory arrest or with continuous antegrade cerebral perfusion (either via a cannula advanced into a carotid artery or via a temporary shunt sewn to the innominate artery). A generous incision in the recipient ascending aorta extends across the transverse arch and down into the descending aorta. This incision extends distally to beyond the recipient's first intercostal artery takeoff, to minimize ductal constriction and subsequent coarctation. The undersurface of the aortic arch is reconstructed with a generous tongue of donor aorta arch (**Figure 64.6**). Patients with less severe forms of aortic hypoplasia, coarctation and interruption are reconstructed with modifications of the above technique as needed.

Abnormalities of the orientation of the ventricular mass (including dextrocardia, dextroversion, mesocardia, mesoversion)

Unilateral or bilateral pericardial release will create space for the cardiac mass and cardiac apex. Great care must be taken to identify and avoid the phrenic nerve(s).

Abnormalities secondary to previous operations that have altered the pathways of systemic venous return, pulmonary venous return, and/or pulmonary arterial anatomy (including previous superior cavopulmonary anastomosis(es), previous Fontan operations, previous atrial switch operations, previous arterial switch operations, and previous double-switch operations)

These cases are very challenging in several domains. Many of the technical strategies mentioned above may be necessary in various combinations. An accurate understanding of the preoperative anatomy is very important. A creative and complex reconstruction will be planned specific to the recipient preoperative anatomy. This plan will determine the specific procurement needs regarding extra tissue to be harvested to yield a successful complex implantation. A typical example is the failed Fontan patient following staged palliation for hypoplastic left heart syndrome (HLHS). Usually, most of the intrapericardial structures are resected and cuffs of tissue are prepared near the pericardial reflection for the SVC, IVC, pulmonary venous confluence, pulmonary arteries just proximal to their branch points, and the previously reconstructed aorta (**Figure 64.7**). The implantation would be on CPB with aortic arterial and bicaval venous cannulation, although circulatory arrest can be utilized if needed or preferred. The sequence of anastomosis would be as follows:

1. left atrium
2. IVC
3. right and left branch pulmonary arteries
4. aorta
5. SVC.

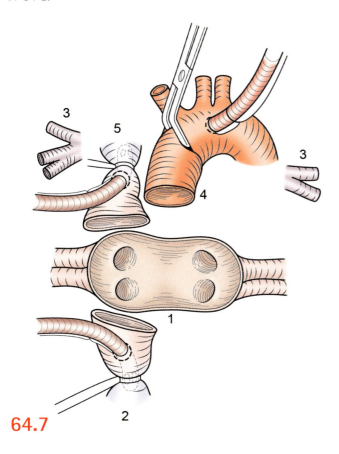

64.7

HEMOSTASIS

Postoperative hemostasis can be very challenging. The age-old adage of "dry in – dry out" is useful but commonly post-bypass coagulopathy and hemorrhage are very problematic. Serious coagulopathies are frequently encountered and aggressive blood product resuscitation is essential. Liberal use of adjuncts such as antifibrinolytics (aminocaproic acid) and recombinant factor seven is encouraged. Often these are very lengthy and difficult procedures performed in the middle of

the night. A team or "multi-surgeon" approach can be very helpful.

SUMMARY

A variety of technical strategies are available to facilitate cardiac transplantation for the recipient with congenital heart disease. A comprehensive working knowledge of these techniques is necessary in order to achieve optimal outcomes. Communication, planning, and excellent teamwork are critical in treating these challenging patients.

REFERENCES

1. Jacobs JP, Asante-Korang A, O'Brien SM, et al. Lessons learned from 119 consecutive cardiac transplants for pediatric and congenital heart disease. *Ann Thorac Surg.* 2011; 91 (4): 1248–55.
2. Mavroudis C, Harrison H, Klein JB, et al. Infant orthotopic cardiac transplantation. *J Thorac Cardiovasc Surg.* 1988; 96(6): 912–24.
3. Jacobs ML, Williams JF. Pediatric heart transplantation. *Cardiol Clin.* 1990; 8(1): 149–57.
4. Allard M, Assaad A, Bailey L, et al. Session IV: Surgical techniques in pediatric heart transplantation. *J Heart Lung Transplant.* 1991; 10(5 Pt 2): 808–27.
5. Backer CL, Zales VR, Idriss FS, et al. Heart transplantation in neonates and in children. *J Heart Lung Transplant.* 1992; 11(2 Pt 1): 311–19.
6. Bailey LL. Heart transplantation techniques in complex congenital heart disease. *J Heart Lung Transplant.* 1993; 12: S168–75.
7. Chiavarelli M, Gundry SR, Razzouk AJ, et al. Operative procedures for infant cardiac transplantation. In: Kapoor AS, Laks H (eds). *Atlas of heart–lung transplantation.* New York: McGraw-Hill; 1994: pp. 75–85.
8. del Nido PJ, Bailey LL, Kirklin JK. Surgical techniques in pediatric heart transplantation. In: Canter CE, Kirklin JK (eds). *ISHLT Monograph Series 2, Pediatric Heart Transplantation.* Philadelphia: Elsevier; 2007: pp. 83–102.
9. Montalvo J, Bailey LL. Operative methods used for heart transplantation in complex univentricular heart disease and variations of atrial situs. *Oper Tech Thorac Cardiovasc Surg.* 2010; 15(2): 172–84.
10. Razzouk AJ, Gundry SR, Chinnock RE, et al. Orthotopic transplantation for total anomalous pulmonary venous connection associated with complex congenital heart disease. *J Heart Lung Transplant.* 1995; 14: 713–17.
11. Vricella LA, Razzouk AJ, Gundry SR, et al. Heart transplantation in infants and children with situs inversus. *J Thorac Cardiovasc Surg.* 1998; 116: 82–9.
12. Bailey L, Concepcion W, Shattuck H, Huang L. Method of heart transplantation for treatment of hypoplastic left heart syndrome. *J Thorac Cardiovasc Surg.* 1986; 92: 1–5.
13. Vricella LA, Razzouk AJ, del Rio M, et al. Heart transplantation for hypoplastic left heart syndrome: modified technique for

reducing circulatory arrest time. *J Heart Lung Transplant.* 1998; 12: 1167–71.

14. Backer CL, Idriss FS, Zales VR, Mavroudis C. Cardiac transplantation for hypoplastic left heart syndrome: a modified technique. *Ann Thorac Surg.* 1990; 50(6): 894–8.

15. Jacobs JP, Quintessenza JA , Soucek RJ, et al. Pediatric cardiac transplantation in children with high panel reactive antibody. *Ann Thorac Surg.* 2004; 78(5): 1703–9.

16. Jacobs JP, Quintessenza JA, Chai PJ, et al. Rescue cardiac transplantation for failing staged palliation in patients with hypoplastic left heart syndrome. *Cardiol Young.* 2006; 16: 556–62.

65

Lung and heart–lung transplantation for congenital heart disease

CHARLES B. HUDDLESTON AND ANDREW C. FIORE

INTRODUCTION

Experimental heart–lung transplantation (HLT) preceded the first clinical success by 25 years. Initial studies in dogs were unsuccessful, probably due to respiratory failure secondary to denervation. Experimental success was achieved by Webb and Lower and in the late 1960s and 1970s, but the first three clinical attempts at HLT made by Cooley and later by Lillehei and Bernard were unsuccessful. The longest survival was for only 23 days, but some patients were able to be extubated and breathe spontaneously, allaying the concern of denervation-induced apnea.

The experimental success of HLT in primates at Stanford coupled with the discovery of cyclosporine as an immunosuppressant led the group at Palo Alto in December 1980 to transplant the heart and lungs into three recipients with pulmonary vascular occlusive disease. Two of them survived beyond 5 years. These patients represented the first long-term lung transplant survivors as clinical isolated lung transplant did not occur until 4 or 5 years later.

HLT transplantation rapidly increased in the 1980s as indications expanded beyond end-stage heart disease with pulmonary vascular occlusive disease to parenchymal lung disease such as cystic fibrosis. While a steep rise in HLT to a level of approximately 250 recipients occurred worldwide in the early 1990s, the numbers have dropped off quite steadily to 50 adult and 8 pediatric (less than 18 years old) HLT in 2009 worldwide. The reasons for this include recognition that cystic fibrosis and idiopathic pulmonary hypertension can be treated with isolated lung transplantation alone. On the other hand, lung transplantation has continued to grow steadily in numbers and now nearly 3000 are performed per year. However, the percentage of lung transplants performed for congenital heart disease remains a very small percentage of the total number.

INDICATIONS

Although cystic fibrosis and chronic obstructive lung disease once made up around one-third of all patients undergoing HLT, these have become a very unusual indication more recently. Idiopathic pulmonary hypertension continues to be a common indication despite of evidence that isolated lung transplantation is suitable. Congenital disease remains the most common indication, with many of these patients having Eisenmenger's syndrome. Isolated lung transplantation has supplanted HLT for cystic fibrosis, obstructive lung disease, and most patients with idiopathic pulmonary hypertension.

The congenital heart disease diagnoses for which HLT has been performed in the past include Eisenmenger's syndrome with associated unrepaired ventricular septal defect (VSD), patent ductus arteriosus (PDA), atrial septal defect (ASD), complete atrioventricular (AV) canal, truncus arteriosus, aortopulmonary window, or any other complex cardiac lesion associated with reversal of shunt flow due to very high pulmonary vascular resistance. It is possible for most of these cardiac lesions to be repaired at the time of isolated lung transplantation. The advantage of this approach is the increased availability of donors and better economical approach to the entire transplant enterprise – two recipients served by a single donor as opposed to one. The disadvantage is the relative complexity of the operation and the potential for left ventricular dysfunction following the intracardiac repair, putting the donor lungs at increased risk for pulmonary edema. Certainly for the non-complex lesions (VSD, ASD, and PDA), isolated lung transplantation with repair of this lesion is the preferred approach at most experienced centers.

Other congenital cardiac lesions for which lung transplantation is performed include pulmonary vein stenosis, severe distal branch pulmonary artery stenosis, and tetralogy of Fallot with pulmonary atresia and associated multiple aortopulmonary collaterals where there is no suitable conventional approach feasible. Isolated lung transplantation with repair of the associated defects and HLT are competing therapies for these entities. The complexity of the repair and the experience of the surgeon dictate which approach is taken at each center. A lesion that requires a very long, complex repair (transposition of the great arteries with VSD, for example) would likely result in a temporary cardiac injury that would make the post-transplant course very risky. Lesions which might result in significant residual valve dysfunction (complete AV canal, for example) might also put the newly transplanted lungs at risk. In both those situations, HLT transplant is probably the better option.

Finally, single ventricle lesions with pulmonary hypertension will definitely require HLT. These patients are particularly challenging, not only technically but also in terms of their management pre- and post-transplant because of the morbidities associated with failing single ventricle circulation.

CONTRAINDICATIONS

The contraindications for isolated lung or heart–lung transplantation include end-stage other organ failure (renal or hepatic), severe neurologic injury, ongoing infection, recently diagnosed malignancy, and a psychosocial evaluation which does not support the commitment necessary for the rigors families must endure for this procedure to be successful.

The issue of previous thoracic operations as a contraindication is somewhat controversial. These patients definitely present technical challenges. There are published reports that suggest no additional risk is imposed by prior operations, however that has certainly not been our experience. Prior operations result in extraordinarily vascular thoracic adhesions in cyanotic patients with pulmonary hypertension. These are very problematic at the time of recipient pneumonectomies. It remains important to carefully evaluate these patients with regard to prior palliative cardiac procedures in the overall assessment of their risks. Performing a heart–lung transplant in a very high risk patient will deprive two other potential recipients of life-saving organ transplants.

The relative complexity of the anatomy is not necessarily a risk factor. Even patients with situs inversus can be successfully transplanted. Prior palliative procedures which alter the anatomy significantly produce challenges, but there are techniques to deal with these variations.

DONOR EVALUATION AND HARVEST

The donor organs individually must meet the same criteria for donation as for isolated heart and lung transplantation. The heart function must be nearly normal on modest inotropic support at most. There should be no significant valvar stenosis or insufficiency. The chest radiograph should be free of significant infiltrates and the arterial PO_2 on oxygen challenge should exceed 350 mmHg. The donor must be free of systemic infection and have no evidence of malignancy. Size matching is often difficult because of the relative malnourished state of recipients with end-stage heart and lung disease. A larger donor may be problematic fitting the organs into the chest of the recipient unless there is significant hyperexpansion of the lungs creating a larger thoracic cavity. Recipients with fibrotic lung diseases typically have contracted chest cavities; one should be very cautious of a larger donor in these instances. The lungs can be trimmed or a lobectomy performed to allow for a better fit in some cases. Smaller donors obviously will fit easily but potentially can suffer hyperexpansion pulmonary edema when the mismatch is significant. In general, one is safe to accept a donor 10% above or below the weight of the recipient with a similar height range. Beyond this very limited range, expansion of the accepted donor size is based upon the recipient characteristics.

The final evaluation of the donor is on-site with flexible bronchoscopy to evaluate the airways for evidence of aspiration or pneumonia as well as looking for other anomalies. A median sternotomy is performed. The donor heart is examined by direct inspection with the chest open. The pleural spaces are opened widely to allow direct visual and tactile examination of the lungs. The trachea is dissected circumferentially between the aorta and the superior vena cava (SVC). Both the SVC and inferior vena cava (IVC) are dissected out. At the appropriate time, heparin is given intravenously and prostaglandin E1 is administered into the main pulmonary artery. The IVC is divided and the left atrial appendage is amputated. This allows complete emptying of the heart. The aorta is cross-clamped and both the heart preservative and lung preservative solutions are delivered via cannulae inserted into the ascending aorta and the main pulmonary artery respectively. Topical cold saline and slush are applied to the organs. A nominal ventilator rate should be maintained throughout this period to enhance the distribution of the pulmoplegia.

For HLT the organs are harvested as a heart–lung bloc. The pericardium is divided down to the diaphragm and posteriorly along the diaphragm. The inferior pulmonary ligaments are divided up to the inferior pulmonary veins on each side. The left lung is flipped medially, effectively out of the pleural space, allowing access to the posterior mediastinum. The pleura there is divided with a knife and the mediastinal contents are bluntly mobilized including the esophagus and descending aorta. A similar procedure is performed in the right pleural space. The aorta is divided at the level of the innominate artery; a longer segment of aorta can be taken if necessary for any reconstructive purposes in the recipient. The trachea is mobilized further and stapled to occlude it distally at least 1 cm above the carina. The lungs should be mildly inflated at low pressure at the time of application of the stapler. It is then divided proximally while occluded with a clamp of some sort. The esophagus is divided with a GIA™ type of stapler proximally and distally. The nasogastric (NG) tube should have been removed and the endotracheal tube pulled back enough to be excluded from the stapling devices. The descending thoracic aorta is divided. The heart–lung bloc can now be removed from the chest and placed in cold solution, usually the cardioplegia solution, and then placed in cold storage for transport.

When retrieving lungs for isolated lung transplantation, the preparation and administration of preservative solution proceeds as noted above. The separation of the heart and lungs is usually done *in situ*. The pulmonary artery is divided at the bifurcation and the left atrium is divided midway between the AV groove and the insertion of the pulmonary veins. The posterior left atrial wall is left with the lung bloc. Once the heart is out of the field the lung retrieval is performed as noted above. The lungs are placed in the pulmonary preservative solution and then into cold storage for transport. When congenital heart disease is the indication, it may be necessary to obtain additional tissue such as more pulmonary artery. This would have to be worked out with the heart retrieval team. The portion of the descending aorta acquired with the mediastinal dissection can also serve as tissue for reconstructive procedures.

RECIPIENT OPERATION

Heart–lung transplant

The incision is a median sternotomy (**Figure 65.1a**). Depending upon the circumstances, as much dissection as possible should be conducted prior to initiating cardiopulmonary bypass (CPB). This includes dissecting out adhesion in each pleural space if present. Care must be taken in preserving the phrenic nerves on each side. The donor lungs will be placed into the pleural spaces posterior to each nerve. At some point it will be necessary to create a wide opening into the pleural space on each side posterior to the phrenic nerve. This may be done in part prior to CPB.

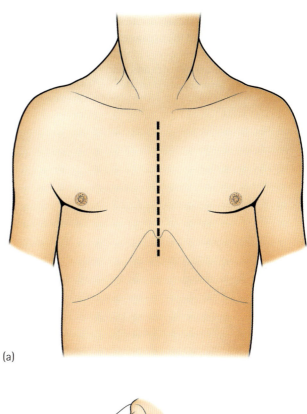

(a)

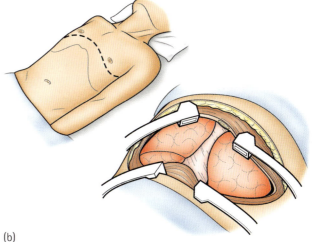

(b)

65.1a, b Initial incisions. (a) For HLT, a median sternotomy incision is employed. This provides excellent exposure for all the dissection necessary including access to the pleural spaces. (b) For isolated lung transplantation, a so-called "clamshell incision" is used. This is a transsternal bilateral anterior thoracotomy incision. It provides better exposure of each hilar region while still allowing for access to the heart for cannulation and performing a cardiac repair should the need arise. In either case, the importance of performing as much dissection as possible prior to initiating cardiopulmonary bypass will pay dividends in obtaining hemostasis.

Bicaval CPB is initiated, cannulating the SVC and IVC relatively distal from the cardiac insertion of each (**Figure 65.2**). The aorta is clamped and the organs excised. The heart comes out first, leaving sufficient aortic length for the anastomosis. The branch pulmonary arteries and veins are merely divided without ligating any vessels near the pericardial reflection (**Figure 65.3**).

Once the heart is out it is a bit easier to create the phrenic nerve pedicles for making the openings into each pleural space (**Figures 65.4 to 65.7**). One should anticipate quite a bit of blood return from the pulmonary veins in those patients with congenital heart disease as extensive aortopulmonary collaterals are the rule. Each lung is dissected out of the pleural space, freeing up the arterial and venous branches from the mediastinum.

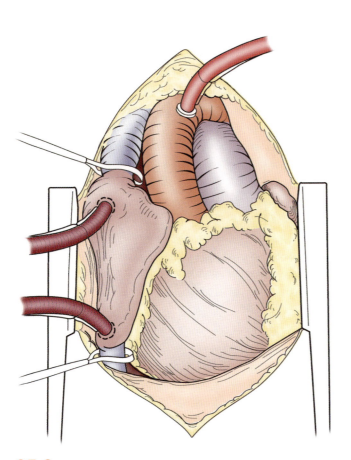

65.2 Cardiopulmonary bypass is achieved using bicaval cannulation, usually cannulating the superior and inferior vena cavae directly. Although bicaval cannulation is not necessary for standard isolated lung transplantation, for those with a diagnosis of congenital heart disease, it is anticipated that an intracardiac repair will be necessary.

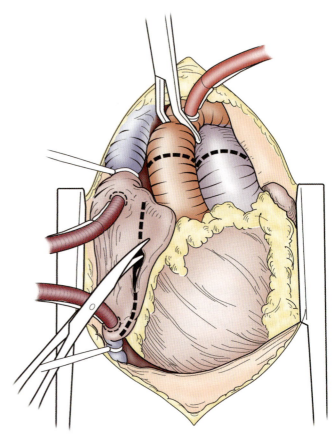

65.3 For HLT once the donor organs have arrived the aorta is cross-clamped and the cardiopneumonectomy is performed, starting with the cardiectomy. The right atrium is incised anteriorly, with this incision carried over the roof of the right atrium. The aorta is transected just above the aortic valve and the pulmonary artery is divided just above the pulmonic valve. The right atrial incision crosses the roof into the left atrium and then this is taken all the way around to the inferior left atrial wall. The atrial septum is divided, taking it down toward the coronary sinus. The inferior portion of the right atrial incision then meets up with this and the heart is removed from the field. The right atrial anastomosis can be either bicaval anastomosis or directly to the right atrium. For bicaval anastomosis, all the excess right atrial tissue is removed leaving sufficient cuff for the caval connections.

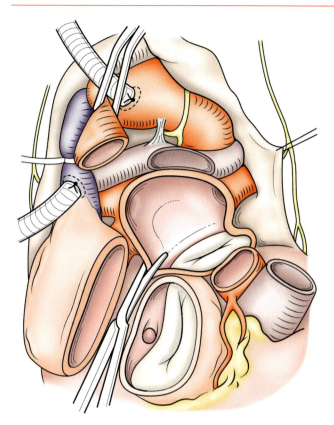

65.4 The posterior left atrial wall is divided in the midline to allow the pericardial dissection of the pulmonary veins, mobilizing both sides back toward the pleural spaces. One should stay close on to the atrial wall to avoid inadvertent injury to the vagus nerves. Some of the right atrium can be excised at this point along with the left atrium on the right.

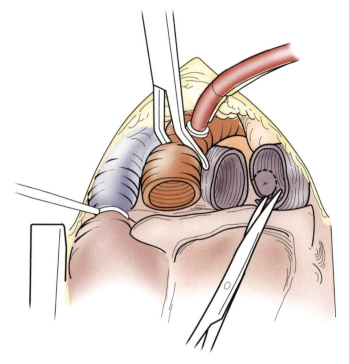

65.5 The pulmonary artery bifurcation is also divided in the midline to excise each pulmonary artery with its respective lung. It is advisable to leave a bit of the pulmonary artery at the insertion of the ligamentum arteriosum to avoid injury to the recurrent laryngeal nerve. The insertion site of the ligamentum is easily identified as a small dimple on the inner aspect of the pulmonary artery bifurcation posteriorly. Both branch pulmonary arteries are then dissected back toward the pleural spaces as was done with the left atrium/pulmonary veins.

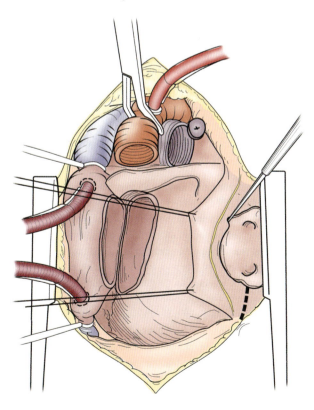

65.6 With the heart out, the left and right lungs are dissected free. Virtually all these patients will have extensive mediastinal and pleural collateral vessels. Liberal use of the electrocautery is necessary to provide hemostasis. The left inferior pulmonary ligament is divided and the hilum is dissected out, freeing up the pulmonary artery and veins from the pleural side, having done that already from the pericardial side. Once all this is accomplished there is a wide opening into the left pleural space from the pericardial space posterior to the phrenic nerve. This can be enlarged further inferiorly to allow ease of passage of the lung from the heart–lung bloc.

To remove the lungs the final step is stapling the bronchus and cutting distal to that (**Figure 65.8**).

At this point, time should be taken to establish hemostasis in the mediastinum and pleural spaces. Bleeding is without doubt one of the major complicating factors in HLT. A focused effort at this point with no organs in the thoracic cavity to obscure the view will save headaches after the implant.

The next step is to identify the location for the tracheal anastomosis. This should be done as distal as possible (**Figure 65.9**).

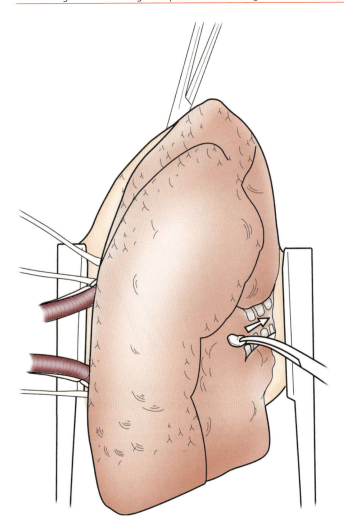

65.7 The left lung is flipped up to allow adequate visualization of the posterior hilum. The posterior bronchus is identified and dissected free. The bronchial arteries may be identified and controlled with hemoclips at this stage.

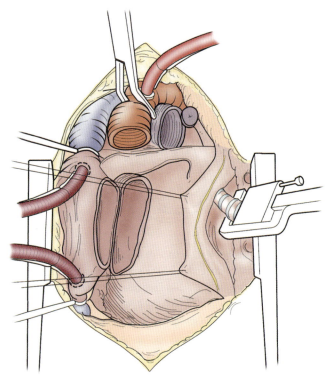

65.8 The left lung is returned to its anatomic location in the chest. The mainstem bronchus is now occluded with a standard TA30 stapling device and the distal bronchus divided. This should allow removal of the left lung from the operative field. Care should be taken to avoid any spillage of bronchial secretions into the chest cavity.

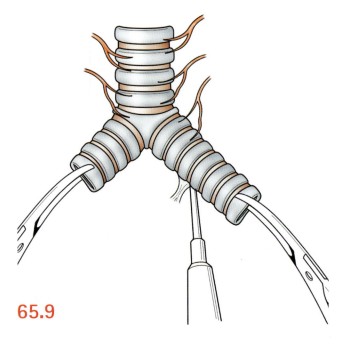

65.9

65.9 Now that the heart and both lungs are out, the trachea is prepared. Both stapled mainstem bronchi are grasped with clamps to allow mobilization to the distal trachea. The right bronchus is dissected out from under the superior vena cava and the left out from under the clamped aorta. Retracting the ascending aorta to the left assists with the exposure at this stage. Anterior and inferior traction on the bronchial stumps allows for adequate exposure of the posterior trachea. Although most of this dissection is done without electrocautery, in fact the vascularity at this point is extensive and hemostasis is paramount. The vagus nerves are primarily at risk for injury. Minimal dissection beyond the distal trachea is necessary, leaving the vascular supply intact. Prior to opening the trachea, some time should be spent assuring hemostasis in the mediastinum and pleural spaces.

Preparation of the heart–lung bloc

The heart–lung bloc is taken out of cold storage at the appropriate time and all excess mediastinal tissue is removed. This includes the portion of esophagus and aorta removed with the organs. The excess pericardium is also removed. The para-tracheal tissue of the donor should be left intact to facilitate post-transplant blood supply to the area of the anastomosis. This comes primarily from coronary artery collaterals. The staple line on the trachea is removed leaving one or two cartilaginous rings above the takeoff of the right mainstem bronchus for the tracheal anastomosis. A culture of the tracheal secretions is taken and all the retained mucous is suctioned with a separate suction device which will be discarded as soon as the tracheal anastomosis is completed (**Figure 65.10**). The amputated left atrial appendage is closed with a pursestring stitch, which is placed on a tourniquet for use during the transplant procedure. A catheter is placed into the left atrium for irrigation using cold saline during the implant.

Preparation of the donor lungs

When isolated lung transplantation is to be performed, the donor lungs are prepared in a similar fashion to the heart–lung bloc. However, each lung is separated by cutting across the posterior wall of the pulmonary artery bifurcation and the posterior wall of the left atrium. Each of these is trimmed back further to accommodate the tissue necessary for the anastomoses. Each bronchus is divided off the trachea to within two cartilaginous rings of the takeoff of the upper lobe bronchus on each side.

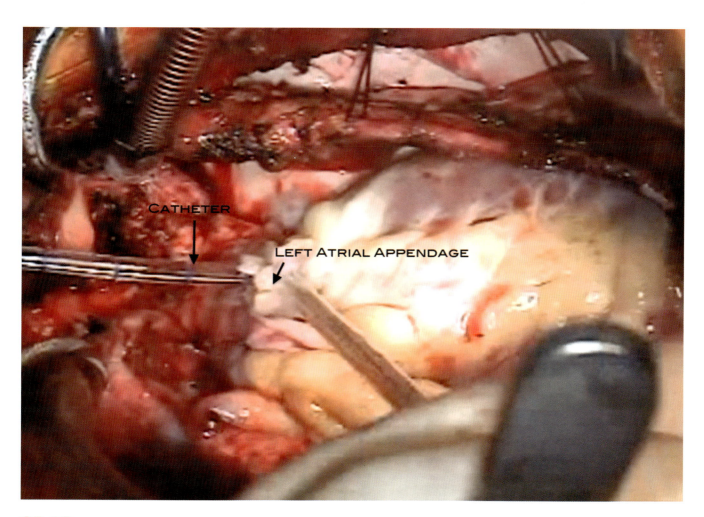

65.10 The heart–lung bloc is then prepared. The mediastinal tissue taken at the retrieval is trimmed away including excess pericardium, the segment of esophagus and descending thoracic aorta, and lymphatic tissue. A pursestring stitch is placed around the previously amputated left atrial appendage; through this a small left ventricular vent is placed for use later. The trachea is trimmed to within one or two cartilaginous rings of the takeoff of the mainstem bronchi. The secretions in the airways are suctioned free and each bronchus is irrigated with saline for complete clearance.

At this point in HLT, the recipient distal trachea is divided and prepared (**Figure 65.11**). The heart–lung bloc is brought up onto the field. The catheter placed into the left atrium is attached to sterile i.v. tubing for the infusion of cold saline solution to run while performing the initial anastomoses (**Figure 65.12**). The left lung is placed into the left pleural space behind the phrenic nerve and then the right lung into its pleural space. This should result in the heart lying comfortably in the mediastinum. The tracheal anastomosis is performed first in an end-to-end fashion with a running monofilament suture such as polypropylene. Some surgeons prefer absorbable suture. Following completion of this, it ought to be covered with some surrounding mediastinal tissue.

Next the aortic anastomosis is performed, also in an end-to-end fashion. While this is going on, the cold saline infusion into the left atrium serves to keep the heart cold as well as providing a means of evacuating air from the heart. There is no pulmonary venous return at all during the implant and there will not be any until the aortic cross-clamp is removed and antegrade flow is initiated via the right ventricle. Some will occur via collaterals from the coronary artery circulation, but that is minimal. When the aortic anastomosis is completed, the cross-clamp can be removed. At this point the cannula in the left atrial appendage can be placed on suction and converted to a vent.

The SVC and IVC anastomoses are performed next. If a right atrial anastomosis is preferred, it is then performed. With completion of these, preparations are made to come off CPB (**Figure 65.13a–d**).

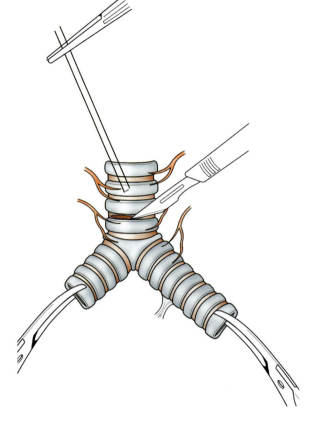

65.11 With the donor heart–lung bloc now prepared, the recipient trachea is trimmed just above the carina. A stay suture (Fiore stitch) should be placed in the anterior wall of the trachea as this will retract back up into the superior mediastinum. The distal trachea with the mainstem bronchi are then removed.

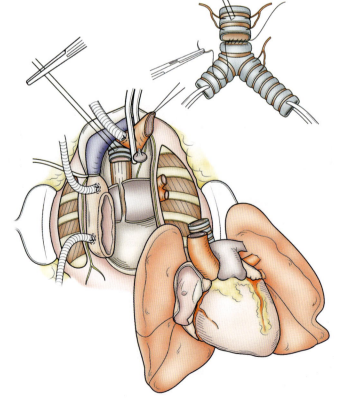

65.12 The heart–lung bloc is delivered into the operative field. The right lung is first passed under the phrenic nerve/pericardium through the defect previously created there. The left lung is then delivered into its pleural space through the corresponding defect created posterior to the phrenic nerve. Care must be taken to assure that the lungs have not twisted on their pedicles in the process of the preparation and placement. The heart and trachea should now be lined up with the recipient trachea and aorta. The left ventricular vent placed into the left atrium via the appendage is now connected to tubing to deliver cold saline into the left heart. This is done to keep the heart cold and to assist with the evacuation of air. The tracheal anastomosis is performed in an end-to-end fashion with running monofilament suture, usually polypropylene. Upon completion of this, the anastomosis is covered by donor and recipient peritracheal tissue.

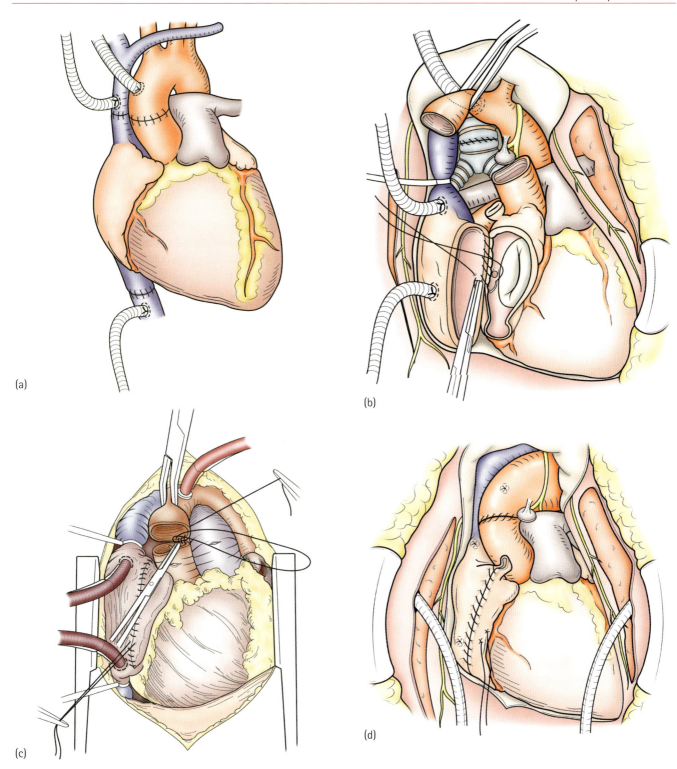

(a)

(b)

(c)

(d)

65.13a–d The cardiac connections are performed now. While this is going on, the irrigation through the left atrial cannula continues although it may need to be slowed somewhat to permit adequate visualization (a). The systemic venous anastomosis can be either right atrial or caval anastomosis (b). Following completion of this the aortic anastomosis is performed in an end-to-end fashion (c). The cross-clamp is removed and de-airing maneuvers may be carried out following this as the heart should still contain some saline from the irrigation. There will also be a limited amount of pulmonary venous return via the trachea–bronchial collateral circulation provided by connections to the coronaries. Once this is done, the vent can be placed on suction to keep the heart decompressed while reperfusing. The final anastomosis is for the systemic venous return. This can be either a right atrial anastomosis (b) or caval anastomoses (c). Caval anastomoses are generally preferable. The lung should be gently ventilated during this part of the procedure. Once rewarming is completed, the left ventricular vent is removed, full ventilation is commenced, and the patient is weaned from CPB (d).

Lung transplant with repair of congenital heart lesion

Each different congenital cardiac lesion requires its own method of treatment. The timing of the repair in the context of the transplant procedure is one factor along with the technical aspects of the repair. In general, the cardiac lesion should be repaired prior to performing the transplant itself. PDA should be repaired after initiating CPB prior to recipient pneumonectomies. In most patients, this will involve clamping the ductus, dividing it, and oversewing each end. In some cases the ductal wall may be calcified and require a brief period of circulatory arrest to deal with it. For any major intracardiac repair, it is probably best to perform the repair after the lungs are removed. This provides for a completely bloodless field to visualization of the defect and expeditious repair.

The approach is the so-called clamshell incision, entering the fourth intercostal space. Bicaval CPB (see **Figure 65.1b**) is initiated following the appropriate dissection. Assuming the transplant is a bilateral lung transplant (as opposed to single lung), the lungs are removed leaving sufficient lengths of pulmonary artery and vein branches for the transplant procedure. The bronchus is dissected out, occluded with a stapling device, and divided distally to remove the lung from the operative field. The congenital defect is then repaired. It is important to note that patients with Eisenmenger's syndrome have severe hypertrophy of the right ventricular outflow tract and can develop dynamic right ventricular outflow tract obstruction post repair. Therefore, it is best to divide muscle bundles in the outflow tract to avoid this post-transplant complication. The aortic cross-clamp is removed and the heart is allowed to reperfuse while the lung transplant proceeds.

The donor lungs are brought up onto the field. The bronchial anastomosis is performed first, followed by the pulmonary artery, and finally the pulmonary venous anastomosis. For patients with severe pulmonary vein stenosis, especially those following repair of total anomalous pulmonary venous return, there may not be adequate left atrial tissue to access to clamp. In that case, a brief period of aortic cross-clamping may be necessary to properly perform a suitable anastomosis for each set of pulmonary veins.

POSTOPERATIVE MANAGEMENT

The care of patients following either HLT or isolated lung transplantation focuses heavily on pulmonary issues rather than cardiac. The management is therefore similar regardless. The most common causes of death following HLT or isolated lung transplantation are technical factors, infection, and graft failure of the heart or lungs or both. Thus, the goals of postoperative management center on prevention and treating these issues. Naturally, technical factors are related to the efficiency of the operation, hemostasis acquired therein, and absence of any technical errors and misadventures. Infection prevention is related to the appropriate choice of prophylactic antibiotics and prompt recognition and treatment of acquired organisms including whatever the donor might have colonizing the airways.

Graft failure is more complicated. Many factors are in play including ischemia/reperfusion phenomenon, ventilator management, fluid balance, hemodynamic stability, the use of multiple blood products, and perhaps others. The hemodynamic management mantra is generally to keep these patients "dry", realizing that optimal management of cardiac output usually involves maintaining filling pressures that are somewhat elevated. The problem is that transplanted lungs develop pulmonary edema at a lower pulmonary capillary wedge pressure than in the normal state. This contributes to graft failure post transplant and thus a balance between these competing factors should be maintained. A combination of modest inotropic/vasotonic support with judicious use of diuretics is generally recommended.

Immunosuppression

The classes of immunosuppressants and the timing of their use are summarized in **Table 65.1**. Induction therapy with polyclonal cytolytic therapy or interleukin-2 receptor blockade is used in approximately half the centers performing heart–lung or lung transplantation. Maintenance immunosuppression generally involves so-called "triple drug therapy" consisting of a calcineurin inhibitor, purine metabolism antagonist, and steroids. A typical combination is tacrolimus, mycophenolate mofetil, and prednisone.

Table 65.1 Immunosuppression

Drug class	Timing
Lymphocyte cytolytic	
Antithymocyte globulin	Induction
Antilymphocyte globulin	Induction
IL-2 receptor antagonists	
Dacluzimab	Induction
Basilixamab	Induction
Calcineurin inhibitors	
Tacrolimus	Maintenance
Cyclosporine	Maintenance
Purine metabolic inhibitors	
Azathioprine	Maintenance
Mycophenolate mofetil	Maintenance
Corticosteroids	Maintenance, acute rejection treatment

Infection prophylaxis

Ganciclovir is commonly used for cytomegaloviral prophylaxis if cytomegalovirus (CMV) titers are found in either recipient or donor. The duration of therapy is controversial but generally lasts for a minimum of 6 weeks. Prophylaxis against *Pneumocystis jiroveci* pneumonia is recommended in all patients with either trimethoprim/sulfamethoxazole or monthly pentamidine inhalations in patients with sulfa allergy. To prevent oral and esophageal candidiasis, nystatin troches are used. Aerosolized amphotericin is administered throughout the post-transplant hospitalization for patients colonized with fungal organisms pre-transplant, especially *Aspergillus*.

Rejection

Surveillance for rejection begins within the first 2 weeks of transplantation. Transbronchial biopsy is performed every 7–10 days for the first month and then at 6 weeks, and 3, 6, and 12 months post transplant or if clinically indicated. Although isolated cardiac rejection is rare, it does occur; therefore, endomyocardial biopsy should be performed at similar intervals.

Biopsy proven acute lung ($\geq A_2$)or heart rejection ($\geq_2 R$; formally A_3) is treated with 500–1000 mg of intravenous methylprednisolone for 3 days followed by a 2-week tapering schedule. Persistent rejection is managed with cytolytic agents, total lymphoid eradiation, or methotrexate along with alteration in the maintenance immunosuppressive regimen.

OUTCOME

Early outcomes

The current operative mortality for HLT is approximately 25%, whereas that for isolated lung transplantation is 10% for all diagnoses. When looking only at those with pulmonary vascular disease (which includes idiopathic pulmonary hypertension and congenital heart disease), the mortality is again around 25% for HLT and 18% for isolated lung transplantation. There may therefore be an inclination to conclude that the type of transplant itself may not be a risk factor. Having said that, it is also likely that the recipient groups are substantially different. If one looks at cystic fibrosis only as an indication for lung transplantation or HLT, the early outcomes with isolated lung transplantation are significantly better.

Late outcomes

MORTALITY

The current 1-, 5-, 10-, and 15-year actuarial survival rates for HLT are 64%, 42%, 31%, and 23% respectively. Interestingly, there is no survival difference between the three most common indications for HLT, i.e. cystic fibrosis, primary pulmonary hypertension, and congenital heart disease. The long-term survival following isolated lung transplantation for congenital heart disease is very similar (65%, 48%, 36%, and 24%).

REJECTION

Early acute rejection and the number of rejection episodes negatively correlates with patient survival. At 5 years, only 34% of patients are free of lung rejection, while 67% are free of cardiac rejection. This actuarial freedom from either heart or lung rejection remains constant out to 20 years.

INFECTION

Only 12% of HLT and lung transplant patients survive the first year without therapy for infection. The most common source is the respiratory tract. The shift in respiratory tract infections over time from *Pseudomonas* has been toward more Gram-positive pathogens (*Staphylococcus*), more fungal infections, and fewer viral infections. CMV infections are now markedly reduced in part because of specific immunoglobulin. However, patients of CMV-positive donors and negative recipients are the most likely category for a CMV infection.

MALIGNANCY

Post-HLT malignancy is noted in 25% of patients surviving to 10 years. Lymphoma is the most common early post-transplant neoplasm, with skin cancer occurring more frequently in 10-year survivors. The acquisition of new Epstein–Barr viral infection is a risk factor for post-transplant lymphoproliferative disease, a variant of lymphoma.

GRAFT VASCULOPATHY AND BRONCHIOLITIS OBLITERANS

Bronchiolitis obliterans is clearly the most significant late morbidity associated with either lung transplantation or HLT. It is also by far the most common cause of death. The underlying etiology remains elusive and the treatment (usually enhanced immunosuppression) is marginally effective. Although transplant coronary arteriopathy occurs in the hearts of HLT recipients, the incidence is lower and the onset later than with isolated heart transplantation.

The high operative mortality combined with bronchiolitis obliterans has resulted in relatively poor long-term results for HLT transplantation. Although the early mortality for isolated lung transplantation in general is acceptable, when the diagnosis is congenital heart disease, the risk is higher, approaching that seen with HLT. The factors which can lower the early mortality are better (lower risk) recipient selection, increasing experience in transplant centers, better organ preservation, and reduction in the incidence and severity of early graft dysfunction. In reality, transplantation for congenital heart disease is producing higher risk potential recipients, the lower numbers for transplantation means that there will be less experience, and there remains no clearly effective preventive or therapeutic measures for early graft dysfunction. Organ preservation may be improved with the use of *ex vivo* perfusion techniques, although this remains unproved. Bronchiolitis obliterans remains an enigma and will continue to plague long-term survivors of lung transplantation, whether or not the heart is transplanted with the lungs. Thus, it is unlikely that the survival for either HLT or isolated lung transplantation will improve over the coming years. However, this does provide emphasis for the notion that these procedures should be carried out only in experienced centers by experienced surgeons.

FURTHER READING

Baumgartner WA, Reitz BA, Achuff SC. *Heart and lung transplantation*. Philadelphia: W.B. Saunders Company; 1990.

Benden C, Edwards LB, Kucheryavaya AY, et al. The Registry of the International Society for Heart and Lung Transplantation: fifteenth pediatric lung and heart–lung transplantation report – 2012. *J Heart Lung Transplant*. 2012; 31: 1087–95.

Deuse T, Sista R, Weill D, et al. Review of heart and lung transplantation at Stanford. *Ann Thorac Surg*. 2010; 90: 329–37.

Huddleston CB, Richey SR. Heart–lung transplantation. *J Thoracic Dis*. 2014; 6(8): 1150–8.

Kuo PC, Davis RD, Dafoe DC, Bollinger RR. *Comprehensive atlas of organ transplantation*. Philadelphia: Lippincott Williams and Wilkins; 2004.

Pasque MK. Standardizing thoracic organ procurement for transplantation. *J Thorac Cardiovasc Surg*. 1010; 139: 13–17.

Shumway SJ, Shumway NE. *Thoracic transplantation*. Oxford: Blackwell; 1995.

66

Ventricular assist devices for congenital heart disease

DAVID L.S. MORALES, FARHAN ZAFAR, AND CHARLES D. FRASER JR.

HISTORY

Hall performed the first ventricular assist device (VAD) implant in 1963 and Michael DeBakey is credited for the first successful VAD implantation in 1966. Since then, the field of mechanical circulatory support (MCS) has continued to grow and progress for adult heart failure patients. At present, there are numerous US Food and Drug Administration (FDA)-approved devices to support adults suffering from heart failure. Unfortunately, the same is not true for pediatric heart failure patients, particularly small children, infants, and neonates. In fact, no pediatric-specific VAD was available in North America prior to 2000 and not more than one was implanted in a given year until 2004 when the Berlin Heart EXCOR® gained widespread use throughout the US.

Recently, there has been a refocus of attention and resources towards the development of pediatric-specific VADs. Industry, government, and clinicians have now begun to address the large number of children who suffer from heart failure. There is an apparent trend towards increased incidence with a rising number of pediatric hospital admissions for heart failure (>30% over 3 years).[1] This may be explained, in part, by the growing success of both palliative and corrective surgeries for congenital heart disease (CHD), which is creating an ever-growing cohort of patients at risk of developing heart failure as children and adolescents. A significant portion is also explained by a better recognition of pediatric cardiomyopathy. Although it is the standard of care for children with end-stage heart failure resistant to medical therapy, heart transplantation is not an ideal therapy secondary to medicinal burden and notable morbidity. Most importantly, heart transplantation is a resource-limited therapy because of the relatively static number of donor organs. The number of pediatric heart transplants has scarcely changed in the face of the rapidly increasing waiting list.[2] For these reasons, MCS is gaining attention as a possible solution for these children. This recognition and refocus led to the first study focused on an FDA-approved VAD (Berlin Heart EXCOR®; approved in December 2011) for children in the US. Similarly, many in the industry are redirecting their resources towards development of pediatric-specific VADs, some of which is also led and supported by the National Heart, Lung and Blood Institute (NHLBI) under the PumpKIN (Pumps for Kids, Infants and Neonates) trial and other federal sources. Even though the first grant awards towards the development of MCS for adults were in 1964, it was not until 2004 that US governmental funding agencies started recognizing the need for the development of pediatric-specific mechanical support options. Also in the early 2000s, there were no US industry-driven initiatives for pediatric VADs; today, all VAD companies have at least one pediatric initiative. Many of the smaller adult VADs are now regularly placed in children because of their lower morbidity profile and the potential to be discharged home. In fact, more intracorporeal continuous flow (CF) VADs were placed in patients less than 18 years of age than any other type of VAD over the last 2 years. There is already evidence that the introduction of VADs to this population has led to significant improvement in outcomes for patients waiting for heart transplantation.[3] Approximately 40% of all pediatric heart transplants in the US are bridge to transplant with VAD support. These are all signs of a fast-growing and emerging field.

PRINCIPLES AND JUSTIFICATION

Patient selection and timing of MCS have been demonstrated to be critical for successful use of VADs. These factors are even more challenging in children who tend to compensate very well and who may not demonstrate symptoms until severe heart dysfunction already exists. Unlike the adult world, the relatively new field of pediatric MCS faces numerous limitations. One of the challenges is that pediatric heart centers are only beginning to gain experience and comfort in using available technology, therefore implant criteria at pediatric centers continue to evolve and are currently less consistent when compared to adult VAD centers. In addition, there are distinct limitations in intracorporeal devices currently available for smaller children (weight <20 kg). Smaller patients cannot be supported at home, and thus are not suitable for DT, and the morbidity profiles of air-actuated VADs are less desirable than those of the second- and third-generation devices. At present, however, the only reasonable alternative to devices like the EXCOR for this younger cohort is extracorporeal membrane oxygenation (ECMO), which has definitively shown to be inferior to the Berlin Heart. However, the use of extracorporeal centrifugal devices (i.e. CentriMag, RotaFlow) with EXCOR cannulae is becoming a popular strategy to bridge neonates/smaller infants as well as congenital heart patients to transplant.

Indications

Criteria for MCS in the authors' practice have evolved over the years with experience. Presently, patients with heart failure requiring an inotrope are evaluated for MCS if the circulation remains suboptimal (as evidenced by a requirement of a second inotrope or mixed venous of <60%) or if there is evidence of other end-organ dysfunction (Table 66.1). At present, the experience of a program and the consistency of results should be factored in when considering a small child stable on a single inotrope, extubated, with preserved organ function, but unable to tolerate enteral nutrition. This may not be an ideal patient for a program which is in the early phases of development of their team and protocols. Device availability is also important with decision-making. For example, a 12-year-old on milrinone awaiting transplant in the hospital is a good candidate if the program can offer a CF device (HeartMate II™, HeartMate III™, or HeartWare™). If, however, the device offered or the management team would not allow discharge, then there may be little advantage to mechanical support. On the other hand, one should not undervalue the opportunity to rehabilitate a patient more aggressively in the form of nutrition, physical therapy, and psychological improvement when that patient can be supported by an intracorporeal device with no i.v. medications, particularly at home.

SPECIAL CONSIDERATION FOR PATIENTS WITH CONGENITAL HEART DISEASE

Appropriate application of MCS in children requires an understanding of the unique pathological features of

Table 66.1 Indications for mechanical circulatory support in children

If patient has cardiac failure requiring an inotrope
AND
Failure of one other organ system:
Respiratory: intubation
Gastrointestinal: inability to tolerate enteral feeds, rising liver function tests
Renal: rising creatinine
Inability to get out of bed (when appropriate), fatigue limiting any activity
Chronically requiring a second inotrope
Myocardial viability <60% despite inotropes
Neurological: mental status changes

pediatric heart failure as compared to adult heart failure. Cannulation represents a distinctive challenge in pediatric MCS patients. There are frequently geometric considerations for cannula placement that must be critically addressed (e.g. situs abnormalities). Further, intracardiac anatomy must be clearly understood with respect to septal defects, hypoplastic chambers, and anomalous systemic and venous connections, as well as extracardiac anatomy (i.e. aortic interruption or coarctation). The identification and management of systemic to pulmonary artery shunts, both surgically created (i.e. Blalock–Taussig shunt) and pathological (i.e. aortopulmonary collateral arteries) is challenging as there will be a need for greater than normal cardiac output. Although reported, these patients have not, in general, done well under chronic MCS. VAD support in children with single ventricles (SV) has been more successful after superior cavopulmonary connection (Glenn) than the first stage. One way to ensure that the Glenn shunt is adequate for oxygenation with a systemic ventricular assist device (SVAD) is to place the child on a temporary centrifugal pump first (common atrium and aortic cannulation), which is a straightforward and quick procedure. If the patient is well supported, one can then return and place a more durable device (i.e. Berlin Heart EXCOR). However, the use of EXCOR cannulae with extracorporeal centrifugal pumps has been gaining momentum in the field in the past few years because of its success. For the first time, neonates with SV physiology are being bridged successfully to transplantation and discharged home. The centrifugal pump's abilities to respond to the ever-changing preload and to meet the very high CO demands in these SV patients are thought to be the key factors in this recent success.

Heart failure in a patient with a previous Fontan operation is a challenging category of SV patients who may present for MCS. Historically, results of VAD support of failing Fontan circulation have been inconsistent. It is important to distinguish between acute and chronic circulatory failure. Chronic circulatory failure will present with arrhythmia, new-onset organ dysfunction, protein-losing enteropathy, cirrhosis, renal failure, and/or plastic bronchitis. It is important to understand that the chronic failure of the Fontan circulation is multifactorial and not all cases are the result of systemic ventricular failure. One must first take an inventory of why a particular patient's Fontan circulation is failing and determine if it is failing predominantly for right-sided (pulmonary) or left-sided (systemic) reasons and, if the former, a SVAD may not help hemodynamics. An SVAD is only effective if systemic ventricular failure is the predominant cause of a failing Fontan circulation, which is why it is important to know the systemic end diastolic pressure (EDP) of a Fontan patient before placing a VAD.[4] If the systemic EDP is not high, say above 12–14 mmHg, then an SVAD will not improve the situation. Fontan conversion is appropriate for patients who have an atriopulmonary Fontan with re-enterant tachycardia or beginning to have signs of failure or Fontans with anatomical issues. However, once early end-organ function begins, referral to cardiac transplantation is suggested before the onset of serious end-organ dysfunction. It is well documented that patients with failing Fontan circulations but preserved ventricular function or significant end-organ dysfunction show an increased risk of poor outcomes post transplantation.[5] Once significant renal and/or hepatic insufficiency has developed along with other end-stage consequences of poor nutrition and protein-losing enteropathy, a total artificial heart (TAH) may be an option. The theoretical advantages of the TAH in this setting include end-organ rehabilitation as well as physical and nutritional health. TAH has been used in a limited number of CHD patients and its use continues to evolve.[6, 7] Technical considerations due to anatomical (e.g. ccTGA) and iatrogenic (e.g. Fontan) variations need to be considered carefully.[8]

Contraindications

Extreme prematurity, very low birth weight (<2 kg), significant neurologic damage, a constellation of congenital anomalies with poor prognosis, and lethal chromosomal aberrations are generally accepted as relative contraindications for MCS. Patients with multisystem organ failure, while also considered a relative contraindication, may be reconsidered if reversal of organ function is predicted with hemodynamic improvement. Hepatic and renal dysfunction have been demonstrated to improve in some patients after restoration of hemodynamic stability with VADs.[9, 10] A theoretical proposition is that application of the TAH, which offers supraphysiologic cardiac output (cardiac index > 3.5 mL/m^2) and low central venous pressure may confer added benefit in multi-organ failure patients. The idea of frailty is now just beginning to be explored in our patient population. This is the idea of defining what components of a patient's illness can be improved upon with a good cardiac output and what cannot. This will be essential to avoid those patients who we support successfully but who still die because there are issues that ail them that a good cardiac output does not resolve. Contraindications to device implantation will be further refined as the field matures and different devices become available to the pediatric population.

Device selection

Device selection is guided by what needs to be supported (systemic ventricle, pulmonary ventricle, respiratory system, or any combination), anticipated length of support (bridge to recovery (BTR); bridge to transplant (BTT); or destination therapy (DT)), and the devices that are available. Unlike the adult population, device options for MCS in certain smaller children are limited and unfortunately this often thus dominates the decision-making for our smaller patients. Devices are usually categorized by expected length of support as short-term or long-term MCS. **Figure 66.1** represents an example of a protocol of device selection from an

independent pediatric VAD program. **Table 66.2** describes commonly used VADs for children in North America. There are other devices in use and in development, particularly in Europe, which are not included in this chapter as they are in preliminary stages of development and/or have very few documented pediatric implants.

The type of support is determined first; our experience suggests that ECMO should be considered only if the patient needs cardiopulmonary or emergent support. ECMO is time-sensitive regarding complications and is converted to other forms of MCS upon recovery of pulmonary function or weaned if cardiopulmonary recovery is achieved. If cardiac support alone is required, there is no need to use ECMO and, based on the anticipated length of support, either a short-term VAD (<2 weeks) or long-term VAD (>2 weeks) may be applied. Patients need to be transitioned from short-term to long-term support if anticipated recovery takes longer or the clinical course is unclear.

In chronic heart failure in a pediatric patient with either end-stage CHD or chronic cardiomyopathy, a long-term device is chosen according to the patient's size, therapeutic strategy (i.e. bridge to destination or transplant), and etiology of heart failure. Current devices being used in the pediatric population and the specific cohorts in which they appear most effective are described in the following sections. A summary is shown in **Figure 66.1**.

SHORT–TERM MCS

Some children with heart failure will require the initiation of MCS emergently or urgently. Some patients with acute cardiac failure may have significant potential for improvement in ventricular function, either with surgical intervention to address a residual or recently discovered hemodynamic lesion or with recovery from acute ischemic or inflammatory insult. The selection of the modality of temporary MCS is guided by the urgency required and whether pulmonary function is also compromised.

The most urgent need for MCS is seen in children with ongoing cardiac arrest who will require venoarterial (VA) ECMO. If the need for MCS is not immediate but is urgent (within hours), such as patients with myocarditis or inability to wean from cardiopulmonary bypass (CPB), one can assess the pulmonary status and, if failure is secondary to isolated cardiac dysfunction, then the use of a temporary VAD should be considered.

While ECMO is a rapidly available, versatile, and familiar technology, it carries several major disadvantages: the duration of effective support is typically limited to a few weeks at most, after which time dependent complications such as thromboembolism, bleeding, and infection begin to increase significantly; the cannulation attachments are generally quite tenuous, mandating heavy sedation for patients, typically with obligatory mechanical ventilation and bed rest; the devices are large and difficult to move. Also it does not provide great decompression of the systemic ventricle even with atrial septostomy, which is why the authors almost always place a left heart vent if the systemic ventricular function is

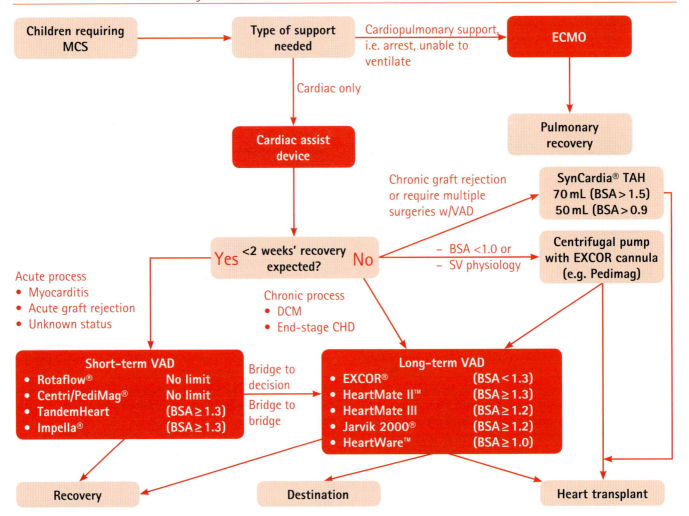

66.1 Protocol for device selection; name of the devices used in the figure are authors' preference for each device type. BSA, body surface area; ECMO, extracorporeal membrane oxygenation; MCS, mechanical circulatory support; VAD, ventricular assist device; DCM, dilated cardiomyopathy; CHD, congenital heart defect; TAH, total artificial heart.

severely compromised to avoid further lung injury. ECMO is therefore most appropriately considered a short-term, temporary form of mechanical cardiopulmonary support. If recovery of cardiac function has not occurred within 10–14 days, conversion to a more durable form of support is appropriate. If the prospects for recovery are clearly negligible, then conversion should be undertaken even earlier, after stabilization of the patient, to minimize the potential for ECMO-related complications.

In patients who are in need of support and are relatively stable but believed to have recoverable disease, a temporary support strategy can be used. This includes the use of CF blood pumps being placed with bypass cannulae and without using CPB.[11–14] The patient is cannulated through the left atrial appendage with return to the ascending aorta. A variety of centrifugal pumps are available, including the Rotaflow (Maquet Cardiovascular, Wayne, NH), CentriMag/PediMag (Thoratec, Pleasanton, CA), BIO-Pump and Affinity CP (Medtronic, Minneapolis, MN). In a patient not already on

some form of support, a sternotomy approach is typically required although, with left atrial cannulation in particular, the support can be initiated without the need for CPB in most cases. Significant advantages of temporary VADs include the ease and rapidity of cannulation if one undertakes a left atrial/aortic cannulation strategy. One can almost always do this cannulation off bypass as minimal manipulation of the heart is necessary. Adachi reported the utility of this approach in more than 30 children with acute heart failure due to myocarditis, acute graft failure, or acute-on-chronic heart failure. He observed ($n = 35$) an overall survival rate of 91%, and BTR rate for patients with myocarditis of 85% (17/20).[15] Several children ($n = 15$) with acute decompensation of chronic heart failure were also supported with a temporary VAD and 80% (12/15) where bridged to a long-term VAD "bridge to bridge." This support strategy should not be confused with the placement of EXCOR cannulae and the use of centrifugal pumps since the placement of the cannulae requires bypass and is a more involved procedure,

Table 66.2 Commonly used ventricular assist devices for children in North America

Device	Position	Pump type	Flow type	Flow generation	SV (mL) or speed (rpm)	Flow range (L/min)	Body surface area (m²)	Ambulation
Short-term MCS								
Rotaflow	EC	Rotary, radial	Continuous	Electromagnetic	0–5000 rpm	0–10	No minimum	No
PediMag	EC	Rotary, radial	Continuous	Electromagnetic	0–5500 rpm	<1.5	<0.5	No
TandemHeart	EC	Rotary, radial	Continuous	Electric	3000–7500 rpm	<5	>1.3	No
Long-term MCS								
EXCOR	EC	Volume displacement	Pulsatile	Pneumatic	10, 25, 30, 50 mL*	Variable	0.2–1.3	Yes
PVAD/IVAD	EC/IC	Volume displacement	Pulsatile	Pneumatic	65 mL	Up to 7	>0.7	Yes, possible discharge
TAH	EC	Volume displacement	Pulsatile	Pneumatic	50/70 mL	Up to 9.5†	>0.9/ >1.5	Yes, possible discharge
HVAD	IC	Rotary, radial	Continuous	Electromagnetic	2400–3200 rpm	Up to 10	>1.0	Yes, possible discharge
HeartMate II	IC	Rotary, axial	Continuous	Electric	6000–15 000 rpm	>2.5	>1.3	Yes, possible discharge
HeartMate III	IC	Rotary, radial	Continuous	Electromagnetic	3000–9000 rpm	>2.5	>1.2	Yes, possible discharge
HeartAssist 5	IC	Rotary, axial	Continuous	Electric	7500–12 500 rpm	1–10	>0.7–<1.5	Yes

MCS, mechanical circulatory support; EC, extracorporeal; IC, intracorporeal; PVAD, Thoratec Paracorporeal VAD; IVAD, Thoratec Intracorporeal VAD; HVAD, HeartWare VAD; TAH, total artificial heart.
*60 mL and 80 mL pumps are also available but in Europe only; †through both ventricles.

therefore, not fully taking advantage of the ease, speed, and less traumatic implant advantage of temporary support. The strategy with EXCOR cannulae and these pumps is really for longer types of BTT not for myocardial recovery from an inflammatory process such as myocarditis.

In larger children and adolescents, the TandemHeart System is an alternative approach to centrifugal pump support, (CardiacAssist Inc, Pittsburgh, PA). Inflow to the centrifugal pump is obtained utilizing a 21 Fr left atrial cannula, which is inserted percutaneously via the femoral vein, and advanced under fluoroscopic guidance into the left atrium (LA). Arterial return is delivered via a percutaneously inserted 15 Fr or 17 Fr femoral arterial cannula. The device is capable of delivering flows of 4–5 L/min, depending on arterial cannula size. Most of the experience with this device has been in adults with cardiogenic shock (CS) or undergoing percutaneous coronary intervention (duration of support hours to days), and there is limited experience with the device for longer periods of support as either BTT, BTR, or bridge-to-durable-VAD implantation.[16-19] Presumably because of the size of the device, there has been very limited use of the Tandem Heart system in children, though the pump by itself has been used with different cannulae and central cannulation in children.[20] The Tandem system is particularly problematic in children. Maintaining correct positioning of the left atrial cannula may be very challenging, particularly if the atrium is small. In these cases, the patient may become acutely desaturated, which corresponds to cannula malposition in the right atrium.

In larger patients in urgent need of temporary support, but who have not recently undergone sternotomy, placement of an Impella (Abiomed Inc, Danvers, MA), an intraluminal axial flow pump, by peripheral arterial cannulation may be considered. Under fluoroscopic and echocardiographic guidance, this device is passed retrograde across the aortic valve with the inflow port placed in the left ventricular cavity. The rotary pump provides flows of up to 5 L/min with an outflow port distal to the aortic valve. A lower flow version of the device with an upper limit of 2.5 L/min of flow is also available. At the entrance site in the femoral artery, both versions of the pump are 9 Fr, though the pump apparatus is substantially larger (24 Fr and 12 Fr), so either will likely need to be inserted surgically via a pursestring suture in the femoral artery or through a graft sewn onto either the femoral or the axillary artery. An alternative approach to placing either pump is via sternotomy through the ascending aorta, which approach would make irrelevant any concerns about compromise of femoral arterial flow and consequent lower-extremity ischemia. No series of pediatric Impella implants has yet been published, although there are case reports of use of the device in larger children.[21, 22]

In summary, children of all sizes who are acutely decompensating and in need of the most rapidly deployable means of MCS are best supported by ECMO. For smaller children in less urgent need, with an indeterminate projected support time or with hope of recovery within 2 weeks, transsternal cannulation for placement of cannulae to allow centrifugal pump temporary LVAD support is the preferred choice. The use of ECMO for isolated heart failure is declining, as it should.

LONG-TERM MCS

Berlin Heart

The Berlin Heart EXCOR® is the only long-term VAD available (FDA approved December 2011) for infants and smaller children in the US and is the most commonly used pediatric VAD throughout the world.[23-25] It has been implanted in more than 800 pediatric patients in the US and more than 2100 pediatric patients worldwide. The Berlin Heart is a paracorporeal VAD with pulsatile flow and is approved solely as a BTT, although there have been anecdotal reports of BTR with this device. It works with a mobile driving unit and, per current FDA guidelines, in the US patients are not eligible for discharge home. The EXCOR has been used to successfully support all types of heart failure in children.

Before the Berlin Heart, there was no well-accepted pediatric long-term VAD in the US and there were only adult VADs being placed in larger adolescents. The EXCOR is the first pediatric-specific VAD to gain widespread use across the US.[24] It can be used as an LVAD, RVAD, or BiVAD. Pump sizes of 10–60 mL (10, 25, 30, 50, 60 mL) are available and it is capable of supporting children of every age and size. It is currently powered by a bedside driver unit, but an EXCOR Active driver is being tested and will allow for discharge of patients to home with all pump sizes.

The EXCOR Pediatric VAD received Human Device Exemption (HDE) approval on December 16, 2011, for pediatric patients with uni- or biventricular heart failure who are candidates for heart transplant. There are no weight or age restrictions or limitations to the type of patient in whom the device can be implanted. The FDA has therefore thoughtfully allowed the clinician to determine the best application of the EXCOR, since it is the only MCS device available to support smaller children and infants chronically. Since this was an HDE approval, all institutions implanting the device need to have an active institutional review board (IRB) and it is now undergoing post-market approval.[26, 27]

Despite the time-tested success of the Berlin Heart EXCOR, its use in small children (<10 kg), especially those with SV physiology, has not been successful. The size issue (4–10 kg) seems to be complicated by poor patient selection such as the use of the EXCOR as a "salvage VAD" (i.e. a failed congenital palliation then bridged with ECMO to EXCOR). Thus, the issue of SV physiology and very small patients remains a challenge for the EXCOR. Recently, there has been increasing use and success of placing EXCOR cannulae connected to extracorporeal CF pumps as a BTT for smaller children, especially those with CHD. This is a long-term strategy and requires a more involved procedure with placement of EXCOR cannulae on CPB. This is why the phrase "short-term VADs" no longer suffices for these extracorporeal CF pumps. The advantages of this technique include easier management of anticoagulation postoperatively as well as a simpler, cheaper pump to replace should it thrombose. In addition, a centrifugal pump can compensate for changes in preload typical of the perioperative period without adjustments by the provider. This is very important in CHD when the Qp:Qs is constantly changing and is rarely 1:1 due to intracardiac shunting, an operative shunt, or aortopulmonary collaterals. In fact, a 2018 study by Lorts et al. identified 63 devices from the Pedimacs database which were first-time implantations of "temporary" or "short-term VADs."[28] Nonetheless, 40% were placed as a BTT strategy with a median duration of 47 days (interquartile range: 10–227) of support to transplant. Incredibly, five patients lived with a classically "temporary" VAD for longer than 5 months. In all, there was a 71% positive outcome (transplanted, on device, or recovered) with the extracorporeal CF devices.

Thoratec® VAD PVADTM

Thoratec VAD (Thoratec Corporation) is a pneumatic VAD with a 65 mL stroke volume chamber and a maximum output flow of 7 L/min. Thoratec IVAD™ (implantable) and PVAD™ (paracorporeal) are similar in design and mechanics; the difference is that the IVAD™ is slightly smaller in size, weighs 70 g less, and has a smooth, titanium exterior, which contrasts with the polysulfone exterior of PVAD™. The device can be used to assist left ventricular, right ventricular (RV), or biventricular function. The pump is compatible with a mobile console, the TLC-II Plus Driver®, and hence compatible with home discharge. The PVAD can be used for larger children (BSA > 1.5 m^2) if biventricular support is needed. This is a limited patient population and this device is rarely used.

Total Artificial Heart (TAH)

TAH is an implantable single unit biventricular device, which anatomically replaces both ventricles at implant but not the atria. It has a 70 mL pump volume in each chamber; a 50 mL pump for smaller patients is currently under investigational use. Theoretical indications for the TAH which may represent advantages over VAD therapy include patients with chronic rejection after orthotopic heart transplant, end-stage failing Fontan circulation, chronic right heart failure with VAD in place, significant restrictive disease, primary arrhythmia-induced heart failure, or patients with multiple defects (such as residual intracardiac shunting, aortic insufficiency, stenotic RV-to-pulmonary artery conduit) that require repair prior to VAD placement. Since it orthotopically replaces both ventricles and all cardiac valves, it eliminates the problems commonly seen with LVADs and BiVADs, such as right heart failure, valvular regurgitation, cardiac arrhythmias, ventricular clots, intraventricular communications, and low blood flow. Currently, it is only available for patients with BSA of 1.7 m^2 or greater or 10 cm distance between thoracic vertebra 10 and the sternum. Studies such as those by Moore et al. have demonstrated that virtual fit changed the eligibility

of 33% of patients and allowed fit down to a BSA of 0.9 m^2.[29] This has greatly expanded its use in pediatric patients. An ongoing trial with a 50 mL chamber version is testing the device in patients with a BSA of 1.2–1.85 m^2 or those demonstrated to fit by virtual implantation, which will hopefully extend its use down to a BSA of 0.9 m^2. The device has been used 70 times worldwide and has been successful at allowing increased use in underserved populations such as congenital (4% to 9% of TAHs), pediatric (4% to 13%), and female (12% to 70%) patients.

The TAH may offer treatment opportunities for cancer patients in heart failure who are generally not considered transplant candidates. Patients with proven cardiac malignancy may potentially undergo TAH placement as a definitive cancer operation. The patient may be observed for recurrence over a 1–2 year period and, if free of cancer, could theoretically become a transplant candidate. This is, of course, a highly controversial approach and is unproven. Nonetheless, this may represent the only treatment option for some patients.

Patients with chronic rejection after orthotopic heart transplant may benefit from a TAH implantation since we know this population is particularly difficult to support with VADs because of the immunosuppression and because they often have significant restrictive physiology and small ventricular cavities. However, these are not issues with the TAH since immunosuppression can be stopped and restrictive ventricular disease is not an issue.

At the International Society for Heart and Lung Transplantation (ISHLT) 2013, the worldwide use of the TAH 70 mL in the pediatric population was reported as 45 implants with an overall survival of 71%. The use in patients with congenital heart surgery was 24 implants with an overall survival of 67% and 100% survival in adolescents with CHD.[30, 31]

HeartWare HVAD™

The HeartWare HVAD™ (Medtronic, Minneapolis, MN) is a CF LVAD FDA approved for use as a BTT and under IDE-approved clinical trial for DT. It is relatively smaller in size and implantable in the pericardium without the need for a surgical pump pocket. This device now offers the opportunity to discharge children down to a BSA of 1.0 m^2, although careful consideration must be given for use under BSA 1.5 m^2 as clinical efficacy is yet to be established for this group. It is unclear what will be the lower size limit of patients who can be implanted with this device but, by virtual implantation techniques, the authors feel it will be around 20 kg, though patients smaller than this have been successfully supported. This device also offers the concept of chronic therapy in children. Currently, VAD therapy for children can be used to treat medically resistant heart failure in a hospitalized child to allow them to be discharged home without certainty of their transplant status. This has opened up the door to treat patient populations who in the past had no options for their end-stage heart failure (i.e. Duchenne muscular dystrophy patients).

A world report of 205 pediatric patients undergoing HVAD implantation found that over 50% of patients were discharged home and 89% had a positive outcome at 1 year.[32] Unsurprisingly, the discharged patients were typically older and larger than those remaining in the hospital. Presently, this is the most common VAD placed in patients under 18 years of age in the US.

HeartMate II™

HeartMate II™ (HMII) (Thoratec, Pleasanton, CA) is a rotary, axial flow pump with FDA approval for both BTT and DT. Like other axial flow devices, this pump is smaller and simpler than pulsatile pumps and has only one moving component, with no valves, vent, or compliance chamber reducing the complexity. Because of its small size, the HM II LVADs can be used in adolescent patients with BSA of $\geq 1.4\,m^2$. It is the most commonly used LVAD in adult patients and has over 25 000 implants worldwide.

Use of the HeartMate II in the pediatric field has decreased significantly over the last several years because of the use of smaller CF VADs. It does offer better unloading of the ventricle than the HVAD but the HVAD's size has made it the mainstay CF device in pediatric centers. In 2011, the Interagency Registry for Mechanically Assisted Circulatory Support (INTERMACS) data were analyzed and demonstrated that 28 pediatric patients were supported by the HMII. This cohort had a positive outcome (transplanted or being well supported on device) at 6 months of 96%.[33]

HeartMate III™

In late 2017, the HeartMate III, a smaller centrifugal VAD similar to the HVAD, was approved for adults. The results in adults have been outstanding with an even better morbidity profile than current devices, and this device is already being placed in several pediatric institutions, including the authors'.[34] Notably, the extracardiac portion of the device is larger and heavier than the HVAD, but the intraventricular shaft is shorter, which is potentially beneficial in children. This device also appears to decompress the ventricle less than the HMII but more than the HVAD, which may prove important in certain patient populations such as the Fontan group. It is unclear what will be the lower size limit of patients who can be implanted with this device but, by virtual implantation techniques, the authors feel it will be around 30 kg.

PREOPERATIVE ASSESSMENT AND PREPARATION

A thorough understanding of the unique pathologic features of pediatric heart failure is an absolute prerequisite to a successful outcome with MCS. The underlying cardiac condition and its impact on end-organ function, particularly liver and kidney, is important to consider prior to procedure. Hemodynamic stabilization is desired prior to surgery, but it is not always possible, depending upon the degree of decompensation at the time of presentation. If possible, pharmacologic therapy to optimize hemodynamics should be considered in an intensive care unit. It is clear that all patients requiring VAD can decompensate easily from even a transient hemodynamic abnormality (tachycardia, bradycardia, hypercarbia, loss of sinus rhythm, sudden alterations in volume status, hypotension), therefore each patient should be dealt with due diligence.

Management of non-surgical heart failure that is progressive with increasing inotropes is an indication for consideration of MCS. With the variety of VADs available for short-term circulatory support, the need to use large amounts of fluid and inotropes such as epinephrine for acute forms of acute heart failure should be limited. In addition, patients who have been followed for chronic heart failure with progression of their disease requiring intubation and inotropes beyond milrinone should be considered for mechanical support quickly. The preoperative assessment of these children before going onto support is critical. A complete hematological workup to assess their current and congenital coagulation tendencies is important. Also, careful neurological assessment by a neurologist imaging (head computed tomography, CT) is an essential part of caring for these patients. As pediatric programs mature, many centers have a rigorous pre-VAD protocol which activates a host of consults, tests, and labs so that as complete an understanding of the patient as possible can be achieved.

Expanding patient population through virtual implantation

The use of advanced 3D imaging has revolutionized the way patients can be selected for VAD implantation and has the potential to expand greatly, especially in children. The SynCardia 50 mL trial was the first in which the FDA allowed virtual fit as an acceptable criterion for device implantation. This is in part due to studies such as those by Moore et al. discussed earlier.[29] An example of the enhanced visualization provided by 3D imaging is seen in **Figure 66.2**. Similarly, this technology has been used to fit HVADs in patients below the recommended BSA of $1.5\,m^2$ down to a 7 year-old with a BSA of $0.86\,m^2$.[35] Though body imaging is required, this method will supplant the antiquated use of weight and BSA with much greater accuracy and the ability to plan complicated implantations in the growing wave of congenital heart patients presenting with heart failure. In the early days of its use, the surgeon and the imaging cardiologist would sit down at a monitor and perform the virtual fit. However, now at the authors' institution, a patient's CT or MRI is placed in a virtual space where all implanted devices at our institution (HVAD, HMIII, TAH 50/50 and 70/70) are available, and the surgeon can perform a virtual fit and choose which device may be the best for that particular patient. This technology's usefulness for orthotopic heart transplantation (HTx) sizing and complex implantation planning is also being explored.

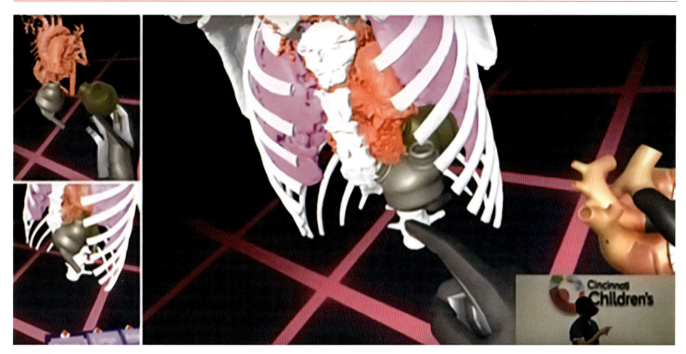

66.2 Demonstration of virtual fit with initial positioning demonstrating chest wall overlap (bottom left) followed by modified position demonstrating appropriate fit (image right). Courtesy of the creator Dr Morales and Dr Ryan Moore at Cincinnati Children's Hospital, Cincinnati, Ohio.

ANESTHESIA

The anesthetic plan must take into consideration the degree of cardiac dysfunction and potential pre-existing organ compromise. Pharmacologic agent-induced cardiac depression and increased myocardial oxygen demand must be avoided. Ketamine induction and remifentanil infusion maintenance remains a useful choice to achieve this goal. Various combinations have been used and examined,[36] the key being to ensure adequate analgesia and amnesia without reducing systemic vascular resistance or myocardial contractility. The authors find it helpful to use a continuous SVO_2 central line in postoperative management, especially when a patient has presented severely compromised and has thus gone for VAD implantation in an unstable or rapidly progressing state.

Another important aspect of anesthetic management in these patients is monitoring the right heart. Increased pulmonary vascular resistance (PVR) and RV failure should always be considered and treated promptly in the presence of unexplained hypotension. Interventions to improve RV function include maintaining a mildly alkalotic environment, use of phosphodiesterase inhibitors (milrinone), diuretics, and inhaled nitric oxide (iNO) or other pulmonary vasodilators. Spontaneous ventilation lowers alveolar pressure and PVR, improves venous return and hemodynamic stability, and should be considered if the procedure allows.

In addition to standard monitoring for any cardiothoracic surgery, transesophageal echocardiographic (TEE) monitoring should be routine during VAD implantation. TEE may detect anatomic variations and pathologies prior to implantation, can confirm proper positioning of cannulae, ascertain adequate de-airing of the device during the implantation, and examine LV decompression and RV function after implantation. Also, the authors encourage leaving the TEE probe in when implanting devices in children, especially when there are plans to close the chest. When placing the EXCOR whose aortic cannulae are stiff or when using intracorporeal VADs in smaller children, it is essential that one makes sure that the settings of the VAD after chest closure remain ideal with regard to decompression of the ventricle and positioning of the interventricular septum.

OPERATION

Children with CHD have intrinsic anatomic variations that can pose significant difficulty in cannulation for MCS (e.g. abnormal size and location of the aorta, SV). Previous surgical procedures may further jeopardize the application of MCS not only anatomically but also physiologically (e.g. systemic–pulmonary artery shunts, surgically disconnected venae cavae after Glenn or Fontan operations). A thorough understanding of the unique pathologic features of heart failure is an absolute prerequisite to successful MCS. This is particularly important for adults with palliated CHD who may have operations and connections that are presently used and may be unfamiliar to the care team. Therefore, preoperative imaging and a very detailed understanding of all connections and shunts is essential.

Surgical techniques for implantable devices and extracorporeal devices that require central cannulation are discussed in detail here. Some devices require peripheral cannulation, which is performed by cannulating a graft sutured to the native vessel (i.e. axillary or femoral) in order to avoid distal ischemia, particularly in smaller children and when accessing smaller vessels.

Temporary support is initiated by using standard CPB cannulae and, as previously noted, may almost always be done off CPB. Decisions concerning cannulation of the aorta should include the assumption that a long-term device may be needed. Therefore, the aortic cannula should be high on the ascending aorta, if not in the arch, so one will be able to place a side-biting clamp on the ascending aorta in the future. This aortic cannula used for temporary VAD support can be used as the aortic cannula for CPB if one needs to place a permanent device. The LA should be cannulated usually with a wired, reinforced "lighthouse" type of cannula that can be formed into a curve to ease its placement through the appendage and into the LA body. In these patients, the LA appendage is quite large and usually hanging over or just lateral to the main pulmonary artery, so it is easily accessible without much or any manipulation of the heart. A pursestring is placed and then a side-biter clamp under the pursestring, so the appendage can be opened and the venous cannula placed under TEE guidance. After this, connection the extracorporeal centrifugal pump allows VAD support to start.

Each of the long-term VADs requires specific methods of insertion and subtleties but there are some general principles common to all. One should always remember that CPB is often the best cardiac output the patient has seen in some time and, via ultrafiltration, it is the best opportunity to remove free water. Unless there is intracardiac shunting, one should not need to arrest the heart and, even if one does (i.e. close an ASD), then after closure, one should take the cross-clamp off to place the device. Minimizing the time the right heart is ischemic may be beneficial in avoiding an RVAD. If the patient is single-ventricular, stopping the heart is of little consequence so always do so if it makes implantation easier. If cardiac arrest is unnecessary, aortic atrial cannulation with an LA vent to a pump sucker will be adequate. This allows the left heart to completely decompress, making positioning easier, and allows the volume in the LV to be controlled when placing the apical cannula. During CPB, continuous ultrafiltration is done, which will help with total body fluid overload, myocardial edema, and reducing the cytokine burden, all of which are thought to improve RV function post-LVAD placement. After VAD placement, establishing excellent hemostasis is essential in avoiding the need for significant postoperative blood products, which will definitely affect lung mechanics, myocardial/body edema, and strain on the RV. It is possible to avoid giving any perioperative blood products completely with VAD placement but this requires a combination of appropriate timing of VAD implantation, meticulous surgical technique, physiologic CPB, and insightful VAD selection; the vast majority of pediatric VAD patients should be able to leave the operating room with their chest closed and with minimal bleeding. This optimizes outcomes in these challenging patients and is the key to a successful postoperative care period.

POSTOPERATIVE CARE

Successful postoperative management of patients on VADs requires a multidisciplinary approach through critical cooperation with other subspecialty consultants (e.g. hematology, infectious disease, nephrology, psychiatry, family support). There are five general phases of recovery for patients after VAD implantation. When separating from CPB, all patients at the authors' institutions are on a combination of epinephrine, iNO, and milrinone.

- *Phase 1* is during the first 24–48 hours and is primarily focused on bleeding and right heart function. During this period, epinephrine may be useful, at least low dose, even if there is hypertension to aid the right heart. The latter can be managed with sodium nitroprusside. The reason for being over aggressive regarding right heart function is that failure of the right heart and the need to return to the OR for RVAD significantly changes the patient's outcome. Once the right heart is clearly functioning adequately and there is minimal bleeding, the next phase begins.
- *Phase 2* (day 2–4). The focus is now on extubation while remaining on all inotropes and iNO. Also, anticoagulation with heparin is started for most patients unless they are extubated earlier than postoperative day 2.
- *Phase 3* (day 3–6). Once extubated, the goal is to wean off all intravenous medications, remove all tubes, and establish a steady anticoagulation regimen, wean off iNO and usually convert to sildenafil, and initiate enteral nutrition and rehabilitation.
- *Phase 4* (day 4–8). Prepare for discharge to floor and intensifying rehabilitation.
- *Phase 5* (day 5–14). Continue with rehabilitation and prepare for patients with TAH and second- and third-generation devices to be discharged home. Patients with the EXCOR should have no central lines, no i.v. medications, minimal blood draws, be enterally fed, and be working with physical and occupational therapy to continue to develop normally. The authors have noted that many of the younger children on the EXCOR often do not completely take all their nutrition orally and require a nasogastric tube for enteral nutrition.

Appropriate anticoagulation remains a critical concern and is difficult in children as the coagulation cascade is continuously changing until approximately the age of 5–7 years. It remains a question as to what is the optimal anticoagulation; however, most agree to start with heparin. Many convert the infants and toddlers to (low molecular weight heparin) lovenox for chronic anticoagulation because of their irregular diet and differences in their coagulation cascade. The use of bivalirudin instead of heparin has significantly increased, especially in smaller infants and those children being supported with extracorporeal centrifugal devices (i.e. CentriMag, RotaFlow). Older children, especially any with the HeartWare, HeartMate, or TAH, are converted to coumadin. Questions include what age patients fare better on lovenox than on coumadin, the optimal antiplatelet therapy for children on different devices, and optimal lab tests to measure the effect of these medications. Whether children are truly anticoagulated is not well established and is beyond the scope of this chapter.[37]

SPECIAL CONSIDERATIONS

Acute versus chronic recovery

The term *recovery* has broad definitions as it pertains to myocardial dysfunction and the role of MCS. Traditionally, the term *bridge to recovery* designates the use of a VAD to improve myocardial function sufficiently to allow decannulation and device removal. In the purest sense, it implies return to a "normal" or even improved state of function after an injury or decline. Ultimately, the type and degree of recovery is heavily influenced by the nature and acuity of the myocardial injury. Acute injury – as in the case of viral myocarditis or post-cardiotomy low cardiac output syndrome – often portends rapid and complete recovery, while long-standing injury, as in the case of chronic congestive heart failure secondary to cardiomyopathy, typically predicts a long period of recovery, or rather "reverse remodeling." The latter is usually not to a "normal" state but to a degree of heart failure that is manageable with medical therapy and that clinically allows the patient to be active. The utility of MCS for myocarditis or acute graft rejection is simply to support the body with a good cardiac output for the time necessary to allow natural or medically treated resolution of the inflammatory storm taking place in the cardiac myocardium. Conversely, the goal of mechanical support strategies in patients with long-standing dilated cardiomyopathy (mechanical decompressive therapy) may be to promote reverse remodeling with normalization of the neurohumoral mileau, and reversal of chamber enlargement.[38–40] The evidence suggesting reverse remodeling is still controversial and should be sought carefully. For patients who present acutely, the challenge is to predict which cardiac insults are likely to recover in a timely manner and which have a low likelihood of improvement, and to choose an MCS modality accordingly. True reverse remodeling usually takes several months and sometimes over a year, which is why those reported cases in which recovery is achieved in 2–3 months may often be cases of subacute myocarditis that can take several weeks to months to resolve. However, the field is still in its infancy regarding our understanding of reverse remodeling. Approaches to MCS as it relates to acute and chronic recovery strategies will be reviewed below.

Acute myocardial depression resulting in systemic hypoperfusion and associated sequelae is the syndrome of CS. It can occur for a variety of reasons in children, including but not limited to:

- post-cardiotomy dysfunction
- myocarditis
- intractable arrhythmia
- graft failure following cardiac transplantation
- acute on chronic heart failure
- unknown patient or reason for circulatory compromise
- resuscitation out of CS as bridge to chronic VAD.

Children with CS refractory to medical management can have swift deterioration, necessitating MCS. VA ECMO has traditionally been the first-line modality for temporary cardiopulmonary support in CS. The goal of ECMO in this setting is to maintain circulation and end-organ perfusion until other cardiopulmonary derangements have been adequately treated. ECMO has the benefit of rapid deployment, high-flow biventricular support, and oxygenation. The ability to cannulate peripherally obviates the need for sternotomy. ECMO remains the traditional form of MCS for children unable to wean from CPB and post-cardiotomy low output, where the expectation of myocardial recovery is high and relatively rapid (days) since lung function and oxygenation are often an issue.[41–43] However, these benefits come at the high cost of circuit-related complications that exponentially increase in frequency and severity with duration of support, especially after 10–14 days. Based on the 2012 Extracorporeal Life Support Organization (ELSO) report, intracranial hemorrhage, surgical and cannula bleeding, and cardiac tamponade occurred at a frequency of 21–52% across neonates and adolescents.[44] Overall, outcomes with cardiac ECMO in pediatrics have shown some improvement over time, with 38% survival reported for 1990–2000, and subsequently, 45% survival for 2001–2011 ($P < 0.0001$).[44] However, considering that the number of cardiac runs and the percentage of all pediatric ECMO patients supported for primary cardiac disease have steadily increased since 1985, it is disappointing that survival outcomes have not improved more substantially with this increasing experience.

As such, many centers are advocating alternative temporary support strategies that will reliably unload the left heart and maximize potential for myocardial recovery. The use of CF devices is gaining popularity for this purpose in children due to ease of implantation/explantation and the ability of such devices to accommodate different patient sizes. Devices that have been used in children for temporary uni- and/or biventricular support include the Rotaflow® (MAQUET Medical System, Wayne, MJ), PediVAS/CentriMag® (Thoratec Corporation, Pleasanton, CA),[45, 46] percutaneous TandemHeart® (CardiacAssist Inc, Pittsburgh, PA),[20] and the percutaneous Impella 2.5/5.0® (ABIOMED Inc, Danvers, MA).[21, 22, 47, 48] The Rotaflow® and PediVAS/CentriMag® are centrifugal CF pumps that can be connected either to standard bypass cannulae or to VAD cannulae (such as Berlin Heart and ABIOMED cannulae) for central cannulation providing uni- or biventricular support.[49–52] Some have proposed a staged approach to MCS, using ECMO as a first-line therapy with acute pulmonary and cardiac failure or cardiac arrest but promptly converting to a paracorporeal CF VAD

(Rotaflow, CentriMag) strategy within days if the pulmonary status improves and cardiac function does not. With experience, one can often implant a short-term CF VAD in a timely fashion prior to cardiac arrest and development of pulmonary dysfunction (i.e. before ECMO support would traditionally be instituted).[47] In the setting of fulminant myocarditis, both ECMO and short-term VADs have been used successfully as a BTR or BTT.[53, 54] In a review of ELSO registry data of 19 348 pediatric ECMO uses from 1995 to 2006, 260 cardiac runs for myocarditis in 255 patients were identified with an overall survival of 61%.[54] Wilmot et al. reported a single-center experience of MCS for myocarditis in 16 children and found no statistically significant difference in survival between patients supported with ECMO (4/6 patients, 67%) versus VADs (8/10 patients, 80% $P = 0.3$) and an overall survival with MCS of 75%, although this study is likely underpowered to detect such a difference.[53] The other issue is that transplant is not the goal and it is very well documented that patients reaching heart transplantation on ECMO do significantly worse post-transplant than VAD patients who have the same outcome as those reaching transplant without a VAD. Adachi demonstrated the usefulness of this technique for more than 30 children who had acute heart failure from myocarditis, acute graft failure, or acute or chronic heart failure. He presented ($n = 35$) an overall survival rate of 91%, and BTR rate for myocarditis of 85% (17/20).[15] Several children ($n = 15$) who had acute decompensation of their chronic heart failure were also supported with a temporary VAD but 80% (12/15) were bridged to a long-term VAD (bridge-to-bridge). There appears to be a growing trend towards the use of short-term support in many but not all scenarios where ECMO was traditionally applied. In certain patients, short-term VADs may offer a lower risk of complications such as bleeding and infection, greater survival, and in the future facilitate extubation, mobilization, and rehabilitation.[55]

Cardiac support strategies for chronic cardiac disease with the goal of reverse remodeling have similar requirements to acute recovery support strategies:

- effective decompression of the LA to protect pulmonary vasculature
- modifying loading conditions of the LV to decrease wall stress
- low adverse event profile
- allow for nutritional and physical rehabilitation at home.

Use of pulsatile and CF extracorporeal/paracorporeal VADs as a long-term BTR in pediatric patients has been reported.[56–61] It is important to note that it is not clear that in the literature many of the patients chronically "bridge to recovery" did not have some inflammatory/acute or subacute cause of the heart failure, where recovery is often expected. Without an endocardial/myocardial biopsy or a prolonged well-documented history of heart failure, it is difficult to discern if a pediatric patient has chronic heart failure from cardiomyopathy. Most programs that are attempting chronic recovery use a combination of medications, physical therapy

regimens, and VAD settings to encourage reverse remodeling and recovery. The medications usually include a beta blocker such as carvediolol (i.e. goal dose 0.8 mg/kg/day or 50 mg/day), an ACE inhibitor such as enalapril (i.e. goal dose 0.5 mg/kg/day or 40 mg/day), and an aldosterone antagonist such as aldactone (i.e. goal dose 5 mg/kg/day or 50 mg/day). Many adult programs use an angiotensin receptor blocker but there has been hesitation in the pediatric population because of hyperkalemia.[62] Also important to note is that there is literature suggesting that, after 3 months of decompression, if the ventricle is not allowed to have some ejection, it may atrophy, which would be counterproductive to reverse remodeling. Therefore, the device is often turned down at about 90 days to allow for ejection. Explantation usually occurs at a time after 9 months of support, and often at over a year.[63] Requirements for explantation vary widely, and in adult protocols this often includes invasive monitoring, but one example of a pediatric set of criteria that have been used successfully is given in **Table 66.3**.

A unique consideration when selecting a MCS strategy for chronic recovery is choosing a device that facilitates improvement in total body conditioning through nutritional support and physical rehabilitation. Advancement in VAD technology, and in particular the development of intracorporeal CF VADs such as the HMII and the HeartWare HVAD™, has allowed patients to become ambulatory, return home, and resume activities of daily living. These durable (long-term) VADs have been used extensively as a BTT and even DT; there are also reports of their use in promoting myocardial recovery.[22, 62]

BiVAD versus LVAD

Device strategy is a difficult topic and one that changes as a program matures. If one looks at the Interagency Registry for Mechanically Assisted Circulatory Support (INTERMACS registry), the use of BiVAD support in adults has significantly decreased from 18% in 2006 to less than 5% of all implants in 2010 while outcomes have continued to improve.[64] This is related to the maturation of decision-making and timing of when to place a patient on support. In the adult VAD field an array of different criteria algorithms has been put forward to determine the need of RV support.[65] However, it is unclear that these sets of criteria apply to the pediatric population. What is clear is that, in the pediatric and adult populations, use of BiVADs is shown to be associated with increased morbidity and mortality.[64–67] In pediatrics, the concept that increased experience decreases the number of BiVADs as well as morbidity and mortality rates has been demonstrated in a few series with the Berlin Heart EXCOR VAD, especially at the Berlin Heart Institute, which has the largest single institutional experience.[61, 68, 69] Hetzer et al. have written extensively about this series and that their need for BiVAD support decreased with experience, despite the patient population remaining the same in regard to etiology of heart failure. They have shown that the

Table 66.3 Overview of Heart Failure Recovery Surveillance Protocol for Children on Mechanical Circulatory Support. Reprinted with permission from *Congenital Heart Disease*[62]

Pharmacotherapy	Carvedilol (goal 0.8 mg/kg/day, max. 50 mg/day)
	Enalapril (goal 0.5 mg/kg/day, max. 40 mg/day)
	Aldactone (goal 5 mg/kg/day, max. 50 mg/day)
VAD support	
Early (0–4 months)	Complete LV unloading (little or no aortic ejection)
Late (4+ months)	Partial LV unloading (increased aortic ejection on echocardiography and, when applicable, an increased pulsatility index)
Surveillance	Monthly evaluations performed on zero net flow device conditions (continuous flow devices are set to 6000 rpm, pulsatile flow devices are off during testing; all patients receive a heparin bolus of 50 units/kg prior to evaluation)
	• 6-minute walk test
	• Exercise treadmill testing
	• Transthoracic echocardiography (before and after treadmill testing)
	• Serum BNP
Other	Physical rehabilitation
	Mental health evaluation
	Nutritional counseling
Consideration for device removal (e.g., myocardial recovery)	Device explant is considered when the following clinical parameters are met:
	• 6-minute walk test: >1 SD below mean for age
	• Transthoracic echocardiography: LVEDD of ≥1 SD below mean for age (55 mm for adult-sized patients), and an LV EF of >50% (before and after treadmill testing)
	• Serum BNP: <100 pg/mL

BNP, B-type natriuretic peptide; LVEDD, left ventricle end-diastolic dimension; LV EF, left ventricle ejection fraction; SD standard deviation.

use of BiVAD support and the need for BiVAD support are different. They also note that this decreasing use of BiVAD support has significantly contributed to improved outcomes. They state that this is a result of the maturation of their program as it improves its patient selection and timing of intervention.[69]

The results of the initial North American experience with the EXCOR also demonstrated significantly worse survival associated with BiVAD support (64% at 6 months) compared to LVAD support (88% at 6 months).[56] However, Almond and colleagues' analysis of the entire Berlin EXCOR pediatric experience still reports BiVAD use at 37% across the US. In the same paper, BiVAD use came out as an independent predictor of early mortality.[66] Another study by Zafar and colleagues reported that BiVAD support was not associated with improved survival in any subset of patients; in fact, some patients supported with BiVAD might have done better with LVADs alone.[67]

There are a number of key factors to reducing RV stress and avoiding BiVAD support:

- attention to surgical technique, particularly aortic cannula placement with the EXCOR
- limiting volume, reducing myocardial edema, and cytokine overload via ultrafiltration throughout CPB
- balancing of the intraventricular septum to allow septal contribution to RV function and minimize tricuspid insufficiency

- ensuring hemostasis to limit postoperative transfusions
- routine use of inhaled nitric oxide and milrinone coming off CPB.

There is a cohort of patients (<10%) who probably would benefit from BiVAD support (i.e. primary arrhythmia-induced heart failure). However, with timely decision-making, the need for BiVAD support in children will not be hemodynamically driven but will be determined by the etiology of heart failure. If the patient is not in CS, then the RV will only be happier after LVAD placement unless the RV is stressed during surgery with unnecessary ischemia or immediately afterwards with excessive products for bleeding. Future studies should focus on identifying those pediatric cohorts which would benefit from BiVAD support rather than LVAD support alone.

Single ventricle

Literature regarding ECMO support for SV physiology,[43, 70–75] and particularly that describing VAD support, is quite limited.[76–83] MCS for SV patients raises particular anatomic and physiologic challenges having a direct impact on outcomes.[75] Booth et al. reviewed the literature of ECMO support for SVs at any stage up to 2004, which demonstrated a survival rate of 30% (16 survivors from a total of 54 patients).[73] Literature on VAD support for SV patients almost exclusively discusses application to a failing Glenn or Fontan circulation, until the recent report by Weinstein et al. on the North American experience with the Berlin Heart EXCOR in SV patients.[81]

In general, the term single ventricle heart (SVH) refers to any patient on the SV pathway before or after any stage of palliation. However, it is best to group patients as pre-bidirectional Glenn (BDG), post-BDG, or post-Fontan when considering how their physiology affects VAD function. Regardless of stage, precise timing and careful patient selection are critical to a successful outcome when contemplating VAD support in SVH.

PRE-BIDIRECTIONAL GLENN

Weinstein et al. reviewed the North American EXCOR experience and identified 26 patients with SVHs which were further analyzed by stage of palliation.[81] Of the nine patients having undergone stage I palliation (pre-BDG), eight died. The lone survivor was unique in being a non-infant who had survived to undergo a Damus–Kaye–Stansel procedure with modified Blalock–Taussig shunt at 19 months of age. The literature has not documented nor is the author aware of any neonatal Norwood patient who has been successfully bridged to transplantation and discharged home by an EXCOR VAD. Therefore, it remains unclear that EXCOR VAD therapy provides any survival benefit for this cohort of patients. Part of the issue is patient selection but, as stated, the constantly changing Qp:Qs, especially in a shunted patient, and the fact that they often need a cardiac index of 4 L/min/m² or more is not something the EXCOR is designed to accommodate. However, the use of EXCOR atrial and aortic cannula with an extracorporeal CF VAD can accommodate these demands and has been showing success. Multiple shunted SVH patients have been successfully bridged to transplant with this strategy. Nonetheless, when attempting to support SVH physiology in very small patients (<3 kg), EXCOR cannulae are probably not preferable, and the use of shunts and bypass cannulae are probably the best strategy. Using this strategy, there have been cases of successfully supporting these children, even down to 2.5 kg, to transplant and discharge home.

POST-BIDIRECTIONAL GLENN

The analysis by Weinstein of patients with BDG was considerably better as 7/12 progressed to transplant after EXCOR support, which compares favorably to ECMO. Post-BDG patients benefit from the fact that their heart failure is typically not post-cardiotomy but over an extended period of time, between the Glenn and Fontan. This is helpful because they are less commonly placed on a VAD as a "salvage" maneuver after a failed operation as is commonly seen in stage 1 palliations. Salvage VADs are known to have poor outcomes.[84] It is the rare Glenn that presents in chronic heart failure without a significant aortopulmonary collateral burden, thus in many ways they are still a "shunted" physiology with a changing Qp:Qs and a greater than normal cardiac

index requirement. Hence, the aforementioned strategy of combining EXCOR cannulae with centrifugal pumps is an effective management strategy that is gaining popularity in these patients. It is important to note that, as opposed to pre-BDG, a post-BDG circulation is not well supported by peripheral ECMO due to inadequate decompression of the heart secondary to inferior vena cava inflow and the high rate of neurological complications with Glenn cannulation. Therefore, after stabilization, peripheral ECMO should swiftly be converted to central ECMO or temporary support with an extracorporeal CF.

POST-FONTAN

The challenge with a failing Fontan circulation is identifying the cause of the failure, which is almost always multifactorial, and thus targeting interventions at correcting it. Therefore, MCS is often not the right answer for these patients. However, in the well-vetted Fontan patient, VAD support can be consistently successful. This is a complex subject and beyond the scope of this chapter but, in short, VADs are most successfully placed in patients with late failure of their Fontan circulation with systolic dysfunction and rising EDP over 12–14 mmHg. If the EDP is not high, then the patient's heart failure is dominated by right-sided issues and VAD placement will not improve their circulation and may even worsen it. Additionally, VAD therapy in these patients, especially, should be applied before the development of the end-stage morbidities of this disease (i.e. liver cirrhosis, protein-losing enteropathy, plastic bronchitis, etc.) have resulted in significant frailty. There are reports of Fontan patients being discharged home with VAD support.[4] Overall, VAD therapy in Fontan circulation has a positive outcome of around 66% in review of case and series reports in the literature with many patients reaching transplantation. However, with proper patient selection this could be improved further.

Some Fontan patients present late with a variety of comorbidities and end-organ dysfunction that make them poor heart transplantation candidates. In these cases, it may be best to avoid heart transplantation and offer the patients a device that can provide both a supraphysiologic cardiac output and a central venous pressure of 3–5 mmHg. This type of support can only be supplied by a TAH. The resultant perfusion and decreased venous congestion surpasses that of a fresh transplant or VAD and potentially allows recovery of end organs such as the liver and kidneys. Though only five TAHs have been placed in Fontan patients, as smaller TAH (50 mL) sizes become available and the use of virtual reality surgery helps establish fit in smaller patients with unique palliated congenital anatomy, this may become an increasingly enticing option for resuscitation and make transplantation a more realistic expectation for these frail patients. Because the Fontan circulation fails at multiple levels, supporting these patients should be a well-thought-out, staged, and multi-therapy approach.

OUTCOME

Corresponding to the age of this field, very little is known about the long-term outcome of pediatric VADs. The first multi-institutional prospective trial of a pediatric VAD (Berlin Heart EXCOR) was carried out for HDE approval, thus to establish safety and probable efficacy.[25] There was a 92% positive outcome (transplant, recovery, or alive on device) at 6 months for both cohorts (<0.7 m² and 0.7–1.5 m²) in the study, which was significantly better than the matched ECMO groups. The incidence of serious side effects (bleeding, infection, and stroke) remains a concern. Bleeding was noted in 42% and 50%, infection in 63% and 50%, and neurologic event in 29% and 29% of cohort 1 and 2 respectively. This was similar to the incidence of adverse events reported in studies where children and adolescents were treated with adult-sized devices.[85]

The EXCOR pediatric VAD received HDE approval in December 2011 for pediatric patients with uni- or biventricular heart failure who are candidates for heart transplant. With no weight or age restriction or limitation on the type of patient in which the device can be implanted, the clinician determines the best application of the EXCOR, since it is the only MCS device available to support smaller children and infants chronically. However, since this study cohort included only the 48 patients who met the inclusion criteria for the investigational device exemption (IDE) study (only 23% of all EXCOR placed during that time period), it was felt by the Berlin Heart EXCOR publications committee not to represent the "real world" or entire US experience with the EXCOR. Therefore, an analysis of all 204 patients who underwent EXCOR implant in the US during the study period between May 2009 and December 2011 without exclusion of any patients was completed.[66] Even though the entire cohort included significantly more patients who were younger, smaller, in CS, were on ECMO, had BiVADs placed, and had worse renal and liver function, the overall positive outcome was 74%. However, the IDE and compassionate use (CU) cohorts had significantly different positive outcomes (92% in the IDE cohort versus 64% in the CU cohort), as did those performed at centers with experience compared to those performed at centers with less experience (89% for centers with more than 10 implants versus 72% for centers with 6–10 implants or 53% for centers with less than 6 implants). Interestingly, the frequency of morbidity in the CU and IDE cohorts did not differ. Therefore, it was not that the IDE or more experienced programs had fewer complications (which many feel is patient driven) but that the IDE sites had experienced teams that were probably able to recognize complications quickly and institute a mitigation plan to avoid poor outcomes. This emphasizes the importance of a multidisciplinary team focused on these patients in order to maximize outcomes.

The second Pediatric Interagency Registry for Mechanical Circulatory Support (Pedimacs) report in 2018 described 432 devices in 364 patients implanted across 42 hospitals. Twenty-one per cent of the cohort had CHD with 48 having SV physiology. The majority (64%) of the devices now are CF devices, highlighting the rapidly changing landscape of this field.[86] This review reported nearly 50% BTT by 6 months and only 19% overall mortality, but a high burden of adverse events, mainly bleeding, infection, and stroke. Pedimacs now includes more than 600 devices and 40 institutions.

SUMMARY

The number of children with medically resistant end-stage heart failure is growing significantly. This has been recognized by government, industry, and clinicians, who are now working together to develop mechanical circulatory technology to treat this rapidly emerging cohort. Industry continues to develop smaller second- and third-generation VADs for smaller adults but now has recognized the potential of these devices to be used in children. The field of pediatric VADs therefore benefits from the adult VAD technological advancements, allowing the number of children (younger age groups) who can benefit from second- and third-generation VAD technology to increase. Pediatric VAD therapy is now being used to treat medically resistant heart failure as a stand-alone therapy more often and is providing hope for certain patient cohorts who in the past did not have options (i.e. Duchenne muscular dystrophy) or do not want transplant. The Berlin Heart EXCOR remains the only pediatric-specific VAD to gain widespread acceptance and has become the standard of care for bridging infants and smaller children to cardiac transplantation.

As well described by our adult colleagues and now by the analysis of the overall Berlin EXCOR cohort, timing of VAD implantation is crucial since the existence of end-organ dysfunction at VAD implantation and being in CS are clearly associated with poor outcomes. Therefore, as the types of VAD available to the pediatric field change and our decision-making matures, outcomes will continue to improve. Analyses have also highlighted that experience and multidisciplinary teams are essential for the best outcomes, which are achieved not by avoiding morbidity but by recognizing complications and responding to them quickly and effectively to mitigate their effects.

In the future, children with end-stage heart failure will hopefully only be selectively transplanted and the vast majority will be mechanically supported with minimal medications and will require VAD or TAH exchange only every 10–20 years. Ultimately, the field strives to develop novel therapies that can be applied during the unique environment of mechanical unloading that will allow for myocardial recovery and device explantation.

REFERENCES

1. Rossano JW, Zafar F, Graves DE, et al. Prevalence of heart failure related hospitalizations and risk factors for mortality in pediatric patients: an analysis of a nationwide sampling of hospital discharges. *Circulation.* 2009; 120: S586.

2. Colvin M, Smith JM, Hadley N, et al. OPTN/SRTR 2016 Annual Data Report: Heart. *Am J Transplant.* 2018; 18 Suppl 1: 291–362.

3. Zafar F, Castleberry C, Khan MS. Pediatric heart transplant waiting list mortality in the era of ventricular assist device. *J Heart Lung Transplant.* 2015; 34: 82–8.

4. Morales DL, Adachi I, Heinle JS, Fraser CD. A new era: use of an intracorporeal systemic ventricular assist device to support a patient with a failing Fontan circulation. *J Thorac Cardiovasc Surg.* 2011; 142: e138–40.

5. Kanter KR. Heart transplantation in children after a Fontan procedure: better than people think. *Semin Thorac Cardiovasc Surg Pediatr Card Surg Annu.* 2016; 19: 44–9.

6. Ryan TD, Jefferies JL, Zafar F, et al. The evolving role of the total artificial heart in the management of end-stage congenital heart disease and adolescents. *ASAIO J.* 2015; 61: 8–14.

7. Morales DL, Lorts A, Rizwan R, et al. Worldwide experience with the SynCardia total artificial heart in the pediatric population. *ASAIO J.* 2017; 63: 518–19.

8. Morales DL, Khan MS, Gottlieb EA, et al. Implantation of total artificial heart in congenital heart disease. *Semin Thorac Cardiovasc Surg.* 2012; 24: 142–3.

9. Helman DN, Addonizio LJ, Morales DL, et al. Implantable left ventricular assist devices can successfully bridge adolescent patients to transplant. *J Heart Lung Transplant.* 2000; 19: 121–6.

10. May LJ, Montez-Rath ME, Yeh J, et al. Impact of ventricular assist device placement on longitudinal renal function in children with end-stage heart failure. *J Heart Lung Transplant.* 2016; 35: 449–56.

11. Karl TR, Horton SB, Brizard C. Postoperative support with the centrifugal pump ventricular assist device (VAD). *Semin Thorac Cardiovasc Surg Pediatr Card Surg Annu.* 2006; 9: 83–91.

12. Thuys CA, Mullaly RJ, Horton SB, et al. Centrifugal ventricular assist in children under 6 kg. *Eur J Cardiothorac Surg.* 1998; 13: 130–4.

13. Duncan BW, Hraska V, Jonas RA, et al. Mechanical circulatory support in children with cardiac disease. *J Thorac Cardiovasc Surg.* 1999; 117: 529–42.

14. Hetzer R, Stiller B. Technology insight: use of ventricular assist devices in children. *Nat Clin Pract Cardiovasc Med.* 2006; 3: 377–86.

15. Adachi I. The use of short-term ventricular assist devices in children. Personal Communication, 2013.

16. Brinkman WT, Rosenthal JE, Eichhorn E, et al. Role of a percutaneous ventricular assist device in decision making for a cardiac transplant program. *Ann Thorac Surg.* 2009; 88: 1462–6.

17. Tempelhof MW, Klein L, Cotts WG, et al. Clinical experience and patient outcomes associated with the TandemHeart percutaneous transseptal assist device among a heterogeneous patient population. *ASAIO J.* 2011; 57: 254–61.

18. Bruckner BA, Jacob LP, Gregoric ID, et al. Clinical experience with the TandemHeart percutaneous ventricular assist device as a bridge to cardiac transplantation. *Tex Heart Inst J.* 2008; 35: 447–50.

19. Chandra D, Kar B, Idelchik G, et al. Usefulness of percutaneous left ventricular assist device as a bridge to recovery from myocarditis. *Am J Cardiol.* 2007; 99: 1755–6.

20. Ricci M, Gaughan CB, Rossi M, et al. Initial experience with the TandemHeart circulatory support system in children. *ASAIO J.* 2008; 54: 542–5.

21. Andrade JG, Al-Saloos H, Jeewa A, et al. Facilitated cardiac recovery in fulminant myocarditis: pediatric use of the Impella LP 5.0 pump. *J Heart Lung Transplant.* 2010; 29: 96–7.

22. Hollander SA, Reinhartz O, Chin C, et al. Use of the Impella 5.0 as a bridge from ECMO to implantation of the HeartMate II left ventricular assist device in a pediatric patient. *Pediatr Transplant.* 2012; 16: 205–6.

23. FDA panel approval: https://www.fda.gov/downloads/AdvisoryCommittees/CommitteesMeetingMaterials/PediatricAdvisoryCommittee/UCM519888.pdf. [Accessed August 3, 2018.]

24. Fraser CD, Jaquiss RD. The Berlin Heart EXCOR pediatric ventricular assist device: history, North American experience, and future directions. *Ann N Y Acad Sci.* 2013; 1291: 96–105.

25. Fraser CD, Jaquiss RD, Rosenthal DN, et al. Prospective trial of a pediatric ventricular assist device. *N Engl J Med.* 2012; 367: 532–41.

26. FDA guideline: https://www.accessdata.fda.gov/cdrh_docs/pdf10/H100004B.pdf. [Accessed July 10, 2018.]

27. Berlin Heart product catalog: https://www.berlinheart.com/fileadmin/user_upload/Berlin_Heart/Bilder/US_Website/Berlin_Heart_Inc_Product_Catalog_MPC21_5_print.pdf. [Accessed August 3, 2018.]

28. Lorts A, Eghtesady P, Mehegan M, et al. Outcomes of children supported with devices labeled as "temporary" or short-term: a report from the Pediatric Interagency Registry for Mechanical Circulatory Support (Pedimacs). *J Heart Lung Transplant.* 2018; 37: 54–60.

29. Moore RA, Lorts A, Madueme PC, et al. Virtual implantation of the 50 cc SynCardia total artificial heart. *J Heart Lung Transplant.* 2016; 35(6): 824–7.

30. Morales DL, Zafar F, Lorts A, et al. Worldwide use of SynCardia total artificial heart in adolescents: a 25 year experience. *J Heart Lung Transplant.* 2013; 32(4): S109.

31. Morales DL, Zafar F, Gaynor JW, et al. The worldwide use of SynCardia total artificial heart in patients with congenital heart disease. *J Heart Lung Transplant.* 2013; 32(4): S142.

32. Conway J, Miera O, Adachi I, et al. Worldwide experience of a durable centrifugal flow pump in pediatric patients. *Semin Thorac Cardiovasc Surg.* 2018 March; doi: 10.1053/j.semtcvs.2018.03.003. [Epub ahead of print.]

33. Cabrera AG, Sundareswaran K, Samayoa AX, et al. Outcomes of pediatric patients supported by the HeartMate II LVAD in the USA. *J Heart Lung Transplant.* 2013; 32: 1107–13.

34. Lorts A, Villa C, Riggs KW, et al. First use of HeartMate 3™ in

a failing Fontan circulation. *Ann Thorac Surg.* 2018 May. doi: 10.1016/j.athoracsur.2018.04.021. [Epub ahead of print.]

35. Moore RA, D'Souza GA, Villa C, et al. Optimizing surgical placement of the HeartWare ventricular assist device in children and adolescents by virtual implantation. *Prog Pediatr Cardiol.* 2017; 47: 11–13.

36. Mossad EB, Motta P, Rossano JW, et al. Perioperative management of pediatric patients on mechanic cardiac support. *Paediatr Anesth.* 2011; 21: 585–93.

37. Rutledge JM, Chakravarti S, Massicotte MP, et al. Antithrombotic strategies in children receiving long-term Berlin Heart EXCOR ventricular assist device therapy. *J Heart Lung Transplant.* 2013; 32: 569–73.

38. Young JB. Healing the heart with ventricular assist device therapy: mechanisms of cardiac recovery. *Ann Thorac Surg.* 2001; 71: S210–19.

39. Madigan JD, Barbone A, Choudhri AF, et al. Time course of reverse remodeling of the left ventricle during support with a left ventricular assist device. *J Thorac Cardiovasc Surg.* 2001; 121: 902–8.

40. Levin HR, Oz MC, Chen JM, et al. Reversal of chronic ventricular dilation in patients with end-stage cardiomyopathy by prolonged mechanical unloading. *Circulation.* 1995; 91: 2717–20.

41. del Nido PJ, Dalton HJ, Thompson AE, Siewers RD. Extracorporeal membrane oxygenator rescue in children during cardiac arrest after cardiac surgery. *Circulation.* 1992; 86: II300–4.

42. Kulik TJ, Moler FW, Palmisano JM, et al. Outcome-associated factors in pediatric patients treated with extracorporeal membrane oxygenator after cardiac surgery. *Circulation.* 1996; 94: II63–8.

43. Salvin JW, Laussen PC, Thiagarajan RR. Extracorporeal membrane oxygenation for postcardiotomy mechanical cardiovascular support in children with congenital heart disease. *Paediatr Anaesth.* 2008; 18: 1157–62.

44. Paden ML, Conrad SA, Rycus PT, Thiagarajan RR. Extracorporeal Life Support Organization Registry Report 2012. *ASAIO J.* 2013; 59: 202–10.

45. Hirata Y, Charette K, Mosca RS, et al. Pediatric application of the Thoratec CentriMag BiVAD as a bridge to heart transplantation. *J Thorac Cardiovasc Surg.* 2008; 136: 1386–7.

46. Kouretas PC, Kaza AK, Burch PT, et al. Experience with the Levitronix CentriMag in the pediatric population as a bridge to decision and recovery. *Artif Organs.* 2009; 33: 1002–4.

47. Jefferies JL, Morales DL. Mechanical circulatory support in children: bridge to transplant versus recovery. *Curr Heart Fail Rep.* 2012; 9: 236–43.

48. Vlasselaers D, Desmet M, Desmet L, et al. Ventricular unloading with a miniature axial flow pump in combination with extracorporeal membrane oxygenation. *Intensive Care Med.* 2006; 32: 329–33.

49. Maat AP, van Thiel RJ, Dalinghaus M, Bogers AJ. Connecting the CentriMag Levitronix pump to Berlin Heart EXCOR cannulae; a new approach to bridge to bridge. *J Heart Lung Transplant.* 2008; 27: 112–15.

50. De Robertis F, Birks EJ, Rogers P, et al. Clinical performance with the Levitronix CentriMag short-term ventricular assist device. *J Heart Lung Transplant.* 2006; 25: 181–6.

51. De Robertis F, Rogers P, Amrani M, et al. Bridge to decision using the Levitronix CentriMag short-term ventricular assist device. *J Heart Lung Transplant.* 2008; 27: 474–8.

52. Bennett MT, Virani SA, Bowering J, et al. The use of the Impella RD as a bridge to recovery for right ventricular dysfunction after cardiac transplantation. *Innovations.* 2010; 5: 369–71.

53. Wilmot I, Morales DL, Price JF, et al. Effectiveness of mechanical circulatory support in children with acute fulminant and persistent myocarditis. *J Card Fail.* 2011; 17: 487–94.

54. Rajagopal SK, Almond CS, Laussen PC, et al. Extracorporeal membrane oxygenation for the support of infants, children, and young adults with acute myocarditis: a review of the extracorporeal life support organization registry. *Crit Care Med.* 2010; 38: 382–7.

55. Duncan BW, Bohn DJ, Atz AM, et al. Mechanical circulatory support for the treatment of children with acute fulminant myocarditis. *J Thorac Cardiovasc Surg.* 2001; 122: 440–8.

56. Morales DL, Almond CS, Jaquiss RD, et al. Bridging children of all sizes to cardiac transplantation: the initial multicenter North American experience with the Berlin Heart EXCOR ventricular assist device. *J Heart Lung Transplant.* 2011; 30: 1–8.

57. Ihnat CL, Zimmerman H, Copeland JG, et al. Left ventricular assist device support as a bridge to recovery in young children. *Congenit Heart Dis.* 2011; 6: 234–40.

58. Grinda JM, Chevalier P, D'Attellis N, et al. Fulminant myocarditis in adults and children: bi-ventricular assist device for recovery. *Eur J Cardiothorac Surg.* 2004; 26: 1169–73.

59. Jones CB, Cassidy JV, Kirk R, et al. Successful bridge to recovery with 120 days of mechanical support in an infant with myocarditis. *J Heart Lung Transplant.* 2009; 28: 202–5.

60. Tschirkov A, Nikolov D, Papantchev V. The Berlin Heart EXCOR in an 11-year-old boy: a bridge to recovery after myocardial infarction. *Tex Heart Inst J.* 2007; 34: 445–8.

61. Rockett SR, Bryant JC, Morrow WR, et al. Preliminary single center North American experience with the Berlin Heart pediatric EXCOR device. *ASAIO J.* 2008; 54: 479–82.

62. Lowry AW, Adachi I, Gregoric ID, et al. The potential to avoid heart transplantation in children: outpatient bridge to recovery with an intracorporeal continuous-flow left ventricular assist device in a 14-year-old. *Congenit Heart Dis.* 2012; 7: E91–6.

63. Birks EJ, Tansley PD, Hardy J, et al. Left ventricular assist device and drug therapy for the reversal of heat failure. *N Engl J Med.* 2006; 355: 1873–84.

64. Kirklin JK, Naftel DC, Kormos RL, et al. The fourth INTERMACS annual report: 4000 implants and counting. *J Heart Lung Transplant.* 2012; 31: 117–26.

65. Fitzpatrick JR, Frederick JR, Hiesinger W, et al. Early planned institution of biventricular mechanical circulatory support results in improved outcomes compared with delayed conversion of a left ventricular assist device to a biventricular assist device. *J Thorac Cardiovasc Surg.* 2009; 137: 971–7.

66. Almond CS, Morales DL, Blackstone EH, et al. Berlin Heart EXCOR® pediatric ventricular assist device for bridge to heart transplantation in US children. *Circulation*. 2013; 127: 1702–11.

67. Zafar F, Jefferies JL, Tjossem CJ, et al. Biventricular Berlin Heart EXCOR pediatric use across the United States. *Ann Thorac Surg*. 2015; 99: 1328–34.

68. Baldwin JT, Borovetz HS, Duncan BW, et al. The National Heart, Lung, and Blood Institute Pediatric Circulatory Support Program: a summary of the 5-year experience. *Circulation*. 2011; 123: 1233–40.

69. Hetzer R, Potapov EV, Stiller B, et al. Improvement in survival after mechanical circulatory support with pneumatic pulsatile ventricular assist devices in pediatric patients. *Ann Thorac Surg*. 2006; 82: 917–24.

70. Allan CK, Thiagarajan RR, del Nido PJ, et al. Indication for initiation of mechanical circulatory support impacts survival of infants with shunted single-ventricle circulation supported with extracorporeal membrane oxygenation. *J Thorac Cardiovasc Surg*. 2007; 133: 660–7.

71. Aharon AS, Drinkwater DC Jr, Churchwell KB, et al. Extracorporeal membrane oxygenation in children after repair of congenital cardiac lesions. *Ann Thorac Surg*. 2001; 72: 2095–101.

72. Meliones JN, Custer JR, Snedecor S, et al. Extracorporeal life support for cardiac assist in pediatric patients: review of ELSO Registry data. *Circulation*. 1991; 84: S168–72.

73. Booth KL, Roth SJ, Thiagarajan RR, et al. Extracorporeal membrane oxygenation support of the Fontan and bidirectional Glenn circulations. *Ann Thorac Surg*. 2004; 77: 1341–8.

74. Kolovos NS, Bratton SL, Moler FW, et al. Outcome of pediatric patients treated with extracorporeal life support after cardiac surgery. *Ann Thorac Surg*. 2003; 76: 1435–41.

75. Jaggers JJ, Forbess JM, Shah AS, et al. Extracorporeal membrane oxygenation for infant postcardiotomy support: significance of shunt management. *Ann Thorac Surg*. 2000; 69: 1476–83.

76. Mackling T, Shah T, Dimas V, et al. Management of single-ventricle patients with Berlin Heart EXCOR ventricular assist device: single-center experience. *Artif Organs*. 2012; 36: 555–9.

77. Prêtre R, Häussler A, Bettex D, Genoni M. Right-sided univentricular cardiac assistance in a failing Fontan circulation. *Ann Thorac Surg*. 2008; 86: 1018–20.

78. Frazier OH, Gregoric ID, Messner GN. Total circulatory support with an LVAD in an adolescent with a previous Fontan procedure. *Tex Heart Inst J*. 2005; 32: 402–4.

79. Vanderpluym CJ, Rebeyka IM, Ross DB, Buchholz H. The use of ventricular assist devices in pediatric patients with univentricular hearts. *J Thorac Cardiovasc Surg*. 2011; 141: 588–90.

80. Sharma MS, Forbess JM, Guleserian KJ. Ventricular assist device support in children and adolescents with heart failure: the Children's Medical Center of Dallas experience. *Artif Organs*. 2012; 36: 635–9.

81. Weinstein S, Bello R, Pizarro C, et al. The use of the Berlin Heart EXCOR in patients with functional single ventricle. *J Thorac Cardiovasc Surg*. 2014; 147: 697–704.

82. Russo P, Wheeler A, Russo J, Tobias JD. Use of a ventricular assist device as a bridge to transplantation in a patient with single ventricle physiology and total cavopulmonary anastomosis. *Paediatr Anaesth*. 2008; 18: 320–4.

83. Irving CA, Cassidy JV, Kirk RC, et al. Successful bridge to transplant with the Berlin Heart after cavopulmonary shunt. *J Heart Lung Transplant*. 2009; 28: 399–401.

84. Morales DL, Zafar F, Rossano JW, et al. Use of ventricular assist devices in children across the United States: analysis of 7.5 million pediatric hospitalizations. *Ann Thorac Surg*. 2010; 90: 1313–18.

85. Reinhartz O, Keith FM, El-Banayosy A, et al. Multicenter experience with the Thoratec ventricular assist device in children and adolescents. *J Heart Lung Transplant*. 2001; 20: 439–48.

86. Blume E, VanderPluym C, Lorts A, et al. Second annual Pediatric Interagency Registry for Mechanical Circulatory Support (Pedimacs) report: pre-implant characteristics and outcomes. *J Heart Lung Transplant*. 2018; 37: 38–45.

67

Congenital mitral valve repair

VLADIMIRO VIDA, MASSIMO A. PADALINO, AND GIOVANNI STELLIN

HISTORY AND CLASSIFICATION

Surgical management of mitral valve (MV) dysplasia remains a therapeutic challenge due to the wide spectrum of different valve malformations, and the high incidence of associated cardiac anomalies in a context of a relatively rare congenital heart disease (CHD).

Congenital MV repair, rather than replacement, has been advocated for many years, mostly because of the undesired deleterious effects of prosthetic valve replacement, particularly in small children.

That said, there is still no optimal classification to fulfil surgical criteria. Using a pathophysiologic classification, Alain Carpentier, in 1976 (**Table 67.1**), divided the MV anomalies into two functional groups: *regurgitation* (or prevalent regurgitation) and *stenosis* (or prevalent stenosis), although it is uncommon that a dysplastic MV shows isolated signs of stenosis or incompetence alone. Stenotic MVs were further divided into two types according to the anatomy of the papillary muscles (PMs) (**Table 67.1**). Regurgitant MVs were further divided into three types, according to the leaflets' motion (normal, restricted, or prolapsed).

More recently, Mitruka and Lamberti (**Table 67.2**) proposed a simpler, albeit less detailed, anatomic classification dividing the whole spectrum of malformations topically into supravalvar, valvar, subvalvar, and mixed lesions. A limitation of such a classification, however, is that many MV lesions fall into the "mixed lesions" category and therefore remain without any specific topic classification.

Despite the availability of more sophisticated preoperative diagnostic tools today than were around at the time of Carpentier's classification, which was based on surgical observation, the preoperative and intraoperative MV classification can still sometimes be complicated, especially when more than one MV anomaly is present.

With the aid of Carpentier's classification, the most common congenital MV malformations are discussed here, together with the related surgical treatment.

INDICATIONS FOR CONGENITAL MITRAL VALVE REPAIR

Indications for MV repair are usually dictated by symptoms. Neonates and young infants can present with severe symptoms. Surgical indication can also be dictated by the association with other congenital cardiac anomalies. In

Table 67.1 Carpentier pathophysiologic classification (Carpentier, et al., 1976)

Mitral valve regurgitation (or prevalent)	Mitral valve stenosis (or prevalent)
Type I (normal leaflet motion)	**Type A** (normal papillary muscles)
● Annular dilatation	
● Cleft anterior leaflet	● Papillary muscle commissure fusion
● Leaflet defect	
Type II (leaflet prolapse)	● Supravalvar membrane
● Elongated chordae	● Double orifice MV
Type III (restricted leaflet motion)	**Type B** (abnormal papillary muscles)
● *Type A* (normal papillary muscles)	● Parachute MV
– Papillary muscle commissure fusion	● Hammock MV
– Short chordae	● Shone complex
● *Type B* (abnormal papillary muscles)	● Arcade MV
– Parachute MV	
– Hammock MV	

Table 67.2 Mitruka–Lamberti contemporary anatomic classification (Mitruka and Lamberti, 2000)

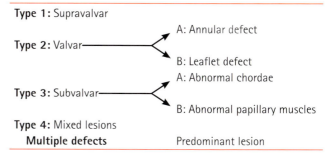

Type 1: Supravalvar
Type 2: Valvar → A: Annular defect / B: Leaflet defect
Type 3: Subvalvar → A: Abnormal chordae / B: Abnormal papillary muscles
Type 4: Mixed lesions
Multiple defects — Predominant lesion

symptomatic neonates and young infants, when possible, interim medical therapy can be preferred to an early surgical repair; it must be remembered that atrioventricular valve development continues into the first few months of life. MV surgery should be deferred as long as the patient's condition permits clinical management, to enhance the chances for a more successful and satisfactory repair later.

The most common symptoms in small children are dyspnea and failure to thrive. Some patients can be admitted on an emergency basis in cardiogenic shock, requiring mechanical ventilation and inotropic support. Bigger children can be admitted for valve repair while still asymptomatic. Stenotic (or prevalent stenotic) valves frequently show onset of early symptoms when compared to incompetent (or prevalent incompetent) valves. Realistically, congenital MV repair, when performed on severely malformed MVs in infancy, remains a palliative temporary treatment, the main aim of surgery being to obtain an improvement of the MV function, which would ameliorate the clinical status and allow deferral of eventual MV replacement to an older age. MV reconstruction needs to be carefully planned and tailored for each patient with the aim of respecting the original conformation of the valve to achieve a "physiologic repair" rather than an "anatomic one."

OPERATION

As a general rule, each operation must be tailored to the peculiar anatomy of each type of congenital MV dysplasia. Regardless of the anatomic and physiologic severity of the MV malformation(s), reconstructive surgery at any age should always be attempted with the aim of avoiding the high incidence of early and late complications, as well as the high mortality and reoperation rate which are related to prosthetic valve replacement, in the pediatric age group.

Intraoperative transesophageal or epicardial 2D and 3D echocardiography is essential for planning the best surgical strategy and for checking the performance of the MV immediately after repair.

The surgical approach is similar to that described in Chapter 16, "Mitral valve repair," for adult patients with acquired MV disease. A transseptal approach is always preferred, especially in small children. Four everting pledgeted stitches can be placed at the annulus site (**Figure 67.1**) to enhance surgical exposure. A hypothermic circulatory arrest is occasionally employed, particularly when dealing with complex malformations, in order to gain a completely bloodless field and to make a thorough MV inspection before planning the detailed surgical strategy.

MITRAL VALVE STENOSIS

Type A (normal papillary muscles)

COMMISSURE FUSION/SHORT CHORDAE

This is a common complex MV malformation. As described by Carpentier, et al. one or two PMs are directly implanted onto the commissure without any (or with very small) chordae tendinae. The commissures are fused and thickened; the motion of the leaflets is restricted (**Figure 67.2**). The functional MV orifice is often very stenotic. The anatomical MV annulus can be normal (type 3 Mitruka–Lamberti).

This condition is treated by commissurotomy (**Figure 67.3**) and splitting of the papillary muscles (**Figure 67.4**). PM fenestration (**Figure 67.5**) with the aim of enhancing the leaflets' motion is also possible in older children.

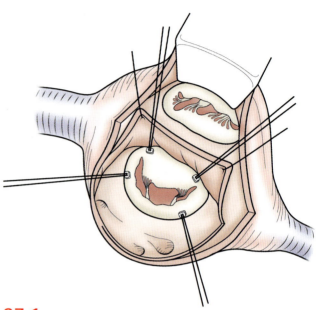

67.1

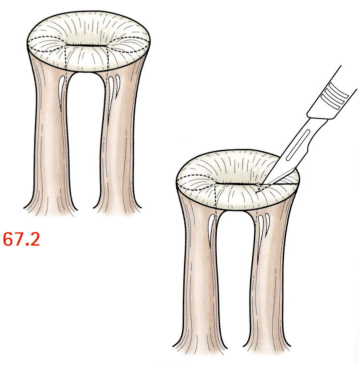

67.2

67.3

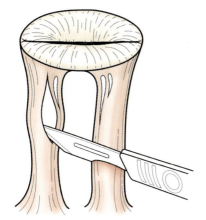

67.4

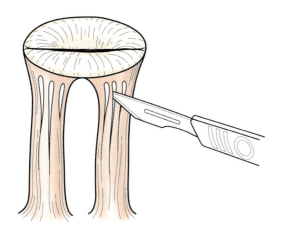

67.5

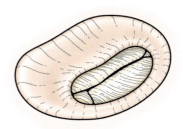

67.6

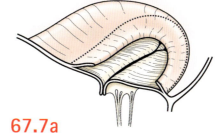

67.7a

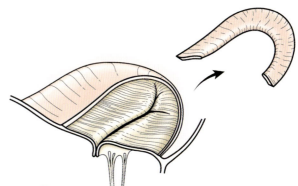

67.7b

SUPRAVALVAR RING

A supravalvar ring is seldom found as an isolated form and very often it reflects a complex malformation of the whole subvalvar apparatus. It consists of a fibrous circumferential ring of different size which lies just above the MV annulus (and often fused with it), creating an obstruction at supravalvar level (type A, Mitruka–Lamberti classification) (**Figure 67.6**). When small, it can be an occasional intraoperative finding.

Surgery consists of a complete resection of the ring, often including other maneuvers in the subvalvular area to treat associated lesions (**Figure 67.7a and b**).

EXCESS VALVAR TISSUE

In some cases excess interchordal tissue is found to be impinging on the proper chordae motion (**Figure 67.8**), often in association with other MV anomalies. Treatment consists of resection of the excess tissue with the aim of freeing the chordae operatus (**Figure 67.9**). A splitting of one or both PMs can be performed in association with the resection (see **Figure 67.4**).

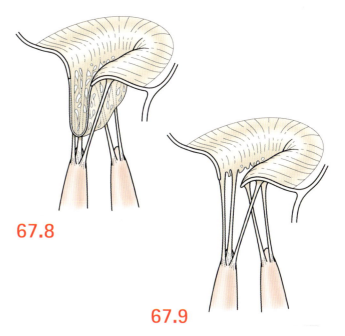

67.8

67.9

Type B (abnormal papillary muscles)

PARACHUTE MITRAL VALVE

Parachute mitral valve is a rather common malformation. All the chordae tendinae are attached to a single PM (**Figure 67.10**). When two PMs are present, only one is receiving chordal attachment. This lesion can often be found in association with other MV malformations, most commonly a supravalvar ring.

Surgery consists of a splitting of the PM-bearing chordae, down to the ventricular wall (**Figure 67.11**). Care must be taken not to disrupt the chordal apparatus or weaken the PM with consequent possible chordal detachment.

HAMMOCK VALVE/MITRAL ARCADE

These complex lesions are similar in that both are characterized by the presence of abnormal PMs in conjunction with the absence of first-degree chordae. Short second-degree chordae tendinae directly attach the MV leaflets to the PMs.

In the Hammock valve, two large cylinder-like PMs are present, impinging on the inlet to the ventricle (**Figure 67.12**). In the mitral arcade, there is a fusion of both PMs creating a "muscle arcade" where small chordae attach (**Figure 67.13**). Other MV malformations are often found in association i.e. commissures fusion and supravalvar ring.

Surgical repair is similar in the two malformations, consisting of a splitting of both PMs in Hammock valve (**Figure 67.14**) or of a longitudinal splitting of the "muscle arcade" in mitral arcade (**Figure 67.15**). In both procedures the aim is to free the leaflets which are anchored to the PMs by the short chordae.

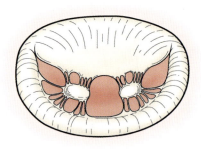

67.12

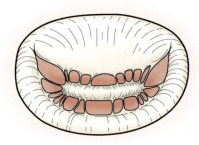

67.13

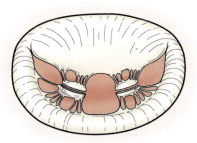

67.14

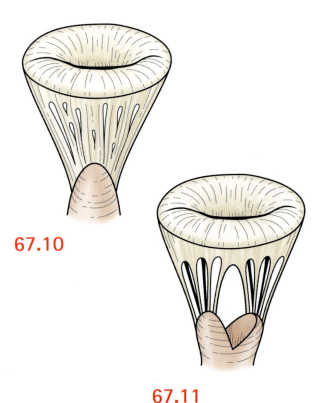

67.10

67.11

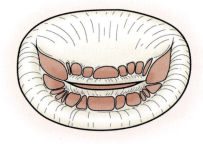

67.15

MITRAL VALVE REGURGITATION

Carpentier classifies these lesions according to the leaflet motion: normal, prolapsed, or restricted.

Type I (normal leaflet motion)

ANNULAR DILATATION

A pure annular dilatation is seldom found as an isolated form of MV deformity. It is often the result of other associated malformations causing MV regurgitation and ventricular dilatation (**Figure 67.16**).

Surgery consists of a posterior annular placation, as described by Kay in 1977 (**Figure 67.17**). No prosthetic rings, including the open one, should be used in children, due to the scar tissue caused by the sutures and the ring itself, which can limit proper annulus growth and leaflet motion.

CLEFT LEAFLET

Cleft leaflet should not be confused with the so-called "cleft" which is found in association with an atrioventricular canal defect. It usually involves the anterior MV leaflet. The MV apparatus is usually normal with the exception of a vertical cleft, which separates the anterior leaflet into two hemileaflets (**Figure 67.18**). Abnormal small chordae can be attached to the free margins of the cleft. The edges of the cleft can often be thickened, as a result of the turbulence created by the regurgitation at that point.

Surgery consists of total closure of the cleft with interrupted fine stitches (single or figure-eight) with particular care taken not to distort the MV anterior leaflet and reduce the coaptation with the posterior one (**Figure 67.19**). An annular placation is often performed in association with this.

LEAFLET DEFECT

This is quite a rare malformation which most commonly involves the posterior MV leaflet (**Figures 67.20 and 67.21**). Repair is usually undertaken by a direct suture or patch

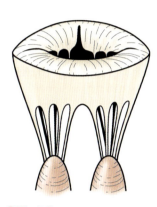

67.18

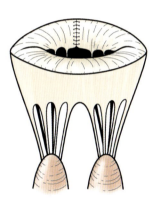

67.19

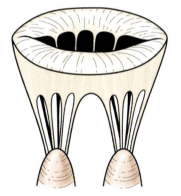

67.16

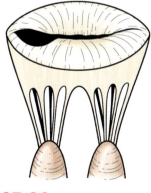

67.20

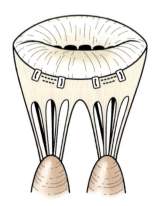

67.17

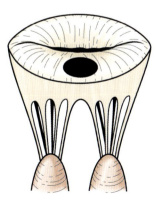

67.21

closure of the gap (**Figures 67.22 and 67.23**), often associated with a hemiannular posterior ring plication.

Type II (leaflet prolapse)

ELONGATED CHORDAE

Elongated chordae can be found in any of the PMs and also in association with other MV malformations (**Figure 67.24**). Congenital forms need to be differentiated from other acquired forms of myxoid degeneration of the whole valve apparatus or forms found in association with anomalous origin of the left coronary artery from the main pulmonary artery where the PMs are infarcted and elongated.

Elongated chordae are treated as described by Carpentier, by creating a groove in the PM, next to the elongated chordate, and by encircling the chordae with a suture, imbricating them into the groove (**Figure 67.25a and b**). Tying of the suture buries the excessive length of the chordae into the groove, which is subsequently closed. This maneuver may be difficult in small children, and therefore a fine, longitudinal suture can be passed over each chorda and anchored onto the PM (**Figure 67.26a and b**).

Artificial chordae can also be utilized, as they are in the treatment of acquired lesions, for treating both the anterior and the posterior leaflet prolapse (**Figure 67.27**).

Type III (restricted leaflet motion)

This is a very rare condition with normal PMs. It is often confused with forms with associated valve stenosis (i.e. commissure fusion/short chordae).

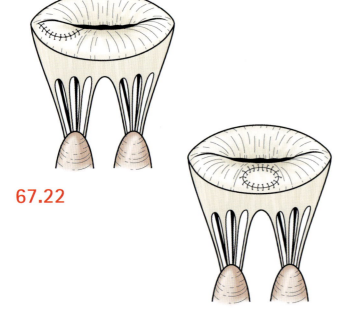

67.22

67.23

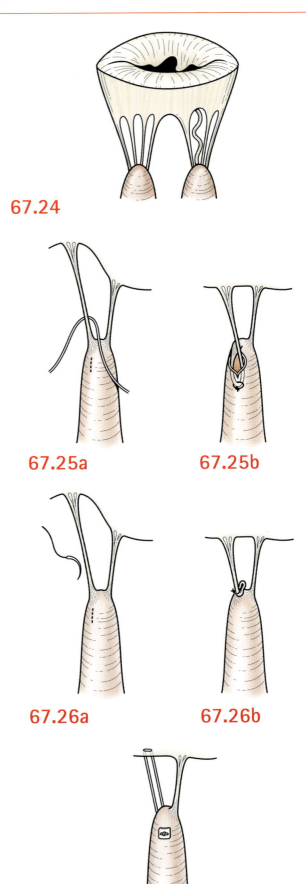

67.24

67.25a   **67.25b**

67.26a   **67.26b**

67.27

PAPILLARY MUSCLE HYPOPLASIA

Chordae tendinae are attached to small PMs (**Figure 67.28**). The mechanism of valve regurgitation is due to a lack of leaflet coaptation. Surgical treatment often includes a posterior leaflet extension (biological tissue is usually employed) in order to favor better leaflet coaptation (**Figures 67.29 and 67.30**). The incision of the small PMs down to the ventricular wall can also be performed. When annular dilatation is present in association with PM hypoplasia, an annulus remodeling can also be performed by a posterior plication (or hemiplication).

PARACHUTE MITRAL VALVE

An incompetent parachute MV can be found in association to signs of MV stenosis (see "Mitral valve stenosis – parachute mitral valve"). The regurgitation is usually due to the hypoplasia of the anterior leaflet near the commissure, usually the anterior one, a malformation also called "cleft commissure" (Carpentier classification). The anterior leaflet can be extended with biological autologous or heterologous tissue (**Figure 67.31a–c**). An annuloplasty (or partial annuloplasty) of the posterior leaflet can also be performed in association.

HAMMOCK VALVE/MITRAL ARCADE

Both malformations can also present with signs of regurgitation due to the restricted leaflet motion. A splitting of the PMs or the muscle arcade usually produces a better leaflet excursion.

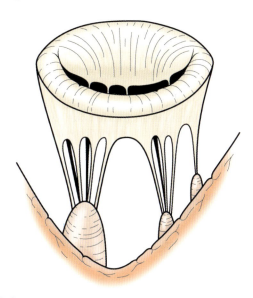

67.28

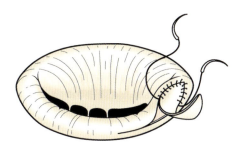

67.29

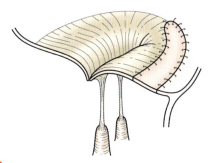

67.30

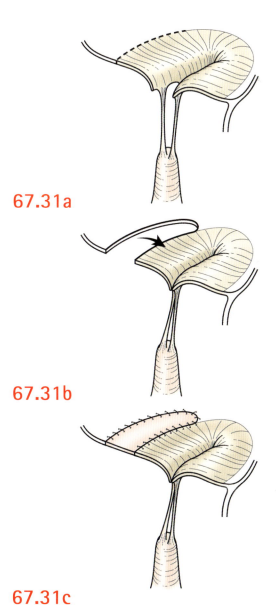

67.31a

67.31b

67.31c

Testing the results of the repair

As for acquired lesions, the result of MV reconstruction is tested intraoperatively by injecting cold saline solution into the left ventricular cavity. During this maneuver, care must be taken not to distort the MV annulus with stay stitches or retractors on the annulus during the injection. This test is important for assessing a proper closure of the MV leaflets after repair of incompetent MVs but also after repair of stenotic MV lesions, where reconstructing maneuvers might have caused MV damage.

Small MV leakages are usually accepted in the presence of a satisfactory leaflets coaptation. In small children, in contrast to adult patients, a perfect MV competence at the hydrodynamic test is often difficult to achieve.

At the end of the cardiopulmonary bypass, MV performance is tested again by means of transesophageal or epicardial echocardiography interrogation. Four- and two-chamber and long-axis views are used for assessing MV anatomy and function, particularly leaflet movements and coaptation and also the anatomy and function of the whole subvalvar apparatus (chordae tendinae and PMs).

With the aid of color Doppler modality flow, after careful adjustment of the color settings, the presence and direction of regurgitation can be detected and the effective regurgitation orifice area measured with the proximal isovelocity surface area (PISA) method. With the use of spectral Doppler, the presence of residual stenosis or regurgitation is tested further, with the measurement of the velocity of the filling pattern of the left ventricle. By rotating the probe at "commissural view" at 90 degrees and 120 degrees, the same interrogation is repeated, as previously described.

POSTOPERATIVE CARE

A left atrial line is often inserted either through the intra-atrial groove or through the left atrial appendix. Valve performance is also checked again by 2D echocardiography in the intensive care unit before removing the left atrial line and weaning the patient off the ventilator. In the presence of preoperative pulmonary artery hypertension, a pulmonary artery line is often inserted through the main pulmonary artery or through the infundibulum.

OUTCOME

Recent series have shown that MV repair in infants and children is an effective and reliable treatment with acceptable mortality and success rates, which have improved considerably in the last few years. MV reconstruction needs to be planned in detail, for each malformation, on the basis of information received preoperatively by 2D and 3D echocardiography. Such information is extremely important for the surgeon, for planning in advance the ideal surgical strategy and at the time of repair. In very dysplastic valves, it must be borne in mind that minimal reconstructing maneuvers are often sufficient to improve MV performance. It has been found that very dysplastic valves which were treated "minimally" in early infancy can still perform adequately after several years.

MV repair must always be attempted as a first line of treatment, especially in infants, despite the frequent severity of MVs dysplasia, to avoid the drawbacks of the currently available prosthesis. It has also been found that anatomical severity of MV malformations influences the long-term freedom from MV replacement. Parachute MVs tend to have worse outcomes and are associated with a high rate of early mortality.

There is an increased risk for perioperative mortality when major cardiac anomalies, such as left outflow track obstruction, ventricular septal defect, or impaired preoperative ventricular function, are present in association with MV malformations. Nevertheless, the durability of valve repair appears to be independent of the presence of associated cardiac anomalies.

FURTHER READING

Carpentier A, Branchini B, Cour JC, et al. Congenital malformations of the mitral valve in children: pathology and surgical treatment. *J Thorac Cardiovasc Surg.* 1976; 72(6): 854–66.

Carpentier A, Brizard C. Congenital malformations of the mitral valve. In: Stark JF, de Leval MR, Tsang VT (eds). *Surgery for congenital heart defects.* 3rd edn. Chichester: John Wiley & Sons; 2006: pp. 573–90.

Castaneda AR, Anderson RC, Edwards JE. Congenital mitral stenosis resulting from anomalous arcade and obstructing papillary muscles: report of correction by use of ball valve prosthesis. *Am J Cardiol.* 1969; 24(2): 237–40.

Layman T, Edwards JE. Anomalous mitral arcade. *Circulation.* 1967; 35: 389–95.

Mitruka SN, Lamberti JJ. Congenital Heart Surgery Nomenclature and Database Project: mitral valve disease. *Ann Thorac Surg.* 2000; 69(4 Suppl): S132–46.

Stellin G, Padalino MA, Vida VL, et al. Surgical repair of congenital mitral valve malformations in infancy and childhood: a single-center 36-year experience. *J Thorac Cardiovasc Surg.* 2010; 140(6): 1238–44.

Thiene G, Frescura C, Daliento L. The pathology of congenitally malformed mitral valve. In: Marcelletti C, Anderson RH, Becker AE, et al. (eds). *Pediatric cardiology.* New York: Churchill Livingstone; 1986: pp. 225–39.

68

Aortic valve repair

EMILE BACHA AND PAUL CHAI

HISTORY

Tuffier is believed to have performed the first aortic valve repair in a patient with aortic stenosis in 1913. The operation consisted of digital invagination of the dilated ascending aorta wall and "dilatation" of the stenotic valve. Following the popularization of Gibbon's and Lillehei's methods for extracorporeal circulation in the mid-1950s, aortic insufficiency, which had largely defied closed efforts at correction, was somewhat more responsive to open plastic procedures. Since then, a variety of reports have been published on repair of aortic insufficiency by suturing two adjacent cusps together to correct prolapse or by excising the non-coronary cusp and its aortic sinus and narrowing of the aortic root and proximal ascending aorta, thus converting the aortic valve into a bicuspid valve. Because only a few patients could have aortic valve repair, various autologous tissues, such as pericardium, aortic wall segments, full-thickness left atrial wall, central tendon of the diaphragm, peritoneum, and fascia lata, were used for reconstruction of heart valves. With the development of prosthetic heart valves, aortic valve repair became a rare operation and was largely limited to pediatric cases of subaortic ventricular septal defect and aortic insufficiency due to prolapse of the right cusp. With the development of transesophageal Doppler echocardiography and better understanding of the functional anatomy of the aortic valve, interest in aortic valve repair was renewed.

PRINCIPLES AND JUSTIFICATION

The aortic root functions as a unit, and a sound knowledge of its anatomical components and their geometrical relationships is indispensable to repair the aortic valve and reconstruct the aortic root. The aortic root has four anatomical components: aortic annulus (AA), aortic cusps, aortic sinuses, and sinotubular junction (STJ). The AA attaches the aortic root to the left ventricle. The AA is attached to the interventricular muscle in approximately 45% of the circumference and to fibrous structures in 55%. Histological examination of the aortoventricular junction reveals that the aortic root has a fibrous continuity with the anterior leaflet of the mitral valve and membranous septum, and it is attached to the muscular interventricular septum through fibrous strands. Because the entire circumference of the aortoventricular junction contains a band of connective tissue, it is reasonable to refer to it as the *aortic annulus*. The AA has a scalloped shape.

The aortic cusps have a semilunar shape, and their bases are attached to the AA in a scalloped fashion. This anatomical arrangement creates three triangles beneath the aortic cusps. These triangles are part of the left ventricle. The triangle beneath the right and left cusps is made of interventricular muscle, whereas the other two triangles are made of fibrous tissue. The highest point of these triangles where two aortic cusps come in contact is called the *commissure*, which is located immediately below the STJ. The STJ is where the aortic root ends and the ascending aorta begins. The segments of arterial wall that are delineated by the AA proximally and by the STJ distally are called *aortic sinuses* or *sinuses of Valsalva*.

The geometric relationships and the function of the various components of the aortic root are interrelated. The areas of the aortic cusps probably determine the size of the aortic root. The aortic cusps are attached to the AA in a scalloped fashion. The length of the base of an aortic cusp is approximately 1.5 times longer than the length of its FM. The FM of an aortic cusp extends from one commissure to the other. Thus, the lengths of the FMs of the aortic cusps are related to the diameter of the AA and STJ.

The transverse diameter of the AA at the lowest level of the aortic cusps is 10–20% larger than the diameter of the STJ in children and young adults, but these diameters tend to equalize in older patients. The lengths of the FMs of the aortic cusp must exceed the diameter of the aortic orifice because, when the aortic valve is closed, each cusp extends from one commissure to the center of the aortic root and to the other commissures (**Figure 68.1**).

The aortic root is attached to contractile and fibrous components of the left ventricle. During systole, the interventricular septum shortens and moves inward, and the anterior leaflet of the mitral valve is pushed away from the center of the left ventricular outflow tract. Thus, during systole, the area of the aortic root that is attached to the anterior leaflet of the mitral valve is exposed to greater tension than the area attached to the muscular interventricular septum. These dynamic changes in the geometry of the AA play a role in the function of the aortic valve. Although all three aortic cusps open synchronously during systole, the non-coronary cusp, its annulus, and the commissures open more than the left side of the aortic valve and consequently are exposed to greater stress (LaPlace's law). This situation may explain why the non-coronary aortic sinus and its annulus tend to dilate more than the other sinuses in patients with degenerative disease of the aortic root.

The aortic sinuses are important to maintain coronary artery blood flow throughout the cardiac cycle as well as to create eddies to close the aortic cusps during diastole. The aortic root is very elastic in young patients, expanding considerably during systole and shortening during diastole. However, the number of elastic fibers decreases with aging, and the aortic root becomes less compliant in older patients. The root expands minimally in elderly patients.

Aortic insufficiency is caused by anatomical abnormalities of one or more components of the aortic root. Dilation of the STJ causes outward displacement of the commissures of the aortic cusps and prevents central coaptation, resulting in aortic insufficiency (**Figure 68.2**). This is the mechanism of aortic insufficiency in patients with ascending aortic

aneurysm, mega-aorta syndrome, and long-standing hypertension causing a dilated and elongated ascending aorta. These patients are usually in their sixth or seventh decade of life.

Dilation of the aortic sinuses does not cause aortic insufficiency if the diameters of the AA and of the STJ remain unchanged. However, in patients with degenerative disease of the aortic root, the STJ eventually dilates, and aortic insufficiency ensues. In patients with more advanced degenerative disease of the media, such as those with Marfan syndrome or its forme fruste, the AA may also dilate, creating so-called annuloaortic ectasia. In this condition, the fibrous components of the left ventricular outflow tract become enlarged, and the normal relationship between muscular (45% of the circumference) and fibrous components (55% of the circumference) is altered in favor of the fibrous component. Most of the dilation occurs beneath the commissures of the non-coronary aortic cusp.

Bicuspid aortic valve causes aortic insufficiency because of prolapse of one or both cusps. The FM of the larger of the two cusps, usually the one that contains a raphe, becomes elongated and prolapses. In addition, these patients often have mild to moderate dilation of the aortic root, particularly of the AA.

Type A aortic dissection causes aortic insufficiency because of detachment of one or both commissures of the non-coronary cusp of the aortic valve, with resulting prolapse. Most of these patients also have pre-existing dilation of the aortic root, which contributes to the pathophysiology of aortic insufficiency.

Rheumatic valvulitis of the aortic valve can cause cusp thickening, scarring with contraction, and commissural fusion. Some degree of aortic stenosis is often present in these cases. Rheumatic aortic valve disease is commonly associated with rheumatic mitral valve disease.

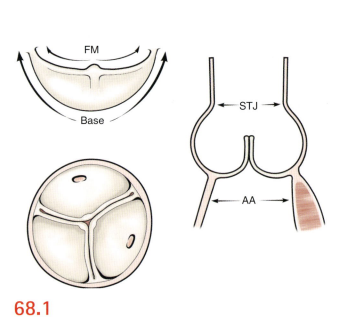

68.1

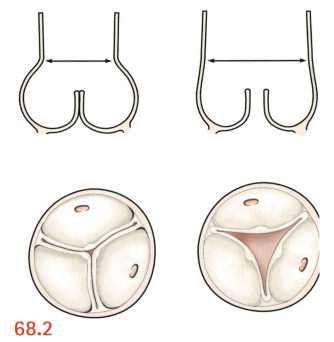

68.2

Ankylosing spondylitis, Reiter's syndrome, osteogenesis imperfecta, rheumatoid arthritis, systemic lupus erythematosus, and idiopathic giant cell aortitis are connective tissue disorders that can be associated with aortic insufficiency, usually because of scarring of the aortic cusps.

Subaortic membranous ventricular septal defect causes aortic insufficiency because of down-and-outward displacement of the AA along the right cusp, which, with time, may become elongated and increase the degree of cusp prolapse.

SELECTION OF PATIENTS FOR AORTIC VALVE REPAIR

Earlier operation is probably justifiable in patients with severe aortic insufficiency if the aortic valve is reparable. Aortic valve repair can be satisfactorily performed only in a small proportion of patients with aortic valve disease. In adult patients, repair is seldom useful in patients with aortic stenosis. Mechanical debridement of mildly calcified tricuspid aortic valves is sometimes performed in elderly patients in whom the primary indication for cardiac surgery is coronary artery disease. The calcific deposits should be limited to the AA and base of the cusps and should be removed manually. If the calcium extends into the body of the cusp, the aortic valve should be replaced with a bioprosthetic valve, preferably a stentless porcine valve to minimize transvalvular gradients.

Open aortic valvotomy for congenital aortic stenosis in children has been largely replaced by percutaneous balloon valvotomy as a palliative procedure. However, several centers have kept up the practice of open neonatal valvotomy with results as least comparable to percutaneous balloon valvotomy.

Aortic valve repair is a valuable operative procedure for certain patients with aortic insufficiency due to prolapse of an aortic cusp or due to dilation of the aortic root with normal aortic cusps. Dilation of the aortic root is the most common cause of aortic insufficiency in North America.

Transesophageal echocardiography is currently the best diagnostic tool to study the aortic root and the mechanism of aortic insufficiency. Each component of the aortic root must be carefully assessed to determine the cause of aortic valve dysfunction. Dilation of the aortic root or ascending aorta, or both, and bicuspid aortic valve disease are the most common entities that are suitable for aortic valve repair. In both instances, the number of aortic cusps, their thickness, the appearance of the FMs, and cusp excursion during the cardiac cycle represent the most important information needed to determine reparability of the valve. Information regarding the morphology of the aortic sinuses, STJ, and ascending aorta is also important. The diameters of the AA, aortic sinuses, STJ, and the heights of the cusps should be measured. The lengths of the FMs of the cusps should be estimated if possible. Dilation of the STJ is easily diagnosed by echocardiography. If the aortic sinuses, cusps, and annulus appear to be normal, and the aortic insufficiency is central, simple adjustment of

the STJ restores valve function. This situation is frequently the case in patients with ascending aortic aneurysm and mega-aorta syndrome. Individuals with dilated STJ and aortic sinuses but with echocardiographically normal aortic cusps may also have aortic valve repair, although a more complex reconstruction of the aortic root is needed. This case occurs in patients with Marfan syndrome or its forme fruste. In our experience the probability of aortic valve repair decreases as the diameter of the STJ increases. When the diameter of the STJ exceeds 50 mm, the aortic cusps often are thinned, are overstretched, and contain stress fenestrations in the commissural areas. The diameters of the aortic sinuses or of the ascending aorta are less important. We have found patients with normal aortic cusps and ascending aortic aneurysms of 6 cm or greater in diameter. Dilation of the aortic sinuses may be associated with dilation of the AA and STJ; for this reason, patients with aortic root aneurysms and echocardiographically normal aortic cusps should be operated on when the diameter of aortic sinuses reaches 50 mm.

Patients with aortic insufficiency due to prolapse of a bicuspid aortic valve are also candidates for aortic valve repair, providing that echocardiography demonstrates pliable, thin, and mobile cusps without calcification and prolapse of only one of the two cusps. Children with subaortic ventricular septal defect and aortic insufficiency are also candidates for aortic valve repair. Rheumatic valvulitis and other nonrheumatic inflammatory diseases of the aortic valve are less suitable for valve repair.

PREOPERATIVE ASSESSMENT AND PREPARATION

Patients younger than 50 years of age and without coronary artery risk factors do not need coronary angiography before surgery, but it should be performed in older patients. It is imperative that candidates for aortic valve repair understand before surgery that repair may not be feasible once the aorta is opened at operation and that aortic valve replacement may be necessary. For this reason, alternative procedures must be discussed with the patient before surgery. As with any valve operation, poor dental hygiene and other potential sources of postoperative bacteremia must be corrected before elective operations.

ANESTHESIA

The anesthetic agents and techniques are the same as for any open heart procedure that uses cardiopulmonary bypass (CPB).

OPERATION

Aortic valve repair is usually performed through a median sternotomy, particularly in patients with extensive vascular disease such as those with aneurysm and coronary artery disease. Isolated repair of the aortic valve can also be performed through an 8–10 cm skin incision and partial or full midline sternotomy.

CPB is established by cannulating the distal ascending aorta or transverse aortic arch, depending on the extent of the aneurysm. Regardless of the aortic valve or aortic root pathology, the best approach to expose the aortic valve for repair is through a generous transverse aortotomy that is at least 1 cm above the commissures. In cases of aneurysm, the aorta should be transected completely. In congenital patients, one must always be careful to pay attention to an anomalous artery origin while dividing the aorta.

Myocardial protection during the aortic cross-clamp is provided by intermittent shots of cold-blood cardioplegia that are delivered directly into the coronary artery orifices by inserting soft, self-inflating balloon cannulae and securing them to the adjacent aortic wall. A ventricular vent is inserted through the interatrial groove.

The components of the aortic root are then carefully assessed. The principal determinant of aortic valve repair is the quality of the aortic cusps. The number of cusps, their thickness, their pliability, and the presence of fenestrations are observed. The motion of the cusps is best appreciated by suspending the commissures to a normal position. If there is prolapse of one cusp, it is corrected by one of the methods described below. Next, the lengths of the FMs of the three cusps are measured. The diameters of the AA and of the STJ should be smaller than the average length of the FMs of the aortic cusps. If not, surgical reduction should be part of the valve repair. For patients who are status post balloon valvotomy, the location and extent of the tear is noted.

Repair of cusp prolapse

Prolapse of an aortic cusp is corrected by shortening the FM. This maneuver can be done by plicating the central portion of the cusp with full-thickness sutures. If the cusp is very thin, horizontal mattress sutures with a fine strip of pericardial pledget on each side can be used (**Figure 68.3**). The degree of shortening of the length of the FM depends on the lengths of the FMs of the other cusps.

Minor prolapse of a thinned-out cusp or of a cusp with a fenestration along its commissural attachment can be corrected by weaving a double layer of a 6-0 expanded polytetrafluoroethylene (PTFE) suture along the FM from commissure to commissure (**Figure 68.4**).

In bicuspid aortic valve disease, the anterior cusp is usually the one that prolapses. That cusp often contains a raphe, which should be excised. After the length of the FM of the prolapsing cusp is corrected, the subcommissural triangles can be plicated to increase the coaptation area of the cusps. This plication is accomplished by passing a horizontal mattress suture from the outside of the aortic root to the inside, including the AA immediately beneath the commissural areas (**Figure 68.5a and b**).

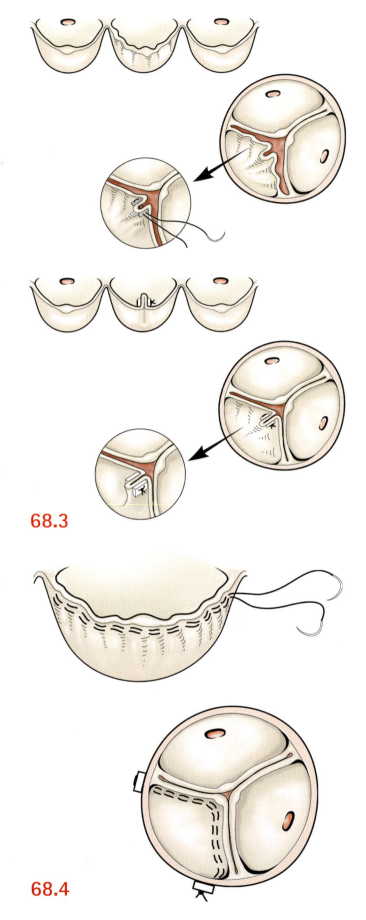

68.3

68.4

Remodeling of the aortic root

Most patients with ascending aortic aneurysm and aortic insufficiency have normal or near-normal aortic cusps and aortic sinuses. Correction of the aortic insufficiency is accomplished by replacement of the ascending aorta, with adjustment of the diameter of the STJ (**Figure 68.6a–c**). The diameter of the STJ is estimated by approximating the three commissures to a point where all three cusps coapt centrally. The ascending aorta should be transected 5 mm above the STJ and a tubular Dacron® graft sutured at the level of the STJ. It is important to space the three commissures in the graft according to the length of the FM of the cusps. Thus, if one cusp is longer than the others, the distance between its commissures should be proportionally longer. Another important consideration is the diameter of the graft in relation to the size of the patient. Large patients should have proportionally larger grafts because a small graft may increase left ventricular afterload. We avoid grafts that are smaller than 26 mm in large patients. If the STJ should be smaller than 26 mm, the graft is reduced in diameter only at the anastomotic area.

If one or more aortic sinuses are dilated or involved by dissecting aneurysm (**Figure 68.7a**), they should be replaced with a properly tailored tubular Dacron graft. The aortic root is dissected circumferentially down to just below the level of the AA. The coronary arteries are detached from their respective aortic sinuses with a rim of arterial wall

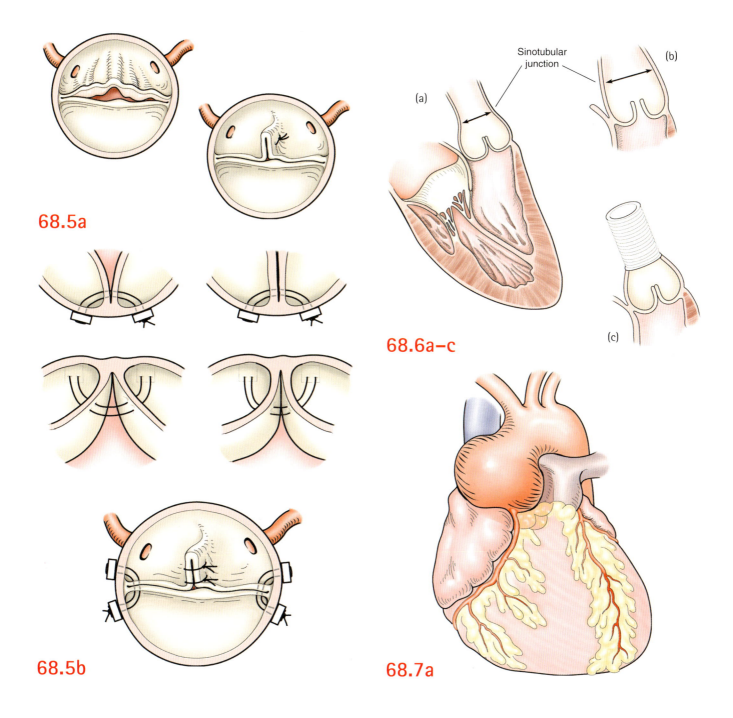

68.5a

68.5b

Sinotubular junction

(a)

(b)

(c)

68.6a–c

68.7a

around their orifices. The aortic sinuses are excised, leaving 4–8 mm of arterial wall attached to the AA (4 mm around the commissures and 8 mm on the bottom of the aortic cusps) (**Figure 68.7b**). A tubular Dacron graft of a diameter equal to or slightly smaller than the average length of the FMs of the cusps is tailored to create three neoaortic sinuses. These neoaortic sinuses are tailored in one end of the graft by making three longitudinal incisions in the graft at least as long as the diameter of the graft. The edges are trimmed to make them semicircular in shape. The commissures of the aortic valve are secured on the outside of the upper part of the neosinuses with 4-0 polypropylene sutures that are passed from the inside to the outside of the graft and from the inside to the outside of the commissures of the aortic valve (**Figure 68.7c**). Before these sutures are tied, they can be passed through a Teflon felt pledget and left on the outside of the aortic wall. The neoaortic sinuses made of Dacron fabric are then sutured to the AA and remnants of arterial wall, with those sutures used to suspend the commissure (**Figure 68.7d**). The graft should lie on the inside of the remnants of the arterial wall. Once all three sinuses have been reconstructed, the coronary arteries are reimplanted.

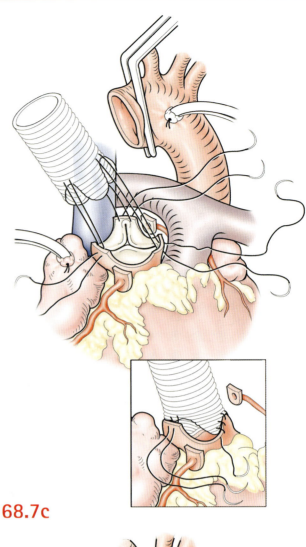

68.7c

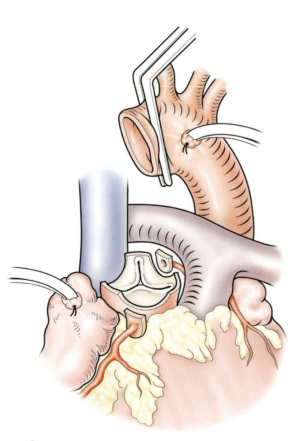

68.7b

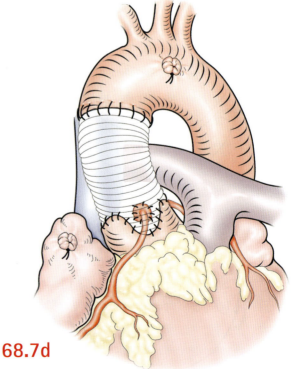

68.7d

Reimplantation of the aortic valve

Reimplantation of the aortic valve is an alternative procedure to remodeling of the aortic root for patients with aortic root aneurysm. Reimplantation is particularly useful in patients with annuloaortic ectasia, Marfan syndrome, or acute type A aortic dissection. It places the entire aortic valve inside a tubular Dacron graft. The aortic sinuses are excised as described for the remodeling procedure. Next, multiple horizontal mattress sutures (3-0 or 4-0 polyester) are placed from the inside to the outside of the left ventricular outflow tract. These sutures should be placed on a single horizontal plane along the fibrous components of the outflow tract and follow the scalloped shape of the AA along the muscular ventricular septum (**Figure 68.8a**). Teflon felt pledgets should be used if the fibrous component is thin. A tubular Dacron graft with a diameter of 2–4 mm larger than the average lengths of the FMs of the cusps is chosen. Three equidistant marks are created in one of its ends, and an 8–10 mm triangular excision is made in one of the thirds to correspond to the commissure subtended by the interventricular muscle. Three plicating sutures are placed in between the spaces marked to align the commissures to reduce the diameter of the graft by 2–4 mm. The sutures that were passed through the left ventricular outflow tract are then passed from the inside to the outside of this tailored end of the graft. It is important to distribute these sutures evenly, particularly along the muscular septum. Most of the reduction in the diameter of the AA should be accomplished beneath the commissures of the non-coronary aortic cusp. The valve is placed in the inside of the graft, and all sutures are tied on the outside. This suture line stabilizes

the AA and reduces its diameter (**Figure 68.8b**). The reduction in diameter should be strictly beneath the commissures of the non-coronary aortic cusp. The three commissures are then resuspended inside the graft and secured to it using horizontal mattress sutures of 4-0 polypropylene with pledgets. These sutures are also used to secure the remnants of the aortic wall and AA to the graft (**Figure 68.8c**). The coronary arteries are reimplanted into their respective neo-aortic sinuses. Because the diameter of the graft is larger than the average lengths of the aortic cusps, the spaces between the commissures are plicated with polypropylene sutures to

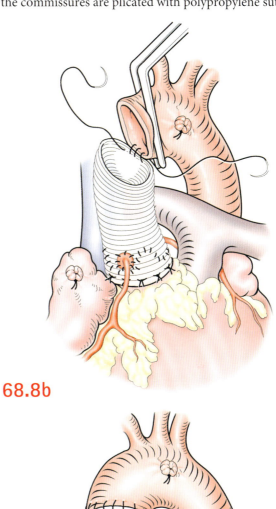

68.8b

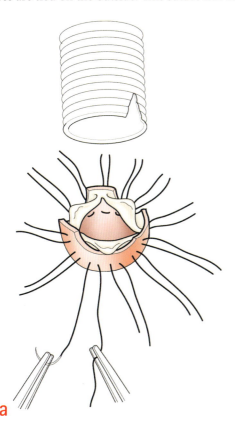

68.8a

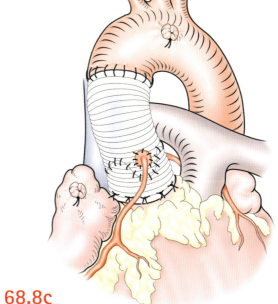

68.8c

create neoaortic sinuses and reduce the diameter of the STJ. The coaptation level of the aortic cusps is inspected again and their FMs shortened as needed.

Cusp extension of deficient cusps

This technique can be used in trileaflet or bileaflet valves. Congenital patients often have deficient cusps, which can be the result of rheumatic heart disease ("rolled" cusps), balloon valvotomy, or simply congenital cusp deficiency in congenital aortic regurgitation (AR). This can be repaired with cusp extensions. The choice of patch material can vary from native pericardium (glutaraldehyde-treated or not) to artificial material such as Gore-Tex to bioengineered patches. No one patch material has proven superior to the other. In general, the more complex the repair is, the less durable it will be. Patch extensions are considered complex aortic valve repairs.

Aortic valve repair must be performed with intraoperative Doppler echocardiography. At the completion of the procedure, no more than trace aortic insufficiency is acceptable. In addition, the morphology of the repaired valve is very important. Persistent prolapse of one cusp may progress with time and causes recurrent aortic insufficiency. It is better to correct the prolapse with a second pump run and further shortening of the FM of the cusp. Central aortic insufficiency without prolapse is usually due to inadequate coaptation of the cusps. This situation can be corrected by further reduction of the diameter of the STJ without placing the patient back on CPB and with echocardiographic guidance. A temporary plication of the graft at the level of the STJ is done and the valve function assessed by Doppler echocardiography.

POSTOPERATIVE CARE

Patients who have had aortic valve repair or aortic valve-sparing procedures receive the same care as any patient who undergoes heart surgery under CPB. Patients are usually extubated for 3–4 hours of observation for hemodynamic stability and hemostasis. Most patients are cared for in an intensive care setting during the first day. They are then discharged to a cardiac surgical ward. They receive analgesic and cardiac medications as needed. We do not anticoagulate these patients, but they all receive aspirin during the first 3 months postoperative or permanently if they also had coronary artery bypass graft. Most patients are discharged from hospital within 5–7 days.

OUTCOME

Clinical experience has shown that it is important to leave no aortic insufficiency or only a trace after the repair of bicuspid aortic valves. Uncorrected prolapse is associated with a high risk of early recurrent aortic insufficiency. The long-term results of aortic valve repair of the bicuspid aortic valve have also been very good.

For pediatric or congenital repairs, outcomes are very much dependent on the etiology of the valve pathology. Where aortic valve repair is for aortic insufficiency due to ventricular septal defect, results have been durable. For complex repairs in combined aortic insufficiency/aortic stenosis lesions, or repairs using patch extensions, results have been less good with freedom from reoperations of about 70% at 5 years postoperative. Here again, as for adult patients, leaving the operating room with more than mild aortic regurgitation will result in poorer long-term results.

FURTHER READING

Bacha EA, McElhinney DB, Guleserian KJ, et al. Surgical aortic valvuloplasty in children and adolescents with aortic regurgitation: acute and intermediate effects on aortic valve function and left ventricular dimensions. *J Thorac Cardiovasc Surg.* 2008; 135(3): 552–9.

Boodhwani M, El Khoury G. Aortic valve repair: indications and outcomes. *Curr Cardiol Rep.* 2014; 16(6): 490.

David TE. Surgery of the aortic valve. *Curr Probl Surg.* 1999; 36: 421–504.

David TE, Armstrong S, Ivanov J, et al. Results of aortic valve-sparing operations. *J Thorac Cardiovasc Surg.* 2001; 122(1): 39–46.

Hraška V, Sinzobahamvya N, Haun C, et al. The long-term outcome of open valvotomy for critical aortic stenosis in neonates. *Ann Thorac Surg.* 2012; 94(5): 1519–26.

Kunzelman KS, Grande J, David TE, et al. 1994. Aortic root and valve relationships: impact on surgical repair. *J Thorac Cardiovasc Surg.* 1994; 107: 162–70.

Myers PO, Tissot C, Christenson JT, et al. Aortic valve repair by cusp extension for rheumatic aortic insufficiency in children: long-term results and impact of extension material. *J Thorac Cardiovasc Surg.* 2010; 140(4): 836–44.

Yacoub MH, Gehle P, Chandrasekaran V, et al. Late results of a valve-preserving operation in patients with aneurysm of the ascending aorta and root. *J Thorac Cardiovasc Surg.* 1998; 115: 1080–90.

Index